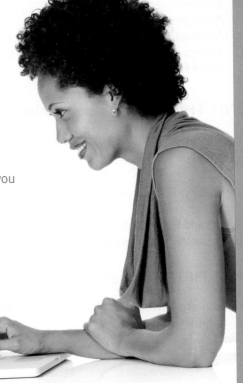

Pharmacology

A Patient-Centered Nursing Process Approach

EDITION **9**

Linda E. McCuistion, PhD, MSN
NCLEX® Live Review Presenter
Mandeville, Louisiana

Kathleen Vuljoin-DiMaggio, RN, MSN
Assistant Professor of Nursing
University of Holy Cross New Orleans
New Orleans, Louisiana

Mary B. Winton, PhD, RN, ACANP-BC
Assistant Professor
Tarleton State University
Stephenville, Texas

Jennifer J. Yeager, PhD, RN, AGNP
Assistant Professor and Director of the Graduate Nursing Program
Tarleton State University
Stephenville, Texas

ELSEVIER

ELSEVIER

3251 Riverport Lane
St. Louis, Missouri 63043

PHARMACOLOGY: A PATIENT-CENTERED NURSING PROCESS APPROACH   ISBN: 978-0-323-39916-6
NINTH EDITION

Notices

Knowledge and best practice in this field are constantly changing. As new research and experience broaden our understanding, changes in research methods, professional practices, or medical treatment may become necessary.

Practitioners and researchers must always rely on their own experience and knowledge in evaluating and using any information, methods, compounds, or experiments described herein. In using such information or methods they should be mindful of their own safety and the safety of others, including parties for whom they have a professional responsibility.

With respect to any drug or pharmaceutical products identified, readers are advised to check the most current information provided (i) on procedures featured or (ii) by the manufacturer of each product to be administered, to verify the recommended dose or formula, the method and duration of administration, and contraindications. It is the responsibility of practitioners, relying on their own experience and knowledge of their patients, to make diagnoses, to determine dosages and the best treatment for each individual patient, and to take all appropriate safety precautions.

To the fullest extent of the law, neither the Publisher nor the authors, contributors, or editors, assume any liability for any injury and/or damage to persons or property as a matter of products liability, negligence or otherwise, or from any use or operation of any methods, products, instructions, or ideas contained in the material herein.

Library of Congress Cataloging-in-Publication Data
Names: McCuistion, Linda E., author. | Vuljoin-DiMaggio, Kathleen, author.
|
   Winton, Mary B., author | Yeager, Jennifer J., author. | Preceded by
   (work): Kee, Joyce LeFever. Pharmacology.
Title: Pharmacology : a patient-centered nursing process approach / Linda
   McCuistion, Kathleen Vuljoin-DiMaggio, Mary B. Winton, Jennifer J.
Yeager.
Description: 9th edition. | St. Louis, Missouri : Elsevier, [2018] | Preceded
   by Pharmacology / Joyce LeFever Kee, Evelyn R. Hayes, Linda E.
McCuistion.
   8th edition. 2015. | Includes bibliographical references and index.
Identifiers: LCCN 2016052177 | ISBN 9780323399166 (pbk. : alk. paper)
Subjects: | MESH: Pharmacological Phenomena | Pharmaceutical Preparations |
   Drug Therapy | Patient-Centered Care | Nurses' Instruction
Classification: LCC RM301 | NLM QV 4 | DDC 615.5/8--dc23 LC record available at
   https://lccn.loc.gov/2016052177

Executive Content Strategist: Sonya Seigafuse
Content Development Manager: Lisa Newton
Senior Content Development Specialist: Tina Kaemmerer
Publishing Services Manager: Jeff Patterson
Senior Project Manager: Tracey Schriefer
Design Direction: Maggie Reid

Printed in China

Last digit is the print number: 9   8   7   6   5   4   3

To Dr. Gerald DeLuca for his expert guidance; to Joyce LeFever Kee, who originated this book; to Evelyn R. Hayes for her efforts; and in memory of my parents, Otto and Pauline Schmidt.

Linda E. McCuistion

To Dr. Linda McCuistion, for her friendship and guidance, and to my daughters, Christina Boudreaux, Maria DiMaggio, and Katie Leboutillier for their constant love and encouragement.

Kathleen Vuljoin-DiMaggio

To my Lord and Savior for the gift of nursing and teaching, to Dr. Richard A. Winton for his love and support for many years, and in loving memory of my parents, Matthew and Mary Wagner.

Mary B. Winton

To Tracy L. Yeager, my husband, my rock, and support; and to my boys, Jacob and Joshua, for just being boys.

Jennifer J. Yeager

LINDA E. MCCUISTION

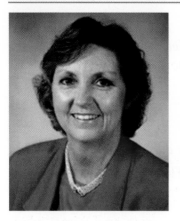

Dr. Linda E. McCuistion received a Diploma of Nursing from the Lutheran Hospital School of Nursing in Fort Wayne, Indiana; Bachelor of Science in Nursing from William Carey College in Hattiesburg, Mississippi; Masters in Nursing from Louisiana State University Medical Center, New Orleans; and PhD in Curriculum and Instruction from the University of New Orleans. She was licensed as an Advanced Practice Nurse in Louisiana and has many years of nursing experience that include acute care and home health nursing. For 20 years, Linda was a Nursing Professor at Our Lady of Holy Cross College in New Orleans, Louisiana. She received an Endowed Professorship Award in 2000 and 2003. Linda worked as a nursing professor at South University, Richmond, Virginia, for 3 years. Currently, Linda teaches NCLEX® review courses for Elsevier.

Linda has served as a past president, vice president, and faculty advisor of the Sigma Theta Tau International Honor Society in Nursing, Xi Psi chapter-at-large. She is a past associate editor of the *NODNA Times,* a New Orleans District Nurses Association newsletter. She has been a member of Phi Delta Kappa and the American Society of Hypertension.

Linda was coordinator for the Graduate Plus internship program, a preceptorship program for new nursing graduates in the state of Louisiana. She has served as a legal nurse consultant; a member of a medical review panel; advisory board member, consultant, and reviewer of a software preparation company focused on the state licensure examination; advisory board member for a school for surgical technicians; and consultant to a local hospital to improve the quality of nursing care and assist acute care facilities in preparation for accreditation.

Linda was chosen as a "Great One-Hundred Nurse" by the New Orleans District Nurses Association in 1993. She is also listed in the 2005/2006 edition of the Empire Who's Who Executive and Professional Registry.

Linda has given numerous lectures and presentations regionally and nationally on a variety of nursing topics. She has published articles in nursing journals and has authored many chapters in several nursing textbooks, including *Pharmacotherapeutics: Clinical Decision Making in Nursing* (1999), *Saunders Manual of Medical-Surgical Nursing: A Guide for Clinical Decision Making* (2002), and *Saunders Nursing Survival Guide: Pathophysiology* (2007). She is author and coauthor of many chapters and coeditor of *Saunders Nursing Survival Guide: Pharmacology* (2007).

Linda enjoys cruises and other travel. When at home, she enjoys family, friends, golf, crafts, playing bridge, and writing.

KATHLEEN VULJOIN-DIMAGGIO

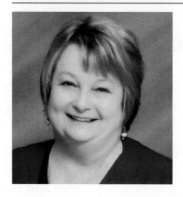

Kathleen Vuljoin-DiMaggio received her Bachelor of Science in Nursing from Our Lady of Holy Cross College of New Orleans and her Master of Science in Nursing from Loyola University of New Orleans, with a focus on Healthcare Systems Management. She completed a preceptorship in palliative care at Ochsner Foundation Hospital through Loyola University. She received Level I designation from the National Hospice and Palliative Care Organization in hospice management and development. She is certified with the Louisiana Department of Health and Hospitals Developmental Disabilities as a Registered Nurse Instructor in medication administration. Kathleen has over 20 years of clinical nursing experience and over 9 years of baccalaureate nursing education. Her professional practice experience includes medical-surgical nursing, neurologic nursing, and home health and hospice nursing. She has experience in nursing management and has worked as director of nursing for a facility specializing in developmental disabilities. In addition, Kathleen has worked as director of nursing in home health and hospice care. She has worked in quality improvement, disease management, and case management.

Kathleen teaches medical-surgical nursing at both junior and senior levels. She teaches in Perspectives of Nursing, a senior launching course, and serves as coordinator of Professional Dimensions of Nursing. She is an academic nursing advisor and serves on the Curriculum Committee, Administrative Council Committee, and Diversity Committee.

Kathleen has served as a volunteer for Junior Achievement of New Orleans, has volunteered for a local hospice agency, and has served in the homeless ministry through her church.

Kathleen is a member of the American Nurses Association, Louisiana State Nurses Association, and Sigma Theta Tau International Honor Society of Nursing, and she is a member of the Alpha Sigma Nu Jesuit Honor Society.

Kathleen is a recipient of the 2011 and 2015 Endowed Professorship from Eminent Eye, Ear, Nose and Throat Hospital. She has received the Order of St. Louis Award through the Archdiocese of New Orleans and has also received the Florence Nightingale Society Award for Nursing.

Kathleen enjoys time with her friends, daughters, and grandchildren. She enjoys golfing, quilting, and cooking.

MARY B. WINTON

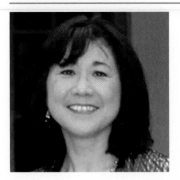

Dr. Mary B. Winton received her Associate Degree in Nursing from Tarleton State University in Stephenville, Texas, a member of the Texas A&M University System; her Bachelor and Master of Science in Nursing from the University of Texas at Arlington; and her PhD in Nursing from the University of Texas at Tyler. Additionally, she is board certified through the American Nurses Credentialing Center as an Acute Care Adult Nurse Practitioner. Mary has many years of hospital nursing experience that include critical care and nursing supervisor. Additionally, she was employed with a hospitalist group as an Acute Care Nurse Practitioner for many years. She is currently an Assistant Professor in the College of Health Sciences and Human Services, Department of Nursing, at Tarleton State University. Mary has experience in teaching graduate-level pharmacology and pathophysiology and nursing informatics and has vast experience teaching at all levels of the undergraduate nursing program, including nursing pathophysiology and pharmacology.

Mary has served as faculty advisor for the Student Nurses Association at Tarleton. She is a member of several organizations, including Sigma Theta Tau International Honor Society in Nursing, Tau Chi chapter; American Nurses Association/Texas Nurses Association; and Rural Nurse Organization. She is actively involved in various university, college, and departmental committees.

During her career as a nurse educator, Mary was the recipient of the Texas A&M Student Evaluation Teaching Excellence Award and the O.A. Grant Excellence in Teaching Award. She is involved in teaching English as a Second Language at her church of membership.

Mary's research interests include health disparity among minorities, especially among Korean immigrants; student learning outcomes; and the use of technology in classrooms. She has presented at several conferences and has published on the health care of Korean immigrants.

During her spare time, Mary enjoys spending time with her husband, daughters, and grandchildren. She also enjoys traveling, reading, crocheting, and snow skiing.

JENNIFER J. YEAGER

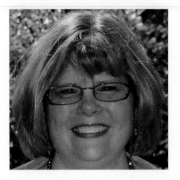

Dr. Jennifer J. Yeager graduated from the University of Portland, Oregon, in 1987 with her Bachelor of Science in Nursing degree; she attended the university on an Air Force ROTC nursing scholarship. Following graduation, she began her nursing career as an Air Force officer, assigned to Wilford Hall USAF Medical Center in San Antonio, Texas. The Air Force provided Jennifer with excellent experience as a transplant/nephrology nurse, and after 6 years of active duty she entered the civilian world as a transplant coordinator at Methodist Medical Center in Dallas, Texas. While there, Jennifer began her Master of Science in Nursing degree at the University of Texas at Arlington, and she completed her degree as an Adult/Gerontological Nurse Practitioner with Educator Role in 1998. After completing ANCC certification in both specialty areas, she went to work in the Baylor Health Care System as a nurse practitioner in Long-term Care and Elder House Calls.

Jennifer moved to Stephenville, Texas, in 2007 and began teaching at Tarleton State University, where she is now Director of the Graduate Nursing Program and RN-BSN Liaison. Since then, she has taught nursing care of the older adult, pharmacology, and research to undergraduate students and RN-BSN students as well as teaching nursing theory, informatics, teaching methods and strategies, pharmacology, and assessment at the master's level. She completed her PhD in Nursing at the University of Texas at Tyler in fall 2013. The findings from her dissertation research were presented at the National Gerontological Nursing Association's annual convention in San Antonio, Texas, in 2014. Currently, she is project director on a research grant funded through the Texas Higher Education Coordinating Board, Nursing Innovation Grant Program, titled "Enhancing Simulation Realism and Building Lab and Simulation Capacity in a Rural BSN Program." Along with a coworker, Jennifer presented the findings from a previous simulation grant at the International Meeting on Simulation in Health Care in San Diego, California, in 2016.

Jennifer currently serves as President of the Tau Chi chapter of Sigma Theta Tau International and as Book Salon Chair for the Society for Simulation in Health Care. She has been involved with revising and reviewing Lehne's *Pharmacology for Nursing Care,* including online components and the study guide, since 2007. She revised chapters for the fifth edition of Meiner's *Gerontologic Nursing.*

To relax, Jennifer enjoys spending time with her family, including multiple dogs. She is a strong advocate for dog rescue organizations and is a member of Pets Are Worth Saving in Stephenville, Texas. Additionally, she enjoys reading, food, and watching television.

IN RECOGNITION

Joyce LeFever Kee taught a pharmacology course to student nurses for 10 years from 1980 to 1990 at the University of Delaware. At the time, there were very few pharmacology texts available and what was published was not appropriate for some BSN and ADN nursing programs. Daniel Ruth from W.B. Saunders approached Kee in 1990 to write a pharmacology book for nurses. With experience in teaching the subject, Kee developed the contents and format for a pharmacology text.

The chapter, Drug Action: Pharmaceutic, Pharmacokinetics, and Pharmacodynamics phases, became the first chapter. These drug phases appear both in the Prototype Drug Charts and within the contents in most of the current chapters. There are many drug tables Kee developed which have been updated by co-authors through the years. The important part that Kee established in the chapters were the five steps of the Nursing Process.

Dr. Evelyn R. Hayes joined Kee starting with the first edition. Hayes developed certain chapters and took the responsibility to work with contributors for the book such as the six chapters on Reproductive and Gender-Related Agents among others.

Linda McCuistion joined Kee and Hayes in 2005. McCuistion has updated many of Kee's chapters with new drugs and content.

Christina DiMaggio Boudreaux, RN, BSN, IBCLC
Director of Nursing
Elba Medical Distributors
Metairie, Louisiana

Linda Laskowski-Jones, MS, APRN, ACNS-BC, CEN, FAWM, FAAN
Vice President
Emergency and Trauma Services
Christiana Care Health System
Newark, Delaware

Bettyrae Jordan, BSN, MA, MEd
Adjunct Faculty
Allied Health Division
Delgado Community College
New Orleans, Louisiana

Suzanne Riche, MSN, RN, BC
Director
Health-Wellness Education Program
Riche Scientific
Denham Springs, Louisiana

Jared Robertson, BSN, MN
Certified Respiratory Nurse Anesthetist
Anesthesia
U.S. Army

CONTRIBUTORS

Christina DiMaggio Boudreaux, RN, BSN, IBCLC
Director of Nursing
Elba Medical Distributors
Memphis, Louisiana

Linda Laskowski-Jones, MS, APRN, ACNS-BC, CEN, FAWM, FAAN
Vice President
Emergency and Trauma Services
Christiana Care Health System
Newark, Delaware

Bettyree Jordan, BSN, MA, MEd
Adjunct Faculty
Allied Health Division
Delgado Community College
New Orleans, Louisiana

Suzanne Riche, MSN, RN, BC
Director
Health Wellness Education Program
Riche Scientific
Denham Springs, Louisiana

Jared Robertson, BSN, MN
Certified Respiratory Nurse Anesthetist
Anesthesia
U.S. Army

Nancy W. Ebersole, PhD, RN
Associate Professor of Nursing
Salem State University
Salem, Massachusetts

Kathy Ham, EdD, RN
Associate Professor, School of Nursing
Southeast Missouri State University
Cape Girardeau, Missouri

Jackie Harris, MSN, APRN
Instructor, School of Nursing
Benedictine College
Atchison, Kansas

Jennifer Hebert, MSN, RN-BC
Education Nurse Specialist
Chesapeake Regional Medical Center
Chesapeake, Virginia

Anita Hornacky, BS, CST, RN
Instructor
Lakeland Community College
Kirtland, Ohio

Janis McMillan, RN, MSN, CNE
Associate Clinical Professor, School of Nursing
Northern Arizona University
Flagstaff, Arizona

Darla K. Shar, MSN, RN
Faculty
Hannah E. Mullins School of Practical Nursing
Salem, Ohio

Harsha Sharma, PhD
Professor, Arts and Sciences
Nebraska Methodist College
Omaha, Nebraska

Amy Winslow, RN
Assistant Professor, School of Nursing
Tarleton State University
Stephenville, Texas

Wanda Wagner, MSN, CNS, RN
Assistant Professor, School of Nursing
University of Holy Cross
New Orleans, Louisiana

The ninth edition of *Pharmacology: A Patient-Centered Nursing Process Approach* is written for nursing students who can benefit from presentation of the principles of pharmacology in a straightforward, student-friendly manner. It focuses on need-to-know content and helps students learn to administer drugs safely and eliminate medication errors through extensive practice of dosage calculations and evidence-based application of the nursing process.

Organization

Pharmacology: A Patient-Centered Nursing Process Approach is organized into 18 units and 55 chapters. **Unit I** is an introduction to pharmacology and includes thoroughly updated chapters on drug action, the drug approval process, cultural and pharmacogenetic considerations, drug interactions, over-the-counter drugs, drugs for substance use disorder, complementary and alternative therapies, lifespan issues, patient collaboration in community settings, and the role of the nurse in drug research.

Unit II focuses on patient care and safety, with completely revised and updated chapters on the nursing process in patient-centered pharmacotherapy, safety and quality in pharmacotherapy, and medication administration. **Unit II** features an introduction to the Quality and Safety Education for Nurses (QSEN) initiative, with special emphasis on patient-centered care and on the QSEN competencies of safety and quality. **Unit II** also features a comprehensive review of drug dosage calculations for adults and children and is a unique strength of this book. This unit, tabbed for quick reference, consists of five sections: Systems of Measurement with Conversion Factors, Calculation Methods: Enteral and Parenteral Drug Dosages, Calculation Methods: Drugs That Require Reconstitution, Calculation Methods: Insulin Dosages, and Calculation Methods: Intravenous Flow Rates. Five methods of dosage calculation are presented, with color coding for easy identification: basic formula, ratio and proportion/fractional equation, dimensional analysis, body weight, and body surface area. Integral to the sections on dosage calculations are clinical practice problems that feature actual drug labels in full color, which provides extensive practice in real-world dosage calculations. With this wide array of practice problems in a variety of health care settings, this unit eliminates the need to purchase a separate dosage calculations book.

Unit III addresses nutrition, fluids, and electrolytes with separate chapters that cover vitamin and mineral replacement, fluid and electrolyte replacement, and nutritional support.

Units IV through XVIII make up the core of *Pharmacology: A Patient-Centered Nursing Process Approach* and covers the drug classifications that students must understand to practice effectively. Each drug family chapter includes a chapter outline, learning objectives, key terms, at least one prototype drug chart, a drug table, and an extensive nursing process section.

- The **prototype drug charts** are a unique tool that students can use to view the many facets of a prototype drug through the lens of the nursing process. Each prototype drug is one of the common drugs in its drug class. The charts include drug class, contraindications, dosage, drug-lab-food interactions, pharmacokinetics, pharmacodynamics, therapeutic effects/uses, side effects, and adverse reactions. With these charts, students can see how the steps of the nursing process correlate with these key aspects of drug information and therapy.
- The **drug tables** provide a quick reference to routes, dosages, uses, and key considerations for the most commonly prescribed medications for a given class. They list the drug's generic names, dosages, uses and considerations, pregnancy categories, and specific information on half-life and protein binding.
- The **nursing process sections** provide a convenient summary of patient assessments, potential nursing diagnoses, plan of care, and outcomes. These sections also include cultural content, nursing interventions, suggestions for patient teaching, and relevant herbal information.

Additional Features

Throughout this edition, we have retained, enhanced, and added a variety of features that teach students the fundamental principles of pharmacology and the role of the nurse in drug therapy:

- **NCLEX study questions** at the end of each chapter help prepare students for the NCLEX examination with its increasing emphasis on pharmacology; answers are listed upside down below the questions for quick feedback.
- **Patient safety boxes** include information on medication safety, complementary and alternative therapies, and more.
- **Key terms** include page numbers and are defined in the text to enhance this "built-in glossary" feature for students.
- **Critical thinking case studies** conclude most chapters. These clinical scenarios are followed by a series of questions that challenge students to carefully consider the scenario and apply their knowledge and analytical skills to respond to the situations.
- **Complementary and alternative therapies** appear throughout the text to provide students with a quick reference to information on popular herbs and their side effects, drug interactions, and more.
- **Anatomy and physiology** unit openers for all drug therapy chapters include illustrated overviews of normal anatomy and physiology. These introductions give students the foundation for understanding how drugs work in various body systems.
- **High-alert drugs** (denoted with the symbol ❶) and **safety concerns** (denoted with the symbol ⚡) are identified within the text with distinctive icons that make it easy to find crucial information.

Teaching and Learning Resources

The ninth edition of *Pharmacology: A Patient-Centered Nursing Process Approach* is the core of a complete teaching and learning package for nursing pharmacology. Additional components of this package include resources for students, resources for faculty members, and resources for both students and faculty.

For Students

A comprehensive *Study Guide,* available for purchase separately, provides thousands of study questions and answers, including clinically based situational practice problems, drug calculation problems and questions (many with actual drug labels), and case studies to help students master textbook content. Answers are provided at the end of the *Study Guide.*

A completely updated Evolve website (http://evolve.elsevier. com/McCuistion/pharmacology) provides additional resources for students, including the following:

- **Review questions for the NCLEX® Examination** organized by chapter
- **Downloadable key points** for content review on the go
- **Pharmacology animations** and **videos**
- **Unfolding case studies** with review questions

For Faculty Members

The updated faculty Evolve website (http://evolve.elsevier. com/McCuistion/pharmacology) includes all of the student resources mentioned previously plus the following instructor-only resources:

- *TEACH for Nurses* **lesson plans** focus on the most important content from each chapter and provide innovative strategies for student engagement and learning. The lesson plans include strategies for integrating nursing curriculum standards (QSEN, concept-based learning, and BSN essentials), links to all relevant student and instructor resources, and an original instructor-only case study in each chapter.
- **ExamView Test Bank** features more than 1000 NCLEX® Examination–format questions that include alternate-item questions as well as rationales and page references for each question.
- **PowerPoint Collection** features customizable slides with images, integrated audience response system questions, and new unfolding case studies with questions.
- **Image Collection** provides approximately 125 full-color images from the book.

This textbook may be supplemented with the drug content found on government agency websites, which supply the latest information regarding changes to drug brand names.

It is our hope that *Pharmacology: A Patient-Centered Nursing Process Approach* and its comprehensive ancillary package will serve as a dynamic resource for teaching students the basic principles of pharmacology and their vital role in drug therapy.

Linda E. McCuistion
Kathleen Vuljoin-DiMaggio
Mary B. Winton
Jennifer J. Yeager

ACKNOWLEDGMENTS

We wish to extend our sincere appreciation to the many professionals who assisted in the preparation of the ninth edition of *Pharmacology: A Patient-Centered Nursing Process Approach* by reviewing chapters and offering suggestions.

We wish to especially thank Joyce LeFever Kee, who originated this pharmacology textbook, and her coauthor Evelyn R. Hayes, who worked tirelessly on many editions of this book.

We wish to thank the current contributors: Christina DiMaggio Boudreaux, Bettyrae Jordan, Linda Laskowski-Jones, Suzanne Riche, and Jared Robertson.

We wish to thank those who created and updated the previous established chapters: Margaret Barton-Burke, Joseph Boullata, Jacqueline Rosenjack Burchum, Katherine L. Byar, Michelle M. Byrne, Karen Carmody, Robin Webb Corbett, Sandy Elliott, Linda Goodwin, Janice Heinssen, Marilyn Herbert-Ashton, Judith W. Herrman, Kathleen J. Jones, Bettyrae Jordan, Robert J. Kizior, Paula R. Klemm, Anne E. Lara, Linda Laskowski-Jones, Ronald J. LeFever, Patricia S. Lincoln, Patricia O'Brien, Laura K. Williford Owens, Byron Peters, Lisa Ann Plowfield, Larry D. Purnell, Nancy C. Sharts-Hopko, Jane Purnell Taylor, Donald L. Taylor, Lynette M. Wachholz, Marcia Welsh, Gail Wilkes, and M. Linda Workman.

Of course, we are deeply indebted to the many patients and students we have had throughout our many years of professional nursing practice. From them we have learned many fine points about the role of therapeutic pharmacology in nursing practice.

Our deepest appreciation goes to pharmaceutical companies for use of their drug labels. Pharmaceutical companies that extended their courtesy to this book include the following:

- Abbott Laboratories
- AstraZeneca Pharmaceuticals
- Aventis
- Bayer Corporation
- Bristol-Myers Squibb (including Apothecon Laboratories and Mead Johnson Pharmaceuticals)
- DuPont/Merck Pharmaceuticals
- Eli Lilly and Company
- Elkins-Sinn, Inc.
- Glaxo-Wellcome
- Marion Merrell Dow, Inc.
- McNeill Laboratory, Inc.
- Merck and Co., Inc.
- Parke-Davis Co.
- Pfizer Inc.
- Rhone-Poulenc Rorer
- SmithKline Beecham Pharmaceutical
- Wyeth-Ayerst Laboratories

Thanks to Becton, Dickinson and Company for the syringe displays. Thanks to CareFusion Corporation for the photos of the infusion pumps.

Our sincere thanks to Elsevier, especially Jamie Blum and Sonya Seigafuse, Content Strategists; Tina Kaemmerer, Senior Content Development Specialist; Tracey Schriefer, Senior Project Manager–Book Production; and Charlene Ketchum, Freelance Content Development Specialist, for their suggestions and assistance.

Linda E. McCuistion
Kathleen Vuljoin-DiMaggio
Mary B. Winton
Jennifer J. Yeager

CONTENTS

Introduction to Pharmacology

When administering drug therapy, it is important that nurses have an understanding of the drug development process and their responsibilities related to drug development and ethical research practices. These topics are discussed in Chapter 1, Drug Development and Ethical Considerations.

Assessing a patient's response to drug therapy is an ongoing nursing responsibility. To adequately assess, plan, intervene, and evaluate drug effects, the nurse must have knowledge of the pharmacokinetic and pharmacodynamic phases of drug action as well as current advances in pharmacogenetics, which are described in Chapter 2, Pharmacokinetics, Pharmacodynamics, and Pharmacogenetics.

Chapter 3, Cultural Considerations, helps the nurse understand and respond to unique cultural factors that may influence adherence to drug therapy for a particular patient. Factors such as heritage, communication styles, family organization, spirituality and religion, health beliefs and practices, and traditional medicine are discussed.

Chapter 4, Complementary and Alternative Therapies, explores herbal supplements that are available over the counter. It covers the most commonly used herbs and discusses their indications, potential hazards, and tips for safe and effective use.

Chapter 5, Pediatric Considerations, and Chapter 6, Geriatric Considerations, cover pharmacokinetic and pharmacodynamic effects specific to these age groups. They also discuss the special attention required when administering drugs to these age groups.

Whereas most drugs are used safely and within prescribed guidelines, it is possible for all drugs to be misused. Drugs that are misused cause serious and complex social and health issues with negative consequences for both the individual and society. This is the topic of Chapter 7, Drugs in Substance Use Disorder.

Drug Development and Ethical Considerations

http://evolve.elsevier.com/McCuistion/pharmacology

OBJECTIVES

- Identify the three core ethical principles.
- Relate the core ethical principles that govern informed consent and risk-benefit ratio.
- Discuss the 2015 American Nurses Association Code of Ethics and its nine provisions.
- Describe the objectives of each phase of human clinical experimentation.
- Discuss federal legislation acts related to U.S. Food and Drug Administration drug approvals.

- Explain the Canadian schedules for drugs sold in Canada.
- Describe the function of state nurse practice acts.
- Differentiate between chemical, generic, and brand names of drugs.
- Define "over the counter" as it relates to drugs.
- Identify three useful drug reference resources.

OUTLINE

KEY TERMS

Approval of new drugs by the U.S. Food and Drug Administration (FDA) has been steady since the early 2000s, reaching an all-time high in 2014 with the approval of 44 new drugs. To facilitate this increase, in 2004 the FDA established its Critical Path Initiative, a national strategy "to drive innovation in the scientific processes through which medical products are developed, evaluated, and manufactured." One focus of this initiative

is on "improving the prevention, diagnosis, and treatment of rare and neglected disorders." Initiative successes include developing biomarkers and other scientific tools, streamlining clinical trials, and ensuring product safety.

The process of drug discovery and manufacturing takes 10 to 12 years, with a cost of more than $1 billion for each drug. Out of every 5000 to 10,000 compounds that begin preclinical testing, only one makes it through the FDA approval process. The steps of the process are shown in Fig. 1.1. Drug research and development is a complex process that is of particular interest and importance to professional nursing practice.

This chapter is devoted to a description of basic ethical principles that govern drug development and the nurse's role in this process.

CORE ETHICAL PRINCIPLES

Three core ethical principles are relevant to research involving human subjects: respect for persons, beneficence, and justice. Derived from the Belmont Report, the World Medical Association Declaration of Helsinki set out ethical principles for medical research that involves human subjects. These ethical principles are integral to the issues of informed consent and risk-benefit ratio in such research.

Respect for Persons

Patients should be treated as independent persons who are capable of making decisions in their own best interests. Patients with diminished decision-making capacity are entitled to protection. When making health care decisions, patients should be made aware of alternatives available to them as well as the consequences that stem from those alternatives. The patient's choice should be honored whenever possible. It is imperative that nurses recognize when patients are not capable of making decisions in their own best interest and are therefore entitled to protection. The nurse can assist with the determination of decision-making capacity through frequent assessment of the patient's cognitive status.

Autonomy is an integral component of respect for persons. Autonomy is the right to self-determination. In health care settings, health care personnel must respect the patient's right to make decisions in their own best interest, even if the decision is not what the health care personnel want or think is best for the patient. Generally, patients can refuse any and all treatments (right of autonomy) except when the decision poses a threat to others—such as with tuberculosis, when taking medications is legally mandated. Autonomy is as relevant to the conduct of research as it is in health care decision making; Patients have the right to refuse to participate in a research study and may withdraw from studies at any time without penalty.

Informed Consent

Informed consent has its roots in the 1947 Nuremberg Code. The two most relevant aspects of the Code are the right to be informed and that participation is voluntary, without coercion. If coercion is suspected, the nurse is obligated to report this suspicion promptly. Informed consent has dimensions beyond protection of the individual patient's choice:

- It is a mutual sharing of information, a process of communication.
- It expresses respect for the person.
- It gains the patient's active involvement in their care.
- It respects the patient's right to self-determination.

It is the role of the health care provider, *not* the nurse, to explain the study and what is expected of the patient to the patient and to respond to questions from the patient. While giving written consent, the patient must be alert and able to comprehend; consent forms should be written at or below the eighth-grade reading level, and words should be kept to fewer than three syllables.

Nurses are patient advocates. In collaboration with the health care provider and the pharmacist, the nurse must be knowledgeable about all aspects of a drug study—including all inclusion and exclusion criteria for participants (Box 1.1), study protocol, and study-related documentation—in order to promote participant safety and quality study results.

Fig. 1.2 shows a sample of an informed consent form for a clinical drug trial, and Box 1.2 shows an informed consent checklist.

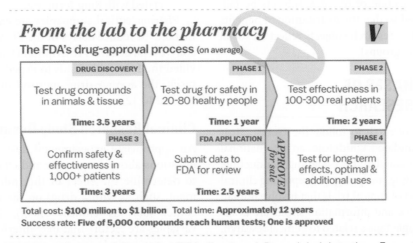

FIG. 1.1 The Drug Approval Process. *FDA,* Food and Drug Administration. From Belluz, J. (2015). This new bill would add $9 billion for medical research. Here are 5 reasons critics are terrified. *VOX Science & Health.* Retrieved from http://www.vox.com/2015/7/14/8961923/21st-century-cures-act

BOX 1.1   Sample Inclusion and Exclusion Criteria

Inclusion
- Persons between the ages of 18 and 65
- Persons weighing between 50 and 100 kg
- Persons on a stable dose (i.e., no dose change in the previous 3 months) of cardiac medications (e.g., anticoagulants, angiotensin-converting enzyme inhibitors [ACEIs], angiotensin II–receptor blockers [ARBs], beta blockers, and diuretics)
- Persons adhering to a no-added-salt diet

Exclusion
- Women who are pregnant or nursing
- Women of childbearing age who do not use oral contraceptives
- Persons with symptomatic cardiac disease, hepatic dysfunction, chronic kidney disease, neurologic disorders, or musculoskeletal disorders
- Persons with clinically significant abnormal laboratory values (chemistry and hematology)

Beneficence

Beneficence is the duty to protect research subjects from harm. It involves assessing potential risks and possible benefits and ensuring the benefits are greater than the risk.

Risk-Benefit Ratio

The risk-benefit ratio is one of the most complex problems faced by the researcher. All possible consequences of a clinical study must be analyzed and balanced against the inherent risks and the anticipated benefits. Physical, psychological, and social risks must be identified and weighed against the benefits. A requirement of the Department of Health and Human Services (DHHS) is that institutional review boards (IRBs) determine that risks to subjects be reasonable in relation to the anticipated benefits, if any, for subjects. No matter how noble the intentions, the calculation of risks and benefits by the researcher cannot be totally accurate or comprehensive.

Justice

Justice requires that the selection of research subjects be fair. Research must be conducted so that the distribution of benefits and burdens is equitable (i.e., research subjects reflect all social classes and racial and ethnic groups).

OBJECTIVES AND PHASES OF PHARMACEUTICAL RESEARCH

The FDA requires clinical research to follow the Good Clinical Practice (GCP) Consolidated Guideline, an international ethical and scientific quality standard for designing, conducting, monitoring, auditing, recording, analyzing, and reporting clinical research. It is the foundation of clinical trials that involve human subjects. Additional guidance and information sheets are available from the FDA on multiple topics related to clinical research.

Preclinical Trials

Prior to the implementation of clinical research, the FDA requires preclinical trials to determine a drug's toxic and pharmacologic effects through in vitro and in vivo animal testing in the laboratory. Through these trials, drug developers are able to determine genotoxicity, the ability of a compound to damage genetic information in a cell, in addition to drug absorption, distribution, metabolism, and excretion.

Human Clinical Experimentation

Historically, drug research was done only with Caucasian males, causing uncertainty as to the validity of research results for people of other ethnicities and for women and children. In 1993, Congress passed the National Institutes of Health (NIH) Revitalization Act, which helped to establish guidelines to include women and minorities in clinical research. Additionally, the Best Pharmaceuticals for Children Act (BPCA) of 2002 and the Pediatric Research Equity Act (PREA) of 2003 encourage pharmaceutical companies to study their drugs in children.

Clinical experimentation in drug research and development encompasses four phases, each with its own objectives (see Fig. 1.1). A multidisciplinary team approach that includes nurses, physicians, pharmacologists, statisticians, and research associates is required to ensure safety and quality in all phases of clinical research. A brief description of each phase follows.

Phase I: Researchers test a new drug or treatment in a small group of people for the first time to evaluate its safety, determine a safe dosage range, and identify side effects.

Phase II: The drug or treatment is given to a larger group of people to see if it is effective and to further evaluate its safety.

Phase III: The drug or treatment is given to large groups of people to confirm its effectiveness, monitor side effects, compare it to commonly used treatments, and collect information that will allow the drug or treatment to be used safely.

Phase IV: Studies are done after the drug or treatment has been marketed to gather information on the drug's effects in various populations and to assess any side effects associated with long-term use.

Pharmaceutical companies are eager to bring new drugs to market. To reduce delays in the FDA approval process, in 1992 congress passed the Prescription Drug User Fee Act, which provided the FDA with funds to expedite the review process. As a result, the average drug approval time has decreased from 30 months to 12.

Clinical Research Study Design

An appropriate experimental design is important to answer questions about drug safety and efficacy. Studies are designed to determine the effect of the independent variable (treatment, such as with a drug) on the dependent variable (outcome, such as clinical effect). Intervening (extraneous) variables are factors that may interfere with study results, and these may include age, sex, weight, disease state, diet, and the subject's social environment. It is important to control for as many of the intervening variables as possible to increase study validity.

Sample Informed Consent Form for Randomized Clinical Trial of a Drug

Title of study: Comparison of a new drug [A] with an existing drug [B} used in treatment of disease X

Principal investigator: Dr. ABC

Institute: Department of Pediatrics, Aga Khan University

Introduction:

I am Dr. [SAK] from Department of Pediatrics, the Aga Khan University and doing a research on treatment of disease [X, for example malaria]. There is a new drug [A] which is being recommended for its treatment. I want to see if the new drug [A] is as good as or better than the commonly used drug [B] for the treatment of disease [malaria]. Since you are a patient of (or suffering from) disease [malaria], I would like to invite you to join this research study.

Background information

Disease X (Malaria) is a common disease in Pakistan, Asia and Africa, caused by a germ (parasite) spread by mosquito. It causes high grade fever. Some patients may have complications and even die. The commonly used drugs are losing their effectiveness and germs are getting resistant to it. A new drug known as [A] is supposed to be effective in treatment of disease (malaria) but there is not enough evidence that it is as good as other drugs used for treatment of disease (malaria).

Purpose of this research study

The purpose of study is to find out if the new drug is as good as or better than other drugs used for treatment of malaria in our population and; also to see if germs are not resistant to it.

Procedures

In this study, all patients aged 15 to 50 years of age, presenting at the clinic with fever for less than one week duration and having no other diagnosis will be registered and screened for malaria. For diagnosis of disease (malaria), one ml of blood will be taken from the patients and checked for presence of germs (malarial parasite). Those patients having positive test for the disease (malaria), will be included in the study. They will be divided randomly in to two groups by a computer draw. One group will get the new drug (A) and the other group will get the commonly used drug (B). Neither the doctor nor the patient will know which drug he/she is getting for treatment of his/her disease. A record will be kept for the duration of fever and other symptoms including any other side effect. Other necessary treatment will also be provided if needed.

Possible risks or benefits

No significant side effects have been reported for this new drug (A). However, some patients may feel nausea or may have vomiting. Drawing of blood may cause some discomfort or blue discoloration at the site of bleeding. Lowering of white blood cells and platelet is a common feature of the disease.

There is no direct financial or other benefit for the participant of the study. However, all the investigations will be done free of cost to the patients and; the drugs (A) or (B) will be provided free. Treatment of any side effect will also be provided free of cost. Sponsor of the study will bear the cost of drugs, investigations and treatment of side effects related to the study drugs.

Right of refusal to participate and withdrawal

You are free to choose to participate in the study. You may refuse to participate without any loss of benefit which you are otherwise entitled to. You child will receive the same standard care and treatment which is considered best for him irrespective of your decision to participate in the study. You may also withdraw any time from the study without any adverse effect on management of your child or any loss of benefit which you are otherwise entitled to. You may also refuse to answer some or all the questions if you don't feel comfortable with those questions.

Confidentiality

The information provided by you will remain confidential. Nobody except principal investigator will have an access to it. Your name and identity will also not be disclosed at any time. However the data may be seen by Ethical review committee and may be published in journal and elsewhere without giving your name or disclosing your identity.

Available Sources of Information

If you have any further questions you may contact Principal Investigator (Dr. SAK), department of pediatrics at Aga Khan University on following phone number 486xxxx

FIG. 1.2 Sample Informed Consent for a Clinical Trial of a Drug. From Sample Informed Consent for a Randomized Clinical Trial of a Drug. (n.d.) Aga Khan University. Retrieved from http://www.aku.edu/research/urc/ethicalreviewcommittee/sampleconsentforms/Pages/sampleconsentforms.aspx

Continued

1.   **AUTHORIZATION**

I have read and understand this consent form, and I volunteer to participate in this research study. I understand that I will receive a copy of this form. I voluntarily choose to participate, but I understand that my consent does not take away any legal rights in the case of negligence or other legal fault of anyone who is involved in this study. I further understand that nothing in this consent form is intended to replace any applicable Federal, state, or local laws.

Participant's Name (Printed or Typed):
Date:

Participant's Signature or thumb impression:
Date:

Principal Investigator's Signature:
Date:

Signature of Person Obtaining Consent:
Date:

FIG. 1.2, cont'd

BOX 1.2   Informed Consent Checklist: Basic Elements

- A statement that the study involves research
- An explanation of the purposes of the research
- The expected duration of the subject's participation
- A description of the procedures to be followed
- Identification of any experimental procedures
- A description of any reasonably foreseeable risks or discomforts to the subject
- A description of any benefits to the subject or to others that may reasonably be expected from the research
- A disclosure of appropriate alternative procedures or courses of treatment, if any, that might be advantageous to the subject
- A statement describing the extent, if any, to which confidentiality of records identifying the subject will be maintained
- For research that involves more than minimal risk, an explanation as to whether any compensation will be paid and whether any medical treatments are available if injury occurs, and if so, what the treatments consist of or where further information may be obtained
- **Research, Rights or Injury**: An explanation of whom to contact for answers to pertinent questions about the research and research subjects' rights and whom to contact in the event of a research-related injury to the subject
- A statement that participation is voluntary, refusal to participate will involve no penalty or loss of benefits to which the subject is otherwise entitled, and the subject may discontinue participation at any time without penalty or loss of benefits to which the subject is otherwise entitled

From Office for Human Research Protections (OHRP). (2014). U.S. Department of Health & Human Services. Retrieved from http://www.hhs.gov/ohrp/policy/consentckls.html

The *experimental group* in drug trials is the group that receives the drug being tested. The *control group* in drug trials may receive no drug; a different drug; a placebo (pharmacologically inert substance); or the same drug with a different dose, route, or frequency of administration.

AMERICAN NURSES ASSOCIATION CODE OF ETHICS

The **American Nurses Association (ANA) Code of Ethics** "was developed as a guide for carrying out nursing responsibilities in a manner consistent with quality in nursing care and the ethical obligations of the profession." It was first adopted in 1950 and most recently was revised with interpretive statements in 2015. The ANA Code of Ethics is founded on the principles first identified by Florence Nightingale, who believed that a nurse's ethical duty was first and foremost to care for the patient. It contains nine provisions (Box 1.3). The 2015 update addresses advances in nursing leadership, social policy and global health, and the challenges nurses face related to social media, electronic health records, and the nurse's expanded role in clinical research.

The Nurse's Role in Clinical Research

Nurses are at the forefront of clinical research. Regardless of the setting (inpatient or outpatient), nurses are likely to encounter patients who are eligible to participate, considering participation, or actively participating in clinical research. As such, nurses are responsible for both the safety of the patient and the integrity of the research protocol.

◎ NURSING PROCESS
Patient-Centered Collaborative Care

Clinical Research

Assessment
- Identify patients who are eligible to participate in or who are participating in clinical research.
- Assess response to the study agent and identify adverse events (an unfavorable or unintended sign, symptom, or disease that was not present at the time of study enrollment and is associated with the treatment or procedure).

Planning

- Have a process in place to identify persons who are eligible to participate in a clinical research or to identify participants actively participating in clinical research studies.
- Have a process in place to facilitate education and informed consent of eligible study participants.
- Plan educational programming for staff who provide direct care to study participants.
- Plan participant care to ensure integrity and compliance with study protocol.

Nursing Interventions

- Support the process of informed consent in a culturally competent manner.
  - Provide an interpreter when necessary.
  - Provide enough time for the person to read the consent and ask questions.
  - Serve as a witness to informed consent.
- After reviewing the study protocol, administer study agent(s).
- Accurately document all participant care, assessment findings, and study agent administration.
- Accurately and safely collect biospecimens.
- Act as advocate, educator, and collaborator in the research process.
  - Ensure safe care.
  - Ensure integrity of study data.
  - Communicate clearly.

Evaluation

- Determine if the potential participant understands what it means to participate in the study by asking open-ended questions.
- Monitor response to the study agent or other interventions.
- Determine whether participants understand how to take their study agents, what to do if they miss a dose, how to store the study agent, and when to call their health care provider.

DRUG STANDARDS AND LEGISLATION

Drug Standards

The set of drug standards used in the United States is the United States Pharmacopeia (USP). The *United States Pharmacopeia and the National Formulary* (USP-NF), the authoritative source for drug standards (dosage, forms, drug substances, excipients, biologics, compounded preparations, and dietary supplements), is published annually. Experts in nursing, pharmaceutics, pharmacology, chemistry, and microbiology all contribute. Drugs included in the USP-NF have met high standards for therapeutic use, patient safety, quality, purity, strength, packaging safety, and dosage form. Drugs that meet these standards have the initials "USP" following their official name, denoting global recognition of high quality.

The *International Pharmacopeia*, first published in 1951 by the World Health Organization (WHO), provides a basis for standards in strength and composition of drugs for use throughout the world. The book is published in English, Spanish, and French.

BOX 1.3 Provisions of the American Nurses Association Code of Ethics

Provision 1
The nurse practices with compassion and respect for the inherent dignity, worth, and unique attributes of every person.

Provision 2
The nurse's primary commitment is to the patient, whether an individual, family, group, community, or population.

Provision 3
The nurse promotes, advocates for, and protects the rights, health, and safety of the patient.

Provision 4
The nurse has authority, accountability, and responsibility for nursing practice; makes decisions; and takes action consistent with the obligation to promote health and to provide optimal care.

Provision 5
The nurse owes the same duties to self as to others, including the responsibility to promote health and safety, preserve wholeness of character and integrity, maintain competence, and continue personal and professional growth.

Provision 6
The nurse, through individual and collective effort, establishes, maintains, and improves the ethical environment of the work setting and conditions of employment that are conducive to safe, quality health care.

Provision 7
The nurse, in all roles and settings, advances the profession through research and scholarly inquiry, professional standards development, and the generation of both nursing and health policy.

Provision 8
The nurse collaborates with other health professionals and the public to protect human rights, promote health diplomacy, and reduce health disparities.

Provision 9
The profession of nursing, collectively through its professional organizations, must articulate nursing values, maintain the integrity of the profession, and integrate principles of social justice into nursing and health policy.

From American Nurses Association. (2015). Code of ethics for nurses with interpretive statements. Retrieved from http://nursingworld.org/DocumentVault/Ethics_1/Code-of-Ethics-for-Nurses.html

---

Federal Legislation

Federal legislation attempts to protect the public from drugs that are impure, toxic, ineffective, or not tested before public sale. The primary purpose of the legislation is to ensure safety. America's first law to regulate drugs was the Food and Drug Act of 1906, which prohibited the sale of misbranded and adulterated drugs but did not address drug effectiveness and safety.

1912: The Sherley Amendment

This act prohibited false therapeutic claims on drug labels. It came about as a result of Mrs. Winslow's Soothing Syrup, a product advertised to treat teething and colic, which contained morphine and led to the death of many infants. Under the Sherley Amendment, the government had to prove intent to defraud before a drug could be removed from the market.

1914: The Harrison Narcotic Act

This act required prescriptions for drugs that exceeded set narcotic limits. It also mandated increased record keeping by physicians and pharmacists.

1938: The Federal Food, Drug, and Cosmetic Act

The Federal Food, Drug, and Cosmetic Act of 1938 empowered the FDA to ensure a drug was safe prior to marketing. It is the FDA's responsibility to ensure that all drugs are tested for harmful effects; it also required that drugs be labeled with accurate information and have detailed literature in the drug packaging that explains adverse effects. The FDA can prevent the marketing of any drug it judges to be incompletely tested or dangerous. Only drugs considered safe by the FDA are approved for marketing.

1951: Durham-Humphrey Amendment

The Durham-Humphrey Amendment distinguished between drugs that could be sold with or without prescription by a licensed health care provider.

1962: Kefauver-Harris Amendment to the 1938 Act

The Kefauver-Harris Amendment resulted from the widely publicized thalidomide tragedy of the 1950s in which European patients who took the sedative-hypnotic thalidomide during the first trimester of pregnancy gave birth to infants with extreme limb deformities. The Kefauver-Harris amendment tightened controls on drug safety, especially experimental drugs, and required that adverse reactions and contraindications must be labeled and included in the literature. The amendment also included provisions for the evaluation of testing methods used by manufacturers, the process for withdrawal of approved drugs when safety and effectiveness were in doubt, and the establishment of effectiveness of new drugs before marketing.

1965: Drug Abuse Control Amendments

Enacted in 1965, the Drug Abuse Control Amendments attempted to control the abuse of depressants, stimulants, and hallucinogens.

1970: The Comprehensive Drug Abuse Prevention and Control Act

In 1970, Congress passed the Comprehensive Drug Abuse Prevention and Control Act. This act, designed to remedy the escalating problem of drug abuse, included several provisions: (1) promotion of drug education and research into the prevention and treatment of drug dependence; (2) strengthening of enforcement authority; (3) establishment of treatment and rehabilitation facilities; and (4) designation of schedules, or categories, for controlled substances according to abuse liability.

Based on their abuse potential and acceptable medical use practices, controlled substances are categorized into five schedules, which are listed in Table 1.1. Schedule I drugs are not approved for medical use and have high abuse potential; schedule II through V drugs have acceptable medical use and decreasing potential for abuse leading to psychological and/or physiologic dependence.

Nurses are key to creating a culture of safety and accountability related to controlled substances. As such, nurses must:
- Verify orders prior to drug administration.
- Account for all controlled drugs.
- Maintain a controlled-substance log that ensures all required information is documented accurately.
- Document all discarded or wasted medication; wastage must be witnessed by another nurse.
- Ensure timely documentation in the patient record following drug administration, including patient response to drug administration.
- Keep all controlled drugs in a locked storage area; keep narcotics under double lock. Be certain that only authorized persons have access to the keys, including keys for patient-controlled analgesia and epidural pumps. Medication may also be administered via an automated dispensing cabinet, with bioidentical identifiers used for access.
- The ANA recognizes the significant threat to patient safety and liability to health care organizations caused by nurse drug diversion and recommends that all states have a peer-to-peer assistance program for addicted nurses. Reporting is mandatory if suspected or known diversion occurs.

1983: The Orphan Drug Act

The Orphan Drug Act was designed to promote the development and manufacture of drugs used in the treatment of rare diseases (orphan drugs). The act's three primary incentives are (1) federal funding of grants and contracts to perform clinical trials of orphan products; (2) a 50% tax credit for costs of clinical testing; and (3) exclusive rights to market the drug for 7 years from the marketing approval date.

1994: Dietary Supplement Health and Education Act

This act established labeling requirements for dietary supplements and authorized the FDA to promote safe manufacturing practices. It classified dietary supplements as food.

1996: Health Insurance Portability and Accountability Act

The Health Insurance Portability and Accountability Act (HIPAA) of 1996 protects health insurance coverage for workers who change or lose their jobs and sets the standard for the privacy of individually identifiable health information. The act provides patients more control over their health information, including boundaries on the use and release of health records.

1997: The Food and Drug Administration Modernization Act

The five provisions in this act are (1) review and use of new drugs is accelerated; (2) drugs can be tested in children before

TABLE 1.1	Schedule Categories of Controlled Substances	
Schedule	**Examples**	**Description**
I	Some examples of substances listed in Schedule I are heroin, lysergic acid diethyl-amide (LSD), *Cannabis*, peyote, methaqualone, and methylenedioxymethamphet-amine (MDMA)	Substances in this schedule have no currently accepted medical use in the United States, a lack of accepted safety for use under medical supervision, and a high potential for abuse.
II	Examples of Schedule II narcotics include hydromorphone (Dilaudid), methadone (Dolophine), meperidine (Demerol), oxycodone (OxyContin, Percocet), and fentanyl (Sublimaze, Duragesic). Other Schedule II narcotics include morphine, opium, codeine, and hydrocodone. Examples of Schedule IIN stimulants include amphetamine (Dexedrine, Adderall), methamphetamine (Desoxyn), and methylphenidate (Ritalin). Other Schedule II substances include amobarbital, glutethimide, and pentobarbital.	Substances in this schedule have a high potential for abuse that may lead to severe psychological or physical dependence.
III	Examples of Schedule III narcotics include products containing not more than 15 mg of hydrocodone per dosage unit (acetaminophen with hydrocodone) or 90 mg of codeine per dosage unit (acetaminophen with codeine), and buprenorphine and naloxone. Examples of Schedule IIIN nonnarcotics include benzphetamine, phendimetrazine, ketamine, and anabolic steroids such as Depo-Testosterone.	Substances in this schedule have a potential for abuse less than substances in Schedules I or II, and abuse may lead to moderate or low physical dependence or high psychological dependence.
IV	Examples of Schedule IV substances include alprazolam, carisoprodol, clonazepam, clorazepate, diazepam, lorazepam, midazolam, temazepam, and triazolam.	Substances in this schedule have a low potential for abuse relative to substances in Schedule III.
V	Examples of Schedule V substances include cough preparations containing not more than 200 mg of codeine per 100 mL or per 100 g (guaifenesin with codeine, promethazine with codeine), and ezogabine.	Substances in this schedule have a low potential for abuse relative to substances listed in Schedule IV and consist primarily of preparations containing limited quantities of certain narcotics.

From Controlled substance schedules. (n.d.). U.S. Department of Justice, Drug Enforcement Administration, Office of Diversion Control. Retrieved from http://www.deadiversion.usdoj.gov/schedules/#define

marketing; (3) clinical trial data are necessary for experimental drug use for serious or life-threatening health conditions; (4) drug companies are required to give information on off-label (non–FDA-approved) use of drugs and their costs; and (5) drug companies that plan to discontinue drugs must inform health professionals and patients at least 6 months before stopping drug production.

2002: Best Pharmaceuticals for Children Act

The BPCA gives manufacturers a 6-month extension of patents to evaluate drugs on the market for their safety and efficacy in children.

2003: Pediatric Research Equity Act

This act authorizes the FDA to require that drug manufacturers test certain drugs and biologic products for their safety and effectiveness in children, noting that "children are not small adults." Additionally, studies that involve children must be conducted with the same drug and in the same disease process as adults.

2007: Food and Drug Administration Amendments Act

This act allows the FDA to do more comprehensive reviews of potential new drugs, mandates postmarketing safety studies, and affects the distribution of drugs found to be not as safe as premarket studies indicated.

2010: Patient Protection and Affordable Care Act

This act was signed into law in 2010 and became effective January 1, 2014. Essential provisions of the reform include (1) quality, affordable health care for all Americans; (2) improved quality and efficiency of health care; (3) prevention of chronic disease and improved public health; (4) improved access to innovative medical therapies; and (5) community living services and supports.

2012: Food and Drug Administration Safety and Innovation Act (FDASIA)

This act was signed into law on July 9, 2012. It strengthens the FDA's ability to safeguard and advance public health by:

- Collecting fees from industry to fund reviews of drugs with the "breakthrough therapy" designation, medical devices, generic drugs, and biosimilar biologic products
- Expediting development of innovative, safe, and effective products
- Increasing stakeholder engagement in FDA processes
- Enhancing the safety of the global drug supply chain

NURSE PRACTICE ACTS

All states and territories have rules and regulations in place to provide guidance and govern nursing practice, which includes drug administration by nurses. Generally, nurses cannot prescribe or administer drugs without a health care provider's order. Practicing nurses should be knowledgeable about the nurse practice act in the state where they are licensed. (Information can be found through the National Council of State Boards of Nursing at www.ncsbn.org.) Nurses are responsible for knowing their state's law and administrative code. Nurses who administer a drug without a licensed health care provider's order are in violation of the Nurse Practice Act and can have their licenses revoked.

In a civil court, the nurse can be prosecuted for giving the wrong drug or dosage, omitting a drug dose, or giving the drug by the wrong route.

CANADIAN DRUG REGULATION

In Canada, prior to approval and becoming available to patients, drugs must be reviewed for safety, efficacy, and quality by the Health Products and Food Branch (HPFB) of Health Canada. Health Canada is a federal department tasked with the mission of improving the quality of life of all Canadians. (Further information can be found at www.hc-sc.gc.ca).

In 1996, the Canadian government passed the Controlled Drugs and Substances Act. This act broke controlled drugs and substances into eight schedules and two classes of precursors (Table 1.2). In 2012, the Safe Streets and Communities Act was passed in Canada, which reclassified amphetamines—including methylenedioxyamphetamine (MDA) and methylenedioxymethamphetamine (MDMA)—and also flunitrazepam and gamma hydroxybutyrate (GHB) from Schedule III to Schedule I drugs. This change imposed stiffer penalties for dealers and those in possession.

INITIATIVES TO COMBAT DRUG COUNTERFEITING

Distribution of counterfeit drugs is a worldwide problem; it is estimated that more than 10% of all drugs available are counterfeit. Counterfeit drugs may contain the incorrect ingredients, insufficient amounts of active ingredients, or no active ingredients. Additionally, they may contain impurities and contaminants or may be distributed in fake packaging.

The most common drugs counterfeited are those used to treat erectile dysfunction, high cholesterol, hypertension, infections, cancer, and HIV/AIDS. The high cost of drugs, combined with the need for prescription drugs to treat chronic diseases—as well as the desire by consumers to misuse drugs (e.g., steroid-containing drugs for body building)—generate a constant demand easily filled by criminals via rogue Internet drug sites. The FDA and consumer groups are working on strategies to combat this problem, including tougher oversight of distributors, a rapid alert system, and better-informed consumers.

The role of the nurse is critical in consumer education. The nurse must advise patients to report any differences in taste or appearance of a drug or in its packaging. Patients should be alert to slight variations in packaging or labeling (e.g., color, package seal), note any unexpected side effects, and buy drugs from reputable sources. Reputable online pharmacies carry the designation of Verified Internet Pharmacy Practice Site (VIPPS; a list of VIPPS-verified pharmacies can be found at www.nabp.net) and display an approval seal. If any suspicion of counterfeit arises, the patient, family, or nurse should contact the FDA at www.fda.gov/Safety/MedWatch/HowToReport.

TABLE 1.2	Canadian Controlled Drugs and Substances Schedule	
Schedule	**Examples**	**Description**
I	Codeine, hydrocodone, oxycodone, coca, cocaine, levomethorphan, ketamine, sufentanil, methamphetamine, amphetamine, gamma hydroxybutyrate (GHB)	Opium poppy, coca leaves, phenylpiperidines, phenazepines, amidones, methadols, phenalkoxams, thiambutenes, moramides, morphinans, benzazocines, ampromides, benzimidazoles, phencyclidine, fentanyls, tilidine, methamphetamine, amphetamine, flunitrazepam, and GHB and its derivatives, alkaloids, and salts
II	*Cannabis*, nabilone, tetrahydrocannabinol	*Cannabis*, its derivatives, and similar synthetic preparations
III	Thirty-three compounds including methylphenidate, lysergic acid diethylamide (LSD), psilocybin, and mescaline	
IV	Twenty-six parent compounds including chlorphentermine, butorphanol, nalbuphine, meprobamate, and zolpidem	Barbiturates, thiobarbiturates, benzodiazepines, and their salts and derivatives; anabolic steroids and their derivatives
V		Propylhexedine and any of its salts
VI	Class A includes 23 compounds such as ephedrine, ergotamine, and pseudoephedrine. Class B includes six compounds such as acetone and sulfuric acid.	Part 1 – Class A precursors Part 2 – Class B precursors Part 3 – Preparations and mixtures
VII		*Cannabis* resin 3 kg *Cannabis* 3 kg
VIII		*Cannabis* resin 1 g *Cannabis* 30 g

For more detailed information, please see the Canadian Legal Information Institute at http://www.canlii.org/.

DRUG NAMES

Drugs have several names. The **chemical name** describes the drug's chemical structure. The **generic name** is the official, *nonproprietary* name for the drug; this name is not owned by any drug company and is universally accepted. Nearly 80% of all prescription drugs in the United States are ordered by generic name. The **brand (trade) name**, also known as the *proprietary* name, is chosen by the drug company and is usually a registered trademark. Drug companies market a compound using its brand name. For example, Lunesta is the (proprietary) brand name of a drug whose generic name is eszopiclone.

Throughout this text, only generic names for each drug will be used because many brand names may exist for a single generic name—for example, the generic drug ibuprofen carries the brand names Advil, Medipren, Motrin, and Nuprin. Generic names are given in lowercase letters, whereas brand names always begin with a capital letter. An example of a generic and brand-name drug listing is *furosemide (Lasix)*.

Generic drugs must be approved by the FDA before they can be marketed. If the generic drug is found to be *bioequivalent* to the brand-name drug, the generic drug is considered *therapeutically equivalent* and is given an "A" rating. If there is less than a 20% variance in drug absorption, distribution, metabolism, and excretion, a generic drug is considered *equivalent* to the brand-name drug.

A list of FDA-approved drug products can be found at www.accessdata.fda.gov/scripts/cder/drugsatfda. The FDA also publishes a list of approved generic drugs that are bioequivalent to brand-name drugs. Generic drugs have the same active ingredients as brand-name drugs but are usually less expensive because manufacturers do not have to do extensive testing; these drugs were clinically tested for safety and efficacy by the pharmaceutical company that first formulated the drug. However, all drugs have varying inert fillers, binders, and excipients used to shape tablets and control how fast or slow the drug is released in the body, and these factors may result in variations in drug bioavailability.

Health care providers and patients must exercise care when choosing generic drugs because of possible variations in their action or in the patient's response to them. In order to maintain stable drug levels, patients should be cautioned *not* to change generic drug manufacturers; this is particularly true when patients are prescribed phenytoin or warfarin. Nurses should check with the health care provider or the pharmacist when generic drugs are prescribed. Health care providers must note on prescriptions whether the pharmacist may substitute the generic drug when the brand name is prescribed.

OVER-THE-COUNTER DRUGS

Although all drugs carry risk, **over-the-counter (OTC)** drugs have been found to be safe and appropriate for use without the direct supervision of a health care provider. They are available for purchase without a prescription in many retail locations. Other OTC drugs (e.g., pseudoephedrine, emergency contraception) are available with some restrictions and must be kept behind the pharmacy counter; prior to dispensing, patient age and identify are verified, and education is provided.

More than $23 billion is spent annually on OTC drugs, which include vitamin supplements, cold remedies, analgesics, antacids, laxatives, antihistamines, sleep aids, nasal sprays, weight-control drugs, drugs for dermatitis and fungal infections, fluoride toothpaste, corn and callus removal products, and herbal products. Information related to OTC drugs available on the market can be found at http://www.drugs.com/otc.

In 2002, the FDA standardized OTC labeling to provide consumers with better information and to describe the benefits and risks associated with taking OTC drugs. It is an important nursing responsibility to ensure that patients are able to read and understand OTC labels. All OTC drugs must have labels that provide the following information in this specific order (Fig. 1.3).

- The product's active ingredients, including the amount in each dosage unit
- The purpose of the product
- The uses (indications) for the product
- Specific warnings, including when the product should not be used under any circumstances, substances or activities to avoid, side effects that could occur, and when it is appropriate to consult with a doctor or pharmacist
- Dosage instructions that include when, how, and how often to take the product
- The product's inactive ingredients and important information to help consumers avoid ingredients that may cause an allergic reaction

Nurses must be aware of OTC drugs and the implications of their use. OTC drugs provide both advantages and potential serious complications for the consumer. The nurse needs to emphasize that many of these drugs are potent and can cause moderate to severe side effects, especially when taken with other drugs. Additionally, many OTC drugs contain the same active ingredients, potentially leading to overdose. Self-diagnosis and self-prescribing OTC drugs may mask the seriousness of clinical conditions. See Box 1.4 for nursing considerations related to OTC drugs.

Interactions between prescription drugs and OTC drugs are potentially dangerous. Many individuals routinely reach for aspirin, acetaminophen, and ibuprofen to relieve discomfort or pain without being aware of these interactions. For example, ibuprofen can increase fluid retention, which can worsen heart failure; use of ibuprofen on a daily basis may decrease the effectiveness of antihypertensive drugs. Ibuprofen has also been linked with cardiovascular events, such as myocardial infarction and stroke; this risk increases with long-term use.

Some OTC drugs, such as cough medicine, are a combination product of two to four drugs. It is conceivable that there could be a drug-drug interaction with a cough medicine and one of the drugs prescribed by the patient's health care provider.

Patients with asthma should be aware that aspirin can trigger an acute asthma episode. Patients may be allergic to aspirin, or aspirin may act as a deregulator of leukotrienes. Aspirin is also not recommended for children with influenza symptoms or chickenpox because it has been associated with Reye syndrome. Patients with kidney disease should avoid aspirin, acetaminophen, and

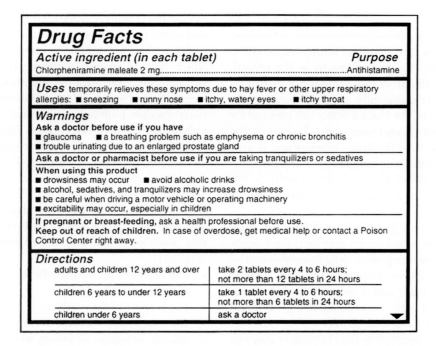

Drug Facts

Active ingredient (in each tablet)	Purpose
Chlorpheniramine maleate 2 mg..Antihistamine	

Uses temporarily relieves these symptoms due to hay fever or other upper respiratory allergies: ■ sneezing ■ runny nose ■ itchy, watery eyes ■ itchy throat

Warnings
Ask a doctor before use if you have
■ glaucoma   ■ a breathing problem such as emphysema or chronic bronchitis
■ trouble urinating due to an enlarged prostate gland

Ask a doctor or pharmacist before use if you are taking tranquilizers or sedatives

When using this product
■ drowsiness may occur   ■ avoid alcoholic drinks
■ alcohol, sedatives, and tranquilizers may increase drowsiness
■ be careful when driving a motor vehicle or operating machinery
■ excitability may occur, especially in children

If pregnant or breast-feeding, ask a health professional before use.
Keep out of reach of children. In case of overdose, get medical help or contact a Poison Control Center right away.

Directions

adults and children 12 years and over	take 2 tablets every 4 to 6 hours; not more than 12 tablets in 24 hours
children 6 years to under 12 years	take 1 tablet every 4 to 6 hours; not more than 6 tablets in 24 hours
children under 6 years	ask a doctor

Drug Facts (continued)

Other information ■ store at 20-25°C (68-77°F)   ■ protect from excessive moisture

Inactive ingredients D&C yellow no. 10, lactose, magnesium stearate, microcrystalline cellulose, pregelatinized starch

FIG. 1.3 Sample Over-the-Counter Drug Label. From U.S. Food and Drug Administration. (2014). The current over-the-counter medicine label: Take a look. U.S. Food and Drug Administration. Retrieved from http://www.fda.gov/drugs/emergencypreparedness/bioterrorismanddrugpreparedness/ucm133411.htm

---

BOX 1.4   Nursing Considerations Related to Over-the-Counter Drugs

Nurses should advise patients of the following when over-the-counter (OTC) drugs are considered:
- Always read the instructions on the label.
- Do not take OTC medicines in higher dosages or for a longer time than the label states.
- If you do not get well, stop treating yourself and talk with a health care professional.
- Side effects from OTCs are relatively uncommon, but it is your job to know what side effects might result from the medicines you are taking.
- Because every person is different, your response to the medicine may be different than another person's response.
- OTC medicines often interact with other medicines, and with food or alcohol, or they might have an effect on other health problems you may have.
- If you do not understand the label, check with the pharmacist.
- Do not take medicine if the package does not have a label on it.
- Throw away medicines that have expired (are older than the date on the package).
- Do not use medicine that belongs to a friend.
- Buy products that treat only the symptoms you have.
- If cost is an issue, generic OTC products may be cheaper than brand name items.

- Avoid buying these products online, outside of well-known Internet insurance company sites, because many OTC preparations sold through the Internet are counterfeit products. These may not be what you ordered and may be dangerous.

Parents should know the following special information about using OTCs for children:
- Parents should never guess about the amount of medicine to give a child. Half an adult dose may be too much or not enough to be effective. This is very true of medicines such as acetaminophen (Tylenol) or ibuprofen (Advil), in which repeated overdoses may lead to poisoning of the child, liver destruction, or coma.
- If the label says to take 2 teaspoons and the dosing cup is marked with ounces only, get another measuring device. Don't try to guess about how much should be given.
- Always follow the age limits listed. If the label says the product should not be given to a child younger than 2 years, do not give it.
- Always use the child-resistant cap, and relock the cap after use.
- Throw away old, discolored, or expired medicine or medicine that has lost its label instructions.
- Do not give medicine containing alcohol to children.

From Edmunds MW: *Introduction to Clinical Pharmacology*, ed 8, St. Louis, 2016, Mosby.

ibuprofen because these can further decrease kidney function, especially with long-term use. Also, patients taking moderate to high doses of aspirin, ibuprofen, or naproxen concurrently with an oral anticoagulant may be at increased risk for bleeding.

The previous examples are not all inclusive. Caution is advised before using any OTC preparation, including antacids, decongestants, and laxatives. Patients should check with their health care providers and read drug labels before taking OTC medications so they are aware of possible contraindications and adverse reactions.

The acronym *SAFER* is a mnemonic for the instructions that the FDA recommends before taking any medicine: **s**peak up, **a**sk questions, **f**ind the facts, **e**valuate your choices, and **r**ead labels.

DRUG RESOURCES

Many drug references are available, including nursing texts that identify related nursing implications and areas for health teaching. Some recommended resources follow.

American Hospital Formulary Service (AHFS) Drug Information is published by the American Society of Health-System Pharmacists in Bethesda, Maryland. It provides accurate and complete drug information for both the health care provider and the consumer on nearly all prescription drugs marketed in the United States. This text contains drugs listed according to therapeutic drug classification. The information given for each drug includes chemistry and stability, pharmacologic actions, pharmacokinetics, uses, cautions, contraindications, acute toxicity, drug interactions, dosage and administration, and preparations.

This reference is updated yearly with monthly supplements that provide information on new drugs such as dosage forms and strengths, uses, and cautions. The text is unbiased. Drug information from the AHFS is available online or in print format.

United States Pharmacopeia—Drug Information (USP-DI) is available in most hospitals and pharmacies either online or in print format. It provides drug information for the health care provider, including pharmacology, precautions to consider, side effects and adverse effects, patient consultation, general dosing information, and dosage forms. The USP-DI also contains patient information presented in a way that is easily understood. The topics include administration of drugs, drug effects, indications, adverse reactions, dosage guidelines, and what to do for missed doses.

The *Medical Letter* on drugs and therapeutics is a nonprofit publication for physicians, nurse practitioners, and other health professionals. Each biweekly issue provides reviews of new FDA-approved drugs and comparisons of drugs available for common diseases.

Prescriber's Letter is a newsletter published monthly by the Therapeutic Research Center in Stockton, California. It provides concise updates and advice concerning new FDA-approved drugs, various uses of older drugs, and FDA warnings.

MedlinePlus is a service of the U.S. National Library of Medicine. Available at www.nlm.nih.gov/medlineplus/druginformation.html, it offers extensive information on prescribed drugs, as well as herbs and supplements, indexed by generic and brand names.

A good source for OTC drug information is *The Handbook of Nonprescription Drugs*, published by the American Pharmacists Association in Washington, DC. This resource is available online and in text. The Internet can be another great resource, but only if credible websites are used.

CRITICAL THINKING CASE STUDY

Miguel, a 53-year-old Hispanic male, is seen by his health care provider for chronic pain in his knees. He states the pain is a dull, constant ache in both knees that happens in the evenings after he's been working as a cashier all day.

1. It is important for the nurse to gather what information about Miguel's medications?
2. Miguel has taken ibuprofen for an extended period of time to control his pain. What risk does this over-the-counter (OTC) drug pose for him?

3. What patient education should the nurse provide Miguel concerning OTC drugs?
4. Miguel is advised by his health care provider to stop taking ibuprofen and begin taking acetaminophen. Prior to leaving the office, he asks the nurse how he will be able to remember the possible side effects of this drug. The nurse tells him he can read the label on his bottle. What is the standardized order of information on OTC drug labels?

NCLEX STUDY QUESTIONS

1. The nurse in the clinical research setting is knowledgeable about ethical principles and protection of human subjects. What principle is demonstrated by ensuring the patient's right to self-determination?
   a. Beneficence
   b. Respect for persons
   c. Justice
   d. Informed consent

2. The research nurse is meeting with a patient and determines, based on the assessment, that the patient meets inclusion criteria for clinical research. The patient agrees to participate in the clinical trial. The nurse advises the patient that which member of the health care team has the responsibility to explain the study and respond to questions?
   a. Registered nurse
   b. Pharmacist
   c. Research associate
   d. Health care provider

3. The clinical research nurse knows that only a small proportion of drugs survive the research and development process. An appreciation of the process and associated costs grows when the nurse is aware that approximately one in how many potential drugs is approved by the U.S. Food and Drug Administration?
   a. 100
   b. 1000
   c. 10,000
   d. 100,000

4. The nurse is interviewing a patient in a Phase I clinical trial. Which patient statement indicates an understanding of this trial phase?
   a. I am doing this to be sure this drug is safe.
   b. I am doing this to be sure this drug is effective.
   c. I hope this drug is better than the current treatment.
   d. I can be part of demonstrating a cure.

5. The foundation of clinical trials, Good Clinical Practice, is a helpful resource for nurses. The nurse is correct in choosing Good Clinical Practice as a reference for standards in which areas? (Select all that apply.)
   a. Design
   b. Monitoring and auditing
   c. Analyses
   d. Reporting
   e. Outcomes evaluation

6. The nurse researcher reviews the proposed informed consent form for a future clinical trial. The nurse expects to find which in the document? (Select all that apply.)
   a. Description of benefits and risks
   b. Identification of related drugs, treatments, and techniques
   c. Description of outcomes
   d. Statement of compensation for participants, if any
   e. Description of serious risks

7. The nurse knows that the patient should be informed about the risks and benefits related to clinical research. What ethical principle does this describe?
   a. Respect for persons
   b. Justice
   c. Beneficence
   d. Informed consent

8. The nurse is reviewing a patient's list of medications and notes that several have the highest abuse potential. According to U.S. standards, the highest potential for abuse of drugs with accepted medical uses is found in drugs included in which schedule?
   a. II
   b. III
   c. IV
   d. V

9. The nurse is reviewing the drug-approval process in the United States and learns that the Food and Drug Administration Modernization Act of 1997 contains which provisions? (Select all that apply.)
   a. Review of new drugs is accelerated.
   b. Drug companies must provide information on off-label use of drugs.
   c. Privacy of individually identifiable health information must be protected.
   d. Drug companies must offer advanced notice of plans to discontinue drugs.
   e. Drug labels must describe side effects and adverse effects.

10. The patient has questions about counterfeit drugs. Which factors alert the patient or nurse that a drug is counterfeit or adulterated? (Select all that apply.)
    a. Variations in packaging
    b. Unexpected side effects
    c. Different taste
    d. Different chemical components
    e. Different odor

11. The nurse knows the importance of administering the right medication to the patient and that drugs have many names. It is therefore most important that drugs be ordered by which name?
    a. Generic
    b. Brand
    c. Trade
    d. Chemical

12. What provisions from the Controlled Substances Act of 1970 were designed to remedy drug abuse?
    a. The act established treatment and rehabilitation facilities.
    b. The act tightened controls on experimental drugs.
    c. The act required clinical trial data on drugs.
    d. The act required drug companies to give information on off-label use of drugs.

Answers: 1, b; 2, d; 3, c; 4, a; 5, a, b, c, d; 6, a, b, c, d, e; 7, c; 8, a; 9, a, b, d; 10, a, b, c; 11, a; 12, a.

2

Pharmacokinetics, Pharmacodynamics, and Pharmacogenetics

http://evolve.elsevier.com/McCuistion/pharmacology

OBJECTIVES

- Differentiate the three phases of drug action.
- Describe the four processes of pharmacokinetics.
- Identify the four receptor families.
- Describe the influence of protein binding on drug bioavailability.
- Check drugs for half-life, percentage of protein binding, therapeutic index, and side effects in a drug reference book.
- Anticipate potential unique responses to drugs based on biologic variations.

- Differentiate the four types of drug interactions.
- Explain the three mechanisms involved with drug-drug interactions.
- Describe the effects of drug-nutrient interactions.
- Explain the meaning of drug-induced photosensitivity.
- Describe the nursing implications of pharmacokinetics and pharmacodynamics.

OUTLINE

Pharmacokinetics
Drug Absorption
Drug Distribution
Drug Metabolism
Drug Excretion
Pharmacodynamics
Dose-Response Relationship
Onset, Peak, and Duration of Action
Therapeutic Drug Monitoring
Receptor Theory
Agonists and Antagonists
Nonspecific and Nonselective Drug Effects
Mechanisms of Drug Action
Side Effects, Adverse Drug Reactions,
    and Drug Toxicity

Pharmacogenetics
Biologic Variations
Tolerance and Tachyphylaxis
Placebo Effect
Drug Interactions
Pharmacokinetic Interactions
Pharmacodynamic Interactions
Drug-Nutrient Interactions
Drug-Laboratory Interactions
Drug-Induced Photosensitivity
Nursing Process: Patient-Centered Collaborative Care
    —Pharmacokinetic, Pharmacodynamic, and
    Pharmacogenetic Considerations
Critical Thinking Case Study
NCLEX Study Questions

KEY TERMS

absorption, p. 16
active transport, p. 16
additive effect, p. 25
adverse drug reactions (ADRs), p. 22
agonists, p. 21
antagonistic effects, p. 26
antagonists, p. 21
bioavailability, p. 17
biotransformation, p. 18
blood-brain barrier (BBB), p. 18
diffusion, p. 16
distribution, p. 17
dose-response relationship, p. 19
drug interaction, p. 24
drug toxicity, p. 23
duration of action, p. 20
excipients, p. 16

excretion, p. 19
facilitated diffusion, p. 16
first-pass effect, p. 17
free drugs, p. 18
half-life, p. 19
ligand-binding domain, p. 20
loading dose, p. 19
maximal efficacy, p. 19
metabolism, p. 18
nonselective, p. 21
nonspecific, p. 21
onset, p. 20
passive transport, p. 16
peak, p. 20
peak drug level, p. 20
pharmacodynamics, p. 19
pharmacogenetics, p. 23

Once a drug is administered, it goes through two phases, the pharmacokinetic phase and the pharmacodynamic phase. The *pharmacokinetic phase*, or what the body does to the drug, describes the movement of the drug through the body. It is composed of four processes: (1) absorption, (2) distribution, (3) metabolism (biotransformation), and (4) excretion (elimination). The *pharmacodynamic phase,* or what the drug does to the body, involves receptor binding, postreceptor effects, and chemical reactions. A biologic or physiologic response results from the pharmacodynamic phase.

PHARMACOKINETICS

Pharmacokinetics is the process of drug movement throughout the body that is necessary to achieve drug action. The four processes are absorption, distribution, metabolism (or biotransformation), and excretion (or elimination).

Drug Absorption

Drug absorption is the movement of the drug into the bloodstream after administration. Approximately 80% of drugs are taken by mouth (enteral). For the body to utilize drugs taken by mouth, a drug in solid form (e.g., tablet or capsule) must disintegrate into small particles and combine with a liquid to form a solution, a process known as *dissolution* (drugs in liquid form are already in solution), in order to be absorbed from the gastrointestinal (GI) tract into the bloodstream. Unlike drugs taken by mouth, parenteral drugs such as eyedrops, eardrops, nasal sprays, respiratory inhalants, transdermal drugs, and sublingual drugs do not pass through the GI tract.

Tablets are not 100% drug. Fillers and inert substances—such as simple syrup, vegetable gums, aromatic powder, honey, and various elixirs—called excipients are used in drug preparation to allow the drug to take on a particular size and shape and to enhance drug dissolution. Some excipients, such as the ions potassium (K+) in penicillin potassium and sodium (Na+) in penicillin sodium, increase the absorbability of the drug. Penicillin is poorly absorbed by the GI tract because of gastric acid. However, by adding potassium or sodium salts, penicillin can be absorbed.

Disintegration is the breakdown of an oral drug into smaller particles. The rate of dissolution is the time it takes the drug to disintegrate and dissolve to become available for the body to absorb it. Drugs in liquid form are more rapidly available for GI absorption than are solids. Generally, drugs are both disintegrated and absorbed faster in acidic fluids with a pH of 1 or 2 rather than in alkaline fluids (those with a pH greater than 7). Both the very young and older adults have less gastric acidity, therefore drug absorption is generally slower for those drugs absorbed primarily in the stomach.

Enteric-coated (EC) drugs resist disintegration in the gastric acid of the stomach, so disintegration does not occur until the drug reaches the alkaline environment of the small intestine. EC tablets can remain in the stomach for a long time, therefore their effect may be delayed in onset. EC tablets or capsules and sustained-release (beaded) capsules should not be crushed because crushing alters the place and time of absorption of the drug. Food in the GI tract may interfere with the dissolution of certain drugs. Some drugs irritate the gastric mucosa, so fluids or food may be necessary to dilute the drug concentration and provide protection.

Most oral drugs enter the bloodstream following absorption across the mucosal lining of the small intestine. The epithelial lining of the small intestine is covered with villi, fingerlike protrusions that increase the surface area available for absorption. Absorption is reduced if the villi are decreased in number because of disease, drug effect, or the removal of some or all of the small intestine.

Absorption across the mucosal lining of the small intestine occurs through passive transport, active transport, or pinocytosis. Passive transport occurs through two processes, diffusion and facilitated diffusion. In diffusion drugs move across the cell membrane from an area of higher concentration to one of lower concentration. Facilitated diffusion relies on a carrier protein to move the drug from an area of higher concentration to an area of lower concentration. Passive transport does not require energy to move drugs across the membrane. Active transport requires a carrier, such as an enzyme or protein, to move the drug against a concentration gradient. Energy is required for active absorption (Fig. 2.1). Pinocytosis is a process by which cells carry a drug across their membrane by engulfing the drug particles in a vesicle.

The mucous membrane that lines the GI tract is composed of lipids (fat) and protein such that lipid-soluble drugs are able

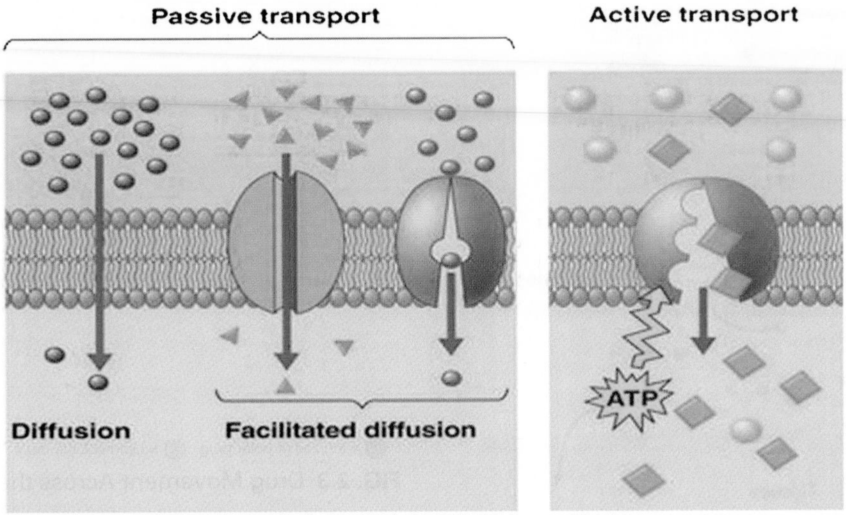

FIG. 2.1 Passive and Active Transport. *ATP,* Adenosine triphosphate. Copyright 2008 Pearson Education, Inc., publishing as Pearson Benjamin Cummings.

to pass rapidly through the mucous membrane. Water-soluble drugs need a carrier, either an enzyme or a protein, to pass through the mucous membrane. Large particles are able to pass through the mucous membrane if they are nonionized (have no positive or negative charge). Drugs that are lipid soluble and nonionized are absorbed faster than water-soluble and ionized drugs.

Blood flow, pain, stress, hunger, fasting, food, and pH affect drug absorption. Poor circulation to the stomach as a result of shock, vasoconstrictor drugs, or disease hampers absorption. Pain, stress, and foods that are solid, hot, or high in fat can slow gastric emptying time, so drugs remain in the stomach longer. Exercise can decrease gastric blood flow by shunting blood flow to peripheral muscles, thereby decreasing blood circulation to the GI tract.

Drugs given intramuscularly are absorbed faster in muscles that have increased blood flow (e.g., deltoid) than in those that do not (e.g., gluteus maximus). Subcutaneous tissue has decreased blood flow when compared with muscle, so absorption is slower when drugs are given subcutaneously. However, drugs that are given subcutaneously have a more rapid and predictable rate of absorption than those given by mouth.

Drugs given rectally are absorbed slower than drugs administered by the oral route. Absorption is slower because the surface area in the rectum is smaller than the stomach, and it has no villi. Additionally, the composition of the suppository base (e.g., fatty bases or water-soluble bases) affects drug absorption.

Following absorption of oral drugs from the GI tract, they pass from the intestinal lumen to the liver via the portal vein. In the liver, some drugs are metabolized to an inactive form and are excreted, thus reducing the amount of active drug available to exert a pharmacologic effect. This is referred to as the **first-pass effect** or *first-pass metabolism.* Most oral drugs are affected to some degree by first-pass metabolism. Lidocaine and some nitroglycerines, for example, are not given orally because they have extensive first-pass metabolism, and most of the drug is inactivated.

Bioavailability refers to the percentage of administered drug available for activity. For orally administered drugs, bioavailability is affected by absorption and first-pass metabolism. The bioavailability of oral drugs is always less than 100% and varies based on the rate of first-pass metabolism (i.e., the bioavailability of rosuvastatin is 20%, whereas the bioavailability of digoxin ranges from 70% to 85%). The bioavailability of intravenous (IV) drugs is 100%.

Factors that alter bioavailability include the (1) drug form, such as tablet, capsule, sustained-release beads, liquid, transdermal patch, suppository, or inhalation; (2) route of administration (e.g., enteral, topical, or parenteral); (3) gastric mucosa and motility; (4) administration with food and other drugs; and (5) changes in liver metabolism caused by liver dysfunction or inadequate hepatic blood flow. A decrease in liver function or a decrease in hepatic blood flow can increase the bioavailability of a drug, but only if the drug is metabolized by the liver. Less drug is destroyed by hepatic metabolism in the presence of a liver disorder.

Drug Distribution

Distribution is the movement of the drug from the circulation to body tissues. Drug distribution is influenced by the rate of blood flow to the tissue, the drug's affinity to the tissue, and **protein binding** (Fig. 2.2).

Protein Binding

As drugs are distributed in the plasma, many bind with plasma proteins (albumin, lipoproteins, and alpha-1-acid-glycoprotein [AGP]). Acidic drugs such as aspirin and methotrexate and neutral drugs such as nortriptyline bind with albumin or lipoproteins; however, basic drugs (morphine, amantadine) bind to AGP. Drugs that are more than 90% bound to protein are known as *highly protein-bound drugs* (e.g., warfarin, glyburide, sertraline, furosemide, and diazepam); drugs that are less than 10% bound to protein are *weakly protein-bound drugs* (e.g., gentamycin, metformin, metoprolol, and lisinopril). The

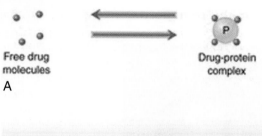

A

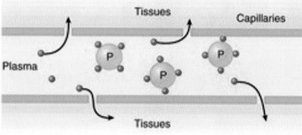

B

FIG. 2.2 Protein Binding. *P*, Protein. From *Pharmacokinetics —objectives* (chap. 4). Retrieved January 1, 2016, from https://quizlet.com/21147360/pharmacology-4-pharmacokinetics-objectives-flash-cards/

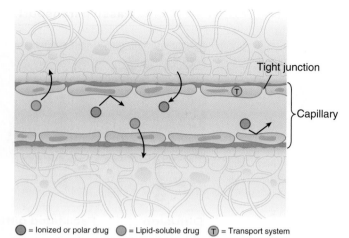

= Ionized or polar drug   = Lipid-soluble drug   (T) = Transport system

FIG. 2.3 Drug Movement Across the Blood-Brain Barrier.

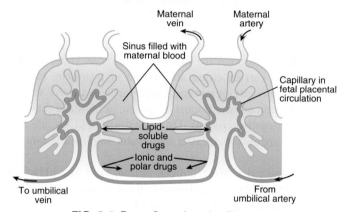

FIG. 2.4 Drug Crossing the Placenta.

portion of the drug bound to protein is inactive because it is not available to interact with tissue receptors and therefore is unable to exert a pharmacologic effect. The portion that remains unbound is free, active drug. Free drugs are able to exit blood vessels and reach their site of action, causing a pharmacologic response.

When two highly protein-bound drugs are administered together, they compete for protein-binding sites, leading to an increase in free drug being released into the circulation. For example, if warfarin (99% protein bound) and furosemide (95% protein bound) were administered together, warfarin—the more highly bound drug—could displace furosemide from its binding site. In this situation, it is possible for drug accumulation to occur and for toxicity to result. Another factor that may alter protein binding is low plasma protein levels, which potentially decrease the number of available binding sites and can lead to an increase in the amount of free drug available, resulting in drug accumulation and toxicity. Patients with liver or kidney disease and those who are malnourished may have significantly lower serum albumin levels. Additionally, older adults are more likely to have hypoalbuminemia, particularly if they have multiple chronic illnesses. With these factors in mind, it is important for nurses to understand the concept of protein binding and check their patient's protein and albumin levels when administering drugs.

Blood vessels in the brain have a special endothelial lining where the cells are pressed tightly together (*tight junctions*); this lining is referred to as the blood-brain barrier (BBB). The BBB protects the brain from foreign substances, which includes about 98% of the drugs on the market. Some drugs that are highly lipid soluble and of low molecular weight (e.g., benzodiazepines) are able to cross the BBB through diffusion, and others cross via transport proteins. Water-soluble drugs

(e.g., atenolol and penicillin) and drugs that are not bound to transport proteins (free drugs) are not able to cross the BBB, which makes it difficult for these drugs to reach the brain (Fig. 2.3).

During pregnancy, drugs can cross the placenta much as they do across other membranes, and this affects both the fetus and the mother (Fig. 2.4). Drugs taken during the first trimester can lead to spontaneous abortion. During the second trimester, drugs can lead to spontaneous abortion, teratogenesis, or other subtler defects. During the third trimester, drugs may alter fetal growth and development. The risk-benefit ratio should be considered before any drugs are given during pregnancy. During breastfeeding, drugs can pass into breast milk, which can affect the nursing infant. Nurses must teach women who breastfeed to consult their health care provider prior to taking any drug—whether over the counter (OTC) or prescribed—or any herb or supplement.

Drug Metabolism

Metabolism, or biotransformation, is the process by which the body chemically changes drugs into a form that can be excreted. The liver is the primary site of metabolism. Liver enzymes—collectively referred to as the *cytochrome P450 system*, or the *P450 system*, of drug-metabolizing enzymes—convert drugs to metabolites. A large percentage of drugs are lipid soluble, thus the liver metabolizes the lipid-soluble drug substance to a water-soluble substance for renal excretion. However, some drugs are transformed into active metabolites, causing an increased pharmacologic response. Liver diseases such as cirrhosis and hepatitis alter drug metabolism by inhibiting the drug-metabolizing enzymes in the liver. When the drug metabolism rate is decreased, excess drug accumulation can occur and can lead to toxicity.

The drug half-life ($t\frac{1}{2}$) is the time it takes for the amount of drug in the body to be reduced by half. The amount of drug administered, the amount of drug remaining in the body from previous doses, metabolism, and elimination affect the half-life of a drug. For example, with liver or kidney dysfunction, the half-life of the drug is prolonged, and less drug is metabolized and eliminated.

A drug goes through several half-lives before complete elimination occurs, and drug half-life is used to determine dosing interval. This is best understood with an example: Ibuprofen has a half-life of about 2 hours. If a person takes 200 mg, in 2 hours, 50% of the drug will be gone, leaving 100 mg. Two hours later, another 50% of the drug will be gone, this time leaving 50 mg; in another 2 hours, 50% more will be gone, so only 25 mg will remain. This process continues such that 10 hours after 200 mg of ibuprofen has been taken, if no additional doses are administered, 6.25 mg of the drug remains.

By knowing the half-life, the time it takes for a drug to reach a steady state (plateau drug level) can be determined. A steady state occurs when the amount of drug being administered is the same as the amount of drug being eliminated; a steady state of drug concentration is necessary to achieve optimal therapeutic benefit. This takes about four half-lives, if the size of all doses is the same. For example, digoxin—which has a half-life of 36 hours with normal renal function—takes approximately 6 days to reach a steady state concentration.

Loading Dose

However, in the case of drugs with long half-lives, it may not be acceptable to wait for a steady state to be achieved. Take, for example, the case of a person with seizures receiving phenytoin. The half-life of phenytoin is approximately 22 hours; if all doses of the drug were the same, steady state would not be achieved for about 3½ days. By giving a large initial dose, known as a loading dose, that is significantly higher than maintenance dosing, therapeutic effects can be obtained while a steady state is reached.

Drug Excretion

The main route of drug excretion, elimination of drugs from the body, is through the kidneys. Drugs are also excreted through bile, the lungs, saliva, sweat, and breast milk. The kidneys filter free drugs (in healthy kidneys, drugs bound to protein are not filtered), water-soluble drugs, and drugs that are unchanged. The lungs eliminate volatile drug substances, and products metabolize to carbon dioxide (CO_2) and water (H_2O).

The urine pH influences drug excretion. Normal urine pH varies from 4.6 to 8.0. Acidic urine promotes elimination of weak base drugs, and alkaline urine promotes elimination of weak acid drugs. Salicylic acid (aspirin), a weak acid, is excreted rapidly in alkaline urine. Treatment of salicylate toxicity includes IV administration of sodium bicarbonate to increase urine pH to 8.0 or higher (alkaline); maintaining alkaline urine promotes the excretion of salicylate at 18 times the normal rate.

Prerenal, intrarenal, and postrenal conditions affect drug excretion. Prerenal conditions, such as dehydration or hemorrhage, reduce blood flow to the kidney and result in decreased glomerular filtration. Intrarenal conditions, such as glomerulonephritis and chronic kidney disease (CKD), affect glomerular filtration and tubular secretion and reabsorption. Postrenal conditions that obstruct urine flow—such as prostatic hypertrophy, stones, and neurogenic bladder—adversely affect glomerular filtration. With any of these situations, drug accumulation may occur, resulting in adverse drug reactions.

Common tests used to determine renal function include creatinine and blood urea nitrogen (BUN). Creatinine is a metabolic by-product of muscle that is excreted by the kidneys; urea nitrogen is the metabolic breakdown product of protein metabolism. Based on National Kidney Foundation recommendations, the estimated glomerular filtration rate (eGFR) is now calculated as part of routine comprehensive metabolic panels (CMPs) and basic metabolic panels (BMPs). The eGFR is calculated using the person's creatinine level, age, body size, and gender. Decreased eGFR is expected in older adult and female patients because of their decreased muscle mass. It is important for nurses to know their patient's kidney function to ensure correct drug dosage.

PHARMACODYNAMICS

Pharmacodynamics is the study of the effects of drugs on the body. Drugs act within the body to mimic the actions of the body's own chemical messengers. Drug response can cause a primary or secondary physiologic effect or both. A drug's primary effect is the desirable response, and the secondary effect may be desirable or undesirable. An example of a drug with a primary and secondary effect is diphenhydramine, an antihistamine. The primary effect of diphenhydramine is to treat the symptoms of allergy; the secondary effect is a central nervous system (CNS) depression that causes drowsiness. The secondary effect is undesirable when the patient drives a car, but at bedtime it could be desirable because it causes mild sedation.

Dose-Response Relationship

The dose-response relationship is the body's physiologic response to changes in drug concentration at the site of action. Two concepts further describe this relationship. Potency refers to the amount of drug needed to elicit a specific physiologic response to a drug. A drug with high potency, such as fentanyl, produces significant therapeutic responses at low concentrations; a drug with low potency, such as codeine, produces minimal therapeutic responses at low concentrations. The point at which increasing a drug's dosage no longer increases the desired therapeutic response is referred to as maximal efficacy (Fig. 2.5).

Closely related to dose-response and efficacy is the therapeutic index (TI), which describes the relationship between the *therapeutic dose* of a drug (ED_{50}) and the *toxic dose* of a drug (TD_{50}). ED_{50} is the dose of a drug that produces a therapeutic

▶ Dose-Response Curve

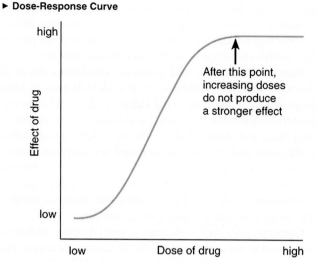

FIG. 2.5 Dose-Response Relationship. From Carlson, N. R. (2010). *Foundations of behavioral neuroscience* (8th ed.). Upper Saddle River, NJ: Pearson.

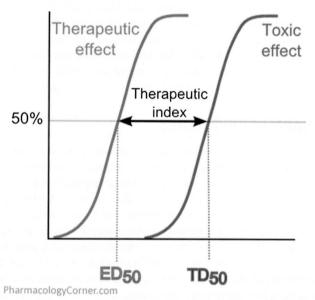

FIG. 2.6 The Therapeutic Index. The therapeutic index is the ratio between the toxic dose of a drug and the therapeutic dose of a drug. From Guzman, F. (n.d.). *Pharmacology corner.* Retrieved on January 1, 2016, from http://pharmacologycorner.com /therapeutic-index/.

response in 50% of the population; TD_{50} is the dose of a drug that produces a toxic response in 50% of the population. The therapeutic index is the difference between these two points (Fig. 2.6). If the ED_{50} and TD_{50} are close, the drug is said to have a narrow therapeutic index. Drugs with a narrow therapeutic index—such as warfarin, digoxin, and phenytoin—require close monitoring to ensure patient safety.

Onset, Peak, and Duration of Action

Other important aspects of pharmacodynamics to understand include a drug's onset, peak, and duration of action. **Onset** is the time it takes for a drug to reach the minimum effective concentration (MEC) after administration. A drug's **peak** occurs when it reaches its highest concentration in the blood. **Duration of action** is the length of time the drug exerts a therapeutic effect. Fig. 2.7 illustrates the areas in which onset, peak, and duration of action occur.

It is necessary to understand this information in relation to drug administration. Some drugs produce effects in minutes, but others may take hours or days. If the drug plasma concentration decreases below the MEC, adequate drug dosing is not achieved; too high of a drug concentration can result in toxicity.

Therapeutic Drug Monitoring

Once steady state has been achieved, drug concentration can be determined by measuring peak and trough drug levels. Peak and trough levels are requested for drugs that have a narrow therapeutic index and are considered toxic.

The **peak drug level** is the highest plasma concentration of drug at a specific time, and it indicates the rate of drug absorption. If the peak is too low, effective concentration has not been reached. If the drug is given orally, the peak time is usually 2 to 3 hours after drug administration. If the drug is given intravenously, the peak time is usually 30 to 60 minutes after the infusion is complete. If the drug is given intramuscularly, the peak time is usually 2 to 4 hours after injection. If a peak drug level is ordered, a blood sample should be drawn at the appropriate peak time based on the route of administration.

Most drugs only require trough concentration levels to be drawn (the exception is aminoglycoside antibiotics, which require both peak and trough levels). The **trough drug level** is the lowest plasma concentration of a drug, and it measures the rate at which the drug is eliminated. Trough levels are drawn just prior to the next dose of drug regardless of route of administration.

Receptor Theory

Drugs act by binding to receptors. Binding of the drug may activate a receptor, producing a response, or it may inactivate a receptor, blocking a response. The activity of many drugs is determined by the ability of the drug to bind to a specific receptor. The better the drug fits at the receptor site, the more active the drug is. Drug-receptor interactions are similar to the fit of the right key in a lock. Fig. 2.8 illustrates a drug binding to a receptor.

Most **receptors**, which are protein in nature, are found on cell surface membranes or within the cell itself. Drug-binding sites are primarily on proteins, glycoproteins, proteolipids, and enzymes. The four receptor families (Fig. 2.9) include (1) cell membrane–embedded enzymes, (2) ligand-gated ion channels, (3) G protein–coupled receptor systems, and (4) transcription factors. The **ligand-binding domain** is the site on the receptor at which drugs bind.

- *Cell membrane–embedded enzymes.* The ligand-binding domain for drug binding is on the cell surface. The drug activates the enzyme inside the cell, and a response is initiated.
- *Ligand-gated ion channels.* The channel crosses the cell membrane. When the channel opens, ions flow into and out of the cells. This primarily affects sodium and calcium ions.
- *G protein–coupled receptor systems.* The three components to this receptor response are (1) the receptor, (2) the G protein

Onset-Peak-Duration

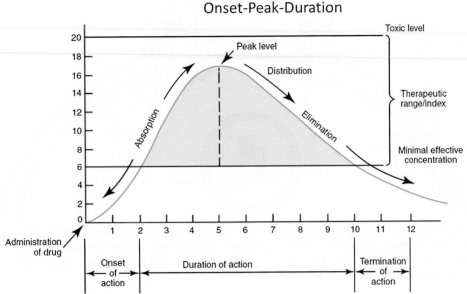

FIG. 2.7 **Onset, Peak, and Duration of Action.** From McKenry, L. M., Tessier, E., & Hogan, M. A. (2006). *Mosby's pharmacology in nursing* (22nd ed). St. Louis: Elsevier.

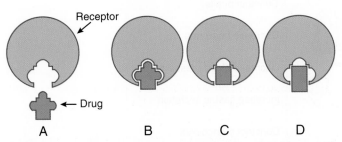

FIG. 2.8 A, Drugs act by forming chemical bonds with specific receptor sites, similar to a key and lock. B, The better the fit, the better the response. Drugs with complete attachment and response are called *agonists*. C, Drugs that attach but do not elicit a response are called antagonists. D, Drugs that attach and elicit a small response but also block other responses are called partial agonists. From Clayton, B. D. & Willihnganz, M. J. (2017). *Basic pharmacology for nurses* (17th ed). St. Louis: Elsevier.

that binds with guanosine triphosphate (GTP), and (3) the effector, which is either an enzyme or an ion channel. The system works as follows:

$$\text{drug} \xrightarrow{\text{activates}} \text{receptors} \xrightarrow{\text{activates}} \text{G protein} \xrightarrow{\text{activates}} \text{effect}$$

- *Transcription factors.* Found in the cell nucleus on DNA, not on the surface. Activation of receptors through transcription factors regulates protein synthesis and is prolonged. With the first three receptor groups, activation of the receptors is rapid.

Agonists and Antagonists

Drugs that activate receptors and produce a desired response are called **agonists**. Drugs that prevent receptor activation and block a response are called **antagonists**. Blocking receptor activation either increases or decreases cellular action, depending on the endogenous action of the chemical messenger that is blocked.

Nonspecific and Nonselective Drug Effects

Many agonists and antagonists lack specific and selective effects. Receptors produce a variety of physiologic responses, depending on where the receptor is located. Cholinergic receptors are located in the bladder, heart, blood vessels, stomach, bronchi, and eyes. A drug that stimulates or blocks the cholinergic receptors affects all anatomic sites. Drugs that affect multiple receptor sites are considered **nonspecific**. For example, bethanechol may be prescribed for postoperative urinary retention to increase bladder contraction. This drug stimulates cholinergic receptors located in the bladder, and urination occurs by strengthening bladder contraction. However, because bethanechol is nonspecific, other cholinergic sites are also affected: the heart rate decreases, blood pressure decreases, gastric acid secretion increases, the bronchioles constrict, and the pupils of the eye constrict (Fig. 2.10). These other effects may be either desirable or harmful.

Some drugs affect multiple receptors, and these are considered **nonselective** drugs. For example, epinephrine, which is used for treatment of anaphylaxis or severe asthma exacerbations, acts on the $alpha_1$, $beta_1$, and $beta_2$ receptors (Fig. 2.11), affecting multiple body systems.

Mechanisms of Drug Action

Mechanisms of drug action include (1) stimulation, (2) depression, (3) irritation, (4) replacement, (5) cytotoxic action, (6) antimicrobial action, and (7) modification of immune status. A drug that stimulates enhances intrinsic activity (e.g., adrenergic drugs that increase heart rate, sweating, and respiratory rate during fight-or-flight response). Depressant drugs decrease neural activity and bodily functions (e.g., barbiturates and opiates). Drugs that irritate have a noxious effect, such as astringents. Replacement drugs such as insulins, thyroid drugs, and hormones replace essential body compounds. Cytotoxic drugs selectively kill invading parasites or cancers. Antimicrobial drugs prevent, inhibit, or kill infectious organisms. Drugs that

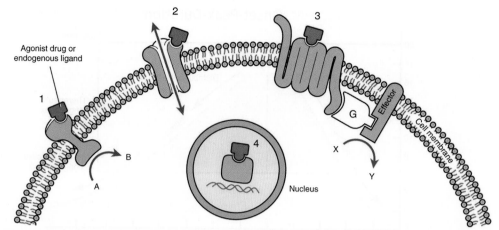

FIG. 2.9 The Four Receptor Families. The four receptor families are (1) cell membrane–embedded enzymes, (2) ligand-gated ion channels, (3) G protein–coupled receptor systems, and (4) transcription factors. From Burchum, J. & Rosenthal, L. (2016). *Lehne's pharmacology for nursing care* (9th ed). St. Louis: Elsevier.

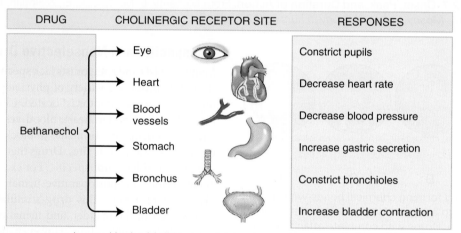

DRUG	CHOLINERGIC RECEPTOR SITE		RESPONSES
Bethanechol	Eye		Constrict pupils
	Heart		Decrease heart rate
	Blood vessels		Decrease blood pressure
	Stomach		Increase gastric secretion
	Bronchus		Constrict bronchioles
	Bladder		Increase bladder contraction

FIG. 2.10 Cholinergic receptors are located in the bladder, heart, blood vessels, stomach, bronchi, and eyes.

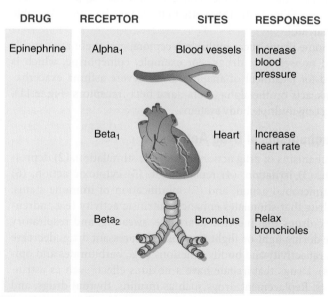

DRUG	RECEPTOR	SITES	RESPONSES
Epinephrine	Alpha₁	Blood vessels	Increase blood pressure
	Beta₁	Heart	Increase heart rate
	Beta₂	Bronchus	Relax bronchioles

FIG. 2.11 Epinephrine affects three different receptors: alpha₁, beta₁, and beta₂.

modify immune status modify, enhance, or depress the immune system (e.g., interferons and methotrexate).

Side Effects, Adverse Drug Reactions, and Drug Toxicity

Side effects are secondary effects of drug therapy. All drugs have side effects. Even with correct drug dosage, side effects occur that can be predictable and range from inconvenient to severe or life threatening. In some instances, the side effects may be desirable (e.g., using diphenhydramine at bedtime, when its side effect of drowsiness is beneficial). Chronic illness, age, weight, gender, and ethnicity all play a part in drug side effects.

It is important to know that the occurrence of side effects is one of the primary reasons patients stop taking their prescribed medications. An important role of the nurse includes teaching patients about a drug's side effects and encouraging them to report side effects. Many can be managed with dosage adjustments, changing to a different drug in the same class, or implementing other interventions.

Adverse drug reactions (ADRs) are unintentional, unexpected reactions to drug therapy that occur at normal drug dosages. The reactions may be mild to severe and include anaphylaxis (cardiovascular collapse). Adverse drug reactions are always undesirable and must be reported and documented because they represent variances from planned therapy.

Drug toxicity occurs when drug levels exceed the therapeutic range; toxicity may occur secondary to overdose (intentional or unintentional) or drug accumulation. Factors that influence drug toxicity include disease, genetics, and age.

PHARMACOGENETICS

Pharmacogenetics refers to the study of genetic factors that influence an individual's response to a specific drug. Genetic factors can alter drug metabolism, resulting in either enhanced or diminished drug response. Nurses must integrate knowledge of pharmacogenetics into their practice in order to identify patients at increased risk for adverse drug reactions, and they must effectively monitor patients for therapeutic drug responses and prevent complications to drug therapy.

Biologic Variations

Through the work of the *Human Genome Project,* an international collaborative research program, the field of pharmacogenomics is rapidly expanding. In the United States, the project is managed by the National Human Genome Research Institute, which is part of the National Institutes of Health (NIH). Pharmacogenomics refers to the study of how genetics play a role in a person's response to drugs (absorption, distribution, metabolism, and excretion). Through the use of pharmacogenomics, the goal is to develop *precision medicine,* which uses the person's genetic makeup to determine appropriate drug therapy, thereby improving patient outcomes and safety (Table 2.1).

In 2005, IBM and the National Geographic Society launched the *Genographic Project.* Since then, the Project has performed DNA testing on populations all over the world. Findings reveal that human beings are 99.9% genetically identical; this implies that there are not multiple races but multiple genotypes (an individual's genetic identity).

Certain classifications of medications have different effects in individuals with specific genetic markers. For example, 10% of Caucasians have no CYP2D6 enzyme activity (identified as poor metabolizers), the enzyme responsible for metabolizing drugs in a variety of therapeutic categories, such as antidepressants, antipsychotics, and beta blockers. A lack of this enzyme becomes important, for example, when a patient who is a poor metabolizer is prescribed codeine. The CYP2D6 enzyme is necessary to convert codeine to the active metabolite, morphine. Individuals lacking this enzyme will have little to no pain relief when prescribed codeine. Conversely, 30% of Ethiopians are ultrarapid metabolizers, individuals who could experience severe, toxic consequences from taking codeine.

Researchers conducting clinical trials for development of new drugs are now required to obtain genetic testing of the participants in the study. The U.S. Food and Drug Administration (FDA) includes pharmacogenomics information in package inserts of more than 150 drugs. The information relates to "dosage guidance, possible side effects or differences in effectiveness for people with certain genomic variations."

Issues to be resolved before widespread genetic testing can occur include cost-benefit ratio and ethical considerations. Genetic testing is expensive and is generally not covered by third-party payers. Genetic information can affect employment, insurability, and family relationships.

Tolerance and Tachyphylaxis

Tolerance refers to a decreased responsiveness to a drug over the course of therapy; an individual with drug tolerance requires a higher dosage of drug to achieve the same therapeutic response. In contrast, tachyphylaxis refers to an acute, rapid decrease in response to a drug; it may occur after the first dose or after several doses. Tachyphylaxis has been demonstrated with drugs such as centrally acting analgesics, nitroglycerine, and ranitidine, to name a few. To provide safe and effective care, nurses must be aware of these potential reasons a patient may fail to respond therapeutically to drug administration.

Placebo Effect

Placebo effect is a drug response not attributed to the chemical properties of the drug. The response can be positive or negative and may be influenced by the beliefs, attitudes, and expectations of the patient. Although the placebo effect is psychological in origin, the response can be physiologic, resulting in changes in heart rate, blood pressure, and pain sensation.

DRUG INTERACTIONS

Seventy percent of Americans are taking one or more prescription drugs. Drug therapy is complex because of the great number of drugs available. Drug-drug, drug-nutrient (e.g., food, supplements, alcohol), drug-disease, and drug-laboratory interactions (when a drug interferes with laboratory testing) are an increasing problem. Because of the possibility of numerous

TABLE 2.1 Terminology Used in Pharmacogenetics	
Term	**Definition**
Genome	Complete genetic material present in a cell
Genotype	The complete genetic constitution of an individual as determined by the specific combination and location of the genes on the chromosomes
Pharmacogenetics	Study of the effect genetic factors have on response to certain drugs.
Pharmacogenomics	A larger scale study of how variations in the human genome affect the response to medications
Phenocopy	An environmentally induced, nonhereditary variation in an organism, closely resembling a genetically determined trait
Phenotype	The observable physical or biochemical characteristics of an organism as determined by both genetic makeup and environmental influences
Polymorphism	The occurrence of different forms, stages, or types in individuals independent of sexual variations

interactions, the nurse must be knowledgeable about drug interactions and must closely monitor patient response to drug therapy. Thorough and timely communication among members of the health team is essential. Patients at high risk for interactions include those who have chronic health conditions, take multiple medications, see more than one health care provider, and use multiple pharmacies. Older adults are at especially high risk for drug interactions because 20% of older adults take five or more medications. Multiple drug-interaction checker websites are available on the Internet for both health care personnel and consumer use, such as Drugs.com at www.drugs.com/drug_interactions.html or *Web*MD at www.webmd.com/interaction-checker.

A drug interaction is defined as an altered or modified action or effect of a drug as a result of interaction with one or multiple drugs. It should not be confused with drug incompatibility or an adverse drug reaction, an undesirable drug effect that ranges from mild untoward effects to severe toxic effects that include hypersensitivity reaction and anaphylaxis. Drug incompatibility is a chemical or physical reaction that occurs among two or more drugs in vitro. In other words, the reaction occurs between two or more drugs within a syringe, IV bag, or other artificial environment outside of the body.

Drug interactions can be divided into two categories, pharmacokinetic and pharmacodynamic interactions.

Pharmacokinetic Interactions

Pharmacokinetic interactions are changes that occur in the absorption, distribution, metabolism, and excretion of one or more drugs.

Absorption

When a person takes two drugs at the same time, the rate of absorption of one or both drugs can change. A drug can block, decrease, or increase the absorption of another drug. It can do this in one of three ways: (1) by increasing or decreasing gastric emptying time, (2) by changing the gastric pH, or (3) by forming drug complexes.

Drugs that increase the speed of gastric emptying, such as laxatives, may cause an increase in gastric and intestinal motility and a decrease in drug absorption. Most drugs are absorbed primarily in the small intestine; exceptions include barbiturates, salicylates, and theophylline, which undergo gastric absorption. Opioids and anticholinergic drugs such as atropine decrease gastric emptying time and GI motility, causing an increase in absorption rate. For drugs that undergo gastric absorption, the amount or extent of absorption increases the longer the drug remains in the stomach.

When the gastric pH is decreased, a weakly acidic drug such as aspirin is less ionized and is more rapidly absorbed. Drugs that increase the gastric pH decrease absorption of weak-acid drugs. Antacids such as magnesium hydroxide and aluminum hydroxide raise the gastric pH and block or slow absorption. Some drugs may react chemically. For example, tetracycline and the heavy-metal ions calcium, magnesium, aluminum, and iron found in antacids or iron supplements may lead to the formation of a drug complex and thus prevent the absorption of tetracycline. This phenomenon may also be observed when products that contain calcium, magnesium, or iron are ingested

with fluoroquinolone antibiotics such as ciprofloxacin. Consequently, dairy products, multivitamins, and antacids should be avoided 1 hour before and 2 hours after tetracycline or ciprofloxacin administration. The nonabsorbable, cholesterol-lowering drug cholestyramine binds with multiple drugs and fat-soluble vitamins (e.g., vitamin K) in the GI tract, resulting in reduced absorption. Vitamin supplementation may be necessary when cholestyramine is prescribed.

At times, the formation of drug complexes is desired; for example, in the case of acute iron poisoning. In this situation, the chelating agent deferoxamine is administered; it binds to the excess iron in the blood so it can be excreted from the body via the kidneys.

GI bacteria account for 70% of the body's microbes. They play a major role in the absorption of drugs and nutrients and in the metabolism of bilirubin, bile acids, cholesterol, and steroid hormones as well as the synthesis of vitamins B and K. GI bacteria help to maintain homeostasis and factor into the overall health and immune status of an individual. Alteration of bacteria normally found in the GI tract (caused by patient genotype, antibiotic treatment, diet, and environment) can affect drug pharmacokinetics. Orally administered drugs can be metabolized by intestinal microbial enzymes, resulting in toxic compounds or reduced drug absorption, which leads to decreased therapeutic response. For example, administration of antibiotics can alter the synthesis of vitamin K, interfering with therapeutic blood levels of the anticoagulant warfarin.

Metabolism

Many drug interactions of metabolism occur with the induction or inhibition of the hepatic microsomal system. A drug can increase the metabolism of another drug by stimulating liver enzymes. These enzymes produce a cascade effect in drug function. Drugs that promote induction of enzymes are called *enzyme inducers*. Some drugs—such as phenobarbital, carbamazepine, and rifampin—are enzyme inducers. Phenobarbital increases the metabolism of most antipsychotics and methylxanthine; phenobarbital, carbamazepine, and rifampin increase the metabolism of warfarin. Increased metabolism promotes drug elimination and decreases plasma concentration of the drug; the result is a decrease in therapeutic drug action. Care must be taken when enzyme inducers are discontinued because less drug is eliminated by hepatic metabolism, and toxicity can result.

Some drugs are enzyme inhibitors. The antiulcer drug cimetidine is an enzyme inhibitor that decreases metabolism of certain drugs (e.g., theophylline, warfarin, phenytoin) and causes an increase in the plasma concentration of these drugs. To avoid toxicity, dosage of these drugs must be reduced. If cimetidine or any enzyme drug inhibitor is discontinued, the dosage of other drugs affected by its administration should be adjusted, and blood levels should be closely monitored.

The use of tobacco and alcohol may have variable effects on drug metabolism. Polycyclic aromatic hydrocarbons found in cigarette smoke induce production of the specific family of enzymes responsible for theophylline metabolism. Chronic cigarette smoking leads to an increase in hepatic enzyme activity and can increase theophylline clearance. Asthmatics who smoke and take theophylline to manage their disease may require an increase in theophylline dosage. With chronic alcohol use, hepatic enzyme activities are increased; with acute alcohol use, metabolism is inhibited.

Natural or herbal products can also impact drug metabolism. St. John's wort, an OTC herbal product used to manage symptoms of depression, induces the metabolism of certain drugs (e.g., warfarin, digoxin, and theophylline). This action potentially decreases the effectiveness of these medications, possibly necessitating a dose increase to sustain efficacy. Flavonoids, a group of naturally occurring compounds found in the juice and pulp of citrus fruits, are potent inhibitors of the metabolism of certain drugs (e.g., carbamazepine, calcium channel blockers, and drugs for erectile dysfunction). Patients who are stabilized on therapeutic doses of these drugs may subject themselves to adverse effects from greater-than-expected drug levels if they eat or drink grapefruit products concurrently with the drug. Table 2.2 describes the effects of drug enzyme inducers and inhibitors.

Excretion

Most drugs are filtered through the glomeruli and are excreted in the urine. With some drugs, excretion occurs in the bile, which passes into the intestinal tract. Drugs can increase or decrease renal excretion and can have an effect on the excretion of other drugs. Drugs that decrease cardiac output decrease blood flow to the kidneys; decreased blood flow results in decreased glomerular filtration rate, which can decrease or delay drug excretion.

Diuretics promote water and sodium excretion from the renal tubules. Furosemide acts on the loop of Henle, and hydrochlorothiazide acts on the distal tubules. Both diuretics decrease reabsorption of water, sodium, and potassium. The renal loss of potassium can result in *hypokalemia,* which can alter the action of some drugs; for example, it can enhance the action of digoxin and can lead to toxicity.

Two or more drugs that undergo the same route of excretion may compete with one another for elimination from the body. Probenecid, a drug for gout, decreases penicillin excretion by inhibiting the secretion of penicillin in the renal tubules of the kidneys. In some cases, this effect may be desirable to increase or maintain the plasma concentration of penicillin—which has a short half-life—for a prolonged period of time.

Changing urine pH affects drug excretion. The antacid sodium bicarbonate causes the urine to be alkaline. Alkaline urine promotes the excretion of drugs that are weak acids (e.g., aspirin, barbiturates). Drugs that acidify the urine, such as ascorbic acid, promote the excretion of drugs that are weak bases (e.g., amphetamine).

With decreased renal or hepatic function, there is usually an increase in free drug concentration. It is essential to closely monitor these patients for drug toxicity when they take multiple drugs. Checking serum drug levels, a practice known as **therapeutic drug monitoring (TDM),** is especially important for drugs that have a narrow therapeutic range and are highly protein bound. Digoxin and phenytoin are two drugs that require TDM.

Pharmacodynamic Interactions

Pharmacodynamic interactions are those that result in additive, synergistic, or antagonistic drug effects.

Additive Drug Effects

When two drugs are administered in combination, and the response is increased beyond what either could produce alone, the drug interaction is called an **additive effect**; it is the sum of the effects of the two drugs. Additive effects can be desirable or undesirable. For example, a desirable additive drug effect occurs when a diuretic and a beta blocker are administered for the treatment of hypertension. In combination, these two drugs use different mechanisms to have a more pronounced blood pressure–lowering effect. As another example, aspirin and codeine are two analgesics that work by different mechanisms but can be given together for increased pain relief.

An example of an undesirable additive effect is that from two vasodilators, hydralazine prescribed for hypertension and nitroglycerin prescribed for angina. The result could be a severe hypotensive response. Another example is the interaction of aspirin and alcohol. Aspirin is directly irritating to the stomach; it causes platelet dysfunction, and it inhibits prostaglandin-mediated mucus production of the gastric mucosa that protects the underlying tissues of the stomach. Alcohol disrupts the gastric mucosal barrier and suppresses platelet production. Both aspirin and alcohol can prolong bleeding time and, when taken together, may result in gastric bleeding.

Synergistic Drug Effects and Potentiation

When two or more drugs are given together, one drug can have a **synergistic effect** on another. In other words, the clinical effect of the two drugs given together is substantially greater than that of either drug alone. An example of this is the use of two cytotoxic drugs to reduce individual drug dosing, thereby decreasing side effects. An example of an undesirable effect occurs

TABLE 2.2	**Drugs: Enzyme Inducers and Enzyme Inhibitors**
Drug Category	**Drug Effect**
Drug enzyme inducer	Onset and termination of drug effect is slow, approximately 1 week.
	Drug dosage may need to be increased with use of drug inducer.
	Drug dosage should be adjusted after termination of drug inducer.
	Monitor serum drug levels, especially if the drug has a narrow therapeutic drug range.
Drug enzyme inhibitor	Onset of drug effect usually occurs rapidly.
	Half-life ($t\frac{1}{2}$) of the second drug may be increased, causing a prolonged drug effect.
	Interaction may occur related to the dosage prescribed.
	Disease entities affect drug dosing.
	Monitor serum drug levels, especially if the drug has a narrow therapeutic range.

when alcohol and a sedative-hypnotic drug such as diazepam are combined. The resultant effect of this example is increased CNS depression.

Some antibiotics have an enzyme inhibitor added to the drug to potentiate the therapeutic effect. Examples are ampicillin with sulbactam and amoxicillin with clavulanate, in which sulbactam and clavulanate potassium are bacterial enzyme inhibitors. Ampicillin and amoxicillin can be given without these inhibitors; however, the desired therapeutic effect may not occur because of the bacterial beta-lactamase, which inactivates the drugs and causes bacterial resistance. The combination of the antibiotic with either sulbactam or clavulanate inhibits bacterial enzyme activity and enhances the effect, or broadens the spectrum of activity, of the antibacterial agent.

Antagonistic Drug Effects

When drugs with antagonistic effects are administered together, one drug reduces or blocks the effect of the other. In some situations, antagonistic effects are desirable. In morphine sulfate overdose, naloxone is given as an antagonist to block the narcotic effects of morphine sulfate. This is a beneficial drug interaction of an antagonist. Likewise, in the case of heparin overdose, protamine sulfate is administered to block the effects of heparin.

The most common symptoms of drug-drug interactions include nausea, heartburn, headache, and lightheadedness. Patients should contact their pharmacist or health care provider if they experience any unusual reaction. The most feared interactions are those that result in a dramatic drop in blood pressure or cause a rapid or irregular heart rate. Also of concern are drug interactions that produce toxins capable of damaging vital organs such as the heart or liver. Fortunately, most interactions are not severe or life threatening. Patients should be aware that prescription drugs, OTC drugs, and herbal products can interact with each other. It is a myth that interactions occur only with prescription medications. Severe adverse reactions are highlighted with a boxed warning in the product literature.

DRUG-NUTRIENT INTERACTIONS

Food may increase, decrease, or delay the body's pharmacokinetic response to drugs. A classic drug-food interaction occurs when a monoamine oxidase inhibitor (MAOI) antidepressant (e.g., phenelzine) is taken with tyramine-rich foods such as cheese, wine, organ meats, beer, yogurt, sour cream, or bananas. Tyramine is a potent vasoconstrictor, and when taken in conjunction with an MAOI, the result could be a hypertensive crisis. These foods must be avoided when taking MAOIs.

Grapefruit alters the metabolism of many drugs through inhibition of the CYP450-3A4 drug-metabolizing enzyme. This is important because the CYP3A4 substrate is involved in metabolism of roughly 50% of the drugs on the market; grapefruit is known to effect more than 44 drugs, inhibiting metabolism and potentially causing serious adverse drug reactions.

Nutritional deficiencies such as protein-energy malnutrition (PEM) may alter pharmacokinetic processes and drug responses, resulting in toxicity. There are two forms of PEM, kwashiorkor and marasmus. Persons with either form of PEM may have altered pharmacokinetics, such as decreased drug absorption and decreased protein binding, altered volume of distribution and biotransformation, and decreased drug elimination. Because of the risk for toxicity, persons with PEM require careful monitoring and possible changes in drug dosing.

DRUG-LABORATORY INTERACTIONS

Drugs often interfere with clinical laboratory testing by cross-reaction with antibodies, interference with enzyme reactions, or alteration of chemical reactions. Drug-laboratory interactions may lead to misinterpretation or invalidation of test results, resulting in additional health care costs associated with unnecessary repeat laboratory testing or additional testing. Drug-laboratory interactions may also lead to missed or erroneous clinical diagnosis. Health care personnel and consumers can find information related to drug-laboratory interactions on several websites on the Internet, such as RxList at http://www.rxlist.com/script/main/hp.asp.

DRUG-INDUCED PHOTOSENSITIVITY

A drug-induced photosensitivity reaction is a skin reaction caused by exposure to sunlight. It is caused most often by the interaction of a drug and exposure to ultraviolet A (UVA) light, which can cause cellular damage; however, ultraviolet B (UVB) light may also contribute to drug-induced photosensitivity reactions.

The two types of photosensitivity reactions are photoallergic and phototoxic. A *photoallergic reaction* occurs when a drug (e.g., sulfonamide) undergoes activation in the skin by ultraviolet light to a compound that is more allergenic than the parent compound. Because it takes time to develop antibodies, photoallergic reactions are a type of delayed hypersensitivity reaction. With a *phototoxic reaction,* a photosensitive drug undergoes photochemical reactions within the skin to cause damage. This type of reaction is not immune mediated. The onset of a phototoxic reaction with erythema can be rapid, occurring within 2 to 6 hours of sunlight exposure.

Both types of reactions are the result of light exposure, but they differ according to the wavelength of light and the photosensitive drug. A phototoxic reaction may be the result of the drug dose, whereas a photoallergic reaction is not and only requires previous exposure, or sensitization, to the offending agent. Examples of drugs that can induce photosensitivity are listed in Table 2.3.

Most photosensitive reactions can be avoided by using sunscreen with a sun protection factor (SPF) greater than 15; avoiding excessive sunlight, especially at the height of the daylight hours; and wearing protective clothing. Decreasing the drug dose may decrease the risk of photosensitivity if treatment is required. It may be necessary, however, to discontinue use of the offending drug.

TABLE 2.3 Examples of Drugs That Cause Drug-Induced Photosensitivity

Oral Drugs

Antibiotics	Tetracyclines
	Fluoroquinolones (e.g., ciprofloxacin)
	Sulfonamides
Nonsteroidal antiinflammatory drugs (NSAIDs)	Ibuprofen
	Naproxen
	Ketoprofen
	Celecoxib
Diuretics	Furosemide
	Bumetanide
	Hydrochlorothiazide
Retinoids	Isotretinoin
	Acitretin
Hypoglycemics	Sulfonylureas (e.g., glipizide, glyburide)
Anticonvulsants	Phenothiazines (e.g., chlorpromazine, fluphenazine)
	Thioxanthenes (e.g., chlorprothixene)
Other drugs	Amiodarone
	Diltiazem
	Quinine
	Quinidine
	Hydroxychloroquine
	Enalapril
	Dapsone

Topical Agents

Sunscreens	Benzophenones
	Para-aminobenzoic acid (PABA)
	Cinnamates
	Salicylates
Fragrances	Musk
	6-Methylcoumarin
Miscellaneous	5-Fluorouracil (oral and topical)
	Coal tar

From DermNet NZ. *Drug-induced sensitivity*. Retrieved from http://www.dermnetnz.org/reactions/drug-photosensitivity.html.

NURSING PROCESS
Patient-Centered Collaborative Care

Pharmacokinetic, Pharmacodynamic, and Pharmacogenetic Considerations

Assessment
- Assess family patterns, economic issues, and cultural patterns that influence compliance with the medical regimen.
- Assess language spoken, literacy level, cognitive level, and use of glasses or other aids.
- Check peak levels and trough levels of drugs as appropriate.
- Detect possible interactions and cumulative or other adverse effects among prescribed medications, self-administered over-the-counter (OTC) products, culturally based home treatments, herbal remedies, and foods.
- Determine whether the patient participates in traditional health practices or complementary and alternative medical practices.
- Determine renal function by checking for adequate urine output; the guideline is 30 mL/hr for adults.
- Determine the potential for drug interaction problems related to an increased or decreased absorption rate of drugs.
- Determine whether the patient smokes cigarettes.
- Identify all of the patient's current drugs, including prescription and OTC drugs, supplements, herbs, and teas.
- Inquire about the patient's preferences regarding touch, modesty, and personal space.
- Perform a physical exam to identify problems that may affect pharmacokinetics and pharmacodynamics.
- Review all literature provided by drug companies and pharmacies; be sure to check the protein-binding percentage of the drug and any need for therapeutic monitoring.
- Take a thorough patient history to identify factors that may affect drug pharmacokinetics and pharmacodynamics.

Nursing Diagnoses
- Anxiety related to health status, unmet needs, role function and status, heredity
- Deficient Knowledge related to information misinterpretations, unfamiliarity with information resources and cultural differences
- Ineffective Self–Health Management related to complexity of therapeutic regimen, economic difficulties, complexity of health care system and cultural differences
- Ineffective Health Maintenance related to deficient communication skills, insufficient resources, ineffective coping
- Ineffective Protection related to pharmaceutical agents and treatment-related side effects

Planning
- The patient will demonstrate behaviors that decrease the risk for injury.
- The patient will describe the rationale for the therapeutic regimen.

- The patient will discuss blocks to implementing a therapeutic regimen or related fears.
- Effective communication techniques will be utilized.
- The patient will follow a mutually agreed on health maintenance plan.
- The patient will be aware of drug interactions, will avoid drugs that may cause a severe reaction, and will know what to report immediately to the health care provider.
- The patient will effectively manage the therapeutic regimen.
- The patient will not take any OTC drugs without consultation with the health care provider.
- The patient's health care needs will be met within a culturally competent framework.
- The patient will express confidence in his or her personal ability to manage the health situation and remain in control of life.

Nursing Interventions
- Advise patients not to eat high-fat foods before ingesting an enteric-coated tablet; high-fat foods decrease the drug absorption rate.
- Allow patients adequate time with significant members of the social group.
- Anticipate unique responses to drugs based on social, cultural, and biologic influences.
- Consult a pharmacist about the use of a drug-interaction computer program.
- Consult with persons who are knowledgeable about both the patient's culture and mainstream culture.
- Contact the health care provider to assess the need for a drug dose adjustment if one has not been ordered after a drug enzyme inducer has been discontinued.
- If negative side effects of prescribed drugs are a problem, explain that many side effects can be controlled or eliminated.
- Include significant members of the social group in the planning and implementation of patient care.
- Monitor the therapeutic range of drugs that are more toxic or that have a narrow therapeutic range.
- Notify the health care provider of drugs ordered that have antagonistic or opposite effects, such as beta stimulants and beta blockers.

- Recognize drugs of the same category that might have an additive effect. The additive drug effect might be undesirable and could cause a severe physiologic response.
- Recognize the need for patients to exercise control in their environment.
- Reconcile all drugs at discharge and provide a list to the patient; ensure that accurate drug information is available to all health care personnel involved in patient care.
- Simplify therapy.
- Use appropriate persons as translators.
- Use therapeutic communication.

Patient Teaching
- Advise patients not to take OTC drugs with prescribed drugs without first notifying the health care provider.
- Encourage the patient to use one pharmacy.
- Include significant members of the social group, when appropriate, in the drug regimen.
- Remind patients to be cautious about taking herbal products, especially if taking OTC or prescription medications; advise that they check with their health care provider first.
- Use illustrations to explain the drug regimen.

🌐 Cultural Considerations
- Assess for adverse effects that may result from pharmacogenomic variances.
- Incorporate traditional health practices with mainstream prescriptive therapies when appropriate.
- Facilitate adherence to mainstream prescriptive therapies within the patient's social and cultural contexts.
- Provide health information written in the patient's primary language. Medline, an online service of the National Institutes of Health, offers a variety of patient education materials in a number of languages online at www.nlm.nih.gov/medlineplus/languages/languages.html.

Evaluation
- Assess for signs and symptoms of drug side effects and toxicity.
- Evaluate physical, social, and psychological outcomes of prescriptive therapies.
- Evaluate the effectiveness of the drugs.
- Monitor for patient adherence to prescriptive therapies.

CRITICAL THINKING CASE STUDY

The nurse is caring for JM, a patient who was admitted to the hospital with severe migraines. JM has been taking warfarin, a highly protein-bound anticoagulant, for atrial fibrillation. After a thorough evaluation, the neurologist has ordered valproic acid, an antiseizure medication. Valproic acid is also highly protein bound.

1. What nursing diagnosis would be appropriate for this patient?

2. What information needs to be included in the interdisciplinary health/teaching plan for this patient?
3. During a teaching session, the patient shares that he plans to start taking over-the-counter products to boost his energy. What is the nurse's best response to the patient's comment? Explain your answer.

NCLEX STUDY QUESTIONS

1. Which components of pharmacokinetics does the nurse need to understand before administering a drug? (Select all that apply.)
   a. Drugs with a smaller volume of drug distribution have a longer half-life.
   b. Oral drugs are dissolved through the process of pinocytosis.
   c. Patients with kidney disease may have fewer protein-binding sites and are at risk for drug toxicity.
   d. Rapid absorption decreases the bioavailability of the drug.
   e. When the drug metabolism rate is decreased, excess drug accumulation can occur, which can cause toxicity.

2. The nurse will question the health care provider if a drug with a half-life ($t\frac{1}{2}$) of more than 24 hours is ordered to be given more than how often?
   a. Once daily
   b. Every other day
   c. Twice weekly
   d. Once weekly

3. The nurse is explaining drug action to a nursing student. Which statement made by the nurse is correct?
   a. Water-soluble and ionized drugs are quickly absorbed.
   b. A drug not bound to protein is an active drug.
   c. Most receptors are found under the cell membrane.
   d. Toxic effects can result if the trough level is low.

4. A Native American patient is newly diagnosed with type 2 diabetes mellitus and is prescribed the antidiabetic drug metformin 500 mg per os with morning and evening meals. Which statement best indicates to the nurse that the patient will adhere to the therapeutic regimen?
   a. I will no longer put sugar on my cereal because that will help me be healthier.
   b. If I take this medicine, I will feel better soon and won't have to take it anymore.
   c. To reduce the possibility of damage to my body, I must take the medicine as scheduled.
   d. I have diabetes because of my ancestry, so there's not much I can do about it.

5. The nurse is aware that the rate of absorption can be changed by which actions? (Select all that apply.)
   a. Modifying gastric emptying time
   b. Changing gastric pH
   c. Decreasing inflammation
   d. Forming drug complexes
   e. Eating too slowly

6. The nurse is reviewing a patient's medications as part of patient teaching. The nurse is aware that which drug is least likely to cause photosensitivity?
   a. Penicillins
   b. Sulfonamides
   c. Sulfonylureas
   d. Thiazides

7. The nurse is meeting with a community group about medication safety. The nurse must emphasize that patients at high risk for drug interactions include which groups? (Select all that apply.)
   a. Older patients
   b. Patients with chronic health conditions
   c. Patients taking three or more drugs
   d. Patients dealing with only one pharmacy
   e. Patients covered by Medicare or Medicaid

8. The nurse recognizes that when a patient takes a hepatic enzyme inducer, the dose of warfarin is usually modified in which way?
   a. It is increased.
   b. It is decreased.
   c. It remains the same.
   d. It is unpredictable.

9. The nurse is describing to a patient the synergistic effects of two of his medications. Which statement by the nurse is correct about synergistic drug effects?
   a. Two drugs have antagonistic effects on each other.
   b. The action of a drug is nullified by another drug.
   c. One drug acts as an antidote to the side effects of another drug.
   d. A greater effect is achieved when two drugs are combined.

10. A patient asks the nurse about drug interactions with over-the-counter preparations. What is the nurse's best response?
    a. Discuss this with the health care provider.
    b. There are not many interactions, so don't worry about it.
    c. Read the labels carefully, and check with your health care provider.
    d. Avoid over-the-counter preparations.

Answers: 1, c, e; 2, a; 3, b; 4, a; 5, a, b, d; 6, a; 7, a, b, c; 8, a; 9, d; 10, c.

3

Cultural Considerations

http://evolve.elsevier.com/McCuistion/pharmacology

OBJECTIVES

- Recognize verbal and nonverbal communication practices of various social and cultural groups.
- Explain appropriate spatial configurations for patients when delivering nursing care.
- Discuss the importance of including significant members of the social group in the planning and implementation of patient care.

- Compare patients' perception of time based on cultural constructs.
- Describe patients' need to exercise control in their environment.
- Anticipate potential unique responses to drugs based on social, cultural, and biologic influences.
- Safeguard patients' rights to confidentiality during inclusion of significant others in the plan of care.

OUTLINE

Ethnomedicine
Ethnopharmacology
Pharmacogenetics
Transcultural Nursing
The Giger and Davidhizar Transcultural Assessment Model
   Communication
   Space
   Social Organization

Time
Environmental Control
Biologic Variations
Nursing Process: Patient-Centered Collaborative Care
   —Cultural and Pharmacogenetic Considerations
Critical Thinking Case Study
NCLEX Study Questions

KEY TERMS

alternative health therapies, p. 31
assimilation, p. 31
complementary health therapies, p. 31
culture, p. 31
ethnomedicine, p. 30

ethnopharmacology, p. 30
genomes, p. 33
healers, p. 30
pharmacogenetics, p. 31
polymorphisms, p. 33

ETHNOMEDICINE

Ethnomedicine, sometimes referred to as *folk medicine* or *traditional medicine,* is a focus within medical anthropology that examines the ways in which people in different cultures conceptualize health and illness. These cultural constructs dictate healing practices. In many non-Western cultures, there is the belief that illness is spiritually based rather than biologically based. In some cultures, illness is thought to be caused by spirit possession or by a loss of balance within the body. Healing techniques may be based on astrology, magic, rituals, and indigenous medicinal compounds.

Traditional **healers** play a role in health practices worldwide and can include priests, shamans, bone setters, herbalists, curanderos, and midwives. Some cultural groups perceive that certain practitioners have specialized knowledge and skills. Traditional practitioners usually have some practical understanding of human anatomy and physiology

and of pharmaceutical substances. Rituals may be performed to seek the assistance of otherworldly forces such as deities or spirits. Every cultural group has its own traditions, superstitions, and belief systems. Throughout history, healing practices, religious ideology, and spirituality have been tightly intertwined.

ETHNOPHARMACOLOGY

Ethnopharmacology is a subdivision of ethnomedicine and focuses on the use of herbs, powders, teas, and animal products as healing remedies (Guest, 2016). These traditional health practices can have neutral, beneficial, or deleterious effects on a patient's health. The emergence of ethnopharmacology highlights the need for nurses to use research from the social sciences, as well as the biological and physical sciences, to provide holistic nursing care within a culturally competent context. Culture is based on learned beliefs and behaviors that are shared by a group of people. Symbols, artifacts, institutions, values, mores, and rules are the products of culture. Culture is not biologically inherited. There are certain universals that are biologically driven, such as the need to eat, but what is eaten and how it is eaten is culturally driven.

PHARMACOGENETICS

Pharmacogenetics refers to the study of all the different genes that determine drug behavior within the human body. Culturally competent care integrates pharmacogenetics with the social and cultural attributes of the patient, which helps to predict variations in drug responses.

TRANSCULTURAL NURSING

The concept of transcultural nursing was formalized by Madeleine Leininger, a nurse anthropologist who founded the Transcultural Nursing Society in 1974. A challenge for nurses worldwide is the degree of cultural diversity owing to migration across the globe. To provide culturally competent care, it is imperative that nurses be sensitive to the beliefs and practices of immigrant and indigenous groups concerning health and illness. As part of the health history, it is important to determine all the pharmacotherapeutic agents the patient is using. Obtaining a thorough history is more difficult than it seems. Patients may not reveal pertinent information, assuming that such things as herbs and teas are natural substances and therefore are not drugs. They may also be reluctant to share this information with a conventional Western health care practitioner.

Varying degrees of assimilation occur within and among cultural groups, such as when a minority group changes its ways to blend in with the dominant cultural group. Adults who immigrate into a new region usually take longer to assimilate than children or adolescents. Minority groups often practice the life-ways of the dominant culture while maintaining their ethnic identity. This sets the stage for complementary health therapies that combine traditional and conventional Western health practices. However, it is essential that nurses not make generalizations about an individual's beliefs or behaviors based on membership in a certain cultural group.

Adding to the challenges faced by nurses in countries with a high degree of cultural diversity is the phenomenon of the dominant cultural group borrowing traditional health practices from less dominant groups, resulting in alternative health therapies. This often involves the use of a traditional therapy in place of a conventional therapy. Use of complementary and alternative health therapies is growing in the United States. A major impetus for this movement is the difficulty many patients experience when attempting to access conventional Western health care. This difficulty may stem from a lack of faith in the system, a lack of funds, or the lack of services in a particular geographic location. Conversely, individuals who have access to conventional

Western health care may perceive that it is not personalized or effective. The vast amount of teas and herbs available in drug stores, health stores, and supermarkets and the increased use of acupuncture, acupressure, and therapeutic massage serve as evidence to this trend.

COMPLEMENTARY AND ALTERNATIVE THERAPIES 3.1
Gender-Specific Herb Protocols

Women have traditionally sought substitutes for hormonal replacement therapy. More women are now using phytoestrogens like those found in flaxseed, licorice, black cohosh, and soybeans. Health care providers should ask patients about the use of these naturally occurring phytoestrogens because they are contraindicated in women with a history of or risk for hormonally mediated cancers and benign tumors.

THE GIGER AND DAVIDHIZAR TRANSCULTURAL ASSESSMENT MODEL

The Transcultural Assessment model, developed by Giger and Davidhizar in 1998, depicts the six cultural phenomena of (1) communication, (2) space, (3) social organization, (4) time, (5) environmental control, and (6) biologic variation. These cultural phenomena flow from a culturally unique individual (Fig. 3.1). This model has been frequently reviewed for relevancy and is clinically useful for nurses and other members of the health care team.

Communication

Communication occurs verbally and nonverbally. Nurses must be alert to different types of communication styles among patients to provide culturally competent care. A myriad languages are spoken in pluralistic societies. When the patient and the health care provider speak different languages, professional translators should be used whenever possible to safeguard a patient's confidentiality. If a professional translator is not available, it is important that the nurse select an alternative person carefully. For example, asking the teenage son of a patient with gynecologic health issues to translate may create an uncomfortable situation that is better avoided. Even with the use of a translator, nuances in languages are unique and may not lend themselves to accurate translation in another language. There can be miscommunication between the patient, the translator, and the nurse.

Vernacular English and Standard English

There can be miscommunication between speakers of the same language when there is a pervasive use of words and phrases that are popular in particular social or cultural groups. This is evidenced by multiple regional dialects within a population. The term *African-American Vernacular English* has been used to describe a style of English speaking used among some African Americans. This vernacular is thought to be a mixture of

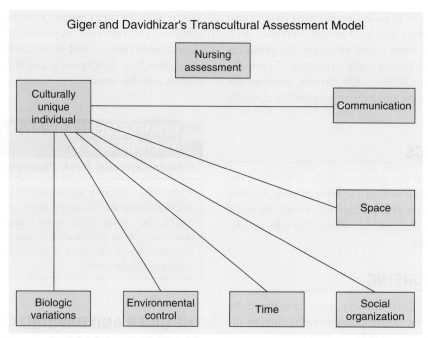

FIG. 3.1 The Giger and Davidhizar Transcultural Assessment Model. From Newman Giger, J. (2016). *Transcultural nursing: assessment and intervention* (7th ed.). St Louis: Elsevier.

English and the West African languages spoken by slaves. More generally, vernacular English is any style of speaking that varies from standard English.

Greetings and Communication Styles

All cultures have prescribed norms for greeting and addressing others. Americans of European descent may be more informal when greeting and addressing others than descendants of non-European cultures. Nurses must keep in mind that patient-nurse interactions in health care settings are considered formal and that informal styles of communication should be used only after careful consideration.

A communication style that might hinder culturally competent nursing care can be found in some patients of Asian descent, who might speak in a soft tone of voice and avoid direct eye contact. This type of communication is intended to be respectful of the health care practitioner. The nurse who is unaware of this may miss cues that care is needed. Asian Americans and Native Americans may be comfortable with periods of silence, whereas persons of Latin American, African, Middle Eastern, or European descent may be uneasy during periods of silence. Being cognizant of these preferences will help the nurse provide a comfortable environment for the patient. Nurses should not confuse politeness with meaningful communication. Many patients will nod in agreement to statements made by the nurse even if the statements are not well understood.

Space

The amount of space around a person's body is an important psychological consideration. Americans often desire a great deal of personal space and value privacy. In other cultures, population density dictates limited personal space. Patients who are used to dense living quarters may feel insecure in a hospital room. It is important that the nurse have frequent contact with these patients and allow significant members of the social group to remain with the patient as much as possible.

A major challenge in caring for patients is the use of touch and the protection of modesty. Although nurses must touch patients to administer care, all cultures have taboos regarding touch. There are added considerations when the patient is of a different gender than the nurse. This is a particularly sensitive issue for those within Muslim, Orthodox Jewish, Amish, and Roma groups. For example, a Muslim woman will likely prefer to be cared for by a female nurse rather than a male nurse. East Asians consider a pat on the head to be offensive due to the belief that the head is sacred. Nurses should consider inquiring about patients' preferences regarding touch before implementing nursing care. If possible, it may be best to have a family member of the same gender as the patient present during procedures. There may also be apparent paradoxes within cultures; for example, persons of Hispanic descent may value human contact but also value modesty.

Social Organization

Families are basic social units. The definition of *family* and the criteria for inclusion vary among individuals and among cultures. Americans of Western European descent are likely to have small, nuclear families, whereas other cultural groups living in the United States may have larger, extended families. Nurses are in a position to advocate for inclusion of the family in health care settings. Limiting the amount of time a patient can visit with members of the social group is a long-standing practice in American health care settings, but in some other countries, such as the Philippines, it is expected that family members will stay by the patient's bedside and participate in his or her care.

Time

Nurses and patients are likely to have different perceptions of time. Time moves slowly for a patient who is anxious or in pain but moves quickly for a nurse who has a demanding workload. The use of vague terms to denote time may also cause a disparity between nurses' and patients' perceptions of time. Words like *soon, about,* or *later* may have vastly different nuances among individuals and groups.

Adding to the complexity of time perception are the concepts of *linear* time and *circular* time. When time is perceived as linear, the present flows into the future and is irretrievably lost. Viewing time as linear is likely to prompt thinking such as "I must do this now." When time is perceived as circular, the present has more stability, and the need to do things at a particular moment has less urgency. Viewing time as circular is likely to prompt thinking such as, "I will have the opportunity to do this later." The cultural aspect of time perception has a profound effect on pharmacotherapeutic adherence, especially if dosing is more than once a day. All cultures have a concept of time as it is related to the past, present, and future. It is the *relative importance* placed on the past, present, and future that directs the use of time.

People of Western European descent are likely to exhibit future orientation. Future orientation promotes health practices perceived to prevent illness, such as adhering to a low-fat diet to prevent high cholesterol levels or wearing a condom during sex to prevent disease. Concern for the future also serves as motivation to take steps to control chronic illness, which is likely to lead to greater adherence to long-term pharmacotherapy. A possible explanation for this phenomenon is that people of Western European descent have historically experienced longevity and expect to have a long future ahead of them. Also to be considered is that their economic and social lives have revolved around calendars and clocks for centuries.

Non-European cultural groups such as those of African, Asian, Native American, Latin American, and Middle Eastern descent have exhibited less dependence on strict time schedules for economic and social activities. The perception of time for these groups may be rooted in agrarian cultures that use daily and seasonal rhythms of the earth and the sun to direct activities. This could result in emphasis being placed on the present. Measures to ease the discomfort of a current illness may take precedence over measures to promote long-term wellness or to treat a chronic illness. Patients with a present-oriented perception of time are more likely to discontinue conventional prescriptive therapies when they feel well. It must be noted, however, that agrarian cultures are shrinking and European-style economic practices are spreading, therefore the perception of time is changing among these groups.

Environmental Control

A major aspect of some cultures is the desire to enlist the assistance of nature to facilitate the needs of human beings. The concept of "nature" may include otherworldly forces or beings, such as deities and spirits.

Healers and spiritual advisors can be beneficial in health care settings; examples include the practice of clergy (e.g., ministers,

priests, rabbis) visiting ill members of a congregation or the inclusion of a traditional healer in the plan of care.

The Indian Health Service is a federal agency within the U.S. Department of Health and Human Services that oversees the health care of approximately 2 million Native Americans who belong to federally recognized tribes. Similarly, the Canadian health care system has developed many initiatives to improve the health care of its indigenous peoples, known as the *First Nations, Inuit,* and *Metis.* In both systems, the use of traditional healers and spiritual guides is incorporated into conventional prescriptive therapies.

Biologic Variations

The *Genographic Project* was conducted by National Geographic scientists and performed DNA testing on populations all over the world. Findings reveal that human beings are 99.9% genetically identical. This implies that there are not multiple races but multiple genotypes that define an individual's genetic identity.

Through the work of the *Human Genome Project,* an international collaborative research program, the field of pharmacogenetics has rapidly expanded. In the United States, the project was managed by the National Human Genome Research Institute, which is part of the National Institutes of Health (NIH). A significant finding is the effect of the cytochrome P450 (CYP450) enzymes on drug response, drug-drug interactions, and adverse drug events.

To illustrate the significance of these findings in patient care settings, it is necessary to review additional terms used in the field of pharmacogenetics. **Genomes** are a complete set of chromosomes and make up a cell's DNA. **Polymorphisms** are DNA variants that occur within a specific population at a frequency greater than 1%. A *substrate* is a substance that binds to and is metabolized by one or more enzymes. Drugs are chemical substances and a type of substrate. The CYP450 enzyme system either induces or inhibits the action of substrates. Induction or inhibition of a substrate accounts for the variations in drug metabolism in individuals and groups.

Human migration around the world has been so vast over such a long period of time that most people have a variety of genetic markers. The study of pharmacogenetics can pave the way for pharmacotherapy that yields greater therapeutic benefits and causes fewer adverse reactions. The application of pharmacogenetics should be approached with caution. A person who is dark skinned and appears to be of African descent is likely to have some European genetic markers.

Certain classifications of medications have different effects in individuals whose genetic markers are predominantly characteristic of a certain biologic group. For example, in the United States, Caucasians are more likely than people of Asian or African heritage to have abnormally low levels of the CYP2D6 enzyme that metabolizes drugs belonging to a variety of therapeutic areas, such as antidepressants, antipsychotics, and beta blockers.

African Americans respond poorly to several classes of antihypertensive agents such as beta blockers and angiotensin-converting enzyme (ACE) inhibitors. Differences in skin structure and physiology can affect response to dermatologic and topically applied products. Clinical trials have demonstrated lower responses to interferon-alfa used in the treatment of hepatitis C among African Americans compared with other racial subgroups.

The U.S. Food and Drug Administration (FDA) has entered into an agreement with the manufacturers of drugs containing carbamazepine to include product labeling recommending that patients of Asian ancestry be genetically tested before treatment with this agent begins. There is a strong association between serious skin reactions and an inherited variant of the *H 1502LA-B* gene found in Asians. These intrinsic biologic factors must be considered, along with extrinsic factors such as diet and environmental and sociocultural issues, to prescribe effective therapies and provide holistic health care.

Researchers conducting clinical trials for development of new drugs are now required to obtain genetic testing of the participants in the study. Issues to be resolved concerning widespread genetic testing are the cost-benefit ratio and ethical considerations. Genetic testing is expensive and is generally not covered by third-party payers. Genetic information can affect employment, insurability, and family relationships. There is also the danger of genetic stereotyping.

Table 3.1 applies the Giger and Davidhizar Transcultural Assessment model to six broad cultural categories of people of European, African, Latin American, Native American, Asian, and Middle-Eastern descent. It is important to keep in mind that there is no generic prototype for any of these categories. Italian Americans are likely to have different customs than German Americans in spite of both groups being of European descent. There is often a perception in the United States that most Asians are Chinese and most Hispanics are Mexican, but in fact there is great variation among these broad groups regarding geography of origin, language, customs, and spiritual systems. Another misperception in the United States is that people of African descent are a homogenous group from one country, but Africa comprises 54 countries over a large geographic area. Language, customs, and spiritual systems vary extensively.

TABLE 3.1   Selected Cultural Groups and Components of the Giger and Davidhizar Transcultural Assessment Model*

Cultural Group	Communication Styles	Spatial Preferences	Social Organization	Perception of Time	Environmental Control	Biologic Variations
People of European descent	• Prefer direct eye contact • Use moderate to loud vocal volume • Use many words to describe symptoms • Uncomfortable with silence	• Prefer a large amount of personal space • Value privacy • Exhibit low to moderate amount of touching among group members	• Small, nuclear families • Extended family members often live a far distance away • Increasing number of single-parent families headed by a female • High degree of individualism	Future oriented	• Believe that healthy behaviors prevent or control illness • Believe in being united with a deity in the afterlife	Poor metabolizers of antidepressants, antipsychotics, cardiovascular agents, and isoniazid, which can lead to toxicity
People of African Descent	• Prefer direct eye contact • Use moderate to loud vocal volume • Uncomfortable with silence	• Comfortable with smaller personal spaces • Exhibit moderate amount of touching among group members	• Small, nuclear families in household but have large extended family networks • Increasing number of single parent families headed by a female • May include unrelated persons as family • Strong church affiliations	Present oriented	• Spiritually oriented • Important to include clergy in plan of care • Believe in being united with a deity in the afterlife	Diminished therapeutic effects from beta blockers, ACE inhibitors, and warfarin
People of Latin American descent	• May avoid direct eye contact with persons perceived to be in a position of authority • Uncomfortable with long periods of silence	• Comfortable with smaller personal spaces • Value touching • Like the physical presence of other people	• Extended, multigenerational family important • Godparents play important roles in an individual's life.	Present oriented	• Spiritually oriented • Use traditional healers and folk medicine • Believe in being united with a deity in the afterlife	There is great biologic diversity among Latin Americans, who can have European, Native American, and Asian biomarkers.

TABLE 3.1   Selected Cultural Groups and Components of the Giger and Davidhizar Transcultural Assessment Model*—cont'd

Cultural Group	Communication Styles	Spatial Preferences	Social Organization	Perception of Time	Environmental Control	Biologic Variations
People of Native American descent	• Value silence • Sensitive to body language • Wish to keep tribal languages alive	• Value personal space • Engage in light touch	• Tribal affiliation valued • Traditional kinship patterns are valued.	Present oriented	• Spiritually oriented • Use traditional healers and folk medicine	Increased vasomotor response to alcohol
People of Asian descent	• Value silence • Sensitive to body language	• Comfortable with smaller personal spaces • Exhibit low amount of touching among group members	• Hierarchic social structure • Traditional kinship patterns are valued.	Present oriented	• Many religious systems; some are polytheistic and believe in reincarnation.	Diminished therapeutic effects of codeine; rapid metabolizers of isoniazid
People of Middle-Eastern descent	• Patient may appear quiet and docile while family members ask many questions about the diagnosis and plan of care.	• Comfortable with smaller personal spaces • Displays of public affection strongly discouraged • Gender separation in social settings	• Males are strong heads of household. • Extended family important • Sharing with others highly valued	Present oriented	• Spiritually oriented • Although the majority of Middle Easterners are of the Muslim faith, minority groups practice Christianity and Judaism. • Use traditional healers and folk medicine but consider Western health care institutions to be more prestigious • Believe in being united with a deity in the afterlife	Many genetic diseases such as thalassemia

*This table is limited in scope and does not necessarily reflect an individual's beliefs, behaviors, or biologic functioning.

◎ NURSING PROCESS
Patient-Centered Collaborative Care
Cultural and Pharmacogenetic Considerations

Assessment

- Assess the patient's ability to communicate using standard English.
- Determine if the patient participates in traditional health practices or uses complementary or alternative medical therapies.
- List the patient's use of pharmacotherapeutic agents, including prescription medications, over-the-counter (OTC) medications, herbs, teas, and ointments.
- Ascertain whether a patient's belief system includes a traditional faith healer, and if so, if the presence of a healer would facilitate the patient's adherence to the prescriptive therapies.
- Inquire about the patient's preferences regarding touch, modesty, and personal space.
- Gauge the patient's perception of time.

Nursing Diagnoses

- Anxiety related to unfamiliarity with conventional Western health care practices
- Impaired Verbal Communication related to limited fluency in the English language
- Spiritual Distress, Risk for
- Ineffective Self–Health Management related to limited knowledge of health care resources

Planning

- The patient's health care needs will be met within a culturally competent framework.
- The patient will effectively manage self–health care.

Nursing Interventions

- Use appropriate translators when the patient's use of standard English is limited.
- Anticipate that therapeutic communication with the patient and significant others will require additional time with each encounter.

- Provide appropriate spatial configurations for the patient when delivering nursing care.
- Include significant members of the social group in the planning and implementation of patient care.
- Allow the patient adequate time with significant members of the social group.
- Recognize the need for the patient to exercise control of the environment.
- Anticipate unique responses to drugs based on social, cultural, and biologic influences.
- Consult with persons who are knowledgeable about the patient's culture.
- Incorporate traditional health practices with conventional prescriptive therapies when appropriate.
- Facilitate adherence to conventional prescriptive therapies within the patient's social and cultural contexts.

Patient Teaching
- Include significant members of the social group, when appropriate, while teaching about prescriptive therapies.
- Provide health information written in the patient's primary language. Medline, an online service of the National Institutes of Health, offers a variety of patient-education materials in a number of languages online at www.nlm.nih.gov/medlineplus/languages/languages.html.
- Use illustrations to explain prescriptive therapies.

Evaluation
- Monitor for patient adherence to prescriptive therapies.
- Evaluate physical, social, and psychological outcomes of prescriptive therapies.

CRITICAL THINKING CASE STUDY

NS is a 72-year-old woman who immigrated to the United States from Egypt 5 years ago. She is a widow, has five grown children, and follows Islamic doctrine. She lives with her oldest daughter, and a younger daughter and three sons live near her home. NS is currently hospitalized due to a recent cerebral vascular accident. She has left-sided paralysis. The attending physician tells the patient she should go to a rehabilitation unit for 3 weeks for physical therapy. The oldest daughter is present for the physician's visit. Both the patient and her daughter appear anxious but do not ask the physician any questions.
1. What cultural factors could explain the apparent anxiety?
2. Which nursing interventions would help decrease the anxiety?
3. How might the patient view the idea of physical therapy?
4. How can other members of the family be included in the plan of care?

NCLEX STUDY QUESTIONS

1. The nurse is performing a health assessment on a newly admitted patient of Asian descent. The patient looks at the floor whenever the nurse asks a question. Communication is enhanced when the nurse does which action?
   a. Frequently touches the patient
   b. Asks questions that require only "yes" or "no" answers
   c. Discontinues the health assessment
   d. Uses eye contact sparingly
2. The nurse has been measuring the blood pressure of an African-American patient every 4 hours for the past 3 days in a hospital setting. The blood pressure is consistently above 140/90. The patient has been adherent to the antihypertensive drug therapy while hospitalized. The nurse will initially perform which action?
   a. Determine if the patient has been given high sodium foods from visitors.
   b. Withhold the antihypertensive drug until the physician can be notified.
   c. Increase blood pressure measurements to every 2 hours.
   d. Place the patient on a restricted fluid intake.
3. A male nurse is caring for a young married woman who is an observant Muslim. It is important that the nurse initially perform which action?
   a. Delay any care that requires touching until a female nurse is available.
   b. Identify the patient's preference regarding touch.
   c. Touch the patient only when her spouse is present.
   d. Inform the patient that she must allow him to touch her.
4. A nurse is teaching a 16-year-old female patient about a newly prescribed medication. The patient is bilingual in Spanish and English. Which behavior best indicates the patient's understanding of the instructions?
   a. The patient frequently nods her head while listening to the nurse's instructions.
   b. The patient states that she understands the instructions.
   c. The patient repeats the nurse's instructions to her parents.
   d. The patient does not ask the nurse for clarification of the instructions.
5. A Native American patient is newly diagnosed with diabetes mellitus type 2 and is prescribed the antidiabetic drug metformin 500 mg per os with morning and evening meals. Which statement best indicates to the nurse that the patient will adhere to the pharmacotherapy?
   a. I will be healthier if I don't eat sugar anymore.
   b. When I feel better, I won't have to take this medicine.
   c. I must take the medicine as scheduled to prevent damage to my body.
   d. I have diabetes because of my ancestry, so there's not much I can do about it.

Answers: 1, d; 2, a; 3, b; 4, c; 5, c.

Complementary and Alternative Therapies

http://evolve.elsevier.com/McCuistion/pharmacology

OBJECTIVES

- Discuss at least six important points associated with the use of complementary and alternative medicine.
- Compare at least six common herbs and their associated toxicity.
- Differentiate at least eight of the most common herbal therapies and the potential use for each.

- Describe the recommendations for labels on herbal products.
- Discuss the nursing implications, including patient teaching, related to herbal products.

OUTLINE

KEY TERMS

Complementary and alternative medicine (CAM) is used by 40% of adults to either augment or replace traditional medical therapies. CAM practices include, but are not limited to, botanicals, nutritional products, and herbal supplements. It is critical for nurses to know about alternative medicine and to note its use in their assessment. CAM products can have both positive and negative effects, and they can interact with prescription and over-the-counter (OTC) medications. Nurses are in an excellent position to educate patients about these interactions.

Botanicals are additive substances that come from plants; an **herb** is "any plant that is used for culinary or medicinal purposes." Plants have been the source of old and new drugs for some time: foxglove is the source of digitalis, from snakeroot we get reserpine, willow bark is the source of aspirin, and Taxol comes from the Pacific yew tree, just to name a few. The therapeutic value of plants is the basis of **phytomedicine**. Research into the effects of CAM continues to grow.

Many Americans use botanical dietary supplements for therapeutic or preventive reasons, and herbal therapy has surged in popularity; marketing and media have fueled the demand, with advertisements and promotions on television, in magazines, and on the Internet. In the United States alone, sales have topped the $6 billion mark and are expected to continue to grow.

Few pharmacy schools in the United States offer courses in botanical remedies, but herbal therapy is being addressed in the professional literature with increasing frequency and seriousness. Health care providers and consumers are asking questions about herbal therapy's effectiveness, potential toxicity, and reactions with conventional medications. Consumers are right to question advertisements that imply that herbs will cure anything. Herbs can be useful, but they can also be ineffectual or even dangerous (Complementary and Alternative Therapies 4.1).

🌿 COMPLEMENTARY AND ALTERNATIVE THERAPIES 4.1

Patient Responsibility

To optimize the therapeutic regimen, the patient has the responsibility to (1) consult with the health care provider before taking any herbal preparation, (2) report all herbal preparations taken to all health care providers, (3) inform health care providers of any allergy or sensitivity to any herbal products, (4) use caution if pregnant or lactating, and (5) not take a greater dose than recommended.

In 1992 the U.S. Congress instructed the National Institutes of Health (NIH) to develop an Office of Alternative Medicine to support studies of alternative therapies. This office is now called the *National Center for Complementary and Integrative Health* (NCCIH), which lists current clinical trials with herbal products on their website (www.nccam.nih.gov/research/clinicaltrials). The Natural Standard research collaboration also reviews global literature on herbal studies. These studies are important because CAM cannot be patented, so their manufacturers generally cannot justify the expenses associated with safety and efficacy testing in an already booming conventional medicine economy.

This chapter describes selected aspects of herbal therapy, including (1) the Dietary Supplement Health and Education Act (DSHEA) of 1994, (2) varieties of herbal preparations, (3) the most commonly used herbs, (4) herbs used to treat selected common ailments, (5) potential hazards of herbs, (6) tips for consumers and health care providers, and (7) herbal resources.

DIETARY SUPPLEMENT HEALTH AND EDUCATION ACT OF 1994

In 1994 the U.S. Congress enacted the Dietary Supplement Health and Education Act (DSHEA), which defined dietary supplements as the following:

- Is intended to supplement the diet
- Contains one or more dietary ingredients (including vitamins, minerals, herbs or other botanicals, amino acids, and certain other substances) or their constituents
- Is intended to be taken by mouth, in forms such as tablet, capsule, powder, softgel, gelcap, or liquid
- Is labeled as being a dietary supplement

Although dietary supplements are regulated through the Food and Drug Administration (FDA), oversight is limited compared with prescription drugs (see http://www.fda.gov/Food/DietarySupplements/default.htm). Manufacturers are required to ensure that their products are safe and that the label information is truthful and not misleading; however, they are not required to demonstrate product safety before the product is sold. Packaging of all dietary supplements must bear the wording "This statement has not been evaluated by the U.S. Food and Drug Administration (FDA). This product is not intended to diagnose, treat, cure, or prevent any disease."

Additionally, all labels are required to have the following five components:

1. Name of the supplement
2. Amount of the supplement (net quantity)
3. Nutrition labeling
4. Ingredient list
5. Name and place of the manufacturer, packer, or distributor

Manufacturers of dietary supplements are allowed to make three types of claims: (1) health claims, (2) structure and function claims, and (3) nutrient content claims. To make these claims, manufacturers must have supporting data. The Federal Trade Commission (FTC) is responsible for regulating the truth in advertising related to dietary supplements. Herbal supplements can be marketed with suggested dosages. The physiologic effects of the product can be noted, but no claims can be made about preventing or curing specific conditions. For example, a product label cannot claim that the agent "prevents heart disease," but it can say that the agent "helps increase blood flow to the heart." Health maintenance claims (e.g., "maintains a healthy immune system") and claims for relief of minor symptoms related to life stages (e.g., "alleviates hot flashes") are acceptable because they do not relate to disease. Herbal products using a "may be beneficial" disclaimer, rather than claims of definite benefit, are appropriate legally. Dietary supplement manufacturers are still required to substantiate any claims they make. Consumers are reminded that premarket testing for safety and efficacy is not required, and manufacturing is not standardized.

CURRENT GOOD MANUFACTURING PRACTICES

The FDA proposed standards for marketing and labeling dietary supplements in 2003. Known as the Current Good Manufacturing Practices (CGMPs), these standards are multifaceted and require that package labels give the quality and strength of all contents and that products be free of contaminants and impurities (Table 4.1). Manufacturing quality control procedures are part of the CGMPs.

Additionally, a *seal of approval* is awarded to products that meet criteria similar to that of the CGMPs by four organizations: the U.S. Pharmacopeial Convention (USP), ConsumerLab.com, National Products Association, and NSF International. The fee-based tests provide information on an herbal product's identity, potency, dissolution, purity, and labeling accuracy. However, the seal of approval is no indication of the product's safety or efficacy.

COMMONLY USED HERBAL REMEDIES

Most herbal therapies are used to maintain or improve health. This section discusses the most commonly used herbs. The National Center for Complementary and Integrative Health (https://nccih.nih.gov/) is an excellent resource for information on herbal therapies not discussed here.

Astragalus (A. membranaceus and *A. mongholicus)*

Astragalus membranaceus and *Astragalus mongholicus* have been used as an adjunct to boost the immune system, such as for hepatitis and cancer, and to limit the effects of cold and flu symptoms. There is no strong evidence to support the use of *Astragalus* to support the immune system; however, preliminary evidence supports such benefits. *Astragalus* is considered safe, but little is known about its side effect profile because it is commonly used as adjunctive therapy. The herb may interact with

TABLE 4.1 Definitions of Herbal Preparations

Preparation	Definition
Decoction	A tea made from boiling plant material—usually the bark, rhizomes, roots, or other woody parts—in water. May be used therapeutically. Natural dyes are often made this way.
Infusion	A tea made by pouring water over plant material (usually dried flowers, fruit, leaves, and other parts, although fresh plant material may also be used); the mixture is then allowed to steep. The water is usually boiling, but cold infusions are also an option. May be used therapeutically; hot tea is an excellent way to administer herbs.
Tincture	An extract of a plant made by soaking herbs in a dark place with a desired amount of either glycerine, alcohol, or vinegar for two to six weeks. The liquid is strained from the plant material and then may be used therapeutically.
Liniment	Extract of a plant added to either alcohol or vinegar and applied topically for therapeutic benefits.
Poultice	A therapeutic topical application of a soft moist mass of plant material (such as bruised fresh herbs), usually wrapped in a fine woven cloth.
Essential oils	Aromatic volatile oils extracted from the leaves, stems, flowers, and other parts of plants. Therapeutic use generally includes dilution of the highly concentrated oil.
Herb-infused oils	A process of extraction in which the volatile oils of a plant substance are obtained by soaking the plant in a carrier oil for approximately 2 weeks and then straining the oil. The resulting oil is used therapeutically and may contain the plant's aromatic characteristics.
Percolation	A process to extract the soluble constituents of a plant with the assistance of gravity. The material is moistened and evenly packed into a tall, slightly conical vessel; the liquid (menstruum) is then poured onto the material and allowed to steep for a certain length of time. A small opening is then made in the bottom, which allows the extract to slowly flow out of the vessel. The remaining plant material (the *marc*) may be discarded. Many tinctures and liquid extracts are prepared this way.

From American Botanical Council. (2013). *Terminology*. Retrieved from http://abc.herbalgram.org/site/PageServer?pagename=Terminology

drugs used to alter immune function, such as cyclosporine. Persons using CAM need to be aware that not all species of *Astragalus* are safe for human consumption; some species contain the neurotoxin swainsonine, others contain toxic levels of selenium.

Chamomile (*Matricaria recutita* and *Chamomilla recutita*)

Chamomile is used primarily to treat sleeplessness, anxiety, and stomach or intestinal ailments. Little research has been conducted on chamomile; however, early studies indicate some benefit in the use of chamomile for some skin conditions and oral ulcers secondary to chemotherapy or radiation treatment. Side effects include allergic reaction from mild skin reactions to anaphylaxis. Allergic reactions are more likely to occur in persons who are allergic to ragweed or other members of the daisy family.

Cinnamon (*Cinnamomum zeylanicum* and *C. cassia*)

Cinnamon has a long history of use as a treatment for bronchitis, gastrointestinal (GI) problems, anorexia, and diabetes. However, little evidence is available to support any of these claims. Although some people have allergic reactions to cinnamon, in general it is usually safe if taken in amounts of no more than 6 g a day for no longer than 6 weeks. Both species of cinnamon contain coumarin; however, cassia cinnamon contains much larger amounts and may decrease blood clotting.

Echinacea (*Echinacea purpurea*)

Echinacea is commonly used for colds, flu, and infections. It has also been used for skin problems, such as acne. It is thought to stimulate the immune system to fight infection. Research regarding the benefits of *Echinacea* as treatment for cold and flu symptoms is inconclusive. Few side effects are reported by persons taking the herb, the most common being GI effects and allergic reactions, particularly in those who are allergic to ragweed.

Garlic (*Allium sativum*)

Garlic is reported to lower cholesterol, decrease blood pressure, and reduce heart disease. It has also been used to prevent cancer of the stomach and colon. Inconclusive evidence supports the use of this herb as a treatment for elevated cholesterol, hypertension, and heart disease; no evidence supports its use in the prevention of cancer. Garlic has few side effects but may cause heartburn and upset stomach; it has also been associated with body odor. Because it also reduces blood clotting, patients should be advised to notify their health care provider about taking garlic if they are having surgery or dental work. Patients should be cautioned not to take garlic if they have a bleeding disorder or if they are taking the drug saquinavir (a protease inhibitor used in the treatment of HIV). Garlic reduces the effectiveness of saquinavir.

Ginger (*Zingiber officinale*)

Ginger has been used to treat postoperative, pregnancy-related, and chemotherapy-related nausea as well as motion sickness and diarrhea. In addition, it may provide relief from pain, swelling, and stiffness of both osteoarthritis and rheumatoid arthritis. Available research suggests it is effective for the short-term treatment of nausea associated with pregnancy. Evidence is inconclusive concerning its use for motion sickness, as treatment of chemotherapy-induced or postoperative nausea, and in the treatment of arthritis. Side effects of ginger include gas, bloating, heartburn, and nausea.

Ginkgo (*Ginkgo biloba*)

Ginkgo has been used for thousands of years to treat ailments such as asthma, bronchitis, fatigue, and tinnitus. In more recent times, it has been used to improve memory, prevent Alzheimer disease and other dementias, decrease intermittent claudication, and as a treatment for sexual dysfunction and multiple sclerosis. In a study following older adult subjects for an average of 6 years, *Ginkgo* was shown to be ineffective in the prevention of Alzheimer and other dementias. Other studies have shown it to be ineffective in improving memory in older adults. There is conflicting evidence of the benefit of *Ginkgo* for treatment of intermittent claudication and tinnitus. Side effects include headache, nausea, GI upset, dizziness, and allergic reactions that include severe reactions leading to death. In patients taking blood thinners, *Ginkgo* has been shown to increase bleeding risk. Animal studies have shown that rats and mice given *Gingko* develop tumors; however, more research is needed to determine if this is true for humans.

Ginseng *(Panax ginseng)*

Ginseng has been said to boost the immune system, increase a person's sense of well-being, and increase stamina. It has also been used to treat erectile dysfunction, hepatitis C, and menopausal symptoms and to lower glucose and blood pressure. The active component in the herb is thought to be a chemical called *ginsenoside*. Some evidence supports the use of ginseng in the treatment of hypertension and as an immune system booster. Short-term use of the herb appears to be safe; however, long-term use is associated with side effects such as headaches, GI problems, and allergic reactions. There have also been reports of breast tenderness, menstrual irregularities, and high blood pressure, although it is not known if it is the herb causing these effects or other components. Diabetics should use caution when taking ginseng, especially if used in conjunction with other herbs or drugs, because hypoglycemia may result.

Hawthorn *(Crataegus laevigata* and *C. monogyna)*

Hawthorn has predominantly been used in the treatment of heart disease (e.g., heart failure and angina). It has also been used to treat digestive issues and kidney disease. Although some evidence supports its use in mild heart failure, study results are conflicting. Side effects of hawthorn include nausea, headache, and dizziness. Hawthorn may interact with multiple drugs, including those used for erectile dysfunction (hypotension), nitrates (dizziness and lightheadedness), and antihypertensives (hypotension).

Licorice Root *(Glycyrrhiza glabra* and *G. uralensis)*

Licorice has been used to treat stomach ulcers, bronchitis, sore throat, and viral hepatitis. However, there is not enough research to show the benefit of licorice in the treatment of any condition. In large amounts, licorice can elevate blood pressure, cause salt and water retention, and lower potassium levels. When taken with diuretics, corticosteroids, or other medications that lower potassium, life-threatening hypokalemia may result. People with heart disease or hypertension and those who are pregnant (some data associate licorice with preterm labor) should not take licorice in large amounts.

Milk Thistle *(Silybum marianum)*

Milk thistle has been used widely to treat cirrhosis, chronic hepatitis, and gallbladder disorders. It has also seen use in the treatment of elevated cholesterol and insulin resistance in type 2 diabetes. Although laboratory study has indicated that milk thistle may promote the growth of liver cells and

may fight oxidation and inhibit inflammation, two rigorous human studies found no benefit when compared with standard therapy and no change in viral activity or inflammation. Milk thistle may cause stomach upset, and in persons allergic to ragweed, milk thistle may trigger an allergic reaction. When combined with drugs for diabetes, milk thistle may lead to hypoglycemia. Nurses should caution diabetics using milk thistle to closely monitor their blood sugars and to watch for symptoms of hypoglycemia.

Peppermint *(Mentha x piperita)*

Peppermint has been used to treat a wide variety of ailments, from nausea, indigestion, and irritable bowel syndrome (IBS) to cold symptoms, headaches, and muscle and nerve pain. Some evidence supports the use of peppermint in the treatment of IBS and possibly the use of peppermint oil to relieve indigestion; however, no current evidence supports the use of peppermint to treat other ailments. Side effects include possible allergic reaction and heartburn.

St. John's Wort *(Hypericum perforatum)*

St. John's wort has been used extensively throughout history to treat mental disorders and nerve pain. It has also been used as a treatment for malaria, sleep disorders, and wounds. Current research indicates St. John's wort is no more effective than placebo as treatment for depression, whether mild, moderate, or severe. Patients must be informed that this herb is not effective in the treatment of depression, and that for adequate treatment to take place, they must see their health care provider. St. John's wort interacts with multiple drugs including antidepressants, which can lead to serotonin syndrome; birth control pills, cyclosporine, digoxin, indinavir, irinotecan, drugs for seizure control, and anticoagulants. Side effects include sensitivity to sunlight, anxiety, dry mouth, dizziness, GI problems, fatigue, headache, and sexual dysfunction.

Turmeric *(Curcuma longa)*

Turmeric has been used for heartburn, stomach ulcers, gallstones, inflammation, and cancer. However, little research has been conducted on the use of turmeric to treat health conditions. Preliminary research in the lab suggests that it may have antiinflammatory, anticancer, and antioxidant properties, but human studies have not been conducted to confirm such properties outside of the lab. Turmeric is generally safe, although high doses may cause nausea or diarrhea. Persons with gallbladder disease should avoid the herb because it may worsen their condition.

Valerian *(Valeriana officinalis)*

Valerian has seen wide use in the treatment of insomnia; it has also been used to treat anxiety, headaches, depression, irregular heartbeat, and tremors. Although early research indicates valerian may be useful in the treatment of insomnia, there is not enough evidence to recommend the herb for this treatment. Multiple research studies are in progress, but no available evidence supports the use of valerian for any other medical condition at this time. Valerian is generally safe when used for short periods of time (4 to 6 weeks). Side effects include fatigue, headaches, dizziness, and stomach upset.

POTENTIAL HAZARDS OF HERBS

Consumers and health care providers must be alert to potential hazards with herbal therapy; although herbs are natural substances, *natural* does not mean safe. Patients may not disclose use of herbal products to health care providers for a variety of reasons, including the sense that the health care provider is biased against or not knowledgeable about herbal products or the belief that these products are not considered medications. However, it is essential that health care providers obtain a complete listing of all of the herbal preparations the patient takes in all forms—teas, infusions, tinctures, tablets, and dried herbs—the reason they are taken, and their perceived effectiveness to ensure that they do not interfere with the use and actions of prescribed medications. This assessment should be updated regularly along with information on the patient's OTC and prescription drug use.

Health care providers must be alert for possible herb-drug interactions. For example, Asian ginseng induces the drug-metabolizing enzyme CYP3A; when taken in combination with other CYP3A substrates with a narrow therapeutic index, drug levels and therapeutic response should be monitored carefully. Goldenseal has a high potential for herb-drug interaction because it is a potent inhibitor of both CYP3A4 and CYP2D6. St. John's wort has significant documented interactions with cyclosporine, indinavir, oral contraceptives, warfarin, digoxin, and benzodiazepines, among other drugs; it is also a potent inducer of CYP-450 enzymes and intestinal p-glycoprotein.

Some herbal products can also directly affect laboratory test results. Two Chinese alternative therapies, Dan Shen and Chan Su, are known to interfere with tests to determine digoxin levels. It is *extremely important* that patients taking digoxin avoid these two products!

Not all compounds are safe via all routes. For example, comfrey has both internal and external preparations. Internal use is discouraged because hepatic damage may be fatal. For external use, comfrey is used as an ointment for relief of swelling associated with abrasions and sprains.

Many products have significance for patients facing surgery because they may interfere with the absorption, breakdown, and excretion of anesthetics, anticoagulants, and other surgery-related medications (Complementary and Alternative Therapies 4.2). The American Society of Anesthesiologists suggests patients discontinue herbal therapy beginning 2 to 3 weeks prior to surgery.

COMPLEMENTARY AND ALTERNATIVE THERAPIES 4.2

Anticoagulants

The following commonly used herbal products have been reported to interfere with anticoagulants: bilberry, cat's claw, chamomile (German), Dong Quai, feverfew, garlic, ginseng, ginger, *Ginkgo*, and licorice.

TIPS FOR CONSUMERS AND HEALTH CARE PROVIDERS

The following are guidelines for prudent use of herbs:
- Do not take herbs without talking to your health care provider first if you are taking any prescription drugs.
- Do not take herbal supplements if you are pregnant, attempting to become pregnant, or are nursing.
- Do not give herbs to infants or young children.
- Follow the label instructions!
- If you experience any side effects that concern you, stop taking the herb and contact your health care provider.
- *Natural* does not mean safe!
- Herbal supplements may contain many compounds, and all of the ingredients may not be known; what is on the label may not be what is in the bottle.

HERBAL RESOURCES

It is the responsibility of consumers to educate themselves about herbs before use and to purchase products only from reputable dealers. Determination of the purity and concentration of a particular product can be done only through assays, a costly process; thus most products have not had appropriate human toxicologic analysis. Many herbal resources are available on the Internet and from print sources, and the reader must evaluate each independently and decide whether the information is credible and appropriate.

◎ NURSING PROCESS
Patient-Centered Collaborative Care
Complementary and Alternative Therapies

In the provision of holistic nursing care, it is important that nurses understand both conventional drug therapy and complementary and alternative practices.

Assessment
- Assess for the influence of cultural beliefs, norms, and values in the patient's therapeutic regimen.
- Using culturally sensitive, nonjudgmental, and unbiased questioning, assess the following:
  - Which herbs are being used and how long ago were they started?
  - Why is the herb being used?
  - Who recommended the herb?
  - How often and how much of the herb is being taken?
- Assess use of other prescribed and over-the-counter (OTC) drugs and supplements, and include the reason for and duration of use.
- Assess for potential or actual side effects of any drug, herb, or supplement being used.
- Assess for potential or actual drug-drug, drug-herb, or drug-supplement interactions.
- Assess the patient's readiness to learn and literacy skill.

Nursing Diagnoses
- Deficient Knowledge related to treatment regimen
- Readiness for Enhanced Knowledge related to complementary and alternative therapies

Planning
- The patient and family will verbalize understanding of herbal therapy, prescription and OTC drugs, interaction

between herbal therapy and prescription and OTC drugs, and strategies for optimal participation in the therapeutic regimen.

Nursing Interventions
- Engage patients in the care-planning process; provide information supportive of self-management and mutual goal setting; support patients and family choices.
- Consult a dietitian and other specialists as necessary.

Patient Teaching
- Use an individualized, culturally appropriate approach when discussing the therapeutic regimen.
- Use open-ended questions.
- Due to inconsistencies in manufacturing, advise patients to continue with the same brand of herbal therapy, and advise them to notify their health care provider if considering changing brands or preparations.
- Advise patients to first notify their health care provider before substituting any herbal product for a prescription or OTC medication.

- Encourage patients to read labels and heed the recommended information displayed on the label.
- Teach patients about foods that enhance or diminish the action of specific herbs.
- Advise patients about foods to avoid, if any, while taking herbs.
- Advise patients of potential side effects of herbal therapy.
- Counsel patients about symptoms that require prompt reporting to the health care provider.

Evaluation
- Evaluate perceived effectiveness of herbal remedies for alleviating symptoms.
- Evaluate adherence to the therapeutic regimen.
- Evaluate drug-herb interactions or side effects.
- Evaluate the patient's use of resources.

▌CRITICAL THINKING CASE STUDY

JR, a 55-year-old white male, is seen in follow-up after being diagnosed with type 2 diabetes. He was prescribed metformin 500 mg twice daily at his last visit. When talking to JR, he admits he never filled his prescription but took his neighbor's advice instead and began taking cinnamon. He states he Googled the spice and found that it is effective at lowering blood sugar. Upon further questioning, he states he just grabs a spoon from the drawer and uses his wife's baking cinnamon.

1. What additional information is needed prior to developing a mutually agreed upon plan of care?
2. What information should JR be given concerning the use of cinnamon to treat diabetes?

▌NCLEX STUDY QUESTIONS

1. What provisions of the Dietary Supplement Health and Education Act of 1994 are most important for the nurse to know related to patient health teaching? (Select all that apply.)
   a. Clarified marketing regulations
   b. Reclassified herbs as dietary supplements
   c. Stated that herbal products can be marketed with suggested dosages
   d. Required that package labels give quality and strength of all contents
   e. Stated that herbs can be used as drugs

2. The nurse discovers that a patient has recently decided to take four herbal preparations. Which action will the nurse take first?
   a. Discuss the cost of herbal products.
   b. Instruct the patient to inform the health care provider of all products taken.
   c. Instruct the patient to stop taking all herbal products immediately.
   d. Suggest that the patient taper off use of herbal products over the next 2 weeks.

3. Labeling of herbal products is important. Which is an appropriate claim for an herbal product?
   a. Prevents diabetes
   b. Helps increase blood flow to the extremities
   c. Cures Alzheimer disease
   d. Is safe for all

4. The nurse is reviewing a patient's current medications. Which herbal products interfere with the action of anticoagulants? (Select all that apply.)
   a. *Astragalus*
   b. Garlic
   c. Ginger
   d. Licorice root
   e. *Gingko*

5. A patient being seen at a cardiovascular clinic mentions he takes garlic, which is reported to decrease cholesterol, blood pressure, and heart disease. Which patient statement indicates a need for further teaching? (Select all that apply.)
   a. I can just take garlic for my heart problems.
   b. Garlic may provide some decrease in blood pressure.
   c. Garlic is very effective in preventing depression.
   d. Garlic will not cure impotence.

Answers: 1, a, b, c; 2, b; 3, b; 4, b; 5, a, b, c.

Pediatric Considerations

5

http://evolve.elsevier.com/McCuistion/pharmacology

OBJECTIVES

- Apply principles of pharmacokinetics and pharmacodynamics to pediatric drug administration.
- Differentiate components of pharmacology unique to pediatric patients.
- Synthesize knowledge about pediatric drug safety and administration with current or potential nursing practice.

OUTLINE

Pharmacokinetics
  Absorption
  Distribution
  Metabolism
  Excretion
Pharmacodynamics
Nursing Implications
  Pediatric Drug Dosing and Monitoring
  Pediatric Drug Administration

Considerations for the Adolescent Patient
Nursing Process: Family-Centered Collaborative Care
  Nursing Process: Family-Centered Collaborative Care—Pediatrics
Critical Thinking Case Study
NCLEX Study Questions

KEY TERMS

family-centered care, p. 46
off label, p. 44
pharmacodynamics, p. 45

pharmacokinetics, p. 44
Principle of Atraumatic Care, p. 47

A nurse who is providing care to children must make certain adaptations in assessment, treatment, and evaluation of nursing care because of the physiologic, psychological, and developmental differences inherent in the pediatric population. This is especially true in the science of pharmacology, in both the administration of drugs to children and evaluation of the therapeutic and adverse effects of a drug. This chapter addresses pediatric nursing adaptations and discusses the impact of a child's growth and development on many aspects of pharmacology: pharmacokinetics, pharmacodynamics, dosing and monitoring, methods of drug administration, and nursing implications.

Pediatric pharmacology is limited to available research in the provision of dosing protocols, safe practices, key assessments, and important nursing implications. Most available information about drugs is derived from studies that use adult samples, small sample sizes, or samples with healthy children. Few studies have been conducted to determine the effectiveness of drugs in the pediatric population. Generalizing the results of studies using adult patients to pediatric populations may result in serious errors and ignores the impact of growth and development on pharmacology.

⚡ PATIENT SAFETY

Preventing Drug Administration Errors in Pediatric Pharmacology

- Owing to developmental factors and smaller body size, infants and young children may receive drug dosages much different from those of adults. Careful calculations, double-checking math, and checking with another registered nurse can prevent errors in drug administration.
- Ensure that families understand the units of measurement for a drug. Confusion may occur with the discussion of metric, household, and other measurement systems.
- For safety when administering injectable drugs to children, use the smallest syringe that ensures the most exact measurement of the drug.
- Use the correct drug and procedure to ensure safe dosing. Dilutions, different concentrations, and different solutions of a prescribed drug can complicate administration of appropriate pediatric dosages.
- Infants and children may not be able to confirm identity, allergies, or drugs. The nurse must be positive of such information before drug administration.
- Nurses must be vigilant for severe side effects or adverse reactions to drugs because information on pediatric drug response is limited.
- Regulatory agencies caution that drug administration errors are more common in pediatric patients, which warrants increased precautions in drug administration.

43

Research related to pediatric patients is limited because of several factors. Research risks and obtaining informed consent make it difficult to recruit a pediatric sample. Parents and guardians are reluctant to provide permission for children to participate in research studies because of the risk involved and the potentially invasive nature of data gathering. Pharmaceutical companies invest fewer resources in pediatric drug research because of the smaller market share afforded to pediatric drugs. However, many contend that lack of pediatric data reflects lack of due diligence, especially when drugs are administered to pediatric patients without supporting research data on which to base safe practices. As a result, less is known about the effects, uses, and dosages of pediatric drugs, and nurses must investigate pediatric drugs carefully to provide knowledgeable nursing care for children.

Closely aligned with the conflicts that affect pediatric pharmacologic research are those associated with drug labeling and dosing instructions. Because many drugs have not undergone the clinical trials required for federal approval, they have not been approved for pediatric use. Safe use for children may be guided by small studies or the judgment of the clinician and may be based on anecdotal evidence rather than scientific study. These conflicts have generated new legislation designed to protect pediatric patients and provide health care professionals with better information and resources.

Despite the permanent reauthorization of the Pediatric Research Equity Act (PREA) in 2012, which requires drug manufacturers to study pediatric drug use and offers incentives for pediatric pharmacology research, only half of all drugs carry federally approved indications for use in children. This means many drugs prescribed for children are being prescribed off label, which means the drug is being used for some purpose for which it has not been approved. Current research agendas reinforce the need for pediatric drug research and establishment of safe guidelines for pediatric drug dosing, administration, and evaluation.

PHARMACOKINETICS

Significant differences exist in drug pharmacokinetics for pediatric patients versus adults. These distinctions stem from differences in body composition and organ maturity and appear to be more pronounced in neonates and infants but less significant in school-age and adolescent children. Pharmacokinetics may be defined as the study of the time course of drug absorption, distribution, metabolism, and excretion.

Absorption

The degree and rate of drug absorption are based on factors such as age (Table 5.1), health status, weight, and route of administration. As children grow and develop, the absorption of drugs generally becomes more effective; therefore less developed absorption in neonates and infants must be considered in dosage and administration. In contrast, poor nutritional habits, changes in physical maturity, and hormonal differences during the adolescent years may cause slowing of drug absorption. Hydration status, presence of underlying disease, and

TABLE 5.1	Pediatric Age Classification
Classification	Age
Term neonate	Birth at 38 or more weeks' gestation to 27 days
Infant/toddler	28 days to 23 months
Children	24 months to 11 years
Adolescent	12 years to 16 or 18 years (regional difference)

From U.S. Food and Drug Administration. (2014). *Pediatric exclusivity study age group* (C-DRG-00909). Retrieved from http://www.fda.gov/Drugs/DevelopmentApprovalProcess/FormsSubmissionRequirements/ElectronicSubmissions/DataStandardsManualmonographs/ucm071754.htm

gastrointestinal (GI) disorders in the child may be significant factors in the absorption of drugs.

Drug absorption is initially influenced by the route of administration. For oral drugs, conditions in the stomach and intestine such as gastric acidity, gastric emptying, gastric motility, GI surface area, enzyme levels, and intestinal flora all mediate drug absorption. Lack of maturation of the GI tract is most pronounced in infancy, making the neonatal and infancy periods those most affected by changes in absorption physiology. Gastric pH is alkaline at birth; acid production begins in the neonatal period, and gastric acid secretion reaches adult levels around 2 to 3 years of age. A low pH, or acidic environment, favors acidic drug absorption, whereas a high pH, or alkaline environment, favors basic drug formulations; therefore differences in pH may hinder or enhance drug absorption. Gastric emptying and GI motility are unpredictable in neonates and infants; however, it approaches that of adults between 6 and 8 months of age. Gastric emptying is affected by feeding, and breast-fed infants have faster gastric emptying than formula-fed infants. Unpredictable GI motility may hinder or enhance absorption of oral drugs, depending on the usual site of chemical absorption.

Intestinal surface area in neonates does not reach that of adults until 20 weeks; prior to this, the reduced surface area leads to reduced drug absorption. Immature enzyme function may also affect drug absorption; neonates have inadequate production of bile salts and pancreatic enzymes, which leads to reduced absorption of lipid-soluble drugs. Intestinal microbial colonization begins in the first few hours after birth and is influenced by gestational age and whether the neonate is breast or formula fed; GI microbial colonization reaches adult levels in adolescence. All of these factors must be considered when assessing the effectiveness of drugs administered by the oral route.

For drugs administered via the subcutaneous (subcut) or intramuscular (IM) routes, absorption occurs at the tissue level. The level of peripheral perfusion and effectiveness of circulation affects drug absorption. Conditions that alter perfusion—dehydration, cold temperatures, and alterations in cardiac status—may impede absorption of drugs in the tissues. Intravenous (IV) drugs are administered directly into the bloodstream and are immediately absorbed and distributed.

The skin of infants and young children is thinner than that of adults; additionally, the ratio of body surface area to body mass of infants and children is proportionately higher than for adults such that many drugs are more readily absorbed in children, and toxicity may result.

Distribution

Drug distribution is affected by factors such as body fluid composition, body tissue composition, protein-binding capability, and effectiveness of various barriers to drug transport. In neonates and infants, the body is about 75% water, compared with 60% in adults. This increased body fluid proportion allows for a greater volume of fluid in which to distribute drugs, which results in a lower drug concentration. Until about age 2 years, the pediatric patient requires higher doses of water-soluble drugs to achieve therapeutic levels. Younger patients also have higher levels of extracellular fluids, which increases the tendency for children to become dehydrated and changes the distribution of water-soluble drugs. Compared with older children, neonates and infants have fat stores with an increased ratio of water to lipids, which alters the distribution of some lipid-soluble drugs. Close monitoring of drug levels (e.g., anti-epileptic drugs) can help ensure drug safety.

To varying degrees, drugs become bound to circulating plasma proteins in the body. Only drugs that are free, or unbound, are available to cross the cell membrane and exert their effect. Neonates and infants have decreased protein concentrations compared with adults, and they have fewer protein receptor sites with an affinity for drug binding in the first 12 months after birth; this results in higher levels of unbound drug and an increased risk of drug toxicity.

In neonates, high bilirubin levels may pose a health risk related to drug administration. Bilirubin molecules may bind with protein receptor sites, which makes the sites unavailable to drugs or displaces drugs from binding sites, allowing large amounts of drug to remain free and available for effect. When drugs are prescribed to neonates, dosages must be decreased and closely monitored to both avoid adverse effects and ensure therapeutic effectiveness.

Anatomic barriers to drug distribution, such as the blood-brain barrier (BBB), must be considered when drugs are administered to pediatric patients. This barrier in neonates is relatively immature and allows drugs to pass easily into central nervous system (CNS) tissue, thereby increasing the likelihood for toxicity. As a child matures, the BBB becomes more impervious to drugs, and drug dosages must be titrated accordingly.

Metabolism

The metabolism of drugs depends greatly on the maturation level of the pediatric patient and varies from child to child. Metabolism is carried out primarily in the liver, with the kidneys and lungs playing a small part in metabolism. Infants have reduced hepatic blood flow and drug-metabolizing enzymes; however, by the time they reach 1 year of age, hepatic blood flow has reached that of an adult. Whereas drug-metabolizing enzymes reach an adult level at around age 11, it is important to understand that the isoenzymes involved in the cytochrome P450 system—CYP1, CYP2, and CYP3 (Table 5.2)—develop at different rates and demonstrate individual variation. Drug prescribing should be based on therapeutic effect and drug concentration. Such differences in drug metabolism, as with other pharmacokinetic factors, reinforce the importance of the nurse evaluating therapeutic effects and monitoring the adverse effects of drugs.

Excretion

Renal excretion is the predominant means of drug elimination. The glomerular filtration rate (GFR) in term neonates is roughly 30% that of adults. During infancy, the GFR rises, and by 12 months, it reaches adult levels. Nurses must carefully monitor renal function, urine flow, and drug effectiveness to evaluate the impact of drug administration on patient status.

PHARMACODYNAMICS

Pharmacodynamics refers to the mechanisms of action and effects of a drug on the body and includes the onset, peak, and duration of effect of a drug. It can also be described as the intensity and time course of therapeutic and adverse effects of drugs. The variables of pharmacokinetics—absorption, distribution, metabolism, and excretion—all affect the parameters of pharmacodynamics. These processes determine the time a drug begins to function, reaches its peak, and sustains its length of action. Variables such as organ function, developmental factors, and administration issues affect drug pharmacodynamics and drug half-life in pediatric patients (Table 5.3), and these have an impact on drug dosing.

NURSING IMPLICATIONS
Pediatric Drug Dosing and Monitoring

Because of the changes in pharmacokinetics and pharmacodynamics inherent in pediatric patients, a key nursing role is to monitor the patient for therapeutic effect and adverse reactions. The processes described earlier in the chapter may be measured using plasma or serum drug levels, which indicate the amount of drug in a patient's body. The therapeutic ranges established for many drug levels are based on adult studies; therefore close monitoring of serum drug levels can assist in establishing appropriate dosages, schedules, and routes of administration. Monitoring can also assist in indicating when the dose is subtherapeutic or becomes toxic. Serum blood levels are not available for all drugs, so patient clinical responses to drugs are especially important when monitoring drug effects.

The calculation of pediatric dosages is based in part on U.S. Food and Drug Administration (FDA) recommendations; as a result of the Best Pharmaceuticals for Children Act (BPCA) and PREA, pediatric dosing is now available for over 450 drugs. For those drugs without pediatric dosing schedules, dosing is based on approved protocols, research studies, and provider experience. Drugs for pediatric patients are ordered based on either the child's weight in kilograms (mg/kg) or body surface area (BSA; or mg/m²). Body surface is based on a percentage of adult surface area (1.73 m²). Dosing must also consider the individual child's status, including age, organ function, health, and route of administration.

TABLE 5.2   Isoenzyme Activity in the Pediatric Population Compared With Adults

Isoenzyme	Pediatric Activity	Drug Class	Examples
CYP1A2	↓ Until 2 y	Antidepressant Bronchodilator Diuretic	Duloxetine Theophylline Triamterene
CYP2C9	↓ Until 1-2 y	Anticoagulant Antidepressant Nonsteroidal antiinflammatory	Warfarin Phenytoin Diclofenac, ibuprofen, naproxen, tolbutamide
CYP2C19	↓ Until 10 y	Antidepressant Benzodiazepine Proton pump inhibitor	Citalopram, sertraline Diazepam Lansoprazole, omeprazole, pantoprazole
CYP2D6	↓ Until 12 y	Analgesic Antidepressant Antihistamine Antipsychotic Beta blocker	Codeine, tramadol amitriptyline, desipramine, doxepin, imipramine, fluoxetine, nortriptyline, paroxetine, venlafaxine Diphenhydramine Risperidone Labetalol, metoprolol
CYP3A4	↓ Until 2 y	Analgesic Antiepileptic Antifungal Antihistamine Antiretroviral Benzodiazepine	Alfentanil, fentanyl Carbamazepine Itraconazole, ketoconazole Loratadine Indinavir, lopinavir/ritonavir, saquinavir Alprazolam, midazolam
MAO A	↑ Until 2 y		
MAO B	≈		
N-methyltransferases	≈		
UGTs	↓ Until 7-10 y	Analgesic Antiepileptic Benzodiazepine	Morphine Lamotrigine Clonazepam, lorazepam
NAT2	↓ Until 1-4 y	Antihypertensive Antibacterial	Hydralazine Isoniazid

CYP, Cytochrome P450; *MAO,* monoamine oxidase; *y,* years.
From Fernandez, E., Perez, R., Hernandez, A., Tejada, P., Arteta, M., & Ramos, J. T. (2011). Factors and mechanisms for pharmacokinetic differences between pediatric population and adults. *Pharmaceutics, 3,* 53-72. http://dx.doi.org/10.3390/pharmaceutics3010053

TABLE 5.3   Different Drug Half-Lives* Among Neonates, Infants, Children, and Adults

Isoenzyme	Drug	Neonate	Infant	Child	Adult
CYP1A2	Caffeine	95	7	3	4
	Theophylline	24-36			3-9
CYP2C9	Phenytoin	30-60	2-7	2-20	20-30
CYP2C19	Phenobarbital	70-500	20-70	20-80	60-160
	Diazepam	22-46	10-12	15-21	24-48
CYP3A	Carbamazepine	8-28	–	14-19	16-36
	Lidocaine	2,9-3,3	–	1-5	1-2,2

*Half-lives are given in hours.
From Fernandez, E., Perez, R., Hernandez, A., Tejada, P., Arteta, M., & Ramos, J. T. (2011). Factors and mechanisms for pharmacokinetic differences between pediatric population and adults. *Pharmaceutics, 3,* 53-72. http://dx.doi.org/10.3390/pharmaceutics3010053

Pediatric Drug Administration

Developmental and cognitive differences must always be considered in pediatric drug administration. It is important for the nurse to differentiate the child's developmental age from chronologic age, because this difference has an impact on the child's response to drug administration. The pediatric patient's ability to understand the process, the reason for drug administration, and the need to cooperate with the procedure must always figure prominently in the nurse's plan of care. The child's temperament may influence understanding and level of cooperation. The concept of family-centered care is essential to ensuring safety during and after health care interventions, especially drug administration. Teaching is directed toward both family members or caregivers and patients, commensurate with the cognitive level of the child. When possible, family members or caregivers should be solicited to assist in drug administration. These significant persons in the child's life, individuals who see the child on a day-to-day basis, are usually in the best position to evaluate the effectiveness of a drug and observe for adverse reactions. Some adverse drug reactions in children, such as ringing in the ears and nausea, may be difficult to evaluate; those closest to the child may be in the best position to assess for these reactions. However, family members or caregivers may request not to participate in invasive procedures such as injections. This request should be respected, and family members or caregivers should be encouraged to provide comfort to the child after drugs are administered. Family members or caregivers should always be supported in their caring function so that the child feels safe and secure.

Pediatric patients must be assessed for the ability to understand the reason for the drug, the need for the drug despite unpleasant taste or method of administration, and the need to complete all doses and courses of the drug. When the family is taught about pediatric drug administration, education for the child at a developmentally appropriate level must also be included. Communication with the child and family members or caregivers must always consider level of knowledge, developmental age, cultural factors, and anxiety levels. The nurse should use optimal interpersonal skills to ensure the best outcome in drug administration to pediatric patients.

The primary concerns in drug administration to infants are maintaining safety and providing care while ensuring as much comfort as possible. Family members or caregivers must be able to practice and repeat the psychomotor skills associated with drug administration. The following are tips to enhance safe drug administration and facilitate comfort:

- Toddlers may react violently and negatively to drug administration. Simple explanations, a firm approach, and enlisting the imagination of a toddler through play may enhance success.
- Preschoolers are fairly cooperative and respond well to age-appropriate explanations. Allowing some level of choice and control may facilitate success with preschool children.
- School-age children, although often cooperative, may fear bodily injury and should be permitted even more control, involvement in the process, and information.
- Age-appropriate fears related to pain, changes in body image, and injury are prevalent among older school-age and adolescent patients. The nurse should establish a positive rapport with the patient, develop the plan of care in collaboration with the patient, and ensure privacy in all aspects of drug administration.

Atraumatic care principles should be used when possible. Donna Wong's **Principle of Atraumatic Care** is "the philosophy of providing therapeutic care through the use of interventions that eliminate or minimize the psychologic and physical distress experienced by children and families." Atraumatic care is achieved by decreasing the separation of children from their family members or caregivers, identifying family and patient

TABLE 5.4	Dosage Form Variability for Pediatric Age Groups
Neonates: 0-4 weeks	???
Infants: 1 month-2 years	Liquids—small volumes (syrups, solutions)
Children: 2-5 years	Liquids; effervescent tablets dispersed in liquids; sprinkles on food
Children: 6-11 years	Solids (chewable tablets, orally disintegrating tablets, oral films)
Adolescents: 12-18 years	Solids (typical adult dosage forms—tablets, capsules)

From Pinto, J. C. (n.d.). *Pediatric dosage development: Where are we?* [PowerPoint slides]. Retrieved from http://www.fda.gov/downloads/NewsEvents/MeetingsConferencesWorkshops/UCM415217.pdf

stressors, decreasing pain, and providing care within the framework of a collaborative partnership.

Most pediatric drugs are administered via the oral route (Table 5.4). This route is the least invasive and easiest to use and can be used by family members or caregivers. Topical, rectal, and parenteral routes are also used to deliver drugs to pediatric patients for whom the oral route is contraindicated. Because of tissue differences among children, the IV route is more predictable than other routes.

Most oral drugs administered to children under the age of 6 are given using an oral syringe. Oral syringes ensure more exact dosing and are relatively easy to use. Syringes may be marked to ensure correct dosages. The syringe is inserted into either side of the mouth and is pointed toward the buccal mucosa. Depositing the drug too close to the front of the mouth increases the likelihood that it will be spit out. Pointing the syringe directly toward the back of the mouth may increase the risk for gagging or choking. Infants may suck drugs from a bottle nipple into which the measured drug has been squirted from an oral syringe. Preschool and school-age children are usually able to inject oral drugs into their own mouths, enhancing their sense of control over what can be an anxiety-provoking situation.

Nurses may need to crush pills or dissolve the contents of capsules in fluid for administration to pediatric patients. The nurse should work closely with the pharmacist and in compliance with hospital policies to determine the advisability of crushing or dissolving a drug before administration; some drugs, particularly timed-release and enteric-coated drugs, should *not* be crushed or dissolved. Some drugs may be made more palatable by adding jam, yogurt, or honey (although infants younger than 1 year should not be given honey because of the risk of botulism). Small volumes (10 mL) should be used to dilute drugs so the patient is ensured the full dose. For children who require tube feeding, oral drugs can be administered via nasogastric, orogastric, or gastrostomy tubes, if the drugs can be crushed or dissolved prior to administration.

When drug injection or venipuncture is necessary, topical anesthetic protocols may be followed to reduce the pain associated with the procedure. Agents such as eutectic mixture of local anesthetics (EMLA), topical liposomal 4% lidocaine cream

(LMX4), or a vapocoolant spray may be effective in reducing the pain and fear associated with invasive procedures, such as injection or venipuncture, in children.

Based on the cognitive level of the child, other nonpharmacologic methods of pain and anxiety control such as distraction, diversion, relaxation, and creative imagery can also be used to decrease the perception of pain. Injections should *never* be given to a sleeping child with the intent to surprise the child with a quick procedure. The child may subsequently experience a lack of trust and may be reluctant to sleep in the future.

IV infusion sites must be protected, especially in infants and toddlers, who do not understand the rationale or importance of maintaining the IV site. Commercial products are available to protect the IV site and maintain an intact IV infusion set. Stocking-like covers may hide the IV site from infants before they master the concept of object permanence. The patency of an IV site should be checked prior to each drug administration to avoid infiltration and extravasation. Any injection site on a preschooler should be covered with a bandage, preferably a decorated one, so that the child does not fear "leakage" from the area. Selection of injection and IV sites is made based on developmental variables, site of preference, and access to administration sites. The ventrogluteal or vastus lateralis are preferred sites for pediatric IM injections. The length of the needle depends on the child's muscle mass, subcutaneous tissue, and the site of injection. Children may prefer subcutaneous injections in the leg or upper arm rather than in the abdomen. IV sites may be difficult to find in children. The amount of fatty tissue, hydration status of the child, and ability to isolate and immobilize veins are all mitigating factors.

When administering drugs to children, follow these basic principles: honesty, respect, age-appropriate teaching and explanations, attention to safety, atraumatic care, use of the least amount of restraint necessary (e.g., swaddling a neonate), providing positive reinforcement for age-appropriate cooperation, refraining from use of negative messages or behaviors, and upholding family-centered principles. These standards may be used throughout the pediatric life span and highlight the need for nursing interventions that are sensitive, individualized, and caring.

CONSIDERATIONS FOR THE ADOLESCENT PATIENT

Adolescent patients need individualized nursing care specific to their developmental stage. Age-oriented developmental considerations include physical changes, cognitive level and abilities, emotional factors, and impact of chronic illness.

Physically, adolescence is a highly diverse period of growth and development. Growth rates during these years may be affected by nutrition, factors within the environment, genetics and heredity, and gender. A group of adolescents of similar ages may manifest very different sizes, height-to-weight proportions, timing of secondary sex characteristics, and other indicators of physical maturity. These differences may warrant individualization of drug dosage based on weight or body surface area,

even when the adolescent meets or exceeds the size of standard adults. For example, an adjustment may be required in the dosage of a lipid-soluble drug because of the changes in lean-to-fat body mass, especially in young adolescent males, that coincide with physical maturation. Hormonal changes and growth spurts may necessitate changes in drug dosages; many children with chronic illnesses require dosage adjustments in the early teen years as a result of these transitions. Sleep requirements and metabolic rates may greatly increase during the teen years, along with appetite and food consumption, which may affect the scheduling of and response to drugs. Although adolescents' physical appearance and organ structure and function resemble those of adults, their bodies continue to grow and change; this requires increased vigilance in monitoring therapeutic and toxic drug levels.

The cognitive level and abilities of adolescents may pose additional considerations. Cognitive theorists have posited that adolescents progress from concrete to abstract reasoning. Individuals who are still in the concrete operational stage may have difficulty comprehending how a drug exerts its effects on the body and the importance of meticulous dosing and administration. Adolescents may also have difficulty understanding such concepts as drug interactions, side effects, adverse reactions, and therapeutic levels. For example, the patient taking birth control pills may or may not be able to comprehend the reduced action of birth control pills caused by antibiotics taken during an acute infection and may fail to take extra precautions to prevent pregnancy.

An understanding of the adolescent brain and the ongoing development of social, reasoning, and decision-making skills can be used to guide nursing assessment and interventions with the pediatric patient. As adolescents learn to reason in an abstract manner, teaching may be based on more complex information. Potentially, adolescent perception of invulnerability and difficulty relating future consequences to current actions may dictate that the nurse adapt teaching to address specific adolescent thought processes. An adolescent who is told that an insulin injection schedule must be adhered to in order to avoid long-term complications may not understand the rationale for treatment if it is only substantiated by abstract, future-oriented risks. The same patient may find the relationship between using insulin to maintain normoglycemia and the ability to participate in sports more immediate and relevant. Allowing the adolescent to verbalize concerns about the drug and its regimen may offer opportunities for clarifying misconceptions and teaching new concepts.

Emotional development of the adolescent also occurs on an individual basis. The adolescent years are characterized by sensation seeking, risk taking, questioning, formation of identity, and increasing influences exerted by peer groups. To avoid potential drug interactions, the nurse should assess for high-risk behaviors that include use of alcohol, tobacco, and recreational drugs. Other issues, including sexual practices and stressful family and social situations, may affect the patient's response to drugs. Nurses must be respectful of the emotional needs of adolescence while attending to the mental health issues that may surface during these years. A comprehensive history must be solicited from adolescent patients to ensure appropriate drug administration. The nurse must also be conscious of the need to exercise care in offering confidentiality in the event that information needs to be divulged to other health care providers, family members, or caregivers to ensure patient safety.

As adolescents attain greater levels of independence from their parents, self-care behaviors increase. The nurse should assess the patient's abilities to self-administer drugs and monitor therapeutic and adverse reactions. Adolescents spend less time with family members and caregivers and may need increased instruction about their drug regimen and the key observations that are needed. Although adolescents frequently display "breaking away" behaviors in response to parental bonds, they often continue to use family members or caregiver drug habits as models for their own drug behaviors.

For the pediatric patient with a chronic illness, issues may change during adolescence. Engaging peers in the plan of care for drug administration, allowing the adolescent to make safe choices and have flexibility within that plan, setting up mutual drug contracts, and permitting the patient to design their own adult-monitored drug regimen may facilitate adherence. The nurse can facilitate required adaptations and support both the patient and family members during these times.

NURSING PROCESS: FAMILY-CENTERED COLLABORATIVE CARE

In working with pediatric patients, key developmental differences must be considered when administering and monitoring drugs. The nursing process provides the framework to guide nursing practice in administering drugs, planning and evaluating nursing care, providing patient and family teaching, and incorporating the family into all aspects of treatment.

Family and patient teaching is a key role for the nurse. Issues such as indications for the drug, the side effects, the dose, how to measure the dose, how to administer the dose, the therapeutic effect, adverse effects to monitor for, the duration, and the frequency are all important information needed by the family or caregiver. Specifics such as the need for refrigeration, the need to shake the medicine, the difference between household and prescriptive measurements, and other issues should be addressed to ensure patient safety. Adherence to the drug regimen is of paramount importance with children and families; providing written instructions or a drug calendar may facilitate this through concrete reminders.

Nurses should also be aware of the tendency for parents to treat infants and children with over-the-counter (OTC) analgesics. Parents may provide frequent analgesia to their children and may be largely unaware of the potential for misuse and overuse in the pediatric population. Additional concern has arisen regarding the inappropriate use of OTC cough and cold remedies with children. Deaths and significant illness have been attributed to lack of label recommendations, misuse of adult drugs, poor drug instructions, and overdose, which warrants rigid restrictions on the use of these drugs in the pediatric population.

NURSING PROCESS
Family-Centered Collaborative Care
Pediatrics

Assessment
- Assess the context and meaning of illness.
- Assess developmental age, health status, nutritional status, and hydration status.
- Assess family member and caregiver health literacy level and the child's cognitive level.
- Assess family patterns, economic issues, and cultural patterns that influence adherence to a therapeutic regimen.
- Assess learning style.
- Assess readiness to learn.
- Assess the allergy history of the child and determine family allergy history.
- Identify all of the patient's drugs (prescriptions, over-the-counter [OTC], and herbal).
- Record the age, weight, and height of the child. Drug calculations are based on these three factors.

Nursing Diagnoses
- Knowledge, Deficient related to cognitive limitation or decreased health literacy, misinterpretation of available information or unfamiliarity with available resources, lack of interest in learning
- Health Maintenance, Ineffective related to cognitive limitations, insufficient resources, and unachieved developmental tasks
- Knowledge, Readiness for Enhanced
- Injury, Risk for

Planning
- Family members and caregivers, as well as the pediatric patient if appropriate, will recognize the need for drug administration.
- Family members and caregivers, as well as the pediatric patient if appropriate, will describe the rationale for drug therapy.
- Family members and caregivers, as well as the pediatric patient if appropriate, will incorporate the drug treatment regimen into their lifestyle.
- Family members and caregivers, as well as the pediatric patient if appropriate, will demonstrate safe drug administration practices.
- Family members and caregivers, as well as the pediatric patient if appropriate, will state with confidence their ability to manage the treatment regimen and remain in control of their life.
- The pediatric patient will remain free of drug-related injuries.

Nursing Interventions
- Assist the patient, family members, and caregivers with appropriate follow-up resources and support.
- Avoid the use of restraints.

- Engage the patient, family members, and caregivers as partners in the educational process.
- Follow all rights of safe drug administration.
- Help patients, their family members, and caregivers manage complex drug schedules.
- Reconcile the drug list at discharge, and provide the list to the patient, family members, and caregivers as appropriate.
- Support patient, family member, and caregiver priorities, preferences, and choices.
- Use at least two methods of patient identification.
- Use open-ended questions and encourage two-way communication.

Patient Teaching

- Consider the use of alternative settings for teaching the chronically ill pediatric patient, their family members, and caregivers.
- Provide a developmentally appropriate environment when addressing the health education needs of adolescents.
- Provide information to support self-efficacy, self-regulation, and self-management of the drug regimen.

- Use educational strategies that are interactive and engaging for younger children and toddlers.
- Use family-centered approaches when teaching children and adolescents.
- Use strategies to promote motivation and sustain learning.

Cultural Considerations

- Assess for cultural/ethnic self-care practices.
- Assess the influence of cultural beliefs and values on the knowledge base.
- Provide educational materials in the native language of patients, family members, and caregivers.

Evaluation

- Evaluate the child's physiologic and psychological response to the drug regimen.
- Evaluate the family member's knowledge about the drug, the dosage, the schedule for administration, and the side effects.
- Evaluate the therapeutic and adverse effects of the drug(s).

CRITICAL THINKING CASE STUDY

A 9-month-old infant weighing 20 pounds comes to the emergency department with a 3-day history of vomiting, fever greater than 102.5°F, and significant pain. Physical assessment reveals acute otitis media, for which the doctor prescribed amoxicillin 500 mg three times a day for 5 days and ibuprofen 2.5 mL every 6 hours.

1. Prior to administration of amoxicillin, what must the nurse assess for?

2. If the safe dose of amoxicillin for a child under the age of 2 is 80 mg/kg/day in divided doses, is the prescribed dose safe? How do you know?

3. How will you instruct the family member to safely administer the drugs?

NCLEX STUDY QUESTIONS

1. A 4-year-old patient is discharged on an oral liquid drug suspension of 4 mL per dose. Which device will the nurse recommend to ensure the highest level of accuracy in home administration of the drug?
   a. Measuring spoon
   b. Graduated medicine cup
   c. Household teaspoon
   d. Oral syringe

2. A child is ordered to receive naloxone intravenously STAT. The child's weight is 20 kg, and the recommended child's dosage is 0.01 mg/kg. Naloxone is available in a 400 mcg/mL solution. How much drug will the nurse plan to administer?

3. A child who weighs 88 pounds is ordered to receive 3 mg/kg of a drug. The drug is available in a 15 mg/mL elixir. How much drug will the patient receive?

4. The nurse understands the differences between drug excretion in children and that in adults. With this knowledge, what does the nurse consider when administering drugs to children?
   a. Most children need a higher dose of drug, so the nurse will contact the physician for an increase in the ordered dose.
   b. Children excrete drugs rapidly, so the nurse must assess carefully for therapeutic effects of the drug.
   c. The most important assessment is to evaluate for drug accumulation, because the excretion of drugs is slower in children.
   d. Excretion of most drugs is the same in children as in adults, but assessments are important to avoid side effects.

5. A parent is learning to administer drug to a school-age child. Which strategy will the nurse teach the parent to achieve cooperation in a child of this age?
   a. Enlisting physical restraint
   b. Establishing drug contracts
   c. Providing age-appropriate explanations
   d. Tolerating violent reactions

6. A nurse caring for a child with developmental delay prepares to teach the patient about prescribed drugs. Which actions are essential to ensure patient safety? (Select all that apply.)
   a. Assess the child's developmental age.
   b. Assess for side effects the same as those experienced by adults.
   c. Consider the actions and uses of the drug.
   d. Focus on the child's chronologic age.
   e. Involve the family in teaching sessions.

7. The Principle of Atraumatic Care includes (select all that apply):
   a. Pain management
   b. Collaborative care with family members
   c. Restraining infants to administer drugs
   d. Keeping the child apart from family members when administering drugs

8. Which of the following strategies are helpful when working with adolescent patients to promote adherence? (Select all that apply.)
   a. Allow flexibility in the treatment plan.
   b. Use future-oriented examples and consequences to support the need for drug therapy.
   c. Guarantee the adolescent patient privacy when obtaining history.
   d. Set up a mutually developed drug contract.

Answers: 1, d; 2, 0.5 mL; 3, 8 mL; 4, c; 5, c; 6, a, c, e; 7, a, b; 8, a, d.

6

Geriatric Considerations

http://evolve.elsevier.com/McCuistion/pharmacology

OBJECTIVES

- Explain how the physiologic changes associated with aging impact drug therapy.
- Describe two ways the Beers criteria can be used to improve the care of older adults.
- Discuss issues that affect older adults' adherence to therapeutic regimens.
- Describe nursing implications related to drug therapy in the older adult.

OUTLINE

KEY TERMS

By 2033, persons over the age of 65 will outnumber those under the age of 18 in the United States. There are expected to be over 98 million older adults by the year 2060, with close to 20 million over the age of 85. These numbers are staggering, more so considering 92% of older adults have at least one chronic illness, and over 75% of older adults have two chronic illnesses. Typically, persons with two or more chronic conditions take five or more prescription drugs.

Over half of all older adults use at least one over-the-counter (OTC) drug, and nearly three-quarters of older adults use at least one supplement to augment their prescription drugs; however, older adults are more likely to experience adverse reactions or drug interactions related to OTC drugs and supplements, many times resulting in hospitalization.

Administration of drugs in the older adult population requires special attention to age-related factors that influence drug absorption, distribution, metabolism, and excretion. Drug dosages are often adjusted according to the older adult's weight, laboratory results (e.g., liver enzymes and glomerular filtration), and comorbid health problems. Because of altered organ function in the older adult, the effects of drug therapy must be closely monitored to prevent adverse reactions and possible toxicity.

Drug toxicity may develop in the older adult for drug doses that are within the therapeutic range for the younger adult. These therapeutic drug ranges are usually safe for young and middle-aged adults but are not always within the safe range for older adults. It has been suggested that drugs for older adults should initially be prescribed at low dosages with a gradual increase in dosage based on therapeutic response; this practice is commonly stated as *start low and go slow*. This approach to drug prescribing reduces the chance of drug toxicity.

Common characteristics in older adults that increase the risk for problems with drug administration include lack of coordinated care, recent discharge from the hospital, self-treatment, multiple diagnoses, sensory and physical changes associated with aging, multiple health care providers, and cognitive impairment.

PHYSIOLOGIC CHANGES

Physiologic changes associated with aging can influence absorption, distribution, metabolism, and excretion of drugs as well as pharmacodynamic responses at receptors and target organs. These physiologic changes include the following:

- A reduction in total body water and lean body mass, resulting in increased body fat, which alters the volume of distribution of drugs.
- A reduction in kidney mass and lower kidney blood flow, leading to a reduced glomerular filtration rate (GFR) and reduced clearance of drugs excreted by the kidneys.
- A reduction in liver size and blood flow, resulting in reduced hepatic clearance of drugs.

A decline in the physiologic processes that maintain equilibrium in the older adult may mean a higher incidence of adverse effects. Examples of this include:

- Postural hypotension in response to drugs that reduce blood pressure
- Volume depletion and electrolyte imbalance in response to diuretics
- Excessive bleeding with anticoagulant and antiplatelet drugs
- Altered glycemic response to antidiabetic drugs
- Gastrointestinal (GI) irritation with nonsteroidal antiinflammatory drugs (NSAIDs)

Physiologic changes with aging affect the determination of risk versus benefit underlying drug choice, dose, and frequency.

PHARMACOKINETICS

Pharmacologic processes have not received adequate study in the older adult, therefore a thorough understanding of pharmacokinetics is necessary for the safe administration of drugs in this population.

Absorption

Adults experience several GI changes with aging that may influence drug absorption. These include a decrease in small-bowel surface area, slowed gastric emptying, reduced gastric blood flow, and a 5% to 10% decrease in gastric acid production. These changes are not always clinically relevant; however, calcium carbonate is affected by the decreased gastric acidity. Older adults should be prescribed calcium citrate, which requires a less acidic environment for dissolution. Other common problems that occur in older adults that can significantly influence drug absorption include swallowing difficulties, poor nutrition, and dependence on feeding tubes.

Distribution

Aging can significantly alter drug distribution. With aging, adults experience a decline in muscle mass and a 20% to 40% increase in fat. The increase in body fat means lipid-soluble drugs have a greater volume of distribution, increased drug storage, reduced elimination, and a prolonged period of action. Older adults have a 10% to 15% reduction in total body water, which affects water-soluble drugs, and a 10% reduction in albumin. Reduced albumin levels can result in decreased protein binding of drugs and increased free drug available to exert therapeutic effects, but it also increases the risk for drug toxicity.

Metabolism

Hepatic blood flow in the older adult may be decreased by 40%; aging also results in a 15% to 30% decrease in liver size and a reduction in cytochrome P450 (CYP450) enzyme activity that is responsible for the breakdown of drugs. Drug clearance by hepatic metabolism can be reduced by these age-related changes. A reduction in hepatic metabolism can decrease first-pass metabolism and can prolong drug half-life, resulting in increased drug levels and potential drug toxicity. Nurses must be aware of these metabolic changes and must monitor response to drug therapy to avoid adverse reactions.

To assess liver function, liver enzymes must be checked. Elevated levels of alanine aminotransferase (ALT) and aspartate aminotransferase (AST) may indicate possible liver dysfunction. However, an older adult can have normal liver function test (LFT) results and still have impaired hepatic enzyme activity.

Excretion

Renal excretion of drugs decreases with age. Excretion is altered by age-related changes in kidney function, such as decreased renal size and volume, which differ for each individual. However, it is generally accepted that the GFR declines by 1 mL/min after the age of 40 (normal GFR is 100 to 125 mL/min). Despite a decline in kidney function, an individual's creatinine may remain normal as he or she ages due to a decline in muscle mass and activity. Changes in kidney function affect many drugs, leading to a prolonged half-life and elevated drug levels. Changes in kidney function require dosage adjustment, especially if the drug has a narrow therapeutic range.

GFR can be calculated using the Cockroft-Gault formula, which is the formula recommended by the U.S. Food and Drug Administration (FDA) and therefore used by pharmaceutical manufacturers when determining dosage adjustments:

$$C_{Cr} = [(140 - age) \times weight) / (72 \times S_{Cr}) \times 0.85 \text{ (if female)}$$

Abbreviations/Units: C_{Cr} (creatinine clearance) = mL/minute; Age = years; Weight = kg; S_{Cr} (serum creatinine) = mg/dL.

However, it can also be estimated by many calculators found on the Internet (www.globalrph.com/crcl.htm).

Nurses must have a general understanding of drug classifications that require dosage adjustment in patients with chronic kidney disease (CKD). The mnemonic *BANDD CAMP* (Table 6.1) may be helpful in remembering the drug classifications; however, nurses should not rely on their memory for drug administration. Package inserts, up-to-date drug reference books, and reputable websites (www.globalrph.com/index_renal.htm) maintain current dosing information.

PHARMACODYNAMICS

Pharmacodynamic responses to drugs are altered with aging as a result of changes in the number of receptor sites, which affects the affinity of certain drugs. These changes are seen most clearly in the cardiovascular and central nervous systems.

	Drug Class	Adjust Dose	Avoid in Stages 4 and 5
B	Beta blockers	Acebutolol, atenolol, bisoprolol, nadolol, sotalol	Sotalol
A	ACEIs/ARBs	All ACEIs	Olmesartan
N	NSAIDs, opioids	Codeine, morphine, oxycodone, tramadol	All NSAIDs, meperidine
D	Diuretics	Potassium-sparing diuretics, thiazide diuretics	Potassium-sparing diuretics, thiazide diuretics
D	Diabetic medications	Gliclazide, acarbose, insulin, gliptins	Glyburide, metformin, exenatide
C	Cholesterol medications	Pravastatin, rosuvastatin, fibrates	—
A	Antimicrobials (dose reductions are often delayed for 24-48 h to allow for aggressive dosing and for the drug to reach steady state)	Antibiotics: Most antibiotics except cloxacillin, clindamycin, metronidazole, erythromycin, azithromycin Antifungals: Fluconazole, itraconazole Antivirals: Acyclovir, famciclovir, valacyclovir	Nitrofurantoin
M	Miscellaneous	Allopurinol, colchicine, digoxin, H_2RAs	New anticoagulants
P	Psychotropics	Lithium, gabapentin, pregabalin, topiramate, vigabatrin; bupropion, duloxetine, paroxetine, venlafaxine	—

TABLE 6.1   Drug Classes That Require Dosage Adjustment in Chronic Kidney Disease

ACEI, Angiotensin-converting enzyme inhibitor; *ARB,* angiotensin II-receptor blocker; *h,* hours; *H_2RAs,* histamine-2 receptor antagonists; *NSAID,* nonsteroidal antiinflammatory drug.
From Meyer, D., Damm, T., & Jensen, K. (2012). Drug dosage adjustments in chronic kidney disease: The pharmacist's role. Saskatchewan Drug Information Services College of Pharmacy and Nutrition, University of Saskatchewan. Retrieved from www.rxfiles.ca/rxfiles/uploads/documents/ltc/HCPs/CKD/SDIS.Renal_newsletter.pdf

Older adults experience a loss of sensitivity in adrenergic receptors, affecting both agonists and antagonists; this results in a reduced response to beta blockers and beta$_2$ agonists. Older adults also experience a blunting in compensatory reflexes leading to orthostatic hypotension and falls.

With age, there is a reduction in dopaminergic and cholinergic receptors, neurons, and available neural connections in the brain. There is reduced blood flow to the brain, and the blood-brain barrier also becomes more permeable. This puts the older adult at risk for central nervous system (CNS) drug side effects, which include dizziness, seizures, confusion, sedation, and extrapyramidal effects.

NURSING IMPLICATIONS: OLDER ADULT DRUG DOSING AND MONITORING

Polypharmacy

Polypharmacy refers to the use of more medications than is medically necessary. There is little agreement on the actual number of drugs that constitutes polypharmacy, but researchers use five drugs because this number has been associated with increased incidence of adverse drug reactions, geriatric syndromes, and increased mortality.

Risk factors associated with polypharmacy include advanced age, female sex, multiple health care providers, use of herbal therapies and OTC drugs, multiple chronic diseases, and the number of hospitalizations and care transitions. Polypharmacy can cause an increase in geriatric syndromes (cognitive impairment, falls, decreased functional status, urinary incontinence, and poor nutrition) as well as an increased incidence of adverse drug reactions and poor adherence.

Pharmacotherapy in older adults is complex. In order to reduce the risk for and incidence of polypharmacy, nurses must be involved in the coordination of care for older adults. Older adults should be encouraged to use only one pharmacy and should give the pharmacist a list of all the drugs taken—prescribed, herbal, and OTC. A properly informed pharmacist will be able to conduct a clinical review of the patient's drugs to ensure the appropriateness of therapy. A pharmacist can also confirm patient understanding of individual therapy and can monitor responses to drug therapy. All of this is done to improve the overall quality of life of patients in their care.

Beers Criteria for Potentially Inappropriate Medication Use in Older Adults

The American Geriatrics Society Beers Criteria for Potentially Inappropriate Medication Use in Older Adults is a document developed by a consensus panel of 12 experts in geriatric care to aid health care providers in the safe prescription and administration of drugs to older adults (available free from http://onlinelibrary.wiley.com/doi/10.1111/jgs.13702/epdf). First developed in 1991, it has been revised four times, most recently in 2015. The 2015 Beers Criteria added new information on renal dosing of drugs and drug-drug interactions; as in previous editions, it continues to provide safety information based on best available evidence to use in decision making for drug therapy. Although the document provides information on drugs to avoid in older adults and drugs to use with caution, it is not designed for use in isolation. All drug therapy decisions should be made taking into consideration an individual's preferences, values, and needs. It is very important that the nurse advocate for the patient in these areas to ensure safety and promote adherence.

TABLE 6.2 Barriers to Effective Drug Use by Older Adults

Causes	Nursing Actions
Taking too many drugs at different times	Develop a chart indicating times to take drugs. Provide space to place a mark for each drug taken. Coordinate the drug regimen with activities of daily living (e.g., meals) and events. Use an organizer container (daily or weekly). Have the patient bring all drugs—including over-the-counter drugs and herbal, vitamin, and mineral supplements—to all health appointments.
Failure to understand the purpose or reason for a drug	Explain the purpose, drug action, and importance of the drug. Provide time for questions and reinforcement. Reinforce with written information.
Impaired memory	Encourage family members or friends to monitor the patient's drug regimen.
Decreased mobility and dexterity	Advise family members or friends to have drugs and water or other fluid accessible and to assist older adults as needed.
Visual and hearing disturbances	Suggest eye and ear examinations (glasses or hearing aids).
High cost of prescriptions	Contact the social services department of your institution and compassionate care programs as appropriate.
Childproof drug bottles	Suggest that the patient request nonchildproof bottle caps.
Side effects or adverse reactions from the drug	Educate the patient and family about side effects to report to the health care provider.

Adverse Drug Events

No drug is safe. Every year, over 775,000 emergency department (ED) visits occur due to adverse drug events (ADEs), and over 125,000 people are hospitalized due to ADEs. Older adults are twice as likely as younger adults to visit the ED with adverse drug events and are seven times as likely to be hospitalized. Most visits and hospitalizations occur due to reactions to blood thinners, drugs used to treat diabetes and seizures, cardiac drugs, and drugs used for pain control.

According to the World Health Organization, ADEs are "unintended and undesired effects of a [drug] at the normal dose." There are five types of adverse drug events: (1) adverse drug reactions, (2) medication errors, (3) therapeutic failures, (4) adverse drug withdrawal events, and (5) overdoses. Older adults have multiple risk factors for ADEs, including frailty, multiple comorbidities, polypharmacy, and cognitive issues.

Adherence

Adherence to a drug regimen is a problem for all patient age groups, but it is especially troublesome in older adult patients. Older adults may fail to ask questions during interactions with health care providers, which leads to the drug regimen not being fully understood or precisely followed. Failure to adhere to a drug regimen can cause underdosing or overdosing that could be harmful to the patient's health. Table 6.2 lists barriers to effective drug use by older adults.

Failure to adhere to a drug regimen can lead to ADEs, resulting in hospital admission, readmission to health care institutions, and even death. Complex drug regimens may be difficult for older adults to follow. Education is the cornerstone of adherence, and this includes education of the patient, family, and formal and informal caregivers.

Working with older adult patients is an ongoing nursing responsibility. The nurse should plan strategies with the patient and family or friends to encourage adherence with prescribed regimens. Daily contact may be necessary at first. Simply ordering the drug does not mean that the patient is able to get the drug or take it correctly. Older adults should have their prescriptions filled at one pharmacy if possible so a relationship can be established with a pharmacist and drug interactions can be identified and monitored closely.

The Medicare Modernization Act of 2003 made it possible for older adults to obtain prescription drug coverage through Medicare, with initial enrollment beginning in 2006. Older adults who are eligible for Medicare Part A or Part B are eligible for the optional Medicare Prescription Drug Plan (Part D) or coverage through a Medicare Advantage Plan (Part C). Each of these plans has its own formulary, copay rate, and in-network pharmacies. No plan is perfect for every older adult; the nurse, as advocate, must be able to assist the older adult to find the plan that is right for him or her and to make the most of the policy.

However, not all older adults have insurance that includes prescription drug coverage, nor are they able to afford their drugs even with insurance. Nurses need to assess the patient's ability to obtain prescriptions prior to sending the patient home. Options for assistance are available, and the nurse can assist patients in navigating the system to obtain their drugs for free or at a reduced cost (see Partnership for Prescription Assistance at www.pparx.org and Extra Help at www.ssa.gov/medicare/prescriptionhelp).

Health care professionals—nurses, pharmacists, and health care providers—need to work collaboratively to enhance safety and adherence of older adult patients and to avoid errors and unwarranted concerns. Nurses are in a unique position to educate patients and to monitor the effectiveness of therapeutic regimens. A handout of tips for patients on talking with their pharmacist can be found at www.fda.gov/downloads/Drugs/ResourcesForYou/UCM163349.pdf.

HEALTH TEACHING WITH THE OLDER ADULT

Specific factors that enhance educational readiness and promote adherence in the older adult include the following:
- Ensure that the patient is wearing eyeglasses and has working hearing aids in place if needed. Check sensory aids to be sure they are clean and working.
- Speak in a tone of voice that the patient can hear; sit facing the patient, and limit distractions.
- Treat the patient with respect; never infantilize (also referred to as "elderspeak"); expect that the patient can learn.
- Use large print and dark type against a light background; use a font with serifs, or "feet and tails" (like this one), which makes letters close together easier to read.

- Review all drugs at each patient visit; ask the patient to bring all drugs to each appointment, and advise use of only one pharmacy.
- Advise the patient to complete the *vial of life* (medical information for emergency personnel to use in the provision of care; www.vialoflife.com) and keep it on the refrigerator door where safety personnel will know to look for it.
- Instruct the patient to keep a list of all drugs taken, bring it to all health appointments, and carry it when out of the house.
- Encourage a simple dosing schedule when possible.
- Suspect recently prescribed drug(s) if new confusion or disorientation occurs.

- Encourage the patient to report if a drug is not improving the condition for which it was prescribed.
- Consider use of memory aids such as pill organizers or planners, alarms, blinking lights, or prerecorded messages.

The National Institutes of Health (NIH) websites on aging are excellent resources for both health care providers and older adults and their families. The website for health care providers is www.nia.nih.gov; it has sections on health information, research, grants, training, news, and events. The website for older adults is www.nihseniorhealth.gov.

◎ NURSING PROCESS
Patient-Centered Collaborative Care
Geriatrics

Assessment
- Assess for allergies.
- Assess for sensory and cognitive barriers.
  - Assess the patient's use of eyeglasses, and check the date of the last eye examination.
  - Is the patient confused or disoriented? If so, is this state transitory?
- Assess laboratory test results, and follow up as appropriate.
  - Decreased kidney and liver function can increase the half-life of drugs.
- Assess weight and vital signs.
- Determine all drugs the patient takes, including illicit, prescription, and OTC drugs and supplements.
  - Assess patient adherence to the drug regimen.
  - Assess patient knowledge of the purpose of each drug, how it works, and its possible side effects.
- Discern whether the patient has difficulty opening drug containers and whether the patient is experiencing side effects or adverse reactions.
- Discern whether the patient lives alone, with or without social support, and if assistance is needed with drugs, including costs or the transportation to acquire them.
- Obtain a history of chronic conditions.

Nursing Diagnoses
- Health Maintenance, Ineffective related to lack of, or alteration in, communication skills (written, verbal, and nonverbal)
- Therapeutic Regimen Management, Ineffective related to the complexity of the regimen
- Knowledge, Deficient related to cognitive limitation, information misinterpretation, and lack of interest in learning
- Constipation, Risk for related to use of drugs (e.g., aluminum-containing antacids, anticholinergics, calcium channel blockers, diuretics, and opiates)

Planning
- The patient will collaborate with health care providers to develop a therapeutic regimen that is congruent with health goals and lifestyle.

- The patient will describe why the drug is needed, how the drug is administered, common adverse reactions, and drug interactions.
- The patient will identify measures to prevent constipation.
- The patient will list resources that can be used for more information or support.
- The patient will verbalize the ability to manage the therapeutic regimen.

Nursing Interventions
- Ascertain whether financial problems are preventing the patient from purchasing prescribed drugs. Assistance programs are available.
- Communicate with the pharmacist or health care provider when a drug dose is in question. Check drug references for recommended drug dosages for older adults.
- Establish a collaborative partnership with the patient in order to meet health-related goals.
- Monitor the patient's laboratory results to ensure that blood urea nitrogen (BUN), serum creatinine, estimated glomerular filtration rate (eGFR), and liver enzymes are within normal range and that drug levels are within the therapeutic range. Discuss findings with the health care provider.
- Observe the patient for adverse reactions when multiple drugs are being taken.
- Recognize a change in usual behavior or an increase in confusion. One of the first signs of drug toxicity is a change in mental status. Report changes to the health care provider.
- Remind the patient and family to tell the pharmacist about OTC preparations the patient is taking when picking up prescriptions.

Patient Teaching
General
- Advise patients and family to request a non–childproof cap from the pharmacy if the patient has arthritis in the hand joint or has difficulty opening childproof bottle caps. The patient may need to sign for this at the pharmacy, and safety of children or pets in the environment must be ensured.
- Advise patients to keep a record of their drugs and when they are to be taken. Consider offering them a sample

log for recording information. This removes barriers, increases drug adherence, and avoids drug errors.

- Advise patients to use one pharmacy to fill prescriptions, and instruct them to inform the pharmacist of all illicit, prescription, and OTC drugs and supplements taken.
- Be available to answer patient questions. Be supportive of the older adult and the family. Discuss problems related to the drugs.
- Counsel patients not to share prescribed drugs with others or to take drugs prescribed for another person.
- Explain to patients and family the importance of adherence to the drug regimen. Emphasize the importance of taking drugs as prescribed.
- Review drugs with patients and family, including the reason the drug was prescribed, route of administration, frequency, common side effects, and when to notify the health care provider.

⊕ Cultural Considerations

- Do not assume that lack of eye contact means the patient is not listening or does not care; it might indicate respect. More traditional or older individuals in some cultures do not maintain eye contact.
- Provide additional time for verbal and written explanations to ensure all questions related to the drug regimen have been asked and answered. This will promote adherence.
- Recognize that language difficulties may interfere with older adults' understanding of the prescribed drug regimen if English is not their first language; provide educational material in the patient's native language.

Evaluation

- Evaluate adherence to the drug regimen, and answer any questions the older adult may have.
- Evaluate therapeutic drug response, and ascertain side effects or adverse reactions.

CRITICAL THINKING CASE STUDY

A 78-year-old woman comes to the clinic for a new-patient examination. She reports that she smokes *Cannabis* several times a week and also takes alprazolam 0.5 mg three times per day, a combination tablet of metoprolol tartrate 50 mg/hydrochlorothiazide 25 mg daily, aspirin 81 mg daily; garlic soft-gels 1000 mg twice a day; and ibuprofen 400 mg four times a day.

1. Do any of these drugs appear on the 2015 American Geriatrics Society Beers Criteria for Potentially Inappropriate Medication Use in Older Adults? If so, what do the criteria say about them?
2. What interactions exist among the drugs and supplements this patient is taking?
3. What is the evidence for taking garlic to reduce cholesterol?

NCLEX STUDY QUESTIONS

1. A patient has nine drugs prescribed to take daily. Which are common reasons for nonadherence to the drug regimen in an older adult? (Select all that apply.)
   a. Taking multiple drugs at one time
   b. Impaired memory
   c. Decreased dexterity
   d. Increased mobility
   e. Increased visual acuity
2. The nurse is reviewing a patient's list of drugs. The nurse understands that the older adult's slower absorption of oral drugs is primarily because of which phenomenon?
   a. Decreased cardiac output
   b. Increased gastric emptying time
   c. Decreased gastric blood flow
   d. Increased gastric acid secretion
3. The older adult patient has questions about oral drug metabolism. Information on what subject is most important to include in this patient's teaching plan?
   a. First-pass effect
   b. Enzyme function
   c. Glomerular filtration rate
   d. Motility

4. An older patient has just started on hydrochlorothiazide and is advised by the health care provider to eat foods rich in potassium. What is the nurse's best recommendation of foods to consume?
   a. Cabbage and corn
   b. Bread and cheese
   c. Avocados and mushrooms
   d. Brown rice and fish
5. The nurse is developing teaching materials for an 82-year-old African-American man with macular degeneration, who is being discharged on two new drugs. Which strategies would be best to use to impart the information? (Select all that apply.)
   a. Limit distractions in the room when teaching.
   b. Wait until discharge to teach so information is fresh in the memory.
   c. Augment teaching with audio material.
   d. Use *Honey* and other terms of familiarity to promote trust.
   e. Use large, dark print on a light background for written material.

6. What changes with aging alter drug distribution? (Select all that apply.)
   a. An increase in muscle mass and a decrease in fat
   b. A decrease in muscle mass and an increase in fat
   c. A decrease in serum albumin levels
   d. An increase in total body water
   e. A decrease in kidney mass

7. What factors contribute to polypharmacy in the elderly? (Select all that apply.)
   a. Multiple health care providers
   b. Multiple chronic diseases
   c. Use of a single pharmacy
   d. Care coordination by a nurse
   e. Few hospitalizations

8. What is the best measure for the nurse to use to determine a patient's kidney function?
   a. Creatinine clearance
   b. Estimated glomerular filtration rate
   c. Serum creatinine level
   d. Blood urea nitrogen level

Answers: 1, a, b; 2, c; 3, a; 4, c; 5, a, c; 6, b, c, e; 7, a, b; 8, b.

7

Drugs in Substance Use Disorder

http://evolve.elsevier.com/McCuistion/pharmacology

OBJECTIVES

- Define substance use disorder and differentiate among mild, moderate, and severe cases.
- Describe the short- and long-term effects of drug use.
- Identify the physical and psychological assessment findings associated with drugs most commonly used.
- Explain the rationale for the use of drug-assisted treatments during toxicity, withdrawal, and maintenance of abstinence from commonly misused drugs.

- Prioritize appropriate nursing interventions to use during the treatment of patients with drug toxicity and withdrawal.
- Identify nursing interventions appropriate during the management of surgical experiences and pain in patients with substance use disorder.
- Describe the nurse's role in recognizing and promoting the treatment of nurses with substance use disorder.
- Implement the nursing process in the care of patients with substance use disorders.

OUTLINE

KEY TERMS

Although most drugs are used safely and within prescribed guidelines, it is possible for all drugs to be misused. It has been reported that over 40 million Americans ages 12 and over use tobacco, alcohol, or illicit drugs. Drug use is a serious and complex social and health issue with negative consequences for both the individual and society that include family dysfunction, loss of employment, failure in school, domestic violence, and child abuse. The economic cost of drug use is staggering: $600 billion annually in costs related to lost productivity, health-related issues, and crime.

SUBSTANCE USE DISORDER

Context

Since 1975, the Monitoring the Future project has been tracking drug use in adolescents and young adults. Current data from the survey indicate that 26.4% of children have tried illicit drugs by the eighth grade, 40% by the tenth grade, and 51.8% by the twelfth grade. Tenth graders had tried alcohol (49.8%), *Cannabis* (28.8%), amphetamines (6.6%), and prescription and over-the-counter (OTC) drugs such as oxycodone or cough medicine (2.6% to 5.9%). Between 15% and 39% used more than one drug, known as polydrug use.

Many factors play into the decision to use drugs and whether an individual develops substance use disorder. Cognitive development at the time drugs are introduced plays a major role; adolescents are in a period of brain development where they are especially vulnerable to stress and risk-seeking behaviors. Other risk factors are also related to substance use disorder:

- *Family-related risk factors*: Between 16% and 29% of children who suffer neglect or abuse—physical, sexual, and emotional—have tried or use drugs.

TABLE 7.1   Substance Use Disorder Categories

Criteria	Subcomponents

• Mild substance use disorder (2-3 criteria required)
• Moderate substance use disorder (4-5 criteria required)
• Severe substance use disorder (6-7 criteria required)
	• The substance is often taken in larger amounts or over a longer period than was intended.
	• There is a persistent desire or unsuccessful effort to cut down on or control use of the substance.
	• A great deal of time is spent in activities necessary to obtain the substance, use the substance, or recover from its effects.
	• Craving, or a strong desire or urge to use the substance, is present.
	• Recurrent use of the substance results in a failure to fulfill major role obligations at work, school, or home.
	• Continued use of the substance occurs despite having persistent or recurrent social or interpersonal problems caused or exacerbated by the effects of its use.
	• Important social, occupational, or recreational activities are given up or reduced because of use of the substance.
	• Recurrent use of the substance occurs in situations in which it is physically hazardous.
	• Use of the substance is continued despite knowledge of having a persistent or recurrent physical or psychological problem that is likely to have been caused or exacerbated by the substance.
	• *Tolerance occurs, as defined by either of the following:
	  • A need for markedly increased amounts of the substance to achieve intoxication or desired effect
	  • A markedly diminished effect with continued use of the same amount of the substance
	• *Withdrawal occurs, as manifested by either of the following:
	  • The characteristic withdrawal syndrome for that substance is evident as specified in the DSM-5.
	  • The substance or a closely related substance is taken to relieve or avoid withdrawal symptoms.

*Does not apply when used appropriately under medical supervision.
DSM-5, Diagnostic and Statistical Manual of Mental Disorders, 5th edition.
From Horvath, A. T., Misra, K., Epner, A. K., & Cooper, G. M. (n.d.). The diagnostic criteria for substance use disorders (addiction). Retrieved from www.amhc.org/1408-addictions/article/48502-the-diagnostic-criteria-for-substance-use-disorders-addiction; and National Institute on Drug Abuse. (2014). The science of drug abuse and addiction: The basics. Retrieved May 16, 2016, from www.drugabuse.gov/publications/media-guide/science-drug-abuse-addiction-basics

- *Social risk factors*: Deviant peer relationships (i.e., the adolescent associates with abusers and uses drugs to feel accepted), peer pressure, popularity, and bullying have all been correlated to drug use. Gang affiliation is associated with higher drug use and delinquent behavior.
- *Individual risk factors*: Individuals with attention-deficit/hyperactivity disorder (ADHD) are three times as likely as the general population to use drugs such as nicotine, alcohol, and drugs other than *Cannabis*; depression is associated with alcohol use, particularly among young men.

It should be noted that positive family relationships are a protective factor that has been related to a decrease in drug use among adolescents.

Definition

According to the *Diagnostic and Statistical Manual of Mental Disorders* (5th edition [DSM-5]), substance use disorder occurs "when the recurrent use of alcohol and/or drugs causes clinically and functionally significant impairment, such as health problems, disability, and failure to meet major responsibilities at work, school, or home." Substance use disorder is categorized along a continuum from mild to severe, based on the number of diagnostic criteria met (Table 7.1). The terms *abuse* and *dependence* are no longer used due to the violence and stigma associated with the term *abuse* and the ambiguity associated with the term *dependence*; gambling is the only condition in the category of behavioral addiction (continued involvement in an activity despite the substantial harm it causes; Table 7.2). Excessive caffeine use is not considered a substance use disorder, even though there appears to be a withdrawal syndrome with cessation of use.

Neurobiology

Drugs that are misused typically increase the availability of dopamine and other neurotransmitters in the limbic system of the brain. This area contains the brain's reward circuit, a structure that regulates our ability to feel pleasure and other emotions, both positive and negative. The drugs interfere with the way neurons in the brain normally send, receive, and process information by mimicking the brain's own neurotransmitters; however, drugs do not copy neurotransmitters exactly, which results in faulty transmission or excessive stimulation. Most of the drugs facilitate an increase of dopamine in the system, leading to mood elevation or euphoria—factors that provide strong motivation to repeat the experience. Some drugs increase the availability of other neurotransmitters, such as serotonin and gamma-aminobutyric acid (GABA), but dopamine's effect on the reward system appears to be pivotal to substance use disorder.

Repeated use of drugs remodels the neural circuitry of the brain cells and reduces the responsiveness of receptors. This decreased responsiveness leads to tolerance, the need for a larger dose of a drug to obtain the original euphoria. Drug use results in levels of dopamine that do not naturally occur; tolerance also reduces the sense of pleasure from experiences that previously resulted in positive feelings, such as food, sex, or relationships. Without the drug, the individual may experience depression, anxiety, and/or irritability (Table 7.3; see also Table 7.2).

Current research is focused on epigenetics, the study of environmental influences on genetics. How a person responds to their social and cultural environment affects drug use. Altering environmental factors that increase the risk for drug use can discourage drug-seeking behavior. Studies have shown that drug use alters DNA proteins, those that affect both gene expression and function, and this influences drug-seeking behavior.

TABLE 7.2 Terminology Related to Substance Use Disorder

Term	Definition
Abstinence	Refraining from drug use
Craving	Strong desire for a drug or for the intoxicating effects of that drug
Intoxication	A condition that results in disturbances in the level of consciousness, cognition, perception, judgment, affect or behavior, or other psychophysiological functions and responses
Stabilization	Acute treatment for substance use disorder involving supervision, observation, support, intensive education, and counseling that involves multidisciplinary treatment interventions
Tolerance	Requiring a significantly increased amount of a drug to achieve the desired effect
Withdrawal syndrome	A group of symptoms of varying severity that occur upon cessation or reduction of use of a drug that has been taken repeatedly, usually for a prolonged period and/or in high doses; may be accompanied by signs of physiological disturbance
Remission	None of the 11 criteria for substance use disorder for at least three months (early remission, 3 to 12 months; sustained remission, after 12 months)
Controlled environment	Environment where access to any drug is restricted (e.g., treatment center or halfway house)
Impaired control	Diminished ability of an individual to control his or her use of a drug in terms of onset, level, or termination
Social impairment	Recurrent drug use despite problems at work or school, interpersonal problems, or the cessation of social and recreational activities
Risky use	Recurrent drug use despite the difficulty it is causing (e.g., driving while intoxicated, liver damage)
Recovery	A process of change through which an individual improves health and wellness, lives a self-directed life, and strives to reach full potentials
Relapse	A return to drug use after a period of abstinence, often accompanied by reinstatement of substance use disorder

From Substance Abuse and Mental Health Services Administration. (2015). Substance use disorders. Retrieved May 17, 2016, from www.samhsa.gov/disorders/substance-use; and World Health Organization. (n.d.). Lexicon of alcohol and drug terms published by the World Health Organization. Retrieved May 18, 2016, from http://www.who.int/substance_abuse/terminology/who_lexicon/en/

Understanding these processes may lead to new treatments for substance use disorders.

Types of Substance Use Disorders

Alcohol Use Disorder (AUD)

People drink for many reasons, including socializing, celebrating, and relaxing; people also drink to cope, because of low self-esteem and a need for approval, or because of peer pressure. Alcohol affects everyone differently, depending on the amount consumed, the frequency of consumption, age, health status, and family history. People of all ages drink, and 15% of all alcohol sales in the United States are to teens. Alcohol use is the underlying cause in 88,000 deaths per year. Additionally, the Centers for Disease Control and Prevention report that AUD may shorten a person's life by up to 30 years!

Alcohol use inhibits the effects of GABA, thereby reducing neurotransmission in the brain. Short-term effects of alcohol use include nausea, vomiting, headaches, slurred speech, impaired judgment, memory loss, hangovers, and blackouts. Box 7.1 discusses alcohol toxicity.

Long-term problems associated with heavy drinking include stomach ailments, heart problems, cancer, brain damage, serious memory loss, immune system compromise, and liver cirrhosis. Persons with AUD increase their chances of dying from automobile accidents, homicide, and suicide. Spouses and children of persons with AUD may face family violence, and children may suffer physical and sexual abuse and neglect and may develop psychological problems. Women who drink during pregnancy run a serious risk of their fetus developing fetal alcohol spectrum disorder. To intervene promptly and avoid long-term problems associated with AUD, nurses should question all patients about their drinking habits with every encounter, using plain language, without bias (Fig. 7.1).

Treatment. AUD can be treated through a variety of options. However, very few people with the disorder seek care. Alcohol treatment centers offer inpatient-type care, where the person undergoes stabilization in a controlled environment that includes group therapy. Persons with AUD are provided the tools they need to become abstinent and go into remission. Outpatient treatment is also available. People with AUD who participate in outpatient therapy are given the tools to become abstinent and go into remission (Table 7.4).

Drug-assisted treatment. Several drugs have been approved by the U.S. Food and Drug Administration (FDA) to treat AUD. Disulfiram, acamprosate, and naltrexone are the most commonly used (Table 7.5). Disulfiram inhibits aldehyde dehydrogenase, the enzyme involved in metabolizing alcohol. It is best used in people who are newly abstinent. Disulfiram is administered in tablet form; dosage ranges from 125 to 500 mg daily. It is contraindicated in persons who are intoxicated and should not be taken within 12 hours of alcohol consumption (including use of mouthwash, cough medicine, or eating desserts that contain alcohol or eating foods cooked in alcohol). Side effects occur within 10 minutes of alcohol consumption and can last for over an hour. These side effects include nausea, headache, vomiting, chest pains, and difficulty breathing. Disulfiram keeps patients from drinking because of the unpleasant side effects that occur if alcohol is consumed while taking the drug. Patients who have recently been treated with metronidazole or paraldehyde should not take disulfiram because these same side effects will occur, as if

TABLE 7.3 Most Commonly Used Illicit Drugs

Drug	Street Name	Desired Effects by the User	Short-Term Effects	Long-Term Health Effects	Treatment
Inhalants are compounds that can be breathed in without smoking or using heat to vaporize them. Includes solvents, aerosols, and gases found in household products such as spray paints, markers, glues, and cleaning fluids; also nitrites (e.g., amyl nitrite), which are prescription medications for chest pain.	Poppers, snappers, whippets, laughing gas	Generally, people experience mild highs that last for a short time—normally on the order of minutes—so they tend to be taken repeatedly to extend the high.	Confusion; nausea; slurred speech; lack of coordination; euphoria; dizziness; drowsiness; disinhibition, lightheadedness, hallucinations, delusions; headaches	Liver and kidney damage; bone marrow damage; limb spasms due to nerve damage; brain damage from lack of oxygen that can cause problems with thinking, movement, vision, and hearing; sudden death due to heart failure (from sniffing butane, propane, and other chemicals in aerosols); death from asphyxiation or suffocation, convulsions or seizures, coma, or choking	There are no FDA-approved medications to treat inhalant addiction. More research is needed to find out if behavioral therapies can be used to treat inhalant addiction.
Ketamine is a dissociative drug used as an anesthetic in veterinary practice. Dissociative drugs are hallucinogens that cause the user to feel detached from reality. It is typically injected or snorted, but it can be smoked or taken in pill form.	Cat valium, K, Special K, Vitamin K	Ketamine produces an abrupt high that lasts for about an hour. Large doses of ketamine can result in what some describe as the "K-hole," which can include intense and unpleasant visual and auditory hallucinations coupled with marked de-realization and a frightening detachment from reality.	Problems with attention, learning, and memory; dreamlike states, hallucinations; sedation; confusion and problems speaking; loss of memory; problems moving to the point of being immobile; raised blood pressure; unconsciousness; slowed breathing that can lead to death	Ulcers and pain in the bladder; kidney problems; stomach pain; depression; poor memory	There are no FDA-approved medications to treat ketamine addiction. More research is needed to find out if behavioral therapies can be used.
Cocaine hydrochloride is a powerfully addictive stimulant drug made from the leaves of the coca plant. It is usually snorted, smoked, or injected.	Blow, Bump, C, Candy, Charlie, Coke, Crack, Flake, Rock, Snow, Toot	Users claim to feel euphoric or high when using crack; some paradoxical drawbacks exist to using crack for any length of time—the initial euphoria can quickly turn to feelings of depression and paranoia. People who experience drug-induced paranoia might imagine someone is following them or trying to get into their house or that others are trying to attack them.	Narrowed blood vessels; enlarged pupils; increased body temperature, heart rate, and blood pressure; headache; abdominal pain and nausea; euphoria; increased energy and alertness; insomnia, restlessness; anxiety; erratic and violent behavior, panic attacks, paranoia, psychosis; heart rhythm problems, heart attack, inflammation of the heart muscle, deterioration of the ability of the heart to contract, and aortic ruptures; stroke, seizure, coma	Loss of sense of smell, nosebleeds, nasal damage and trouble swallowing from snorting; infection and death of bowel tissue from decreased blood flow; poor nutrition and weight loss from decreased appetite. Movement disorders, including Parkinson's disease, may also occur after many years of cocaine use. Smoking cocaine damages the lungs and can worsen asthma.	There are no FDA-approved medications to treat cocaine addiction. CBT, a community reinforcement approach, plus vouchers, contingency management, motivational incentives, the matrix model (an intensive, structured, 16-week outpatient treatment program), and 12-step therapy may facilitate recovery.
Methamphetamine is a central nervous system stimulant drug with high potential for addiction, easily made in small clandestine laboratories, with relatively inexpensive over-the-counter ingredients such as pseudoephedrine, a common ingredient in cold medicines. It is typically swallowed, snorted, smoked, or injected.	Crank, Chalk, Crystal, Fire, Glass, Go Fast, Ice, Meth, Speed ("Crystal meth" is methamphetamine in the form of a rocklike crystal.)	Methamphetamine is a wildly addictive and dangerous substance. Users can rapidly develop a dependency on its effects (increased wakefulness and physical activity). The illegal production and distribution of meth is one of the leading reasons for crime within some areas of the United States.	Decreased appetite; increased breathing, heart rate, blood pressure, temperature; irregular heartbeat	Anxiety, confusion, insomnia, mood problems, violent behavior, paranoia, hallucinations, delusions, weight loss, severe dental problems ("meth mouth"), intense itching leading to skin sores from scratching	There are no FDA-approved medications to treat methamphetamine addiction. CBT, contingency management, or motivational incentives along with matrix model 12-step therapy may facilitate recovery.

MDMA is an abbreviation for 3,4-methylenedioxymethamphetamine. It is a synthetic chemical with complex effects that mimic both methamphetamine stimulants and mescaline hallucinogens. It is typically swallowed or snorted.	Adam, Clarity, Ecstasy, Eve, Molly, Lover's Speed, Peace, Uppers, E, X, XTC, Scooby snacks, Roll, Beans	A perceived increase in energy levels and a euphoric state of being; distorted perception of time; higher pleasure from and desire for physical touch; increased levels of sexuality and sexual arousal; elevated alertness, increased energy and focus	Lowered inhibition, enhanced sensory perception, confusion, depression, sleep problems, anxiety; increased heart rate and blood pressure; muscle tension, teeth clenching; nausea; blurred vision; faintness; chills or sweating. Taking more than one dose at a time or taking a series of pills over time to maintain the desired effects (*piggybacking*) can lead to overdose, which presents with high blood pressure, seizures, loss of consciousness, and a sharp rise in body temperature that leads to liver, kidney, or heart failure and death.	Long-lasting confusion, depression, problems with attention, memory, and sleep; increased anxiety, impulsiveness, aggression; loss of appetite; decreased libido	There are no FDA-approved medications to treat MDMA addiction. More research is needed to find out if behavioral therapies can be used; however, psychosocial and behavioral interventions and participation in a 12-step group or other support fellowship may be effective.
Synthetic cathinones (bath salts) are typically made from a synthetic version of an amphetamine-like stimulant in the cathinone class, α-PVP. Bath salts can be swallowed, snorted, or injected.	Bloom, Cloud Nine, Cosmic Blast, Flakka, Ivory Wave, Lunar Wave, Scarface, Vanilla Sky, White Lightning	Use results in a flood of dopamine in the brain leading to an intense feeling of euphoria.	Increased heart rate and blood pressure, euphoria, increased sociability and sex drive, paranoia, agitation, hallucinations, psychotic or violent behavior, nosebleeds, sweating, nausea and vomiting, insomnia, irritability, dizziness, depression, suicidal thoughts, panic attacks, reduced motor control, cloudy thinking	Breakdown of skeletal muscle tissue, kidney failure, death	There are no FDA-approved medications to treat addiction to synthetic cathinones. Behavioral therapy includes CBT, contingency management, and motivational incentives such as motivational enhancement therapy (MET) and behavioral treatments geared to teens.
Kratom comes from the leaves of a tropical deciduous tree, *Mitragyna speciosa*, that contains mitragynine, a psychoactive opioid. The leaves may be chewed, eaten (mixed in food or brewed as tea), or smoked.	Herbal Speedball, Biak-biak, Ketum, Kahuam, Ithang, Thom	Kratom is consumed for mood-lifting effects and pain relief and as an aphrodisiac	Sensitivity to sunburn, nausea, itching, sweating, dry mouth, constipation, increased urination, loss of appetite. *Low doses:* Increased energy, sociability, alertness. *High doses:* Sedation, euphoria, decreased pain	Anorexia, weight loss, insomnia, skin darkening, dry mouth, frequent urination, constipation; with long-term use at high doses, hallucination and paranoia	No clinical trials have been conducted on medications for kratom addiction. More research is needed to find out if behavioral therapies can be used.
Heroin is an opioid drug processed from morphine, a naturally occurring opiate extracted from the seedpod of certain varieties of poppy plants. It can be injected, smoked, or snorted.	Brown sugar, China White, Dope, H, Horse, Junk, Skag, Skunk, Smack, White Horse	Heroin binds to opioid receptors in the body, prompting a release of dopamine and creating intensely pleasurable feelings.	Euphoria, warm flushing of skin, dry mouth, heavy feeling in the hands and feet, clouded thinking, alternating wakeful and drowsy states, itching, nausea and vomiting, slowed breathing and heart rate	Collapsed veins, abscesses, infection of the lining and valves in the heart, constipation and stomach cramps, liver or kidney disease, pneumonia, and hypoxic brain injury	Medications approved to treat heroin addiction and aid withdrawal include methadone, buprenorphine, and naltrexone. Behavioral therapy includes contingency management, motivational incentives, and 12-step facilitation therapy.

Continued

TABLE 7.3 Most Commonly Used Illicit Drugs—cont'd

Drug	Street Name	Desired Effects by the User	Short-Term Effects	Long-Term Health Effects	Treatment
Phencyclidine (PCP) is a dissociative drug that causes the user to feel detached from reality. It can be injected, snorted, swallowed, or smoked.	Angel Dust, Boat, Hog, Love Boat, Peace Pill	Produces visual and auditory distortions and perceptual changes that result in an individual feeling detached from themselves or the world around them; users may feel that their body is not their own.	Delusions, hallucinations, paranoia, problems thinking, a sense of distance from one's environment, anxiety *Low doses:* A slight increase in breathing rate, increased blood pressure and heart rate, shallow breathing, face redness and sweating, numbness of the hands or feet; problems with movement *High doses:* Lowered blood pressure, pulse rate, breathing rate; nausea and vomiting; blurred vision; flicking up and down of the eyes; drooling; loss of balance, dizziness; violence or suicidal thoughts; seizures, coma, death	Impaired memory, thinking, and decision-making abilities; speech problems; severe depression, suicidal thoughts; higher anxiety, paranoia, and isolation; extreme weight loss; "flashback" phenomena and continuous hallucinations and delusional thinking even when not using the substance	There are no FDA-approved medications to treat addiction to PCP. More research is needed to find out if behavioral therapies can be used to treat addiction to dissociative drugs.
Synthetic cannabinoids; may be smoked or swallowed	K2, Spice, Black Mamba, Bliss, Bombay Blue, Fake Weed, Fire, Genie, Moon Rocks, Skunk, Smacked, Yucatan, Zohai	Euphoric feelings, altered perception, feelings of relaxation	Increased heart rate, vomiting, agitation, confusion, hallucinations, anxiety, paranoia, increased blood pressure	Kidney failure and heart attacks; severe and lasting heart conditions, seizure activity in frequent users	There are no FDA-approved medications to treat synthetic cannabinoid addiction. More research is needed to find out if behavioral therapies can be used.
Rohypnol (flunitrazepam); an intermediate-acting benzodiazepine typically swallowed (as a pill or dissolved in a drink) or snorted	Circles, Date Rape Drug, Forget Pill, Forget-Me Pill, La Rocha, Lunch Money, Mexican Valium, Mind Eraser, Pingus, R2, Reynolds, Rib, Roach, Roach 2, Roaches, Roachies, Roapies, Rochas Dos, Roofies, Rope, Rophies, Row-Shay, Ruffies, Trip-and-Fall, Wolfies	Because of the strong amnesia produced by the drug, it has been used for it its ability to sedate and incapacitate unsuspecting rape victims when placed in their drinks. It has also been used illegally to lessen the depression caused by the use of stimulants, such as cocaine and methamphetamine, and by heroin and cocaine users to produce profound intoxication and boost the high of heroin.	Drowsiness, sedation, sleep; amnesia, blackout; decreased anxiety; muscle relaxation, impaired reaction time and motor coordination; impaired mental functioning and judgment; confusion; aggression; excitability; slurred speech; headache; slowed breathing and heart rate; in combination with alcohol, severe sedation, unconsciousness, and slowed heart rate and breathing can lead to death.	Unknown	There are no FDA-approved medications to treat addiction to flunitrazepam. More research is needed to find out if behavioral therapies can be used to treat addiction.

Substance	Street Names	Effects	Intoxication / Health Effects	Potential Health Consequences	Treatment Options
GHB (gamma-hydroxybutyrate) is a depressant approved for use in the treatment of narcolepsy. It is swallowed.	G, Georgia Home Boy, Goop, Grievous Bodily Harm, Liquid Ecstasy, Liquid X, Soap, Scoop	Euphoria, increased sex drive, and tranquility; has been used for sexual assault as victims become incapacitated due to the sedative effects and they are unable to resist. GHB may also induce amnesia in its victims.	Euphoria, drowsiness, decreased anxiety, confusion, memory loss, hallucinations, excited and aggressive behavior, nausea, vomiting, unconsciousness, slowed heart rate and breathing, lower body temperature. *High doses:* Even without other illicit substances or alcohol, high doses may result in profound sedation, seizures, coma, severe respiratory depression, and death.	Unknown	Withdrawal may be treated with benzodiazepines. More research is needed to find out if behavioral therapies can be used to treat GHB addiction.
LSD (lysergic acid diethylamide) is a hallucinogen that is swallowed or absorbed through mouth tissues	Acid, Blotter, Blue Heaven, Cubes, Microdot, Yellow Sunshine	Users experience impaired depth and time perception and a distorted perception of the size and shape of objects, movements, color, sound, touch, and body image; sensations may seem to "cross over," giving the feeling of hearing colors or seeing sounds (synesthesia, also called "tripping").	Rapid emotional swings; distortion of a person's ability to recognize reality, think rationally, or communicate with others; raised blood pressure, heart rate, body temperature; insomnia; loss of appetite, dry mouth, sweating, numbness, weakness, tremors, dizziness, enlarged pupils	Frightening flashbacks (called *hallucinogen persisting perception disorder* [HPPD]); ongoing visual disturbances, disorganized thinking, paranoia, and mood swings	There are no FDA-approved medications to treat addiction to LSD. More research is needed to find out if behavioral therapies can be used to treat addiction.

α-*PVP*, Alpha-pyrrolidinopentiophenone; *CBT,* cognitive behavioral therapy; *FDA,* U.S. Food and Drug Administration.

Information obtained from DrugAbuse.com. (n.d.). http://drugabuse.com/library/drugs-a-z/; www.drugs.com; and National Institute on Drug Abuse. (2016). Commonly abused drugs. Retrieved May 15, 2016, from www.drugabuse.gov/drugs-abuse/ Drugs.com. (2016). Drugs A-Z. Retrieved May 15, 2016, from www.drugs.com; and National Institute on Drug Abuse. (2016). Commonly abused drugs. Retrieved May 15, 2016, from www.drugabuse.gov/drugs-abuse/

BOX 7.1 Alcohol Toxicity

Alcohol toxicity is a life-threatening condition that can occur by drinking large amounts of alcohol over a short period of time. A standard drink contains 10 g of alcohol. This is equal to 10 ounces of beer with 5% alcohol, 3.25 ounces of wine with 12% alcohol, or 1 ounce of hard liquor with 40% alcohol (or 80 "proof"). Roughly 20% of alcohol is absorbed from the stomach, and the remainder is absorbed in the small intestine. Food intake slows absorption. Alcohol is metabolized in the liver and is excreted by the lungs and kidneys, and the average person can only metabolize 10 g of alcohol per hour.

Complications of alcohol toxicity include aspiration of vomitus, asphyxiation, severe dehydration, seizures, hypothermia, brain damage, and death. Treatment involves airway management and supplemental oxygenation, correction of hypoglycemia if present, supportive care, and intravenous (IV) hydration. If the person chronically uses alcohol, thiamine 100 mg may be administered intramuscularly to prevent neurologic damage. Patients with impaired hepatic function may require hemodialysis to remove alcohol from the blood; however, this invasive treatment is only used in persons whose condition is rapidly deteriorating.

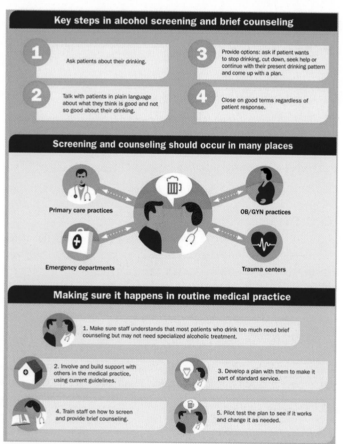

FIG. 7.1 Alcohol Screening and Brief Counseling. From Centers of Disease Control and Prevention.

TABLE 7.4 Nonpharmacological Therapy for Substance Use Disorders: Individual and Group Counseling

Therapy	Description
Cognitive behavioral therapy (CBT)	CBT teaches people to recognize and stop negative patterns of thinking and behavior and helps enhance self-control. For instance, therapy might help a person become aware of the stressors, situations, and feelings that lead to substance use so that the person can avoid them or act differently when they occur.
Contingency management	This approach is based on frequent monitoring of behavior and removal of rewards for drug use and was designed to provide incentives to reinforce positive behavior and help the person remain abstinent from drug use.
Motivational enhancement therapy (MET)	MET helps people with substance use disorders develop internally motivated changes and commit to specific plans to engage in treatment and seek recovery. It is often used early in the process to engage people in treatment.
Twelve-step facilitation therapy	Seeks to guide and support engagement in 12-step programs such as Alcoholics Anonymous or Narcotics Anonymous.

From Substance Abuse and Mental Health Services Administration. (2015). Treatments for substance use disorders. Retrieved June 3, 2016, from www.samhsa.gov/treatment/substance-use-disorders

they had been drinking. Because of the risk for drug toxicity, disulfiram should *never* be used in combination with eliglustat or ritonavir.

Other side effects of disulfiram include rash, drowsiness, impotence, acne, and a metallic aftertaste. Serious reactions include psychosis, hepatotoxicity, peripheral neuropathy, and optic neuritis. Patients taking disulfiram should have baseline liver function studies obtained; liver function studies should be repeated after 2 weeks of therapy. For disulfiram to be effective,

persons with AUD also need to participate in behavior modification, psychotherapy, and counseling. Disulfiram was designated pregnancy category C, and whether it will harm the fetus is unknown; however, it is excreted into breast milk. Therefore a decision should be made to either discontinue breastfeeding or discontinue the drug, taking into account the importance of the drug to the mother.

Acamprosate is a GABA analogue thought to work in the brain to restore the balance between neuronal excitation and inhibition via GABA and glutamate. It should only be used in persons who are abstinent; however, acamprosate may be continued through a relapse. Usual dosing is 666 mg orally three times per day. Dosing is adjusted in kidney disease, and a serum creatinine level should be obtained at baseline. Persons with a creatinine clearance of 30 mL/min to 50 mL/min should only take 333 mg three times per day. Acamprosate is contraindicated in people with a creatinine clearance less than 30 mL/min. Common side effects include pain, loss of appetite, nausea, diarrhea, dizziness, anxiety, pruritus, depression, insomnia, xerostomia, and paresthesia. Patients should be assessed for suicide ideology prior to beginning treatment. This drug is used in conjunction with behavior modification and counseling. Naltrexone increases acamprosate levels. No dosage adjustment is needed, but patients should be monitored closely. Acamprosate was designated pregnancy category C; it is not known if it will harm the fetus or if it is excreted into breast milk. Therefore a decision should be made to either discontinue breastfeeding or discontinue the drug, taking into account the importance of the drug to the mother.

TABLE 7.5   Pharmacokinetics of Drug-Assisted Treatments

Drug Name	Absorption	Distribution	Metabolism	Excretion
Acamprosate	Peak plasma time: 3-8 h Bioavailability: 11%, decreased by food but not clinically important	Protein binding: Negligible	Not metabolized	In urine as unchanged drug Half-life: 20-33 h
Buprenorphine	Extensive first-pass effect if taken orally; 31% bioavailability (SL) Time to peak plasma varies from 40 min-3.5 h.	Highly lipophilic Highly protein bound (96%)	Extensive hepatic	In bile and feces, 70%; urine, 30% Half-life: SL, 37 h
Disulfiram	Absorbed from the GI tract (80%-90%), onset is 3-12 h after administration. Effects may persist up to 14 d after the last dose.	Highly lipophilic	Hepatic	In urine primarily but also in feces (5%-20% unchanged) and lungs
Methadone	Oral administration: Bioavailability ranges from 36%-100%, and peak plasma concentrations are achieved between 1 and 7.5 h.	Lipophilic; 85%-90% protein bound	Hepatic, into inactive metabolite	Renal and fecal Half-life is highly variable.
Naloxone	Onset: Administered IV, 2 min; subcut and IM, 5 min Duration of action is 30-60 min.	Plasma protein binding occurs but is relatively weak.	Hepatic	In urine Half-life is 1-1.5 h.
Naltrexone	96% absorbed from the GI tract; extensive first-pass metabolism; 5%-40% reaches the systemic circulation. Onset is 15-30 min; duration is 24 h and is dose dependent.	Protein bound: 21%-28%	Hepatic, into active metabolite	In urine
Varenicline	Well absorbed from the GI tract and unaffected by food Time to peak plasma: 3-4 h	Less than 20% protein binding	Minimal hepatic (<10%)	In urine, 92% unchanged Half-life: 24 h

d, Day; *GI*, gastrointestinal; *h*, hours; *IM*, intramuscular; *IV*, intravenous; *min*, minutes; *SL*, sublingual; *subcut*, subcutaneous.
From Drugs.com for Healthcare Professionals. (n.d.). Retrieved from www.drugs.com/professionals.html; and Medscape.com. (n.d.). Drugs, OTCs & Herbals. Retrieved from http://reference.medscape.com/drugs

Naltrexone is a competitive opioid antagonist with a high affinity for mu receptors. Oral forms absorbed through the gastrointestinal (GI) tract undergo up to 40% first-pass metabolism. Onset occurs in 15 to 30 minutes with peak occurring in 1 hour. Naltrexone is used in persons who are abstinent. If there is concern about comorbid opioid use disorder (OUD), a naloxone challenge test may be done prior to initiating treatment, in which a test dose of 25 mg is administered orally, and the patient is observed for an hour. If no withdrawal is observed, dosing may begin the following day at 50 mg per day for 12 weeks or less. Dosing using 380 mg intramuscularly (IM) once every 4 weeks can be used for maintenance therapy. Common side effects include insomnia, nausea, vomiting, anxiety, headache, abdominal pain, myalgia, arthralgia, rash, dizziness, fatigue, constipation, and increased creatine phosphokinase (CPK). Serious reactions include suicidality, depression, hepatotoxicity, and hypersensitivity reaction. Patients should be assessed for suicide ideology prior to beginning treatment. This drug should *not* be taken in conjunction with any drugs that bind to opioid receptors because withdrawal may be precipitated in persons with OUD. Naltrexone was designated pregnancy category C; it is not known if it will harm the fetus, and it is excreted into breast milk. Therefore a decision should be made to either discontinue breastfeeding or discontinue the drug, taking into account the importance of the drug to the mother.

Cannabis Use Disorder

Cannabis is the most commonly used recreational drug in the United States. Over 4.2 million people ages 12 and over meet the criteria for *Cannabis* use disorder. *Cannabis* use disorder is more common among people in their late teens and early 20s. Users report feeling an alteration in their senses and an altered sense of time as well as changes in mood. *Cannabis* goes by many street names, including Marijuana, Blunt, Bud, Dope, Ganja, Grass, Green, Herb, Joint, Mary Jane, Pot, Reefer, Sinsemilla, Skunk, Smoke, Trees, and Weed; names for various forms of hashish include Boom, Gangster, Hash, and Hemp. *Cannabis* contains more than 60 related psychoactive chemicals known as *cannabinoids*; however, the most abundant of these is delta-9-tetrahydrocannabinol (THC).

When smoked, THC rapidly crosses the blood-brain barrier and binds to cannabinoid receptors in many areas of the brain, overwhelming the endocannabinoid system and making it difficult for the user to respond appropriately to incoming stimuli. The drug impairs short-term memory, learning, and ability to focus, and it can cause problems with balance and coordination. In addition, *Cannabis* increases heart rate and may cause hallucinations, anxiety, panic attacks, and psychosis in some people. When smoked, *Cannabis* may harm the lungs, and concurrent use of alcohol increases blood pressure in addition to heart rate and further slows mental processes and reaction times.

Long-term use of *Cannabis* is associated with chronic cough, frequent respiratory infections, and exposure to cancer-causing compounds because the smoke has many of the same irritating and lung-damaging properties as tobacco. Ingestion of the drug increases the heart rate for hours, increasing risk for heart attack and stroke. When repeated use begins in adolescence, there is an association with decreased motivation and decreased performance on memory-related tasks. The drug has also been linked to mental health problems and increased symptoms in persons with schizophrenia. Babies born to women who use *Cannabis* have behavioral issues and problems with attention, memory, and problem solving.

Many have supported the nationwide legalization of *Cannabis* to treat medical conditions; however, rigorous scientific evidence to show that the benefits of *Cannabis* outweigh its health risks is limited and does not support approval. Despite the current evidence, 24 states have legalized medical use of *Cannabis* to treat pain (e.g., cancer pain, headaches, glaucoma, and nerve pain), muscle spasms related to multiple sclerosis, chemotherapy-induced nausea and vomiting, anorexia and weight loss associated with HIV, seizure disorders, and Crohn disease. Four states—Alaska, Colorado, Oregon, and Washington—have legalized the recreational use of *Cannabis,* leading to sales upward of $2.7 billion.

Cognitive behavioral therapy (CBT), contingency management, and motivational enhancement therapy (MET) may be effective in the treatment of *Cannabis* use disorder; however, no medications are currently approved or indicated for this use.

Opioid Use Disorder

Opioids (e.g., oxycodone, hydrocodone, morphine, methadone, and fentanyl) are controlled substances legally prescribed to treat moderate to severe pain. These drugs interact with opioid receptors in the brain and nervous system to reduce pain. In addition to reducing pain, this receptor interaction floods the brain's reward system with dopamine, producing a sense of euphoria and tranquility.

Short-term effects of opioid use include drowsiness, mental confusion, nausea, constipation, and dose-dependent respiratory depression. When taken with alcohol, users may experience dangerous slowing of heart rate and breathing leading to coma or death. When taken with serotonergic drugs (e.g., selective serotonin reuptake inhibitors [SSRIs], serotonin-norepinephrine reuptake inhibitors [SNRIs], and antimigraine agents), serotonin syndrome may occur. Symptoms of serotonin syndrome include agitation, hallucinations, coma, tachycardia, hypertension, hyperthermia, and rigidity.

In addition to the oral route, when misused, opioids are smoked, snorted, or administered parenterally. Prescription opioids are also known by numerous street names, including Vikes, Cody, China White, Fizzies, M, Demmies, Blue Heavens, Juice, Smack, Hillbilly Heroin, and Roxy.

Nonmedical use of prescription opioid drugs has reached epidemic proportions; over 1.9 million people in the United States meet criteria for OUD. Close to 19,000 people with OUD die each year secondary to overdose of prescription opioids. Over 50% of people who misuse prescription opioids obtain them from a friend or relative for free, and 22.1% obtain them from a doctor. With repeated use, tolerance to the euphoric effects of the drug increase, and users may not be able to obtain the drug from friends, relatives, or any doctor; this causes them to turn to the street for drugs. Some users switch from prescription drugs to cheaper and riskier substitutes, like heroin.

⚡ The FDA has toughened the safety warnings on opioids, including adding a boxed warning about the potentially lethal risks associated with misuse. The safety warning includes a caution regarding the use of opioids during pregnancy and the risk of neonatal opioid withdrawal syndrome (NOWS), which can be life threatening.

Contingency management therapy or 12-step facilitation therapy may be useful in treating prescription opioid addiction. Treatment approaches are tailored to each patient and are often combined with medication therapy.

Drug-Assisted Treatment. Naloxone (see Table 7.6) is the drug of choice in the treatment of respiratory depression associated with opioid overdose. Naloxone is a short-acting opioid antagonist that competitively attaches to opioid receptors in the central nervous system (CNS), thereby blocking activation by opioid drugs. In emergency situations, it is administered IV; however, it may also be administered IM or subcutaneously (subcut). In persons with suspected opioid use disorder, dosing begins at 0.1 to 0.2 mg every 2 to 3 minutes until the patient responds. Careful monitoring is required to prevent opioid withdrawal. Symptoms of withdrawal include nausea and vomiting, abdominal cramps, hyperthermia, hypertension, and restlessness.

Naltrexone is approved by the FDA to treat opioid use disorder. (See the previous discussion under alcohol use disorder.) Dosing begins at 50 mg daily after the patient has been opioid free for 7 to 10 days. It is also available in an injectable, extended-release form, with dosing at 380 mg each month. Once treated with naltrexone, patients may have reduced tolerance to opioids; if they relapse after a period of abstinence and resume opioid use at previous doses, they may experience life-threatening consequences, including respiratory arrest and circulatory collapse.

Since the 1950s, methadone has been prescribed to treat persons with OUD. When taken as prescribed and combined with counseling and behavioral therapies, administration of this long-acting opioid drug is safe and effective. Methadone has a boxed warning concerning the risk of cardiac and respiratory-related deaths due to QT prolongation and cardiac arrhythmias. Methadone used for stabilization and maintenance of persons with OUD may only be administered by programs certified by the Substance Abuse and Mental Health Services Administration (SAMHSA) and approved by state authority. Opioid treatment programs must follow federal guidelines and standards for medically monitored withdrawal and treatment.

Methadone works by changing the way a person's brain responds to pain; it is an opioid receptor agonist at the mu receptor and an antagonist at the N-methyl-D-aspartate (NMDA) receptor. Taken daily, it blocks the sense of euphoria and tranquility caused by opioid use and prevents opioid withdrawal and craving. Concurrent administration of rifampin, phenytoin, St. John's wort, phenobarbital, and carbamazepine can reduce serum methadone levels and precipitate withdrawal. Administration with zidovudine may lead to toxicity.

Initial dosing ranges from 15 mg to 30 mg, followed by 5 mg to 10 mg, adjusting the dose to suppress withdrawal and block the euphoric effects of opioids. Maximum dosage is 40 mg on the first day of stabilization. Maintenance therapy is based on patient assessment and ranges from 80 to 120 mg a day. Tapering methadone should only be done under medical supervision, with dose reductions of less than 10% every 14 days.

Common methadone side effects include lightheadedness, constipation, dizziness, sedation, nausea, and vomiting. Patients should be educated to prevent theft and misuse of methadone by friends, family, and others. Methadone was designated pregnancy category C; whether it will harm the fetus is unknown, but it is excreted into breast milk, therefore a decision should be made to either discontinue breastfeeding or discontinue the drug, taking into account the importance of the drug to the mother.

Buprenorphine is a long-acting, mixed narcotic agonist-antagonist. It binds to various opioid receptors in the brain, producing partial agonism at mu receptors and antagonism at kappa receptors, resulting in decreased withdrawal symptoms and cravings. Although it does produce some euphoria, there is a ceiling effect: increasing the dose beyond a moderate level (8 to 16 mg) does not increase euphoria, therefore it has a low potential for misuse. To further deter people from misusing buprenorphine, naloxone is added. Because of the almost complete first-pass metabolism of naloxone, it has minimal pharmacologic activity when the drug is used appropriately as a sublingual tablet. However, if the tablet is crushed and injected, the effects of naloxone lead to opioid withdrawal.

This drug may be administered in qualified outpatient settings (e.g., office, health department, or correctional facility) after providers have received training. When taken as prescribed and used in combination with counseling and behavioral therapies, it is safe and effective. Initial dosing begins when the person with OUD has been opioid free for at least 12 hours and is beginning to experience withdrawal. Dosing starts at 2 to 8 mg sublingual (SL) for the first day, then it is raised to 8 to 16 mg SL for 1 to 2 days. Once the patient is stable and is not experiencing cravings or significant side effects, dosing is tailored to the individual; the maximum daily dose of buprenorphine is 44 mg.

Side effects of buprenorphine include nausea, vomiting, and constipation; muscle aches and cramps; and cravings, sedation, headache, depression, anxiety, and withdrawal symptoms. Buprenorphine was designated pregnancy category C; whether it will harm the fetus is unknown, but it is excreted into breast milk. Therefore a decision should be made to either discontinue breastfeeding or discontinue the drug, taking into account the importance of the drug to the mother.

Tobacco Use Disorder

In 2014, nearly 70 million Americans aged 12 and older used tobacco products. The largest group of users (35%) were those in the 18- to 25-year-old group, followed by adults aged 26 or older (25.8%). American Indians and Alaska Natives made up the largest group of users in 2014, followed by Caucasians and African Americans.

When smoked, nicotine is absorbed from the lungs into the pulmonary venous circulation. It then enters the arterial circulation and moves quickly to the brain. Once across the blood-brain barrier, nicotine stimulates the release of dopamine, norepinephrine, GABA, glutamate, and endorphins, resulting in stimulation and pleasure and a reduction in stress and anxiety. These sensations fuel the brain's reward circuit.

According to the Centers for Disease Control and Prevention (CDC), more than 480,000 deaths each year are caused by cigarette smoking. Short-term effects of tobacco use include increased blood pressure, breathing, and heart rate. Tobacco use does long-term damage to nearly every organ in the human body, often leading to a variety of cancers, respiratory disorders, heart disease, stroke, immune dysfunction, and type 2 diabetes. Women who smoke while pregnant may experience miscarriage, premature delivery, and stillbirth and may have infants of lower birthweight. Children born to women who used tobacco while pregnant may be born with learning and behavior problems. Persons with tobacco use disorder (TUD) have increased health care utilization and higher health care costs compared with nonusers, and they are frequently absent from work.

Since 2002, the number of persons with TUD in sustained remission has outnumbered those actively using nicotine; the CDC reported that 70% of smokers want to quit. Within 1 to 2 years of quitting, persons with TUD significantly reduce their risk for cancer, heart disease, stroke, and respiratory illness. Quitting is difficult. Persons attempting to quit experience irritability, anger, anxiousness, difficulty thinking, cravings, and increased hunger. Support is a very important part of the process and is often combined with pharmacologic measures.

Cognitive behavioral therapy (CBT) is a goal-directed and problem-focused therapy designed to help the person with TUD identify negative thought patterns and inaccurate beliefs to learn new ways of coping and develop new ways of thinking. It helps the person increase their self-confidence in the ability to quit. CBT helps people identify their triggers and learn to either avoid them or respond differently to them. It also helps with any ambivalence people may feel about quitting.

Self-help materials in the form of Internet-based aids or cell phone apps are available to assist the person with TUD. For example, the American Lung Association offers *Freedom From Smoking Online* (www.ffsonline.org/?referrer=http://www.lung.org/stop-smoking/join-freedom-from-smoking), which offers modules with lessons and activities that reinforce the person's commitment to quit. Phone apps are available as well. Some require a small fee, such as *Butt Out—Quit Smoking Forever*, which monitors progress and helps the person stay focused on the goal to quit by providing motivational pictures and messages. Other apps are free, such as *Get Rich or Die Smoking*, which shows the person how much money they are saving each day by not smoking. It also monitors their health progress and shows what the person could buy with the money they have saved, and it rewards the app user with trophies.

Telephone-based resources link persons with TUD with counselors trained to assist the caller in developing an individualized plan to quit smoking. Telephone-based counseling is easy to use because it does not require the person to drive or find child care in order to attend a meeting in person; additionally, it is available nights and weekends.

Combining a nonpharmacologic support measure with drug-assisted treatment is the most effective means to quit smoking.

Drug-Assisted Treatment. Nicotine replacement drugs—sold as a gum, patch, spray, inhaler, or lozenge—mimic the nicotine effects of tobacco by binding to nicotine receptors in the CNS. They are used to relieve the withdrawal symptoms associated with smoking cessation and provide some of the stimulation and stress-relief effects the user gained from smoking (see Table 7.6). Those who choose to use nicotine-replacement gums, sprays, inhalers, or lozenges dose themselves when they feel the urge to smoke; those who use the patch have a sustained nicotine level throughout the day (see Nursing Process: Patient-Centered Collaborative Care—Tobacco Use Disorder). Side effects include hypertension, tachycardia, dizziness, insomnia, irritability, anorexia, dyspepsia, nausea, vomiting, hiccups, and cough. In 2013 the FDA relaxed warnings about patients who relapse while using nicotine-replacement products; it was determined there are no significant safety concerns. Designated pregnancy category D, nicotine has been shown to cause adverse fetal outcomes in animals; however, nicotine replacement is believed to be safer during pregnancy than smoking. Nicotine is excreted into breast milk and may increase infant heart rate, therefore a decision should be made to discontinue breastfeeding or discontinue the drug, taking into account the importance of the drug to the mother.

Bupropion, an antidepressant drug, increases levels of dopamine and norepinephrine in the brain, mimicking the effects of nicotine. It also has some neuronal nicotinic receptor–blocking activity, reducing reinforcement from the brain's reward circuit. When used for smoking cessation, the dosage is 150 mg/day for 7 to 12 weeks. When starting the drug, smokers continue to smoke for the first week but have a stop date set for the second week. If patients have not quit smoking by week seven, providers may add a nicotine-replacement drug. Bupropion should not be used by those who have seizures or eating disorders. Additionally, it should not be taken within 14 days of taking a monoamine oxidase inhibitor (MAOI). Bupropion should not be stopped suddenly, rather the patient should be weaned off the drug to avoid withdrawal symptoms. The drug can cause a false-positive drug screen; when providing urine for a drug screen, laboratory personnel should be told of bupropion use. Bupropion was designated pregnancy category C; whether it will harm the fetus is unknown, but it is excreted into breast milk, therefore a decision should be made to either discontinue breastfeeding or discontinue the drug, taking into account the importance of the drug to the mother.

Varenicline is a partial alpha-4–beta-2 nicotinic receptor agonist that stimulates dopamine activity in the brain but not to the extent of nicotine, thereby reducing cravings and withdrawal. Dosing begins 1 week before an identified quit date at 0.5 mg daily for 3 days, then 0.5 mg are taken twice daily for 4 days, then maintenance therapy begins at 1 mg twice daily for 11 weeks. Dosage is adjusted for patients with a creatinine clearance (CrCl) less than 30 mL/min (maximum dosage, 0.5 mg twice daily). Common side effects include nausea and vomiting, insomnia, headache, abnormal dreams, constipation or diarrhea, fatigue and malaise, upper respiratory tract infection, dyspnea, chest pain, abdominal pain, xerostomia, appetite changes, rash, and emotional disturbances. ⚡ Varenicline carries a

---

BOX 7.2 Electronic Cigarettes (e-Cigarettes)

Electronic cigarettes are a tobacco product often marketed as a tool to stop smoking; however, marketing is also aimed at children and adolescents. A reported 2.4 million middle and high school students use e-cigarettes, also known as *Hookah Pens, e-Hookahs,* and *Vape Pipes.* E-cigarettes aerosolize "e-juice," a mixture of flavorings, propylene glycol (a toxic component of antifreeze), glycerin, and nicotine. The vapor from e-cigarettes contains heavy metals and formaldehyde, a breakdown product of propylene glycol. Because of this, the second-hand aerosol from e-cigarettes is also potentially harmful. Some of the flavors used in e-cigarettes contain carcinogens and other harmful chemicals. For example, the butter flavoring may contain diacetyl, the chemical used to give popcorn a buttery flavor and which causes irreversible lung disease when inhaled, a disease referred to a *popcorn lung.*

According to the CDC, e-cigarettes are no safer than traditional tobacco cigarettes, nor are they a more effective method of quitting smoking than counseling and drug-assisted treatments. When users try to quit e-cigarettes, they experience the same withdrawal symptoms as users of traditional tobacco cigarettes, including irritability, depression, restlessness, and anxiousness. E-cigarettes increase the risk for myocardial infarction due to hypertension, tachycardia, and hardening of the arteries secondary to nicotine. Nicotine has been shown to adversely affect adolescent brain development, leading to cognitive and behavioral issues. There are over 500 brands of e-cigarettes, each of which contains *some* level of nicotine—even those that claim they do not. E-juice refill cartridges often contain more nicotine than is indicated on the label.

In August 2016, the FDA began regulation of all tobacco products, including e-cigarettes, cigars, hookah tobacco, and pipe tobacco. The sale of all tobacco products, including e-cigarettes, will be prohibited to those under the age of 18; packaging and marketing of all tobacco products, including e-cigarettes, will require the display of health warnings; and the FDA will be able to stop manufacturers from making statements about their products that have not been proven by research.

Nurses who work with children and adolescents must be diligent in asking about the use of e-cigarettes and providing counseling concerning the dangers of using them. Related to this, they must ask about media and Internet usage and teach young people critical viewing skills; that is, they must help young people understand that what appears in the media does not always represent reality; often, it is a representation of someone or something's special interest. Nurses must urge children and adolescents who use e-cigarettes to quit, and they must provide the help needed to achieve sustained remission.

---

black-box warning for serious neuropsychiatric symptoms including behavior changes, hostility, agitation, depression, and suicidality. Nurses must caution patients and their family about this warning and advise them to contact their provider immediately if suicidal thoughts or actions occur. Varenicline was designated pregnancy category C; it is unknown whether it will harm the fetus or if it is excreted in breast milk, therefore a decision should be made to either discontinue breastfeeding or discontinue the drug, taking into account the importance of the drug to the mother.

To advocate for their patients, nurses must keep in mind that 80% of those with TUD who attempt to quit relapse in the first month; only 3% remain abstinent at 6 months. Patients with TUD require multiple attempts at quitting before they achieve sustained remission.

Box 7.2 discusses e-cigarettes (electronic cigarettes).

Other Substance Use Disorders

Cough and Cold Products. One in 10 adolescents has used cough and cold products to get high. Cough and cold products contain ingredients that are psychoactive when taken in higher-than-recommended amounts (sometimes up to 25 times the recommended dose). Dextromethorphan (DXM), an antitussive that can be purchased without a prescription, and promethazine-codeine cough syrup, available by prescription only, are the products most frequently misused. Using DXM is known on the street as "robotripping" or "skittling"; when taken in higher-than-recommended amounts, users may experience euphoria, dissociative effects, or hallucinations. Side effects of DXM include nausea and vomiting, stomach pain, confusion, dizziness, double or blurred vision, slurred speech, impaired coordination, tachycardia, drowsiness, numbness, and disorientation. Many of the DXM-containing products that are used to get high also contain other drugs, such as antihistamines, analgesics, or decongestants. High doses of these drugs can lead to hepatic damage or failure, cardiovascular effects, and coma.

Promethazine-codeine cough syrup can result in relaxation and euphoria when taken in higher-than-recommended amounts; when combined with soda, it is referred to as *Syrup, Sizzurp, Purple drank, Barre,* or *Lean.* Hard candy may be added for flavor. (See the previous section on OUD for information concerning codeine, an opioid drug).

There are no FDA-approved medications to treat substance use disorders related to cough and cold products. More research is needed to find out if behavioral therapies can be used to treat such misuse.

Anabolic-Androgenic Steroids. An anabolic-androgenic steroid (AAS) is a synthetic agent used to treat conditions caused by low levels of testosterone in the body, such as delayed puberty, hypogonadism, and cachexia related to chronic disease states. By binding to androgen receptors, these prescription drugs (e.g., danazol, fluoxymesterone, nandrolone, and oxandrolone) exert *anabolic effects,* such as growth of muscle and bone and red blood cell production, and *androgenic effects,* such as production of primary and secondary sexual characteristics. Anabolic-androgenic steroids have been used to enhance athletic and sexual performance and physical appearance in all age groups. Evidence indicates AAS use by athletes ranges from 1% to 6%. Street names of these drugs include Juice, Gym Candy, Pumpers, Stackers, and Roids. The drug may be taken orally or may be administered IM in doses 10 to 100 times higher than what would be recommended for medical conditions.

Short-term effects of AAS use include headache, acne, fluid retention in the hands and feet, oily skin, yellowing of the skin and whites of the eyes, aggression, extreme mood swings, anger, paranoid jealousy, extreme irritability, delusions, impaired judgment, and infection at the injection site. Long-term effects include kidney damage or failure, liver damage, high blood pressure, enlarged heart, or changes in cholesterol leading to increased risk of stroke or heart attack. Additionally, men may experience shrunken testicles, infertility, baldness, development of breasts, and an increased risk for prostate cancer. Women may experience excess facial and body hair, male-pattern baldness, menstrual cycle changes, enlargement of the clitoris, and deepened voice. Adolescents who use anabolic steroids may experience stunted bone growth and height.

Withdrawal from AAS use may lead to mood swings, fatigue, restlessness, loss of appetite, and decreased sex drive. ⚡ Nurses must be alert when caring for persons withdrawing from AAS use because withdrawal may cause depression lasting up to a year, which can result in suicide attempts. Antidepressants and behavioral therapy may be helpful.

Box 7.3 discusses dehydroepiandrosterone (DHEA) and its risks and benefits.

BOX 7.3 Dehydroepiandrosterone

Dehydroepiandrosterone (DHEA), a precursor to testosterone and estrogen, can be found in many dietary supplements. Many people take supplements that contain DHEA in the belief that it will slow aging, increase energy levels, and build bone and muscle strength. However, there is no evidence to support these claims. Small studies have noted that DHEA may be effective in the relief of mild depression and skin changes associated with aging. Side effects include oily skin and acne, hair loss, nausea, hypertension, menstrual changes, deepening of the voice in women, fatigue, headache, irregular heartbeat, insomnia, and hypercholesterolemia. Long-term effects include stunting of growth, aggressive behavior, mood swings, and hepatic toxicity. Nurses who care for patients who take dietary supplements containing DHEA should be sure to counsel them about the risks and benefits associated with DHEA use.

SPECIAL NEEDS OF PATIENTS WITH SUBSTANCE USE DISORDER

Surgical Patients

Patients with substance use disorder are at high risk for drug interactions, postoperative complications, and death when surgery is required. An assessment of drug use and application of the CAGE questionnaire, a screening tool for alcohol misuse, should be part of all patient histories. Respiratory changes in persons with TUD make introduction of endotracheal and suction tubes more difficult and increase the risk for postoperative respiratory problems. During the postoperative period, nurses should be alert for signs and symptoms of drug interactions with pain medications or anesthesia and for signs of withdrawal.

Special precautions must be taken for the patient with AUD who requires surgery. Alcohol use may be overlooked in an accident victim if there are injuries that cause CNS depression. In addition, many persons are undiagnosed as persons with AUD at the time of admission for elective surgery. The patient with AUD may require an increased level of anesthesia, which can increase the risk for cardiovascular instability in susceptible patients. Delirium may be triggered by surgery and abstinence. After surgery, patients with AUD may develop withdrawal syndrome, indicated by tremors, mild anxiety, gastric distress, and headache; left untreated, withdrawal may progress to withdrawal seizures or delirium tremens (DT), manifested by hallucinations, disorientation, tachycardia, hypertension, hyperthermia, agitation, and diaphoresis. Symptoms may develop anywhere from 6 hours to 5 days after the last drink; left untreated, alcohol withdrawal syndrome can be fatal. The goal of treatment is the alleviation of symptoms and the provision of supportive care with fluids and nutrition.

Pain Management

Although health care personnel may be reluctant to administer narcotic analgesics to persons with substance use disorder, there is no evidence that providing narcotic analgesia to these patients in any way worsens their disease. *When patients experience pain, the goal is to treat the pain.* All patients should be treated with dignity and respect. Withholding adequate analgesia due to misconceptions leads to unnecessary suffering and harm and is a breach of the ethical principles central to nursing care. Addressing substance use disorder is *not* a priority when a patient is in pain.

When patients acknowledge substance use disorder, it is important to determine which drug is used and the amount taken each day. If the patient misuses opioids, it is often best to avoid further exposure to the drug of choice because recommended opioid doses do not provide adequate pain relief due to tolerance. Paradoxically, significantly increasing the dose of opioid in an effort to achieve pain control can induce hyperalgesia, where patients become abnormally sensitive to pain. Effective doses of other analgesics can be determined if daily doses of the drug of choice are known. Nonopioid and adjuvant analgesics and nonpharmacologic pain relief measures may also be used, particularly when the person with opioid use disorder is on drug-assisted treatment with buprenorphine or naltrexone.

THE NURSE WITH SUBSTANCE USE DISORDER

Substance use disorder is no more prevalent among nurses than it is among the rest of the population. However, nurses care for others during the most vulnerable times of their life; nurses literally have the lives of others in their hands, and they are therefore held to a higher standard than other professionals. Drug use is a serious concern in health care professions. The most commonly used drugs include *Cannabis,* cocaine, narcotics, opiates, alcohol, and nicotine. It is estimated that 10% to 15% of nurses have substance use disorder.

Contributing Factors

Factors that contribute to drug use among nurses have been identified as job stress, the emotional demands of nursing, long hours and shift rotations, and easy access to drugs. Additionally, nurses internalize their feelings in order to stay in control during crisis and have little to no time to decompress. Nurses take care of others before themselves.

Characteristics

Signs and symptoms of substance use disorder may be indicated by changes in personality and behavior, including alterations in job performance, unexplained absence from the unit, arriving to work late and leaving early, poor judgment and errors (e.g., medication errors), alteration of verbal and telephone orders and illogical documentation.

Signs and symptoms of substance use disorder also include physical changes. Behaviors related to influence of the drug or signs of withdrawal may also be present, such as subtle changes in appearance, self-imposed isolation, inappropriate responses to situations (i.e., both verbal and emotional), confusion, lapses in memory and decreased levels of alertness.

Discrepancies in controlled-drug handling and records may indicate **drug diversion**, the deliberate redirecting of a drug from a patient or facility to the employee for personal use. Indications of drug diversion include frequent narcotic wastage, multiple corrections to medication records and other documentation, and frequent reports of uncontrolled pain from patients.

Nurses often enable drug use among coworkers by covering up their mistakes or tardiness, excusing their behavior, or simply ignoring obvious signs and symptoms. When it is recognized that a nurse is impaired, help for the nurse requires sharing observations and concerns with the nurse and supervisor to provide the means for rehabilitation. For more information related to substance use disorder among nurses, please go to the National Council of State Boards of Nursing (NCSBN) website at www.ncsbn.org.

Management

In most states, nurses may enter nondisciplinary programs designed for evaluation and treatment. These programs include compliance monitoring during treatment and recovery as well as abstinence monitoring upon the nurse's return to work. These programs allow nurses to maintain their licenses. The goals of these programs are to protect the safety of the public, to maintain the integrity of the profession, and to ensure that the nurse is offered the possibility of treatment and rehabilitation before the license to practice is revoked or the job is terminated. Further information can be found at www.ncsbn.org/substance-use-in-nursing.htm.

Given the prevalence of drug use, all nurses care for patients who use drugs, regardless of whether the use has been identified as substance use disorder. Therefore, it is important for nurses to identify patients who misuse drugs and to intervene. Knowledge of the most commonly misused drugs and their treatments are critical to sustained remission and promotion of healthy lifestyles.

 NURSING PROCESS
Patient-Centered Collaborative Care

Tobacco Use Disorder

Assessment

- Ask the patient to identify any barriers or impediments to quitting.
- Assess current smoking status and smoking history.
- Assess for feelings of hopelessness, depression, and apathy.
- Assess health history.
- Assess the patient's decision-making capacity.
- Determine the willingness of the patient to attempt to quit.
- Have the patient identify negative consequences of smoking and the potential benefits of quitting.
- Identify the cultural context of the patient's smoking pattern.
- Identify the patient's locus of control.
- Identify what rewards for quitting are most important to the patient.

Nursing Diagnoses

- Health Maintenance, Ineffective related to the presence of adverse personal habits (smoking)
- Powerlessness related to perceived lack of control over the ability to give up nicotine
- Decision-Making, Readiness for Enhanced in expressing a desire to enhance understanding and meaning of choices
- Health Management, Readiness for Enhanced in expressing desire to learn measures to stop smoking
- Health Behavior, Risk-Prone related to smoking

Planning

- The patient begins to identify ways to achieve control over nicotine use.
- The patient demonstrates positive health maintenance behaviors as evidenced by keeping scheduled appointments and participating in a tobacco cessation program.
- The patient identifies and uses available resources.

Nursing Interventions

- Advise the patient to keep a list of "slips" and "near-slips" to learn to avoid their causes.

- Assist the patient with problem solving.
- Define your role as the patient's advocate.
- Encourage the patient to avoid environments and activities previously associated with smoking.
- Enhance the patient's sense of autonomy by involving the patient in decision making.
- Help the patient choose the best method to quit smoking based on patient preferences and anticipated benefits.
- Refer the patient to support groups or programs available in the community.
- Schedule frequent follow-up contacts with the patient to offer encouragement and help the patient deal with relapses.
- Set a quit date with the patient, ideally within 1 to 2 weeks.
- Teach the patient about drug-assisted treatment available to assist in smoking cessation.
- Teach the patient to anticipate the withdrawal symptoms and challenges of quitting.

Evaluation

- To avoid relapse, evaluate the effectiveness of the cessation plan, including the use of drug-assisted treatment and support systems.

CRITICAL THINKING CASE STUDY

LM, a 57-year-old man, is admitted to the surgical unit in preparation for back surgery after conservative treatment for a recent back injury failed to relieve his pain. His wife tells the nurse she hopes the surgery will be successful. She confides that her husband has just been sitting around the house drinking more beer than usual because he has not been able to work. LM appears relaxed and unconcerned about his anticipated surgery. He jokes with the nurse, telling her that he would be cured if "a cute young thing like her would only rub his back."

1. What assessments of LM's alcohol use should the nurse make and communicate to the surgeon and anesthesiologist before he is further prepared for surgery?
2. During LM's postoperative period, when will the nurse expect signs of withdrawal syndrome to occur?
3. What early signs and symptoms would alert the nurse to the development of withdrawal syndrome?
4. What goal of treatment during LM's postoperative period is related to alcohol withdrawal syndrome?

NCLEX STUDY QUESTIONS

1. When caring for a patient recovering from an episode of opioid toxicity, the nurse determines that the patient has opioid use disorder based on which finding?
   a. Withdrawal symptoms
   b. A history of daily use
   c. Craving that results in drug-seeking behaviors
   d. Intravenous, rather than oral, use of the drug
2. A patient hospitalized with a fractured femur following an automobile accident develops nausea and vomiting, abdominal cramps, and restlessness. The nurse suspects that the patient is experiencing which reaction?
   a. Opioid withdrawal
   b. Alcohol toxicity
   c. Flashbacks from LSD use
   d. Nicotine withdrawal

3. Which treatments will the nurse anticipate administering to a patient who has been admitted with alcohol toxicity? (Select all that apply.)
   a. Naloxone
   b. Thiamine
   c. Intravenous fluids
   d. Naltrexone
   e. Intravenous glucose solution
   f. Flumazenil

4. A nurse observes another nurse taking oral opioids from the medication room at the hospital. Which is the best action for the nurse who observes drug diversion to take?
   a. Report the finding to the nursing supervisor to enable the nurse's participation in a nondisciplinary program.
   b. Ignore the situation to protect the nurse from dismissal and possible loss of licensure.
   c. Confront the nurse and demand that the drugs be returned before someone notices their absence.
   d. Ask the nurse to request pain medications from a physician rather than stealing them from the hospital.

5. A patient is to start disulfiram to help with alcohol use disorder. The nurse providing medication education about the drug will include which topics in the education plan? (Select all that apply.)
   a. Importance of taking the medication every day
   b. That better results are experienced when a support group helps with treatment adherence
   c. Common food and hygiene products that contain alcohol
   d. That disulfiram treatment should be stopped 1 day before alcohol consumption
   e. That disulfiram works by disrupting the metabolism of alcohol
   f. That use of alcohol with disulfiram may cause nausea and vomiting and may even be fatal

Answers: 1, c; 2, a; 3, b, c, e; 4, a; 5, a, b, c, e, f.

Pharmacotherapy and Drug Administration

The nursing process is utilized by nurses for the appropriate delivery of patient care and for drug administration. Chapter 8 discusses the nursing process and patient-centered care. It supports the nurse in prioritizing medication delivery by following the steps of the nursing process. Chapter 9 discusses safety and quality in drug administration. The nursing student will discuss the patients' and nurses' rights and the culture of safety in drug administration. Chapter 10 provides current guidelines of drug routes used by the nurse. Chapter 11 provides practice in drug calculation and dosage. This information is vital in the study of nursing and for the safe delivery of patient care.

8

The Nursing Process and Patient-Centered Care

http://evolve.elsevier.com/McCuistion/pharmacology

OBJECTIVES

- Discuss Quality and Safety Education for Nurses (QSEN) and Nursing Alliance for Quality Care (NAQC) guidelines in relation to medication safety.
- Differentiate the steps of the nursing process and their purpose in relation to drug therapy.

- Develop patient-centered goals.
- Discuss at least eight principles for health teaching related to drug therapy plans.
- Describe at least six culturally sensitive health-teaching tips.
- Analyze the nurse's role related to drug therapy plans.

OUTLINE

Nursing Process: Patient-Centered Collaborative Care
Assessment
Nursing Diagnosis
Planning

Implementation of Nursing Interventions
Evaluation
Critical Thinking Case Study
NCLEX Study Questions

KEY TERMS

In their everyday practice, nurses have many important tasks; however, drug administration is at the top of the list. It is estimated that about 40% of the nurse's time is spent on drug administration, and knowledge of these drugs is essential to patient safety. If unsure about a patient's medication, consult the health care provider for clarification.

Nurses are often the first line of defense against drug errors in patient care. Federal, state, and local authorities issue regulations and guidelines for practice, and each state has a nurse practice act that defines the scope and function under which the nurse practices. Health care institutions also have policies that help nurses follow federal and state guidelines and regulations.

This chapter focuses on the nursing process as it relates to pharmacology and the safe administration of patient drugs with a focus on patient- and family-centered care. Chapter 9 offers additional information on safety in pharmacotherapy.

QSEN The Quality and Safety Education for Nurses (QSEN) initiatives guide nurses in the practice of safe, comprehensive care. QSEN offers competencies to provide structure and encourages professional development while advocating for safe patient care. QSEN equips nurses with competencies to improve the quality and safety of the health care system in which they work.

QSEN The QSEN competencies are as follows:

1. *Patient- and family-centered care:* Recognize the patient as the source of control and full partner in providing compassionate and coordinated care based on respect for patient preferences, values, and needs.
2. *Collaboration and teamwork:* Function effectively in nursing and inter-professional teams, fostering open communication, mutual respect, and shared decision-making to achieve quality patient care.
3. *Evidence-based practice:* Integrate best current evidence with clinical expertise and patient/family preferences and values for delivery of optimal health care.
4. *Quality improvement:* Continuously improve the quality and safety of health care systems by using data to monitor outcomes of care processes and improvement methods to design and test changes.
5. *Safety:* Minimize risk of harm to patients and providers through both system effectiveness and individual performance.
6. *Informatics:* Use information and technology to communicate, manage knowledge, mitigate error, and support decision making.

QSEN QSEN competencies are integrated throughout the book and are highlighted in special features such as "Patient Safety" boxes and high-alert drug icons.

The Nursing Alliance for Quality Care (NAQC) is an organization that supports quality patient-centered health care. The NAQC in partnership with the American Nurses Association

(ANA) has published guidelines that support the core principles of patient-centered quality care. These guidelines aim to foster "the patient relationship as the cornerstone of patient safety and quality." The NAQC's mission is to advance the highest quality, safety, and value of consumer-centered health care for all individual patients, their families, and their communities. NAQC believes it is the nurse's role to cultivate successful patient and family engagement, and that fostering family engagement is an essential component in reducing drug errors. The nurse serves as a patient advocate by supporting the patient's right to practice informed decision making and by maintaining patient-centered engagement in the health care setting. These guidelines include nurses at all levels of education and across all health care settings. Both QSEN and NAQC principles are fundamental to patient-centered practice and safety in pharmacotherapy.

NURSING PROCESS: PATIENT-CENTERED COLLABORATIVE CARE

The nursing process is a five-step decision-making approach that includes (1) assessment, (2) diagnosis, (3) planning, (4) implementation, and (5) evaluation. The purpose of the nursing process is to identify, diagnose, and treat human responses to health and illness. The nursing process is the essential core of practice for nurses. It supports the nurse in prioritizing the safe, timely delivery of drug administration. The nursing process is continuous and moves back and forth between the various steps. Careful attention to each phase of the process promotes the patient's success with the prescribed medication regimen. These steps are discussed as each relates to health teaching and drug therapy.

Assessment

During the assessment phase, the nurse is gathering information from the patient about the patient's health and lifestyle. Assessment includes both subjective and objective data. Always perform a complete, systemic assessment of the patient's body systems. In this assessment, the nurse asks the patient questions about the illness and about the drug regimen. The nurse can also get information from family members, health professionals, and the medical record. The assessment phase is paramount because the nurse will use the information gathered to form the basis of the patient's plan of care, which includes drug administration. Careful attention to each phase of the nursing process encourages the patient's success with the prescribed medication regimen.

Subjective Data

Subjective data include information provided verbally by the patient, family members, friends, or other sources. The patient must verbalize subjective data, which are imperceptible by the nurse's senses. The nurse may ask open-ended questions that allow the patient to answer directly, such as "Please tell me about your current medications." The nurse may help the patient explain or describe subjective data but must never speak for the patient. Subjective data comprise what the patient personally has to say about his or her medications, health problems, and

lifestyle. Examples of pertinent information that the nurse can use to help solicit subjective data from the patient concerning medication administration include the following:

- Current health history, including family history
- Swallowing problems (dysphagia)
- Signs and symptoms of the patient's illness verbalized by the patient
- Current concerns about the patient's:
  - Knowledge about medications and side effects
  - Over-the-counter (OTC) remedies, nutritional supplements, herbal remedies, and contraceptives
  - Knowledge of side effects to report to the physician
  - Attitude and beliefs about taking medications
- Allergies
- Financial barriers
- Use of tobacco, alcohol, and caffeine
- Cultural dietary barriers
- The patient's home safety needs
- Caregiver needs and support system

Enhancing the patient's adherence to the drug therapy regimen is an essential component of health teaching. The patient's attitudes and values about taking medication are important considerations when determining readiness to learn. Attitudes and values should be considered when planning interventions to support the patient's decision to adopt healthy behaviors related to medications. In addition, the patient's social support system should be emphasized. This special support system is unique to the individual and may be composed of persons who assist in preparing drugs, organizing pills, and ordering medications. A support system can alert a patient to side effects, encourage actions that promote medication compliance, and notify the health care provider if a problem arises.

Objective Data

Objective data are what the nurse directly observes about the patient's health status. It involves collecting the patient's health information by using the senses: seeing, hearing, smelling, and touching. Objective data collection provides additional information about the patient's symptoms and also targets the organs most likely to be affected by drug therapy. For example, if a drug is nephrotoxic, the patient's creatinine clearance should be assessed.

The following are examples of objective data concerning medication administration:

- Physical health assessment
- Laboratory and diagnostic test results
- Data from the physician's notes (i.e., health history)
- Measurement of vital signs
- The patient's body language

Nursing Diagnosis

A nursing diagnosis is made based on analysis of the assessment data, and it determines the type of care the patient will receive. When data show an abnormality during the assessment, it can serve as the defining characteristic of a problem to support the appropriate nursing diagnosis; and more than one applicable nursing diagnosis may be generated. The nurse formulates nursing diagnoses and uses them to guide the development of a care plan to provide patient-centered quality care.

Common nursing diagnoses related to drug therapy include the following:

- Pain, Acute or Chronic, related to surgery
- Confusion, Acute related to an adverse reaction to medication
- Health Maintenance, Ineffective related to not receiving recommended preventive care
- Knowledge, Deficient related to effects of anticoagulant medication
- Noncompliance related to forgetfulness
- Health Management, Ineffective related to lack of finances

Use of nursing diagnoses is beneficial to patient care because it facilitates the development of an individualized care plan for each patient. It is important to note that a *nursing diagnosis* is different from a *medical diagnosis,* which identifies a disease condition and the results of diagnostic tests and procedures.

To review the complete list of NANDA nursing diagnoses please see http://faculty.mu.edu.sa/public/uploads/1380604673 .6151NANDA%202012.pdf.

Planning

During the **planning** phase, the nurse uses the data collected to set goals or expected outcomes and interventions. Goals or expected outcomes should address the problems in the patient's nursing diagnosis. Goals are patient centered, describe the specific activity, and include a time frame for achievement and reevaluation. Planning includes the development of nursing interventions used to assist the patient in meeting goals. In order to develop patient-centered goals and outcomes, collaboration with the patient and/or family is necessary. Effective **goal setting** has the following qualities:

- The expected change is realistic, measurable, and includes reasonable deadlines.
- The goal is acceptable to both the patient and nurse.
- The goal is dependent on the patient's decision-making ability.
- The goal is shared with other health care providers, including family or caregivers.
- The goal identifies components for evaluation.

Examples of well-written comprehensive goals include the following:

- The patient will independently administer the prescribed dose of 4 units of regular insulin by the end of the fourth session of instruction.
- The patient will prepare a 3-day medication recording sheet that correctly reflects the prescribed medication schedule by the end of the second session of instruction.

Implementation of Nursing Interventions

The **implementation** phase is the part of the nursing process in which the nurse provides education, drug administration, patient care, and other interventions necessary to assist the patient in accomplishing the established goals. In most practice settings, administration of drugs and assessment of the drug's effectiveness are important nursing responsibilities. (See Chapter 9 for more information.)

Patient Teaching

It is important for the nurse to keep in mind factors that help promote patient learning. The patient must be ready to learn and must make an investment in learning. If the patient buys into wanting to practice good health principles, learning can be successful. The nurse and patient together must become fully engaged in the learning process. Timing is another important factor. What is the best time for the patient to learn? Is the patient a morning or night person? People seem to learn best if the time between the learning and use is short. The environment should be conducive to learning with a temperature that is comfortable and an environment that is quiet. It is important for the nurse to recognize that certain barriers to learning exist. Pain is an obstacle, and the patient's teaching should be postponed until pain is relieved. Be mindful of language barriers. If the patient does not speak the same language as the nurse, an interpreter may be needed. The patient's age may be another important obstacle. If the patient is young, or perhaps elderly and forgetful, a family member or significant other will need to be present.

Patient teaching is essential to the patient's recovery. It allows the patient to become informed about his or her health problems and to participate in creating interventions that can lead to good health outcomes. It is within the scope and practice of the nurse to embrace patient education and to use health-teaching strategies.

Nurses have a primary role in teaching both patients and families about drug administration. It is important that all teachings be tailored to the patient's educational level and that the patient trusts the nurse for learning to begin. When possible, it is always important to include a family member or friend in the teaching to provide support to the patient with reminders and encouragement; they can also detect possible side effects that may occur in the patient. The following are important principles to remember when teaching patients about their medications:

- *General.* Instruct the patient to take the drug as prescribed. Consistency in adhering to the prescribed drug regimen is important.
  - Provide simple written instructions to the patient with the doctor and pharmacy names and telephone numbers.
  - Instruct the patient to notify the health care provider if any of the following occur:
    - The dose, frequency, or time of the drug is adjusted.
    - A female patient becomes pregnant.
    - An OTC medication or supplement is added.
- *Side effects.* Give the patient instructions that will help minimize any side effects (e.g., avoid direct sunlight with drugs that can cause photosensitivity or sunburn). Advise patients of any expected changes in the color of urine or stool, and counsel the patient who has dizziness caused by orthostatic hypotension to rise slowly from a sitting to a standing position.
- *Self-administration.* Perform an ongoing assessment of the patient's motor skills and abilities. Remember that modifications may be necessary to the teaching plan based on the assessment.

BOX 8.1 Patient Teaching Card

Name of drug: Acetaminophen 325 mg
Reason for taking the drug: Minor aches, pains, and fever
Dosage: One or two tablets as needed every 4-6 hours; max 4 g/day or 6 tabs/day
Time to take the drug: 8:00 am/2:00 pm/8:00 pm
Possible side effects: Nausea, upper stomach pain, itching, loss of appetite, dark urine, and jaundice
Possible adverse effects: Overdosage can affect the liver and cause hepatotoxicity.
Notify health care provider: If side effects occur
Health care provider's telephone #: _____
Warning:
- *Never* take this medication with alcohol.
- If pregnant or nursing, notify the health care provider prior to taking the medication.

BOX 8.2 Culturally Sensitive Health-Teaching Tips

- Prior to the teaching, learn the ethnicity of the patient and arrange for an interpreter who speaks the patient's language. The use of family members as interpreters should be avoided because they may not be able to interpret medical terminology and may hinder communication on the part of the patient.
- Allow time for patients to respond to questions. Ask open-ended questions, and have patients demonstrate their understanding of treatments rather than verbalizing them.
- Be flexible in the timing of medication administration, such as with patients who are praying or fasting.
- Always be culturally sensitive when providing fluids to patients when administering medications. Ask in advance, and provide warm water when requested.
- Does your patient's culture have specific laws to follow concerning food preparation?
- Be mindful of body language. Many cultures are uncomfortable with too much eye contact, touching, or hugging.

- Instruct the patient on drug administration according to the prescribed route: eye or nose instillation, subcutaneous injection, suppository, oral/mucosal (e.g., swish-and-swallow suspensions), and inhaled via a metered-dose inhaler with or without a spacer. Include a return demonstration in the instructions when appropriate.
- The use of drug cards is a helpful teaching tool (Box 8.1). Drug cards can be obtained from the health care provider or from the drug manufacturer. They are helpful components for teaching. Drug cards may include the name of the drug, the reason for taking the drug, the drug dosage, times to take the drug, possible side effects, possible adverse effects and when to notify the care provider, and specific things that should or should not be done while taking the medication (e.g., take with food, do not crush tablets).
- *Diet.* Advise the patient about foods to include in their diet and foods to avoid. Many foods interact with certain drugs. Depending on the nature of the interaction, certain foods have the ability to decrease drug absorption, increase the risk of drug toxicity, or create other problems that make them an important safety concern.
- *Cultural considerations.* The nurse must apply knowledge of cultural considerations to individualize a teaching plan (Box 8.2). A **culturally sensitive** nurse is alert to the patient's cultural expectations. Begin by identifying your own cultural beliefs, practices, and values in order to keep them separate from those of the patient.

Additional suggestions include the following:
- Space instruction over several sessions if appropriate.
- Review community resources related to the patient's nursing and medical diagnoses.
- Collaborate with the patient and family and other health care staff and agencies to mobilize resources to meet the patient's needs.
- Identify patients at risk for noncompliance with the regimen. Alert the health care provider and pharmacist so they can develop a plan to minimize the number of drugs and the number of times drugs are administered.

BOX 8.3 Points for Patients and Families to Remember

- Medications should be taken as prescribed by your health care provider. If problems arise with the dose or timing, or if side effects occur, contact your medical provider.
- If drugs are placed in a drug box, keep the original labeled container.
- Keep all drugs out of the reach of children.
- Before using any over-the-counter drugs, including vitamins and nutritional supplements, check with your health care provider. This includes the use of aspirin, ibuprofen, and laxatives. Consider asking the pharmacist before buying or using a product.
- Bring all drugs with you when you visit the health care provider.
- Know the purpose of each medication and under what circumstances to notify the health care provider.
- Do not drink alcoholic beverages around the time you take your medications. Alcohol is absolutely contraindicated with certain medications, and it may alter the action and absorption of medications.
- Be aware that smoking tobacco also alters the absorption of some medications (e.g., theophylline-type drugs, antidepressants, pain medications). Consult your health care provider or pharmacist for specific information.

- Evaluate the patient's understanding of the medication regimen on a regular basis.
- Empower the patient to take responsibility for drug management.
- General points to remember and tips for successful patient education are presented in Box 8.3.

Many people take multiple drugs simultaneously several times each day, which presents a challenge to patients, their families, and nurses. This complex activity of taking several drugs can be segmented into several simple tasks that include the following:
- Drug boxes obtained from a local pharmacy can be used to prepare a day's or week's supply of medication. The boxes sort the drugs according to the time of day each pill is to be taken.

- A recording sheet may be helpful. When the drug is administered, the patient or family member marks the sheet, which is designed to meet the patient's individual needs. For example, the time can be noted by the patient, or it can be entered beforehand, with the patient marking the designated time the dose should be taken. A generic format follows:

Medication	Dosage (mg Daily)	S	M	T	W	Th	F	S
Captopril	12.5							
Digoxin	0.25							
Furosemide	40							

DAY OF WEEK

- Alternatives to recording sheets are also available, and alarm reminder devices may be used.

Throughout the teaching plan, the nurse promotes patient independence (e.g., self-administering, safely storing, and ordering of the drug regimen). Always keep in mind patients' goals and outcomes when teaching. Box 8.4 presents a checklist for health teaching in drug therapy.

BOX 8.4   Checklist for Health Teaching in Drug Therapy

- Reinforce the importance of drug adherence.
- Prior to giving the patient written material, ensure the patient can read.
- Always complete a health history and physical assessment on the patient.
- Assess all of the drugs on the patient's profile for possible drug interactions.
- Explain the reason the patient is taking the drug, the time it should be administered, and whether it should be taken with or without food.
- Review the side effects and adverse reactions, and make sure the patient has the doctor's telephone number and knows when to notify the health care provider or pharmacist.
- Discern whether the patient needs baseline and monthly lab work to monitor drug levels.
- Keep in mind that patient validation of learning may include a return demonstration of psychomotor skills (insulin administration).
- Show the patient how to record drug administration on a sheet of paper by indicating time of day.
- Discuss the patient's financial resources, and if needed, consult a social worker for resources.
- Discuss the patient's support system, such as family or friends as caregivers.
- Provide the patient with a list of community resources.

Evaluation

In the evaluation phase of the nursing process, the nurse determines whether the goals and teaching objectives are being met. The nurse continues to use ongoing assessment data to evaluate the successful attainment of the patient's objectives and goals. If the objectives and goals are not met, the nurse will revise the objectives, goals, and interventions to ensure success. If the objectives, goals, and interventions are met, the nurse will document the successful attainment in the nursing plan of care.

CRITICAL THINKING CASE STUDY

Mr. J.S. is a 66-year-old man who just arrived on the medical surgical unit following an appendectomy. He is complaining of pain. You are the nurse assigned to care for Mr. J.S.
1. What critical assessment data do you need to identify and collect?
2. Formulate a nursing diagnosis based on your assessment data.
3. Describe two nursing interventions to assist the patient.
4. What criteria would you use to evaluate the effectiveness of the nursing interventions?

NCLEX STUDY QUESTIONS

1. During a medication review session, a patient says, "I just do not know why I am taking all of these pills." Based on this piece of subjective data, which diagnosis will the nurse identify?
   a. High risk for injury
   b. Knowledge deficit
   c. High risk for aspiration
   d. Anxiety
2. The nurse is developing goals in collaboration with a patient. Which is the best goal statement?
   a. The patient will self-administer albuterol by tomorrow.
   b. The patient will self-administer the prescribed dose of albuterol by the end of the second teaching session.
   c. The patient will independently self-administer the prescribed dose of albuterol by the end of the second teaching session.
   d. The patient will organize his or her medications by tomorrow.
3. When developing an effective medication teaching plan, which component will the nurse identify as most essential?
   a. Written instructions
   b. The patient's readiness to learn
   c. Use of colorful charts
   d. A review of community resources
4. When developing an individualized medication teaching plan, which topics will the nurse include? (Select all that apply.)
   a. The importance of adherence to the prescribed drug regimen
   b. How to administer medication(s) according to the prescribed route
   c. The side/adverse effects that should be reported to the health care provider
   d. If a drug is inadvertently missed, whether to double the next dose
   e. Notifying the physician prior to taking over-the-counter drugs or supplements

5. The Nursing Alliance for Quality Care's focus is for health care providers to strive for which goal?
   a. Safety in medication administration
   b. Confidentiality as determined by the patient
   c. Development of a patient relationship and family engagement
   d. Patient independence within the family
6. The Quality and Safety Education for Nurses' focus on safety is *best* exemplified by which competency?
   a. Patient advocacy
   b. Technology-enhanced medication administration
   c. Infection control
   d. Patient- and family-centered collaborative care

7. Which teaching strategy is most likely to succeed in health teaching with the patient and family?
   a. Have the patient verbalize why they are taking the drug.
   b. Have the patient answer closed-ended questions.
   c. Have the patient demonstrate information.
   d. Have the patient identify pills by color.

Answers: 1, b; 2, c; 3, b; 4, a, b, c, e; 5, c; 6, d; 7, c.

9

Safety and Quality

e http://evolve.elsevier.com/McCuistion/pharmacology

OBJECTIVES

- Describe the original "five-plus-five" rights of medication administration.
- Analyze safety risks with medication administration.
- Discuss the culture of safety and include the Institute of Medicine's "To Err is Human" and the American Nurses Association's "Just Culture" impact on nursing.
- Discuss safe disposal of medications.

- Discuss high-alert drugs and strategies for safe administration.
- Discuss the nurse's rights when administering medications.
- Discuss safety regulations for pregnancy.
- Apply the nursing process to safe administration of medications.

OUTLINE

KEY TERMS

According to the Institute for Healthcare Informatics, spending on prescription medicines increased by 10.3% in the United States during 2014. A total of $373.9 billion is spent on prescription medications yearly. In 2014, over 4.3 billion prescriptions were filled in the United States. Recently, the *Journal of Patient*

Safety published a study that concluded that as many as 440,000 people die each year from preventable medical errors.

The focus of this chapter is quality and safety. It involves a discussion of safety initiatives and interventions that include the "five-plus-five" rights of medication administration, the nurse's rights when administering medications, the culture of safety, and The Joint Commission (TJC) Patient Safety Goals. Also included are high-alert drugs, look-alike and sound-alike drugs, and dosage forms to crush or not to crush. (See Chapter 8, which reviews the Quality and Safety Education for Nurses [QSEN] initiatives from www.qsen.org.)

"FIVE-PLUS-FIVE" RIGHTS OF MEDICATION ADMINISTRATION

The "five-plus-five" rights of medication administration are important goals for medication safety. The nurse following these guidelines will give (1) the right patient (2) the right drug in (3) the right dose via (4) the right route at (5) the right time. The "plus five" refers to the five additional rights that have been recommended: (1) right assessment, (2) right documentation, (3) the patient's right to education, (4) right evaluation, and (5) the patient's right to refuse. The original five rights and the subsequent additions are important; however, additional interventions are necessary to ensure the patient's positive response to the administered drug. Although nurses work together with health care providers and pharmacists to provide safe medication practices, it is the nurse who works closely with the patient and follows the patient's response to the medication. The rights and interventions necessary for safe drug administration will be reviewed in this chapter.

Right Patient

The **right patient** determination is essential. TJC requires two forms of identification before drug administration.

- Ask the patient to state his or her full name and birth date, and compare these with the patient's identification (ID) band and the medication administration record (MAR).
- Many facilities have electronic health records (EHRs) that allow the nurse to directly scan the bar code from the patient's ID band. Once the band is scanned, the nurse can see the patient's medication record.
  Additional nursing implications include the following:
- Most hospitals have color-coded ID bands that include bands coded for allergy, do not resuscitate (DNR), fall risk, and restricted extremity. Always check facility policies for the use of color-coded bands and their meanings.
- Verify the patient's identification each time a medication is given.
- If the patient is an adult with a cognitive disorder or a child, verify the patient's name with a family member. In the event a family member is unavailable and the patient is unable to self-identify, follow the facility's policy. Many facilities have policies that include a photo ID on the band with the patient's name and birth date affixed to the band.
- Distinguish between two patients with the same first or last name by placing "name-alert" stickers as warnings on the medical records.

Right Drug

The nurse must accurately determine the **right drug** prior to administration. When working with an EHR, once the bar code on the patient's wristband has been scanned, the patient's drug profile will appear on the computer screen. The nurse will then scan the patient's medication label, and it will automatically validate the time, date, and the nurse administering the patient's medication. If it is not the correct medication, the nurse will receive an alert and will be unable to proceed in the MAR until the correct medication is scanned.

Both federal and state legislation governs who can write a prescription order. Medication orders are prescribed by a licensed health care provider (HCP) under authority from the state to prescribe drugs. Those disciplines that have prescriptive authority are medical doctor (MD), dentist (doctor of dental surgery [DDS]), podiatrist (doctor of podiatric medicine [DPM]), certified nurse practitioner (CNP), advanced practice registered nurse (APRN), physician assistant (PA), veterinarian, chiropractor, and optometrist. In addition, medical clinical psychiatrists and pharmacists have prescriptive authority with strict guidelines set by the state. Prescriptions may be handwritten by the HCP, delivered as a telephone order (T/O) or verbal order (V/O), or directly entered into the patient's EHR. Handwritten prescriptions are written on a provider's legal prescription pad and are filled by a pharmacist.

Sometimes providers order medications by directly speaking to the nurse. All telephone orders or verbal orders for medications are either handwritten by the nurse taking the order or entered directly into a computer and "read back" to ensure accuracy. The nurse will write the name of the prescribing provider and will include that the order was read back, and affixing his or her signature to the order will complete it. After dictating a verbal order, the provider must sign it within 24 hours. If the order is a controlled medication, most facilities require two licensed nurses to listen to the order and sign it. Nursing students are not allowed to accept or take provider orders, but they may administer the medication after it has been verified by a registered nurse.

Many hospitals are implementing computerized physician order entry (CPOE) systems to handle HCP medication orders. This method of ordering medications can help decrease drug errors by decreasing transcription errors. HCPs using a CPOE will directly input the prescription into the patient's EHR; the order is electronically signed by the HCP and is sent directly to the pharmacy, and it is recorded as part of the patient's MAR. A strong safety feature is the ability to identify drug interactions with the patient's current drugs and any newly prescribed medications.

The use of computerized ordering systems has added speed and a measure of safety to the order process. Orders can be written from virtually any location and can be sent electronically, but the computer will not process the order unless all necessary information is included. Because the order is computerized, illegible orders or signatures are prevented. Before the nurse can administer the medication, both the pharmacy and the nurse must validate the accuracy of the patient's prescription order in the EHR.

The components of a drug order are as follows (Fig. 9.1):
- Patient name and birth date
- Date the order is written
- Provider signature or name if an electronic order, T/O, or V/O

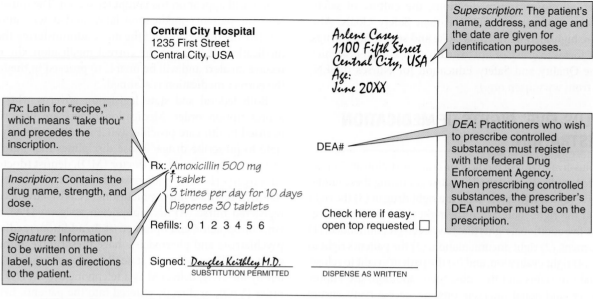

Central City Hospital
1235 First Street
Central City, USA

Arlene Casey
1100 Fifth Street
Central City, USA
Age:
June 20XX

Superscription: The patient's name, address, and age and the date are given for identification purposes.

Rx: Latin for "recipe," which means "take thou" and precedes the inscription.

Inscription: Contains the drug name, strength, and dose.

Signature: Information to be written on the label, such as directions to the patient.

Rx: *Amoxicillin 500 mg*
1 tablet
3 times per day for 10 days
Dispense 30 tablets

Refills: 0 1 2 3 4 5 6

DEA#

DEA: Practitioners who wish to prescribe controlled substances must register with the federal Drug Enforcement Agency. When prescribing controlled substances, the prescriber's DEA number must be on the prescription.

Check here if easy-open top requested ☐

Signed: *Douglas Keithley M.D.*
SUBSTITUTION PERMITTED   DISPENSE AS WRITTEN

FIG. 9.1 Example of a Drug Order. From Medical School Headquarters. (n.d.) *Prescription writing 101.* Retrieved from http://medicalschoolhq.net/prescription-writing-101

- Signature of licensed staff who took the T/O or V/O, if applicable
- HCPs who wish to prescribe controlled drugs must register with the federal Drug Enforcement Agency (DEA). When prescribing controlled substances, the HCP's DEA number must be on the prescription.
- Drug name and strength
- Drug frequency or dose (e.g., once daily)
- Route of administration
- Duration of administration (e.g., × 7 days, × 3 doses, when applicable)
- Number of patient refills
- Number of pills to be dispensed
- Any special instructions for withholding or adjusting dosage based on nursing assessment, drug effectiveness, or laboratory results

It is the nurse's responsibility to administer the drug as ordered by the provider, and if the drug order is incomplete, the drug should not be administered. Verification of a questionable order must be done in a timely manner. The HCP is usually contacted, and the conversation is documented. Nurses must become familiar with the components of a drug order and must question any incomplete or unclear orders. Nurses are legally liable if they give a prescribed drug and the dosage is incorrect, or if the drug is contraindicated for the patient's health status. Once the drug has been administered, the nurse becomes liable for the predicted effects of that drug.

Medication administration is never considered just a process of "passing" drugs. Nurses must use critical thinking skills and assess whether the medication is correct for the patient's diagnosis. The nurse must ask critical questions: Is the dose appropriate? What is the patient's expected response? Also, the nurse must teach the patient about the drug's side effects and when it is necessary for the patient to notify the HCP.

To avoid drug errors, the drug label should be read three times: (1) when you pick up the medication and remove it from the drug cabinet, (2) as you prepare the drug for administration, and (3) when you administer the drug.

Nursing interventions related to drug orders can ensure correct administration of medications:

- The nurse should verify the identity of the patient by comparing the name on the wristband with the name on the MAR for accuracy.
- Always use two patient identifiers, such as having patients repeat their name and date of birth.
- The nurse should be familiar with the patient's health history and should have performed a head-to-toe assessment on the patient, including a complete set of vital signs.
- Always review the patient's lab work prior to the administration of drugs.
- Read the drug order carefully. If the order is unclear, verify it with the HCP before administering the drug.
- Know the patient's allergies.
- Know the reason the patient is to receive the medication.
- Check the drug label by identifying the drug name, the amount of the drug (tablet or volume), and its suitability for administration by the intended route.
- Check the dosage calculations.
- Know the date the medication was ordered and any ending date (e.g., for controlled substances and antibiotics and for limited or a specific number of doses). Some agencies have automatic stop orders that are generally facility specific. Examples of such orders include controlled drugs that need to be renewed every 48 hours, antibiotics to be renewed every 7 to 14 days, and cancellation of all medications when the patient goes to surgery.
- All orders—including first-dose, one-time, and as-needed (PRN) medication orders—should be checked against the original orders.

Right Dose

The **right dose** refers to verification by the nurse that the dose administered is the amount ordered and that it is safe for the patient for whom it is prescribed. The right dose is based on the patient's physical status. Many medications require the patient's weight in order to determine the right dose. Usually pediatrics, medical-surgical, and critical care situations require weight to complete the drug calculation and determine the correct dose (heparin and digoxin drip are examples of medications calculated according to weight). The nurse determines if the drug is safe to administer according to the drug's pharmacodynamics (action) and the patient's vital signs. Renal and hepatic functions are important considerations because many drugs are cleared through the kidneys and metabolized by the liver. Prior to drug administration, it is important that the nurse carefully review the patient's most current lab results. A chemistry panel includes renal and liver function and sodium and potassium levels. Also, the nurse should review the hematology labs, which include a complete blood count (CBC), red blood cells (RBCs), hemoglobin, hematocrit, and platelets. It is most important that the nurse check the drug's correct dose range in a reliable drug resource book or by consulting with a pharmacist. In most cases, the right dose for a specific patient is within the recommended range for the particular drug. Nurses must calculate each drug dose accurately.

Nurses use dimensional analysis or ratio and proportion when calculating a drug dose (see Chapter 11). Always recheck the drug calculation if the dose is within a fraction or if it is an extremely large dose. Consult another nurse or the pharmacist when in doubt.

Today, most drugs are dispensed through automated dispensing cabinets (ADCs), computerized drug storage cabinets that store and dispense medications near the point of care while controlling and tracking drug distribution. The patient's drugs are stocked in the cabinet by the pharmacist and are accessed under the patient's name, and the nurse is able to select and pull the patient's drugs from the cabinet. This technology improves patient care by promoting accurate and quick access to medications, locked storage for all medications, and electronic tracking for controlled substances. Automation of drug administration saves time and decreases costs associated with drug administration.

Another method of dispensing drugs is the **unit dose method**, in which drugs are individually wrapped and labeled for single-dose use for each patient. The unit dose method has reduced dosage errors because no calculations are required. Some facilities still use a multidose vial from the ADC. If this occurs, the nurse will have to complete a calculation in order to retrieve the correct amount ordered by the physician from the vial. If there is any medication left in the vial, it is disposed of according to the facility's policy for disposal of drugs.

An important nursing intervention related to the right dose includes calculating the drug dose correctly. If in doubt about the amount to be administered, consult with a nurse peer to validate the correct amount. In some settings, two registered nurses (RNs) are required to check the dosage for certain medications, such as insulin and heparin.

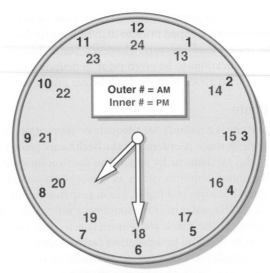

FIG. 9.2 Military Time.

Right Time

The **right time** refers to the time the prescribed dose is ordered to be administered. Daily drug dosages are given at specified intervals, such as twice a day (bid), three times a day (tid), four times a day (qid), or every 6 hours (every 6hrs); this is so the plasma level of the drug is maintained at a therapeutic level. Every drug cannot be given exactly when ordered, therefore health care agencies have policies that specify a range of times within which drugs can be administered (check your agency's policy). When a drug has a long half-life, it is usually given once a day. Drugs with a short half-life are given several times a day at specified intervals. Some drugs are given before meals, whereas others must be given with meals.

Use of military time, which is based on a 24-hour clock (Fig. 9.2), reduces administration errors and decreases documentation. Many nursing settings use military time rather than standard time. Nursing interventions related to the right time include the following:

- Administer drugs at the specified times (refer to agency policy).
- Administer drugs that are affected by food, such as tetracycline, 1 hour before or 2 hours after meals.
- Give food with drugs that can irritate the stomach (gastric mucosa)—for example, potassium and aspirin. Some medications are absorbed better after eating.
- Adjust the medication schedule to fit the patient's lifestyle, activities, tolerances, or preferences as much as possible.
- Check whether the patient is scheduled for any diagnostic procedures that contraindicate the administration of medications, such as endoscopy or fasting blood tests. Determine whether the medication should be given before or after the test based on the policy.
- Check the expiration date. If the date has passed, discard the medication or return it to the pharmacy, depending on the policy.
- Administer antibiotics at even intervals (e.g., every 8 hours rather than three times daily) throughout the 24-hour period to maintain therapeutic blood levels.

- Patients who require dialysis usually have blood pressure medications stopped prior to dialysis because dialysis can decrease blood pressure. However, some doctors order the medications to be given prior to dialysis. If any questions arise, check with the HCP before proceeding.

Right Route

The right route is necessary for adequate or appropriate absorption. The **right route** is ordered by the health care provider and indicates the mechanism by which the medication enters the body. The more common routes of **absorption** include oral, with drug in the form of a liquid, elixir, suspension, pill, tablet, or capsule; sublingual, under the tongue for venous absorption; buccal, between the cheek and gum; via a feeding tube; topical, applied to the skin; by inhalation (aerosol sprays); via otic (eye), ophthalmic (ear), or nasal (spray) instillation; by suppository (rectal or vaginal); and through the five parenteral routes: (1) intradermal, (2) subcutaneous (subcut), (3) intramuscular (IM), (4) intravenous (IV), or (5) intraosseous (IO).

Nursing interventions related to the right route include the following:

- Assess the patient's ability to swallow before administering oral medications; make sure the patient has not been ordered nothing by mouth (NPO).
- Do not crush or mix medications in other substances without consulting a pharmacist or a reliable drug reference. Do not mix medications in an infant's formula feeding.
- If the medication must be mixed with another substance, explain this to the patient. For example, elderly patients may use applesauce or yogurt to mix their medications to make them easier to swallow. Medications should be administered one at a time in the substance.
- Best Practice Guidelines and TJC state that drugs must be identifiable up until the point of delivery. When administering many drugs at one time, it is *not* recommended to mix drugs together. The correct practice is to administer one pill at a time. When a patient has an enteral tube, it is important to follow these guidelines; this allows the nurse to flush the tube before and after each pill or liquid is administered to prevent the tube from clogging. In the event that a patient's drug inadvertently falls to the ground, the nurse will be able to identify, discard, and replace the pill.
- Instruct the patient that medications must be swallowed with water and not juice, which can interfere with the absorption of certain medications; however, it is recommended that iron be taken with orange juice or vitamin C supplements to aid in the absorption of the iron.
- Use aseptic technique when administering drugs. Sterile technique is required with the parenteral routes.
- Administer drugs at the appropriate sites for the route.
- Stay with the patient until oral drugs have been swallowed.

Right Assessment

The **right assessment** requires the collection of appropriate baseline data before administration of a drug. Examples of assessment data include taking a complete set of vital signs and checking lab levels prior to drug administration. This may

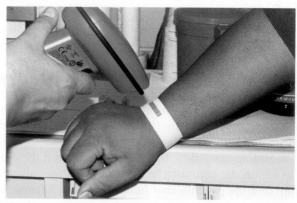

FIG. 9.3 Bar code reader used to scan the patient's wristband. From Kee, J. L. & Marshall, S. M. (2017). *Clinical calculations: With applications to general and specialty areas* (8th ed.). St. Louis: Elsevier.

also include both apical heart rate and potassium level prior to administering digitalis; blood pressure level prior to administering an antihypertensive drug; blood glucose levels before insulin administration; or respirations with blood pressure prior to administering an opioid. It is also important for the nurse to identify high-risk patients, such as patients with medication allergies, patients on dialysis, those with liver disease, diabetic patients, cardiac and pulmonary patients, and the elderly and pediatric populations. If at-risk patients are identified, precautions can be taken to reduce risk.

Right Documentation

The **right documentation** requires the nurse to record immediately the appropriate information about the drug administered. Many systems are available for documenting drug administration. The most common is the paper medication administration record (MAR), which the pharmacy will furnish. Facility policies vary, but when nurses administer a drug, they place their initials next to the name of the drug on the paper MAR. The nurse's initials verify that the medication was administered. Both paper and computerized MARs include information about the drug to be administered, including (1) the name of the drug, (2) the dose, (3) the route, (4) the time and date, and (5) the nurse's initials or signature.

Now popular and becoming common in most facilities is computerized charting, in which the nurse enters a personal identification and password to gain entry into the system. By scanning the patient's identification band (Fig. 9.3), which includes the patient's bar code information, the nurse accesses the patient's personal MAR with the emergency medical record (EMR) system. Once the nurse scans the bar code on the patient's medication package, the administration is validated in the computerized MAR. The computerized system interfaces with other departments, including the pharmacy, laboratory, and sometimes the physician's office.

Documentation of the patient's response to the medication is required with a variety of medications such as (1) opioid and nonopioid analgesics (Ask, how effective was pain relief?); (2) sedatives (How effective was relaxation?); and (3) antiemetics (Was nausea/vomiting decreased or eliminated?). The nurse

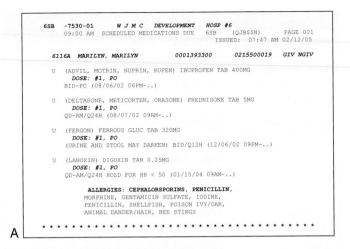

FIG. 9.4 Medication Record. A, Computerized format. B, Written format.

with return demonstration, and laboratory test result monitoring. This right is a principle of informed consent, which is the individual having the necessary knowledge to make a decision. Informed patients and families are critical to preventing medication errors.

Right Evaluation

The right evaluation determines the effectiveness of the drug based on the patient's response to the drug. Evaluation in this context asks whether the medication did for the patient what it was supposed to do. It is essential that the nurse evaluate the therapeutic effect of the medication by assessing the patient for side effects and adverse drug reactions. Evaluation is ongoing and is an important aspect of patient safety.

Right to Refuse

The patient has the right to refuse the medication, and it is the nurse's responsibility to determine the reason for the refusal, explain to the patient the risks involved with refusal, and reinforce the important benefits of and reasons for taking the medication. When a medication is refused, the refusal must be documented immediately, and follow-up is always required. The primary nurse and health care provider should be informed because the omission may pose a specific threat to the patient (e.g., a change in the lab values with insulin and warfarin).

All medication errors are potentially serious. A medication error may involve one or more types of errors such as administration of the wrong medication or IV fluid; the incorrect dose or rate; administration to the wrong patient, by the incorrect route, or at the incorrect scheduled interval; administration of a known allergic drug; omission of a dose; or discontinuation of medication or IV fluid that was not ordered to be discontinued.

NURSES' RIGHTS WHEN ADMINISTERING MEDICATION

In addition to the rights of medication administration, there are six rights for nurses who administer medications. These rights provide an additional layer of safety by ensuring that the nurse has what is needed to provide safe medication administration.

The nurses' six rights are (1) the right to a complete and clear order; (2) the right to have the correct drug, route (form), and dose dispensed; (3) the right to have access to information; (4) the right to have policies to guide safe medication administration; (5) the right to administer medications safely and to identify problems in the system; and (6) the right to stop, think, and be vigilant when administering medications. These rights can assist in increasing the safety of medication administration.

In addition, the American Nurses Association (ANA) published a bill of rights for nurses in 2015 that contains seven premises concerning workplace expectations and environments that nurses from across the United States recognize as necessary for safe nursing practice. The *Bill of Rights* supports nurses in workplace situations and includes issues such as unsafe staffing, mandatory overtime, and health and safety issues in the

continues to assess the patient's response to the medication (Was there any gastrointestinal irritation or skin sensitivity?) and documents this in the patient's plan of care. Keep in mind that patient responses are not necessarily verbal; they could be physiologic (e.g., blood pressure decreasing in response to an antihypertensive). With the paper MAR and a pen, the nurse documents the response in the nursing notes. The computerized MAR allows for documentation of the patient's response directly into the plan of care. Delay in charting may result in forgetting to chart the medication, and another nurse can inadvertently administer the drug, assuming it was not given because it was not charted. Therefore it is important to remember that drugs *must* be signed off on when the drug is administered. Graphic formats or computerized systems (Fig. 9.4) assist in the accurate and timely recording of drugs administered.

Right to Education

The right to education requires that patients receive accurate and thorough information about the drugs they are taking and how each drug relates to their particular condition. Patient teaching also includes why the patient is taking the drug, the expected result of the drug, possible side effects of the drug, any dietary restrictions or requirements, skill of administration

workplace. These issues are essential to meet the responsibilities of patient care, including safe drug administration and the responsibility nurses have to themselves. (For more information, see http://nursingworld.org/DocumentVault/NursingPractice/FAQs.aspx.) Facilities have an obligation to both nurses and patients to educate and to provide guidelines and policies concerning patient safety in all aspects of patient care. Many disciplines are involved in medication administration, and the different departments must work together to provide a method of drug delivery and administration in a safe environment for the patient and the nurse. This can be done by having modern equipment, staff education opportunities, policies and procedures, and communication among the different departments involved in drug administration.

CULTURE OF SAFETY

The National Council for Medication Error Reporting (2009) defines medication error as "any preventable event that may cause or lead to inappropriate medication use or harm to a patient."

Much progress has been made since the landmark Institute of Medicine (IOM) report in 1999, *To Err Is Human: Building a Safer Health Care System*. The report served as a basis for creating an awareness of patient safety systems in health care and led to the development of safety tools that have been instrumental in decreasing the number of drug errors. Over the last 15 years, drug administration and the margin of error have shown some improvement with the development of bar coding, CPOE systems, EHRs, and ADCs. However, there is still much work ahead.

The ANA supports the concept of Just Culture in its position statement (2010), and it encourages organizations to avoid using punitive approaches in reporting drug errors because they focus on punishing individuals for reporting such errors. In a Just Culture, individuals would be encouraged to report drug errors so the system can be repaired and the problem fixed. A Just Culture does not hold individual practitioners responsible for a failing system, although it does not tolerate disregard for a patient or gross misconduct. (For more information on Just Culture, see http://nursingworld.org/psjustculture.)

In a true culture of safety, everyone in the organization is committed and driven to keep patients safe from harm. Risk management is a process that identifies weaknesses in the system. It then allows changes to be made in order to minimize the effects of adverse patient outcomes. Most organizations have a risk management department staffed with nurse managers and risk managers who conduct root cause analysis (RCA), a method of problem solving used to identify potential workplace errors. Such analysis presents opportunities for learning and focuses on strategies that can be put in place to correct problems.

Drug administration is a vulnerable area where the possibility for error is high. If a patient dies as the result of a drug error, it is called a sentinel event, an unanticipated event in a health care setting that results in death or serious harm to a patient

TABLE 9.1	"Do Not Use" Abbreviations

In 2004, the Joint Commission created a "Do Not Use List" of abbreviations that should be written out to avoid misinterpretation. In 2010, National Patient Safety Goal (NPSG) 02.02.01 was integrated into the Information Management (IM) standards as elements of performance 2 and 3 under IM 02.02.01.

Abbreviation	Preferred
q.d., Q.D.	Write "daily" or "every day."
q.o.d., Q.O.D.	Write "every other day."
U	Write "unit."
IU	Write "International Unit."
MS, MSO$_4$	Write "morphine sulfate."
MgSO$_4$	Write "magnesium sulfate."
.5 mg	Use a zero before a decimal point when the dose is less than a whole unit (e.g., write *0.5 mg*).
1.0 mg	Do not use a decimal point or zero after a whole number (write *1 mg*).

Visit www.jointcommission.org and www.ismp.org for more detailed safety information concerning "Do Not Use" abbreviations.

unrelated to the natural course of the patient's illness. TJC tracks these events in a database to ensure they are adequately analyzed and that unsafe processes are caught and resolved. The most common occurrence of sentinel events is medication errors, and of those, the most frequently implicated drug was potassium chloride (KCl). Most often, KCl was mistaken for sodium chloride, heparin, or furosemide (See http://www.ismp.org/Tools/jcahosentinelevent.asp).

The Joint Commission National Patient Safety Goals

Additionally, TJC has taken steps to support safety and quality care in the workplace. In 2004, they first announced their National Patient Safety Goals (NPSGs), which focus on problems in health care safety and how to solve them. The goals are written for a variety of health care settings including ambulatory health care, behavioral health care, critical access hospitals, home care, hospitals, laboratory services, long-term care (Medicare/Medicaid), and office-based surgery. These goals are updated and published annually. Once a goal becomes a standard, the goal number is retired and is not used again, and the standard must be adopted by all Joint Commission–accredited agencies. Two important goals that have already become standards for all TJC-accredited organizations are the "do not use" abbreviations (Table 9.1) and the list of acceptable abbreviations (Table 9.2; visit TJC's website at http://www.jointcommission.org and the Institute for Safe Medication Practices website at http://www.ismp.org for current detailed safety information).

Another safety feature is the U.S. Food and Drug Administration's (FDA) black-box warning system. When a prescription drug is known to be effective for some patients but may cause serious side effects in others, the FDA will require the drug's printed materials to carry a warning about the adverse effects surrounded by a black box. A black-box warning is the

TABLE 9.2 Acceptable Abbreviations

These abbreviations are frequently used in drug therapy and must be known by the nurse, but also check your facility's list of medical abbreviations. It is now a Joint Commission standard that each facility have a list of acceptable medication abbreviations.

Abbreviation	Meaning
DRUG MEASUREMENTS AND DRUG FORMS	
cap	Capsule
elix	Elixir
ER	Extended Release
g	Gram
gtt	Drops
kg	Kilogram
L	Liter
m^2	Square meter
mcg	Microgram
mEq	Milliequivalent
mg	Milligram
mL	Milliliter
NKA	No known allergies
NKDA	No known drug allergies
oz	Ounce
SR	Sustained release
One-Half tablet	Half-tablet
supp	Suppository
susp	Suspension
Tbsp, tbs, or T	Tablespoon
tsp	Teaspoon
ROUTES OF MEDICATION ADMINISTRATION	
ID	Intradermal
Inj	Injection
IM	Intramuscular

ROUTES OF MEDICATION ADMINISTRATION	
IV	Intravenous
IVPB	Intravenous piggyback
KVO	Keep vein open
PO	By mouth
subQ, subcut, or subcutaneous	Subcutaneous
Subling	Sublingual (under tongue)
TKO	To keep open
vag	Vaginal

TIMES OF ADMINISTRATION	
PRIOR USAGE	**CURRENT USAGE**
ā	before
ac	before meals
ad lib	as desired
bid (Twice a day)	bid
c̄	with
hr (hour)	hr or hrs
hs	bedtime
NPO (nothing by mouth)	NPO
pc	after meals
PCA (patient-controlled analgesia)	PCA
per (Through, by [route])	per
prn (As needed)	PRN
q	every or each
qh or q1h	every hr or every 1 hr
qid (Four times daily)	qid
q2h, q4h, etc.	every 2 hrs, every 4 hrs, etc.
s̄ (Without)	without
stat	immediately, at once
tid (Three times a day)	tid

Please visit www.jointcommission.org and www.ismp.org for more detailed safety information concerning "Acceptable Abbreviations."

strongest form of warning issued by the FDA about a drug. (For more information on the use of black-box warnings, see https://www.verywell.com/black-box-warnings-1124107 and for specific drug information, see www.fda.gov and insert black-box into the site's search box.)

Drug Reconciliation

Drug reconciliation is an important component of the culture of safety. It is defined as the process of identifying the most accurate list of all medications that the patient is taking at transitions in care, which includes admissions and discharges from a hospital to another health care setting such as long-term care. Correct drug reconciliation is important because it prevents discrepancies that can cause a drug error. One in five patients experience an adverse event transitioning from hospital to home (see https://www.jointcommission.org/sentinel_event_alert_issue_35_using_medication_reconciliation_to_prevent_errors/).

Drug reconciliation was created to provide drug continuity during care transitions, thereby promoting patient safety. For this reason, the nurse should advise patients to do the following:
- Always carry a list of personal drug information in case of an emergency.
- Update this list of drugs whenever a change occurs.
- Bring a list of medications to each doctor appointment.

The Agency for Healthcare Research and Quality (AHRQ) has published a list of patient tools and resources that can help patients play an active role in their own safety. It can be accessed at http://www.ahrq.gov/professionals/quality-patient-safety/patient-safety-resources/index.html.

NPSG 03.06.01 from TJC requires facilities to find out, record, and share information on any drugs patients are taking, and it requires them to compare that list of drugs with a list of any new drugs being given (see http://www.jointcommission.org/assets/1/6/2015_npsg_hap.pdf) and, for patient teaching, (see www.ahrq.gov/consumer/20tips.pdf).

BOX 9.1   Medications Recommended for Disposal by Flushing

Medicine	Active Ingredient	Medicine	Active Ingredient
Abstral, tablets (sublingual)	Fentanyl	Morphine sulfate, tablets (immediate release)	Morphine sulfate
Actiq, oral transmucosal lozenge	Fentanyl citrate	Morphine sulfate, oral solution	Morphine sulfate
Avinza, capsules (extended release)	Morphine sulfate	MS Contin, tablets (extended release)	Morphine sulfate
Belbuca, soluble film (buccal)	Buprenorphine hydrochloride	Nucynta ER, tablets (extended release)	Tapentadol
Buprenorphine Hydrochloride, tablets (sublingual)	Buprenorphine hydrochloride	Onsolis, soluble film (buccal)	Fentanyl citrate
Buprenorphine Hydrochloride; Naloxone Hydrochloride, tablets (sublingual)	Buprenorphine hydrochloride; Naloxone hydrochloride	Opana, tablets (immediate release)	Oxymorphone hydrochloride
Butrans, transdermal patch system	Buprenorphine	Opana ER, tablets (extended release)	Oxymorphone hydrochloride
Daytrana, transdermal patch system	Methylphenidate	Oxecta, tablets (immediate release)	Oxycodone hydrochloride
Demerol, tablets	Meperidine hydrochloride	Oxycodone hydrochloride, capsules	Oxycodone hydrochloride
Demerol, oral solution	Meperidine hydrochloride	Oxycodone hydrochloride, oral solution	Oxycodone hydrochloride
Diastat/Diastat AcuDial, rectal gel	Diazepam	Oxycontin, tablets (extended release)	Oxycodone hydrochloride
Dilaudid, tablets	Hydromorphone hydrochloride	Percocet, tablets	Acetaminophen; oxycodone hydrochloride
Dilaudid, oral liquid	Hydromorphone hydrochloride	Percodan, tablets	Aspirin; oxycodone hydrochloride
Dolophine hydrochloride, tablets	Methadone hydrochloride	Suboxone, film (sublingual)	Buprenorphine hydrochloride; Naloxone hydrochloride
Duragesic, patch (extended release)	Fentanyl		
Embeda, capsules (extended release)	Morphine sulfate; naltrexone hydrochloride	Targiniq ER, tablets (extended release)	Oxycodone hydrochloride; Naloxone hydrochloride
Exalgo, tablets (extended release)	Hydromorphone hydrochloride	Xartemis XR, tablets	Oxycodone hydrochloride; Acetaminophen
Fentora, tablets (buccal)	Fentanyl citrate		
Hysingla ER, tablets (extended release)	Hydrocodone bitartrate	Xtampza ER, capsules (extended release)	Oxycodone
Kadian, capsules (extended release)	Morphine sulfate	Xyrem, oral solution	Sodium oxybate
Methadone hydrochloride, oral solution	Methadone hydrochloride	Zohydro ER, capsules (extended release)	Hydrocodone bitartrate
Methadose, tablets	Methadone hydrochloride	Zubsolv, tablets (sublingual)	Buprenorphine hydrochloride; Naloxone hydrochloride
Morphabond, tablets (extended release)	Morphine sulfate		

From U.S. Food and Drug Administration. (n.d.). *Medicines recommended for disposal by flushing: Listed by medicine and active ingredient.* Retrieved from http://www.fda.gov/downloads/drugs/resourcesforyou/consumers/buyingusingmedicinesafely/ensuringsafeuseofmedicine/safedisposalofmedicines/ucm337803.pdf

Disposal of Medications

The FDA and DEA issue guidelines for appropriate disposal of prescription drugs based on the Secure and Responsible Disposal Act issued by Congress in 2010, which encourages both public and private entities to develop secure, convenient, and responsible methods for collecting and destroying medications and controlled substances. It also recommends a decrease in the amount of controlled substances released into the environment, especially into water and sewage systems.

General guidelines include take-back events, mail-back programs, and collection receptacles. Facilities may contract with an independent or local collection program authorized by the state and the DEA to dispose of medical waste and hazardous materials. The drugs are disposed of in a receptacle that must comply with strict security and record-keeping requirements as established by the FDA and DEA. The waste is then incinerated by the company.

Consumers who do not have DEA-authorized collectors or medicine take-back programs can follow these simple steps:
1. Remove medications from the original packaging and mix them (do not crush tablets or capsules) with an unpalatable substance such as dirt, kitty litter, or used coffee grounds. This method is intended to make medications less attractive to people and animals.
2. Place the mixture in a container such as a sealed plastic bag.
3. Throw the container in the household trash.
4. Scratch out all personal information on the prescription label before disposing of the empty container.

Unless specifically instructed, do not flush drugs down the toilet, where they will pollute the environment and pose a danger to humans and animals. (Exceptions to this rule are listed in Box 9.1.) Nurses and patients can consult a pharmacist with questions related to medication disposal. Pharmacists are always available to answer questions on how to properly dispose of unused medications.

Sharps Safety

U.S. hospital-based health care professionals experience over 384,000 needlestick injuries each year (see http://www.cdc.gov/sharpssafety/index.html). The Occupational Safety and Health Administration (OSHA) Needlestick Safety and Prevention Act (NSPA) of 2000 resulted from the ANA's campaign Safe Needles Save Lives. The NSPA requires that employers implement safer medical devices for their employees, provide a safe and secure workplace environment with educational opportunities, and develop written policies to help prevent sharps injuries.

Twelve years after the NSPA, the University of Virginia's International Healthcare Worker Safety Center, in collaboration with the ANA and many health care colleagues, issued a consensus statement and call to action (2012) to increase awareness of the risk of needlesticks, a hazard health care workers face daily in the line of duty. The consensus statement and call to action provides a framework of the progress made and a look at what is needed in the future to continue to protect health care workers from the risk of needlesticks (see http://www.medical center.virginia.edu/safetycenter/Consensus_statement_sharps_ injury_prevention.pdf).

SAFETY RISKS WITH MEDICATION ADMINISTRATION

Every year in the United States, 1.5 million preventable drug errors occur. Data support that a hospitalized patient is subject to one medication administration error per day. The majority of medication errors occur in the transcription stage (56%), followed by the nurse administration stage (41%), and finally the doctor prescribing stage (39%).

Examples of risks to safety include the following:

- *Tablet splitting.* In an effort to counteract steeply rising drug costs, some patients are cutting their pills in half. However, this is not recommended by the FDA. The only time tablet splitting is advisable is when it is specified by the pharmacist on the label. Splitting tablets is risky because the patient may not receive an equal distribution of the medication with each dose. Some tablets are not recommended for splitting and are difficult to split. The FDA recommends that a patient get advice directly from the pharmacist to determine whether tablet splitting is appropriate for a particular drug.
- *Buying drugs over the Internet.* Consumers may find it convenient to order drugs over the Internet, but precautions must be taken because drugs sold online may be too old, too strong, or too weak to be effective. Online sources may sell expired medications without the consumer knowing. The FDA suggests drugs obtained from these sites may not be made using safe standards, are unsafe to use with other medications, and may be expired. Patients should look for websites that (1) require a prescription from a health care provider; (2) have a licensed pharmacist to answer questions and a contact person to consult if problems arise; (3) are located in the United States; and (4) are licensed by the state board of pharmacy. Some sites may sell counterfeit drugs.

Counterfeit Drugs

Counterfeit drugs look like the desired drug but may have no active ingredient, the wrong active ingredient, or the wrong amount of active ingredient. Improper packaging and contamination can also be problems. Counterfeit drugs may look remarkably like the real thing! To report suspected counterfeit products, call the FDA Office of Counterfeit Issues at 1-800-551-3989 or email DrugSupplyChainIntegrity@fda.hhs.gov.

TABLE 9.3	**Abbreviations for Sustained- or Extended-Release Medications**
Abbreviation	**Meaning**
CD	Controlled delivery
CR	Controlled release
DR	Delayed release
ER	Extended release
IM	Immediate release
LA	Long acting
MR	Modified release
SA	Sustained action (Ambiguous, can also mean short acting)
SR	Sustained release
TR	Timed release
XR	Extended release
XT	Extended release

To reduce the risk of exposure to counterfeit drugs, patients should purchase drugs only from licensed pharmacies. Refer to the National Association of Boards of Pharmacy (NABP) at www.nabp.net for information.

Dosage Forms: To Crush or Not to Crush

Although some drugs can be used crushed, some should not be crushed. Always consult with the pharmacist or, when possible, the health care provider prior to crushing a patient's drug. Also, consult a reliable drug guide to confirm the medication is crushable. Do not crush any extended- or sustained-release drugs because this will change the pharmacokinetic phase of the drug. There is no industry standard for sustained- or extended-release abbreviations, which can cause confusion and drug errors. Table 9.3 includes abbreviations for sustained- and extended-release drugs. For a current complete listing of drugs that should not be crushed, see Do-Not-Crush-List, Institute for Safe Medication Practices at http://www.ismp.org/tools/donotcrush.pdf.

❶ HIGH-ALERT MEDICATIONS

High-alert drugs can cause significant harm to the patient. If a high-alert medication is given in error, it can have a major effect on the patient's organs; this includes cardiac, respiratory, vascular, and neurologic systems. A medication can also affect the sympathetic and parasympathetic nervous systems. Specific high-alert medications as listed by the Institute for Safe Medication Practices (ISMP) include epinephrine, subcutaneous; epoprostenol, IV; insulin; magnesium sulfate injection; methotrexate, nononcologic oral use; opium tincture; oxytocin, IV; nitroprusside sodium for injection; potassium chloride concentrate for injection; potassium phosphate injection; promethazine, IV; and vasopressin, IV or IO. Please note that all forms of insulin, subcutaneous and IV, are considered high-alert medications. For additional classes and categories of high-alert medications, visit the Institute for Safe Medication Practice's website at http://www.ismp.org/. These lists are provided to reduce the risk of errors, but specific strategies can optimize safety when dealing with high-alert drugs:

1. Simplify the storage, preparation, and administration of high-alert drugs.
2. Write policies concerning safe administration.
3. Improve information and education.
4. Limit access to high-alert medications.
5. Use labels and automated alerts.
6. Use redundancies (automated or independent double-checks).
7. Closely monitor the patient's response to the medication (possibly the most important step).

⚡ LOOK-ALIKE AND SOUND-ALIKE DRUG NAMES

Nurses should be aware that certain drug names sound alike and are spelled similarly. Examples of drugs involved in medication errors and recognized as confusing drug names include *Amaryl* (glimepiride) with *Reminyl* (galantamine); *captopril* with *carvedilol*; *Depakote* (valproic acid) with *Depakote ER* (divalproex sodium); *Depo-medrol* with *Solu-medrol* (methyprednisolones); *ephedrine* with *epinephrine*; and *Humalog* mix 75/25 with *Humulin* 70/30 (insulins). The FDA, ISMP, and TJC advocate the use of "tall-man" letters as a safety strategy to reduce confusion between similar-sounding drugs. For example, rispiridone is written as *rispiriDONE,* and ropinirole is written as *rOPINIRole* to call attention to differences in spelling. Tall-man letters should be used for computer listing and storage labeling for look-alike and sound-alike drug names, and this is now standard; the list may be found at https://www.ismp.org/tools/confuseddrugnames.pdf. Nursing students must familiarize themselves with this list.

OTHER FACTORS IN THE PREVENTION OF MEDICATION ERRORS

Creating a distraction-free environment is critical to safe administration of medications. Data show that interruptions are responsible for 45% of medication errors (https://www.ismp.org/newsletters/acutecare/articles/20081204.asp). To avoid drug errors, many facilities are creating medication safety zones by implementing policies that provide for a medication room or safety area. When a nurse enters this safety zone, he or she is not to be disturbed. The zone offers a quiet atmosphere in which nurses can dispense medications from a Pyxis system and prepare them for administration. The patient's medical record is available to the nurse in the safety zone, which has proper lighting and a design conducive to safe preparation of medications. Overall, the nurse's role is best achieved by the application of the nursing process.

◎ NURSING PROCESS
Patient-Centered Collaborative Care
Medication Safety

Assessment
- Assess the patient's vital signs and perform a head-to-toe physical assessment.
- Assess the patient's current laboratory results such as hematology labs, chemistry panel, and other pertinent labs pertaining to the patient's diagnosis and designated medication profile.
- Assess the patient's history, including current diagnostics and ability of the patient to swallow (for oral medications).
- Assess medication orders for completeness. Know the purpose and the expected effect of medications and interactions, including over-the-counter (OTC) and herbal preparations. Question the primary care provider if the prescription is unclear or seems inappropriate for the client's condition.
- ⚡ Make a determination using critical thinking skills when applying the assessment data and lab values in regard to whether it is safe to administer the patient's medications. Report to the provider any abnormal findings in regard to any medications along with the medications not administered.
- ⚡ Refuse to give a medication if you believe it to be unsafe, and notify the patient's provider and nurse manager.

Planning
- ⚡ Calculate doses accurately, and if necessary, verify dosages with a colleague or pharmacist.
- Measure doses accurately and double-check high-alert medications.
- Avoid distractions during drug preparation.

Nursing Interventions
- Use relevant resources appropriately.
- ⚡ Calculate doses correctly.
- Avoid skin contamination or inhalation of substances to minimize your own exposure.
- Wash your hands.
- ⚡ Administer only medications you prepared.
- ⚡ Identify the patient using two forms of identification.
- ⚡ Administer medications according to the five-plus-five rights: right patient, right drug, right dose, right time, and right route plus right assessment, right documentation, right evaluation, right to education, and right to refuse.
- Remain with the patient until the medication has been taken.
- Discard needles and syringes in appropriate containers; be alert to sharps safety.
- Use aseptic/sterile technique appropriate for the route of administration.
- Thoroughly document drug administration in the designated format in a timely manner.
- Document a patient's refusal to take a medication, and notify the health care provider.

Patient Teaching
- Counsel patients and families on anticipated effects of medications.
- Counsel patients on side effects and adverse reactions and what to report promptly to a health care provider.
- Advise patients what foods to eat or avoid.
- Advise patients whether to take medications before, with, or after meals to promote optimal absorption.

Evaluation
- Evaluate the patient's response to the medication, recognize side effects, and document and report these appropriately.
- Evaluate the patient's understanding of the expected results from the medication and what to report to the health care provider.
- Evaluate the effectiveness of medications administered to treat the condition for which they were prescribed.
- Omit or delay doses as indicated by the patient's condition, and if not administered, report this to the provider.

RESOURCES FOR PREVENTING ERRORS IN MEDICATION ADMINISTRATION

Several resources address medication errors and their prevention:
- The Institute for Safe Medication Practices provides accurate medication safety information. The ISMP also provides knowledge and understanding of the system-based causes of medication errors, based largely on interdisciplinary reviews of thousands of reports to its national Medication Error Reporting Program (MERP) as well as hundreds of visits to health care organizations nationwide.
- The FDA database of medication errors and "near misses" assists all health care personnel to identify, implement, and evaluate strategies to prevent medication errors. It is strongly suggested that health care workers report errors and near misses to the FDA. Reports are confidential.

- When the nurse is unsure about a dosage, potential side effects, expected therapeutic effects, contraindications, or adverse reactions, an external resource—a drug reference book, pharmacist, or an acceptable technology resource (e.g., Micromedex, Epocrates)—should be consulted to determine the correct answer.
- The FDA MedWatch Program, through their official site found at http://www.fda.gov/safety/medwatch/default.htm, provides current information on notifications for drug recalls, counterfeit products, and safety alerts.

PREGNANCY CATEGORIES AND SUBSECTIONS

In 2015, the FDA replaced the lettered pregnancy categories A, B, C, D, and X on prescription drug labeling. After much research, the FDA decided that the previous lettering did not effectively communicate the risk a drug may have during pregnancy and lactation and in females and males with reproductive potential. It was thought to be overly simplistic and could easily be misinterpreted. The new labeling system provides a broader explanation based on current available information of the benefits and risks medications can have to the mother, the fetus, and the breastfeeding child. The new subsections are listed as Pregnancy (includes Labor and Delivery), Lactation (includes Nursing Mothers), and Females and Males of Reproductive Potential (Fig. 9.5). The Pregnancy subsection provides information relevant to the use of the drug in pregnant women, such as dosing, potential risks to the fetus, information about whether a registry collects and maintains data on how pregnant women are affected when they use the drug, and relevant information to help health care providers make prescribing and counseling decisions. The Lactation subsection provides information about using the drug while breastfeeding, such as the amount of the drug in breast milk and potential effects on the breast-fed child. The Females and Males of Reproductive Potential subsection includes information about pregnancy testing, contraception, and infertility as it relates to the drug. For more information, see http://www.fda.gov/Drugs/DevelopmentApprovalProcess/DevelopmentResources/Labeling/ucm093307.htm.

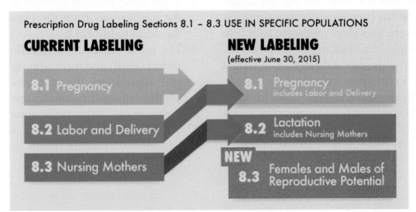

FIG. 9.5 U.S. Food and Drug Administration Pregnancy Categories. From U.S. Food and Drug Administration. (2014). *Pregnancy and lactation labeling (drugs) final rule.* Retrieved at http://www.fda.gov/Drugs/DevelopmentApprovalProcess/DevelopmentResources/Labeling/ucm093307.htm

GUIDELINES FOR MEDICATION ADMINISTRATION

General guidelines for correct administration of medications are listed in Box 9.2. Nurses should follow these guidelines to enhance safety when administering medications. Application of the nursing process to medication administration is presented in Chapter 8.

BOX 9.2   Guidelines for Correct Administration of Medications

Preparation
1. Perform hand hygiene.
2. Access patient's medication administration record (MAR) via chart or electronic health record (EHR).
3. Check patient medications with the health care provider's order for accuracy.
4. Obtain the patient's medications from Pyxis, remote stock, or pharmacy while checking the medication label with the patient's drug order for accuracy.
5. Check drug allergies.
6. Prepare medications for only one patient at a time.
7. Calculate the medication dose and perform a double check of the calculation.
8. Check the expiration date on the drug label, and use the drug only if the date is current.
9. While preparing the medication, check the drug label against the MAR for accuracy.
10. If a unit dose is prescribed, open the packet at the patient's bedside.
11. If a liquid is prescribed, measure it in a calibrated syringe and put it into a drug cup (see Fig. 10.2).
12. Never leave medications unattended.

Administration
13. Administer only drugs that you have prepared.
14. Identify patients using at least two patient identifiers (e.g., name and birth date). Compare the patient's name and birth date on the MAR, computer printout, or EHR with the information on the patient's identification (ID) bracelet. If possible, ask patients to state their name and birth date.
15. Assist patients into an appropriate position, depending on the route of administration.
16. Compare labels on medications with the MAR prior to administering drugs to a patient.
17. Explain each medication and its action to the patient.
18. For patients who cannot hold medications, place the cup to their lips. Introduce one drug at a time, and do not rush the patient.
19. Stay with the patient until all the medications have been taken.
20. Dispose of used supplies and perform hand hygiene.
21. Evaluate the patient's response to the medications.
22. Educate patients and family members about medication actions and side effects.

Recording
23. Report any drug errors immediately to the patient's health care provider and to the nurse manager; complete an incident report per your facility's policy.
24. Record effectiveness and results of medication administered, especially medications administered as needed (prn).
25. Record drugs that were refused and report these to the patient's health care provider along with the reason given for the refusal.
26. Record the amount of fluid taken with medications on an input and output chart.

CRITICAL THINKING CASE STUDY

Ms. C.J., a patient on the medical-surgical unit, was admitted 2 days before with a diagnosis of exacerbation of heart failure. This morning her blood pressure is 175/80 mm Hg. She denies chest pain but states that she has been experiencing shortness of breath. She tells the nurse she uses three pillows to be able to breathe at night while sleeping. Her baseline weight at admission was 170 lb, but this morning's scale indicates a 4-lb weight gain, and +3 pitting edema to the lower extremities is evident. The nurse telephones the doctor and receives an order for furosemide 40 mg by mouth (PO) twice daily and metoprolol 25 mg PO daily to start immediately.

1. How will the nurse identify Ms. C.J. prior to administering medications?

2. Which labs should the nurse review prior to administering furosemide and metoprolol?
3. What safety measures should the nurse use when obtaining the medications from the Pyxis system and administering the drugs to Ms. C.J.?
4. The nurse scans the medications in the electronic health record (EHR) and medication administration record (MAR) and administers the metoprolol. When she attempts to administer the furosemide, the patient states, "I don't want the water pill." What is the nurse's next action?
5. What important information should the nurse document into Ms. C.J.'s medical record 30 minutes after administering the medications?

NCLEX STUDY QUESTIONS

1. A patient asks about disposal of medications. What are the nurse's best responses? (Select all that apply.)
   a. Mix medications with coffee grounds or cat litter before disposal.
   b. Pour medications down the sink.
   c. Remove identifying information on the original container.
   d. Pulverize all tablets before disposal.
   e. Dilute the medication with bleach before disposal.

2. The nurse educator on the unit receives a list of high-alert drugs. Which strategy is recommended to decrease the risk of errors with these medications? (Select all that apply.)
   a. Store medications alphabetically on an easy-access shelf for quick retrieval.
   b. Limit access to these drugs.
   c. Use special labels for these drugs.
   d. Provide increased information to staff.
   e. Standardize the ordering and preparation of these drugs.

3. The nurse is aware that The Joint Commission has recommended which abbreviation be on the "Do Not Use" list for ordering or documenting medications?
   a. qd
   b. NPO
   c. Subling
   d. bid

4. A patient refuses to take the prescribed medication. Which is the nurse's best response to this patient?
   a. Explain the benefits and side effects of the drug.
   b. Leave the medication at the patient's bedside to be taken later.
   c. Persuade the patient to take the medication.
   d. Explain the risks of not taking the medication.

5. What information is essential for the nurse to know related to right documentation? (Select all that apply.)
   a. The necessity to document all medications given at the end of a shift
   b. The correct site of injectable medication
   c. Patient response to an antiemetic
   d. Patient's blood pressure prior to giving an antihypertensive
   e. Date and time of dose and necessity for the nurse's initials/signature

6. The nurse prepares to administer medications. Which are complete drug orders? (Select all that apply.)
   a. Aspirin 81 mg PO daily
   b. Multivitamin
   c. Vitamin D 2000 units PO
   d. Ciprofloxacin hydrochloride (Cipro) 500 mg PO q12h × 7d
   e. Promethazine 50 mg IV q3-6h PRN for nausea

Answers: 1, a, c; 2, b, c, d, e; 3, a; 4, d; 5, b, c, d, e; 6, a, d, e.

10

Drug Administration

http://evolve.elsevier.com/McCuistion/pharmacology

OBJECTIVES

- Identify the different routes of administration.
- Compare and contrast the various sites for parenteral therapy.
- Explain the equipment and technique used in parenteral therapy.
- Explain the Z-track intramuscular injection technique.
- Analyze the nursing interventions related to administration of medications by various routes.
- Apply the nursing process to the administration of medication.

OUTLINE

KEY TERMS

Administration of medications is a complex but routine nursing activity, and nurses play a significant role in preparing, administering, teaching, and evaluating their patients' responses to the drugs they administer. Whether in an acute care, clinic, restorative, or home setting, nurses work closely with patients and their family members. Patients must receive adequate training to self-administer medications upon discharge, therefore nurses must be knowledgeable about the many aspects of drug administration that include pharmacology, pharmacokinetics, safety practices, and legal aspects of medication administration along with anatomy and physiology and dosage calculations. Nurses must have specific knowledge concerning their patients' diagnoses, allergies, diagnostics, and laboratory results (see Chapter 9).

SELF-ADMINISTRATION OF MEDICATION

The Institute for Safe Medication Practices (ISMP) website offers a booklet for safe practices in self-medication administration for consumers and the health care professionals responsible for teaching and evaluating consumers. The free booklet is called "Your Medicine: Play It Safe," available at https://www.ismp.org/consumers/safemeds.pdf.

FORMS AND ROUTES OF DRUG ADMINISTRATION

A variety of forms and routes are used for the administration of drugs. These include sublingual, buccal, oral (tablets, capsules,

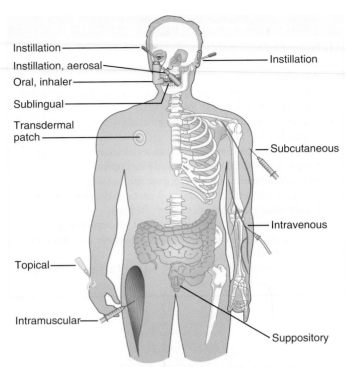

Instillation
Instillation, aerosal
Oral, inhaler
Sublingual
Transdermal patch
Topical
Intramuscular

Instillation
Subcutaneous
Intravenous
Suppository

FIG. 10.1 Routes for Medication Administration.

liquids, suspensions, and elixirs), transdermal, topical, instillation (drops and sprays), inhalation, nasogastric and gastrostomy tubes, **suppositories**, and parenteral forms (Fig. 10.1).

Tablets and Capsules

- Tablets and capsules are the most common drug forms; they are convenient and less expensive and do not require additional supplies for administration.
- Oral drugs are not given to patients who are vomiting, who lack a gag reflex, or who are comatose.
- Do not mix a drug with large amounts of foods or beverages. Patients may not be able to consume them and will not get the full dose of medication. Do not mix drugs in infant formula.
- Enteric-coated and timed-release capsules must be swallowed whole to maintain a therapeutic drug level. If crushed, the initial excessive drug release poses a risk of toxicity such that it could lead to a potentially fatal overdose. Crushing can increase the rate of absorption, and it can cause oropharyngeal irritation. To maintain a therapeutic drug level, enteric-coated and timed-release medications must be swallowed whole so the drug is released gradually. These medications should never be cut in half or crushed for administration. Advise the patient or family member to notify the health care provider or pharmacist if the patient is having difficulty swallowing the medication. Instruct the patient to never cut or crush medications unless advised by the health care provider or pharmacist that cutting or crushing is safe. In acute care settings, the nurse should follow the agency's policy for changing or altering drugs. Most policies indicate to notify the health care provider or pharmacist if the patient is unable to swallow the drug. Many drugs can be given in liquid or intravenous (IV) form or in a non–extended-release form.

- Be aware of medications with "extended release" in the name that should never be cut in half or crushed (e.g., guaifenesin tablets can be changed to liquid form).
- Administer irritating drugs with food to decrease gastrointestinal (GI) discomfort.
- Administer drugs on an empty stomach if food interferes with medication absorption.
- Drugs given via **sublingual** (under the tongue) or **buccal** (between the cheek and gum) routes remain in place until fully absorbed, therefore no food or fluid should be taken while the medication is in place.
- If patients have difficulty opening child-resistant caps, have them request non–child-resistant caps from the pharmacist.

Liquids

- Forms of liquid medication include elixirs, emulsions, and suspensions. *Elixirs* are sweetened, hydroalcoholic liquids used in the preparation of oral liquid medications. *Emulsions* are a mixture of two liquids that are not mutually soluble. *Suspensions* are liquids in which particles are mixed but not dissolved.
- Read the labels to determine whether diluting or shaking is required.
- Make sure your facility has plastic dosing cups that measure in milliliters and not the archaic drams. One dram is equivalent to 3.7 mL. To avoid mix-ups, it is always best to measure the prescribed dose of liquid medication in a syringe calibrated for milliliters (mL) and to then squirt the medication into the oral measuring cup. According to the U.S. Pharmacopeial Convention (USP), a proposed change is required for all facilities to supply dosing cups with legible markings in metric units (Fig. 10.2).

Transdermals

- **Transdermal** medication is stored in a patch placed on the skin and is absorbed through the skin to produce a systemic effect. A patch may be left in place for as little as 12 hours or as long as 7 days depending on the drug. Transdermal drugs provide more consistent blood levels than oral and injectable forms, and they avoid GI absorption problems associated with oral products. To prevent skin breakdown, transdermal patches should be rotated to different sites and should not be reapplied over the exact same area every time. Additionally, the area should be thoroughly cleansed before administration of a new transdermal patch.
- Perform hand hygiene and apply gloves when administering medicated patches to prevent transfer of medication; advise the patient to do the same for self-administration. Never cut the patch in half.
- Advise patients to secure the patch with tape, being careful not to apply the tape too tightly, which could alter the drug delivery.

Topicals

- **Topical** medications are most frequently applied to the skin by painting or spreading the medication over an area and applying a moist dressing or leaving the area exposed to air. Such medications can be applied to the skin in several ways,

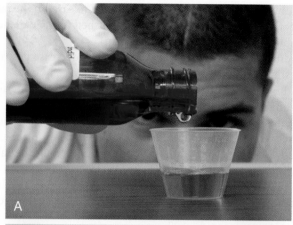

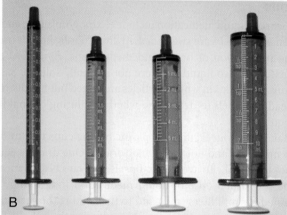

FIG. 10.2 A, Pour desired volume of liquid so base of meniscus is level with mL increment on plastic dosing cup. B, Measure liquid medication in a mL syringe and squirt liquid into dosing cup. From Potter, P. A., et al. (2017). *Fundamentals of nursing* (9th ed.). St. Louis: Elsevier.

such as with a glove, tongue blade, or cotton-tipped applicator. Nurses should never apply a topical medication without first protecting their own skin with gloves.

- Use the appropriate technique to remove the medication from the container, and apply it to clean, dry skin when possible. Do not contaminate the drug in a container; instead, use gloves or an applicator.
- Gloves and applicators that come in contact with a patient should not be reinserted into the container. Estimate the amount needed and remove it from the container, or use a fresh sterile applicator each time the container is entered.

Instillations

Instillations are liquid medications usually administered as drops, ointments, or sprays in the following forms:
- Eyedrops (Box 10.1 and Fig. 10.3)
- Eye ointments (Box 10.2 and Fig. 10.4)
- Eardrops (Box 10.3 and Fig. 10.5)
- Nose drops and sprays (Box 10.4 and Figs. 10.6 and 10.7)

Inhalations

- Metered-dose inhalers (MDIs) are handheld devices used to deliver a number of commonly prescribed asthma and

---

BOX 10.1   Administration of Eyedrops

1. Perform hand hygiene and wear gloves.
2. Instruct patients to lie down or sit back in a chair, and have them look at the ceiling.
3. Remove any discharge by gently wiping from the inner to outer canthus. Use a separate cloth for each eye.
4. Gently draw the skin down below the affected eye to expose the conjunctival sac (see Fig. 10.3).
5. Notify patients immediately before drops are administered so they are prepared to avoid blinking when drops hit the conjunctiva.
6. Administer the prescribed number of drops into the center of the sac. If the drug is placed directly on the cornea, it can cause discomfort or damage. Avoid touching eyelids or eyelashes with the dropper.
   a. Gently press on the lacrimal duct with a sterile cotton ball or tissue for 1 to 2 minutes after instillation to prevent systemic absorption through the lacrimal canal.
   b. Instruct patients to keep their eyes closed for 1 to 2 minutes after application to promote absorption.

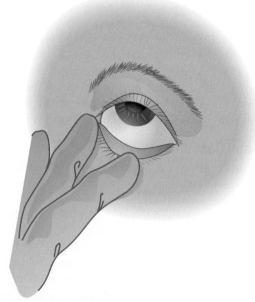

FIG. 10.3 Administering Eyedrops. Gently pull down on the skin below the eye to expose the conjunctival sac. Apply drops to the middle third of the sac, and apply gentle pressure over the lacrimal duct after administration.

bronchitis drugs to the lower respiratory tract (Box 10.5) via inhalation. When the airway becomes constricted, the drug is needed quickly. When properly used, MDIs get up to 12% to 14% of the drug deep into the lungs with each puff. MDIs act faster than drugs taken by mouth, and fewer side effects occur because the drug goes right to the lungs and not to other parts of the body. Some MDIs have a counter to indicate the number of inhalations used. For those that do not, ask the pharmacist the number of inhalations the inhaler will provide, then count the number of inhalations used. Every effort should be made to have the patient know how much medication is in the canister and to anticipate and obtain refills in a timely manner.

BOX 10.2 Administration of Eye Ointment

1. Perform hand hygiene and wear gloves.
2. Instruct patients to lie down or sit down, and have them look at the ceiling.
3. Remove any discharge by gently wiping outward from the inner canthus. Use a separate cloth for each eye.
4. Gently draw the skin down below the affected eye to expose the conjunctival sac.
5. Prepare patients by explaining that ointment will be placed in the eye so they can help by not blinking.
6. Squeeze a strip of ointment (about ¼ inch unless stated otherwise) onto the conjunctival sac (see Fig. 10.4). Medication placed directly on the cornea can cause discomfort or damage. Avoid touching eyelids or eyelashes with the applicator tip.
7. Instruct patients to close their eyes for 2 to 3 minutes.
8. Instruct patients to expect blurred vision for a short time. If possible, apply at bedtime.

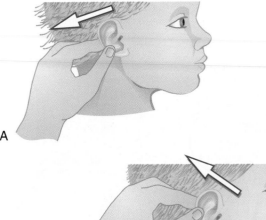
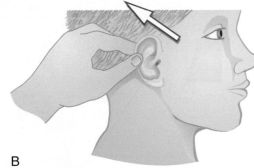

A

B

FIG. 10.5 Administering Eardrops. A, Straighten the external ear canal by pulling the auricle down and back in children under 3 years of age. B, In patients older than 3 years of age, including adults, pull the auricle upward and outward.

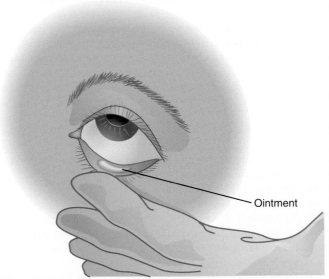

Ointment

FIG. 10.4 Administering Eye Ointment. Squeeze a ¼-inch–wide strip of ointment into the conjunctival sac.

BOX 10.4 Administration of Nose Drops and Sprays

1. Perform hand hygiene and wear gloves.
2. Advise patients to blow their nose.
3. Advise patients to tilt the head back for drops to reach the frontal sinus and to tilt the head to the affected side to reach the ethmoid sinus (see Figs. 10.6 and 10.7).
4. Administer the prescribed number of drops or sprays without touching the tip of the medication applicator to the nasal passages.
5. Some sprays have instructions to close one nostril, tilt the head to the closed side, and hold the breath or breathe through the nose for 1 minute.
6. If a patient is using a nasal spray to reach the sinuses, proper head position is with the patient looking down at the feet with the spray tip aimed toward the eye.
7. Advise the patient to keep the head tilted back for 5 minutes after instillation of drops.

BOX 10.3 Administration of Eardrops

1. Perform hand hygiene and wear gloves.
2. Ensure the medication is at room temperature.
3. Instruct patients to sit up with the head tilted slightly toward the unaffected side. This position straightens the external ear canal for better visualization. Maintain this position for 2 to 3 minutes to facilitate drops reaching the affected area (see Fig. 10.5).
4. Pull down and back on the auricle for a child younger than 3 years of age. For a child older than 3 years or an adult, pull upward and outward on the auricle.
5. Instill the prescribed number of drops. Take measures to avoid allowing drops to fall directly on the tympanic membrane. Drops should be aimed at the side of the ear canal and should be allowed to run down into the ear.
6. Do not contaminate the dropper.

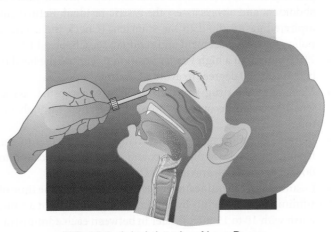

FIG. 10.6 Administering Nose Drops.

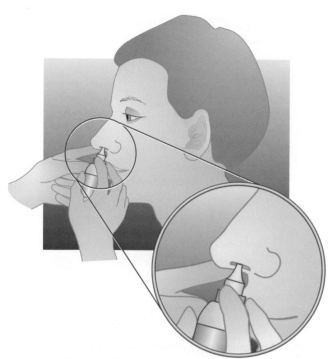

FIG. 10.7 Administering Nasal Spray.

- Take special measures when handling the capsules used in some MDIs to prevent the transfer of medication (e.g., powder from a punctured capsule can get on the nurse's hands and transfer to the eyes or absorb into the skin).
- Spacers are devices used to enhance the delivery of medications from the MDI (Fig. 10.8). A *nebulizer* is a device that changes a liquid medication into a fine mist or aerosol that has the ability to reach the lower, smaller airways. Handheld nebulizers deliver a very fine particle in a spray of medication.
- When administering drugs via an MDI or nebulizer, the preferred patient position is the semi-Fowler or high Fowler position.
- Instruct the patient on the correct use and cleaning of MDIs or nebulizers.

Nasogastric and Gastrostomy Tubes

- Before administering drugs, always check for proper tube placement of any feeding tube that enters the mouth, nose, or abdomen, and always assess the gastric residual. Return any aspirated gastric fluid to the stomach. (Check the agency's policy for tube placement and residual; see Chapter 14.)
- Place patient in a high Fowler position or elevate the head of bed at least 30 degrees to avoid aspiration.
- Make sure the drug is crushable. If it is a capsule, assess whether it can be opened to be administered through the tube.
- Remove the plunger from the syringe and attach it to the feeding tube, release the clamp, and allow the medication to flow in properly by gravity.
- Ensure proper identification of each drug up until the time of administration. Do this by administering one drug at a time. Flush with 10 to 15 mL of water in between each administration to maintain patency of the tubing.

BOX 10.5   Correct Use of a Metered-Dose Inhaler

1. Explain what a metered dose is, and warn the patient about overuse and side effects of the drug.
2. Explain the steps for administering drug using a squeeze-and-breathe metered-dose inhaler (MDI), and demonstrate the steps when possible. Consult a pharmacist for details if necessary.
3. Insert the medication canister into the plastic holder.
4. If a spacer is used, insert the MDI into the end of the spacer.
5. Shake the inhaler vigorously five or six times before using. Remove the cap from the mouthpiece.
6. Have the patient breathe out through the mouth and exhale.
7. An MDI may be positioned in one of two ways:
   a. With the mouth closed around the MDI with the opening toward the back of the throat
   b. With the device positioned 1 to 2 inches from the mouth
   c. If a spacer is used, the patient closes the mouth around the mouthpiece of the spacer. Avoid covering the small exhalation slots with the lips.
8. With the inhaler properly positioned, have the patient hold the inhaler with the thumb at the mouthpiece and the index finger and middle finger at the top (see Fig. 10.8).
9. Instruct the patient to take a slow, deep breath through the mouth and during inspiration, to push the top of the medication canister once.
10. Have patients hold the breath for 10 seconds then exhale slowly through pursed lips.
11. If a second dose is required, wait 1 to 2 minutes, and repeat the procedure by first shaking the canister in the plastic holder with the cap on.
12. When it is first used or if it has not been used recently, test the inhaler by spraying it into the air before administering the metered dose.
13. If a glucocorticoid inhalant is to be used with a bronchodilator, wait 5 minutes before using an inhaler that contains a steroid.
14. Teach patients to self-monitor their pulse rate.
15. Caution against overuse because side effects and tolerance may result.
16. Teach patients to monitor the amount of medication remaining in the canister. Advise patients to ask a health care provider or pharmacist to estimate when a new inhaler will be needed based on the dosing schedule.
17. Teach patients to rinse their mouth after using an MDI. This is especially important when using a steroid drug. Rinsing the mouth helps to prevent irritation and secondary infection to oral mucosa.
18. Advise patients to avoid smoking.
19. Teach patients to do daily cleaning of equipment; this should include (1) washing the hands; (2) taking apart all the washable parts of the equipment and washing them with warm water; (3) rinsing; (4) placing the parts on a clean towel and covering them with another clean towel to air dry; and (5) storing the parts in a clean plastic bag once completely dry. Alternate two sets of washable equipment to make this process easier.

- When finished with drug administration, flush tubing with 30 mL of water or whichever amount is recommended by the agency's policy. Always record the amount of water used with the administration of drugs on the patient's input sheet.
- Clamp the tube and remove the syringe.
- If the patient has a nasogastric tube to suction, clamp the tube for 30 minutes to allow medication to be absorbed before placing the patient back on suction.

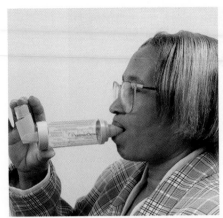

FIG. 10.8 Metered-Dose Inhaler With a Spacer. (From Potter, P. A., et al. (2017). *Fundamentals of nursing* (9th ed.). St. Louis: Elsevier.)

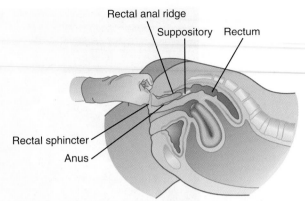

FIG. 10.9 Inserting a Rectal Suppository.

Suppositories

A suppository is a solid medical preparation that is cone- or spindle-shaped for insertion into the rectum, globular or egg-shaped for use in the vagina, or pencil-shaped for insertion into the urethra. Suppositories are made from glycerinated gelatin or high-molecular weight polyethylene glycols and are common vehicles for a variety of drugs. A suppository is a useful route in babies, in uncooperative patients, and in cases of vomiting or certain digestive disorders.

Rectal Suppositories

- Medications administered as suppositories or enemas can be given rectally for local and systemic absorption. The numerous small capillaries in the rectal area promote medication absorption.
- The foil around the suppository is removed, and the suppository may be lubricated before insertion.
- During insertion, place the suppository past the internal anal sphincter; otherwise, the suppository will be expelled before it can dissolve and be absorbed into the mucosa.
- Some suppositories tend to soften at room temperature and therefore may be refrigerated before use.
- Explain administration procedures to the patient and provide for patient privacy.
- Use gloves for insertion.
- Instruct the patient to lie in the Sims position and to breathe slowly through the mouth to relax the anal sphincter.
- Apply a small amount of water-soluble lubricant to the tip of the unwrapped suppository, and gently insert the suppository beyond the internal sphincter (Fig. 10.9).
- Ask the patient to remain flat or on one side for at least 30 minutes to prevent expulsion of the suppository.
- Observe for effects of the suppository that correlate with the medication's onset, peak, and duration.

Vaginal Medications

Vaginal drugs are available as suppositories, foams, jellies, or creams. They are individually packaged in foil wrappers and are sometimes stored in the refrigerator to prevent the solid,

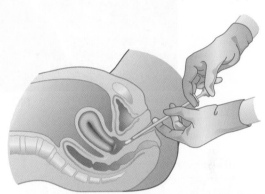

FIG. 10.10 Inserting a Vaginal Suppository.

oval-shaped suppositories from melting. Foams, jellies, creams, and suppositories are generally inserted into the vagina with an applicator supplied with the medication (Fig. 10.10); gloves should be worn, and the patient should be in the lithotomy position. Advise patients to remain lying for a time sufficient to allow medication absorption; times vary depending on the medication. After insertion, provide the patient with a sanitary pad. If the patient is able, she may want to insert vaginal drugs herself.

Parenteral Administration of Medications

Safety is a special concern with parenteral drugs, which are administered via injection. Manufacturers have responded with safety features to help decrease or eliminate needlestick injuries and possible transfer of blood-borne diseases such as hepatitis and human immunodeficiency virus (HIV; Fig. 10.11 shows examples of safety needles). Methods of parenteral administration include intradermal, subcutaneous, intramuscular, Z-track technique, intravenous, and intraosseous administration. A description of each follows with special considerations noted for the pediatric patient.

Intradermal (ID)

Action
- Local effect
- Administered for skin testing (e.g., tuberculin screening, allergy testing and testing for other drug sensitivities, some immunotherapy for cancer).

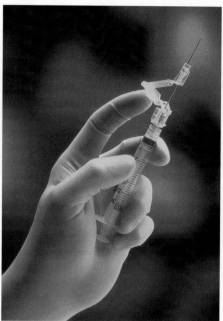
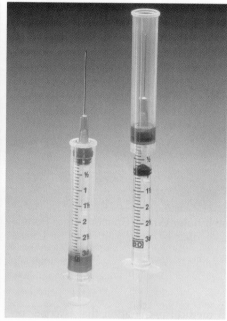

FIG. 10.11 Safety Needles.

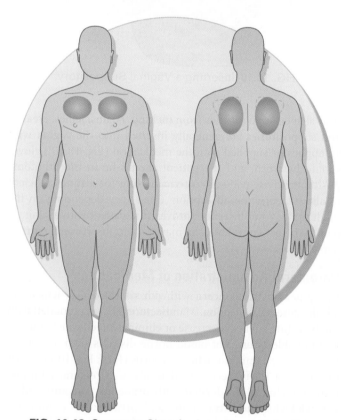

FIG. 10.12 Common Sites for Intradermal Injection.

Sites

- Locations are chosen so an inflammatory reaction can be observed. Preferred areas are lightly pigmented, free of lesions, and hairless such as the ventral mid-forearm, clavicular area of the chest, or scapular area of the back (Fig. 10.12).

Equipment

- Needle: 25 to 27 gauge, ¼ to ½ inch long, tuberculin syringe
  Syringe: 1 mL calibrated in increments of (0.01) hundredth mL represented on syringe as 0.1 mL to 1 mL. Syringe holds up to 1 mL of solution; however, tuberculin skin tests require injection of a small amount of solution (usually 0.01 to 0.1 mL) to ensure formation of bleb.

Technique

- Perform hand hygiene and wear gloves.
- Cleanse the area with a circular motion using aseptic technique.
- Hold the skin taut.
- Insert the needle, bevel up, at a 10- to 15-degree angle; the outline of the needle should be visible under the skin (Fig. 10.13).
- Inject the medication slowly to form a bleb (or wheal). A small amount is injected so the volume will not interfere with bleb formation or cause a systemic reaction. If the bleb does not appear, the needle has been injected subcutaneously. Document according to facility policy and inform the health care provider. The nurse may need to obtain orders to repeat the procedure.
- Remove the needle slowly, and do not recap it.
- Do *not* massage the area, and also instruct the patient not to do so.
- Mark the area with a pen, and ask the patient not to wash it off until the response can be "read" by a health care provider.
- It is not recommended to put an adhesive bandage over the testing site because it can alter the results of the test.
- Assess for allergic reaction in 24 to 72 hours; measure the diameter of any local reaction. For tuberculin testing, measure only the indurated area; do not include the area of erythema in the measurement.

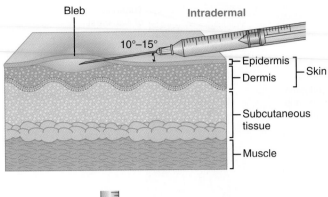

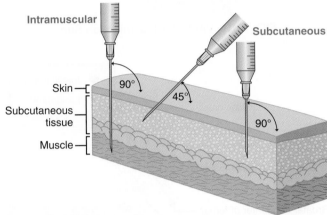

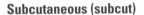

FIG. 10.13 Needle Angles for Intradermal, Subcutaneous, and Intramuscular Injections.

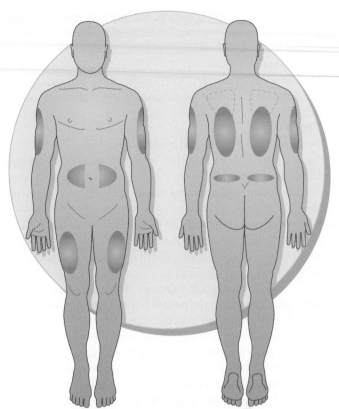

FIG. 10.14 Common Sites for Subcutaneous Injections.

Subcutaneous (subcut)

Action

- Systemic effect
- Sustained effect; absorbed mainly through capillaries; usually slower in onset than with the intramuscular (IM) route.

Sites

- Locations for subcut injections are chosen for adequate fat-pad size. Areas such as the upper outer aspect of the arms; the abdomen, at least 2 inches from the umbilicus, and the anterior thighs are important subcut sites (Fig. 10.14). Sites should be rotated with subcut injections, such as with insulin and heparin.
- Usually, 0.5 to 1 mL of solution is given subcutaneously. A larger amount (2 mL) of medication may have to be divided and administered at two sites. Larger amounts add to the patient's discomfort and predispose to poor absorption. Refer to agency policy for the maximum amount of medication to be administered via this route.

Equipment

- Needle: 25 to 27 gauge; ⅜ to ⅝ inch long
- The length of the needle and the angle of the needle insertion are based on the amount of subcutaneous tissue present. The shorter, ⅜-inch needle should be inserted at a 90-degree angle, and the longer, ⅝-inch needle is inserted at a 45-degree angle (see Fig. 10.13).
- Syringe: 1 to 3 mL (injection of solution is usually 0.5 to 1 mL)
- Insulin syringe measured in units for use with insulin only

Technique

- Perform hand hygiene and wear gloves.
- Cleanse the area with a circular motion using aseptic technique.
- Grasp or gently pinch the area of the patient's loose fatty tissue with the fingers of your nondominant hand.
- Insert the needle quickly.
- Release the pinch and use the hand to stabilize the syringe.
- Do not aspirate.
- Inject the medication slowly.
- Remove the needle quickly; do not recap.
- Apply gentle pressure to the injection site to prevent bleeding or oozing into the tissue with subsequent bruising and tissue damage, especially if the patient is on anticoagulant therapy.
- Apply a bandage if needed.

Intramuscular (IM)

Action

- Systemic effect
- Usually a more rapid effect of drug than with a subcut route
- Used for solutions that are more viscous and irritating for adults, children, and infants
- IM injections are associated with many risks, so the nurse should use accurate, careful technique when administering an IM injection and should check the agency's policy.

Sites. Locations are chosen for adequate muscle size and minimal major nerves and blood vessels in the area. Other considerations include the volume of drug administered, needle size, angle of injection, patient position, site location, and advantages and disadvantages of the site. Underweight patients should be evaluated for sites with adequate muscle.

Equipment
- Needle: 18 to 25 gauge; ⅝ to 1½ inches long. Patient's weight, age, and the amount of adipose tissue influence needle length.

Technique
- Perform hand hygiene and apply gloves.
- Same as for subcut injection with two exceptions: Flatten the skin area using the thumb and index finger and inject between them, and insert the needle at a 90-degree angle into the muscle (see Fig. 10.13).
- Syringe: 1 to 3 mL (usually no more than 1 to 1.5 mL of solution is injected), although this varies based on the intended site, the age of the patient, and the developed muscle site. (Check the agency's policy.)

Preferred Intramuscular Injection Sites. Table 10.1 shows the four sites along with the patient positioning and advantages and disadvantages of each injection site.

- *Ventrogluteal* (Fig. 10.15). Located near the gluteus medius, a deep muscle, and away from major nerves, this site is well suited for Z-track injections. Volume of drug is 1 to 1.5 mL, administered with an 18- to 25-gauge, 1½-inch needle. The gauge and length of the needle depends on the medication to be administered and the size of the patient. Slightly angle the needle toward the iliac crest. The ventrogluteal is the preferred site for most injections given to adults and all children, including infants of any age.
- *Dorsogluteal* (Fig. 10.16). Do not use this site for IM injections. Studies have demonstrated that the exact location of the sciatic nerve varies from person to person, and if a needle hits the sciatic nerve, the client can experience an adverse outcome, including permanent or partial paralysis of the involved leg.
- *Deltoid* (Fig. 10.17). This muscle is easy to find, but it is not well developed in many adults. The volume of drug administered is 0.5 to 1 mL, with a 23- to 25-gauge, ⅝- to 1½-inch needle. Place the needle at a 90-degree angle to the skin or slightly toward the acromion. There is risk for injury because of the nerves and arteries that lie within the upper arm along the humerus. Use this site for small medication volumes or when other sites are inaccessible. This site is not used in infants or children due to underdeveloped muscles.
- *Vastus lateralis* (Fig. 10.18). The vastus lateralis is a good site for multiple injections. It is frequently used in infants (less than 12 months) receiving immunizations and is often used in older children and toddlers receiving immunizations. If a long needle is used, insert it with caution to avoid sciatic nerve or femoral structures. The volume of drug administered is 0.5 mL in infants (maximum [max] 1 mL), 1 mL in pediatric patients, and 1 to 1.5 mL in adults (max 2 mL).

Z-Track Injection Technique. The Z-track injection technique shown in Fig. 10.19 is recommended when administering IM injections to help minimize local skin irritation by

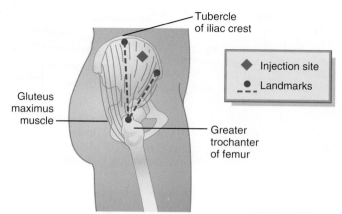

FIG. 10.15 Ventrogluteal Injection Site.

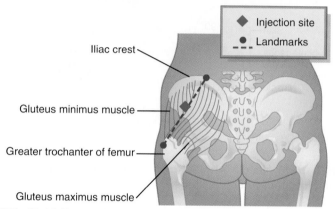

FIG. 10.16 Dorsogluteal Injection Site. This site is no longer used.

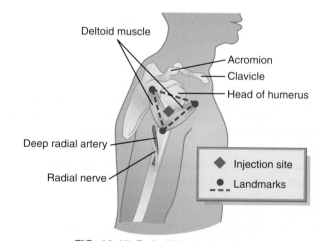

FIG. 10.17 Deltoid Injection Site.

sealing the medication in the muscle tissue. The ventrogluteal site is preferred. Using aseptic technique, draw up the medication. Replace the first needle with a second needle of appropriate gauge and length to penetrate the muscle tissue and to deliver the medication to the selected site. Holding the skin taut, inject the needle deep into the muscle, and if there is no blood return on aspiration, slowly inject the medication. Allow the needle to remain inserted for 10 seconds for the

TABLE 10.1   Intramuscular Injection Sites: Patient Position, Advantages, and Disadvantages

Site	Patient Position	Anatomic Landmark
Ventrogluteal	Supine, lateral	Locate the ventrogluteal muscle by placing the heel of the hand over the greater trochanter of the patient's hip with the wrists perpendicular to the femur. Use the right hand for the patient's left hip and the left hand for the right hip. Point the thumb toward the patient's groin, the index finger toward the anterior superior iliac spine, and extend the middle finger back along the iliac crest toward the buttock. The index finger, the middle finger, and the iliac crest form a V-shaped triangle; the injection site is the center of the triangle (see Fig. 10.15). The ventrogluteal is the preferred site for most injections given to adults and all children, including infants of any age.
Dorsogluteal	Prone	This site is no longer used because it is detrimental to the patient.
Deltoid	Lateral, prone, sitting, supine	Palpate the lower edge of the patient's acromion process, which forms the base of a triangle in line with the midpoint of the lateral aspect of the upper arm. The injection site is in the center of the triangle, about 1 to 2 inches below the acromion process. Or locate the site by placing four fingers across the deltoid muscle with the top finger along the acromion process. The injection site is then three fingerwidths below the acromion process (see Fig. 10.17).
Vastus lateralis	Sitting, supine Flex knee to help relax muscle if supine	Located on the anterior lateral aspect of the thigh, it extends in an adult from a handbreadth above the knee to a handbreath below the greater trochanter of the femur. Use the middle third of the muscle for injection. With young children or cachectic patients, it helps to grasp the body of the muscle during injection to ensure delivery of the drug into the muscle. Vastus lateralis is frequently used in infants (less than 12 months) receiving immunizations and is often used in older children and toddlers receiving immunizations. (see Fig. 10.18).

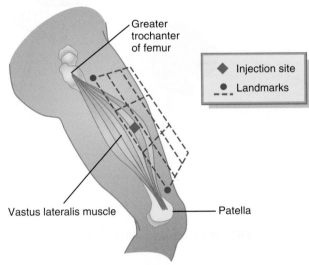

FIG. 10.18 Vastus Lateralis Injection Site in Children.

medication to disperse evenly rather than channeling back up the track of the needle.

Intravenous (IV)

Action
- Systemic effect
- More rapid than IM or subcut routes

Sites. Accessible peripheral veins are preferred (e.g., cephalic or cubital vein of arm, dorsal vein of hand; Fig. 10.20). When possible, ask the patient about his or her preference, and avoid needless body restriction. In newborns, the veins of the feet, lower legs, and head may also be used after other sites have been exhausted.

Equipment
- Needle
  - Adults: 20 to 21 gauge, 1 to 1½ inches
  - Infants: 24 gauge, 1 inch
  - Children: 22 gauge, 1 inch
- Larger bore for viscous drugs and whole blood and a large volume for rapid infusion
- Electronic IV delivery device, an infusion controller, or pump
- May use a mixture of lidocaine/prilocaine anesthetic if appropriate

Technique
- Perform hand hygiene and apply gloves.
- Apply a tourniquet.
- Apply anesthetic 1 hour before the procedure on unbroken skin.
- Cleanse the area using aseptic technique with an appropriate solution.
- Insert a butterfly or catheter, and feed it up into the vein until blood returns. Remove the tourniquet.
- Stabilize the needle or IV catheter, and apply dressing to site.
- Flush the catheter with sodium chloride or sterile water to check for site patency.
- Monitor flow rate, distal pulses, skin color and temperature, and insertion site.
- Consult agency policy regarding IV fluids, intermittent IV (IVPB), and direct IV (IV push) drugs. The pharmacy adds medications to the IV bag to avoid error; except in some specialty areas that allow it, nurses should *never* add medications to the bag.

Intraosseous (IO)

The intraosseous (IO) method of drug administration involves the infusion of medication directly into the bone marrow (Fig. 10.21). IO administration is used when IV access is not possible; it is maintained for 24 to 72 hours, after which another means of access is obtained. It is mostly used in infants and toddlers who have poor IV access and in emergency situations when IV access is impossible. Contraindications include fracture in the insertion limb, infection at the insertion site, severe osteoporosis, and other bone abnormalities.

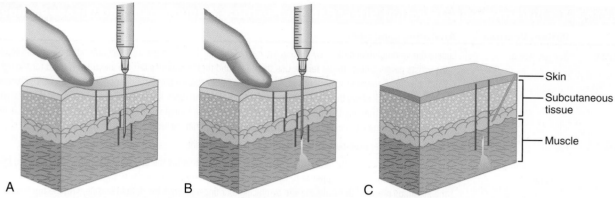

FIG. 10.19 Z-Track Injection. A, Use a deep muscle, such as in the ventrogluteal injection, and pull skin approximately 1 to 1½ inches laterally to one side, and hold it taut with the nondominant hand. B, Inject the needle deep into the muscle, and if no blood returns on aspiration, slowly inject the medication. C, Wait 10 seconds before withdrawing the needle and releasing the skin. This technique prevents medication entering subcutaneous tissue.

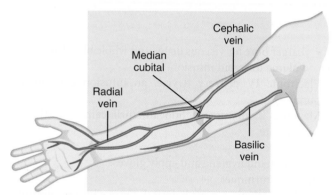

FIG. 10.20 Common Sites for Intravenous Administration.

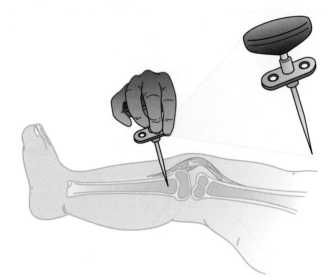

FIG. 10.21 Intraosseous Access.

NURSING IMPLICATIONS FOR ADMINISTRATION OF PARENTERAL MEDICATIONS

Sites

- The ventrogluteal site is preferred for IM injections in adults and children, including infants of any age, because the gluteal muscle is a deep muscle, situated away from major nerves and blood vessels.
- For infants less than 12 months and toddlers not walking alone, the vastus lateralis is the preferred site for immunizations.
- The dorsogluteal muscle is no longer used for IM injections. Research has shown that if this site is used, the patient can experience serious complications.

Equipment

- The syringe size should approximate the volume of medication to be administered.
- Use the tuberculin syringe for amounts less than 1 mL.
- Use the filter needle to draw up drugs taken from a glass vial or ampule. Change the needle before administration to prevent tissue irritation from any glass fragment or drug left on the needle.

Technique

- Perform hand hygiene and apply gloves.
- Correctly identify the patient.
- Explain the procedure to the patient.
- Position the patient.
- Follow the rights of medication administration (see Chapter 9).
- Inspect the site, choose the correct anatomic markers, and assess skin for breakdown.
- Inject the drug slowly to minimize tissue damage.
- Stabilize the skin during needle removal to reduce pain.
- Do not administer injections if sites are inflamed, edematous, or lesioned (e.g., moles, scars).
- Rotate the injection site to enhance absorption of the drug.
- Document the injection site.
- Observe the patient to evaluate drug effectiveness.
- Report any untoward reactions immediately.
- Multiple products are available to reduce the pain of parenteral drug administration (e.g., lidocaine, prilocaine, and benzocaine/tetracaine).

DEVELOPMENTAL NEEDS OF PEDIATRIC PATIENTS

Anticipate patients' developmental needs. Examples of needs associated with administration of medications include the following (refer to Chapter 5 for additional examples):

- Stranger anxiety (infant): Act to instill a sense of safety and security in the infant.
- Hospitalization, illness, or injury viewed as punishment (3 to 6 years of age): Allow control when appropriate; obtain the child's view of the situation; encourage activities, positive relationships, and expression of feelings in an acceptable manner. Include family or support person if appropriate.
- Fear of the procedure (3 to 6 years of age): Explain procedures carefully; use less intrusive routes, such as the oral route, whenever possible; allow children to give "play" injections to a doll or stuffed animal.

TECHNOLOGICAL ADVANCES

Advances in drug administration therapy continue to enhance safety, increase accessibility to sites, promote patient mobility, and improve patient adherence. Examples of these advances include the following:

- Pain-free delivery of insulin through a transdermal patch
- Insulin pumps that deliver insulin based on monitoring of serum glucose level
- Intelligent infusion technology that programs IV infusions based on scanned information
- Aerosolized antibiotics
- Expanding use of medicinal plants in medicine
- Robotic mixing of antineoplastic drugs

Current technological advances found in many facilities today include computerized order entry and electronic medical records systems, electronic medication administration records, bar code administration records, smart pumps, and point-of-care technologies. These advances have been implemented to help reduce medication errors and improve the delivery of safe and effective patient care.

 NURSING PROCESS
Patient-Centered Collaborative Care

Overview of Medication Administration

Assessment
- Obtain appropriate vital signs and relevant laboratory test results for future comparisons and to evaluate therapeutic response.
- Determine the patient's level of consciousness, risk for aspiration, and ability to take medications.
- Obtain a drug history that includes drug allergies.
- Identify patients at high risk for reactions.
- Assess the patient's capability to follow the therapeutic regimen.
- Assess possible contraindications to certain medication regimens.

Nursing Diagnoses
- Injury, Risk for related to possible reaction
- Management, Readiness for Enhanced Learning related to the medication regimen

Planning
- Identify goals.
- Promote therapeutic response and prevent or minimize adverse reactions.
- Identify strategies to promote adherence to the drug regimen.
- Identify interventions that foster patient independence.

Nursing Interventions
- Prepare equipment and environment and perform hand hygiene.
- Check for allergies and other assessment data.
- Check the drug label three times; check the expiration date, and apply the rights of medication administration.
- Be certain of drug calculations; verify the dose with another RN, licensed personnel, or pharmacy as necessary.
- Measure liquids in a milliliter syringe, and squirt the medication into a plastic measuring cup calibrated in milliliters.
- Avoid contact with topical and inhalation preparations by wearing gloves.
- Verify patient by using two patient identifiers.
- Administer only drugs you have prepared.
- Assist the patient into the appropriate position.
- Discard needles and syringes in a sharps container. Do not recap needles.
- Keep all drugs stored properly, especially in regard to temperature, light, and moisture.
- The drug should be identifiable up until the time of patient administration.
- Follow agency policy related to discarding drugs and controlled substances.
- Report drug errors immediately.
- Document all appropriate information in a timely manner.
- Record effectiveness of administered drugs, their side effects or adverse effects, and the reason given when any drug was refused.

Patient Teaching
General
- Emphasize safety.
- Monitor the patient's physical abilities regularly as needed.
- Store medications in original, labeled containers with child-resistant caps when needed.
- Provide patients and family with written instructions about the drug regimen; provide audio instructions if the patient or family are visually impaired or unable to read.
- Advise patients and family about expected therapeutic effects, anticipated onset of action, and expected duration of treatment.
- Educate patients and family on possible side effects or signs of an adverse reaction.

- Instruct patients and family about possible drug–laboratory test interactions.
- Advise patients of nonpharmacologic measures to promote therapeutic response.
- Encourage patients and family to have an adequate supply of necessary medications available.
- Caution against the use of over-the-counter (OTC) preparations, including herbal remedies, without first contacting the health care provider.
- Reinforce the importance of follow-up appointments with a health care provider.
- Encourage patient to wear a medical alert band with drugs or allergies indicated.
- As needed, encourage lifestyle changes associated with drug administration (e.g., smoking cessation, exercise, limiting salt or fat intake).
- Encourage use of community resources to assist with patient and family needs.

Diet
- Advise patients and family about possible drug-food interactions and contraindicated foods, if any.
- Advise patients and family about possible drug-alcohol interactions.

Self-Administration
- Advise patients and family regarding drug dose and dosing schedule.

- Teach patients and family about psychomotor skills related to the drug regimen.
- Provide patients and family with contact information for questions and concerns.

Side Effects
- Counsel patients and family about general side effects and adverse reactions of the medications.
- Teach patients and family to monitor drug effects as appropriate (e.g., check blood pressure if the drug is to treat hypertension).
- Advise patients and family when and how to notify the health care provider.

Cultural Considerations
- Assess personal beliefs of patients and family.
- Modify communications to meet the cultural needs of patients and family.
- Communicate respect for culture and cultural practices of patients and family.

Evaluation
- Evaluate the effectiveness of the drugs administered.
- Identify the expected time frame of the desired response from the drug; consider modification of therapy as needed.
- Determine patient satisfaction with the therapeutic regimen.

CRITICAL THINKING CASE STUDY

Ms. J.B., a diabetic on oral hypoglycemic medication, is being discharged from 24-hour observation care. The health care provider orders regular, subcutaneous (subcut) insulin and syringes. Home health is ordered with instructions for the nurse to provide detailed teaching concerning insulin administration. As the nurse assigned to discharge Ms. J.B., explain the following information included in the discharge teaching about subcut injections:

1. Common subcut injection sites
2. The angle of the needle's insertion
3. How the skin is held prior to inserting the needle
4. Choosing the correct needle gauge for a subcut injection
5. Maximum amounts of solution administered in a subcut site
6. An explanation of what occurs after the needle is inserted
7. The final step after the drug is injected

NCLEX STUDY QUESTIONS

1. The nurse is administering oral medications to a patient. Which are important considerations? (Select all that apply.)
   a. Administer irritating drugs with food.
   b. Avoid mixing medications in infant formula.
   c. Enteric-coated capsules may be chewed or crushed.
   d. Oral medication should be stopped if the patient is vomiting.
   e. Cut all transdermal patches to the correct dose.
2. The clinic nurse is preparing to administer an intradermal injection. Which supplies are most appropriate for this procedure?
   a. A 21-gauge, ⅝-inch needle
   b. A 27-gauge, ⅝-inch needle and a 3-mL syringe
   c. A 25-gauge needle and an insulin syringe
   d. A 25-gauge needle and a tuberculin syringe

3. The nurse is administering an intramuscular injection to a 5-year-old child. Choose the correct site the nurse will use.
   a. Intravenous
   b. Dorsogluteal
   c. Deltoid
   d. Ventrogluteal
4. The nurse administers a variety of drugs to a patient. Which statement by the patient indicates a need for further teaching?
   a. I do not eat or drink when I have sublingual nitroglycerin in place.
   b. I mix all of these meds in my dessert and hope I am not too full to finish it.
   c. I keep the meds in their original labeled containers.
   d. I store medications away from children and pets.

5. The nurse is teaching a patient to use an inhaler. What common teaching point is essential for the nurse to include?
   a. Cleaning the metered-dose inhaler or nebulizer is not recommended.
   b. The semi-Fowler or high Fowler position is recommended.
   c. Spacers decrease delivery of medication.
   d. Nebulizers change medications to a large-particle powder mist.

6. A 3-year-old patient has an intramuscular medication ordered. What is the most appropriate approach to gain the child's cooperation?
   a. Engage the help of a second nurse to hold the child.
   b. Give a pretend injection to a toy animal.
   c. Restrain the patient's upper extremities.
   d. Ask family members to leave the room.

7. The nurse prepares to administer oral medications to a patient. What nursing intervention is needed in addition to the "five-plus-five" rights to ensure safety?
   a. Assess the patient for risk of aspiration.
   b. Mix two of the four medications into the meal.
   c. Administer drugs on a full stomach if food interferes with medication absorption.
   d. Administer irritating drugs without food to decrease gastrointestinal discomfort.

8. A patient is to start on a lidocaine transdermal patch. What is essential for the nurse to include in the patient's teaching? (Select all that apply.)
   a. Wear gloves when applying the patch.
   b. Cut the patch in half if a reduced dose is needed.
   c. Wear gloves when removing the patch.
   d. Rotate placement of patch to different sites.
   e. Remove the patch if it becomes loose.

Answers: 1, a, b, d; 2, d; 3, d; 4, b; 5, b; 6, b; 7, a; 8, a, c, d.

11

Drug Calculations

OVERVIEW

Nurses perform basic mathematical operations on a regular basis when preparing drugs for administration. To accurately calculate drug dosages, a systematic process is used. The same process should be used for every drug calculation so that a step is not missed. Missed steps could lead to errors that may cause serious harm or death to the patient.

This chapter is subdivided into five sections: 11A, Systems of Measurement With Conversion Factors; 11B, Calculation Methods—Enteral and Parenteral Drug Dosages; 11C, Calculating Dosages—Drugs That Require Reconstitution; 11D, Calculation Methods—Insulin Dosages; and 11E, Calculation Methods—Intravenous Flow Rates. Five calculation methods are explained. The three methods generally used are (1) the basic formula, (2) a ratio and proportion/fractional equation, and (3) dimensional analysis. The nurse should select one of these methods for the calculation of drug dosages. The other two methods are used to individualize drug dosing by body weight and body surface area (BSA). Numerous drug labels are used in the drug calculation problems to familiarize the reader with the information on a typical drug label. Answers for the practice problems can be found at the end of each section in this chapter.

To calculate correct dosages, knowing how to convert from one unit to another is essential because this is the basis for most drug calculations. Two systems of measurement, metric and household, are used to measure drugs and solutions. The metric system, also known as the *International System of Units (SI)*, is the internationally accepted system of measure, although the household system is commonly used for community and home settings. Chapter 9 lists and discusses currently approved abbreviations used in drug dosages.

Keeping in mind that the goal is to prepare and administer drugs in a safe and correct manner, the following recommendations are offered:

- Think. Focus on each step of the problem. This applies to both simple and difficult problems.
- Read accurately. Pay particular attention to the location of the decimal point and to the operation to be performed, such as conversion from one system of measurement to another.
- Picture the problem.
- Identify an expected range for the answer. The dose should be *reasonable*.
- Seek to understand the problem. Do not merely master the mechanics of the mathematical operations. Seek a second opinion to ensure that the calculation is correct.
- To decrease drug errors, always perform *three checks* prior to administering a drug: (1) when retrieving the drug from a dispensing system, (2) when preparing the drug, and (3) just prior to administering the drug to the patient.

SECTION 11A: Systems of Measurement With Conversion Factors

ⓔ http://evolve.elsevier.com/McCuistion/pharmacology

OBJECTIVES

- Discuss the metric and household systems of measurement.
- Convert larger units to smaller units and smaller units to larger units within the metric system.
- Convert larger units to smaller units and smaller units to larger units within the household system.
- Convert between metric and household measurements.

OUTLINE

Metric System
  Conversions Within the Metric System
  Practice Problems: Metric System Conversions

Household System
  Conversions Within the Household System
  Practice Problems: Household System Conversions

KEY TERMS

METRIC SYSTEM

The **metric system** is a decimal system based on the power of 10. The basic units of measure used in dosage calculations include the **gram** (g, gm, G, Gm) for weight, **liter** (L) for volume, and **meter** (m, M) for linear measurement or length. Prefixes such as *nano, micro, milli, centi,* and *kilo* indicate the size of the units in powers of 10 of the base unit and stand for a specific degree of magnitude: for instance, *kilo* stands for thousands, *milli* for one thousandth, and *centi* for one hundredth. To be able to convert a quantity, one of the values must be known, such as a gram (g, G), liter (l, L), meter (m), milligram (mg), milliliter (mL), millimeter (mm), or microgram (mcg). Grams, liters, and meters are larger units, whereas milligrams, milliliters, millimeters, and micrograms are smaller units. Because the conversion between degrees of magnitude always involves multiplying by a power of 10, converting from one magnitude to another is relatively easy.

Conversions Within the Metric System

Common conversions used to calculate drug dosages using the metric system are listed in Table 11A.1.

Grams and milligrams are related by three factors of 10 according to this relationship. In the first illustration below, the larger unit (gram) is converted to the smaller unit (milligram). In the second illustration, the smaller unit is converted to the larger unit.

$$1\,g = 1\,mg \times 10^3 = 1000\,mg$$

and

$$1000\,mg = 1\,g \times 10^{-3} = 1\,g$$

The easiest way to convert larger units to smaller units is to move the decimal point the appropriate number of spaces to the *right*. In the illustration below, grams have been converted to milligrams by moving the decimal point three spaces to the right:

$$1\,g = 1.000 = 1000\,mg$$

To convert smaller units to larger units, move the decimal point the appropriate number of spaces to the *left*. In the illustration below, milligrams have been converted to grams by moving the decimal point three spaces to the left (thousandths):

$$1000\,mg = 1.000 = 1\,g$$

Remember: When changing larger units to smaller units, move the decimal point to the *right*; when changing smaller units to larger units, move the decimal point to the *left*. There should always be a zero (0) placed before the decimal point, called a *leading zero,* to alert the reader that the number is less than 1. For example, *0.5* clearly indicates a value of ½. If the number was to be written as *.5,* the reader could mistake the number for *5.* Do not leave extraneous zeroes after a decimal point (trailing zeroes). The reader may perceive a number that is many times larger than the desired dose. For example, *1.0* could be misread as *10.*

TABLE 11A.1 Metric and English Units of Measurement

Units	Equivalent Units of Measurement		
Weight	1 kilogram (kg, Kg)	=	1000 g = 2.2 lb
	1 gram (g, gm, G, Gm)	=	1000 mg
	1 milligram (mg)	=	1000 mcg
	1 microgram (mcg)	=	1000 ng (nanograms)
Volume	1 liter (L)	=	1000 mL (milliliters)
Length	1 kilometer (km)	=	1000 m
	1 meter (m, M)	=	100 cm
	1 centimeter (cm)	=	10 mm
	2.54 cm	=	1 inch
	25.4 millimeters (mm)	=	1 inch

						Decimal point					
(100,000)	(10,000)	(1000)	(100)	(10)	(1)		(0.1)	(0.01)	(0.001)	(0.0001)	(0.00001)
Hundred-thousands	Ten-thousands	Thousands	Hundreds	Tens	Ones (Units)		Tenths	Hundredths	Thousandths	Ten-thousandths	Hundred-thousandths
6	5	4	3	2	1	.	1	2	3	4	5

Whole Numbers to the Left · **Decimal Numbers to the Right**

PRACTICE PROBLEMS

Metric System Conversions

Larger to Smaller Units	Smaller to Larger Units
1. Change 2 g to mg	4. Change 1500 mg to g
2. Change 0.5 g to mg	5. Change 3000 mcg to mg
3. Change 2.5 L to mL	6. Change 500 mL to L

HOUSEHOLD SYSTEM

Because of the lack of standardization of spoons, cups, and glasses, **household measurement** is not as accurate as the metric system, therefore measurements are approximate (Table 11A.2). According to the official U.S. Pharmacopeia, a teaspoon (t) is considered to be equivalent to 5 mL in the metric system. Three teaspoons equal 1 tablespoon (T), therefore 1 T equals 15 mL. **Ounces** (oz) are fluid ounces in the household measurement system, and there are 2 T in 1 oz therefore 1 ounce equals 30 mL in the metric system.

TABLE 11A.2	**Household Equivalents**	
1 measuring cup	=	8 oz or 240 mL (1 oz = 30 mL)
1 medium-size glass (tumbler size)	=	8 oz or 240 mL
1 ounce (oz)	=	2 tablespoons or 30 mL
1 tablespoon (T)	=	3 teaspoons or 15 mL
1 teaspoon (t)	=	60 drops (60 gtt)

Conversions Within the Household System

When converting larger units to smaller units within the household system, multiply the requested number by the basic equivalent value.

EXAMPLES: Household System Conversions

Larger Units to Smaller Units
1. Convert 2 T to t.
   The equivalent value of 1 T is 3 t.
   To solve the problem, multiply 2 T with 3 t to get 6 t.
2. Convert 2 T to milliliters (mL).
   The equivalent value of 1 T is 15 mL.
   To solve the problem, multiply 2 T with 15 mL to get 30 mL.

When converting smaller units to larger units in the household system, divide the requested number of units by the basic equivalent value.

Smaller Units to Larger Units
1. Convert 6 t to T.
   The equivalent value of 3 t is 1 T.
   To solve the problem, divide 6 t by 3 t to get 2 T.
2. Convert 30 mL to T.
   The equivalent value of 15 mL is 1 T.
   To solve the problem, divide 30 mL by 15 mL to get 2 T.

Because household measurements are not as accurate as the metric measurements, instruct patients and caregivers to obtain an approved drug-measuring device to dispense liquid medicine, such as the following:

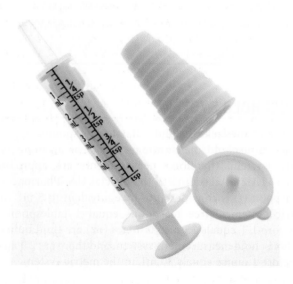

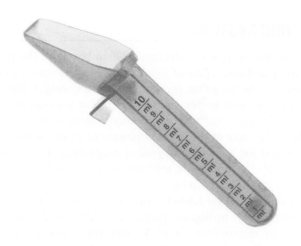

PRACTICE PROBLEMS
Household System Conversions

Remember: To change larger units to smaller units, *multiply* the requested number of units by the basic equivalent value. To change smaller units to larger units, *divide* the requested number of units by the basic equivalent value.

Larger to Smaller Units
1. Change 3 oz to T
2. Change 5 T to t
3. Change 2 T to mL

Smaller to Larger Units
4. Change 3 T to oz
5. Change 12 t to T
6. Change 45 mL to t

ANSWERS TO PRACTICE PROBLEMS

METRIC SYSTEM CONVERSIONS

Converting From Larger Units to Smaller Units
The gram is three factors of 10 greater than the milligram, so the decimal point is moved three spaces to the right.
1. If 1 g = 1000 mg; then
   $2 g = 2 \times 10^3 = 2000$ mg
   or
   2 g = 2000. = 2000 mg
2. If 1 g = 1000 mg; then
   $0.5 g = 0.5 \times 10^3 = 500$ mg
   or
   0.5 g = 0500. = 500 mg
3. If 1 L = 1000 mL; then
   $2.5 L = 2.5 \times 10^3 = 2500$ mL
   or
   2.5 L = 2500. = 2500 mL

Moving From Smaller Units to Larger Units

The milligram is three factors of 10 smaller (less) than the gram, so the decimal point is moved three spaces to the left.

4. If 1000 mg = 1 g; then

$$1500 \text{ mg} = 1500 \times 10^{-3} = 1.5 \text{ g}$$

or

$$1500 \text{ mg} = 1.500 = 1.5 \text{ g}$$

(Note there are no trailing zeroes [no 00] after the decimal.)

5. If 1000 mcg = 1 mg; then

$$3000 \text{ mcg} = 3000 \times 10^{-3} = 3 \text{ mg}$$

or

$$3000 \text{ mcg} = 3.000 = 3 \text{ mg}$$

(Note there are no trailing zeroes [no 000] after the decimal.)

6. If 1000 mL = 1 L; then

$$500 \text{ mL} = 500 \times 10^{-3} = 0.5 \text{ L}$$

or

$$500 \text{ mL} = 0.500 = 0.5 \text{ L}$$

(Note that a leading zero was placed before the decimal.)

HOUSEHOLD SYSTEM CONVERSIONS

Converting From Larger Units to Smaller Units

1. If 1 oz = 2 T, then

$$3 \text{ oz} = 3 \times 2 \text{ T} = 6 \text{ T}$$

2. If 1 T = 3 t, then

$$5 \text{ T} = 5 \times 3 \text{ t} = 15 \text{ t}$$

3. If 1 T = 15 mL, then

$$2 \text{ T} = 2 \times 15 \text{ mL} = 30 \text{ mL}$$

Converting From Smaller Units to Larger Units

4. If 2 T = 1 oz, then

$$3 \text{ T} = 3 \div 2 \text{ T} = 1.5 \text{ oz}$$

5. If 3 t = 1 T, then

$$12 \text{ t} = 12 \div 3 \text{ t} = 4 \text{ T}$$

6. If 15 mL = 1 T and 1 T = 3 t, then

$$15 \text{ mL} = 3 \text{ t; so}$$

$$(45 \text{ mL} \div 15 \text{ mL}) \times 3 \text{ t} = 3 \times 3 \text{ t} = 9 \text{ t}$$

SECTION 11B: Calculation Methods—Enteral and Parenteral Drug Dosages

OBJECTIVES

- Interpret drug labels.
- Calculate drug dosages using the basic formula, the ratio and proportion/fractional equation method, and the dimensional analysis method.
- Convert all measures to the same system and unit of measure within the system before calculating final drug dosages.

- Calculate drug dosages according to body weight.
- Calculate drug dosages according the body surface area using the West nomogram.
- Calculate drug dosages according the body surface area using the square root method.

OUTLINE

KEY TERMS

INTERPRETING DRUG LABELS

Pharmaceutical companies usually label their drugs with the brand name, also called the trade name, first in large letters with the generic name, then in smaller letters. Labels for generic drugs may have only the generic name of the drug listed. The formulation or the drug amount per tablet, capsule, or unit of liquid (for oral and parenteral doses) is printed on the drug label. Other information found on drug labels includes lot number, expiration date, proper storage of the drug, and whether it is a controlled substance. Two examples of drug labels are given below, the first for an oral drug and the second for a parenteral drug. The third example shows additional information provided on drug labels.

EXAMPLES: Interpreting Enteral Drug Labels

1. *Tylenol* is the brand (trade) name, *acetaminophen* is the generic name, and the formulation is 500 mg per caplet. That the container holds 100 caplets is irrelevant when calculating the drug dosage.

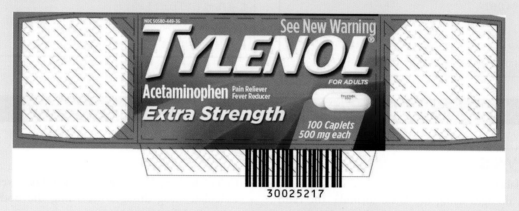

2. This label lists the generic name only (folic acid). The formulation is 5 mg per mL. There are 10 mL in the vial, which is an irrelevant number when calculating the drug dosage.

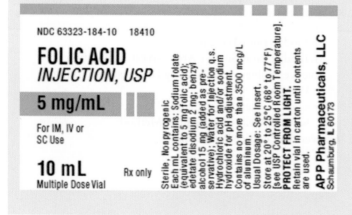

3. *Kadian*[1] is the brand (trade) name and *morphine sulfate*[2] is the generic name. The formulation[3] is 60 mg per capsule, and the container holds 100[4] capsules. It is a schedule II[5] drug, which is a controlled substance because of its potential for abuse. The label indicates how the drug is to be stored[6], and the lot number[7] also appears.

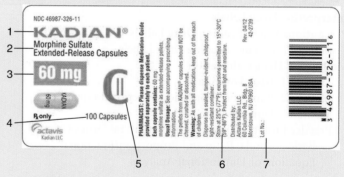

PRECAUTIONS WHEN READING DRUG LABELS

Be aware of drug names that sound or look alike; for example, note the similarity between the trade names *Percodan* and *Percocet*. Percocet, which contains oxycodone and acetaminophen, is the preparation most commonly prescribed. Percodan contains oxycodone and aspirin, and a patient may be allergic to aspirin or should not take aspirin because of a stomach ulcer. Acetaminophen can cause liver toxicity; in persons with normal liver function, the maximum dosage of acetaminophen is 3000 mg per 24 hours.

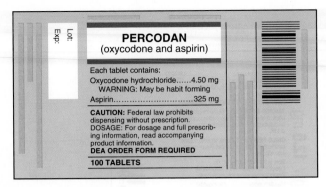

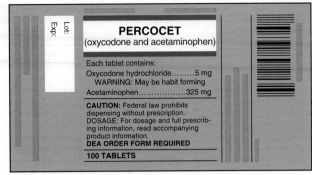

Note the similarity between *quinine sulfate* and *quinidine gluconate*. These drugs differ greatly. Quinine is prescribed for malaria, whereas quinidine is prescribed for cardiac arrhythmias.

To decrease medication errors, the nurse administering the drug should perform a minimum of three label checks with the patient's medication administration record (MAR).

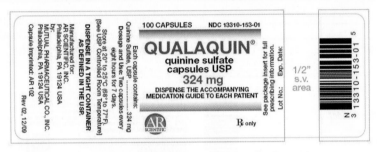

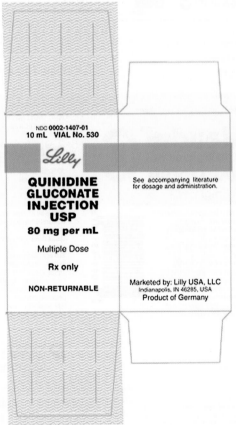

PRACTICE PROBLEMS

Reading Drug Labels

1.

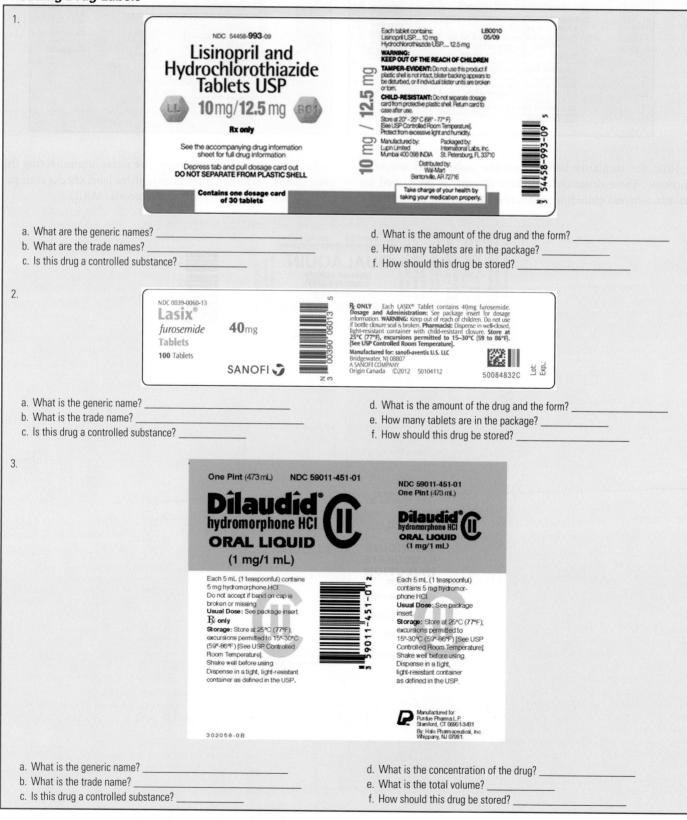

a. What are the generic names? _____

b. What are the trade names? _____

c. Is this drug a controlled substance? _____

d. What is the amount of the drug and the form? _____

e. How many tablets are in the package? _____

f. How should this drug be stored? _____

2.

a. What is the generic name? _____

b. What is the trade name? _____

c. Is this drug a controlled substance? _____

d. What is the amount of the drug and the form? _____

e. How many tablets are in the package? _____

f. How should this drug be stored? _____

3.

a. What is the generic name? _____

b. What is the trade name? _____

c. Is this drug a controlled substance? _____

d. What is the concentration of the drug? _____

e. What is the total volume? _____

f. How should this drug be stored? _____

METHODS OF DRUG CALCULATION

Generally, calculations are made for one dose. For example, if the order states that a patient is to be given 500 mg of a drug three times a day, you would calculate the amount of drug that is equivalent to 500 mg. Occasionally, nurses calculate the full daily dose, which in this case would be 1500 mg (500 mg times three doses).

The three general methods for the calculation of drug dosages are the (1) basic formula (BF), (2) ratio and proportion/fractional equation (RP/FE), and (3) dimensional analysis (DA). These methods are used to calculate most enteral and parenteral drug dosages. The nurse should select one of the methods to calculate drug

dosages and use that method consistently. All but the dimensional analysis requires using the same units of measure. It is most helpful to convert to the system used on the **drug label**. If the drug is ordered in grams (g, G) and the drug label gives the dose in milligrams (mg), convert grams to milligrams (the measurement on the drug label) and proceed with the drug calculation.

For drugs that require individualized dosing, calculation by body weight (BW) or by body surface area (BSA) may be necessary. These last two methods are mostly used for the calculation of pediatric dosages and for drugs used in the treatment of cancer (antineoplastic drugs). BW and BSA methods of calculation are also useful for individuals whose BW is low, who are obese, or who are older adults.

METHOD 1

Basic Formula

The **basic formula (BF)** is easy to recall:

$$\frac{D}{H} \times V = A$$

Where:

D is the *desired* dose (as ordered)
H is the drug on *hand* (available)
V is the *vehicle* or *volume* of a drug form (tablet, capsule, liquid [mL])
A is the *amount* calculated to be given to the patient.

Examples Using the Basic Formula

1. Order: Cefaclor 0.5 g PO bid
   Available: Cefaclor 500 mg capsule

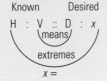

Each capsule contains:
Cefaclor Monohydrate equivalent to 500 mg anhydrous Cefaclor

NDC 61442-**172**-05

CEFACLOR

Capsules USP

500 mg

Rx Only

Usual Adult Dose: 250 mg three times a day. For severe infections, this dosage may be doubled. See accompanying literature.

Dispense in a tight, light-resistant container.

Store at 20° to 25°C (68° to 77°F). [See USP Controlled Room Temperature]. Protect from moisture.

Rev. 08/14
KRC5y USA 2182394-003

Carlsbad Technology, Inc.

500 Capsules

How many capsules should the patient receive per dose? (This is a two-step process.)

a. The unit of measure that is ordered (grams) and the unit of measure on the label (milligrams) are from the same system of measurement—the metric system. Conversion to the same unit as on the label is necessary to solve the problem. Because the label is in milligrams, convert grams to milligrams.

To convert grams (large value) to milligrams (smaller value), move the decimal point three spaces to the right as discussed earlier:
   0.5 g = 500 mg (0.500 is converted to 500 mg); then

b. $\frac{D}{H} \times V$; where D = 500 mg, H = 500 mg, and V = 1 capsule; then

$$\frac{D}{H} \times V = \frac{500 \text{ mg}}{500 \text{ mg}} \times 1 \text{ capsule} = 1 \text{ capsule}$$

Answer: 500 mg, or 1 tablet
The nurse will administer 1 tablet per dose.

2. Order: Phenobarbital 30 mg PO STAT
   Available: Phenobarbital 15 mg per tablet

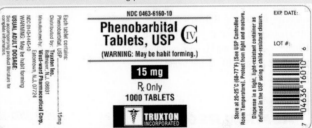

NDC 0463-6160-10

Phenobarbital Tablets, USP (IV)

(WARNING: May be habit forming.)

15 mg

Rx Only
1000 TABLETS

TRUXTON
INCORPORATED

How many tablets should the patient receive per dose?
The dosage is ordered in milligrams and the unit of measure on the label is also expressed in milligrams. There is no need for conversion.

$$\frac{D}{H} \times V; \text{ then}$$

$$\frac{30 \text{ mg}}{15 \text{ mg}} \times 1 \text{ tablet} = 2 \text{ tablets}$$

Answer: 30 mg = 2 tablets
The nurse will administer 2 tablets per dose.

METHOD 2

Ratio and Proportion/Fractional Equation

Ratio and Proportion: Linear Method

The **ratio and proportion (RP)** method can be expressed linearly or as a fraction (a fractional equation). The linear setup is as follows:

Known   Desired

H : V :: D : x
    ⌣means⌣
    ‿extremes‿
        x =

Where:

D is the *desired* dose (as ordered)
H is the drug on *hand* (available)
V is the *vehicle* or *volume* of a drug form (tablet, capsule, liquid [mL])
x is the *unknown amount* to give to the patient
The double colon symbol (::) stands for "as" or "equal to"

Continued

Multiply the extremes and the means ($Hx::VD$). Solve for $x \left(\dfrac{Hx}{H} :: \dfrac{VD}{H} \right)$; H is the divisor $\left(x = \dfrac{VD}{H} \right)$.

Examples Using Ratio and Proportion: Linear Method

1. Order: Amoxicillin 100 mg PO qid
   Available: Amoxicillin 250 mg per 5 mL

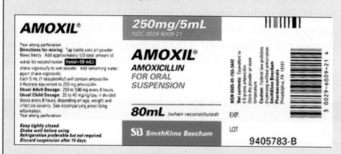

How many milliliters should the patient receive per dose?

Conversion is not needed because both are expressed in the same unit of measure.

$$H \quad : \quad V \quad :: \quad D \quad : \quad x$$
$$250\,mg \quad : \quad 5\,mL \quad :: \quad 100\,mg \quad : \quad x\,mL$$

means

extremes

$$250x = 500$$
$$x = 2\,mL$$

Answer: Amoxicillin 100 mg = 2 mL
The nurse will administer 2 mL per dose.

2. Order: Aspirin 162 mg PO once daily
   Available: Aspirin 81 mg per tablet

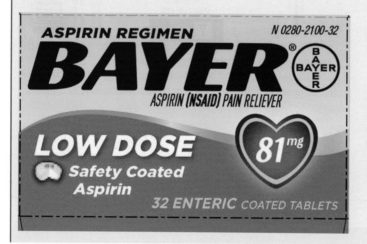

How many tablets should the patient receive per dose?

$$H \quad : \quad V \quad :: \quad D \quad : \quad x$$
$$81\,mg \quad : \quad 1\,tab \quad :: \quad 162\,mg \quad : \quad x$$

means

extremes

$$81x = 162\,mg$$
$$x = 2\,tablets$$

Answer: Aspirin 162 mg = 2 tablets
The nurse will administer 2 tablets per dose.

Fractional Equation

The **fractional equation (FE)** setup is written as a fraction and is more commonly used than the linear setup. This setup will be used to illustrate RP/FE for the rest of this chapter.

$$\frac{H}{V} = \frac{D}{x}; \text{ where } \frac{H \text{ (dosage on hand)}}{V \text{ (vehicle)}} \quad \frac{D \text{ (desired dosage)}}{x \text{ (unknown)}}$$

Cross-multiply and solve for x, where $Hx = VD$; then $x = \dfrac{VD}{H}$.

Examples Using the Fractional Equation—Fraction Method

1. Order: Ciprofloxacin 500 mg PO q12h
   Available: Ciprofloxacin 250 mg per tablet

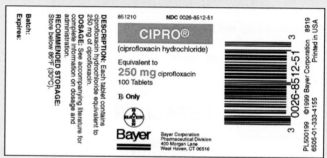

How many tablet(s) should the patient receive per dose?

$$\frac{H}{V} = \frac{D}{x}$$

Where:

H = 250 mg

V = tablet (tab)

D = 500 mg

x = unknown number of tablets

$$\frac{250\,mg}{1\,tab} = \frac{500\,mg}{x\,tab}$$

Cross-multiply and solve for x.

$250x = 500$

$x = 2$

Answer: 500 mg = 2 tablets
The nurse will administer 2 tablets per dose.

2. Order: Citalopram 10 mg PO once daily
   Available: Citalopram 20 mg per tablet

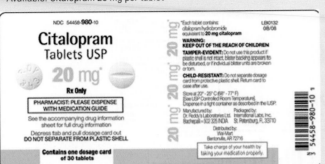

$$\frac{H}{V} = \frac{D}{x}$$

$$\frac{20\ mg}{1\ tab} = \frac{10\ mg}{x\ tab}$$

Cross-multiply and solve for x.

$20x = 10$

$x = 0.5$ tablet (1/2 tab)

(Note that this tablet is scored to allow it to be split in half.)

Answer: $x = 0.5$ tablet

The nurse will administer 0.5 tablet per dose.

(For the duration of this chapter, any RP or FE calculation will be shown using the FE method.)

METHOD 3

Dimensional Analysis

Dimensional analysis (DA) is a calculation method known as *units and conversions*. The D, H, and V are still used in DA. The advantage of DA is that all the steps for calculating drug dosages are conducted in one equation without having to remember various formulas. However, conversion factors still need to be memorized.

Steps for Dimensional Analysis

1. Identify the unit/form (tablet, capsule, mL) of the drug to be calculated. Place the unit/form to one side of the equal sign (=). *This is your desired unit/form.*
2. Determine the *known* dose and unit/form from the drug label that matches the unit/form of the desired dosage. Place this on the other side of the equal sign.
3. Continue with additional fractions using a multiplication operation between each fraction until all but that one unit you want is eliminated.
4. Multiply the numerators and multiply the denominators.
5. Solve for x (the unknown).

Examples Using Dimensional Analysis

1. Order: Amoxicillin 500 mg PO q8h
   Available: 250 mg per capsule

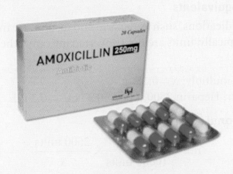

How many capsules (cap) will the nurse administer per dose?

a/b. $cap = \dfrac{1\ cap}{250\ mg}$ (H = on-*hand*)

c. Notice that the drug form "cap" to the left of the equal sign is the same as the "cap" in the numerator to the right of the equal sign. (We must

determine how many capsules need to be administered for the dose to be 500 mg). The available capsule is 250 mg; this is placed in the denominator.

d. The available strength (250 mg) is the denominator, and the unit/form "mg" must match the next numerator, which is the ordered dose of 500 mg (*desired dose*). The next *denominator* would be *x cap* (*unknown*) or it would be left blank.

$$cap = \frac{1\ cap}{250\ mg} \times \frac{500\ mg}{x\ cap}$$

e. Cancel out the *mg*, multiply the numerators, then multiply the denominators.

f. Solve for x by isolating x, reduce the resulting fraction. (Reducing fractions could be done earlier). What remain are *cap* and *2*.

$$\frac{500}{250x}; \text{ then } x = 2\ cap$$

Answer: 2 capsules

When conversions are needed (e.g., between milligrams and grams) a conversion factor (CF) is needed to calculate dosages using the basic formula or RP/FE, requiring a multistep process. When using DA, there should *only* be the one unknown value in the equation (x). This will be especially important when calculating dosages that involve milligrams per kilogram (mg/kg) or milligrams per meters squared (mg/m²).

2. Order: Amoxicillin 0.5 g PO q8h
   Available: 250 mg per capsule

How many capsules will the nurse administer?

A conversion is needed between grams and milligrams. Following the steps for DA, the equation looks like this:

$$H \times CF \times \frac{D}{unknown} =$$

$$cap = \frac{1\ cap}{250\ mg} \times \frac{1000\ mg}{1\ g} \times \frac{0.5\ g}{x\ cap} = \frac{1000 \times 0.5}{250}$$

$$= \frac{500}{250} = 2\ capsules\ of\ amoxicillin$$

As with other methods of calculation, the three components are D, H, and V as indicated in the above problem. With dimensional analysis, the conversion factor (CF) is built into the equation and is included when the ordered drug's unit of measurement and the drug available differ. If the same units of measurement are used, the conversion factor is eliminated from the equation, as shown in the first example.

Continued

3. Order: Acetaminophen 1 g PO q6h PRN for headache
   Available: Acetaminophen 325 mg per tablet

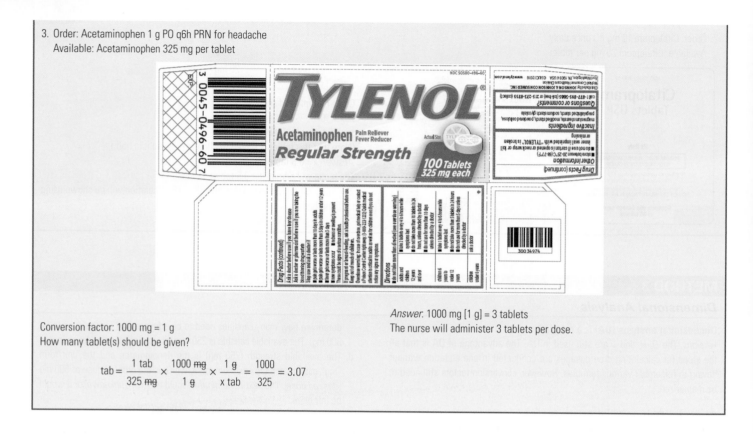

Answer: 1000 mg [1 g] = 3 tablets
The nurse will administer 3 tablets per dose.

Conversion factor: 1000 mg = 1 g
How many tablet(s) should be given?

$$\text{tab} = \frac{1\ \text{tab}}{325\ \text{mg}} \times \frac{1000\ \text{mg}}{1\ \text{g}} \times \frac{1\ \text{g}}{x\ \text{tab}} = \frac{1000}{325} = 3.07$$

Rounding Rules

Notice when to round. Tablets and caplets can be rounded to the nearest half if they are scored (see the image for citalopram). Some tablets are scored in fourths. In this case, the dosage can be rounded to the nearest fourth. However, tablets and caplets that are extended release, sustained release, controlled release, or enteric coated should not be split because splitting or crushing these preparations destroys the properties that render the drug long lasting. For this reason, capsules are rounded to the nearest whole number. Liquid drugs can be rounded to the nearest tenth; the exception to this rule is when calculating dosages of drops, which are rounded to the nearest whole number.

When rounding, determine how many places beyond the decimal point are appropriate. The general rounding rules are:

1. If a number to the right of the digit needs to be rounded and is 4 or less, round down. For example, when rounding 1.343 to the hundredth place, the number becomes 1.34. Rounding 1.343 to the tenth place, it becomes 1.3. Rounding 1.343 to a whole number, it becomes 1.
2. If a number to the right of the digit needs to be rounded and is 5 or greater, round up. For example, when rounding 1.745 to the hundredth place, the number becomes 1.75. Rounding 1.745 to the tenth place, it becomes 1.7. Rounding 1.745 to a whole number, it becomes 2.

Calculating Dosages for Drugs Measured in Units or Milliequivalents

Some medications, such as heparin and insulin, are measured in units. Typically, units are not converted into any other measure.

EXAMPLE: Drug Measured in Units

1. Order: Heparin 2500 units subcut daily
   Available: Heparin 10,000 units per mL in a multiple-dose vial (10 mL)

Basic Formula

$$\frac{D}{H} \times V = \frac{2500\ \text{units}}{10000\ \text{units}} \times 1\ \text{mL} = \frac{25}{100} = 0.25\ \text{mL}$$

Ratio and Proportion/Fractional Equation Methods

$$\frac{H}{V} = \frac{D}{x} = \frac{10000\ \text{units}}{1\ \text{mL}} = \frac{2500\ \text{units}}{x\ \text{mL}}$$

$$10000\ x = 2500$$

Cross-multiply: $x = 0.25$ mL
Answer: Heparin 2500 units = 0.25 mL = 0.3 mL

Dimensional Analysis

$$\text{mL} = \frac{1\ \text{mL}}{10000\ \text{units}} \times \frac{2500\ \text{units}}{x}$$

$$= \frac{2500}{10000}$$

$$= 0.25\ \text{mL} = 0.3\ \text{mL}\ \text{(per the rounding rule)}$$

Electrolytes are often ordered in milliequivalents (mEq). An example is pictured below.

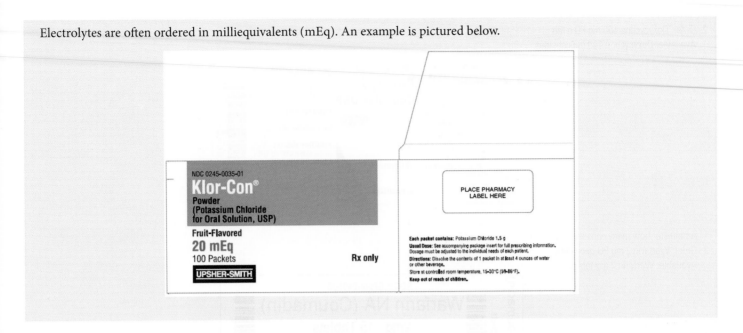

PRACTICE PROBLEMS

Enteral and Parenteral Drugs Using Basic Formula, Ratio and Proportion/Fractional Equation, or Dimensional Analysis

1. Order: Ranitidine 150 mg PO q12h

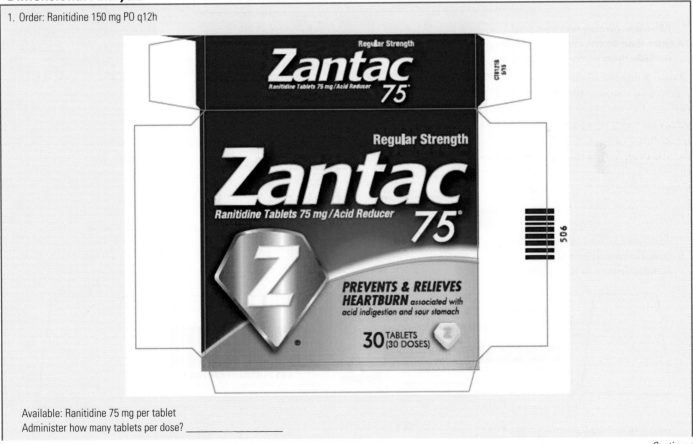

Available: Ranitidine 75 mg per tablet

Administer how many tablets per dose? _____

Continued

2. Order: Doxycycline 100 mg PO q12h
   Available: Doxycycline 100 mg capsules

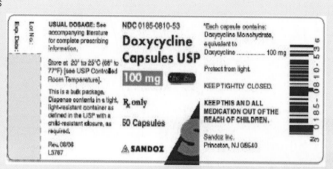

Administer how many capsules per dose? _____

3. Order: Warfarin 2 mg PO once daily
   Available: Warfarin 2 mg tablets

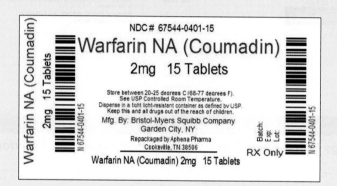

Administer how many tablets per dose? _____

4. Order: Hydrochlorothiazide 12.5 mg PO every morning
   Available: Hydrochlorothiazide 25 mg tablets

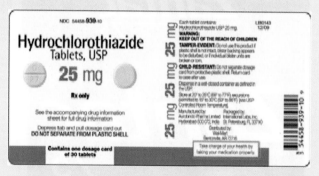

Administer how many tablets per dose? _____

5. Order: Furosemide 20 mg IM STAT
   Available: Furosemide 10 mg per mL

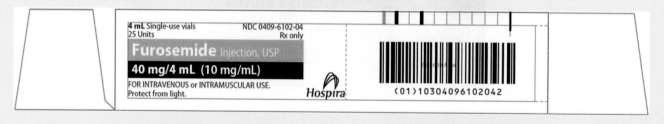

Administer how many milliliters per dose? _____

(Note that this label can be confusing to the reader. The concentration is 10 mg per mL, and it is a 4 mL vial, so the vial contains 40 mg.)

6. Ordered: Atropine sulfate 0.4 mg subcut STAT
   Available: Atropine sulfate 1 mg per mL

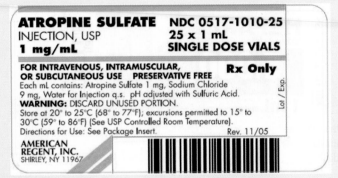

Administer how many milliliters for the STAT dose? _____
(There could be a point of confusion with this label. The concentration is 1 mg/mL in each vial, and there are 25 vials in the package.)

7. Ordered: Lactulose solution 20 g by mouth tid
   Available: Lactulose solution 10 g per 15 mL

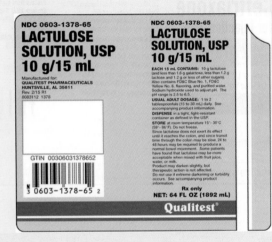

Administer how many milliliters per dose? _____

8. Ordered: Phenytoin oral solution 0.25 g PO bid
   Available: Phenytoin oral solution 125 mg per 5 mL

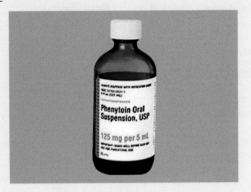

Administer how many milliliters per dose? _____

Continued

9. Order: Heparin 7500 units subcut now; 3500 units subcut daily
   Available: 5000 units per mL single-dose vial

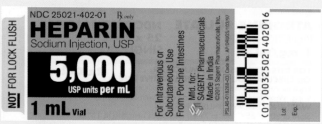

a. Administer how many milliliters for the now dose? _____
b. Administer how many milliliters for the daily dose? _____
c. How many vial(s) of heparin are needed? _____

10. Order: Ceftriaxone 1.5 g IM now
    Available: Ceftriaxone 2 g vial

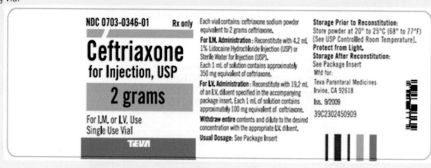

a. How many milliliters of diluent is needed for reconstitution? _____
b. What is the final drug concentration? _____
c. How many milliliters will the nurse administer for the now dose? _____

METHOD 4

Body Weight

The **body weight (BW)** method of calculation allows for individualization of the drug dosage and involves the following three steps:
1. Convert pounds to kilograms; 2.2 lb is equivalent to 1 kg.
2. Determine the drug dose for the body weight by multiplying as follows:

Drug dose × body weight = patient's dose

3. Follow the basic formula, ratio and proportion/fractional equation, or dimensional analysis method to calculate the drug dosage.

Examples of Using Body Weight for Drug Calculation
1. Order: Fluorouracil 12 mg per kg per day intravenous (IV) for a patient who weighs 176 lb
   Available: Two vials of fluorouracil 50 mg per mL

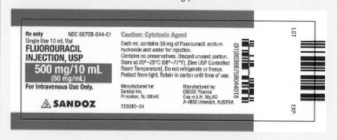

How many milliliters should the nurse administer per day?

Basic Formula
a. The first step is to convert pounds to kilograms by dividing the number of pounds the patient weighs by 2.2 (1 kg = 2.2 lb).

$$176 \text{ lb} \div 2.2 = 80 \text{ kg}$$

b. The second step is to multiply the ordered dose by the patient's weight in kilograms.

$$\text{mg} \times \text{kg} = \text{patient dose}$$
$$12 \text{ mg} \times 80 \text{ kg} = 960 \text{ mg per day}$$

c. The third step is to determine the volume in milliliters to administer 960 mg.

$$\frac{D}{H} \times V = \frac{960 \text{ mg}}{50 \text{ mg}} \times 1 \text{ mL}$$
$$= 19.2 \text{ mL}$$

Dimensional Analysis
(Notice that the conversion factors are included in this one equation.)

$$\text{mL} = \frac{1 \text{ mL}}{50 \text{ mg}} \times \frac{12 \text{ mg}}{1 \text{ kg}} \times \frac{1 \text{ kg}}{2.2 \text{ lbs}} \times \frac{176 \text{ lbs}}{x \text{ mL}}$$
$$= \frac{2112 \text{ mL}}{110}$$
$$= 19.2 \text{ mL}$$

(Because you can administer tenths of liquid medications, round to the nearest tenth.

2. Order: Cefaclor oral suspension 20 mg per kg per day in three divided doses for a pediatric patient who weighs 66 lb
   Available: Cefaclor oral suspension 125 mg per 5 mL

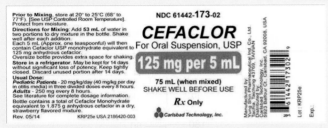

How many milliliters will the nurse administer per dose? _____

Basic Formula
   a. Convert pounds to kilograms.
      66 lb ÷ 2.2 lb = 30 kg
   b. Multiply the desired dosage with the patient's weight in kg
      20 mg × 30 kg = 600 mg per day

   c. Divide by the number of doses needed for the day.
      600 mg ÷ 3 doses = 200 mg per dose
   d. Using the basic formula, determine the mL per dose.

$$\frac{D}{H} \times V = \frac{200 \text{ mg}}{125 \text{ mg}} \times 5 \text{ mL}$$

$$= 8 \text{ mL}$$

Dimensional Analysis

$$mL = \frac{5 \text{ mL}}{125 \text{ mg}} \times \frac{20 \text{ mg}}{1 \text{ kg}} \times \frac{1 \text{ kg}}{2.2 \text{ lbs}} \times \frac{66 \text{ lbs}}{3 \text{ doses}}$$

$$= \frac{6600 \text{ mL}}{825 \text{ mg}}$$

$$= 8 \text{ mL per dose}$$

METHOD 5

Body Surface Area—West Nomogram

The measurement of **body surface area (BSA)** is the most precise method for calculating drug dosages. BSA can be measured using the West nomogram or the square root method.

The BSA by the West nomogram (Fig. 11B.1) is measured in square meters (m^2) and is determined by the patient's height and weight. Determine where the height and weight intersect on the nomogram scale; the height and weight can be in inches and pounds or centimeters and kilograms depending on the column used, but the systems of measurement must match. Centimeters and kilograms are both within the metric system and are most commonly used for the calculation of BSA. To calculate a drug dosage, multiply the dose ordered with the patient's BSA.

Examples of Using Body Surface Area: Drug Calculation
1. Drug dosage will be determined using the West nomogram and the square root calculations for a patient who is 70 inches tall and weighs 160 lb.

Determining Body Surface Area Using the West Nomogram
Using Inches and Pounds
Draw a straight line from *70* in the *inches* column to *160* in the *pounds* column (Fig. 11B.2). Note that the line intersects between 1.9 and 2 square meters.

Using Centimeters and Kilograms
The patient is 178 cm tall (1 in = 2.54 cm) and weighs 73 kg (2.2 lb = 1 kg). The height and the weight were rounded to whole numbers. Draw a straight line from 178 in the *centimeters* column to 73 in the *kilograms* column (Fig. 11B.3). Note that the line also intersects between 1.9 and 2. For the purposes of calculation, 1.95 can be used.

Determining Body Surface Area Using the Square Root Method
The most precise way to determine BSA is to use the **square root method** for the calculation. When calculating the BSA in household measurement (inches and pounds), the following formula applies:

$$BSA = \sqrt{\frac{\text{height (inches)} \times \text{weight (pounds)}}{3131 \text{ (constant)}}}$$

$$= \sqrt{\frac{70 \text{ in} \times 160 \text{ lb}}{3131}}$$

$$= \sqrt{\frac{11200}{3131}}$$

$$= \sqrt{3.6}$$

$$\sqrt{3.6} = 1.9 \text{ m}^2$$

When calculating the BSA using the metric system (centimeters and kilograms), the following formula applies:

$$BSA = \sqrt{\frac{\text{height (centimeters)} \times \text{weight (kilograms)}}{3600 \text{ (constant)}}}$$

$$= \sqrt{\frac{178 \text{ cm} \times 73 \text{ kg}}{3600}} = \sqrt{\frac{12994}{3600}} = \sqrt{3.6}$$

$$\sqrt{3.6} = 1.9 \text{ m}^2$$

(Numbers have been rounded to the nearest tenth, which is common for adults.)

Note that both results using the square root method agree and are more precise than using the West nomogram. The variance of 0.05 from the lowest calculated BSA to the highest calculated BSA is negligible.

2. The following drug dosage for this patient is calculated using a BSA of 1.9 m^2
   Order: CISplatin 20 mg per m^2 intravenous (IV) today
   Available: CISplatin 1 mg per mL

Continued

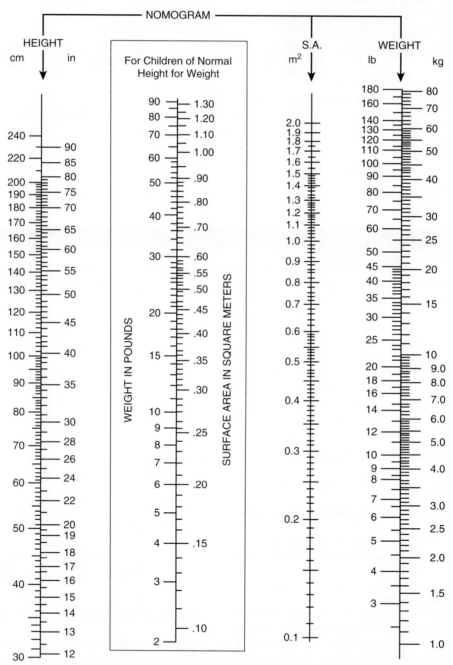

FIG. 11B.1 West Nomogram. The outside columns are used to calculate the meters squared (m²) of adults. The middle column is used to calculate the meters squared of children. (Modified from data by Boyd, E., & West, C. D. [2011]. In R. M. Kliegman, B. F. Stanton, J. W. St. Geme III, et al. [Eds.], *Nelson textbook of pediatrics* [19th ed]. Philadelphia, PA: Saunders.)

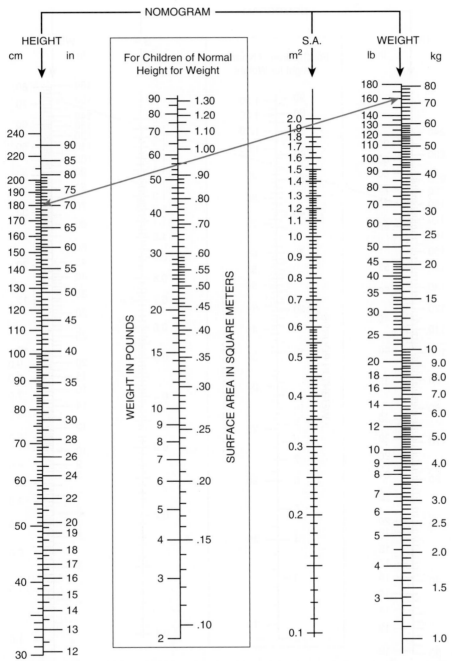

FIG. 11B.2 West Nomogram Using Inches and Pounds. (Modified from data by Boyd, E., & West, C. D. [2011]. In R. M. Kliegman, B. F. Stanton, J. W. St. Geme III, et al. [Eds.], *Nelson textbook of pediatrics* [19th ed]. Philadelphia, PA: Saunders.)

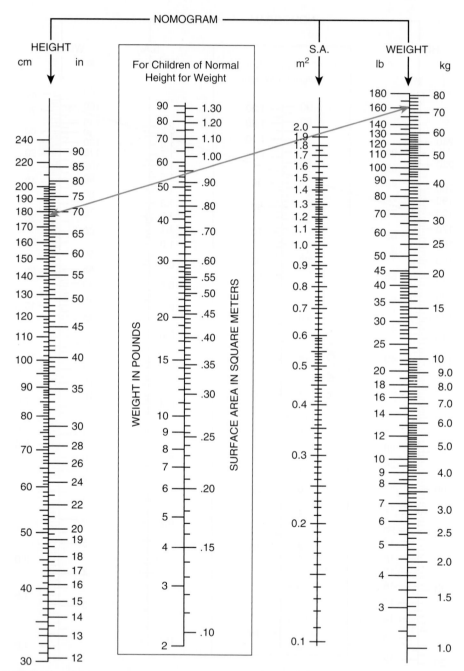

FIG. 11B.3 West Nomogram Using Centimeters and Kilograms. (Modified from data by Boyd, E., & West, C. D. [2011]. In R. M. Kliegman, B. F. Stanton, J. W. St. Geme III, et al. [Eds.], *Nelson textbook of pediatrics* [19th ed]. Philadelphia, PA: Saunders.)

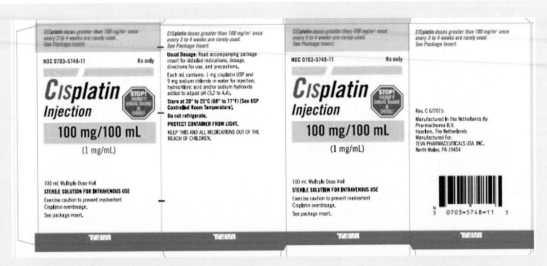

(Note that the label also states 100 mg per 100 mL. Using the lowest numbers listed on a drug label helps to prevent errors by eliminating extraneous zeroes.)

  a. How many milligrams are ordered?

    To calculate the child's dose, multiply 20 mg with 1.9 m² to get 38 mg

  b. How many milliliters will the nurse administer?

Basic Formula

$$\frac{D}{H} \times V$$

$$= \frac{38 \text{ mg}}{1 \text{ mg}} \times 1 \text{ mL}$$

$$= 38 \text{ mL}$$

Ratio and Proportion/Fractional Equation

$$\frac{H}{V} = \frac{D}{x}$$

$$\frac{1 \text{ mg}}{1 \text{ mL}} = \frac{38 \text{ mg}}{x}$$

$$x = 38 \text{ mL}$$

Dimensional Analysis

$$mL = \frac{1 \text{ mL}}{1 \text{ mg}} \times \frac{1000 \text{ mg}}{1 \text{ g}} \times \frac{38 \text{ mg}}{x}$$

$$x = 38 \text{ mL}$$

Answer: The nurse will administer 38 mL of CISplatin intravenously.

3. Calculating a pediatric dose based on BSA using the West nomogram and the square root method is illustrated below:

  Ordered: Vincristine 2 mg per m² today

  Available: Vincristine 1 mg per mL

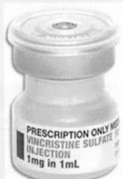

How many milliliters will the nurse administer?

This pediatric patient's height and weight fall within the normal percentiles. The child weighs 44 lb (20 kg).

  a. Using the center column on the West nomogram, the child's BSA is *0.8 m²*.

  b. Use the square root method to calculate BSA using inches and pounds if the child is 36 inches tall.

$$BSA = \sqrt{\frac{36 \text{ in} \times 44 \text{ lb}}{3131}} = \sqrt{\frac{1584}{3131}} = \sqrt{0.51}$$

$$= 0.71 \text{ m}^2$$

(Rounding numbers to the hundredth place is common when calculating pediatric dosages.)

  c. Use the square root method to calculate BSA using centimeters and kilograms.

Continued

$$BSA = \sqrt{\frac{91.4\ cm \times 20\ kg}{3600}} = \sqrt{\frac{1828}{3600}} = \sqrt{0.51}$$

$$= 0.71\ m^2$$

d. The more precise number, 0.71 m², will be used to calculate the drug dosage.

Basic Formula

e. Determine desired dose based on the above BSA.
f. The desired dose is calculated by multiplying 2 mg with 0.71 m² to get 1.42 mg.
g. Solve for the desired unit of measure.

$$\frac{D}{H} \times V$$

$$\frac{1.42\ mg}{1\ mg} \times 1\ mL$$

$$= 1.4\ mL$$

The dose was rounded to the tenth place to accommodate the calibrations on a syringe.

Dimensional Analysis

h. Determine BSA (we will use the calculated BSA from above, 0.71 m²).
i. Solve for the desired unit of measure.

$$mL = \frac{1\ mL}{1\ mg} \times \frac{2\ mg}{1\ m^2} \times \frac{0.71\ m^2}{x}$$

$$= 1.4\ mL$$

The dose was rounded to the tenth place to accommodate the calibrations on a syringe.

PRACTICE PROBLEMS

Calculating Dosages Based on Body Weight

1. Order: Valproic acid oral solution PO 15 mg per kg per day in two divided doses for a pediatric patient who weighs 66 lb
Available: Valproic acid oral solution 250 mg per 5 mL

a. How many kilograms does the child weigh? _____
b. How many milligrams per *day* should the child receive? _____
c. How many milligrams per *dose* should the child receive? _____
d. How many *milliliters* per dose should the child receive? _____

2. Order: Gentamicin 2.5 mg per kg q8h IM for a pediatric patient who weighs 33 lb
Available: Gentamicin 10 mg per mL

a. How many kilograms does the child weigh? _____
b. How many milligrams per dose will the child receive? _____
c. How many milliliters per dose will the child receive? _____

PRACTICE PROBLEMS

Calculating Dosages Based on Body Surface Area—Square Root Method

1. Order: Carboplatin 300 mg per m² per intravenous (IV) infusion today for a patient 66 inches tall who weighs 176 lb

    Available: Carboplatin 10 mg/mL

a. Use the square root method to determine the patient's square meters based on inches and pounds.

b. What is the dosage in milligrams? _____

c. How many milliliters will the patient receive? _____

2. Order: Fluorouracil 350 mg per m² per day IV for a patient 164 cm tall who weighs 66.8 kg.

a. Use the square root method to determine the patient's square meters based on centimeters and kilograms.

b. How many milligrams would the patient receive? _____

ANSWERS TO PRACTICE PROBLEMS

READING DRUG LABELS

1. a. Lisinopril and hydrochlorothiazide
   b. There is no trade name
   c. No
   d. Lisinopril 10 mg; hydrochlorothiazide 12.5 mg per tablet
   e. 30 tablets
   f. At room temperature (68° to 77° F)
2. a. Furosemide
   b. Lasix
   c. No
   d. 40 mg per tablet
   e. 100 tablets
   f. Room temperature (59° to 86° F)
3. a. Hydromorphone
   b. Dilaudid
   c. Yes, Schedule II
   d. 1 mg per mL (oral)
   e. 473 mL = 473 mg
   f. Room temperature (59° to 86° F)

ENTERAL AND PARENTERAL DRUGS

All answers will be shown using dimensional analysis.

1. $\text{tab} = \dfrac{1\,\text{tab}}{75\,\text{mg}} \times \dfrac{150\,\text{mg}}{x} = 2\,\text{tabs}$

2. $\text{cap} = \dfrac{1\,\text{cap}}{100\,\text{mg}} \times \dfrac{100\,\text{mg}}{x} = 1\,\text{cap}$

3. $\text{tab} = \dfrac{1\,\text{tab}}{2\,\text{mg}} \times \dfrac{2\,\text{mg}}{x} = 1\,\text{tab}$

4. $\text{tab} = \dfrac{1\,\text{tab}}{25\,\text{mg}} \times \dfrac{12.5\,\text{mg}}{x} = 0.5\,\text{tab}$

5. $\text{mL} = \dfrac{1\,\text{mL}}{10\,\text{mg}} \times \dfrac{20\,\text{mg}}{x} = 2\,\text{mL}$

6. $\text{mL} = \dfrac{1\,\text{mL}}{1\,\text{mg}} \times \dfrac{0.4\,\text{mg}}{x} = 0.4\,\text{mL}$

7. $\text{mL} = \dfrac{15\,\text{mL}}{10\,\text{g}} \times \dfrac{20\,\text{g}}{x} = 30\,\text{mL}$

8. $\text{mL} = \dfrac{5\,\text{mL}}{125\,\text{mg}} \times \dfrac{1000\,\text{mg}}{1\,\text{g}} \times \dfrac{0.25\,\text{g}}{x} = 10\,\text{mL}$

9. a. $\text{mL} = \dfrac{1\,\text{mL}}{5000\,\text{units}} \times \dfrac{7500\,\text{units}}{x} = 1.5\,\text{mL}$

(Note that units is spelled out rather than using only U, which could be mistaken for a zero.)

b. $\text{mL} = \dfrac{1\,\text{mL}}{5000\,\text{units}} \times \dfrac{3500\,\text{units}}{x} = 0.7\,\text{mL}$

(Note "units" is spelled out rather than using "U," which could be mistaken for a zero.)

c. 1.5 mL + 0.7 mL = 2.2 mL, so 2 vials are needed

10. a. 4.2 mL
    b. 50 mg per mL
    c. $\text{mL} = \dfrac{1\,\text{mL}}{350\,\text{mg}} \times \dfrac{1000\,\text{mg}}{1\,\text{g}} \times \dfrac{1.5\,\text{g}}{x} = 4.28$

= 4.3 mL per rounding rule (administer in two separate injections)

CALCULATING DOSAGES BASED ON BODY WEIGHT

1. a. 66 lb ÷ 2.2 = 30 kg
   b. 15 mg × 30 kg = 450 mg/day
   c. 450 mg ÷ 2 = 225 mg/dose
   d. $\text{mL} = \dfrac{5\,\text{mL}}{250\,\text{mg}} \times \dfrac{225\,\text{mg}}{x} = 4.5\,\text{mL}$

Dimensional analysis

$\text{mL} = \dfrac{5\,\text{mL}}{250\,\text{mg}} \times \dfrac{15\,\text{mg}}{1\,\text{kg}} \times \dfrac{1\,\text{kg}}{2.2\,\text{lb}} \times \dfrac{66\,\text{lb}}{2\,\text{dose}} = 4.5\,\text{mL/dose}$

2. a. 33 lb ÷ 2.2 = 15 kg
   b. 2.5 mg × 15 kg = 37.5 mg
   c. $\text{mL} = \dfrac{1\,\text{mL}}{10\,\text{mg}} \times \dfrac{37.5\,\text{mg}}{x} = 3.8\,\text{mL}$

Dimensional analysis

$\text{mL} = \dfrac{1\,\text{mL}}{10\,\text{mg}} \times \dfrac{2.5\,\text{mg}}{1\,\text{kg}} \times \dfrac{1\,\text{g}}{2.2\,\text{lb}} \times \dfrac{33\,\text{lb}}{x} = 3.8\,\text{mL}$

CALCULATING DOSAGES BASED ON BODY SURFACE AREA—SQUARE ROOT METHOD

1. a. $\text{BSA} = \sqrt{\dfrac{66\,\text{in} \times 176\,\text{lbs}}{3131}} = \sqrt{\dfrac{11{,}616}{3131}} = 1.93\ \text{m}^2$

   b. $\text{mg/m}^2 = 300\,\text{mg} \times 1.93\ \text{m}^2 \quad 579\,\text{mg}$

   c. $\text{mL} = \dfrac{1\,\text{mL}}{10\,\text{mg}} \times \dfrac{300\,\text{mg}}{\text{m}^2} \times \dfrac{1.93\ \text{m}^2}{x} = 57.9\,\text{mL}$

2. $\text{mg/m}^2 = \dfrac{350\,\text{mg}}{\text{m}^2} \times \sqrt{\dfrac{66.8\,\text{kg} \times 164\,\text{cm}}{3600}} = 610.6\,\text{mg}$

SECTION 11C: Calculating Dosages—Drugs That Require Reconstitution

OBJECTIVES

- Identify the information available on drug labels.
- Calculate drug dosages when reconstitution is needed.

- Discuss the difference between enteral and parenteral drugs when reconstituted.
- Identify the difference between an ampule and a vial.

OUTLINE

Calculating Suspensions and Solutions
   Practice Problems: Drug Reconstitution
Considerations When Calculating Dosages of Oral Drugs
   Tablets, Capsules, and Liquids
   Drugs Administered via Nasogastric Tube

Considerations When Calculating Dosages of Parenteral Drugs
   Injectable Preparations
   Syringes
   Vials and Ampules
Answers to Practice Problems

KEY TERMS

CALCULATING SUSPENSIONS AND SOLUTIONS

Both enteral and parenteral drugs may come in powder form due to the drug's instability in liquid. The liquid used to reconstitute a dry powder is called a **diluent**. Diluents can be sterile water intended for injection, 0.9% saline solution, or a special liquid supplied by the manufacturer. The nurse must follow directions for reconstitution on the label exactly. Below is a label of an oral preparation that requires reconstitution.

EXAMPLES: Drug Reconstitution

1. Below is a label for reconstituting cefadroxil.

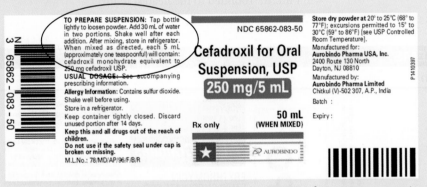

Read the left side of the label that says *To Prepare Suspension*. Note that 30 mL of water in two portions is needed to liquefy the powder. This is an oral drug, so drinking water can be used. The nurse is instructed to shake the powder loose to prevent clumping. Add 15 mL of water and shake well. Add another 15 mL of water and shake well. Now that the powder has been reconstituted into a **suspension**, each 5 mL of liquid contains 250 mg of cefadroxil. The entire bottle has 50 mL when mixed, a number that is irrelevant when calculating a dose. Now the equation can be set up for calculation of a dosage.

Order: Cefadroxil oral solution 1 g PO q12h
Available: Cefadroxil oral solution 250 mg per 5 mL
How many milliliters will the nurse administer per dose?

Dimensional Analysis

$$mL = \frac{5\ mL}{250\ mg} \times \frac{1000\ mg}{1\ g} \times \frac{1\ g}{x} = 20\ mL\ per\ dose$$

2. Below is a label of a parenteral drug that requires reconstitution.

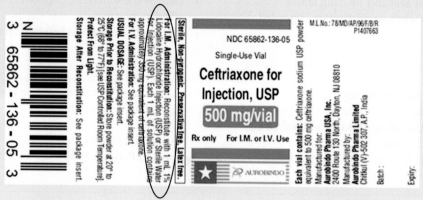

Read the left side of the label. For intramuscular (IM) injection, it states to reconstitute with 1 mL of 1% lidocaine hydrochloride (this diluent is sometimes used when a medication is very painful when given IM) *or* 1 mL sterile water for injection. After this preparation is reconstituted and shaken, each milliliter contains 350 mg. The figure *500 mg* in the center of the label is the dose contained in the *whole vial*. If the medication is to be given intravenously, the instructions are written in the package insert. The nurse will need to read the drug insert to determine proper reconstitution for the intravenous (IV) route.

Order: Ceftriaxone 250 mg IM q12h
Available: Ceftriaxone 350 mg per 1 mL
How many milliliters will the nurse administer per dose? _____
How many milliliters will be administered every 24 hours? _____

Dimensional Analysis

$$mL/dose = \frac{1\ mL}{350\ mg} \times \frac{250\ mg}{x} = 0.7\ mL/dose$$
(rounded to the nearest tenth)

$$mL/d = \frac{1\ mL}{350\ mg} \times \frac{250\ mg}{x} \times \frac{24\ h}{1\ day} \times \frac{1}{12\ h}$$
$$= 1.4\ mL/d\ (rounded\ to\ the\ nearest\ tenth)$$

PRACTICE PROBLEMS

Drug Reconstitution

1.

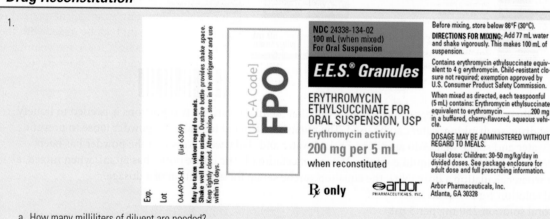

a. How many milliliters of diluent are needed?
b. What is the final concentration?
c. How many milliliters are administered for an order to give 500 mg?

2.

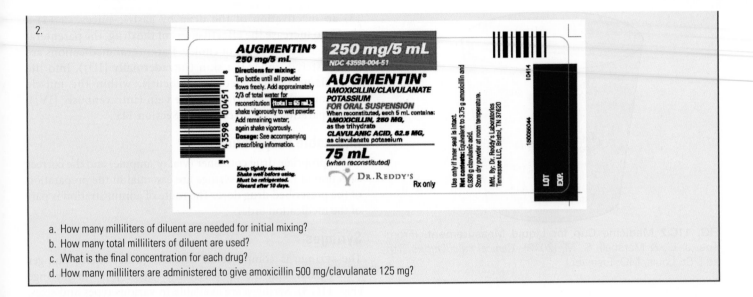

a. How many milliliters of diluent are needed for initial mixing?
b. How many total milliliters of diluent are used?
c. What is the final concentration for each drug?
d. How many milliliters are administered to give amoxicillin 500 mg/clavulanate 125 mg?

CONSIDERATIONS WHEN CALCULATING DOSAGES OF ORAL DRUGS

Most drugs are administered orally. Oral drugs are available in tablet, caplet, capsule, powder, and liquid forms. Oral medications are absorbed by the gastrointestinal (GI) tract, mainly from the small intestine.

Oral medications have several advantages: (1) the patient can often take oral medications without assistance, (2) the cost of oral medications is usually less than that of parenteral preparations, and (3) oral medications are easy to store. The disadvantages include (1) variation in absorption as a result of food in the GI tract and pH variation of GI secretions, (2) irritation of the gastric mucosa by certain drugs (e.g., potassium chloride), and (3) destruction or partial inactivation of the drugs by liver enzymes. Oral drugs (tablets, capsules, liquids) that may irritate the gastric mucosa should be taken with 6 to 8 ounces of fluids or should be taken with food.

Tablets, Capsules, and Liquids

Tablets come in different forms and drug strengths. Many tablets are scored and thus can be readily broken when half of the drug amount is needed. Capsules are gelatin shells that contain powder or timed-release pellets (beads). Capsules that are sustained release (pellet) or controlled release *should not* be crushed and diluted because the medication will be absorbed at a much faster rate than indicated by the manufacturer. Many medications sold in tablet form are also available in liquid form. When the patient has difficulty taking tablets, the oral liquid form of the medication is given. The liquid form can be in a suspension, syrup, elixir, or tincture. Some liquid medications that irritate the stomach, such as potassium chloride, are diluted. The tincture form is always diluted.

Tablets that are enteric coated (with a hard shell) must *not* be crushed because the medication could irritate the gastric mucosa. Enteric-coated drugs pass through the stomach into

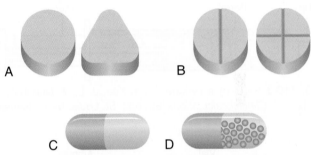

FIG. 11C.1 Shapes of Tablets and Capsules.

the small intestine where the drug's enteric coating dissolves, and then absorption occurs. Fig. 11C.1 shows the different forms of tablets and capsules.

Liquid medications are poured into a medicine cup that is calibrated (i.e., ounces, teaspoons, tablespoons, and milliliters). Fig. 11C.2 shows the markings on a medicine cup.

Drugs Administered via Nasogastric Tube

Oral medications can be administered through a nasogastric or other feeding tube for enteral administration. If the patient is receiving a tube feeding, the drug should *not* be mixed with the feeding solution. Mixing the medications in a large volume of tube feeding solution decreases the amount of drug the patient receives for a specific time. The medication (but *not* timed-release or sustained-release capsules and psyllium hydrophilic mucilloid) should be diluted in 15 to 30 mL of water or other desired fluid unless otherwise instructed. The medication is administered through the tube via a syringe, followed by another 15 to 30 mL of water to ensure that the drug reaches the stomach and is not left in the tube. Check the policy at your institution.

CONSIDERATIONS WHEN CALCULATING DOSAGES OF PARENTERAL DRUGS

When medications cannot be taken by mouth because of (1) an inability to swallow, (2) a decreased level of consciousness,

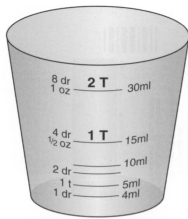

FIG. 11C.2 Medicine Cup for Liquid Measurement. (From Kee, J. L., & Marshall, S. M. [2013]. *Clinical calculations* [7th ed.]. St. Louis, MO: Elsevier.)

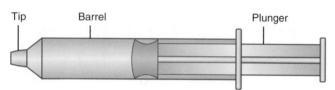

FIG. 11C.3 Parts of a syringe (From Kee, J. L., & Marshall, S. M. [2015]. *Clinical calculations* [8th ed.]. St. Louis, MO: Elsevier.)

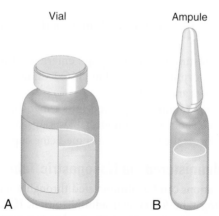

FIG. 11C.4 Vial and Ampule. (From Kee, J. L., & Marshall, S. M. [2013]. *Clinical calculations* [7th ed.]. St. Louis, MO: Elsevier.)

(3) an inactivation of the drug by gastric juices, or (4) a desire to increase the effectiveness of the drug, the parenteral route may be the route of choice. **Parenteral** medications are administered under the skin (intradermally [ID]), into the fatty tissue (subcutaneously [subcut]), within the muscle (intramuscularly [IM]), or in the vein (intravenously [IV]). IV preparations are discussed in Section 11E.

Injectable Preparations

The appropriate drug container (vial or ampule) and the correct selection of needle and syringe are essential in the preparation of the prescribed drug dose. The route of administration is part of the medication order.

Syringes

The **syringe** is composed of a barrel (outer shell), plunger (inner part), and the tip where the needle joins the syringe (Fig. 11C.3). Syringes are available in various types and sizes, including tuberculin and insulin syringes. Syringes prefilled with drugs may be glass, plastic, or metal. The tip of the syringe, inside of the barrel, and the plunger should remain sterile.

Vials and Ampules

A **vial** is usually a small glass vacuum container with a self-sealing rubber top. Some are multiple-dose vials, and when properly stored, they can be used over time. An **ampule** is a glass container with a tapered neck for snapping open and using only once. Caution is advised when snapping an ampule to prevent skin laceration. Also, glass fragments can occur, therefore a filter needle must be used to withdraw medication. Fig. 11C.4 shows a vial and an ampule. Drugs that deteriorate readily in liquid form are packaged in powder form in vials for storage. Once the dry form of the drug is reconstituted (usually with sterile or bacteriostatic water or 0.9% saline), the drug is used immediately or must be refrigerated. Check the accompanying drug circular for specific storage lengths and other instructions. Once the drug in a multidose vial is reconstituted, the vial should be labeled with the date and time of reconstitution and the initials of the person who reconstituted the drug. The shelf life of a reconstituted drug is determined by the manufacturer and can be found on the drug label.

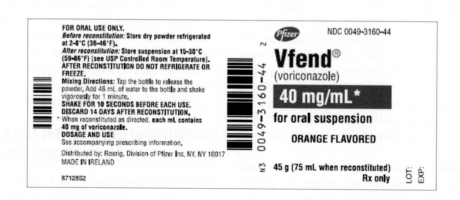

Drug labels on vials and ampules provide the (1) generic and brand name of the drug; (2) drug dose in weight (in milligrams [mg], grams [g], or milliequivalents [mEq]) and volume (milliliters [mL]); (3) expiration date; and (4) directions for administration. If the drug is in powdered form, mixing instructions and dose equivalents (e.g., milligrams per milliliter) may be given.

ANSWERS TO PRACTICE PROBLEMS

DRUG RECONSTITUTION

1. a. 77 mL

   b. 200 mg per 5 mL

   c. $mL = \dfrac{5mL}{200mg} \times \dfrac{500\ mg}{x} = 12.5\ mL$

2. a. $65 \div 3 = 21.6 \times 2 = 43.3mL \left(\dfrac{2}{3}\ of\ 65\ mL\right)$

   b. 65 mL

   c. Amoxicillin 250 mg and Clavulanic acid 62.5 mg per 5 mL

   d. Amoxicillin : $mL = \dfrac{5mL}{250mg} \times \dfrac{500mg}{xmL} = 10mL$

   Clavulanic acid : $mL = \dfrac{5mL}{62.5mg} \times \dfrac{125mg}{xmL} = 10mL$

   (Note that the amoxicillin and clavulanic acid were both 10 mL, therefore a total of 10 mL will be given for a 500 mg/250 mg dose.)

SECTION 11D: Calculation Methods—Insulin Dosages

OBJECTIVES

- Discuss the difference between syringes calibrated in units and milliliters.
- Identify the different types of insulin syringes.
- Calculate drug dosages in units.
- Correlate the dosages in units with the appropriate syringe.

OUTLINE

Drug Calculation in Units
   Practice Problems: Insulin
Answers to Practice Problems

KEY TERMS

tuberculin syringe, p. 137

units, p. 137

DRUG CALCULATION IN UNITS

Drugs are most commonly measured in grams, milligrams, or micrograms. However, some are measured in **units**. This includes insulin and heparin. Typically, units are not converted to any other measure. Heparin infusions are discussed in Section 11E.

Insulin is prescribed and measured in U.S. Pharmacopeia (USP) units. Most insulins are produced in concentrations of 100 units per mL. Insulin should be administered with an insulin syringe, which is calibrated to correspond with the concentration of 100 units of insulin per mL in the vial. For example, if the prescribed insulin dosage is 30 units, using an insulin syringe calibrated to 100 units per mL, withdraw insulin from the vial to the 30-unit mark (Fig. 11D.1). ❶ *(Note that 30 units is not interchangeable with 30 mL or 0.3 mL.)*

U-100 insulin syringes are available in various sizes, such as low-dose insulin syringes that hold a total of 0.3 mL or 0.5 mL. The size of the insulin syringe does not alter the calibration of 100 units per mL. The U.S. Food and Drug Administration (FDA) has now approved a U-500 insulin syringe specifically dedicated to be used with regular U-500 insulin. The U-100 and U-500 insulin syringes are *not* interchangeable. Some insulin is available in insulin pen injectors and insulin pumps. These are further illustrated in Chapter 47.

Administering insulin with a tuberculin syringe should be *avoided*. Although both syringes have 1 mL capacities, the **tuberculin syringe** is calibrated in milliliters rather than units. It is critical that the correct type and dose of insulin is administered to avoid severe aberrations of the patient's blood glucose. Chapter 47 provides information on the different types of insulin.

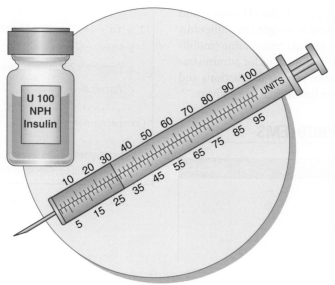

FIG. 11D.1 Vial U-100 Insulin and U-100 Syringe. (From Kee, J. L., & Marshall, S. M. [2013]. *Clinical calculations* [7th ed.]. St. Louis, MO: Elsevier.)

PRACTICE PROBLEMS

Insulin

1. Order: NPH insulin 45 units subcutaneous (subcut)
   Available: NPH insulin 100 units per mL and insulin syringe 100 units per mL
   Indicate on the insulin syringe the amount of insulin that should be withdrawn.

   10 20 30 40 50 60 70 80 90 100
   UNITS
   5 15 25 35 45 55 65 75 85 95

2. Order: Regular insulin 23 units subcut
   Available: Regular insulin 100 units per mL and insulin syringes 100 units per mL as 1-mL and 0.5-mL syringes
   Specify which insulin syringe is best to use, and indicate on the appropriate syringe the amount of insulin to be withdrawn.

   Lo-Dose
   5   15   25   35   45
   10   20   30   40   50   units

   Insulin
   20   40   60   80   100   units
   10   30   50   70   90

ANSWERS TO PRACTICE PROBLEMS

INSULIN

1. Answer:

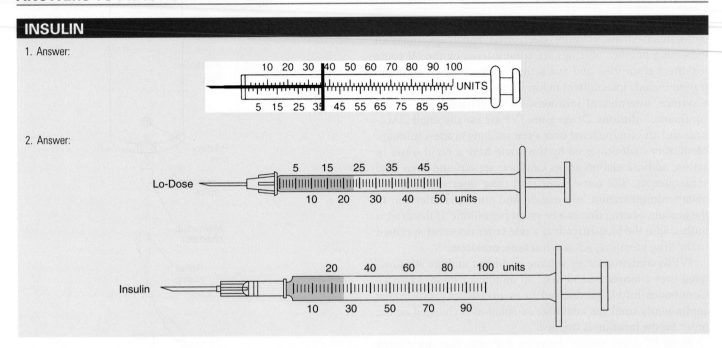

2. Answer:

SECTION 11E: Calculation Methods—Intravenous Flow Rates

OBJECTIVES

- Describe the differences between continuous intravenous (IV) infusion and intermittent IV infusion.
- Describe macrodrip and microdrip sets
- Define to *keep vein open* (KVO) and *to keep open* (TKO).
- Discuss safety considerations during IV therapy.

- Calculate drugs for direct IV injection.
- Calculate IV flow rate in milliliters per hour.
- Calculate IV flow rate in drops per minute.
- Calculate the flow rate of heparin infusions.
- Calculate dosages of critical care drugs.

OUTLINE

KEY TERMS

INTRAVENOUS THERAPY

Intravenous (IV) therapy is used to administer fluids that contain water, dextrose, vitamins, electrolytes, and drugs. Today an increasing number of drugs are administered by the IV route for direct absorption and fast action. Methods of IV administration include intermittent bolus; **IV push (IVP)**, usually with a syringe; intermittent infusions; **IV piggyback (IVPB)**; and continuous infusions. Drugs given IVP are usually small in volume and are administered over a few seconds to a few minutes. Medications administered by this route have a rapid onset of action, and calculation errors can have serious and even fatal consequences. The nurse must read drug inserts carefully to obtain administration information and must give attention to the amount of drug that can be given per minute. If the drug is pushed into the bloodstream at a rate faster than that specified in the drug literature, adverse reactions can occur.

IVPBs contain a larger volume of diluent and are administered over a longer period (e.g., 30 minutes, 1 hour, 3 hours). Continuous infusions, referred to as **primary IV fluid**, flow continuously until the container of solution is changed or the order for the infusion is stopped.

Many IV drugs irritate the veins, therefore they are diluted prior to administration. The amount of diluent used depends on the drug; drugs given by IVP can be diluted in small amounts of diluent, whereas other drugs are diluted in a large volume of fluid given over a specific period, such as 4 to 8 hours. Continuous IV infusion replaces fluid loss, maintains fluid balance, and serves as a vehicle for IV drugs.

The current trend in IV medication administration is the use of premixed IV drugs in 50- to 500-mL containers. These premixed IV medications are prepared by the manufacturer or by the hospital pharmacy. The problems of contamination and drug errors are decreased with the use of premixed IV medications. Each IV solution container has separate tubing to prevent admixture. With the use of premixed IV solution containers, the cost is higher, but the risk of medication error is lower. Because not all medication can be premixed in the solution, nurses will continue to prepare some drugs for IV administration.

Nurses have an important role in the preparation and administration of IV solutions such as 0.9% sodium chloride (normal saline, [NS]), 0.45% sodium chloride (½NS), 5% dextrose in water (D_5W), and Lactated Ringer's solution (LR) and also IV drugs. Chapter 12 further discusses different types of IV solutions. The nursing functions and responsibilities during IV preparation include the following:

- Gathering equipment
- Knowing IV sets, including drop factors
- Calculating appropriate IV flow rates
- Mixing and diluting drugs in IV fluids
- Knowing the pharmacokinetics and pharmacodynamics of drugs and their adverse effects

Nursing responsibilities continue with assessment of the patient for expected outcomes and adverse effects of the therapy in addition to assessment of the IV site. The nurse calculates the **IV flow rate** according to the IV tubing's drop factor, the volume of fluids to be administered, the length of time for infusion, and whether an electronic infusion device will be used. IV

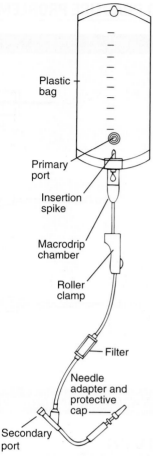

FIG. 11E.1 Intravenous Infusion Sets. (From Morris, D. G. [2014]. *Calculate with confidence* [6th ed.]. St. Louis, MO: Elsevier.)

infusions are ordered to be delivered in some unit of measure over time (e.g., mL/h, mcg/kg/min, unit/h, drops per minute [gtt/min]). Nurses calculate the rate of infusion in milliliters per hour when using an electronic infusion device. If the nurse needs to manually regulate the rate, the flow rate is calculated in drops per minute. The type and size of IV administration tubing must be known when calculating drops per minute.

⚡ Intravenous Administration Sets

IV administration sets (Fig. 11E.1) include printed information on the packaging cover, such as the **drop factor**, or the number of drops per milliliter (Fig. 11E.2). A set that delivers large drops (10 to 20 gtt/mL) is a **macrodrip set**, and one that delivers small drops (60 gtt/mL) is a **microdrip (minidrip) set** (see Fig. 11E.2). A macrodrip IV set is commonly used for adults, and a microdrip IV set is used when small amounts of drug or more precise administration is warranted.

At times, primary IV fluids are given at a slow rate, ordered to **keep vein open (KVO)**, also called **to keep open (TKO)**. The reasons for KVO include a suspected or potential emergency situation for rapid administration of fluids and drugs and the need for an open line to give IV drugs at specified hours. For KVO, a microdrip set (60 gtt/mL) and a 250-mL IV solution bag may be used. KVO is usually regulated to deliver 10 to 30 mL/h.

Drugs prescribed as IVPB (Fig. 11E.3) are administered via separate tubing for IV drugs, the **secondary IV line set**, which

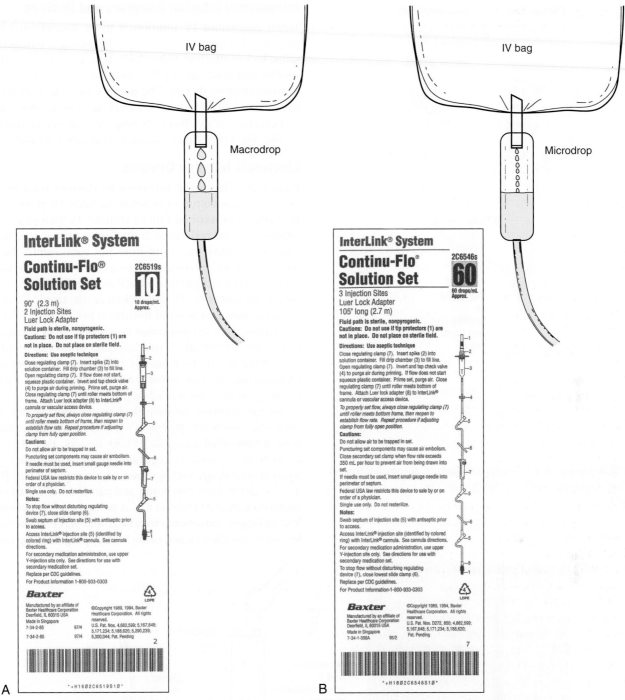

FIG. 11E.2 Macrodrip and Microdrip Intravenous Sets. (From Morris, D. G. [2014]. *Calculate with confidence* [6th ed.]. St. Louis, MO: Elsevier.)

is connected into a port (rubber stopper) on the IV connector on the continuous or **primary IV line set**; the port should be above the IV pump.

Secondary Intravenous Administration Sets

Two secondary IV administration sets available to administer IV drugs are the calibrated cylinder (volume-controlled chamber) with tubing (Fig. 11E.4)—such as the Buretrol, Volutrol, and Soluset—and the secondary IV set, which is similar to a regular IV set except the tubing is shorter. The cylinder can be used with a primary or secondary line and when measurement

of small-volume IV therapy needs to be more accurate, such as in pediatric or critical care settings. The volume-controlled chamber holds up to 150 mL of solution. The secondary IV line set is primarily used to **piggyback** onto a primary line (IVPB). The cylinder and some secondary IV tubing contain a port to inject medications.

When using a calibrated cylinder, such as the Buretrol, add 15 mL of IV solution, such as 0.9% sodium chloride, to flush the drug out of the IV line after the drug infusion is completed. The flush volume is added to the patient's intake. Check hospital policy for guidance.

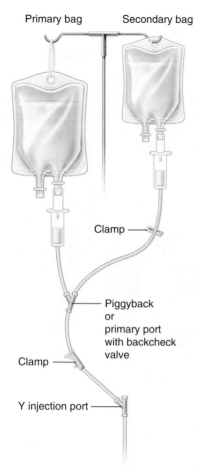

Primary bag   Secondary bag

Clamp

Piggyback
or
primary port
with backcheck
valve

Clamp

Y injection port

FIG. 11E.3 Intravenous Piggyback Setup. (From Morris, D. G. [2014]. *Calculate with confidence* [6th ed.]. St. Louis, MO: Elsevier.)

Intermittent Infusion Adapters and Devices

When continuous IV infusion is to be discontinued but the patient still requires IV access, the IV tubing is removed and a saline lock is attached. Saline locks have ports (stoppers) where needles and needleless or IV tubing can be inserted as needed to continue drug therapy. The use of a saline lock increases the patient's mobility by not having an IV line tagging along, and it is cost effective because less IV tubing, solution, and equipment are needed. Fig. 11E.5 shows examples of needleless infusion devices.

Electronic Infusion Devices

Pumps are **electronic intravenous devices** used in hospitals and some community settings. Such IV pumps are set to deliver a prescribed rate of volume. IV pumps deliver IV solution against resistance. If the flow is obstructed, an alarm sounds, however the alarm does not sound until the pump has exerted its maximum pressure to overcome resistance. Pumps do not recognize infiltration , therefore the nurse must frequently assess the IV site. When an electronic IV device is used, the flow rate is set in milliliters per hour (mL/h).

IV pumps are recommended for use with all IV therapy, however some noncritical IV solutions and drugs can be administered using gravity by manually calculating drops per minute. Ongoing nursing assessment is essential with any IV therapy to ensure proper duration of administration.

Several electronic infusion devices are available that include electronic volumetric pumps (IV pumps), syringe pumps, and **patient-controlled analgesia (PCA)** devices. Fig. 11E.6 shows a variety of electronic IV regulators for the administration of IV solutions and drugs. Part A shows a syringe pump, part B shows a single-channel infusion pump, and part C shows a dual-channel infusion pump. Part D shows a PCA pump, part E shows the Alaris System large-volume pump with PCA, and part F shows the Medley pump module attached to the Medley programming module.

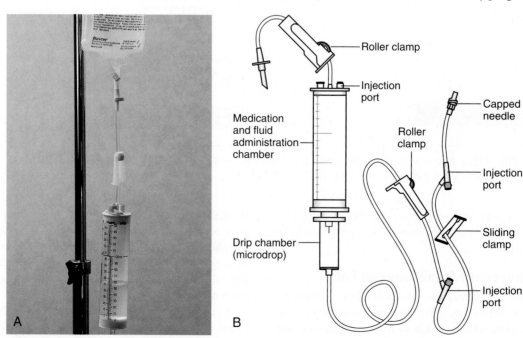

Medication and fluid administration chamber

Drip chamber (microdrop)

Roller clamp

Injection port

Roller clamp

Capped needle

Injection port

Sliding clamp

Injection port

A   B

FIG. 11E.4 Volume-Controlled Chamber. (From Morris, D. G. [2014]. *Calculate with confidence* [6th ed.]. St. Louis, MO: Elsevier.)

Safety Considerations for Intravenous Infusions

All IV infusions and sites should be checked frequently. Common problems associated with IV infusions are kinked tubing, infiltration, and so-called free-flow IV rates. If IV tubing kinks, the flow is interrupted and the prescribed amount of fluid will not be given. The access site can also clog, which obstructs the flow. When infiltration occurs, IV fluid extravasates into the tissues and not into the vascular space. Trauma occurs to the tissues around the IV site. A free-flow IV rate refers to a rapid infusion of IV fluids that is faster than prescribed, which can cause fluid overload due to rapid infusion. Because of the possibility of a free-flow IV rate, electronic infusion pumps with multiple safety features are commonly used today.

Electronic infusion pumps are not without flaws, and mechanical problems can occur. Also, incorrectly programming an infusion pump can result in an incorrect infusion rate. Frequent monitoring of IV infusions can prevent complications of IV therapy such as fluid overload, thrombus formation, and infiltration.

PCA is another method used to administer drugs intravenously (see Fig. 11E.6). The objective of PCA is to provide a

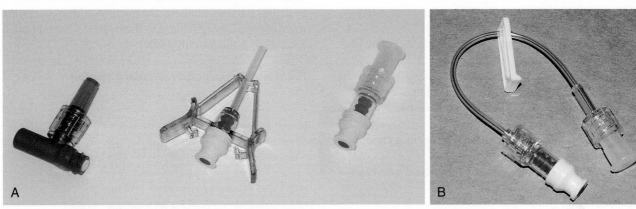

FIG. 11E.5 Needleless Infusion Devices. (From Kee, J. L., & Marshall, S. M. [2013]. *Clinical calculations* [7th ed.]. St. Louis, MO: Elsevier.)

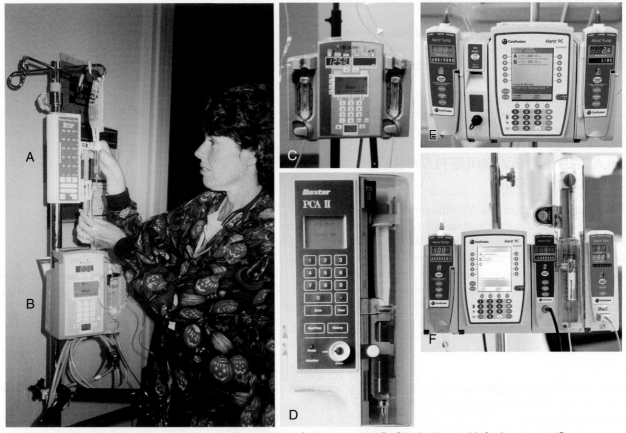

FIG. 11E.6 Electronic Infusion Devices. A, Syringe pump. **B,** Single-channel infusion pump. **C,** Dual-channel infusion pump. **D,** Patient-controlled analgesia (PCA) pump. **E,** Alaris System large-volume pump with PCA. **F,** Medley pump module attached to Medley programming module. (From Kee, J. L., & Marshall, S. M. [2013]. *Clinical calculations* [7th ed.]. St. Louis, MO: Elsevier.)

uniform serum concentration of the medication, thus avoiding drug peaks and valleys. This method is designed to meet the needs of patients who require at least 24 to 48 hours of frequent intramuscular (IM) or IV narcotic injections.

Several reasons for the use of PCA include (1) effective pain control without the patient feeling oversedated, (2) considerable reduction in the amount of narcotic used (approximately one half that of IM delivery), and (3) patients' feelings of having greater control over their pain.

Choices are available in the delivery of PCA. The pump can be programmed to administer the prescribed medication (1) at patient demand, (2) continuously, or (3) continuously and supplemented by patient demand (see Chapter 25).

The health care provider's order must include the following:
- Drug ordered
- Loading dose, administered by the health care provider to obtain a baseline serum concentration of analgesic
- PCA dose, administered each time the patient activates the button
- Lockout interval, the time during which the drug cannot be administered
- Dose limit, the maximum amount the patient can receive during a specified time
Patient Teaching.
- Inform the patient that the pain should be tolerable but not necessarily absent.
- Advise the patient of the pump's safety features, including the alarms.
- Instruct the patient in the use of the control button (medication is administered when the button is *released*).
- Instruct the patient to report any side effects or adverse reactions to the drug.
- Have naloxone, the reversal agent for opioids, easily accessible.
- Instruct patients, family members, and caregivers that the PCA button is to be depressed only by the patient.

CALCULATING INTRAVENOUS FLOW RATE: MILLILITERS PER HOUR

Regardless of the method used to determine the rate, the nurse should have the following information before calculating the flow rate: (1) the volume to be infused, (2) the drop factor of the infusion set, and (3) the time frame or how long to infuse the fluid. As with previous drug calculations, the nurse should select one method, be familiar with it, and consistently use it to calculate IV flow rate. When delivering IV drugs via electronic devices, the flow rate is calculated for milliliters per hour (mL/h).

EXAMPLE: Calculating Milliliters per Hour
1. Order: 500 mL of 0.45% sodium chloride (½NS) to be infused over 8 hours.
   What is the flow rate?

Basic Formula

$$\frac{\text{Amount of solution}}{\text{Hours to administer}} = \text{milliliters per hour (mL/h)}$$

$$x\,\text{mL/h} = \frac{500\,\text{mL}}{8\,\text{h}}$$

$$= 62.5\,\text{mL/h}$$

If the infusion pump can be programmed to deliver partial milliliters, set the pump to deliver 62.5 mL/h (round to the nearest tenth); if the infusion pump cannot be set to deliver partial milliliters, the nurse would set the pump to infuse at 63 mL/h (round to the nearest whole number, according to the rounding rule).

Ratio and Proportion/Fractional Equation

$$\frac{\text{Total volume}}{\text{time (h)}} = \frac{x\,\text{mL}}{1\,\text{h}}$$

$$\frac{500\,\text{mL}}{8\,\text{h}} = \frac{x\,\text{mL}}{1\,\text{h}}$$

$$8x = 500$$

$$x = 62.5\,\text{mL/h}$$

Dimensional Analysis

$$\text{mL/h} = \frac{\text{amount of solution}}{\text{time in hours}}$$

(Dimensional analysis for this particular problem is set up similar to the basic formula.)

2. Order: 1000 milliliters of 0.9% sodium chloride (NS) to infuse at 75 milliliters per hour.
   What is the total infusion time in hours and minutes?

Dimensional Analysis

$$\text{time (h and min)} = \frac{1\,\text{h}}{75\,\text{mL}} \times \frac{1000\,\text{mL}}{x\,\text{time}}$$

$$= \frac{1000}{75} = 13.33\,\text{h}\,;\text{and}$$

$$0.33\,\text{h} \times 60\,\text{min} = 19.8\,\text{min} = 20\,\text{min}$$

Answer: Total infusion time is 13 h and 20 min.

3. Using the total time in example 2 above, what time will the infusion complete if the initial infusion was started at 2:00 PM?
   Convert 2:00 PM to military time (1400 h), then add 13 h and 20 min.

$$1400 + 1320 = 2720 = 3:20$$

4. Infuse Lactated Ringer's solution (LR) 1000 milliliters over 12 hours.
   What is the flow rate?

$$\textit{Answer: mL/h} = \frac{1000\,\text{mL}}{12\,\text{h}} = 83.3\,\text{mL/h}$$

5. D_5 ½NS has been infusing at 125 mL/h.
   After 5½ hours, the IV infiltrated, and the infusion had to be stopped. How many milliliters are left in the IV bag?

Dimensional Analysis

Answer: If mL $= \dfrac{125 \text{ mL}}{1 \text{ h}} \times \dfrac{5.5 \text{ h}}{x \text{ mL}} = 687.5$ mL used,

then 1000 mL − 687.5 mL = 312.5 mL left in the bag

CALCULATING INTRAVENOUS FLOW RATE: DROPS PER MINUTE

When an electronic device is not used and the nurse manually regulates the IV rate, the nurse must calculate the number of drops per minute (gtt/min). The flow rate in drops per minute is determined by the size of the IV tubing (gtt/mL) as discussed earlier in this chapter. To convert hours to minutes, multiply the hours with 60 minutes.

EXAMPLE: Calculating Drops per Minute

1. Order: 500 milliliters of 0.45% sodium chloride (½NS) to be infused over 8 hours. IV tubing reads 10 drops per milliliter. What is the flow rate in drops per minute?
   (The question is asking for flow rate with a given drop factor. When drop factor is involved in computing flow rate, solve for drops per minute.)

Basic Formula

$$\text{gtt/min} = \frac{\text{amount of solution in mL} \times \text{gtt factor}}{\text{time in h} \times 60 \text{ min}}$$

$$\text{gtt/min} = \frac{500 \text{ mL} \times 10 \text{ gtt/mL}}{8 \text{ h} \times 60 \text{ min}}$$

= 10.4 gtt/min = 10 gtt/min (A partial drop cannot be administered.)

Ratio and Proportion/Fractional Equation

a. Determine milliliters per hour.
b. Determine drops per minute.

$$\frac{500 \text{ mL}}{8 \text{ h}} = \frac{x}{1 \text{ h}}$$

62.5 mL/h; then

$$\frac{62.5 \text{ mL/h}}{60 \text{ min}} = \frac{x}{10 \text{ gtt/mL}}$$

$$62.5 \times 10 = 60 \, x$$

$$x = 10.4 \text{ gtt/min} = 10 \text{ gtt/min}$$

Dimensional Analysis

$$\frac{\text{gtt}}{\text{min}} = \frac{10 \text{ gtt}}{\text{mL}} \times \frac{500 \text{ mL}}{8 \text{ h}} \times \frac{1 \text{ h}}{60 \text{ min}}$$

$$= \frac{10 \text{ gtt}}{8} \times \frac{500}{60 \text{ min}}$$

$$= \frac{5000 \text{ gtt}}{480 \text{ min}}$$

$$= 10.41 \text{ gtt/min} = 10 \text{ gtt/min}$$

2. Order: A client is to receive D_5 ½NS at 75 mL/h. The drop factor is 20 gtt/mL. What is the flow rate?
   (The question is asking for flow rate with a given drop factor. When drop factor is involved in computing flow rate, solve for drops per minute.)

Dimensional Analysis

$$\frac{\text{gtt}}{\text{min}} = \frac{20 \text{ gtt}}{\text{mL}} \times \frac{75 \text{ mL}}{1 \text{ h}} \times \frac{1 \text{ h}}{60 \text{ min}}$$

$$= 25 \text{ gtt/min}$$

3. Order: 1 L of 0.9% sodium chloride (NS) to be infused over 12 hours.
   What is the flow rate with the following IV tubing?

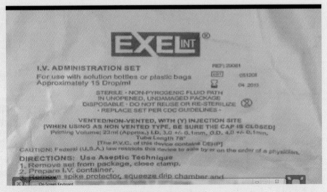

Answer: gtt/min $= \dfrac{15 \text{ gtt}}{1 \text{ mL}} \times \dfrac{1000 \text{ mL}}{12 \text{ h}} \times \dfrac{1 \text{ h}}{60 \text{ min}} = 20.8$

= 21 gtt/min (per the rounding rule)

PRACTICE PROBLEMS

Calculating Intravenous Therapy: Flow Rate

1. Order: 1000 mL of D_5 ½NS to infuse over 12 hours.
   Available: Microdrip set with a drop factor of 60 gtt/mL
   a. Calculate the IV flow rate in drops per minute. _____

2. Order: 3 L of IV solution to infuse over 24 hours: with 1 L of D_5W and 2 L of D_5 ½NS
   a. One liter is equal to how many milliliters? _____
   b. Each liter should infuse for how many hours? _____
   c. The institution uses a set with a drop factor of 15 gtt/mL. How many drops per minute should the patient receive per liter of fluid? _____

3. Order: 250 mL of D_5W over 3 hours
   a. Determine the flow rate. _____

4. Order: 1000 mL of D_5 ½NS, 1 vial of multiple vitamin (MVI), and 10 mEq of potassium chloride (KCl) to be infused over 10 hours
   Available: 1000 mL of D_5 ½ NS; MVI: 1 vial = 10 mL; KCl 20 mEq/20 mL vial
   Macrodrip set, 15 gtt/mL; microdrip set, 60 gtt/mL
   a. What is the total volume of the solution?
   b. How many drops per minute should the patient receive using the macrodrip set and the microdrip set?
   c. The IV pump is set at how many milliliters per hour?

PRACTICE PROBLEMS

⚡ *Calculating Intravenous Therapy: Direct Injection*

1. Order: Protamine sulfate 40 mg IV STAT; IV infusion not to exceed 5 mg per min
Available:

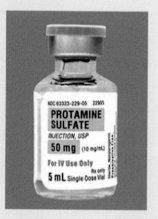

   a. How many milliliters should the patient receive? _____
   b. How many minutes should protamine be administered? _____

2. Order: Morphine sulfate 5 mg IV q3h PRN
Available:

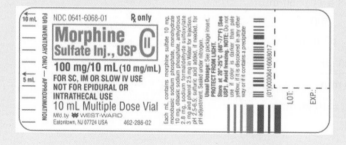

Instructions are to dilute the dose with 5 mL of NS and to administer 2.5 to 15 mg over 5 minutes.

a. How many milliliters of morphine should the patient receive? _____

b. For how many minutes should morphine be administered? _____

3. Order: Furosemide 80 mg IV now
Available:

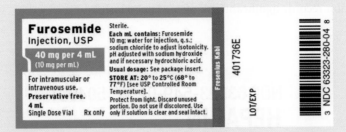

Drug insert states rate of administration is 20 mg/min.

a. How many milliliters will the nurse administer? _____

b. How long should furosemide be given? _____

4. Order: Regular insulin 20 units IV for blood glucose over 600
Available:

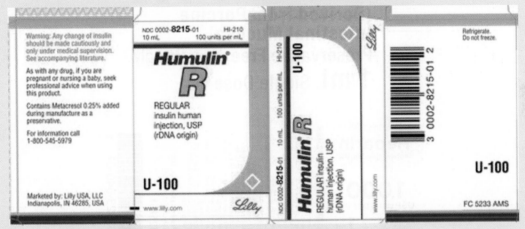

Indicate by shading the appropriate syringe to show the amount of insulin to give.

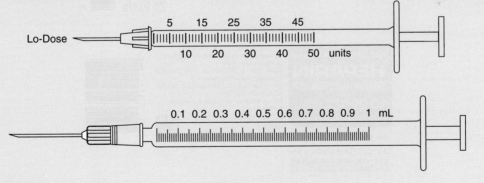

5. Order: Digoxin 0.375 mg IV over 5 min
Available: Digoxin 0.25 mg/mL
How many milliliters will the nurse administer? _____
(When giving drugs by direct IV, always verify the compatibility of the IV solution and the drug; otherwise, precipitation can result. Incompatibility can be avoided if the IV tubing is flushed with a compatible solution of either normal saline or sterile water before and after administration.)

Calculating Intravenous Heparin Infusions

Like insulin, heparin is prescribed in unit dosages. Heparin is a high-alert drug that is available in multiple concentrations from 10 units/mL to 50,000 units/mL. It is important for the nurse to identify the label dosage strength and verify the patient's medication administration record; significant risk of causing serious injury or death can occur with errors. Heparin labels must be read carefully to ensure the correct drug is being administered. The following heparin labels are examples of available strengths. Note that only one is indicated for heparin flush (100 units/mL). All other labels indicate "NOT for Lock Flush."

NDC 63323-549-01   504901

HEPARIN
LOCK FLUSH
SOLUTION, USP

100 USP Units/mL

(Derived from Porcine Intestinal Mucosa)
Preservative Free   Rx only

1 mL Single Dose Vial

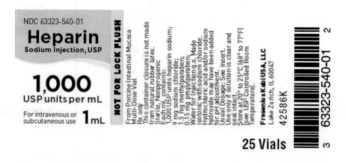

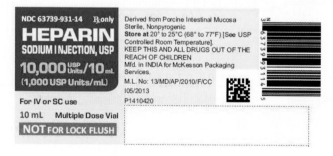

250 mL SINGLE-DOSE CONTAINER   NDC 0409-7794-52

HEPARIN

RX ONLY

12,500 USP Units/250 mL
(50 USP Units/mL)

HEPARIN SODIUM IN
5% DEXTROSE INJECTION

50

WARNING: CONTAINS SULFITES
EACH 100 mL CONTAINS
HEPARIN SODIUM 5,000 USP
UNITS (PORCINE INTESTINAL
MUCOSA); DEXTROSE,
HYDROUS 5 g; CITRIC ACID,
ANHYDROUS 51 mg; SODIUM
CITRATE, DIHYDRATE
334 mg; SODIUM METABISULFITE
20 mg; ELECTROLYTES: SODIUM
38 mEq/L; CITRATE 42 mEq/L.
STERILE. USUAL DOSAGE: SEE
INSERT. **ADDITIVES SHOULD
NOT BE MADE TO THIS
SOLUTION.** LATEX-FREE. SINGLE
DOSE CONTAINER. DISCARD
UNUSED PORTION. FOR
INTRAVENOUS USE ONLY.

100

150

200

OTHER

IM-3490
HOSPIRA, INC., LAKE FOREST, IL 60045 USA   *Hospira*

Heparin can be given as a direct IV injection and as a continuous infusion. Direct IV injection was discussed earlier in this chapter. IV infusion is calculated in units per hour.

EXAMPLE: Calculating Intravenous Heparin Therapy

1. Ordered: 1000 mL D_5W with heparin sodium 20000 units
   to infuse at 30 mL/h
   Calculate the units per hour.

   Answer: $\text{units/h} = \dfrac{20000 \text{ units}}{1000 \text{ mL}} \times \dfrac{30 \text{ mL}}{1 \text{ h}} = 600 \text{ units/h}$

2. Order: Heparin sodium 750 units/h
   Available: Heparin sodium 25000 units in 500 mL D_5W
   Calculate the milliliters per hour.

   Answer: $\text{mL/h} = \dfrac{500 \text{ mL}}{25000 \text{ units}} \times \dfrac{750 \text{ units}}{1 \text{ h}} = 15 \text{ mL/h}$

3. Heparin sodium 80 units/kg IV bolus is ordered followed
   by heparin sodium infusion at 15 units/kg/h for a patient
   who weighs 175 lb.
   Available:

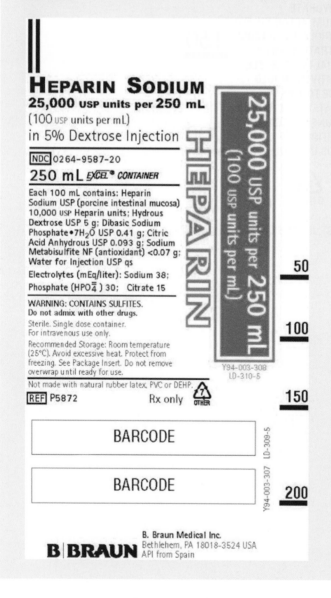

a. Calculate the amount of bolus in units and milliliters to
   administer.
b. Calculate flow rate in units per hour.
c. Calculate flow rate in milliliters per hour.

Answer:

a. $\text{units} = \dfrac{80 \text{ units}}{1 \text{ kg}} \times \dfrac{1 \text{ kg}}{2.2 \text{ lbs}} \times \dfrac{175 \text{ lb}}{x} = 6364 \text{ units bolus}$

   $\text{mL} = \dfrac{1 \text{ mL}}{100 \text{ units}} \times \dfrac{6364 \text{ units}}{x} = 63.6 \text{ mL bolus}$

b. $\text{units/h} = \dfrac{15 \text{ units}}{1 \text{ kg}} \times \dfrac{1 \text{ kg}}{2.2 \text{ lb}} \times \dfrac{175 \text{ lb}}{x} = 1193 \text{ units/h}$

c. $\text{mL/h} = \dfrac{1 \text{ mL}}{100 \text{ units}} \times \dfrac{15 \text{ units}}{1 \text{ kg}} \times \dfrac{1 \text{ kg}}{2.2 \text{ lb}} \times \dfrac{175 \text{ lb}}{x}$

   $= 11.9 \text{ mL/h}$

Intravenous Heparin Therapy

1. Ordered: Heparin sodium 800 units/h

   Available: Heparin sodium 40 units/mL

HEPARIN SODIUM
20,000 USP units per 500 mL
(40 USP units per mL)
in 5% Dextrose Injection

NDC 0264-9567-10 | **500 mL** EXCEL® CONTAINER

Each 100 mL contains: Heparin Sodium USP
(porcine intestinal mucosa) 4,000 USP Heparin units
Hydrous Dextrose USP 5 g
Dibasic Sodium Phosphate•7H$_2$O USP 0.41 g
Citric Acid Anhydrous USP 0.093 g
Sodium Metabisulfite NF (antioxidant) <0.07 g
Water for Injection USP qs

Electrolytes (mEq/liter):   Sodium 38
Phosphate (HPO₄) 30   Citrate 15

WARNING: CONTAINS SULFITES.
Do not admix with other drugs.
Sterile. Single dose container. For intravenous use only.
Recommended Storage: Room temperature (25°C). Avoid
excessive heat. Protect from freezing. See Package Insert.
Do not remove overwrap until ready for use.

REF P5671   Not made with natural rubber latex, PVC or DEHP.   Rx only

BARCODE

BARCODE

B. Braun Medical Inc.
Bethlehem, PA 18018-3524 USA
API from Spain
B|BRAUN

20,000 USP units per 500 mL
(40 USP units per mL)
HEPARIN
LD-306-4 Y94-003-288

-0-
-1-
-2-
-3-
-4-

Calculate the flow rate. _____

2. Order: 250 mL 0.9% sodium chloride (NS) with heparin sodium 25000 units to infuse at 35 mL/h

   Calculate units per hour. _____

3. Order: Heparin flush mediport every 3 days.

   Which heparin product is appropriate?

LOT:

EXP: To open—Cut seal along dotted line.

NDC 0641-0272-25

HEP-LOCK U/P
PRESERVATIVE-FREE
Heparin Lock Flush Solution, USP

10 USP units/mL   Rx only
25 x 1 mL DOSETTE Vials
FOR INTRAVENOUS FLUSH ONLY
NOT FOR ANTICOAGULANT THERAPY

esi

Manufactured by Baxter Healthcare Corporation
Deerfield, IL 60015 USA   462-359-00

SINGLE USE -
DESTROY UNUSED CONTENTS
Each mL contains heparin sodium 10 USP
units, sodium chloride 8 mg, monobasic
sodium phosphate monohydrate 2.3 mg,
and dibasic sodium phosphate anhydrous
0.5 mg in Water for Injection. pH 5.0-7.5.
Intended for maintenance of
patency of intravenous injection
devices only. May alter the
results of blood coagulation
tests.
FROM PORCINE INTESTINES -
NONPYROGENIC
Usual Dosage: See package
insert.
Store at 20°-25°C (68°-77°F)
[see USP Controlled Room
Temperature].

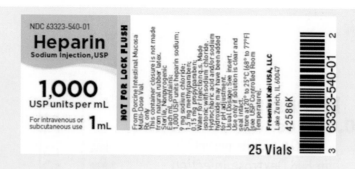

4. Order: Bolus with heparin at 80 units/kg, then initate heparin infusion at 20 units/kg/hour for a patient who weighs 150 lb.

   Available: Heparin sodium 25000 units in 500 mL 5% dextrose in water (D_5W).

   a. Calculate bolus dose in units. _____

   b. Calculate bolus dose in milliliters. _____

   c. What is the flow rate of the heparin infusion? _____

5. Order: Infuse heparin sodium 25000 units in 1000 mL of NS at 30 mL/h.

   Calculate units per hour. _____

Calculating Critical Care Drugs

Most drugs administered in critical care are **titrated** (adjusted) according to the patient's response to the drug therapy. The patient is monitored closely for therapeutic effects and any adverse events. When calculating critical care drugs, any method previously discussed is effective, however dimensional analysis is the best method because units and conversion factors are calculated in one equation.

EXAMPLE: Calculating Critical Care Therapy

1. Order: Infuse dopamine at 5 mcg/kg/min to maintain systolic blood pressure above 110 mm Hg. The patient weighs 130 lb.
   Available: Dopamine hydrochloride (HCl) 200 mg in 250 mL of 5% dextrose in water (D_5W)
   Calculate milliliters per hour.

   $Answer$: $\text{mL/h} = \dfrac{250 \text{ mL}}{200 \text{ mg}} \times \dfrac{1 \text{ mg}}{1000 \text{ mcg}} \times \dfrac{5 \text{ mcg}}{1 \text{ kg}} \times \dfrac{1 \text{ kg}}{2.2 \text{ lb}} \times \dfrac{130 \text{ lb}}{1 \text{ min}} \times \dfrac{60 \text{ min}}{1 \text{ h}} = 22.2 \text{ mL/h}$

   (All the conversion factors for milligrams per microgram, pounds per kilogram, and units are eliminated except for milliliters and hours.)

2. Order: Dobutamine HCl 2 mcg/kg/min, titrated to maintain hemodynamic goals in a patient who weighs 180 lb
   Available: Dobutamine HCl 250 mg in 500 mL of D_5W
   Calculate micrograms per kilograms per minute.
   Calculate milliliters per hour.

   $Answer$: $\text{mcg/kg/min} = \dfrac{2 \text{ mcg}}{1 \text{ kg}} \times \dfrac{1 \text{ kg}}{2.2 \text{ lb}} \times \dfrac{180 \text{ lb}}{x \text{ min}} = 163.6 \text{ mcg/kg/min}$

   $\text{mL/h} = \dfrac{500 \text{ mL}}{250 \text{ mg}} \times \dfrac{1 \text{ mg}}{1000 \text{ mcg}} \times \dfrac{2 \text{ mcg}}{1 \text{ kg}} \times \dfrac{1 \text{ kg}}{2.2 \text{ lb}} \times \dfrac{180 \text{ lb}}{1 \text{ min}} \times \dfrac{60 \text{ min}}{1 \text{ h}} = 19.6 \text{ mL/h}$

   ❶ (Be aware of sound-alike drugs, dopamine and dobutamine. *Dopamine* is an adrenergic agonist that affects dopamine receptors. *Dobutamine* is a beta₁-adrenergic agonist and does *not* affect dopamine receptors. They both have inotropic properties and are used as vasopressors.)

3. Order: Isoproterenol 2 mg in 250 mL of D_5W to infuse at 8 mcg/min
   Calculate milliliters per hour.

   $Answer$: $\text{mL/h} = \dfrac{250 \text{ mL}}{2 \text{ mg}} \times \dfrac{1 \text{ mg}}{1000 \text{ mcg}} \times \dfrac{8 \text{ mcg}}{1 \text{ min}} \times \dfrac{60 \text{ min}}{1 \text{ h}} = 60 \text{ mL/h}$

Additional practice problems for all drug calculations are available in the Study Guide and on the Evolve website.

ANSWERS TO PRACTICE PROBLEMS

CALCULATING INTRAVENOUS THERAPY—FLOW RATE

All answers are provided using dimensional analysis.

1. IV flow rate: $\text{gtt/min} = \dfrac{60\text{gtt}}{1\text{mL}} \times \dfrac{1000\text{mL}}{12\text{hr}} \times \dfrac{1\text{hr}}{60\text{min}} = 83 \text{ gtt/min}$

2. a. 1 L = 1000 mL

   b. 1 L over 8 h each $\left(\dfrac{24\text{ hr}}{3\text{ L}} = 8 \text{ h/L}\right)$

   c. Flow rate: $\text{gtt/min} = \dfrac{15\text{gtt}}{1\text{mL}} \times \dfrac{3000\text{mL}}{24\text{hr}} \times \dfrac{1\text{hr}}{60\text{min}} = \dfrac{45,000\text{gtt}}{1440\text{min}} = 31\text{gtt/min}$

3. Flow rate: $\text{mL/hour} = \dfrac{250\text{ mL}}{3\text{ hr}} = 83.3\text{mL/hr}$

4. a. Total volume = 1030 mL

   b. Macro drip set: $\text{gtt/min} = \dfrac{15\text{gtt}}{1\text{mL}} \times \dfrac{1030\text{mL}}{10\text{h}} \times \dfrac{1\text{h}}{60\text{min}} = \dfrac{15,450\text{gtt}}{600\text{min}} = 25.75 \text{ gtt/min} = 26 \text{ gtt/min after rounding to the nearest whole number}$

   Micro drip set: $\text{gtt/min} = \dfrac{60\text{gtt}}{1\text{mL}} \times \dfrac{1030\text{mL}}{10\text{h}} \times \dfrac{1\text{h}}{60\text{min}} = \dfrac{61,800\text{gtt}}{600\text{min}} = 103 \text{ gtt/min}$

   c. IV pump: $\text{mL/h} = \dfrac{1030\text{mL}}{10\text{h}} = 103\text{mL/h}$

CALCULATING INTRAVENOUS THERAPY—DIRECT INJECTION

All answers are provided using dimensional analysis.

1. a. 4 mL

   b. $\text{min} = \dfrac{1\text{min}}{5\text{mg}} \times \dfrac{40\text{ mg}}{x} = 8 \text{ min or 0.5 mL/min}$

2. a. $\text{mL} = \dfrac{1\text{mL}}{10\text{mg}} \times \dfrac{5\text{mg}}{x} = 0.5\text{mL}$

   b. Because 2.5 to 5 mg can be given over 5 minutes, 5 mg is given over 5 minutes.

3. a. $\text{mL} = \dfrac{1\text{mL}}{10\text{mg}} \times \dfrac{80\text{ mg}}{x} = 8 \text{ mL}$

   b. $\text{min} = \dfrac{1\text{min}}{20\text{mg}} \times \dfrac{80\text{ mg}}{x} = 4 \text{ min or 2 mL/min}$

4.

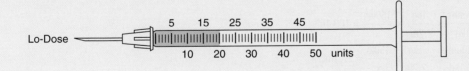

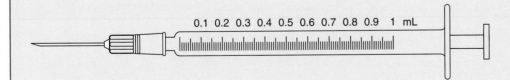

(The top syringe is calibrated in units, the bottom syringe is in milliliters.)

5. Administer: $\text{mL} = \dfrac{1\text{mL}}{0.25\text{mg}} \times \dfrac{0.375\text{mg}}{x} = 1.5\text{mL}$

INTRAVENOUS HEPARIN THERAPY

1. Flow rate in mL/h $= \dfrac{1\text{mL}}{40\text{units}} \times \dfrac{800 \text{ units}}{1\text{ h}} = 20$ mL/h

2. units/h $= \dfrac{25000 \text{ units}}{250 \text{ mL}} \times \dfrac{35 \text{ mL}}{1\text{ h}} = 3500$ units/h

3.

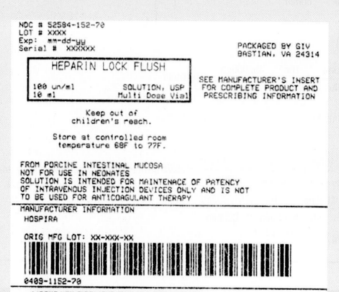

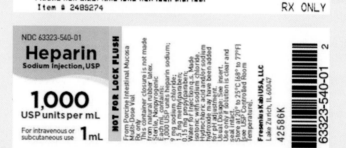

4. a. Bolus in units $= \dfrac{80\text{units}}{1\text{kg}} \times \dfrac{1\text{kg}}{2.2\text{lbs}} \times \dfrac{150\text{lbs}}{x} = 5454.5$ units

   b. Bolus in milliliters $= \dfrac{500\text{mL}}{25000\text{units}} \times \dfrac{80\text{units}}{1\text{kg}} \times \dfrac{1\text{kg}}{2.2\text{lbs}} \times \dfrac{150\text{lbs}}{x} = 109.1$ mL

   c. Flow rate in mL/h $= \dfrac{500\text{mL}}{25,000\text{units}} \times \dfrac{20\text{units}}{1\text{kg}} \times \dfrac{1\text{kg}}{2.2\text{lb}} \times \dfrac{150\text{lb}}{x} = 27.3$ mL/h

5. units/h $= \dfrac{25000\text{units}}{1000\text{mL}} \times \dfrac{30\text{mL}}{1\text{ h}} = 750$ units/h

Central and Peripheral Nervous System Drugs

The nervous system is composed of all nerve tissues: brain, spinal cord, nerves, and ganglia. The purpose of the nervous system is to receive stimuli and transmit information to nerve centers for an appropriate response. There are two types of nervous systems: the central nervous system and the peripheral nervous system.

The central nervous system (CNS), composed of the brain and spinal cord, regulates body functions (Fig. V.1). The CNS interprets information sent by impulses from the peripheral nervous system (PNS) and returns the instruction through the PNS for appropriate cellular actions. Stimulation of the CNS may either increase nerve cell (neuron) activity or block nerve cell activity.

The PNS consists of two divisions: the somatic nervous system (SNS) and the autonomic nervous system (ANS). The SNS is voluntary and acts on skeletal muscles to produce locomotion and respiration. The ANS, also called the *visceral system,* is involuntary; it controls and regulates the functioning of the heart, respiratory system, gastrointestinal system, and glands. The ANS, a large nervous system that functions without our conscious control, has two subdivisions: the sympathetic and the parasympathetic nervous systems.

The sympathetic nervous system of the ANS is called the *adrenergic system* because its neurotransmitter is norepinephrine. The parasympathetic nervous system is called the *cholinergic system* because its neurotransmitter is acetylcholine. Because organs are innervated by both the sympathetic and the parasympathetic systems, they can produce opposite responses. The sympathetic response is excitability, and the parasympathetic response is inhibition.

The sympathetic and the parasympathetic nerve pathways originate from different locations in the spinal cord. These nervous systems send information by two types of nerve fibers, preganglionic and postganglionic, and by the ganglion between these fibers (Fig. V.2). The preganglionic nerve fiber carries

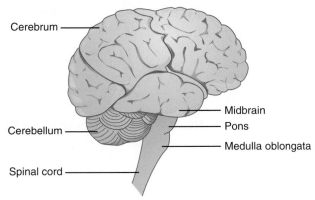

FIG. V.1 Brain and Spinal Cord.

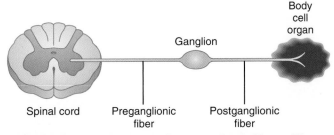

FIG. V.2 Preganglionic and Postganglionic Nerve Fibers.

messages from the CNS to the ganglion, and the postganglionic fiber transmits impulses from the ganglion to body tissues and organs.

The sympathetic nervous system is also called the *thoracolumbar division* of the ANS, because the preganglionic fibers originate from the thoracic segment (T1 to T12) and the upper lumbar segment (L1 and L2) of the spinal cord. The sympathetic preganglionic fibers from the spinal cord to the ganglion are short, and the sympathetic postganglionic fibers from the ganglion to the body cells are long. Fig. V.3 illustrates the sympathetic preganglionic fibers from the spinal cord.

The parasympathetic nervous system is called the *craniosacral division* of the ANS because the preganglionic fibers originate with cranial nerves III, VII, IX, and X from the brainstem and sacral segments S2, S3, and S4 of the spinal cord. The parasympathetic preganglionic fibers are long from the spinal cord to the ganglion, and the parasympathetic postganglionic fibers are short from the ganglion to the body cells. Fig. V.4 illustrates the parasympathetic preganglionic fibers from the spinal cord.

Drugs that stimulate and depress the CNS are discussed in Chapter 17 and Chapter 18, respectively. Drugs used to control seizures are discussed in Chapter 19, and they are also considered CNS depressants. Drugs used to treat neuromuscular disorders such as parkinsonism, myasthenia gravis, multiple sclerosis, and Alzheimer disease have varying effects on the nervous system and muscles. These are discussed in Chapters 20 and 21.

Fig. V.5 shows a schematic breakdown of the nervous systems in the body.

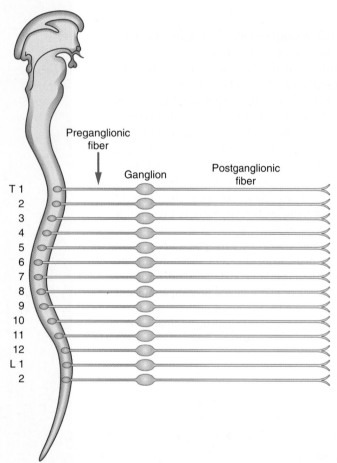

FIG. V.3 Sympathetic Nerve Fibers.

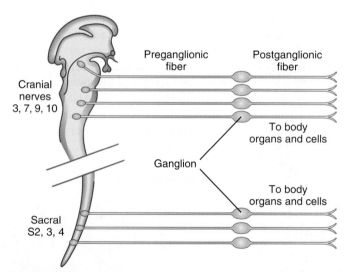

FIG. V.4 Parasympathetic Nerve Fibers.

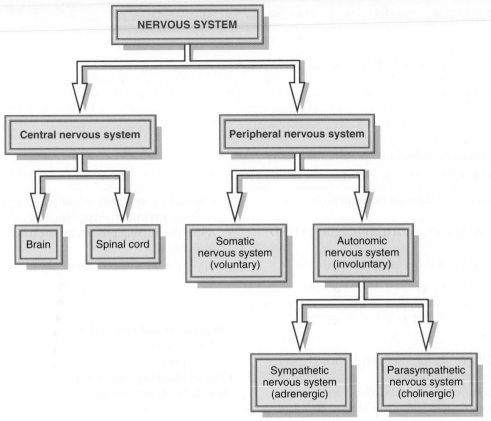

FIG. V.5 The Nervous System.

17

Stimulants

ⓔ http://evolve.elsevier.com/McCuistion/pharmacology

OBJECTIVES

- Explain the effects of stimulants on the central nervous system (CNS).
- Compare attention-deficit/hyperactivity disorder (ADHD) and narcolepsy.
- Differentiate the action of drugs used for ADHD and narcolepsy.

- Contrast the common side effects of amphetamines, anorexiants, analeptics, doxapram, and caffeine.
- Apply the nursing process for the patient taking CNS stimulants.
- Apply the nursing process for the patient taking doxapram.

OUTLINE

KEY TERMS

Numerous drugs can stimulate the central nervous system (CNS), which involves the brain and spinal cord and regulates body functions. Medically approved use of CNS stimulants is limited to the treatment of attention-deficit/hyperactivity disorder in children, narcolepsy, and the reversal of respiratory distress. The major groups of CNS stimulants include amphetamines *and caffeine,* which stimulate the cerebral cortex of the brain; analeptics *and caffeine,* which act on the brainstem and medulla to stimulate respiration; and anorexiants such as diethylpropion, which are thought to suppress appetite by stimulating the satiety center in the hypothalamic and limbic areas of the brain. Amphetamines and related anorexiants are greatly abused. Long-term use of amphetamines can produce psychological dependence or tolerance, conditions in which larger and larger doses of a drug are needed to reproduce the initial response. These medications are recommended for short-term use only (up to 12 weeks). Gradually increasing a drug dose and then abruptly stopping the drug may result in depression and withdrawal symptoms.

PATHOPHYSIOLOGY

Attention-deficit/hyperactivity disorder (ADHD) might be caused by a dysregulation of the transmitter's serotonin, norepinephrine, and dopamine. ADHD occurs primarily in children, usually before the age of 7 years, and may continue through the teenage years. In some cases, it may not be identified until early adulthood. The incidence of ADHD is three to seven times more common in boys than in girls. Characteristic behaviors of the various types of ADHD include inattentiveness, inability to concentrate, restlessness (fidgety), hyperactivity (excessive and purposeless activity), inability to complete tasks, and impulsivity.

The child with ADHD may display poor coordination, and there may be abnormal electroencephalograph (EEG) findings. Intelligence is usually not affected, but learning disabilities are often present. This disorder has also been called *minimal brain dysfunction, hyperactivity in children, hyperkinesis,* and *hyperkinetic syndrome with learning disorder.* Some professionals state that ADHD is often incorrectly diagnosed and results in many children receiving unnecessary treatment for months or years.

Narcolepsy is characterized by falling asleep during normal waking activities, such as driving a car or talking with someone. Sleep paralysis, the condition of muscle paralysis that is normal during sleep, usually accompanies narcolepsy and affects the voluntary muscles. The narcoleptic is unable to move and may collapse.

AMPHETAMINES

Amphetamines stimulate the release of the neurotransmitters norepinephrine and dopamine from the brain and sympathetic nervous system (peripheral nerve terminals) and inhibit the reuptake of these transmitters. Amphetamines ordinarily cause euphoria and increased alertness, but they can also cause insomnia, restlessness, tremors, irritability, and weight loss. Cardiovascular problems such as increased heart rate, palpitations, cardiac dysrhythmia, and increased blood pressure can result from cardiac stimulation and vasoconstriction with continuous use of amphetamines. These drugs have a high potential for abuse, tolerance, and dependence. Excessive use may lead to psychosis.

The half-life of amphetamines varies from 9 to 13 hours. Amphetamines and dextroamphetamine are prescribed for narcolepsy and ADHD when amphetamine-like drugs are ineffective.

Side Effects and Adverse Reactions

Amphetamines can cause adverse effects in the CNS and the cardiovascular, gastrointestinal (GI), and endocrine systems. Side effects and adverse reactions include dizziness, headache, euphoria, confusion, blurred vision, restlessness, insomnia, tachycardia, hypertension, heart palpitations, dysrhythmias, dry mouth, anorexia, weight loss, diarrhea, constipation, seizures, tremors, and erectile dysfunction.

Amphetamine-Like Drugs for Attention-Deficit/Hyperactivity Disorder and Narcolepsy

Methylphenidate and dexmethylphenidate, classed as amphetamine-like drugs, are given to increase a child's attention span and cognitive performance (e.g., memory, reading) and to decrease impulsiveness, hyperactivity, and restlessness. Methylphenidate is also used to treat narcolepsy. Because of the potential for abuse of methylphenidate, it is classified as a Controlled Substance Schedule (CSS) II drug. Prototype Drug Chart 17.1 illustrates the pharmacokinetics, pharmacodynamics, and therapeutic effects of methylphenidate in the treatment of ADHD and narcolepsy. Amphetamine and amphetamine-like drugs should not be taken in the evening or before bedtime because insomnia may result.

PROTOTYPE DRUG CHART 17.1
Methylphenidate

Drug Class	Dosage
Amphetamine-like drug: CNS stimulant CSS II Pregnancy category: C*	ADHD: Immediate release: A/adol: PO: 20-30 mg/d in 2-3 divided doses 30-40 min before breakfast and lunch; *max:* 60 mg/d C 6-12 y: PO: 5-10 mg before breakfast and lunch; *max:* 60 mg/d Extended release: A: PO: 18-36 mg/d in the morning; *max:* 72 mg/d C: PO: 18 mg/d; *max:* 54 mg/d or 2 mg/kg/d Adol/C >6 y: Transdermal patch: Initially 10 mg/9 h patch/d in the morning; *max:* 30 mg/9 h patch/d Narcolepsy: A: PO: 10-60 mg/d in 2-3 divided doses; *max:* 72 mg/d C >6 y: PO: Initially 5 mg bid 30 min before meals; *max:* 60 mg/d
Contraindications Hyperthyroidism, anxiety, Tourette syndrome, glaucoma, psychosis, mental depression, hereditary fructose intolerance *Caution:* Children <6 y, psychosis, depression, substance abuse, MI, alcoholism, bipolar disorder, dysrhythmias, seizures, radiographic contrast administration, pregnancy	**Drug-Lab-Food Interactions** Drug: May increase stimulatory effects of sympathomimetics and psychostimulants; may reduce effect of antihypertensives; increases effects of oral anticoagulants, barbiturates, anticonvulsants, and TCAs; increases hypertensive crisis with MAOIs Food: Caffeine may increase effects.
Pharmacokinetics Absorption: Well absorbed from GI tract Distribution: PB: 10%-33% Metabolism: t½: 1.3-7.7 h Excretion: 90% excreted unchanged in urine	**Pharmacodynamics** PO: Onset: 0.5-1 h Regular release: Peak 1.9 h Duration: 3-6 h Extended release: Peak 4.7 h Duration: 8 h

Therapeutic Effects/Uses
To correct hyperactivity caused by ADHD, increase attention span, and control narcolepsy
Mode of Action: Research suggests modulation of serotonergic pathways occurs by affecting changes in dopamine transport.

Continued

PROTOTYPE DRUG CHART 17.1
Methylphenidate—cont'd

Side Effects	Adverse Reactions
Anorexia, dry mouth, nausea, vomiting, dizziness, insomnia, irritability, tremors, euphoria, blurred vision, headache, abdominal pain, anemia	Tachycardia, hypertension, growth suppression, palpitations, seizures, transient weight loss in children *Life threatening:* Exfoliative dermatitis, stroke, thrombocytopenia, hepatotoxicity

*Pregnancy categories have been revised. See http://www.fda.gov/Drugs/DevelopmentApprovalProcess/DevelopmentResources/Labeling/ucm093307.htm for more information.
>, Greater than; <, less than; *A*, adult; *ADHD*, attention-deficit/hyperactivity disorder; *adol*, adolescent; *bid*, twice a day; *C*, child; *CNS*, central nervous system; *CSS*, Controlled Substances Schedule; *d*, day; *GI*, gastrointestinal; *h*, hour; *MAOI*, monoamine oxidase inhibitor; *max*, maximum; *MI*, myocardial infarction; *min*, minute; *PB*, protein binding; *PO*, by mouth; *t½*, half-life; *TCA*, tricyclic antidepressant; *y*, year.

TABLE 17.1   Amphetamines and Amphetamine-Like Drugs

Drug	Route and Dosage	Uses and Considerations
Amphetamines		
Amphetamine sulfate CSS II	ADHD: Immediate release tab: A/Adol/C >6 y: PO: Initially 5 mg/d or bid, increase by 5 mg/d weekly until desired response; *max.* 60 mg/d C 3-5 y: PO: 2.5 mg/d Extended release: Suspension: A/adol/C >6 y: PO: 2.5-5 mg in morning; *max.* 20 mg/d	For narcolepsy, ADHD, obesity. Dosage should be minimal to control symptoms in ADHD. May cause growth inhibition, agitation, confusion, weight loss, and tremor. Pregnancy category: C*; PB: UK; t½: 10-13 h
Dextroamphetamine sulfate CSS II	ADHD: A/adol: PO: 5 mg/d or bid C 6-12 y: PO: 5 mg/d or bid C 3-5 y: PO: 2.5 mg/d	For ADHD and narcolepsy. May cause headache, anorexia, abdominal pain, euphoria, psychosis, hostility, weight loss, growth inhibition, aggression, and cardiac events. Pregnancy category: C*; PB: UK; t½: 10-12 h
Lisdexamfetamine dimesylate CSS II	ADHD: A: PO: 30 mg/d in the morning, may increase 10-20 mg/d weekly, *max.* 70 mg/d C >6 y: PO: 20-30 mg/d in the morning; *max.* 70 mg/d	For ADHD. May cause anorexia, insomnia, irritability, psychosis, suicidal ideation, aggression, and cardiac events including sudden death. Contraindicated within 14 days of MAOI therapy. Pregnancy category C*; PB: UK; t½: <1 h
Amphetamine-Like Drugs		
Methylphenidate hydrochloride CSS II	See Prototype Drug Chart 17.1.	
Modafinil CSS IV	A: PO: 200 mg/d in the morning; *max.* 400 mg/d	For narcolepsy and sleep apnea. May cause headache, dizziness, anorexia, nausea, diarrhea, agitation, irritability, and nervousness. Pregnancy category: C*; PB: 60%; t½: 15 h
Dexmethylphenidate hydrochloride	Immediate release: A and C >6 y: PO: 2.5 mg bid; *max.* 20 mg/d Extended release: A: PO: 10 mg/d in the morning; *max.* 40 mg/d C >6 y: PO: 5 mg/d in the morning, may increase 5 mg/wk; *max.* 30 mg/d	For ADHD. May cause headache, restlessness, dry mouth, psychosis, aggression, agitation, hostility, insomnia, tremors, anorexia, weight loss, abdominal pain, palpitations, and cardiac events. May cause sudden death in patients with structural cardiac abnormalities. Pregnancy category: C*; PB: UK; t½: 2.2 h
Armodafinil	A and C >17 y: PO: 150-250 mg/d in the morning; *max.* 250 mg/d	For narcolepsy and sleep apnea. May cause headache, nausea, depression, and suicidal ideation. Pregnancy category: C*; PB: 60%; t½: 15 h

*Pregnancy categories have been revised. See http://www.fda.gov/Drugs/DevelopmentApprovalProcess/DevelopmentResources/Labeling/ucm093307.htm for more information.
>, Greater than; <, less than; *A*, adult; *ADHD*, attention-deficit/hyperactivity disorder; *adol*, adolescent; *bid*, twice a day; *C*, child; *CSS*, Controlled Substances Schedule; *d*, day; *h*, hour; *MAOI*, monoamine oxidase inhibitor; *max*, maximum; *PB*, protein binding; *PO*, by mouth; *t½*, half-life; *UK*, unknown; *y*, year.

Modafinil is an amphetamine-like stimulant that increases wakefulness in patients with sleep disorders such as narcolepsy. Its mechanism of action is not fully known.

Methylphenidate is the most frequently prescribed drug used to treat ADHD. Table 17.1 lists the amphetamines and amphetamine-like drugs and their dosages, uses, and considerations, including common side effects and a few serious adverse effects.

Pharmacokinetics Methylphenidate is well absorbed from the GI mucosa and is usually administered to children twice a day before breakfast and lunch. Because food affects its absorption rate, this drug should be given 30 to 45 minutes before meals. Methylphenidate should be given 6 hours or more before sleep because it can cause insomnia. Transdermal patches may be worn for 9 hours. This drug is excreted in the urine, and 40% of methylphenidate is excreted unchanged.

◎ NURSING PROCESS
Patient-Centered Collaborative Care

Central Nervous System Stimulant: Methylphenidate Hydrochloride

Assessment
- Determine whether the patient has a history of heart disease, hypertension, hyperthyroidism, parkinsonism, or glaucoma; in such cases, this drug is usually contraindicated.
- Assess vital signs to be used for future comparisons. Closely monitor patients with cardiac disease because this drug may cause tachycardia, hypertension, and stroke.
- Assess patient mental status, such as mood, affect, and aggressiveness.
- Evaluate height, weight, and growth of children.
- Assess complete blood count (CBC), differential white blood cells (WBCs), and platelets before and during therapy.

Nursing Diagnoses
- Health Behavior, Risk-Prone (e.g., impulsiveness, short attention span, distractibility) that interfere with peer relationships, learning, and discipline
- Family Processes, Interrupted related to dysfunctional behavior
- Development, Risk for Delayed
- Knowledge, Deficient related to inexperience with methylphenidate drug regimen

Planning
- Patient's hyperactivity will be decreased.
- Patient's attention span will increase.
- Patient's blood pressure and heart rate will be within normal limits.
- Patient will behave in a calm manner.

Nursing Interventions
- Monitor vital signs and report irregularities.
- Evaluate height, weight, and growth of children.
- Observe patients for withdrawal symptoms such as nausea, vomiting, weakness, and headache.
- Monitor patients for side effects such as insomnia, restlessness, nervousness, tremors, irritability, tachycardia, and elevated blood pressure. Report findings.

Patient Teaching
General
- Teach patients to take the drug before meals.
- ⚡ Advise patients to avoid alcohol consumption.
- Encourage use of sugarless gum to relieve dry mouth.
- Teach patients to monitor weight twice a week and report weight loss.
- ⚡ Advise patients to avoid driving and using hazardous equipment when experiencing tremors, nervousness, or increased heart rate.
- ⚡ Teach patients not to abruptly discontinue the drug; the dose must be tapered to avoid withdrawal symptoms. Consult a health care provider before modifying doses.

- ⚡ Encourage patients to read labels on over-the-counter (OTC) products because many contain caffeine. A high plasma caffeine level could be fatal.
- Teach nursing mothers to avoid taking all CNS stimulants (e.g., caffeine). These drugs are excreted in breast milk and can cause hyperactivity or restlessness in infants.
- Direct families to seek counseling for children with ADHD. Drug therapy alone is not an appropriate therapy program. Notify school nurse of drug therapy regimen.
- Explain to patients and family that long-term use may lead to drug abuse.

Diet
- Advise patients to avoid foods that contain caffeine (e.g., coffee, tea, chocolate, soft drinks, and energy drinks).
- Encourage parents to provide children with a nutritious breakfast because the drug may have anorexic effects.

Side Effects
- Teach patients about drug side effects and the need to report tachycardia and palpitations.
- Monitor children for onset of Tourette syndrome.

⊕ Cultural Considerations
- Decrease language barriers by decoding the jargon of the health care environment for those who have language difficulties or are not in the health care field.

Evaluation
- Evaluate effectiveness of drug therapy, level of hyperactivity, and presence of adverse effects.
- Monitor weight, sleep patterns, and mental status.
- Evaluate patient knowledge of methylphenidate therapy.

Pharmacodynamics Methylphenidate helps to correct ADHD by decreasing hyperactivity and improving attention span. This drug may also be prescribed for treating narcolepsy. Amphetamine-like drugs are considered generally more effective in treating ADHD than are amphetamines, which are generally avoided because they have a higher potential for abuse, habituation, and tolerance. Sympathomimetics (e.g., pseudoephedrine) and psychostimulants (e.g., caffeine) taken concurrently with methylphenidate increase stimulatory effects of irritability, nervousness, tremors, and insomnia. Concurrent use of monoamine oxidase inhibitors (MAOIs) may cause hypertensive crisis. Methylphenidate potentiates the action of CNS stimulants, such as caffeine, and inhibits the metabolism of some barbiturates, such as phenobarbital, which can lead to increased blood levels and potential toxicity.

ANOREXIANTS AND ANALEPTICS

Anorexiants

Anorexiants cause a stimulant effect on the hypothalamic and limbic regions of the brain to suppress appetite. Most of the anorexiants used to suppress appetite (Table 17.2) do not have the serious side effects associated with amphetamines. For weight-loss attempts, emphasis should be placed on a nutritious diet, exercise, and behavior modification. Reliance on appetite suppressants should be discouraged. Individuals who take anorexiants should be under the care of a health care provider.

Side Effects and Adverse Reactions

Children younger than 12 years should not be given anorexiants, and self-medication with anorexiants should be discouraged. Long-term use of these drugs frequently results in such severe side effects such as nervousness, restlessness, irritability, insomnia, heart palpitations, and hypertension.

Analeptics

Analeptics, which are CNS stimulants, mostly affect the brainstem and spinal cord but also affect the cerebral cortex. The primary use of an analeptic is to stimulate respiration. One subgroup of analeptics is the xanthines (methylxanthines), of which caffeine and theophylline are the main drugs. Depending on the dose, caffeine stimulates the CNS, and large doses stimulate respiration. Newborns with respiratory distress might be given caffeine to increase respiration. Theophylline is used mostly to relax the bronchioles; however, it has also been used to increase respiration in newborns. Refer to Chapter 36 for further discussion of theophylline. Table 17.2 lists the analeptics and their dosages, uses, and considerations, including common side effects and a few serious adverse effects.

Side Effects and Adverse Reactions

Side effects from caffeine are similar to those from anorexiants: nervousness, restlessness, tremors, twitching, palpitations, and

TABLE 17.2 Anorexiants and Analeptics

Drug	Route and Dosage	Uses and Considerations
Anorexiants		
Benzphetamine hydrochloride CSS III	A/adol: PO: 25-50 mg daily; *max:* 150 mg/d	Short-term (8-12 wk) treatment for obesity. Use caution with diabetes mellitus, hypertension, seizures, and Tourette syndrome. A potential for abuse exists. May cause restlessness, dry mouth, dysgeusia, and anorexia. Pregnancy category: X*; PB: UK, t½: UK
Diethylpropion hydrochloride CSS IV	A: PO: 25 mg tid 1 h before meals ; *max:* 75 mg/d Sustained release: A: PO: 75 mg/d mid morning; *max:* 75 mg/d	Short-term use for obesity. Contraindicated within 14 days of MAOI therapy and with severe hypertension or glaucoma. Use caution with psychosis, diabetes mellitus, seizures, hypertension, and Tourette syndrome. May cause headache, insomnia, dry mouth, hypertension, and dependence. Pregnancy category: B*; PB: UK; t½: 4-8 h
Phentermine hydrochloride CSS IV	A/adol >16 y: PO: 15-37.5 mg/d in the morning; *max:* 37.5 mg/d	Short-term use for obesity. Contraindicated with dysrhythmias, heart failure, or glaucoma and within 14 days of MAOI therapy. Use caution with diabetes mellitus, hypertension, Tourette syndrome, seizures, and renal impairment. May cause euphoria, dysphoria, dry mouth, dysgeusia, and constipation. Pregnancy category: X*; PB: 17.5 h; t½: 19-24 h
Phentermine-topiramate	Extended release: A: PO: 3.75 mg phentermine/23 mg topiramate/d for 14 d in the morning, then 7.5 mg phentermine/46 mg topiramate/d; *max:* 15 mg phentermine/92 mg topiramate/d	Used short term for obesity. May cause headache, dry mouth, tachycardia, paresthesia, suicidal ideation, attention difficulty, depression, insomnia, and hypokalemia. Evaluate weight loss in 12 weeks. Pregnancy category: X*; PB: 17.5% phentermine, 15%-41% topiramate; t½: 19-24 h phentermine, 65 h topiramate
Phendimetrazine	A: PO: 17.5-35 mg bid/tid, 1 h before meals; *max:* 210 mg/d Extended release: A: PO: 105 mg/d 30-60 min before breakfast	Used short term for obesity. May cause headache, insomnia, dizziness, restlessness, dry mouth, blurred vision, constipation, tachycardia, palpitations, hypertension, tremor, erectile dysfunction, and tolerance. Pregnancy category: X*; PB: UK; t½: 1.9-9.8 h
Liraglutide	Obesity: A: Subcut: Initially 0.6 mg/d for 1 wk; *max:* 3 mg/d for obesity	Used short term for obesity and type 2 diabetes mellitus. May cause headache, anorexia, nausea, vomiting, constipation, diarrhea, tachycardia, palpitations, suicidal ideation, and hypoglycemia. Use appropriate precautions for handling and disposal of hazardous agent. Pregnancy category: Saxenda (for obesity) X*, Victoza (for diabetes mellitus) C*; PB: >98%; t½: 13 h
Naltrexone hydrochloride/ bupropion hydrochloride	A: PO: 8 mg naltrexone/90 mg bupropion/d in the morning; *max:* 32 mg naltrexone/360 mg bupropion/d	Used short term for obesity. May cause headache, dizziness, insomnia, nausea, vomiting, constipation, psychosis, suicidal ideation, liver dysfunction, hypertension, and tachycardia. Contraindicated with uncontrolled hypertension, seizures, and MAOI therapy. Evaluate weight loss in 12 weeks. Pregnancy category: X*; PB: 21% naltrexone, 84% bupropion; t½: 5 h naltrexone, 21 h bupropion
Serotonin 2C Receptor Agonist		
Lorcaserin	A: PO: 10 mg bid; *max:* 20 mg/d	Used short term for obesity. May cause headache, confusion, back pain, infection, hypertension, peripheral edema, hypoglycemia, and suicidal ideation. Pregnancy category: X*; PB: 70%; t½: 11 h
Analeptics *Methylxanthines*		
Caffeine citrate	Neonatal apnea: Infant: PO/IV: 20-25 mg/kg loading dose, then after 24 h, 5-10 mg/kg/d	For neonatal apnea. Monitor closely for seizures, and intracranial hemorrhage. May cause tachycardia, palpitations, tremors, gastritis, urinary frequency, and withdrawal. Pregnancy category: C*; PB: 36%; t½: A: 3-7 h

TABLE 17.2 Anorexiants and Analeptics—cont'd

Drug	Route and Dosage	Uses and Considerations
Theophylline	A/adol >15 y: IV: 0.4 mg/kg/h; *max.* 900 mg/d Older adults: IV: 0.3 mg/kg/h; *max.* 400 mg/d C >12 y: IV: 0.5 mg/kg/h C 9-11 y: IV: 0.7 mg/kg/h C 1-8 y: IV: 0.8 mg/kg/h Infants 6-52 wk: IV: (0.008) (age in wk) + 0.21 = mg/kg/h	For bronchospasm prophylaxis, COPD, asthma, status asthmaticus, and neonatal apnea. May cause headache, insomnia, nausea, vomiting, seizures, dysrhythmias, hypokalemia, and palpitations. Pregnancy category: C*; PB: 40%; t½: 6.5-10.5 h
Doxapram	A: IV: 0.5 mg-1 mg/kg single injection, may repeat at 5-min intervals; *max.* 4 mg/kg cumulative dose	For postanesthesia respiratory depression. Has narrow margin of safety. Other therapeutic measures used first. May cause headache, dizziness, confusion, tachycardia, flushing, sweating, cough, dyspnea, laryngospasm, and skeletal muscle hyperactivity. Pregnancy category: B*; PB: UK; t½: 2.4-4.1 h

*Pregnancy categories have been revised. See http://www.fda.gov/Drugs/DevelopmentApprovalProcess/DevelopmentResources/Labeling/ucm093 307.htm for more information.

>, Greater than; *A,* adult; *adol,* adolescent; *bid,* twice a day; *C,* child; *COPD,* chronic obstructive pulmonary disease; *CSS,* Controlled Substances Schedule; *d,* day; *h,* hour; *IV,* intravenous; *MAOI,* monoamine oxidase inhibitor; *max,* maximum; *min,* minute; *PB,* protein binding; *PO,* by mouth; *subcut,* subcutaneous; *t½,* half-life; *tid,* three times a day; *UK,* unknown; *wk,* week; *y,* years.

insomnia. Other side effects include diuresis (increased urination), GI irritation (e.g., nausea, diarrhea), and, rarely, tinnitus (ringing in the ears). Excess caffeine affects the CNS and heart and can cause dysrhythmias and convulsions. High doses of caffeine in coffee, chocolate, and cold-relief medications can cause psychological dependence. The half-life of caffeine is approximately 5 hours; however, the half-life is prolonged in patients with liver disease and in patients who are taking oral contraceptives or are pregnant. Caffeine is contraindicated during pregnancy because its effect on the fetus is unknown.

CRITICAL THINKING CASE STUDY

MP, a 7-year-old child, has been diagnosed with attention-deficit/hyperactivity disorder. The physician is considering putting the child on medication.

1. What symptoms does a child with attention-deficit/hyperactivity disorder display?
2. What medication might be prescribed? What class of drugs does the medication fall under?
3. What behavioral improvements might be seen after medication administration?
4. What physical assessment should be completed before medication administration?
5. What teaching should the nurse include related to the use of methylphenidate?

NCLEX STUDY QUESTIONS

1. When a 12-year-old child is prescribed methylphenidate, which is most important for the nurse to monitor?
   a. Temperature
   b. Respirations
   c. Intake and output
   d. Height and weight
2. Several children are admitted for diagnosis with possible attention-deficit/hyperactivity disorder. Which is most important for the nurse to observe?
   a. A girl who is lethargic
   b. A girl who lacks impulsivity
   c. A boy with smooth coordination
   d. A boy with an inability to complete tasks
3. The nurse monitoring a patient for methylphenidate withdrawal should observe the patient for which condition?
   a. Tremors
   b. Insomnia
   c. Weakness
   d. Tachycardia

4. The nurse is teaching a patient to self-administer medications. The nurse knows that which drug is used to treat narcolepsy?
   a. Modafinil
   b. Atomoxetine
   c. Lisdexamfetamine
   d. Phendimetrazine
5. A newborn patient is in respiratory distress. The nurse anticipates preparation for which medication to be given?
   a. Modafinil
   b. Armodafinil
   c. Theophylline
   d. Amphetamine

Answers: 1, d; 2, d; 3, c; 4, a; 5, c.

18

Depressants

http://evolve.elsevier.com/McCuistion/pharmacology

OBJECTIVES

- Differentiate the types and stages of sleep.
- Explain several nonpharmacologic ways to induce sleep.
- Differentiate among these adverse effects: hangover, dependence, tolerance, withdrawal symptoms, and rapid eye movement (REM) rebound.
- Discuss the uses of benzodiazepines.
- Apply the nursing process for the patient taking benzodiazepines for hypnotic use.

- Differentiate nursing interventions related to barbiturates, benzodiazepines, nonbenzodiazepines, and melatonin agonist hypnotics.
- Compare the stages of anesthesia.
- Explain the uses for topical anesthetics.
- Differentiate general and local anesthetics and their major side effects.

OUTLINE

KEY TERMS

Drugs that are central nervous system (CNS) depressants cause varying degrees of depression (reduction in functional activity) within the CNS. The degree of depression depends primarily on the drug and the amount of drug taken. The broad classification of CNS depressants includes sedative-hypnotics, general anesthetics, analgesics, opioid and nonopioid analgesics, anticonvulsants, antipsychotics, and antidepressants. The last five groups of depressant drugs are presented in separate chapters. Sedative-hypnotics and general anesthetics are discussed in this chapter.

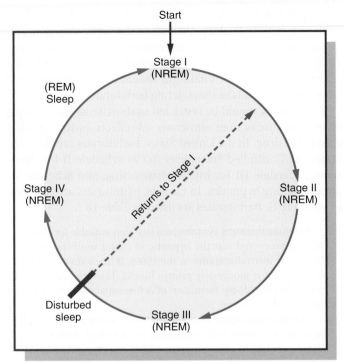

FIG. 18.1 Types and stages of sleep. *NREM*, Nonrapid eye movement (four stages); *REM*, rapid eye movement (dreaming).

TYPES AND STAGES OF SLEEP

Sleep disorders such as insomnia, the inability to fall asleep or remain asleep, occur in 10% to 30% of Americans. Insomnia occurs more frequently in women, and the incidence increases with age.

People spend approximately one third of their lives, or as much as 25 years, sleeping. Normal sleep is composed of two definite phases: **rapid eye movement (REM)** and **nonrapid eye movement (NREM) sleep**. Both REM and NREM sleep occur cyclically at about 90-minute intervals during sleep (Fig. 18.1). The four succeedingly deeper stages of NREM sleep end with an episode of REM sleep, and the cycle begins again. If sleep is interrupted, the cycle begins again with stage 1 of NREM sleep. Individuals perform better during their waking hours if they experience all types and stages of sleep.

During REM sleep, individuals experience most of their recallable dreams. Children have few REM sleep periods and have longer periods of stage 3 and 4 NREM sleep. Older adults experience a decrease in stage 3 and 4 NREM sleep and have frequent waking periods.

It is difficult to rouse a person during REM sleep, and the period of REM sleep episodes becomes longer during the sleep process. Frequently, if a person is roused from REM sleep, a vivid, bizarre dream may be recalled. If these dreams are unpleasant, they may be called *nightmares*. Sleepwalking or nightmares that occur in children take place during NREM sleep.

NONPHARMACOLOGIC METHODS

Before using sedative-hypnotics or over-the-counter (OTC) sleep aids, various nonpharmacologic methods should be used to promote sleep. Once the nurse discovers why the patient cannot sleep, the following ways to promote sleep may be suggested:

1. Arise at a specific hour in the morning.
2. Take few or no daytime naps.
3. Avoid drinks that contain caffeine and alcohol 6 hours before bedtime. Also avoid smoking nicotine products for 6 hours before bedtime.
4. Avoid heavy meals or strenuous exercise before bedtime.
5. Take a warm bath, listen to quiet music, or perform other soothing activities before bedtime.
6. Decrease exposure to loud noises.
7. Avoid drinking copious amounts of fluids before sleep.
8. Drink warm milk before bedtime.

SEDATIVE-HYPNOTICS

Sedative-hypnotics are commonly ordered for treatment of sleep disorders. The mildest form of CNS depression is **sedation**, which diminishes physical and mental responses at lower dosages of certain CNS depressants but does not affect consciousness. Sedatives are used mostly during the daytime. Increasing the drug dose can produce a **hypnotic effect**—not hypnosis but a form of "natural" sleep. Sedative-hypnotic drugs are sometimes the same drug; however, certain drugs are used more often for their hypnotic effect. With very high doses of sedative-hypnotic drugs, anesthesia may be achieved.

Sedatives were first prescribed to reduce tension and anxiety. Barbiturates were initially used for their antianxiety effect until the early 1960s, when benzodiazepines were introduced. Because of the many side effects of barbiturates and their potential for physical and mental dependency, they are now less frequently prescribed.

The Centers for Disease Control and Prevention cite that approximately 70 million Americans have chronic sleep problems and suffer from sleep deprivation. The cost is billions of dollars in lost productivity, and millions of dollars are spent each year on OTC sleep aids. The primary ingredient in OTC sleep aids is an antihistamine such as diphenhydramine.

Hypnotics may be short or intermediate acting. Short-acting hypnotics are useful in achieving sleep because they allow the patient to awaken early in the morning without experiencing lingering side effects. Intermediate-acting hypnotics are useful for sustaining sleep; however, after using one, the patient may experience residual drowsiness, or **hangover**, in the morning. This may be undesirable if the patient is active and requires mental alertness. The ideal hypnotic promotes natural sleep without disrupting normal patterns of sleep and produces no hangover or undesirable effect. Table 18.1 lists the common side effects and adverse reactions associated with sedative-hypnotic use and abuse.

Hypnotic drug therapy should usually be short term to prevent drug **dependence** and **tolerance**. Interrupting hypnotic therapy can decrease drug tolerance, but abruptly discontinuing a high dose of hypnotic taken over a long period can cause **withdrawal symptoms**. In such cases, the dose should be tapered to avoid withdrawal symptoms. As a general rule, the lowest dose should be taken to achieve sleep. Patients with severe respiratory disorders should avoid hypnotics, which could cause an

TABLE 18.1   Common Side Effects and Adverse Reactions of Sedative-Hypnotics

Side Effects and Adverse Reactions	Explanation of the Effects
Hangover	A hangover is residual drowsiness resulting in impaired reaction time. The intermediate- and long-acting hypnotics are frequently the cause of drug hangover. The liver biotransforms these drugs into active metabolites that persist in the body, causing drowsiness.
REM rebound	REM rebound, which results in vivid dreams and nightmares, frequently occurs after taking a hypnotic for a prolonged period then abruptly stopping. However, it may occur after taking only one hypnotic dose.
Dependence	Dependence is the result of chronic hypnotic use. Physical and psychological dependence can result. Physical dependence results in the appearance of specific withdrawal symptoms when a drug is discontinued after prolonged use. The severity of withdrawal symptoms depends on the drug and dosage. Symptoms may include muscular twitching and tremors, dizziness, orthostatic hypotension, delusions, hallucinations, delirium, and seizures. Withdrawal symptoms start within 24 hours and can last for several days.
Tolerance	Tolerance results when there is a need to increase the dosage over time to obtain the desired effect. It is mostly caused by an increase in drug metabolism by liver enzymes. The barbiturate drug category can cause tolerance after prolonged use. Tolerance is reversible when the drug is discontinued.
Excessive depression	Long-term use of a hypnotic may result in CNS depression, which is characterized by lethargy, sleepiness, lack of concentration, confusion, and psychological depression.
Respiratory depression	High doses of sedative-hypnotics can suppress the respiratory center in the medulla.
Hypersensitivity	Skin rashes and urticaria can result when taking barbiturates. Such reactions are rare.

CNS, Central nervous system; REM, rapid eye movement.

increase in respiratory depression. Usually, hypnotics are contraindicated during pregnancy. Ramelteon is the only major sedative-hypnotic approved for long-term use. This drug may be used for treating chronic insomnia.

The category of sedative-hypnotics includes barbiturates, benzodiazepines, and nonbenzodiazepines, among others. Each category is discussed separately. Prototype drug charts are included for benzodiazepines and nonbenzodiazepines.

Barbiturates

Barbiturates were introduced as a sedative in the early 1900s. They are classified as long, intermediate, short, and ultrashort acting.

- The *long-acting* group includes phenobarbital and mephobarbital, which are used to control seizures in epilepsy.
- The *intermediate-acting* barbiturates, such as butabarbital, are useful as sleep sustainers for maintaining long periods of sleep. Because these drugs take approximately 1 hour for

the onset of sleep, they are not prescribed for those who have trouble getting to sleep. Vital signs should be closely monitored in persons who take intermediate-acting barbiturates.

- The *short-acting* barbiturate secobarbital may be used for procedure sedation. Vital signs should be closely monitored in persons who take short-acting barbiturates.

Barbiturates should be restricted to short-term use (2 weeks or less) because of their numerous side effects, including tolerance to the drug. In the United States, barbiturates are classified under the Controlled Substances Act as Schedule II for short-acting, Schedule III for intermediate-acting, and Schedule IV for long-acting hypnotics. In Canada, barbiturates are classified as Schedule G. Barbiturates are listed in Table 18.2.

Pharmacokinetics Pentobarbital has been available for nearly half a century and was the hypnotic of choice until the introduction of benzodiazepines in the 1960s. It has a slow absorption rate and is moderately protein bound. The long half-life is mainly because of the formation of active metabolites resulting from liver metabolism.

Pharmacodynamics Pentobarbital and secobarbital are used primarily for short-term treatment of insomnia. Other uses include control of seizures, preoperative anxiety, and sedation induction. They have a rapid onset with a short duration of action and are considered short-acting barbiturates. The onset of action of pentobarbital is slower when administered intramuscularly (IM) than when administered orally (PO).

⚡ PATIENT SAFETY

Do not confuse:
- **Phenobarbital,** a long-acting barbiturate used to control seizures, with **pentobarbital,** an ultrashort-acting barbiturate used as a general anesthetic.

Many drug interactions are associated with barbiturates. Alcohol, narcotics, and other sedative-hypnotics used in combination with barbiturates may further depress the CNS. Pentobarbital increases hepatic enzyme action, causing an increased metabolism and decreased effect of drugs such as oral anticoagulants, glucocorticoids, tricyclic antidepressants, and quinidine. Pentobarbital may cause hepatotoxicity if taken with large doses of acetaminophen.

❶ Benzodiazepines

Selected benzodiazepines, minor tranquilizers and anxiolytics, were introduced with chlordiazepoxide in the 1960s as antianxiety agents. This drug group is ordered as sedative-hypnotics for inducing sleep. Several benzodiazepines marketed as hypnotics include flurazepam, alprazolam (Prototype Drug Chart 18.1), temazepam, triazolam, estazolam, and quazepam (Table 18.3). Increased anxiety might be the cause of insomnia for some patients, so lorazepam and diazepam can be used to alleviate the anxiety. These drugs are classified as Schedule IV according to the Controlled Substances Act. The benzodiazepines increase the action of the inhibitory neurotransmitter gamma-aminobutyric acid (GABA) to the GABA receptors. Neuron excitability is reduced.

TABLE 18.2 Sedative-Hypnotics: Barbiturates and Other Drugs

Drug	Route and Dosage	Uses and Considerations
Barbiturates: Short-Acting		
Secobarbital sodium CSS II	Sedation induction: A: PO: 200-300 mg 1-2 h before procedure A: PO: 100 mg at bedtime	For sedation induction and insomnia. Use only short term as effectiveness is lost in about 2 weeks. May cause confusion, drowsiness, constipation, withdrawal, sleep-related behaviors, nightmares, and suicidal ideation. Pregnancy category: D*; PB: 30%-45%; t½: 15-40 h
Barbiturates: Intermediate-Acting		
Butabarbital sodium CSS III	Anxiety: A: PO: 15-30 mg tid/qid Insomnia, sedation induction: A: PO: 50-100 mg, 1-1.5 h before procedure or sleep	To manage anxiety, sedation induction, and insomnia. Use short term (<14 days), and avoid alcohol with all barbiturates. May cause ataxia, drowsiness, sleep-related behaviors, confusion, agitation, bradycardia, hypotension, headache, nightmares, depression, and angioedema. This drug is no longer accepted for use in older adults or debilitated adult patients for insomnia. Pregnancy category: D*; PB: 50%; t½: 100 h
Barbiturates: Long-Acting		
Phenobarbital CSS IV	Sedation induction: A: PO/IM: 30-120 mg/d	Used for seizure control, sedation induction, and insomnia. May cause ataxia, depression, bradycardia, hypotension, dizziness, confusion, drowsiness, headache, impaired judgment, nightmares, constipation, and erectile dysfunction. Monitor for respiratory depression. Pregnancy category: D*; PB: 20%-45%; t½: 50-120 h for adults, 37-69 h for children, 47-63 h for infants

*Pregnancy categories have been revised. See http://www.fda.gov/Drugs/DevelopmentApprovalProcess/DevelopmentResources/Labeling/ucm093 307.htm for more information.

<, Less than; *A*, adult; *CSS*, Controlled Substances Schedule; *d*, day; *h*, hour; *IM*, intramuscular; *PB*, protein binding; *PO*, by mouth; *qid*, four times a day; *t½*, half-life; *tid*, three times a day.

PROTOTYPE DRUG CHART 18.1

❶ *Alprazolam*

Drug Class Sedative-hypnotic: benzodiazepine CSS: IV Pregnancy category: D*	**Dosage** Immediate release: A: PO: Initially 0.25-0.5 mg tid, may increase q3-4d; *max:* 4 mg/d Older A: PO: Initially 0.125 bid/tid, may increase q3-4d; *max:* 4mg/d Extended release: A: PO: Initially 0.5-1 mg/d in the morning, may increase q3-4d; *max:* 10 mg/d Older A: PO: Initially 0.5 mg/d, may increase q3-4d; *max:* 10 mg/d
Contraindications Respiratory depression, acute alcohol intoxication, psychotic reactions, recent respiratory depressants, hypersensitivity *Caution:* Older adults, sleep apnea, renal or liver dysfunction, depression, suicidal ideation, drug abuse	**Drug-Lab-Food Interactions** Drug: Decreases respiration with alcohol, CNS depressants; azole antifungals (ketoconazole), antibiotics (erythromycin), aprepitant, cimetidine, diltiazem, and verapamil increase blood levels of alprazolam; rifabutin, rifampin, cortisone, and phenytoin decrease blood levels; alprazolam increases digoxin and lithium levels Food: Grapefruit increases alprazolam levels; green tea decreases alprazolam effects.
Pharmacokinetics Absorption: PO: 90% absorbed from GI tract Distribution: PB: 90% Metabolism: t½: IR, 6.3-26.9 h; ER, 11-16 h; Dtab, 7.9-19.2 h Excretion: In urine as metabolites	**Pharmacodynamics** PO: Onset: 15-30 min Peak: IR, 1-2 h; ER, 9 h; Dtab, 1.5-2 h Duration: UK
Therapeutic Effects/Uses To treat anxiety and panic disorders Mode of Action: CNS depression, binds receptors in limbic system and reticular formation, increases GABA to GABA receptors; shift of chloride ions leads to less excitability and stabilizes neuronal membranes.	
Side Effects Lethargy, drowsiness, dizziness, headache, constipation, anterograde amnesia, memory impairment, fatigue, agitation, ataxia, increased appetite, blurred vision, decreased and increased libido, dry mouth, nausea, edema, weight gain/loss	**Adverse Reactions** Depression, tolerance, dependence, withdrawal, hypotension, tachycardia, seizures *Life threatening:* Hepatic failure, Stevens-Johnson syndrome

*Pregnancy categories have been revised. See http://www.fda.gov/Drugs/DevelopmentApprovalProcess/DevelopmentResources/Labeling/ucm093307.htm for more information.

A, Adult; *CNS*, central nervous system; *CSS*, Controlled Substances Schedule; *d*, day; *Dtab*, disintegrating tablet; *ER*, extended release; *GABA*, gamma-aminobutyric acid; *GI*, gastrointestinal; *h*, hour; *IR*, immediate release; *max*, maximum; *min*, minute; *PB*, protein binding; *PO*, by mouth; *t½*, half-life; *tid*, three times a day; *UK*, unknown.

! TABLE 18.3 Sedative-Hypnotics: Benzodiazepines, Nonbenzodiazepines, and Opioid Agonists

Drug	Route and Dosage	Uses and Considerations
Benzodiazepines		
Alprazolam CSS IV	See Prototype Drug Chart 18.1.	
Estazolam CSS IV	A: PO: 1-2 mg at bedtime; *max.* 2 mg/d Older adults: PO: 0.5-1 mg at bedtime; *max.* 2 mg/d	For treatment of insomnia. Should not be used longer than 6 weeks. May cause tolerance, dizziness, drowsiness, anterograde amnesia, confusion, ataxia, edema, dependence, withdrawal, and sleep-related behaviors. Pregnancy category: X*; PB: 93%; t½: 10-24 h
Lorazepam CSS IV	Insomnia: A: PO: 2-4 mg at bedtime; *max.* 10 mg/d Older adults: PO: 1-2 mg at bedtime; *max.* 10 mg/d	Used for sedation induction and to reduce anxiety, insomnia, and seizures. May cause tolerance, drowsiness, dizziness, hypotension, blurred vision, anterograde amnesia, memory impairment, agitation, nightmares, sleep-related behaviors, and suicidal ideation. Pregnancy category: D*; PB: 91%; t½: 12 h
Temazepam CSS IV	Insomnia: A: PO: 15-30 mg at bedtime; *max.* 30 mg/d Older adults: PO: 7.5 mg at bedtime; *max.* 30 mg/d	To treat insomnia. May cause tolerance, drowsiness, dizziness, confusion, palpitations, hypotension, dependence, withdrawal, anterograde amnesia, and sleep-related behavior. Pregnancy category: X*; PB: 98%; t½: 8-15 h
Triazolam CSS IV	Insomnia: A: PO: 0.125-0.25 mg at bedtime; *max.* 0.5 mg/d Older adults: PO: 0.125 mg at bedtime; *max.* 0.25 mg/d	For management of insomnia. Should not be used longer than 7-10 d at a time to avoid tolerance. Avoid alcohol and smoking when taking triazolam. May cause tolerance, drowsiness, dizziness, ataxia, confusion, visual impairment, headache, tachycardia, depression, dependence, withdrawal, anterograde amnesia, and sleep-related behaviors. Pregnancy category: X*; PB: 90%; t½: 1.5-5.5 h
Benzodiazepine Antagonists		
Flumazenil	A: IV: 0.2 mg over 30 s; may repeat after 45 s, then repeat q1min PRN; *max.* 4 doses	For management of benzodiazepine toxicity and sedation reversal. May cause drowsiness, dizziness, blurred vision, ataxia, seizures, hyperacusis, palpitations, vomiting, and dry mouth. Pregnancy category: C*; PB: 50%; t½: 41 to 79 min
Nonbenzodiazepines		
Zolpidem tartrate CSS IV	See Prototype Drug Chart 18.2.	
Eszopiclone CSS IV	Insomnia: A: PO: Initially 1 mg at bedtime; maint: 2-3 mg at bedtime; *max.* 3 mg/d Older adults: PO: 1-2 mg at bedtime; *max.* 2 mg/d	To treat insomnia. May cause headache, dizziness, drowsiness, unpleasant taste, sleep-related behaviors, infection, depression, and suicidal ideation. Pregnancy category: C*; PB: 52%-59%; t½: 6 h
Zaleplon CSS IV	Insomnia: A: PO: 10 mg at bedtime; *max:* 20 mg Older adults: PO: 5 mg at bedtime; *max:* 10 mg/d	For ultrashort-term treatment of insomnia. May cause headache, dizziness, drowsiness, nausea, abdominal pain, and sleep-related behaviors. Pregnancy category: C*; PB: 60%; t½: 1 h
Melatonin Agonist		
Ramelteon	A: PO: 8 mg within 30 min of bedtime; *max.* 8 mg/d	For treatment of insomnia. May cause dizziness, drowsiness, fatigue, depression, suicidal ideation, and sleep-related behaviors. Pregnancy category: C*; PB: 82%; t½: 1-2.6 h
Opioid Agonists		
Alfentanil CSS II	A: IV: 130-245 mcg/kg over 3 min as induction; maint: 0.5-1.5 mcg/kg/min; *max.* dependent on procedure duration	For general anesthesia induction and maintenance and sedation maintenance. Must be administered by someone trained in general anesthetic administration. May cause dizziness, confusion, dysrhythmias, hypotension or hypertension, respiratory depression, bronchospasm, tachycardia, bradycardia, chest wall rigidity, nausea, and vomiting. Use caution in patients with head trauma and liver dysfunction. Pregnancy category: C*; PB: 88%-92%; t½: 90-111 min
Sufentanil CSS II	A: IV: 8-30 mcg/kg increments or infusion for induction; maint: 0.5-10 mcg/kg intermittent or continuous IV; *max.* dependent on procedure duration	For general anesthesia induction and maintenance, obstetric anesthesia, and severe pain. Must be administered by someone trained in general anesthetic administration. May cause drowsiness, pruritus, bradycardia, hypertension or hypotension, dysrhythmia, chest wall rigidity, bronchospasm, respiratory depression, urinary retention, nausea, and vomiting. Pregnancy category: C*; PB: 93%; t½: 164 min
Remifentanil	A: IV: 0.5-1 mcg/kg/min continuous infusion	For general anesthesia induction and maintenance and moderate to severe pain. Must be administered by someone trained in general anesthetic administration. May cause dizziness, pruritus, confusion, chest wall rigidity, hypotension, bradycardia, dysrhythmias, nausea, and vomiting. Pregnancy category: C*; PB: 70%; t½: 10-20 min

*Pregnancy categories have been revised. See http://www.fda.gov/Drugs/DevelopmentApprovalProcess/DevelopmentResources/Labeling/ucm093307.htm for more information.

A, Adult; *CSS,* Controlled Substances Schedule; *d,* day; *h,* hour; *IV,* intravenous; *maint,* maintenance; *max,* maximum; *min,* minute; *PB,* protein binding; *PO,* by mouth; *PRN,* as needed; *q1min,* once per minute; *s,* second; *t½,* half-life.

NURSING PROCESS
Patient-Centered Collaborative Care
Sedative-Hypnotics: Benzodiazepines

Assessment
- Obtain a drug history of current drugs and complementary and alternative therapies that the patient is taking, especially CNS depressants, which would potentiate respiratory depression and hypotensive effects.
- Assess baseline vital signs for future comparisons.
- Determine whether the patient has a history of insomnia or anxiety disorders.
- Assess renal function. Urine output should be 1500 mL/day. Renal impairment could prolong drug action by increasing the half-life of the drug.

Nursing Diagnoses
- Sleep Deprivation related to adverse effect of insomnia
- Injury, Risk for breathing pattern ineffective
- Breathing Pattern, Ineffective related to CNS depression
- Sexuality Pattern, Ineffective related to adverse effect of erectile dysfunction

Planning
- Patient will receive adequate sleep when taking benzodiazepines.

Nursing Interventions
- Monitor vital signs, especially respirations and blood pressure.
- Use a bed alarm for older adults and for patients receiving a hypnotic for the first time. Confusion can occur, and injury could result.
- Observe the patient for adverse reactions, especially an older adult or a debilitated patient.
- Examine the patient's skin for rashes. Skin eruptions may occur in patients taking benzodiazepines.

Patient Teaching
General
- Teach patients to use nonpharmacologic methods to induce sleep such as taking a warm bath, listening to quiet music, drinking warm fluids, and avoiding drinks with caffeine for 6 hours before bedtime.
- ⚡ Encourage patients to avoid alcohol and antidepressant, antipsychotic, and opioid drugs while taking benzodiazepines. Respiratory depression can occur when these drugs are combined.
- Warn patients that certain complementary and alternative therapy products may interact with benzodiazepines (Complementary and Alternative Therapies 18.1). These products may need to be discontinued, or the prescription drug dose may need to be modified.
- ⚡ Advise patients not to drive a motor vehicle or operate machinery when using benzodiazepines. Caution is always encouraged.
- Encourage patients to check with a health care provider about OTC sleeping aids. Drowsiness may result from taking these drugs, therefore caution while driving is advised.

Side Effects
- Advise patients to report adverse reactions such as cognitive changes and paradoxical reactions to their health care provider. Drug selection or dosage might need to be changed.
- Teach patients that benzodiazepines should be gradually withdrawn, especially if they have been taken for several weeks. Abrupt cessation may result in withdrawal symptoms such as tremors and muscle twitching.

Cultural Considerations
- Use an interpreter as needed, and involve extended family in health teaching and support.
- Provide written instruction or videos in the patient's preferred language.

Evaluation
- Assess the effectiveness of benzodiazepines.
- Evaluate respiratory status to ensure that respiratory depression has not occurred.

⚡ PATIENT SAFETY
Do not confuse:
- **Lorazepam,** a benzodiazepine used to reduce anxiety, with **alprazolam,** a benzodiazepine used to treat anxiety and insomnia.

COMPLEMENTARY AND ALTERNATIVE THERAPIES 18.1
Sedatives

- Kava kava should not be taken in combination with CNS depressants such as barbiturates and opioids. This product may increase the sedative effect.
- Valerian, when taken with alcohol and other CNS depressants such as barbiturates, may increase the sedative effects of the prescribed drug.

Benzodiazepines (except for temazepam) can suppress stage 4 of NREM sleep, which may result in vivid dreams or nightmares and can delay REM sleep. Benzodiazepines are effective for sleep disorders for several weeks longer than other sedative-hypnotics; to prevent REM rebound, however, they should not be used for longer than 3 to 4 weeks.

Triazolam is a short-acting hypnotic with a half-life of 2 to 5 hours. It does not produce any active metabolites. Adverse effects of anterograde amnesia or memory impairment occur more frequently with triazolam than with other benzodiazepines, and the risk increases with higher doses and with concurrent alcohol or opioid ingestion. Currently, it is seldom prescribed and should not be taken longer than 7 to 10 days.

One adverse effect closely associated with benzodiazepines is anterograde amnesia, an impaired ability to recall events that occur after dosing. Associated with anterograde amnesia are sleep-related behaviors, such as preparing and eating meals, sleep driving, engaging in sex, or making phone calls during sleep without any memory of the event. Alcohol and CNS depressants increase the risk of sleep-related behaviors.

Small doses of benzodiazepines are recommended for patients with renal or hepatic dysfunction. For benzodiazepine overdose, the benzodiazepine antagonist flumazenil may be prescribed. Benzodiazepines prescribed as antianxiety drugs are discussed in Chapter 22.

> **Pharmacokinetics** Benzodiazepines are well absorbed through the gastrointestinal (GI) mucosa. They are rapidly metabolized in the liver to active metabolites. Benzodiazepines have an intermediate half-life of usually 8 to 24 hours. These drugs are highly protein bound, and more free drug is available when benzodiazepines are taken with other highly protein-bound drugs, which increases the risk for adverse effects.
>
> **Pharmacodynamics** Benzodiazepines are used to treat insomnia by inducing and sustaining sleep. They have a rapid onset

of action and intermediate- to long-acting effects. The normal recommended dose of a benzodiazepine may be too much for the older adult, so half the dose is recommended initially to prevent overdosing.

Nonbenzodiazepines

Zolpidem is a nonbenzodiazepine that differs in chemical structure from benzodiazepines. It is used for short-term treatment (<10 days) of insomnia. Its duration of action is 6 to 8 hours with a short half-life of 1.4 to 6.73 hours. Zolpidem is metabolized in the liver to three inactive metabolites and is excreted in bile, urine, and feces. When zolpidem is prescribed for older adults, the dose should be decreased. Table 18.3 lists the benzodiazepines and nonbenzodiazepines used as sedative-hypnotics and their dosages, uses, and considerations including common side effects and a few serious adverse effects. Zolpidem is described in Prototype Drug Chart 18.2.

PROTOTYPE DRUG CHART 18.2
Zolpidem Tartrate

Drug Class	Dosage
Sedative-hypnotic: Nonbenzodiazepine CSS IV Pregnancy category: C*	Immediate release: A males: PO: 5-10 mg at bedtime; *max:* 10 mg/d A females/older adults: PO: 5 mg at bedtime; *max:* 5 mg/d SL tabs/oral spray: A: PO: 5-10 mg at bedtime; *max:* 10 mg/d Older adults: PO: 5 mg at bedtime; *max:* 5 mg/d Extended release: A: PO: 6.25-12.5 mg at bedtime; *max:* 12.5 mg/d Older adults: PO: 6.25 mg at bedtime, *max:* 6.25 mg/d
Contraindications	**Drug-Lab-Food Interactions**
Hypersensitivity to benzodiazepine, respiratory depression, lactation *Caution:* Renal or liver dysfunction; mental depression, suicidal ideation; pregnancy; children, older adults, and debilitated individuals	Drug: Decreases CNS function with alcohol, CNS depressants, anticonvulsants, and phenothiazines; increased levels with azole antifungals; decreased levels with rifampin Food: Decreases absorption
Pharmacokinetics	**Pharmacodynamics**
Absorption: PO: well absorbed Distribution: PB: 92% Metabolism: t½: 1.4-8.4 h Excretion: In bile, urine, and feces	PO: Immediate release: Onset: 30 min Peak: 90 min Duration: 6-8 h SL/spray mist: Onset: UK Peak: 35-82 min Duration: UK Extended release: Onset: UK Peak: UK Duration: UK
Therapeutic Effects/Uses	
To treat insomnia Mode of Action: CNS depression, neurotransmitter inhibition	
Side Effects	**Adverse Reactions**
Drowsiness, lethargy, headache, hot flashes, hangover (residual sedation), irritability, dizziness, ataxia, visual impairment, anxiety, nausea and vomiting, edema, erectile dysfunction, anterograde amnesia, memory impairment, nightmares, binge eating	Tolerance, psychological or physical dependence, withdrawal; sleep-related behaviors, hypotension, angioedema, dysrhythmias, depression, suicidal ideation *Life threatening:* Pulmonary edema, renal failure

*Pregnancy categories have been revised. See http://www.fda.gov/Drugs/DevelopmentApprovalProcess/DevelopmentResources/Labeling/ucm093307.htm for more information.
A, Adult; *CNS,* central nervous system; *CSS,* Controlled Substances Schedule; *d,* day; *h,* hour; *max,* maximum; *min,* minute; *PB,* protein binding; *PO,* by mouth; *SL,* sublingual; *t½,* half-life; *UK,* unknown.

Melatonin Agonists

Ramelteon is in the newest category of sedative-hypnotics called *melatonin agonists*. Ramelteon is the first hypnotic approved by the U.S. Food and Drug Administration (FDA) that is *not* classified as a controlled substance. This drug acts by selectively targeting melatonin receptors to regulate circadian rhythms in the treatment of insomnia. Ramelteon has not been shown to decrease REM sleep. This new drug has a half-life of 1 to 2.6 hours. Adverse effects of ramelteon include drowsiness, dizziness, fatigue, headache, nausea, and suicidal ideation.

Sedatives and Hypnotics for Older Adults

Identifying the cause of insomnia in an older adult should be the first diagnostic consideration, and nonpharmacologic methods should be used before sleep medications are prescribed. Because of physiologic changes in older adults, the use of hypnotics can cause a variety of side effects.

Barbiturates increase CNS depression and confusion in older adults and should *not* be taken for sleep. The short- to intermediate-acting benzodiazepines—such as estazolam, temazepam, and triazolam—are considered to be safer than barbiturates. Long-acting hypnotic benzodiazepines such as flurazepam, quazepam, and diazepam should be avoided. In many cases, older adults should be instructed to take the prescribed benzodiazepine no more than four times a week to avoid side effects and drug dependency. They can choose selected nights to take the hypnotic.

The main sleep problem experienced by older adults is frequent nighttime awakening. Reports have shown that older women experience more troublesome sleep patterns than men. Sleep disturbance may be caused by discomfort or pain. Occasionally a nonsteroidal antiinflammatory drug (NSAID) such as ibuprofen may alleviate the discomfort that prevents sleep.

◎ NURSING PROCESS
Patient-Centered Collaborative Care

Sedative-Hypnotics: Nonbenzodiazepines

Assessment
- Assess baseline vital signs and laboratory tests (e.g., aspartate aminotransferase [AST], alanine aminotransferase [ALT], bilirubin) for future comparisons.
- Obtain a drug history. Taking CNS depressants with nonbenzodiazepine hypnotics can depress respirations.
- Ascertain the patient's problem with sleep disturbance.

Nursing Diagnoses
- Sleep Deprivation related to anxiety
- Fatigue related to insomnia
- Injury, Risk for

Planning
- Patient will remain asleep for 6 to 8 hours.

Nursing Interventions
- Monitor vital signs. Check for signs of respiratory depression (slow, irregular breathing patterns).
- Use bed alarm for older adults or patients receiving nonbenzodiazepines for the first time. Confusion may occur, and injury may result.
- Observe patient for side effects of nonbenzodiazepines such as hangover (residual sedation), lightheadedness, dizziness, or confusion.

Patient Teaching
General
- Teach patients to use nonpharmacologic methods to induce sleep (taking a warm bath, listening to music, drinking warm fluids such as milk, avoiding drinks with caffeine after dinner).
- Encourage patients to avoid alcohol, antidepressants, antipsychotics, and narcotic drugs while taking nonbenzodiazepines. Severe respiratory depression may occur when these drugs are combined.
- Advise patients to take nonbenzodiazepine before bedtime. Alprazolam takes effect within 15 to 30 minutes.
- Suggest that patients urinate before taking nonbenzodiazepines to prevent sleep disruption.
- Encourage patients to check with a health care provider about OTC sleeping aids.
- Warn the patient to use caution while driving as drowsiness may occur.
Side Effects
- Advise patients to report adverse reactions such as hangover to a health care provider. Drug selection or dosage may need to be changed if hangover occurs.

⊕ Cultural Considerations
- Ask patients about methods family members have used to promote sleep.
- Suggest nonpharmacologic alternatives that may be effective in inducing sleep.

Evaluation
- Evaluate effectiveness of sedative-hypnotics in promoting sleep.
- Determine whether side effects such as hangover occur after several days of taking a sedative-hypnotic. Another hypnotic may be prescribed if side effects persist.

❶ ANESTHETICS

Anesthetics are classified as *general* and *local*. General anesthetics depress the CNS, alleviate pain, and cause a loss of consciousness. The first anesthetic, nitrous oxide ("laughing gas"), was used for surgery in the early 1800s. It is still an effective anesthetic and is frequently used in dental procedures and surgery.

Pathophysiology

Several theories exist regarding how inhalation anesthetics cause CNS depression and a loss of consciousness. The differing theories suggest the following about inhalation anesthetics:

1. The lipid structure of cell membranes is altered, resulting in impaired physiologic functions.
2. The inhibitory neurotransmitter GABA is activated to the GABA receptor that pushes chloride ions into the neurons. This greatly decreases the fire action potentials of the neurons.
3. The ascending reticular activating system is altered, and the neurons cease to transmit information (stimuli) to the brain.

Balanced Anesthesia

Balanced anesthesia is a combination of drugs frequently used in general anesthesia. Balanced anesthesia may include the following:

1. A hypnotic given the night before
2. Premedication with an opioid analgesic or benzodiazepine (e.g., midazolam) plus an anticholinergic (e.g., atropine) given about 1 hour before surgery to decrease secretions
3. A short-acting nonbarbiturate such as propofol
4. An inhaled gas, often a combination of an inhalation anesthetic, nitrous oxide, and oxygen
5. A muscle relaxant given as needed

Balanced anesthesia minimizes cardiovascular problems, decreases the amount of general anesthetic needed, reduces possible postanesthesia nausea and vomiting, minimizes the disturbance of organ function, and decreases pain. Because the patient does not receive large doses of general anesthetics, fewer adverse reactions occur; and recovery is enhanced by allowing quicker mobility.

Stages of General Anesthesia

General anesthesia proceeds through four stages (Table 18.4). The surgical procedure is usually performed during the third stage. If an anesthetic agent is given immediately before inhalation anesthesia, the third stage can occur without the early stages of anesthesia being observed. However, if the drug is given slowly, all stages of anesthesia are usually observed.

Assessment Before Surgery

The patient's response to anesthesia may differ according to variables related to the health status of the individual. These variables include age (young and older adults), a current health disorder (e.g. cardiovascular, pulmonary, renal, liver), pregnancy, history of heavy smoking, and frequent use of alcohol and drugs. These problems must be identified *before* surgery because the type and amount of anesthetic required may need to be adjusted.

Inhalation Anesthetics

During the third stage of anesthesia, inhalation anesthetics—that is, gas or volatile liquids administered as gas—are used to deliver general anesthesia. Certain gases, notably nitrous oxide, are absorbed quickly, have a rapid action, and are eliminated rapidly. Cyclopropane was a popular inhalation anesthetic from 1930 to 1960, but because of its highly flammable state as ether, it is no longer used. In the late 1950s, halothane was introduced as a nonflammable alternative. Other inhalation drugs used as anesthetics include enflurane, isoflurane, desflurane, and sevoflurane.

Inhalation anesthetics typically provide smooth induction. Upon discontinuing administration of halothane, isoflurane, and enflurane, recovery of consciousness usually occurs in approximately 1 hour. Recovery from desflurane and sevoflurane is within minutes. Inhalation anesthetics are usually combined with a nonbarbiturate, such as propofol; a strong analgesic, such as morphine; and a muscle relaxant, such as pancuronium, for surgical procedures.

Adverse effects from inhalation anesthetics include respiratory depression, hypotension, dysrhythmias, and hepatic dysfunction. In patients at risk, these drugs may trigger malignant hyperthermia. The newer drugs primarily cause less nausea and vomiting than the older anesthetics.

Intravenous Anesthetics

Intravenous (IV) anesthetics may be used for general anesthesia or for the induction stage of anesthesia. For outpatient surgery of short duration, an IV anesthetic might be the preferred form of anesthesia. Propofol, droperidol, etomidate, and ketamine hydrochloride are commonly used to provide a total intravenous anesthetic (TIVA). IV anesthetics have a rapid onset and short duration of action. Table 18.5 describes the inhalation and IV anesthetics used for general anesthesia.

Midazolam and propofol are commonly administered for the induction and maintenance of anesthesia or for conscious

TABLE 18.4	Stages of Anesthesia	
Stage	**Name**	**Description**
1	Analgesia	Begins with consciousness and ends with loss of consciousness; speech is difficult, sensations of smell and pain are lost, dreams and auditory and visual hallucinations may occur; this stage may be called the *induction stage*.
2	Excitement or delirium	Produces a loss of consciousness caused by depression of the cerebral cortex; confusion, excitement, or delirium occur, and induction time is short.
3	Surgical	Surgical procedure is performed during this stage. There are four phases: surgery is usually performed in phase 2 and upper phase 3. As anesthesia deepens, respirations become shallower, and the respiratory rate is increased.
4	Medullary paralysis	Toxic stage of anesthesia in which respirations are lost, and circulatory collapse occurs; ventilatory assistance is necessary.

! TABLE 18.5 Inhalation and Intravenous Anesthetics

Drug	Induction Time	Considerations
Inhalation: Volatile Liquids		
Halothane	Rapid	Highly potent anesthetic; recovery is rapid; could decrease blood pressure, has a bronchodilator effect, and is contraindicated in obstetrics.
Methoxyflurane	Slow	Used during labor; drug dose is usually less than other anesthetics and does not suppress uterine contraction; could cause hypotension. This drug is contraindicated in renal disorders.
Enflurane	Rapid	Can depress respiratory function; ventilatory support may be necessary. This drug should not be used during labor because it could suppress uterine contractions; avoid use in patients with seizure disorders.
Isoflurane	Rapid	Frequently used in inhalation therapy; has a smooth and rapid induction of anesthesia and rapid recovery; could cause hypotension and respiratory depression. This drug should not be used during labor because it suppresses uterine contractions. Cardiovascular effect is minimal.
Desflurane	Rapid	Volatile liquid anesthetic; recovery is rapid after anesthetic administration has ceased; could cause hypotension and respiratory depression.
Sevoflurane	Rapid	For induction and maintenance during surgery; sevoflurane may be given alone or combined with nitrous oxide.
Inhalation: Gas		
Nitrous oxide ("laughing gas")	Very rapid	Must be administered at no less than a mixture of 21% oxygen; potency is low. Recovery is rapid with minimal cardiovascular effect.
Intravenous (Ultrashort-Acting Barbiturates)		
Methohexital sodium	Rapid	Has short duration; frequently used for induction and with other drugs as part of balanced anesthesia; an inhalation anesthesia usually follows.
Thiamylal sodium	Rapid	Used for induction of anesthesia and as anesthesia for electroshock therapy
Benzodiazepines		
Diazepam	Moderate to rapid	For induction of anesthesia; no analgesic effect
Midazolam	Rapid	For induction of anesthesia and for endoscopic procedures; IV drug can cause conscious sedation and should be avoided if a cardiopulmonary disorder is present.
Others		
Droperidol and fentanyl	Moderate to rapid	A neuroleptic analgesic when combined with fentanyl (potent opiate narcotic); frequently used with a general anesthetic, can also be used as a preanesthetic drug and is also used for diagnostic procedures; may cause hypotension and respiratory depression.
Etomidate	Rapid	Etomidate is used for short-term surgery, for induction of anesthesia, or with a general anesthetic to maintain the anesthetic state.
Ketamine hydrochloride	Rapid	Used for short-term surgery or for induction of anesthesia; increases salivation, blood pressure, and heart rate; may be used for diagnostic procedures; avoid use in patients with a history of psychiatric disorders.
Propofol	Rapid	For induction of anesthesia; may be used with general anesthesia; duration of action is short; may cause hypotension and respiratory depression. Pain can occur at the injection site, so a local anesthetic (lidocaine) may be administered intravenously prior to injection of propofol to decrease pain.
Fospropofol	Rapid	For induction and maintenance of anesthesia; may cause hypotension and respiratory depression

sedation for minor surgery or procedures like intubation and mechanical ventilation. Patients are sedated and relaxed but, depending upon the dose, they are responsive to commands.

Adverse effects from IV anesthetics include respiratory and cardiovascular depression. Propofol supports microbial growth and may increase the risk for bacterial infection. Discarding opened vials within 6 hours is a necessary precaution in the prevention of sepsis.

Topical Anesthetics

Use of topical anesthetic agents is limited to mucous membranes, broken or unbroken skin surfaces, and burns. Topical anesthetics come in different forms: solutions, liquid sprays, ointments, creams, gels, and powders. Topical anesthetics decrease the sensitivity of nerve endings in the affected area.

Local Anesthetics

Local anesthetics block pain at the site where the drug is administered by preventing conduction of nerve impulses. Local anesthetics are useful in dental procedures, suturing skin lacerations, short-term (minor) surgery at a localized area, blocking nerve impulses (nerve block) below the insertion of a spinal anesthetic, and diagnostic procedures such as lumbar puncture and thoracentesis. Local anesthetics may also be used to perform regional blocks—such as brachial plexus, axillary, femoral, or sciatic blocks—to provide analgesia for surgery of the upper or lower extremities.

TABLE 18.6 Local Anesthetics

Anesthetics	Type	Uses and Considerations
Short Acting (30 Min to 1 Hour)		
Chloroprocaine hydrochloride	Ester	For infiltration, caudal, and epidural anesthesia; onset of action is 6 to 12 minutes.
Procaine hydrochloride	Ester	For nerve block, infiltration, epidural, and spinal anesthesia; useful in dentistry; use with caution in patients allergic to ester-type anesthetics.
Moderate Acting (1 to 3 Hours)		
Lidocaine hydrochloride	Amide	For nerve block, infiltration, epidural, and spinal anesthesia; allergic reaction is rare. Lidocaine is used to treat cardiac dysrhythmias (see Chapter 37).
Mepivacaine hydrochloride	Amide	For nerve block, infiltration, caudal, and epidural anesthesia; may be used in dentistry
Prilocaine hydrochloride	Amide	For peripheral nerve block, infiltration, caudal, and epidural anesthesia; may be used in dentistry
Long Acting (3 to 10 Hours)		
Bupivacaine hydrochloride	Amide	For peripheral nerve block, infiltration, caudal, and epidural anesthesia
Dibucaine hydrochloride	Amide	For topical use (creams and ointment) to affected areas
Etidocaine hydrochloride	Amide	For peripheral nerve block, infiltration, caudal, and epidural anesthesia
Tetracaine hydrochloride	Ester	For spinal anesthesia (high and low saddle block); also for topical use to affected areas, such as the eye to anesthetize the cornea, the nose and throat for bronchoscopy, and the skin for relief of pain and pruritus (itching)

Most local anesthetics are divided into two groups, the *esters* and the *amides,* according to their basic structures. The amides have a very low incidence of allergic reaction.

The first local anesthetic used was cocaine hydrochloride in the late 1800s. Procaine hydrochloride, a synthetic of cocaine, was discovered in the early 1900s. Lidocaine hydrochloride was developed in the mid-1950s to replace procaine except in dental procedures. Lidocaine has a rapid onset and a long duration of action, is more stable in solution, and causes fewer hypersensitivity reactions than procaine. Since the introduction of lidocaine, many local anesthetics have been marketed. Table 18.6 describes the various types of local anesthetics according to short-, moderate-, and long-acting effects.

Orthopedic joint surgeries, mastectomy, cesarean delivery, hysterectomy, hernia repair, and cholecystectomy frequently use the postoperative pain control provided by an anesthetic pump. For example, the patient who has a bilateral hernia repair has a catheter inserted into the deep fascia of the lower abdomen. A continuous flow of bupivacaine, a local anesthetic, is delivered via a Y-connector to both sides. By controlling pain with this delivery method, the patient is allowed increased mobility; reduced opioid use, which reduces associated drowsiness and nausea; and a reduced hospital stay.

Spinal Anesthesia

Spinal anesthesia requires that a local anesthetic be injected into the subarachnoid space below the first lumbar space (L1) in adults and the third lumbar space (L3) in children. If the local anesthetic is given or spreads too high in the spinal column, the respiratory muscles could be affected, and respiratory distress or respiratory failure could result. A postdural-puncture headache might result following spinal anesthesia (a "spinal"), possibly because of a decrease in cerebrospinal fluid pressure caused by a leak of fluid at the needle insertion point. Encouraging the patient to remain flat following surgery with spinal anesthesia and to take increased fluids usually decreases the likelihood of leaking spinal fluid. Postdural-puncture headaches occur most frequently in females and in younger patients, and obstetric patients have the highest incidence. Hypotension also can result following spinal anesthesia due to the ensuing sympathetic blockade and predisposing factors that include sensory block location, history of hypertension, and chronic alcohol intake.

Various sites of the spinal column can be used for a nerve block with a local anesthetic (Fig. 18.2). A spinal block results from the penetration of the anesthetic into the subarachnoid space, which is the space between the pia mater membrane and the arachnoid membrane. An epidural block is the placement of the local anesthetic in the epidural space just posterior to the spinal cord or the dura mater. The epidural space is located between the posterior longitudinal ligament on the anterior side and the ligamentum flavum posteriorly. A caudal block is an epidural block placed by administering a local anesthetic through the sacral hiatus. A saddle block is given at the lower end of the spinal column to block the perineal area. Blood pressure should be monitored during administration of these types of anesthesia because a decrease in blood pressure resulting from the drug and procedure might occur. Further discussion of labor and delivery drugs can be found in Chapter 50.

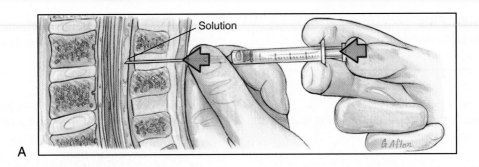

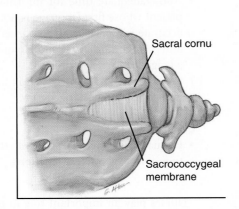

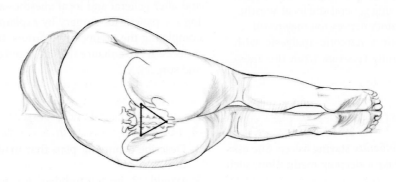

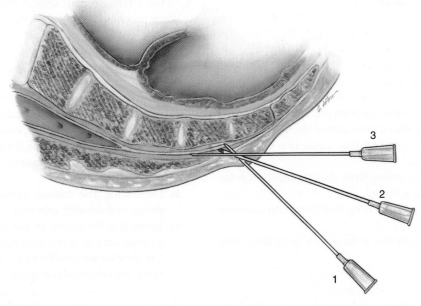

B

FIG. 18.2 A, Administration of solution for epidural placement. B, Caudal anesthesia.

NURSING PROCESS
Patient-Centered Collaborative Care
Anesthetics

Assessment
- Assess baseline vital signs.
- Obtain a drug and health history, noting drugs that affect the cardiopulmonary system.

Nursing Diagnoses
- Pain, Acute related to injury
- Breathing Pattern, Ineffective related to CNS depression

Planning
- Patient will participate in preoperative preparation and will understand postoperative care.
- Patient's vital signs will remain stable following surgery.

Nursing Interventions
- Monitor the postoperative state of sensorium. Report if a patient remains excessively nonresponsive or confused.
- Observe preoperative and postoperative urine output. Report deficit of hourly or 8-hour urine output.
- ⚡ Monitor vital signs following general and local anesthesia; hypotension and respiratory depression may result.
- Administer an analgesic or a narcotic-analgesic with caution until the patient fully recovers from the anes-

thetic. To prevent adverse reactions, the dosage might need to be adjusted if the patient is under the influence of an anesthetic.

Patient Teaching
- Explain to patients the preoperative preparation and postoperative nursing assessment and interventions.

🌐 *Cultural Considerations*
- Allow adequate time for information processing for the patient whose first language is not English to avoid an inaccurate response or no response. Allow time for patients and their families to respond to questions, especially when a language barrier is present.
- Speak clearly and slowly, giving time for translation. Obtain an interpreter if necessary.

Evaluation
- Evaluate the patient's response to the anesthetics. Continue to monitor for adverse reactions.

Nurses play an important role in patient assessment before and after general and local anesthesia is administered. Preparing the patient for surgery by explaining the preparations and completing the preoperative orders, including premedications, is necessary to enhance the safety and effectiveness of anesthesia and surgery.

CRITICAL THINKING CASE STUDY

JZ, a 72-year-old woman, has difficulty staying asleep. She asks the nurse whether she should take a sleeping medication, such as lorazepam, before bedtime.
1. Before JZ takes any sleep aid or hypnotic, what nursing assessments should be made?

2. Describe a nursing plan that may help alleviate JZ's sleep disturbance.
3. Would JZ be a candidate for taking a benzodiazepine? Explain your answer.
4. What follow-up plan should the nurse have related to JZ's sleep problem?

NCLEX STUDY QUESTIONS

1. It is important for the nurse teaching the patient regarding secobarbital to include which information about the drug?
   a. It is a short-acting drug that may cause one to awaken early in the morning.
   b. It is an intermediate-acting drug that frequently causes rapid eye movement rebound.
   c. It is an intermediate-acting drug that frequently causes a hangover effect.
   d. It is a long-acting drug that is frequently associated with dependence.

2. A patient taking lorazepam asks the nurse how this drug works. The nurse should respond by stating that it is a benzodiazepine that acts by which mechanism?
   a. Depressing the central nervous system, leading to a loss of consciousness
   b. Depressing the central nervous system, including the motor and sensory activities
   c. Increasing the action of the inhibitory neurotransmitter gamma-aminobutyric acid (GABA) to GABA receptors
   d. Creating an epidural block by placement of the local anesthetic into the epidural space

3. A patient is taking ramelteon for insomnia. The nurse prepares a care plan that includes monitoring of the patient for side effects/adverse reactions of this drug. Which is a side effect of ramelteon?
   a. Insomnia
   b. Bradycardia
   c. Laryngospasm
   d. Sleep-related behaviors

4. A patient received spinal anesthesia. Which is most important for the nurse to monitor?
   a. Loss of consciousness
   b. Hangover effects and dependence
   c. Hypotension and headaches
   d. Excitement or delirium

5. A nurse is teaching a patient about zolpidem. Which is important for the nurse to include in the teaching of this drug?
   a. The maximum dose is 20 mg/day.
   b. It is used for short-term treatment less than 10 days.
   c. For older adults, the dose is 15 mg at bedtime.
   d. The drug should only be used for 21 days or less.

6. A patient is taking triazolam. Which instructions about this drug are important for the nurse to include?
   a. It may be used as a barbiturate for only 4 weeks.
   b. Use as a nonbenzodiazepine to reduce anxiety.
   c. It may cause agranulocytosis and thrombocytopenia.
   d. Avoid alcohol and smoking while taking this drug.

7. A patient is to receive conscious sedation for a minor surgical procedure. Which drug administration should the nurse expect? (Select all that apply.)
   a. Propofol to reduce anxiety
   b. Lidocaine to provide local anesthesia
   c. Midazolam to promote sedation and following of commands
   d. Ketamine for rapid induction and prolonged duration of action
   e. Phenobarbital for short-acting duration of sleep

Answers: 1, a; 2, c; 3, b; 4, c; 5, b; 6, d; 7, a, b, c.

19

Antiseizure Drugs

🌐 http://evolve.elsevier.com/McCuistion/pharmacology

OBJECTIVES

- Contrast the two international classifications of seizures with characteristics of each type.
- Differentiate between the types of seizures.
- Summarize the pharmacokinetics, side effects and adverse reactions, therapeutic plasma level, contraindications for use, and drug interactions of phenytoin.
- Compare the actions of hydantoins, long-acting barbiturates, succinimides, benzodiazepines, iminostilbenes, and valproate.
- Apply the nursing process to antiseizure drugs, including patient teaching.

OUTLINE

KEY TERMS

Millions of people in the United States have active epilepsy, a **seizure** disorder that results from abnormal electric discharges from the cerebral neurons characterized by a loss or disturbance of consciousness and usually involuntary, uncontrolled movements. The **electroencephalogram (EEG)**, computed tomography (CT), and magnetic resonance imaging (MRI) are useful in diagnosing epilepsy. The EEG records abnormal electric discharges of the cerebral cortex. Of all seizure cases, 75% are considered to be primary, or **idiopathic** (of unknown cause), and the remainder are secondary to brain trauma, brain **anoxia** (absence of oxygen), infection, or cerebrovascular disorders (e.g., cerebrovascular accident [CVA], stroke). Epilepsy is a chronic, usually lifelong disorder. The majority of persons with seizure disorder had their first seizure before 20 years of age.

Seizures that are not associated with epilepsy could result from fever, hypoglycemic reaction, electrolyte imbalance (hyponatremia), metabolic imbalance (acidosis or alkalosis), and alcohol or drug use. When these conditions are corrected, the seizures cease. Recurrent seizures may result from birth and perinatal injuries, head trauma, congenital malformations, neoplasms (tumors), or idiopathic, or unknown, causes.

INTERNATIONAL CLASSIFICATION OF SEIZURES

There are various types of seizures, such as **tonic-clonic** (formerly known as *grand mal*), **absence** (formerly known as *petit mal*), and **psychomotor**. The International Classification of Seizures (Table 19.1) describes two seizure categories: generalized and partial. A person may also have mixed seizures that comprise more than one type.

TABLE 19.1   International Classification of Seizures

Category	Characteristics
Generalized seizure	Seizures involve both cerebral hemispheres of the brain.
Tonic-clonic seizure	Also called *grand mal seizure,* the most common form; in the *tonic phase,* skeletal muscles contract or tighten in a spasm that lasts 3 to 5 seconds; in the *clonic phase,* a dysrhythmic muscular contraction occurs with a jerkiness of legs and arms that lasts 2 to 4 minutes.
Tonic seizure	Sustained muscle contraction
Clonic seizure	Dysrhythmic muscle contraction
Absence seizure	Also called *petit mal seizure;* brief loss of consciousness lasts less than 10 seconds with fewer than three spike waves on the electroencephalogram (EEG) printout. This type usually occurs in children.
Myoclonic seizure	Isolated clonic contraction or jerks that last 3 to 10 seconds may be limited to one limb (focal myoclonic) or may involve the entire body (massive myoclonic); may be secondary to a neurologic disorder such as encephalitis or Tay-Sachs disease.
Atonic seizure	Head drop, loss of posture, and sudden loss of muscle tone occurs. If lower limbs are involved, the patient could collapse.
Infantile spasms	Muscle spasm
Partial seizure	Involves one hemisphere of the brain; no loss of consciousness occurs in simple partial seizures, but there is a loss of consciousness in complex partial seizures.
Simple seizure	Occurs in motor, sensory, autonomic, and psychic forms; no loss of consciousness occurs.
Motor	Formerly called the *Jacksonian seizure,* this type involves spontaneous movement that spreads; it can develop into a generalized seizure.
Sensory	Visual, auditory, or taste hallucinations
Autonomic response	Paleness, flushing, sweating, or vomiting
Psychological	Personality changes
Complex seizure	Loss of consciousness occurs, and the patient does not recall behavior immediately before, during, and immediately after the seizure.
Psychomotor	Complex symptoms include automatisms (repetitive behavior such as chewing or swallowing motions), behavioral changes, and motor seizures.
Cognitive	Confusion or memory impairment
Affective	Bizarre behavior
Compound	May lead to generalized seizures such as tonic or tonic-clonic

ANTISEIZURE DRUGS

Drugs used for epileptic seizures are called antiseizure drugs, *anticonvulsants,* or *antiepileptic drugs* (AEDs). Antiseizure drugs stabilize nerve cell membranes and suppress the abnormal electric impulses in the cerebral cortex. These drugs prevent seizures but do not eliminate the cause or provide a cure. Antiseizure drugs are classified as central nervous system (CNS) depressants.

With the use of antiseizure drugs, seizures are controlled in approximately 70% of patients. These drugs are usually taken throughout the person's lifetime; however, the health care provider might discontinue the medication if no seizures have occurred after 3 to 5 years in some cases.

Many types of antiseizure drugs are used to treat seizures, including the hydantoins (phenytoin), long-acting barbiturates (phenobarbital, mephobarbital, primidone), succinimides (ethosuximide), benzodiazepines (diazepam, clonazepam), carbamazepine, and valproate (valproic acid). Antiseizure drugs are not indicated for all types of seizures. For example, phenytoin is effective in treating tonic-clonic and partial seizures but is not effective in treating absence seizures.

Pharmacophysiology: Action of Antiseizure Drugs

Antiseizure drugs work in one of three ways: (1) by suppressing sodium influx through the drug binding to the sodium channel when it is inactivated, which prolongs the channel inactivation and thereby prevents neuron firing; (2) by suppressing the calcium influx, which prevents the electric current generated by the calcium ions to the T-type calcium channel; or (3) by increasing the action of gamma-aminobutyric acid (GABA), which inhibits neurotransmitters throughout the brain. The drugs that suppress sodium influx are phenytoin, fosphenytoin, carbamazepine, oxcarbazepine, valproic acid, topiramate, zonisamide, and lamotrigine. Valproic acid and ethosuximide are examples of drugs that suppress calcium influx. Examples of drug groups that enhance the action of GABA are barbiturates, benzodiazepines, and tiagabine. Gabapentin promotes GABA release.

Hydantoins

The first antiseizure drug used to treat seizures was phenytoin, a hydantoin discovered in 1938 and still commonly used for controlling seizures. Hydantoins inhibit sodium influx, stabilize cell membranes, reduce repetitive neuronal firing, and limit seizures. By increasing the electrical stimulation threshold in cardiac tissue, it also acts as an antidysrhythmic. It has a slight effect on general sedation, and it is nonaddicting. However, this drug should *not* be used during pregnancy because it can have a teratogenic effect on the fetus.

Drug dosage for phenytoin and other antiseizure drugs is age related. Newborns, persons with liver disease, and older adults require a lower dosage because of a decrease in metabolism that

---

⚡ PATIENT SAFETY

Do not confuse:
- **Cerebyx,** a hydantoin antiseizure drug, with **Celebrex,** a nonsteroidal antiinflammatory drug (NSAID). The names of these drugs look and sound alike but are different in their pharmacology.

results in more available drug. Conversely, individuals with an increased metabolic rate, such as children, may require an increased dosage. The drug dosage is adjusted according to the therapeutic plasma or serum level. Phenytoin has a narrow therapeutic range of 10 to 20 mcg/mL, which is generally considered equivalent to 1 to 2 mcg/mL unbound or free phenytoin. The benefits of an antiseizure drug become apparent when the serum drug level is within the therapeutic range. Typically, if the drug level is below the desired range, the patient is not receiving the required drug dosage to control seizure activity. If the drug level is above the desired range, drug toxicity may result. Monitoring the therapeutic serum drug range is of utmost importance to ensure drug effectiveness. Prototype Drug Chart 19.1 lists the pharmacologic data associated with phenytoin.

Pharmacokinetics Phenytoin is slowly absorbed from the small intestine. It is a highly protein-bound (90% to 95%) drug, therefore a decrease in serum protein or albumin can increase the free phenytoin serum level. With a small to average drug dose, the half-life of phenytoin is approximately 24 hours, but the range can be from 7 to 42 hours. Phenytoin is metabolized to inactive metabolites, and this portion is excreted in the urine.

Pharmacodynamics The pharmacodynamics of orally administered phenytoin include onset of action within 30 minutes to 2 hours, peak serum concentration in 1.5 to 6 hours, steady state of serum concentration in 7 to 10 days, and a duration of action dependent on the half-life of up to 45 hours. Oral phenytoin is most commonly ordered as a sustained-release (SR) capsule. The peak SR concentration time is 4 to 12 hours.

Intravenous (IV) infusion of phenytoin should be administered by direct injection into a large vein via a central line or peripherally inserted central catheter (PICC). The drug may be diluted in saline solution; however, dextrose solution should be avoided because of drug precipitation. The manufacturer recommends use of an in-line filter when the drug is administered as an infusion. IV phenytoin, 50 mg or a fraction thereof, should be administered over 1 minute for adults and at a rate of 25 mg/min for older adults. Infusion rates of more than 50 mg/min may cause severe hypotension or cardiac dysrhythmias, especially for older and debilitated patients. Local irritation at the injection site may be noted, and sloughing—formation of dead tissue that separates from living tissue—may occur. The IV line should always be flushed with saline before and after each dose to reduce venous irritation. Intramuscular (IM) injection of phenytoin irritates tissues and may cause damage. For this reason, and because of its erratic absorption rate, phenytoin is *not* given by the IM route.

PROTOTYPE DRUG CHART 19.1

Phenytoin

Drug Class	Dosage
Anticonvulsant: Hydantoin Pregnancy category: D*	Seizure prophylaxis: A: PO: 4-7 mg/kg/d in 2-3 divided doses Status epilepticus: A/adol/C/infants: IV: LD: 15-20 mg/kg, then in 10 min may give 5-10 mg/kg PRN; *max:* LD: 30 mg/kg, rate: 50 mg/min and 25 mg/min for older adults Therapeutic serum range: 10-20 mcg/mL Toxic level: 30-50 mcg/mL

Contraindications
Hypersensitivity, heart block, bradycardia, Adams-Stokes syndrome
Caution: Hyponatremia, hypotension, hypoglycemia, suicidal ideation,
  myasthenia gravis, thyroid disease, alcoholism, diabetes mellitus,
  renal and hepatic impairment, Asian
	Drug-Lab-Food Interactions
	Drug: Increased effects with cimetidine, isoniazid, chloramphenicol; decreased
	  effects with folic acid, calcium, antacids, sucralfate, vinblastine, cisplatin
	Decreases effects of anticoagulants, oral contraceptives, antihistamines,
	  corticosteroids, theophylline, cyclosporine, quinidine, dopamine, and rifampin
	Food: Decreases effects of folic acid, calcium, and vitamin D because absorption is
	  decreased by phenytoin

Pharmacokinetics Absorption: PO: Slowly absorbed; IM: Erratic rate of absorption Distribution: PB: 90%-95% Metabolism: t½: 7-42 h Excretion: In urine, small amount; in bile and feces, moderate amounts	**Pharmacodynamics** PO: Onset: 0.5-2 h Peak: 1.5-6 h Duration: 6-12 h IV: Onset: Within minutes to 1 h Peak: 2 h moderate amount Duration: >12 h
Therapeutic Effects/Uses To prevent tonic-clonic and partial seizures and status epilepticus Mode of action: Reduces motor cortex activity by altering ion transport	

Side Effects
Headache, diplopia, nystagmus, confusion, dizziness, drowsiness,
  insomnia, fatigue, ataxia, tremor, rash, gingival hyperplasia,
  anorexia, nausea, vomiting, hirsutism, pink-red/brown
  discoloration of urine
	Adverse Reactions
	Leukopenia, hepatic impairment, depression, hyperglycemia, bradycardia, peripheral
	  neuropathy, purple glove syndrome
	Life threatening: Aplastic anemia, thrombocytopenia, agranulocytosis, Stevens-Johnson syndrome, hypotension, ventricular fibrillation, suicidal ideation

*Pregnancy categories have been revised. See http://www.fda.gov/Drugs/DevelopmentApprovalProcess/DevelopmentResources/Labeling/ucm093307.htm for more information.
>, Greater than; *A*, adult; *adol*, adolescent; *C*, child; *d*, day; *h*, hour; *IM*, intramuscular; *IV*, intravenous; *LD*, loading dose; *max*, maximum; *min*, minute; *PB*, protein binding; *PO*, by mouth; *PRN*, as needed; *t½*, half-life.

Side Effects and Adverse Reactions

The adverse effects of hydantoins include psychiatric effects such as depression, suicidal ideation, Stevens-Johnson syndrome, ventricular fibrillation, and blood dyscrasias, such as thrombocytopenia (low platelet count), leukopenia (low white blood cell count), and purple glove syndrome (swollen, discolored, and painful extremities that may require amputation). Patients on hydantoins for long periods might have elevated blood glucose (hyperglycemia) that results from the drug inhibiting the release of insulin. Less severe side effects include nausea, vomiting, gingival hyperplasia (overgrowth of gums or reddened gums that bleed easily), constipation, drowsiness, headaches, slurred speech, confusion, alopecia, hirsutism, and nystagmus (constant, involuntary, cyclical movement of the eyeball).

Drug-Drug Interactions

Drug interaction is common with hydantoins because they are highly protein bound. Hydantoins compete with other drugs (e.g., anticoagulants, aspirin) for plasma protein-binding sites. The hydantoins displace anticoagulants and aspirin, causing more free-drug availability and increasing their activity. Barbiturates, rifampin, and chronic ingestion of ethanol increase hydantoin metabolism. Drugs like sulfonamides and cimetidine can increase the action of hydantoins by inhibiting liver metabolism, which is necessary for drug excretion. Antacids, calcium preparations, sucralfate, and antineoplastic drugs also decrease the absorption of hydantoins. Antipsychotics and certain herbs can lower the seizure threshold, the level at which seizure may be induced, and they increase seizure activity (Complementary and Alternative Therapies 19.1). The patient should be closely monitored for seizure occurrence.

Barbiturates

Phenobarbital, a long-acting barbiturate, is prescribed to treat tonic-clonic, partial, and myoclonic seizures and status epilepticus, a rapid succession of epileptic seizures. Barbiturates reduce seizures by enhancing the activity of GABA, an inhibitory neurotransmitter. Possible teratogenic effects and other side effects related to phenytoin are less pronounced with phenobarbital. The therapeutic serum range of phenobarbital is 20 to 40 mcg/mL. Risks associated with the use of phenobarbital include sedation and tolerance to the drug. Discontinuance of phenobarbital should be gradual to avoid recurrence of seizures.

Succinimides

The succinimide drug group is used to treat absence seizures. Succinimides act by decreasing calcium influx through the T-type calcium channels. The therapeutic serum range of ethosuximide is 40 to 100 mcg/mL. Adverse effects include blood dyscrasias, renal and liver impairment, and systemic lupus erythematosus.

Benzodiazepines

The benzodiazepines that have antiseizure effects are clonazepam, clorazepate dipotassium, lorazepam, and diazepam. Clonazepam is effective in controlling absence and myoclonic seizures, but tolerance may occur 6 months after drug therapy starts; consequently, clonazepam dosage must be adjusted. Clorazepate dipotassium is administered for treating partial seizures.

Diazepam is administered by IV to treat status epilepticus. The drug has a short-term effect; thus other antiseizure drugs, such as phenytoin or phenobarbital, must be given during or immediately after administration of diazepam.

Iminostilbenes

Carbamazepine, an iminostilbene, is used to control tonic-clonic and partial seizures. Carbamazepine is also used for psychiatric disorders (e.g., bipolar disorder), trigeminal neuralgia (as an analgesic), and alcohol withdrawal. The therapeutic serum range of carbamazepine is 4 to 12 mcg/mL.

A potentially toxic interaction can occur when grapefruit juice is taken with carbamazepine, and drug concentrations must be carefully monitored.

Valproate

Valproic acid is prescribed for tonic-clonic, absence, and mixed types of seizures, although the safety and efficacy of this drug has not been established for children younger than 2 years of age. Care should be taken when giving this drug to very young children and to patients with liver disorders because hepatotoxicity is one of the possible adverse reactions. Liver enzymes should be monitored. The therapeutic serum range for a patient with seizures is 50 to 100 mcg/mL.

Table 19.2 lists the various antiseizure drugs and their dosages, uses, and considerations, including common side effects and a few serious adverse effects. Table 19.3 lists selected antiseizure drugs frequently prescribed to treat seizure disorders.

Antiseizure drug dosages usually start low and gradually increase over a period of weeks until the serum drug level is within therapeutic range or the seizures cease. Serum antiseizure drug levels should be closely monitored to prevent toxicity.

Antiseizure Drugs and Pregnancy

During pregnancy, seizure episodes increase 25% in women with epilepsy. Hypoxia that may occur during seizures places both the pregnant woman and her fetus at risk.

Many antiseizure drugs have teratogenic properties that increase the risk for fetal malformations. Phenytoin and carbamazepine have been linked to fetal anomalies such as cardiac defects and cleft lip and palate. It has been reported that valproic acid is known to cause major congenital malformations in infants in 4% to 8% of pregnant women who take the drug. As expected, the highest incidence of birth defects occurs when the woman takes combinations of antiseizure drugs.

🌿 COMPLEMENTARY AND ALTERNATIVE THERAPIES 19.1

Antiseizure Drugs

- Evening primrose and borage may lower the seizure threshold when taken with antiseizure drugs. The antiseizure dose may need modification.
- Ginkgo may decrease phenytoin effectiveness.

TABLE 19.2 Anticonvulsants

Drug	Route and Dosage	Uses and Considerations
Barbiturates		
Phenobarbital CSS IV	Status epilepticus: A/C: IV: 15-18 mg/kg; *max:* 30 mg/kg Adol/C/infants: IV: 15-20 mg/kg; *max.* 40 mg/kg Seizure prophylaxis: A: PO/IM/IV: 1-3 mg/kg/d in 1-2 divided doses Adol/C >7 y: PO/IM/IV: 3-6 mg/kg/d in 1-2 divided doses Infants/C <6 y: PO/IM/IV: 4-8 mg/kg/d in 1-2 divided doses Therapeutic serum range: 15-40 mcg/mL	For tonic-clonic, myoclonic, and partial seizures; status epilepticus; sedation induction and maintenance; and insomnia. May cause dizziness, drowsiness, confusion, hypotension, bradycardia, ataxia, constipation, erectile dysfunction, depression, and suicidal ideation. High doses for adults may lead to dependence, respiratory depression, and coma. Pregnancy category: D*; PB: 20%-45%; t½: A: 50-120 h; C: 37-69 h, Infants: 47-63 h
Primidone	Seizure prophylaxis: A/adol/C >8 y: PO: 125-250 mg/d at bedtime; maint: 750-1500 mg/d; *max:* 2g/d C <8 y: PO: 50-125 mg/d; maint: 10-25 mg/kg/d in 3-4 divided doses; *max:* 25 mg/kg/d Neonates: 12-20 mg/kg/d in 2-4 divided doses; *max:* 20 mg/kg/d Therapeutic serum range: 5-12 mcg/mL	For tonic-clonic and partial seizures. Take with food if drug causes GI distress. May cause confusion, hypotension, respiratory depression, Stevens-Johnson syndrome, dependence, depression, and suicidal ideation. Pregnancy category: D*; PB: 20%-45%; t½: 10-12 h
Benzodiazepines (Anxiolytics)		
Clonazepam CSS IV	Seizure prophylaxis: A/adol >30 kg: PO: Initially 1.5 mg/d in 3 divided doses; gradually increase dose q3d until seizures are controlled *max:* 20 mg/d C <10 y <30 kg: PO: Initially 0.01-0.03 mg/kg/d in 3 divided doses; *max:* 0.2 mg/kg/d	For absence and myoclonic seizures, Lennox-Gastaut syndrome, and panic disorder. May cause dizziness, drowsiness, ataxia, fatigue, dependence, depression, and suicidal ideation. Pregnancy category: D*; PB: 85%; t½: 22-33 h
Clorazepate CSS IV	Seizure prophylaxis: A/adol: PO: 7.5 mg bid/tid; *max:* 60 mg/d C 9-12 y: PO: 3.75-7.5 mg bid; *max:* 60 mg/d	May be used for partial seizures, anxiety, and alcohol withdrawal. May cause blurred vision, amnesia, confusion, dizziness, drowsiness, tolerance, dependence, withdrawal, hypotension, depression, and suicidal ideation. Pregnancy category: D*; PB: 97%; t½: 30-200 h
Diazepam CSS IV	Status epilepticus: A: IV: 5-10 mg at 10-15 min intervals; *max:* 30 mg C >5 y: IV 1 mg/kg q2-5 min slowly; *max:* 10 mg C <5 y: IV: 0.2-0.5 mg q2-5min; *max:* 5 mg Seizure prophylaxis: A: PO: 2-10 mg bid-qid Older A: PO: 2-2.5 mg qd-bid Adol/C/infants >6 mo: PO: 1-2.5 mg tid-qid	For status epilepticus (drug of choice), partial and tonic-clonic seizures, muscle spasms, anxiety, sedation induction, and alcohol withdrawal. May cause confusion, drowsiness, dysarthria, fatigue, tolerance, dependence, withdrawal, paradoxical aggressiveness, and rage. Administer IV slowly to avoid respiratory depression and hypotension; Pregnancy category: D*; PB: 99%; t½: 30-60 h
Lorazepam CSS IV	Status epilepticus: A: IV: 4 mg at 2 mg/min may repeat in 10-15 min	To control status epilepticus, anxiety, and insomnia and for sedation induction. May cause blurred vision, drowsiness, dizziness, headache, respiratory depression, dependence, and suicidal ideation. Pregnancy category: D*; PB: 91%; t½: 12 h
Hydantoins		
Fosphenytoin	Status epilepticus: A: IV: Initially 15-20 mg PE/kg; do not exceed 150 mg PE/min; may give additional 5-10 mg PE/kg PRN; *max:* 30 mg PE/kg	For tonic-clonic and partial seizures and status epilepticus. IV fosphenytoin should only be given if oral phenytoin is not an option. Dilute in D₅W or 0.9% NaCl. May cause dizziness, drowsiness, nystagmus, gingival hyperplasia, tinnitus, ataxia, headache, pruritus, and hypotension. Use mandated precautions for handling and disposal of hazardous agent. Pregnancy category: D*; PB: 95%-99%; t½: 7-42 h
Phenytoin	See Prototype Drug Chart 19.1.	
Iminostilbene		
Carbamazepine	Seizure prophylaxis: A/adol: PO: 200 mg bid; maint: 800-1200 mg/d; *max.* 1600 mg/d C 6-12 y: 100 mg bid; *max:* 1 g/d C <6 y: PO: 10-20 mg/kg/d in divided doses; *max.* 35 mg/kg/d Therapeutic serum range: 4-12 mcg/mL	For tonic-clonic and partial seizures, trigeminal neuralgia, neuropathic pain, and bipolar disorder. May cause dizziness, drowsiness, headache, blurred vision, ataxia, nausea, vomiting, weakness, anemia, agranulocytosis, Stevens-Johnson syndrome, and suicidal ideation. Pregnancy category: D*; PB: 76%; t½: 25-65 h

TABLE 19.2 Anticonvulsants—cont'd

Drug	Route and Dosage	Uses and Considerations
Oxcarbazepine	Immediate release: A/adol >16 y: PO: Initially 300 mg bid; increase to 2400 mg/d C 4-16 y: PO: Initially 8-10 mg/kg/d in 2 divided doses Extended release: A: PO: Initially 600 mg/d; maint: 1200-2400 mg/d	For partial seizures. Drug-level monitoring is not necessary. May cause dizziness, drowsiness, confusion, depression, diplopia, headache, nausea, vomiting, fatigue, ataxia, Stevens-Johnson syndrome, and infection. Use mandated procedure for handling and disposal of hazardous agent. Pregnancy category: C*; PB: 40%; t½: 2 h
Eslicarbazepine	A: PO: Initially 400 mg/d, may increase weekly; maint: 800-1600 mg/d; *max*: 1600 mg/d	For partial seizures. May cause dizziness, drowsiness, fatigue, headache, diplopia, nausea, vomiting, Stevens-Johnson syndrome, and suicidal ideation. Pregnancy category: C*; PB: 40%; t½: 13-20 h
Succinimides		
Ethosuximide	A/adol/C >6 y: PO: Initially 250 mg bid; increase dose gradually; maint: 20-40 mg/kg/d; *max*: 1.5 g/d C 3-6 y: PO: Initially 15 mg/kg/d in 2 divided doses; maint: 15-40 mg/kg/d Therapeutic serum range: 40-100 mcg/mL	For absence seizures. Gastric irritation is common, so this drug may be taken with food. May cause dizziness, drowsiness, headache, nightmares, gingival hyperplasia, dyspepsia, ataxia, Stevens-Johnson syndrome, and suicidal ideation. Pregnancy category: C*; PB: UK; t½: A, 60 h; C, 30 h
Valproate		
Valproate, valproic acid	Seizure prophylaxis: A/C >10 y: PO: 10-15 mg/kg/d in 2-3 divided doses; *max*: 60 mg/kg/d Therapeutic serum range: 50-100 mcg/mL	For partial, myoclonic, absence, and tonic-clonic seizures; bipolar disorder; and migraine prophylaxis. Avoid during pregnancy. Administer with food or increase dosing slowly to avoid GI distress. May cause dizziness, drowsiness, diplopia, asthenia, insomnia, ataxia, nausea, vomiting, diarrhea, suicidal ideation, and thrombocytopenia. Pregnancy category: D*; PB: 90%; t½: 6-16 h
Miscellaneous		
Acetazolamide	Seizure prophylaxis: A: PO: 8-30 mg/kg/d in up to 4 divided doses; maint: 375-1000 mg/d; *max*: 1 g/d	For absence seizures, altitude sickness, glaucoma, and edema. Maintain adequate fluid intake to prevent renal impairment. May cause dizziness, drowsiness, confusion, depression, headache, ataxia, hypokalemia, hyponatremia, hypoglycemia, hyperglycemia, and Stevens-Johnson syndrome. Pregnancy category: C*; PB: 90%; t½: 10-15 h
Gabapentin	Seizure prophylaxis: A/adol: PO: Initially 300 mg tid; maint: 900-1800 mg/d in 3 divided doses; *max*: 3600 mg/d and max time between doses 12 h C 3-12 y: 10-15 mg/kg/d in 3 divided doses; maint: 25-35 mg/kg/d; *max*: 50 mg/kg/d	For partial seizures, restless leg syndrome, and neuropathic pain. May cause dizziness, drowsiness, hostility, nystagmus, fatigue, peripheral edema, and suicidal ideation. Give with food to avoid GI upset. High doses are limited to short-term use. Gradually reduce dose upon discontinuation. Pregnancy category: C*; PB: 3%; t½: 5-7 h
Lamotrigine	Partial seizures: Immediate release: A/adol >16 y: PO: Initially 50 mg/d; maint: 250 mg bid Extended release: A/adol: PO: Initially 50 mg/d; maint: 250-300 mg/d	For partial and tonic-clonic seizures, Lennox-Gastaut syndrome, and bipolar disorder. May cause dizziness, drowsiness, blurred vision, fatigue, nausea, vomiting, diarrhea, abdominal pain, ataxia, and suicidal ideation. Discontinue if rash appears; patient may develop *life-threatening* Stevens-Johnson syndrome. Pregnancy category: C*; PB: 55%; t½: 14-59 h
Levetiracetam	Immediate release: A: PO: Initially 500 mg bid; may increase dose q2wk; maint: 1500 mg bid; *max*: 3 g/d Extended release: A/adol/C >12 y: PO: 1 g/d; *max*: 3 g/d	For partial, tonic-clonic, and myoclonic seizures. May cause drowsiness, irritability, headache, anorexia, weakness, hypertension, Stevens-Johnson syndrome, psychosis, and suicidal ideation. Unlikely to cause drug interactions with commonly prescribed medications. Pregnancy category: C*; PB: <10%; t½: 6-8 h
Brivaracetam	A/adol >16 y: PO/IV: Initially 50 mg bid; *max*: 200 mg/d	For partial seizures. May cause dizziness, drowsiness, weakness, ataxia, nystagmus, psychosis, and suicidal ideation. Pregnancy category: C*; PB: <20%; t½: 9 h
Tiagabine	A/C >12 y: PO: 4 mg/d; maint: 32-56 mg/d; *max*: A, 56 mg/d; C, 32 mg/d	For partial seizures. May cause dizziness, drowsiness, memory impairment, depression, nausea, tremor, weakness, ataxia, infection, Stevens-Johnson syndrome, and suicidal ideation. Pregnancy category: C*; PB: 96%; t½: 7-9 h

Continued

TABLE 19.2 Anticonvulsants—cont'd

Drug	Route and Dosage	Uses and Considerations
Topiramate	Immediate release: A/adol/C >10 y: PO: Initially 25 mg bid; *max:* 400 mg/d Extended release: A/adol/C >10 y: PO: 50 mg/d; *max:* 400 mg/d	For partial and tonic-clonic seizures, Lennox-Gastaut syndrome, and migraine prophylaxis. May cause dizziness, drowsiness, memory impairment, nystagmus, infection, fatigue, dysgeusia, anorexia, paresthesia, Stevens-Johnson syndrome, and suicidal ideation. Pregnancy category: D*; PB: 15%-41%; t½: 21 h
Zonisamide	A/adol >16 y: PO: 100 mg/d; may increase after 2 wk; *max:* 600 mg/d	For partial seizures. May cause dizziness, drowsiness, headache, confusion, insomnia, agitation, memory impairment, depression, fatigue, ataxia, anorexia, nausea, Stevens-Johnson syndrome, and suicidal ideation. Contraindicated for patients sensitive to sulfonamides. Pregnancy category: C*; PB: 40%; t½: 63 h
Magnesium sulfate	Preeclampsia or eclampsia: A: IV: Initially 4-6 g infusion of 1-2 g/h for at least 24 h or 4-5 g IM in alternate buttocks q4h until seizures cease; *max:* 20 g/48 h	For seizures caused by eclampsia or preeclampsia. Monitor Mg levels, BP, respirations, deep tendon reflexes, and urine output. May cause flushing, diaphoresis, hypotension, bradycardia, weakness, hyporeflexia, dysrhythmias, respiratory and cardiac arrest. Use extreme caution with myasthenia gravis. Pregnancy category: A*; PB: 30%; t½: UK
Pregabalin	Partial seizures: A: PO: Initially 150 mg/d in 2-3 divided doses; *max:* 600 mg/d	For partial seizures, neuropathic pain, and fibromyalgia. May cause drowsiness, dizziness, blurred vision, dry mouth, tremor, peripheral edema, weight gain, ataxia, rhabdomyolysis, Stevens-Johnson syndrome, and suicidal ideation. Pregnancy category: C*; PB: 0%; t½: 6 h
Lacosamide	A/adol >17 y: PO/IV: Initially 100 mg bid; maint: 300-400 mg/d in 2 divided doses; *max:* 400 mg/d	For partial seizures. May cause dizziness, drowsiness, blurred vision, nystagmus, headache, ataxia, tremor, fatigue, nausea, and suicidal ideation. Pregnancy category: C*; PB: 15%; t½: 13 h
Ezogabine	A: PO: Initially 150 mg/d in 2-3 divided doses; maint: 200-400 mg tid; *max:* 1200 mg/d Older adult: PO: Initially 50 mg tid; *max:* 750 mg/d	For partial seizures. May cause dizziness, drowsiness, confusion, blurred vision, vision loss, fatigue, skin discoloration, tremor, and suicidal ideation. Pregnancy category: C*; PB: 80%; t½: 7 h
Felbamate	A/adol >14 y: PO: Initially 1200 mg/d in 3-4 divided doses; *max:* 3600 mg/d	For partial seizures and Lennox-Gastaut syndrome. May cause dizziness, diplopia, nervousness, anorexia, nausea, vomiting, constipation, aplastic anemia, and suicidal ideation. Pregnancy category: C*; PB: 22%-35%; t½: 13-23 h
Perampanel	A/C >12 y: PO: Initially 2 mg/d at bedtime; *max:* 12 mg/d	For partial and tonic-clonic seizures. May cause dizziness, drowsiness, headache, fatigue, irritability, psychosis, suicidal ideation. *Black-box warning* cautions *life-threatening* psychiatric and behavioral reactions such as aggression, hostility, anger, and homicidal ideation. Notify health care provider if any changes in mood, behavior, or personality occur. Pregnancy category: C*; PB: 95%-96%; t½: 105 h

*Pregnancy categories have been revised. See http://www.fda.gov/Drugs/DevelopmentApprovalProcess/DevelopmentResources/Labeling/ucm093307.htm for more information.

>, Greater than; <, less than; *A*, adult; *adol*, adolescent; *bid*, twice a day; *BP*, blood pressure; *C*, child; *CSS*, Controlled Substances Schedule; *d*, day; *GI*, gastrointestinal; *h*, hour; *IM*, intramuscular; *IV*, intravenous; *maint*, maintenance; *max*, maximum; *Mg*, magnesium; *min*, minute; *NaCl*, sodium chloride; *PB*, protein binding; *PE*, phenytoin equivalents; *PO*, by mouth; *PRN*, as needed; *q3d*, every three days; *qd*, every day; *qid*, four times a day; *t½*, half-life; *tid*, three times a day; *UK*, unknown; *wk*, weeks; *y*, years.

Antiseizure drugs tend to act as inhibitors of vitamin K, contributing to hemorrhage in infants shortly after birth. Frequently, pregnant women taking antiseizure drugs are given an oral vitamin K supplement during the last week or 10 days of the pregnancy, or vitamin K is administered to the infant soon after birth.

Antiseizure drugs also increase the loss of folate (folic acid) in pregnant women, thus pregnant individuals should take daily folate supplements.

Antiseizure Drugs and Febrile Seizures

Seizures associated with fever usually occur in children between 3 months and 5 years of age. Epilepsy develops in approximately 2.5% of children who have had one or more febrile seizures. Prophylactic antiseizure drug treatment such as phenobarbital or diazepam may be indicated for high-risk patients. Valproic acid should not be given to children younger than 2 years of age because of its possible hepatotoxic effect.

TABLE 19.3 Selected Anticonvulsants For Seizure Disorders

Seizure Disorder	Drug Therapy
Tonic-clonic	Phenytoin
	Carbamazepine
	Fosphenytoin
	Valproic acid
	Lamotrigine
	Primidone
	Phenobarbital
	Diazepam
	Levetiracetam
	Topiramate
Partial (complex secondarily generalized)	Phenytoin
	Carbamazepine
	Oxcarbazepine
	Levetiracetam
	Primidone
	Phenobarbital
	Tiagabine
	Topiramate
	Zonisamide
	Gabapentin
	Valproic acid
	Diazepam
	Fosphenytoin
	Lamotrigine
	Eslicarbazepine
	Clorazepate
	Pregabalin
	Ezogabine
	Lacosamide
	Felbamate
Absence (petit mal)	Ethosuximide
	Valproic acid
	Clonazepam
Myoclonic, atonic, atypical absence	Valproic acid
	Levetiracetam
	Clonazepam
Status epilepticus	Diazepam
	Fosphenytoin
	Lorazepam
	Phenytoin
	Phenobarbital

◎ NURSING PROCESS
Patient-Centered Collaborative Care
Antiseizure Drugs: Phenytoin

Assessment
- Obtain a health history that includes current drugs and herbs the patient uses. Report and document any probable drug-drug or herb-drug interactions.
- Assess the patient's knowledge regarding the medication regimen.
- Check urinary output to determine whether it is adequate (>1500 mL/d).
- Determine laboratory values related to renal and liver function. If both blood urea nitrogen (BUN) and creatinine levels are elevated, a renal disorder should be suspected. Elevated serum liver enzymes (alkaline phosphatase, alanine aminotransferase, gamma-glutamyl transferase, 59-nucleotidase) indicate a hepatic disorder.

Nursing Diagnoses
- Injury, Risk for
- Oral Mucous Membranes, Impaired related to blood dyscrasias
- Nutrition, Imbalanced: Less than Body Requirements related to anorexia
- Falls, Risk for

Planning
- Patient's seizure frequency will diminish.
- Patient will adhere to antiseizure drug therapy.
- Patient's side effects from phenytoin will be minimal.

Nursing Interventions
- Monitor serum drug levels of antiseizure medication to determine therapeutic range (10 to 20 mcg/mL).
- Encourage patient's compliance with medication regimen.
- Monitor patient's complete blood count (CBC) levels for early detection of blood dyscrasias.
- ⚡ Use seizure precautions (environmental protection from sharp objects, such as table corners) for patients at risk for seizures.
- Determine whether the patient is receiving adequate nutrients; phenytoin may cause anorexia, nausea, and vomiting.
- Advise female patients who are taking oral contraceptives and antiseizure drugs to use an additional contraceptive method.

Patient Teaching
General
- Teach patients to shake suspension-form medications thoroughly before use to adequately mix the medication to ensure accurate dosage.

- ⚡ Advise patients not to drive or perform other hazardous activities when initiating antiseizure therapy as drowsiness may occur.
- Counsel female patients contemplating pregnancy to consult with a health care provider because phenytoin and valproic acid may have a teratogenic effect.
- Monitor serum phenytoin levels closely during pregnancy because seizures tend to become more frequent due to increased metabolic rates.
- Warn patients to avoid alcohol and other CNS depressants because they can cause an added depressive effect on the body.
- Explain to patients that certain herbs can interact with antiseizure drugs (see Complementary and Alternative Therapy Box 19.1), and dose adjustment may be required.
- Encourage patients to obtain a medical alert identification card, medical alert bracelet, or tag that indicates their diagnosis and drug regimen.
- ⚡ Teach patients not to abruptly stop drug therapy but rather to withdraw the prescribed drug gradually under medical supervision to prevent seizure rebound (recurrence of seizures) and status epilepticus.
- Counsel patients about the need for preventive dental checkups.
- Warn patients to take their prescribed antiseizure drug, get laboratory tests as ordered, and keep follow-up visits with health care providers.
- Teach patients not to self-medicate with over-the-counter (OTC) drugs without first consulting a health care provider.
- Advise patients with diabetes to monitor serum glucose levels more closely than usual because phenytoin may inhibit insulin release, causing an increase in glucose level.
- Inform patients of the existence of national, state, and local associations that provide resources, current information, and support for people with epilepsy.

Diet

- Coach patients to take antiseizure drugs at the same time every day with food or milk.

Side Effects

- Tell patients that urine may be a harmless pinkish red or reddish brown color.
- Advise patients to maintain good oral hygiene and to use a soft toothbrush to prevent gum irritation and bleeding.
- Teach patients to report symptoms of sore throat, bruising, and nosebleeds, which may indicate a blood dyscrasia.
- Encourage patients to inform health care providers of adverse reactions such as gingivitis, nystagmus, slurred speech, rash, and dizziness. (Stevens-Johnson syndrome begins with a rash.)

🌐 Cultural Considerations

- Communicate respect for cultural beliefs concerning refusal or reluctance to take antiseizure medications daily for life; use an interpreter and the extended family as needed to help the patient understand the importance of keeping to a prescribed drug regimen.
- Use a written drug schedule in the patient's preferred language to support adherence to the prescribed drug regimen.
- Encourage patient compliance with follow-up by a community nurse.
- Show patient videos or pictures in their own cultural group when language barriers exist to help strengthen compliance with health interventions.

Evaluation

- Evaluate effectiveness of drugs in controlling seizures.
- Monitor serum phenytoin levels to determine whether they are within the desired range. High serum levels of phenytoin are frequently indicators of phenytoin toxicity.
- Monitor patients for hydantoin overdose. Initial symptoms are nystagmus and ataxia (impaired coordination). Later symptoms are hypotension, unresponsive pupils, and coma. Respiratory and circulatory support, as well as hemodialysis, are usually used in the treatment of phenytoin overdose.

Antiseizure Drugs and Status Epilepticus

Status epilepticus, a continuous seizure state, is considered a medical emergency. If treatment is not begun immediately, death could result. The choices of pharmacologic agents are diazepam administered by IV or lorazepam followed by IV administration of phenytoin. For continued seizures, midazolam or propofol and then high-dose barbiturates are used. These drugs should be administered slowly to avoid respiratory depression.

The pharmacologic behavior of specific anticonvulsants, including a few common side effects and severe adverse effects, is summarized in Table 19.2.

■ CRITICAL THINKING CASE STUDY

SS, a 26-year-old woman, takes phenytoin 100 mg three times daily to control tonic-clonic seizures. She and her husband are contemplating starting a family.

1. What action should the nurse take in regard to the patient's family planning?

SS complains of frequent upset stomach and bleeding gums when brushing her teeth.

2. To decrease GI distress, what can be suggested?
3. To alleviate bleeding gums, what patient teaching for SS may be included?
4. The nurse checks SS's serum phenytoin level. What are the indications of an abnormal serum level? What appropriate actions should be taken?

NCLEX STUDY QUESTIONS

1. The nurse witnesses a patient's seizure involving generalized contraction of the body followed by jerkiness of the arms and legs. The nurse reports this as which type of seizure?
   a. Myoclonic
   b. Absence
   c. Tonic-clonic
   d. Psychomotor

2. Phenytoin has been prescribed for a patient with seizures. The nurse should include which appropriate nursing intervention in the plan of care?
   a. Report an abnormal phenytoin level of 18 mcg/mL.
   b. Monitor complete blood count levels for early detection of blood dyscrasias.
   c. Encourage the patient to brush teeth vigorously to prevent plaque buildup.
   d. Teach the patient to stop the drug immediately when passing pinkish-red or reddish-brown urine.

3. When administering phenytoin, the nurse realizes more teaching is needed if the patient makes which statement?
   a. "I must shake the oral suspension very well before pouring it in the dose cup."
   b. "I cannot drink alcoholic beverages when taking phenytoin."
   c. "I should take phenytoin 1 hour before meals."
   d. "I will need to get periodic dental checkups."

4. A patient is having absence seizures. Which of the following does the nurse expect to be prescribed for this type of seizure? (Select all that apply.)
   a. Phenytoin
   b. Phenobarbital
   c. Valproic acid
   d. Clonazepam
   e. Ethosuximide

5. A patient is admitted to the emergency department with status epilepticus. Which drug should the nurse most likely prepare to administer to this patient? (Select all that apply.)
   a. Diazepam
   b. Midazolam
   c. Gabapentin
   d. Levetiracetam
   e. Topiramate

6. The nurse should monitor the patient receiving phenytoin for which adverse effect?
   a. Psychosis
   b. Nosebleeds
   c. Hypertension
   d. Gum erosion

7. A nurse administering valproic acid to a patient checks the laboratory values and finds a serum range for valproic acid of 150 mcg/mL. What should the nurse do?
   a. Increase the daily dose to get the patient's level into the therapeutic range.
   b. Hold the morning dose but give the other scheduled dosages for the day.
   c. Ask the patient if he or she is having any adverse effects from the medication.
   d. Hold the medication and notify the health care provider.

Answers: 1, c; 2, b; 3, c; 4, c, d, e; 5, a, b; 6, b; 7, d.

20

Drugs for Parkinson's Disease and Alzheimer Disease

ℹ http://evolve.elsevier.com/McCuistion/pharmacology/

OBJECTIVES

- Summarize the pathophysiology of Parkinson's disease and Alzheimer disease.
- Contrast the actions of anticholinergics, dopaminergics, dopamine agonists, monoamine oxidase B (MAO-B) inhibitors, and catechol-*O*-methyltransferase (COMT) inhibitors in the treatment of Parkinson's disease.
- Compare the side effects of various antiparkinson drugs.

- Apply the nursing process to anticholinergics, dopaminergics, and acetylcholinesterase inhibitors.
- Differentiate the phases of Alzheimer disease with corresponding symptoms.
- Compare the side effects/adverse effects of acetylcholinesterase inhibitors used to treat Alzheimer disease.

OUTLINE

KEY TERMS

Parkinson's disease is a chronic, progressive, neurologic disorder that affects the extrapyramidal motor tract, which controls posture, balance, and locomotion. Parkinson's disease is the most common form of **parkinsonism**, which is considered a syndrome, or a combination of similar symptoms, because of its major features: rigidity (abnormal increased muscle tone), **bradykinesia** (slow movement), gait disturbances, and tremors. Rigidity increases with movement. Postural changes caused by rigidity and bradykinesia include the chest and head thrust forward with the knees and hips flexed, a shuffling gait, and the absence of arm swing. Other characteristic symptoms are masked facies (no facial expression), involuntary tremors of the head and neck, and pill-rolling motions of the hands. The tremors may be more prevalent at rest.

Alzheimer disease is a chronic, progressive, neurodegenerative condition with marked cognitive dysfunction. Various theories exist as to the cause of Alzheimer disease, with neuritic plaques, degeneration of the cholinergic neurons, and deficiency in acetylcholine among them.

PARKINSON'S DISEASE

In 1817, Dr. James Parkinson described six patients as having "shaking palsy." Three symptoms were described by Parkinson: (1) involuntary tremors of the limbs, (2) rigidity of muscles, and (3) slowness of movement. In the United States, approximately one million people have Parkinson's disease, and 60,000 new cases are diagnosed each year. Because Parkinson's disease generally affects patients 50 years of age and older, many consider the health problem to be part of the aging process caused by loss of neurons. The cardinal symptoms are rigidity, tremors, gait disturbance, and bradykinesia. Normally the symptoms have a gradual onset and are usually mild and unilateral in the beginning.

There are different types of parkinsonism. Pseudoparkinsonism frequently occurs as an adverse reaction to chlorpromazine, haloperidol, lithium, metoclopramide, methyldopa, and reserpine. In addition, parkinsonism symptoms could result from poisons, such as carbon monoxide and manganese, or from disorders, such as arteriosclerosis, encephalitis, infections, stroke, trauma, or Wilson disease (hepatolenticular degeneration). Parkinson's disease is the most common type, which is a degeneration of dopaminergic neurons leading to a lack of dopamine.

Nonpharmacologic Measures

Symptoms of Parkinson's disease can be lessened through the use of nonpharmacologic measures such as patient teaching, exercise, nutrition, and group support. Exercise can improve mobility and flexibility; the patient with Parkinson's disease should enroll in a therapeutic exercise program tailored to this disorder. A balanced diet with fiber and fluids helps prevent constipation and weight loss. Patients with Parkinson's disease and their family members should be encouraged to attend a support group to help cope with and understand this disorder.

Pathophysiology

Parkinson's disease is caused by an imbalance of the neurotransmitters dopamine and acetylcholine, and it is marked by degeneration of neurons of the extrapyramidal (motor) tract in the substantia nigra of the midbrain. The reason for the degeneration of neurons is unknown.

The two neurotransmitters within the neurons of the striatum of the brain are dopamine (DA), an inhibitory neurotransmitter, and acetylcholine (ACh), an excitatory neurotransmitter. DA is released from the dopaminergic neurons, and ACh is released from the cholinergic neurons. DA normally maintains control of ACh and inhibits its excitatory response. In Parkinson's disease, an unexplained degeneration of the dopaminergic neurons occurs, and an imbalance between DA and ACh results. With less DA production, the excitatory response of ACh exceeds the inhibitory response of DA. An excessive amount of ACh stimulates neurons that release gamma-aminobutyric acid (GABA). With increased stimulation of GABA, the symptomatic movement disorders of Parkinson's disease occur.

By the time early symptoms of Parkinson's disease appear, 80% of the striatal dopamine has already been depleted. The remaining striatal neurons synthesize DA from levodopa and release DA as needed. Before the next dose of levodopa, symptoms such as slow walking and loss of dexterity return or worsen, but within 30 to 60 minutes of receiving a dose, the patient's functioning is much improved.

Drugs used to treat Parkinson's disease replace the dopamine deficit and reduce the symptoms. These drugs fall into five categories: (1) anticholinergics, which block cholinergic receptors; (2) dopamine replacements, which stimulate DA receptors; (3) dopamine agonists, which stimulate DA receptors; (4) monoamine oxidase B (MAO-B) inhibitors, which inhibit the MAO-B enzyme that interferes with DA; and (5) catechol-O-methyltransferase (COMT) inhibitors, which inhibit the COMT enzyme that inactivates DA. Table 20.1 compares the various drugs for Parkinson's disease.

TABLE 20.1	Comparison of Drugs Used to Treat Parkinson's Disease
Drug	**Purpose**
Dopaminergics	
Carbidopa-levodopa	To decrease symptoms of Parkinson's disease and parkinsonism; carbidopa, a decarboxylase inhibitor, permits more levodopa to reach the striatum nerve terminals, where levodopa is converted to dopamine. With the use of carbidopa, less levodopa is needed.
Dopamine Agonists	
Amantadine	First used as an antiviral drug for influenza A, amantadine decreases symptoms of Parkinson's disease and parkinsonism. It can be used for early treatment of parkinsonism, which could delay the necessity of levodopa. It is effective in treating drug-induced parkinsonism and has fewer side effects than anticholinergics.
Bromocriptine	A D_2-dopamine receptor agonist, bromocriptine can be used for early treatment of Parkinson's disease. With increasing motor symptoms, it can be given with levodopa therapy.
Pramipexole, Ropinirole hydrochloride	These D_2- and D_3-dopamine receptor agonists can be used in combination with carbidopa-levodopa and have fewer side effects than older dopamine agonists.
Monoamine Oxidase B Inhibitors	
Selegiline hydrochloride	Selegiline inhibits catabolic enzymes of dopamine and extends its action. It can be used for early treatment of Parkinson's disease and parkinsonism. If given with carbidopa-levodopa, the dosage of carbidopa-levodopa is usually decreased.
Rasagiline	Rasagiline inhibits the breakdown of dopamine at synapses in the brain and allows neurons to reabsorb more dopamine for use later.
Catechol-O-Methyltransferase (COMT) Inhibitors	
Entacapone, Tolcapone	These inhibit the COMT enzyme and increase the concentration of levodopa. and are used in combination with levodopa-carbidopa. With COMT inhibitors, a smaller dose of levodopa is needed.
Anticholinergics and Antiparkinson Drugs	
	The first group of drugs used to treat Parkinson's disease before levodopa and dopamine agonists were introduced, these were useful in decreasing tremors related to Parkinson's disease. The major use of these agents currently is to treat drug-induced parkinsonism. Treatment starts with a low dosage that is gradually increased. Older adults are more susceptible to the many side effects of anticholinergics, and patients with memory loss or dementia should *not* be on anticholinergic therapy.

Anticholinergics

Anticholinergic drugs reduce the rigidity and some of the tremors characteristic of Parkinson's disease but have a minimal effect on bradykinesia. The anticholinergics are parasympatholytics that inhibit the release of acetylcholine. Anticholinergics are still used to treat drug-induced parkinsonism, or pseudoparkinsonism, a side effect of the antipsychotic phenothiazine drug group. Examples of anticholinergics used for Parkinson's disease include trihexyphenidyl and benztropine.

NURSING PROCESS
Patient-Centered Collaborative Care
Antiparkinson Anticholinergic Agents

Assessment
- Obtain a health history. Report any history of glaucoma, gastrointestinal (GI) dysfunction, urinary retention, angina, or myasthenia gravis. All anticholinergics are contraindicated if a patient has glaucoma.
- Obtain a drug history. Report any probable drug-drug interactions, such as with phenothiazines, tricyclic antidepressants (TCAs), and antihistamines, which increase the effect of trihexyphenidyl.
- Assess baseline vital signs for future comparisons. The pulse rate may increase.
- Assess the patient's knowledge regarding the medication regimen.
- Determine usual urinary output as a baseline for comparison. Urinary retention may occur with continuous use of anticholinergics.

Nursing Diagnoses
- Mobility, Impaired Physical related to muscle rigidity, tremors, and bradykinesia
- Elimination, Impaired Urinary related to urinary retention
- Knowledge, Deficient related to unfamiliarity with drug regimen

Planning
- Patient will have decreased involuntary symptoms caused by Parkinson's disease or drug-induced parkinsonism.

Nursing Interventions
- Monitor vital signs, urine output, and bowel sounds. Increased pulse rate, urinary retention, and constipation are side effects of anticholinergics.
- Observe for involuntary movements.

Patient Teaching
General
- Advise patients to avoid alcohol, cigarettes, caffeine, and aspirin to decrease gastric acidity.
Side Effects
- Encourage patients to relieve a dry mouth with hard candy, ice chips, or sugarless chewing gum. Anticholinergics decrease salivation.

- Suggest that patients use sunglasses in direct sunlight because of possible photophobia.
- Advise patients to void before taking the drug to minimize urinary retention.
- Counsel patients who take an anticholinergic for control of symptoms of Parkinson's disease to have routine eye examinations because anticholinergics are contraindicated in patients with glaucoma.
Diet
- Encourage patients to ingest foods high in fiber and to increase fluid intake to prevent constipation.

Cultural Considerations
- Assess personal beliefs of patients and family, and modify communications to meet cultural needs; use an interpreter and community nurse follow-up as needed.

Evaluation
- Evaluate the patient's response to trihexyphenidyl or benztropine mesylate to determine whether Parkinson's disease symptoms are controlled.

Table 20.2 lists the anticholinergics and their dosages, uses, and considerations. Anticholinergics used to treat Parkinson's disease are also discussed in Chapter 16.

Dopaminergics
Carbidopa and Levodopa

The first dopaminergic drug was levodopa, which was introduced in 1961 but is no longer available in the United States. When introduced, levodopa was effective in diminishing symptoms of Parkinson's disease and increasing mobility; this is because the blood-brain barrier admits levodopa but not dopamine. The enzyme dopa decarboxylase converts levodopa to dopamine in the brain, but this enzyme is also found in the peripheral nervous system and allows 99% of levodopa to be converted to dopamine before it reaches the brain. Therefore only about 1% of levodopa taken is available to be converted to dopamine once it reaches the brain, and large doses are needed to achieve a pharmacologic response. These high doses could cause many side effects, including nausea, vomiting, dyskinesia, orthostatic hypotension, cardiac dysrhythmias, and psychosis.

Because of the side effects of levodopa and the fact that so much levodopa is metabolized before it reaches the brain, an alternative drug, carbidopa, was developed to inhibit the enzyme dopa decarboxylase. By inhibiting the enzyme in the peripheral nervous system, more levodopa reaches the brain. The carbidopa is combined with levodopa in a ratio of 1 part carbidopa to 10 parts levodopa. Fig. 20.1 illustrates the comparative action of levodopa and carbidopa-levodopa.

The advantages of combining levodopa with carbidopa are that more dopamine reaches the basal ganglia and that

TABLE 20.2 Antiparkinson Drugs: Anticholinergics

Drug	Route and Dosage	Uses and Considerations
Benztropine mesylate	Parkinson's disease: A: PO/IM: Initially 0.5-1 mg/d at bedtime; *maint:* 0.5-6 mg/d; *max:* 8 mg/d Drug-induced parkinsonism: A: IV/IM/PO: 1-4 mg qd/bid	For Parkinson's disease, tremor, and drug-induced parkinsonism. Contraindicated in glaucoma and dementia. May cause blurred vision, ocular hypertension, weakness, dry mouth, nausea, constipation, anhidrosis, and urinary retention. Pregnancy category: C*; PB: UK; t½: UK
Trihexyphenidyl hydrochloride	Parkinson's disease: A: PO: Initially 1 mg, then increase by 2 mg q3-5d; maint: 6-10 mg/d; *max:* 15 mg/d Extended release: A: PO: 5-10 mg after breakfast or in 2 divided doses 12 h apart Drug-induced parkinsonism: A: PO: Initially 1 mg; maint: 5-15 mg/d	For Parkinson's disease and drug-induced pseudoparkinsonism. May cause dizziness, drowsiness, increased intraocular pressure, anxiety, headache, insomnia, weakness, paresthesia, dry mouth, nausea, vomiting, constipation, restlessness, and urinary retention. Pregnancy category: C*; PB: UK; t½: UK

*Pregnancy categories have been revised. See http://www.fda.gov/Drugs/DevelopmentApprovalProcess/DevelopmentResources/Labeling/ucm093 307.htm for more information.

A, Adult; *bid*, two times a day; *d*, day; *h*, hour; *IM*, intramuscular; *IV*, intravenous; *maint*, maintenance; *max*, maximum; *PB*, protein binding; *PO*, by mouth; *qd*, every day; *q3-5d*, every 3 to 5 days; *t½*, half-life; *UK*, unknown.

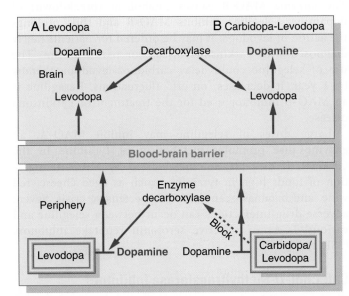

FIG. 20.1 A, When levodopa is used alone, only 1% reaches the brain because 99% converts to dopamine while in the peripheral nervous system. **B,** By combining carbidopa with levodopa, carbidopa can inhibit the enzyme decarboxylase in the periphery, thereby allowing more levodopa to reach the brain.

smaller doses of levodopa are required to achieve the desired effect. The disadvantage of the carbidopa-levodopa combination is that with more available levodopa, more side effects may occur, which may include nausea, vomiting, dystonic movement (involuntary abnormal movement), and psychotic behavior. The peripheral side effects of levodopa are not as prevalent; however, angioedema, palpitations, and orthostatic hypotension may occur. Prototype Drug Chart 20.1 lists the pharmacologic behavior of carbidopa-levodopa.

◎ NURSING PROCESS
Patient-Centered Collaborative Care

Antiparkinson Dopaminergic Agents: Carbidopa-Levodopa

Assessment
- Obtain vital signs to use for future comparisons.
- Assess patients for signs and symptoms of Parkinson's disease, including stooped forward posture, shuffling gait, masked facies, and resting tremors.
- Obtain a patient history that includes glaucoma, heart disease, peptic ulcers, kidney or liver disease, and psychosis.
- Obtain a drug history. Report if drug-drug interaction is probable. Drugs that should be avoided or closely monitored are carbidopa-levodopa, bromocriptine, and anticholinergics.

Nursing Diagnoses
- Mobility, Impaired Physical related to dizziness
- Activity Intolerance, Risk for
- Falls, Risk for
- Knowledge, Deficient related to unfamiliar medications

Planning
- Patient's symptoms of Parkinson's disease will be decreased or absent after 1 to 4 weeks of drug therapy.

Nursing Interventions
- Monitor vital signs and electrocardiogram. Orthostatic hypotension may occur during early use of carbidopa-levodopa and bromocriptine. Instruct patients to rise slowly to avoid faintness.
- Observe for weakness, dizziness, or syncope, which are symptoms of orthostatic hypotension.

- Administer carbidopa-levodopa with low-protein foods. High-protein diets interfere with drug transport to the central nervous system (CNS).
- Observe for symptoms of Parkinson's disease.

Patient Teaching
General
- Urge patients not to abruptly discontinue the medication. Rebound Parkinson's disease (increased symptoms of Parkinson's disease) can occur.
- Inform patients that urine may be discolored and will darken with exposure to air. Perspiration may also be dark. Explain that both are harmless, but clothes may be stained.
- Advise patients to avoid chewing or crushing extended-release tablets.

Side Effects
- Encourage patients to report side effects and symptoms of dyskinesia. Explain that it may take weeks or months before symptoms are controlled.

Diet
- Suggest to patients that taking carbidopa-levodopa with food may decrease GI upset, but food will slow the rate of drug absorption.
- ⚡ Urge patients who take high doses of selegiline to avoid foods high in tyramine such as aged cheese, red wine, cream, yogurt, chocolate, bananas, and raisins to prevent hypertensive crisis.

Amantadine and Bromocriptine
- Urge patients taking amantadine to report any signs of skin lesions, seizures, or depression. A history of these health problems should have been previously reported to a health care provider.
- Advise patients taking bromocriptine to report symptoms of lightheadedness when changing positions, a symptom of orthostatic hypotension.
- Warn patients to avoid alcohol when taking bromocriptine.
- Teach patients to check their heart rate and report rate changes or irregularity.
- Counsel patients not to abruptly stop the drug without first notifying a health care provider.

🌐 Cultural Considerations
- Recognize that various cultural groups will need guidance in understanding the disease process of Parkinson's disease. Support patients and family members who may be dismayed about the symptoms of Parkinson's disease and lack knowledge of the disease process.
- Secure an interpreter for patients who speak little or no English to support understanding of drug doses and schedules and recognition of severe side effects that need to be reported to a health care provider.

Evaluation
- Evaluate effectiveness of drug therapy in controlling symptoms of Parkinson's disease.
- Determine if there is an absence of side effects.
- Determine if the patient and family have increased knowledge of the drug regimen.

Dopamine Agonists

Other dopamine agonists, also called *dopaminergics,* stimulate the dopamine receptors. For example, amantadine hydrochloride is an antiviral drug that acts on the dopamine receptors. It may be taken alone or in combination with carbidopa-levodopa or an anticholinergic drug. Initially, amantadine produces improvement in symptoms of Parkinson's disease and parkinsonism in approximately two-thirds of patients, but this improvement is usually not sustained because drug tolerance develops. Amantadine can also be used to treat drug-induced parkinsonism.

Bromocriptine mesylate acts directly on dopamine receptors in the CNS, cardiovascular system, and GI tract. Bromocriptine is more effective than amantadine and the anticholinergics; however, it is not as effective as carbidopa-levodopa in alleviating Parkinson's disease symptoms. Patients who do not tolerate carbidopa-levodopa are frequently given bromocriptine.

Monoamine Oxidase B Inhibitors

The enzyme MAO-B causes catabolism (breakdown) of dopamine. Selegiline inhibits MAO-B and thus prolongs the action of levodopa. It may be ordered for patients newly diagnosed with Parkinson's disease or parkinsonism. The use of selegiline could delay carbidopa-levodopa therapy by 1 year. It decreases "on-off" fluctuations. Rasagiline is an MAO-B inhibitor used for the treatment of Parkinson's disease.

Large doses of selegiline may inhibit MAO-A, an enzyme that promotes metabolism of tyramine in the GI tract. If they are not metabolized by MAO-A, ingestion of foods high in tyramine—such as aged cheese, red wine, and bananas—can cause a hypertensive crisis. Severe adverse drug interactions can occur between selegiline and various TCAs or selective serotonin reuptake inhibitors (SSRIs).

Catechol-*O*-Methyltransferase Inhibitors

The enzyme COMT inactivates dopamine. When taken with a levodopa preparation, COMT inhibitors increase the amount of levodopa concentration in the brain. Tolcapone was the first COMT inhibitor to be given with levodopa for advanced Parkinson's disease. This drug can affect liver cell function, therefore serum liver enzymes should be closely monitored. Entacapone does not affect liver function. In 2003, the U.S. Food and Drug Administration (FDA) approved a combination drug of dopaminergics (carbidopa and levodopa) and a COMT inhibitor (entacapone). With various dosage strengths available, this drug combination of carbidopa, levodopa, and entacapone provides greater dosing flexibility and individualization to the patient. This drug combination lessens the "wearing off" effects of levodopa that are sometimes experienced prior to the next dose.

Table 20.3 lists dopaminergics, dopamine agonists, MAO-B inhibitors, and COMT inhibitors with their dosages, uses, and considerations.

PROTOTYPE DRUG CHART 20.1

Carbidopa-Levodopa

Drug Class	Dosage
Antiparkinson: Dopamine replacement Pregnancy category: C*	Immediate release: A: PO: Initially 1 tablet containing 25 mg carbidopa/100 mg levodopa tid; maint: 25-250 mg tid/qid; *max:* 200/800 mg/d or 8 tablets/d A: Extended release tablets: Initially 50 mg carbidopa/200 mg levodopa bid; *max:* 1600 mg/d A: Extended release capsules: Initially 23.75 mg carbidopa/95 mg levodopa tid; *max:* 97.5 mg carbidopa/390 mg levodopa tid Enteral suspension: 2000 mg/d over 16 h

Contraindications	Drug-Lab-Food Interactions
Narrow-angle glaucoma; severe cardiac, renal, hepatic disease; suspicious skin lesions (activates malignant melanoma); MAOI therapy *Caution:* Peptic ulcer, impulse control syndrome, orthostatic hypotension, psychosis, seizure disorder, and suicidal ideation	Drug: Increased hypertensive crisis with MAOIs, decreased levodopa effect with anticholinergics and antipsychotics; with TCAs, may cause dyskinesia and hypertension; with methyldopa, may cause psychosis Food: High-protein foods decrease levodopa absorption. Lab: May increase BUN, AST, ALT, ALP, and LDH

Pharmacokinetics	Pharmacodynamics
Absorption: PO: Well absorbed Distribution: PB: Carbidopa: 36%; levodopa: UK Metabolism: t½: 1-2 h Excretion: In urine as metabolites	PO Onset: 15-30 min Peak: 1-3 h Duration: 5 h ER Onset: UK Peak: 2-3 h Duration: 4-5 h

Therapeutic Effects/Uses
To treat Parkinson's disease and parkinsonism and to relieve tremors and rigidity Mode of Action: Transmission of levodopa to brain cells for conversion to dopamine; carbidopa blocks the conversion of levodopa to dopamine in the intestine and peripheral tissues.

Side Effects	Adverse Reactions
Anorexia, nausea, vomiting, dysphagia, dyskinesia, erythema, fatigue, dizziness, headache, dry mouth, constipation, bitter taste, twitching, blurred vision, insomnia, excess dark sweating, urine discoloration (red, brown, or black)	Involuntary movements, angioedema, palpitations, orthostatic hypotension, urinary retention, priapism, psychosis, depression with suicidal ideation, hallucinations, sudden sleep onset, impulse control symptoms *Life threatening:* Agranulocytosis, hemolytic anemia, leucopenia, thrombocytopenia, cardiac dysrhythmias; abrupt discontinuation may cause neuroleptic malignant syndrome

*Pregnancy categories have been revised. See http://www.fda.gov/Drugs/DevelopmentApprovalProcess/DevelopmentResources/Labeling/ucm093 307.htm for more information.

A, Adult; *ALP,* alkaline phosphatase; *ALT,* alanine aminotransferase; *AST,* aspartate aminotransferase; *bid,* two times a day; *BUN,* blood urea nitrogen; *d,* day; *h,* hour; *LDH,* lactic dehydrogenase; *maint,* maintenance; *MAOI,* monoamine oxidase inhibitor; *max,* maximum; *min,* minute; *PB,* protein binding; *PO,* by mouth; *qid,* four times a day; *t½,* half-life; *TCA,* tricyclic antidepressant; *tid,* three times a day; *UK,* unknown.

TABLE 20.3   Antiparkinson Dopaminergics

Drug	Route and Dosage	Uses and Considerations
Dopaminergics Carbidopa-levodopa	See Prototype Drug Chart 20.1	
Dopamine Agonists Amantadine hydrochloride	Parkinson's disease: A: PO: 100 mg bid; *max:* 400 mg/d	For Parkinson's disease, drug-induced parkinsonism, seasonal influenza prophylaxis, and influenza A virus infection. May cause dizziness, drowsiness, headache, anxiety, confusion, fatigue, insomnia, nausea, nightmares, irritability, orthostatic hypotension, and peripheral edema. Pregnancy category: C*; PB: 67%; t½: 11-15 h
Bromocriptine mesylate	A: PO: Initially 1.25 mg bid, gradually increase; *max:* 100 mg/d	For Parkinson's disease. May cause dizziness, drowsiness, orthostatic hypotension, headache, rhinitis, sinusitis, weakness, fatigue, nausea, constipation, and diarrhea. Pregnancy category: B*; PB: 90%-96%; t½: 3 h
Pramipexole dihydrochloride	Parkinson's disease: Immediate release: A: PO: Initially: 0.125 mg tid; *max:* 4.5 mg/d Extended release: A: PO: Initially 0.375 mg/d; *max:* 4.5 mg/d	For Parkinson's disease and restless leg syndrome. May cause dizziness, drowsiness, headache, confusion, abnormal dreams, insomnia, fatigue, weakness, orthostatic hypotension, hallucinations, dyskinesia, nausea, and constipation. Pregnancy category: C*; PB: 15%; t½: 8-12 h

Continued

TABLE 20.3   Antiparkinson Dopaminergics—cont'd

Drug	Route and Dosage	Uses and Considerations
Ropinirole hydrochloride	Parkinson's disease: Immediate release: A: PO: Initially: 0.25 mg tid; titrate up on weekly basis; *max*: 24 mg/d Extended release: A: PO: Initially 2 mg/d for 1-2 wk, titrate up weekly; *max*: 24 mg/d	For Parkinson's disease and restless leg syndrome. May cause dizziness, drowsiness, headache, syncope, dyskinesia, fatigue, weakness, nausea, vomiting, hyperhidrosis, hypertension, and orthostatic hypotension. Pregnancy category: C*; PB: 40%; t½: 6 h
Monoamine Oxidase B Inhibitors		
Selegiline hydrochloride	A: PO: 5 mg bid with breakfast and lunch; *max*: 10 mg/d A: PO: Dtab: 1.25 mg/d for 6 wk, increase to 2.5 mg/d; *max*: 2.5 mg/d	For Parkinson's disease and parkinsonism. May cause dizziness, headache, orthostatic hypotension, dry mouth, nausea, impulse control disorder, and suicidal ideation. Pregnancy category: C*; PB: 85%; t½: 10 h
Rasagiline	A: PO: 0.5-1 mg/d; *max*: 1 mg/d	For Parkinson's disease. May cause headache, orthostatic hypotension, hypertension, dyskinesia, and nausea. Pregnancy category: C*; PB: 88%-94%; t½: 3 h
Catechol-*O*-Methyltransferase Inhibitors		
Tolcapone	A: PO: Initially 100 mg tid; *max*: 600 mg/d	For Parkinson's disease. May cause dizziness, drowsiness, headache, confusion, dyskinesia, dystonic reaction, excess dreams, insomnia, anorexia, nausea, diarrhea, constipation, muscle cramps, orthostatic hypotension, sudden sleep onset, and impulse control symptoms. Monitor liver enzymes frequently because tolcapone may cause fatal hepatotoxicity. Abrupt discontinuation may cause pyrexia, confusion, and NMS. Pregnancy category: C*; PB: 99%; t½: 2-3 h
Entacapone	A: PO: 200 mg with each dose of levodopa-carbidopa; *max*: 1600 mg/d	For Parkinson's disease. Used in combination with levodopa-carbidopa, it prolongs half-life of levodopa and decreases "on-off" fluctuations. Levodopa dose should be decreased when taken with a COMT inhibitor. May cause dizziness, nausea, diarrhea, abdominal pain, dyskinesia, hyperkinesis, sudden sleep onset, and impulse control symptoms. Abrupt discontinuation may cause NMS. Pregnancy category: C*; PB: 98%; t½: 1-2 h

*Pregnancy categories have been revised. See http://www.fda.gov/Drugs/DevelopmentApprovalProcess/DevelopmentResources/Labeling/ucm093307.htm for more information.

A, Adult; *bid*, twice daily; *COMT*, catechol-*O*-methyltransferase; *d*, day; *Dtab*, disintegrating tablet; *h*, hour; *max*, maximum; *NMS*, neuroleptic malignant syndrome; *PB*, protein binding; *PO*, by mouth; *t½*, half-life; *tid*, three times a day; *wk*, weeks.

Precautions for Drugs Used to Treat Parkinson's Disease

Side Effects and Adverse Reactions

The common side effects of anticholinergics include dry mouth and dry secretions, urinary retention, constipation, blurred vision, and an increase in heart rate. Mental effects such as restlessness and confusion may occur in older adults.

The side effects of carbidopa-levodopa are numerous. GI disturbances are common because dopamine stimulates the chemoreceptor trigger zone (CTZ) in the medulla, which stimulates the vomiting center. Taking the drug with food can decrease nausea and vomiting, but food slows the absorption rate. Dyskinesia, impaired voluntary movement, may occur with high levodopa dosages. Cardiovascular side effects include orthostatic hypotension and increased heart rate during early use of levodopa. Nightmares, sudden sleep onset, impulse control symptoms, mental disturbances, and suicidal tendencies may occur.

Amantadine has few side effects, but they can intensify when the drug is combined with other antiparkinson drugs. Orthostatic hypotension, confusion, urinary retention, and constipation are common side effects of amantadine.

Side effects from bromocriptine are more common than from amantadine. These include GI disturbances (nausea), orthostatic hypotension, palpitations, chest pain, lower extremity edema, nightmares, delusions, and confusion. If bromocriptine is taken with carbidopa-levodopa, usually the drug dosages are reduced, and side effects and drug intolerance decrease.

Pramipexole and ropinirole can cause nausea, dizziness, somnolence, weakness, and constipation. These drugs intensify the dyskinesia and hallucinations caused by levodopa. Pramipexole is also FDA approved for treatment of restless legs syndrome.

Large doses of selegiline may inhibit MAO-A. Hypertensive crisis can occur if foods high in tyramine—such as aged cheese, red wine, and bananas—are ingested concurrently.

Tolcapone may cause severe liver damage, and patients with liver dysfunction should *not* take this drug. Entacapone is not known to affect liver function. With entacapone, the urine can have a brownish orange discoloration; with tolcapone, the urine can have a dark discoloration. Both tolcapone and entacapone can intensify the adverse reactions of levodopa (e.g., hallucinations, orthostatic hypotension, constipation, dizziness) because these drugs prolong the effect of levodopa. Both tolcapone and entacapone may lead to intense, uncontrollable urges (sex, gambling, spending money) in addition to suddenly falling asleep. Patients should be warned to avoid driving and other potentially dangerous activities.

Contraindications

Anticholinergics or any drugs that have anticholinergic effects are contraindicated for patients with glaucoma. Those with severe cardiac, renal, or psychiatric health problems should avoid levodopa drugs because of adverse reactions. Patients with chronic obstructive lung diseases such as emphysema can have dry, thick mucous secretions caused by large doses of anticholinergic drugs.

Drug-Drug Interactions

Antipsychotic drugs block the receptors for dopamine. Carbidopa-levodopa taken with a monoamine oxidase inhibitor (MAOI) antidepressant can cause a hypertensive crisis.

ALZHEIMER DISEASE

Alzheimer disease is an incurable dementia illness characterized by chronic, progressive neurodegenerative conditions with marked cognitive dysfunction. Onset usually occurs between 45 and 65 years of age.

Pathophysiology

Many physiologic changes contribute to Alzheimer disease. Currently, theories related to the changes that cause Alzheimer disease include the following:

- Degeneration of the cholinergic neuron and deficiency in acetylcholine
- Neuritic plaques that form mainly outside of the neurons and in the cerebral cortex
- Apolipoprotein E_4 (apo E_4) that promotes formation of neuritic plaques, which binds beta-amyloid in the plaques
- Beta-amyloid protein accumulation in high levels that may contribute to neuronal injury
- Presence of neurofibrillary tangles with twists inside the neurons

Fig. 20.2 illustrates the normal neuron and the neuron affected by Alzheimer disease. The etiology of Alzheimer disease is unknown, although factors thought to influence the occurrence of Alzheimer disease are genetic predisposition, virus, infection, or inflammation that attacks brain cells as well as nutritional, environmental, and immunologic factors.

Alzheimer disease has three stages that include mild, moderate, and severe. The symptoms overlap stages. Generally, in the mild stage, which is the early-stage, the person has memory

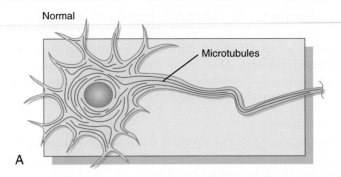

Normal — Microtubules

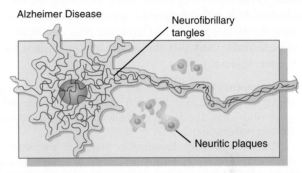

Alzheimer Disease — Neurofibrillary tangles — Neuritic plaques

FIG. 20.2 Histologic changes in Alzheimer disease. **A,** Healthy neuron. **B,** Neuron affected by Alzheimer disease shows characteristic neuritic plaques and cellular neurofibrillary tangles.

lapses, difficulty concentrating, misplaces objects, forgets what was just read, and has increased problems with planning and organizing. At this stage, the person may still drive, work, and interact socially.

The moderate stage (middle-stage) is the longest stage and may last many years. The person may be irritable, moody, withdrawn, display frustration and anger, have personality and behavioral changes (may refuse to bathe), has changes in sleep pattern, confusion regarding what day it is, inability to recall personal information (phone number and address), may wander and become lost, inability to perform routine tasks, and difficulty controlling bowels/bladder. In the severe stage the person forgets recent experiences and previously known individuals, requires high levels of assistance with activities of daily living, inability to respond to their environment or converse, inability to walk, sit, or swallow, becomes vulnerable to infections, especially pneumonia.

Acetylcholinesterase/Cholinesterase Inhibitors

The cure for Alzheimer disease is unknown. FDA-approved medications to treat Alzheimer disease symptoms include acetylcholinesterase (AChE) inhibitors. AChE is an enzyme responsible for breaking down ACh and is also known as *cholinesterase*. The AChE inhibitors are donepezil, memantine, galantamine, and rivastigmine, a drug that permits more ACh in the neuron receptors. Rivastigmine has effective penetration into the CNS, thus cholinergic transmission is increased. These AChE inhibitors increase cognitive function for patients with mild to moderate Alzheimer disease. A reversible AChE inhibitor used to treat mild to moderate Alzheimer disease is galantamine.

Several drugs for treating Alzheimer disease are under investigation. Some of these are certain nonsteroidal antiinflammatory drugs (NSAIDs; piroxicam, indomethacin), calcium channel blockers, MAO-B inhibitors (selegiline), serotonin antagonists, CNS stimulants (methylphenidate), angiotensin-converting enzyme (ACE) inhibitors, and vitamin E.

Rivastigmine

Rivastigmine, an AChE inhibitor, is prescribed to improve cognitive function for patients with mild to moderate Alzheimer disease (Prototype Drug Chart 20.2). This drug increases the amount of ACh at the cholinergic synapses. Rivastigmine tends to slow the disease process and has fewer drug interactions than donepezil. Table 20.4 lists the AChE inhibitors used to treat Alzheimer disease.

Pharmacokinetics Rivastigmine is absorbed faster through the GI tract without food. It has a relatively short half-life and is given twice a day. The dose is gradually increased. The protein-binding power is average.

Pharmacodynamics Rivastigmine has been successful in improving memory in mild to moderate Alzheimer disease. The onset of action is 0.5 to 1.0 hour for topical application; peak action is 8 to 16 hours. When given orally, the peak is 1 hour. This drug is contraindicated for patients with liver disease because hepatotoxicity may occur. Cumulative drug effect is likely to occur in older adults and in patients with liver and renal dysfunction.

📄 PROTOTYPE DRUG CHART 20.2

Rivastigmine

Drug Class	Dosage
Acetylcholinesterase inhibitor Pregnancy category: B*	A: PO: Initially: 1.5 mg bid with food; increase gradually after 2 wk to 3 mg bid; Maintenance: 3-6 mg bid; *max:* 12 mg/d Transdermal: Initially 4.6 mg/24 h; may increase after 4 wk to 9.5 mg/d; *max:* 13.3 mg/24 h

Caution	Drug-Lab-Food Interactions
Liver and renal diseases, urinary tract obstruction, orthostatic hypotension, bradycardia, asthma, COPD, seizures, peptic ulcer disease	Drug: Increased effect of theophylline, general anesthetics; TCAs decrease effect; increased effect with cimetidine; NSAIDs increase GI effects; tobacco increases clearance of rivastigmine. Lab: Increased ALT, AST

Pharmacokinetics	Pharmacodynamics
Absorption: PO: Food decreases absorption rate Distribution: PB: 40% Metabolism: t½: 1 h Excretion: In urine	PO: Onset: UK Peak: 1 h Duration: UK Transdermal: Onset: 30 min-1h Peak: 8-16 h Duration: 24 h

Therapeutic Effects/Uses
Improves memory loss in Alzheimer disease Mode of Action: Elevates acetylcholine concentration

Side Effects	Adverse Reactions
Anorexia, abdominal pain, nausea, vomiting, diarrhea, constipation, weight loss, dizziness, headache, depression, confusion, peripheral edema, dry mouth, dehydration, nystagmus	Seizures, bradycardia, orthostatic hypotension, cataracts, myocardial infarction, heart failure *Life threatening:* Hepatotoxicity, dysrhythmias, suicidal ideation, Stevens-Johnson syndrome

*Pregnancy categories have been revised. See http://www.fda.gov/Drugs/DevelopmentApprovalProcess/DevelopmentResources/Labeling/ucm093307.htm for more information.

A, Adult; *ALT*, alanine aminotransferase; *AST*, aspartate aminotransferase; *bid*, two times a day; *COPD*, chronic obstructive pulmonary disease; *d*, day; *GI*, gastrointestinal; *h*, hour; *max*, maximum; *min*, minute; *NSAID*, nonsteroidal antiinflammatory drug; *PB*, protein binding; *PO*, by mouth; *t½*, half-life; *TCA*, tricyclic antidepressant; *UK*, unknown; *wk*, weeks.

TABLE 20.4   Acetylcholinesterase Inhibitors for Alzheimer Disease

Drug	Route and Dosage	Uses and Considerations
Donepezil	A: PO: Initially 5 mg/d, may increase after 4-6 wk; maint: 5-10 mg/d; *max.* 23 mg/d	For Alzheimer disease. May cause dizziness, insomnia, headache, anorexia, nausea, diarrhea, muscle cramps, weight loss, and infection. Pregnancy category: C*; PB: 95%; t½: 70 h
Rivastigmine	See Prototype Drug Chart 20.2.	
Memantine	Immediate release: A: PO: Initially 5 mg/d, may increase dose slowly over 3 wk in 5-mg increments; *max:* 20 mg/d Extended release: A: PO: Initially 7 mg/d, increase weekly; *max.* 28 mg/d	For Alzheimer disease. May cause dizziness, headache, cough, confusion, diarrhea, and constipation. Pregnancy category: B*; PB: 45%; t½: 60-80 h
Galantamine	Immediate release: A: PO: Initially 4 mg bid with food, may increase 4 mg every 4 wk if well tolerated; maint: 12 mg bid; *max:* 24 mg/d Extended release: A: PO: Initially 8 mg/d in the morning with food; increase at 4-wk intervals; *max.* 24 mg/d	For Alzheimer disease. May cause dizziness, headache, insomnia, fatigue, anorexia, abdominal pain, nausea, vomiting, diarrhea, weight loss, and suicidal ideation. Pregnancy category: C*; PB: 18%; t½: 7 h

*Pregnancy categories have been revised. See http://www.fda.gov/Drugs/DevelopmentApprovalProcess/DevelopmentResources/Labeling/ucm093 307.htm for more information.

A, Adult; *bid*, twice a day; *d*, day; *h*, hour; *maint*, maintenance; *max*, maximum; *PB*, protein binding; *PO*, by mouth; *t½*, half-life; *wk*, week.

 NURSING PROCESS
Patient-Centered Collaborative Care

Drug Treatment for Alzheimer Disease: Rivastigmine

Assessment
- Assess the patient's mental and physical abilities. Note limitation of cognitive function and self-care.
- Obtain a history that includes any liver or renal disease or dysfunction.
- Assess for memory and judgment losses. Elicit from family members a history of behavioral changes such as memory loss, declining interest in people or home, difficulty in following through with simple activities, and a tendency to wander from home.
- Observe for signs of behavioral disturbances such as hyperactivity, hostility, and wandering.
- Examine the patient for signs of aphasia or difficulty in speech.
- Note motor function.
- Determine family members' ability to cope with the patient's mental and physical changes.

Nursing Diagnoses
- Self-Care Deficit, Feeding related to memory loss
- Self-Care Deficit, Bathing related to memory loss
- Self-Care Deficit, Toileting related to memory loss
- Confusion, Chronic related to memory loss
- Family Processes, Interrupted related to decreased cognition
- Coping, Compromised Family related to overwhelming disruption of lifestyle
- Injury, Risk for
- Nutrition, Imbalanced: Less than Body Requirements related to anorexia, nausea, and vomiting

Planning
- Patient's memory will be improved.
- Patient will maintain self-care of body functions with assistance.

Nursing Interventions
- Maintain consistency in care.
- Assist the patient in ambulation and activity.
- Monitor for side effects related to continuous use of acetylcholinesterase inhibitors.
- Record vital signs periodically. Note signs of bradycardia and hypotension.
- Observe any patient behavioral changes, and note any improvement or decline.

Patient Teaching
General
- Explain to the patient and family the purpose for the prescribed drug therapy.
- Clarify times for drug dosing and schedule for increasing drug dosing to the family member responsible for the patient's medications.
- ⚡ Teach family members about safety measures such as removing obstacles in the patient's path to avoid injury when the patient wanders.
- Inform family members of available support groups such as the Alzheimer Disease and Related Disorders Association.

Side Effects
- Inform patients and family members that the patient should rise slowly to avoid dizziness and loss of balance.
- Monitor routine liver function tests because hepatotoxicity is an adverse effect.

Diet
- Inform family members about foods that may be prepared for the patient's consumption and tolerance.

Cultural Considerations
- Recognize that various cultural groups may need guidance in understanding the Alzheimer disease process.
- Communicate respect for variant cultural beliefs and practices; help family members understand that their family member has a neurologic problem that may be part of the aging process. Explain how symptoms may become more progressive.

Evaluation
- Evaluate effectiveness of the drug regimen by determining whether the patient's mental and physical status shows improvement from drug therapy.

CRITICAL THINKING CASE STUDY

TR, a 79-year-old man, was diagnosed with Parkinson's disease 10 years ago. During his early treatment, he took selegiline. The drug dosage was increased to alleviate symptoms.

1. How does selegiline alleviate symptoms of Parkinson's disease?
2. What dietary changes should be made during the time TR takes selegiline?

Because TR developed numerous side effects and adverse reactions to selegiline, the health care provider changed the drug to carbidopa-levodopa. TR asks the nurse why the drug was changed.

3. What are the similarities and differences between selegiline and carbidopa-levodopa?
4. What are the advantages of carbidopa-levodopa?

TR's family says they know a person with Parkinson's disease who takes the antiviral drug amantadine. The family asks whether amantadine is the same as carbidopa-levodopa and, if so, whether TR can take amantadine instead of carbidopa-levodopa.

5. What is the effect of amantadine on symptoms of Parkinson's disease?
6. What would be an appropriate response to the family's question concerning the use of amantadine for TR?
7. What are the uses for dopamine agonists and COMT inhibitors?
8. Certain anticholinergic drugs may be used to control Parkinson's disease symptoms. What is the action of these drugs, and what are their side effects? These anticholinergic drugs are usually prescribed for parkinsonism symptoms resulting from what?

NCLEX STUDY QUESTIONS

1. Which of the following assessment findings could the nurse see in a patient with Parkinson's disease? (Select all that apply.)
   a. An abrupt onset of symptoms
   b. Muscle rigidity
   c. Involuntary tremors
   d. Bradykinesia
   e. Bilateral muscle weakness
2. A patient is receiving carbidopa-levodopa for Parkinson's disease. What should the nurse know about this drug?
   a. Carbidopa-levodopa may lead to hypertension.
   b. Carbidopa-levodopa may lead to excessive salivation.
   c. Dopaminergic and anticholinergic therapy may lead to drowsiness and sedation.
   d. Dopaminergics and anticholinergics are contraindicated in patients with glaucoma.
3. The nurse has initiated teaching for a family member of a patient with Alzheimer disease. The nurse realizes more teaching is needed if the family member makes which statement?
   a. As the disease gets worse, the memory loss will get worse.
   b. There are several theories about the cause of the disease.
   c. Personality changes and hostility may occur.
   d. It may take several medications to cure the disease.
4. A patient is taking rivastigmine. The nurse should teach the patient and family which information about rivastigmine?
   a. Hepatotoxicity may occur.
   b. The initial dose is 6 mg three times a day.
   c. Gastrointestinal distress is a common side effect.
   d. Weight gain may be a side effect.

5. Which is a nursing intervention for a patient taking carbidopa-levodopa for Parkinson's disease?
   a. Encourage the patient to adhere to a high-protein diet.
   b. Inform the patient that perspiration may be dark and may stain clothing.
   c. Advise the patient that glucose levels should be checked with urine testing.
   d. Warn the patient that it may take 4 to 5 days before symptoms are controlled.
6. What would the nurse teach a patient who is taking anticholinergic therapy for Parkinson's disease? (Select all that apply.)
   a. Avoid alcohol, cigarettes, and caffeine.
   b. Relieve dry mouth with hard candy or ice chips.
   c. Use sunglasses to reduce photophobia.
   d. Urinate 2 hours after taking the drug.
   e. Receive routine eye examinations.
7. A patient is taking rivastigmine to improve cognitive function. What should the nurse teach the patient/family member to do? (Select all that apply.)
   a. Rise slowly to avoid dizziness.
   b. Remove obstacles from pathways to avoid injury.
   c. Closely follow the drug dosing schedule.
   d. Have frequent checks for hypertension.
   e. Receive regular liver function tests.

Answers: 1, b, c, d; 2, d; 3, d; 4, c; 5, b; 6, a, b, c, e; 7, a, b, c.

21

Drugs for Neuromuscular Disorders and Muscle Spasms

http://evolve.elsevier.com/McCuistion/pharmacology

OBJECTIVES

- Contrast the pathophysiology of myasthenia gravis and multiple sclerosis.
- Discuss the drug group used to treat myasthenia gravis.
- Discuss the drug group used to treat multiple sclerosis.
- Differentiate between the muscle relaxants used for spasticity and those used for muscle spasms.
- Apply the nursing process to drugs used to treat myasthenia gravis and muscle spasms.

OUTLINE

KEY TERMS

Myasthenia gravis (MG) is an acquired autoimmune disease that impairs the transmission of messages at the neuromuscular junction, resulting in fluctuating muscle weakness that increases with muscle use. MG causes fatigue and muscular weakness of the respiratory system, facial muscles, and extremities. Due to cranial nerve involvement, ptosis (drooping eyelid) and difficulty in chewing and swallowing occur. Respiratory arrest may result from respiratory muscle paralysis. The symptoms of MG are caused by autoimmune destruction of acetylcholine (ACh) sites and a resultant decrease in neuromuscular transmission.

Multiple sclerosis (MS) is a neuromuscular autoimmune disorder that attacks the myelin sheath of nerve fibers, causing lesions known as *plaques*. Although there are no definitive diagnostic tests, the sclerotic plaques are usually detected and measured by magnetic resonance imaging (MRI). Pharmacologic treatment is necessary to control the symptoms of this disorder.

Muscle spasms have various causes, including injury or motor neuron disorders that are associated with conditions such as MS, MG, cerebral palsy, spinal cord injuries (paraplegia [paralysis of the legs]), cerebrovascular accident (CVA [stroke]), or hemiplegia (paralysis of one side of the body). Spasticity of muscles can be reduced with the use of skeletal muscle relaxants.

MYASTHENIA GRAVIS

MG is a chronic autoimmune neuromuscular disease that affects approximately 20 in 100,000 persons. It is estimated that 60,000 Americans are affected. MG can occur in people of any ethnicity and sex; however, MG peaks in women around the childbearing years, whereas the peak onset in men is between 50 and 70 years. MG can also occur in people outside of this age range. Although it is not a genetic disorder, a familial tendency may be apparent.

Pathophysiology

MG results from a lack of acetylcholine receptor (AChR) sites. This autoimmune disorder involves an antibody response against an alpha subunit of the AChR site at the neuromuscular junction. Antibodies attack the AChR sites, obstructing the binding of ACh and eventually destroying the receptor sites. When AChR sites are reduced, ACh molecules are prevented from binding to receptors and stimulating normal neuromuscular transmission. The result is ineffective muscle contraction and muscle weakness. About 90% of patients with MG have anti-ACh antibodies that can be detected through serum testing.

The thymus gland is involved in systemic immunity that is active during infancy and early childhood, but the gland normally shrinks during adulthood. Approximately 60% of MG patients have thymic hyperplasia. It has been suggested in some cases that if the thymus gland is removed during the early onset of MG, clinical symptoms are greatly decreased. Thymectomy has been an option for patients younger than 50 years.

MG is characterized primarily by weakness and fatigue of the skeletal muscles. In 90% of cases, eyelid or extraocular muscles are involved. The patient may experience ptosis and diplopia (double vision). Other characteristics of MG include dysphagia (difficulty chewing and swallowing), dysarthria (slurred speech), and respiratory muscle weakness.

The group of drugs used to control MG are the acetylcholinesterase (AChE) inhibitors. They inhibit the action of the enzyme AChE. As a result of this action, more ACh is available to activate the cholinergic receptors and promote muscle contraction. The AChE inhibitors are classified as parasympathomimetics.

When muscular weakness in the patient with MG becomes generalized, myasthenic crisis may occur. This complication is a severe, generalized muscle weakness that may involve the muscles of respiration, such as the diaphragm and intercostal muscles. Triggers of myasthenic crisis include inadequate dosing of AChE inhibitors, infection, emotional stress, menses, pregnancy, surgery, trauma, hypokalemia, temperature extremes, and alcohol intake. Myasthenic crisis can also occur 3 to 4 hours after taking certain medications (e.g., aminoglycoside and fluoroquinolone antibiotics, calcium channel blockers, phenytoin, and psychotropics; Box 21.1). If muscle weakness remains untreated, death could result from paralysis of the respiratory muscles. Neostigmine, a fast-acting AChE inhibitor, can relieve myasthenic crisis.

Overdosing with AChE inhibitors may cause another complication of MG called cholinergic crisis, which is an acute exacerbation of symptoms. A cholinergic crisis usually occurs within 30 to 60 minutes after taking anticholinergic drugs. This complication is due to continuous depolarization of postsynaptic membranes that creates a neuromuscular blockade. The patient with cholinergic crisis often has severe muscle weakness that can lead to respiratory paralysis and arrest. Accompanying symptoms include miosis (abnormal pupil constriction), pallor, sweating, vertigo, excess salivation, nausea, vomiting, abdominal cramping, diarrhea, bradycardia, and fasciculations (involuntary muscle twitching).

Acetylcholinesterase Inhibitors

The first drug used to manage MG is neostigmine. It is a short-acting acetylcholinesterase inhibitor with a half-life of 0.5 to 1 hour.

BOX 21.1   Medications That May Exacerbate Myasthenia Gravis

Contraindicated Medication
D-Penicillamine

Medications That Exacerbate Symptoms in Most Patients
Aminoglycosides (gentamycin, streptomycin, neomycin)
Phenytoin
Macrolides (erythromycin)
Fluoroquinolones (ciprofloxacin)
Quinine, quinidine, procainamide
Lidocaine
Magnesium salt
Psychotropic medications, (e.g., lithium carbonate, phenothiazine, benzodiazepines, tricyclic antidepressants)
Neuromuscular blocking agents, (e.g., tubocurarine chloride, pancuronium, succinylcholine)

The drug must be given on time to prevent muscle weakness. The AChE inhibitor pyridostigmine has an intermediate action and is given every 4 to 6 hours (Table 21.1). Pyridostigmine is presented in Prototype Drug Chart 21.1.

Pharmacokinetics Pyridostigmine is poorly absorbed from the gastrointestinal (GI) tract. Half of the sustained-release capsule is absorbed readily, but the balance is poorly absorbed. The half-life of oral pyridostigmine is 3 to 7 hours, and it is 2 to 3 hours for intravenous (IV) administration. Because of its short half-life, pyridostigmine must be administered several times a day. The drug is metabolized by the liver and is excreted in the urine.

Pharmacodynamics Pyridostigmine increases muscle strength in patients with muscular weakness resulting from MG. The onset of action of oral pyridostigmine is 30 to 45 minutes, the peak is 1 to 3 hours, and the duration is 3 to 4 hours. Overdosing of pyridostigmine can result in signs and symptoms of cholinergic crisis. This crisis requires emergency medical intervention because of respiratory muscle weakness.

Patients who do not respond to AChE inhibitors may require additional drug treatment such as with prednisone, plasma exchange, IV immune globulin, or immunosuppressive drugs. Prednisone is the drug of choice, but like other immunosuppressants, it reduces the presence of antibodies. Corticosteroids do not produce permanent remission, and the long-term side effects are significant.

The immunosuppressive agent azathioprine can be used in conjunction with a lower dose of prednisone. With azathioprine, the white blood cell (WBC) count and liver enzymes should be closely monitored to avoid leukopenia and hepatotoxicity.

Overdosing and underdosing of AChE inhibitors have similar symptoms: generalized muscle weakness, which can include the muscles of respiration, the diaphragm, and the intercostal muscles resulting in dyspnea (difficulty breathing), and dysphagia. Additional symptoms that may be present with overdosing are increased salivation (drooling), sweating, and bronchial secretions, along with miosis, bradycardia, and abdominal pain. All doses of AChE inhibitors should be administered *on time* because late administration of the drug could result in muscle weakness.

TABLE 21.1 Acetylcholinesterase Inhibitors for Myasthenia Gravis

Drug	Route and Dosage	Uses and Considerations
Edrophonium	A: IV 2 mg over 15-30 s; if no response, administer 8 mg; if cholinergic reaction occurs, administer 0.4-0.5 mg IV atropine. A: IM: 10 mg; if cholinergic reaction occurs, retest after 30 min with 2 mg to rule out false negative. C: <34 kg: IV: 1 mg, repeat in 45 s; if no response, give 1 mg q30-45s until response is seen; *max:* 5 mg C: >34 kg: IV: 2 mg, repeat with 1 mg if no response; *max:* 10 mg	For diagnosing MG. Will distinguish between myasthenic and cholinergic crisis. Ptosis should be absent in 1-5 min. Duration: IV: 5-10 min IM: 5-30 min Onset: Ultra–short-acting drug IV: Rapid 30-60 s IM: Rapid 2-10 min PB: UK; t½: 1.2-2 h Pregnancy category C*
Neostigmine	(The oral drug was discontinued in the United States.) A: IM/subcut: 0.5 mg/mL; 1 mg/mL; *max:* 5 mg A/C: IV: 0.03-0.07 mg/kg/d over 1 min Note: All anticholinesterase drugs should be discontinued 8 h before administration of neostigmine.	For controlling MG. Dose should be individualized to the patient. Must be given on time to prevent myasthenic crisis. Overdose can cause cholinergic reaction: nausea, abdominal cramps, excessive salivation, and sweating. Note: Large parenteral doses should be accompanied with IV atropine to counteract the side effects. PB: 15%-25%; t½: IM: 50-90 min; IV: 24-113 min Pregnancy category C*
Pyridostigmine	See Prototype Drug Chart 21.1.	
IMMUNOSUPPRESSANT		
Azathioprine (for MG poorly controlled with AChE inhibitors)	A: PO: 50 mg daily × 1 wk; gradually increase to 2-3 mg/kg/d; *max:* 250 mg/d Dosage is based on total body weight. A: IV: Used only for those who cannot tolerate PO Dose is determined by a thiopurine methyltransferase (TPMT) test which is done prior to initiation of the drug. Contrainicated in very slow metabolizers (0.3%) and lower doses in slow metabolizers (about 11%).	Onset: 6-8 wk Peak: 12 wk Duration: UK t½: UK PB: 30% Monitor: WBC, AST, and ALT Pregnancy category D*

*Pregnancy categories have been revised. See http://www.fda.gov/Drugs/DevelopmentApprovalProcess/DevelopmentResources/Labeling/ucm093307.htm for more information.
>, Greater than; <, less than; *A*, adult; *AChE*, acetylcholinesterase; *ALT*; alanine aminotransferase; *AST*; aspartate aminotransferase; *C*, child; *d*, day; *h*, hour; *IM*, intramuscular; *IV*, intravenous; *max*, maximum dosage; *MG*, myasthenia gravis; *min*, minutes; *PB*, protein binding; *PO*, by mouth; *q*, every; *s*, second; *subcut*, subcutaneous; *t½*, half-life; *UK*, unknown; *wk*, weeks; *WBC*, white blood count.

Underdosing can result in myasthenic crisis, and overdosing can result in cholinergic crisis. Edrophonium is an ultra–short-acting AChE inhibitor that may be used to distinguish between myasthenic crisis and cholinergic crisis. These two crises have a similar major symptom: severe muscle weakness. After edrophonium is administered, if the symptoms are alleviated because of an increase in ACh, the cause is myasthenic crisis. However, if the muscle weakness becomes more severe, the cause is cholinergic crisis due to drug overdosing. Edrophonium may also be used to diagnose MG. Its ultrashort duration of 5 to 30 minutes increases muscle strength immediately. If ptosis is immediately corrected after administration of this drug, the diagnosis is most likely MG.

Side Effects and Adverse Reactions

Side effects and adverse reactions of AChE inhibitors include GI disturbances (nausea, vomiting, diarrhea, abdominal cramps), increased salivation and tearing, miosis (constricted pupil of the eye), blurred vision, bradycardia, and hypotension.

NURSING PROCESS
Patient-Centered Collaborative Care

Drug Treatment for Myasthenia Gravis: Pyridostigmine

Assessment
- Obtain a drug history from the patient that includes all current medications.
- Observe the patient's drug profile for possible drug interactions.
- Patients should avoid atropine, atropine-like drugs, and muscle relaxants.
- Record baseline vital signs.
- Assess patient for signs and symptoms of myasthenic crisis, such as muscle weakness with difficulty breathing and swallowing.

Nursing Diagnoses
- Breathing Pattern, Ineffective related to weak respiratory muscles

PROTOTYPE DRUG CHART 21.1
Pyridostigmine

Drug Class	Dosage
Acetylcholinesterase (AChE) inhibitors	Myasthenia gravis: A: PO: 60 mg/d in divided doses; average dose is 600 mg/d; max PO route SR: A: PO: 180-540 mg/d or bid with at least 6 h between doses; max PO route A: IM/IV: 2 mg q2-3h C: PO: 1 mg/kg every 4-6 h; compare peak strength and activity 1 h after first dose and immediately before the next dose to individualize dose. C: IV/IM: 0.05-0.15 mg/kg; *max single dose:* 10 mg
Contraindications GI and GU obstructions, ileus, bladder obstruction *Caution:* Asthma, bradycardia, seizure disorder, peptic ulcer, cardiac arrhythmias, renal impairment, hyperthyroidism, pregnancy, breastfeeding	**Drug Interactions** Drug: Corticosteroids, neuromuscular blockers, aminoglycosides, local anesthetics, magnesium salts; increased toxicity with acetylcholinesterase inhibitors, atropine, tetracyclines, polymyxin B, bacitracin, digoxin, quinidine, and insecticides containing malathion; atropine decreases the effect of pyridostigmine.
Pharmacokinetics Absorption: PO: Poorly absorbed SR: 50% absorbed Distribution: PB: UK Metabolism: (short half-life) t½: PO, 3-7 h; IV, 2-3 h	**Pharmacodynamics** PO: Onset: 30-45 min Peak: 1-3 h; Duration: 3-4 h PO SR: Onset: 0.5-1 h Peak: UK; duration: 6-12 h IM: Onset: 15 min Peak: UK; duration: 2-4 h IV: Onset: Within minutes Peak: UK; duration: 2-3 h Pregnancy category C*
Therapeutic Effects/Uses	
Used to control and treat myasthenia gravis, for neuromuscular blockade reversal, and for nerve gas (soman) exposure prophylaxis Mode of Action: Promotes transmission of neuromuscular impulses across the myoneural junctions by preventing destruction of acetylcholine	
Side Effects	**Adverse Reactions**
Nausea, vomiting, diarrhea, headache, blurred vision, dizziness, abdominal pain, excess saliva and sweating, rash, and miosis	Hypotension, bradycardia *Life threatening:* Dyspnea, bronchospasm, respiratory distress, cardiac dysrhythmias, and seizures

*Pregnancy categories have been revised. See http://www.fda.gov/Drugs/DevelopmentApprovalProcess/DevelopmentResources/Labeling/ucm093307.htm for more information.
A, Adult; *bid*, twice a day; *C*, child; *d*, day; *GI*, gastrointestinal; *GU*, genitourinary; *h*, hour; *IM*, intramuscular; *IV*, intravenous; *max*, maximum; *min*, minute; *PB*, protein binding; *PO*, by mouth; *q*, every; *SR*, sustained release; *t½*, half-life; *UK*, unknown.

- Activity Intolerance related to fatigue
- Anxiety related to possible recurrence of myasthenic crisis and dyspnea
- Knowledge, Deficient related to unfamiliar medications

Planning
- Patient's symptoms of muscle weakness and difficulty breathing and swallowing caused by MG will be eliminated or reduced in 2 to 3 days.

Nursing Interventions
- Monitor effectiveness of drug therapy (AChE inhibitors). Muscle strength should be increased. Both depth and rate of respirations should be assessed and maintained within normal range.
- Administer prescribed acetylcholinesterase inhibitor following dosage recommendations and nursing guidelines.
- Observe patient for signs and symptoms of cholinergic crisis caused by overdosing, such as muscle weakness,

respiratory failure, increased salivation, sweating, and bronchial secretions along with miosis.
- Have an antidote for cholinergic crisis (atropine sulfate) readily available.

Patient Teaching
General
- Teach patients to take drugs as ordered to avoid recurrence of symptoms.
- Encourage patients to wear a medical identification bracelet or necklace that indicates health problems.

Side Effects
- Teach patients about the side effects of medication and when to notify the health care provider.
- Advise patients to report recurrence of symptoms of MG to the health care provider.

Diet
- Inform patients to take the drug before meals for best absorption. If gastric irritation occurs, take the drug with food.

- Involve family members in teaching about prescriptive therapies and disease processes using simple and clear instructions.
- Communicate respect for the patient's cultural beliefs.
- Accommodate cultural values and assess the patient's understanding of adhering to the drug regimen. Instruct the patient to notify the health care provider prior to taking any medications other than what the provider has ordered.
- Stress that medications need to be taken as prescribed. Medications are ordered specifically for each ailment. Unused drugs should be discarded, and use of medication by individuals other than the intended patient can have serious consequences.

Evaluation

- Evaluate effectiveness of the drug therapy to maintain muscle strength.
- Determine the absence of respiratory distress.
- Evaluate the correct use of the drug by the patient.

MULTIPLE SCLEROSIS

Multiple sclerosis (MS) is an autoimmune disorder that attacks the myelin sheath of nerve fibers in the brain and spinal cord, which results in lesions called *plaques*. In the United States, MS affects approximately 400,000 persons aged 20 to 40 years, and most are Caucasian women. It is uncommon in African and Asian populations.

Although the cause of MS is unknown, it is thought that the disease develops in a genetically susceptible person as a result of environmental exposure, like an infection. The onset of MS is usually slow. It is a condition in which there are remissions and exacerbations of multiple symptoms. Common manifestations of MS are motor, sensory, neurologic, cerebellar, and emotional problems. Motor symptoms include weakness or paralysis of the limbs, muscle spasticity, and diplopia. Patients with MS experience sensory abnormalities, including numbness and tingling, blurred vision, vertigo, and tinnitus. Patients may experience neuropathic pain particularly in the low thoracic and abdominal areas. Cerebellar signs include nystagmus, ataxia, dysarthria, and dysphagia. Many patients experience severe fatigue. If the sclerotic plaque is located in the central nervous system (CNS), problems with bowel and bladder function and sexual and cognitive dysfunction can occur.

MS is difficult to diagnose. Most physicians use at least one other test besides the medical history and neurologic exam, such as MRI, visual evoked potential (VEP) testing, or analysis of cerebrospinal fluid (CSF), to confirm the diagnosis (see www.multiplesclerosis.net).

Four Classifications of Multiple Sclerosis

MS is classified into four primary patterns for treatment purposes:
- *Relapsing remitting MS (RRMS):* The patient experiences relapse with full recovery and residual deficit on recovery (affects 85%).

- *Primary progressive MS (PPMS):* Slowly worsening neurologic function is evident from the beginning with no relapses or remissions (affects 10%).
- *Secondary progressive MS (SPMS):* The initial course is relapsing remitting, followed by progression with or without occasional relapses, minor remissions, and plateaus (about 50% of people with RRMS develop SPMS within 10 years).
- *Progressive relapsing MS (PRMS):* This form is progressive from the onset, with clear acute relapses with or without full recovery (affects 5%).

There is no known cure for MS.

Immunomodulators

Immunomodulators are disease-modifying drugs (DMDs), also called *disease-modifying therapies* (DMTs), and they are the first line of treatment for patients with MS. DMDs can slow the progression of the disease and prevent relapses.

Immunomodulators include interferon beta-1a and interferon beta-1b (Prototype Drug Chart 21.2), which are popular drugs in the treatment of MS. Beta-1b and glatiramer acetate are administered subcutaneously either once daily or three times a week depending on the health care provider's orders. Teriflunomide is an oral drug that is administered daily. Alemtuzumab is a monoclonal antibody that requires a daily IV dose of 12 mg for 5 consecutive days, and in 12 months, an additional 12-mg dose for 3 consecutive days. It targets the part of the immune system that is thought to be harming people with MS. No two cases of MS are alike, so the drugs are tailored to the disease pattern and manifestations of the patient. See Table 21.2 for medications used in the treatment of MS.

Corticosteroids are used to manage exacerbations of MS. They work by reducing edema and acute inflammation at the site of demyelination.

SKELETAL MUSCLE RELAXANTS

Muscle relaxants relieve muscular spasms and pain associated with traumatic injuries and spasticity from chronic debilitating disorders (e.g., MS, stroke [CVA], cerebral palsy, head and spinal cord injuries). Spasticity results from increased muscle tone from hyperexcitable neurons; this is caused by increased stimulation from the cerebral neurons or lack of inhibition in the spinal cord or at the skeletal muscles. The centrally acting muscle relaxants depress neuron activity in the spinal cord or brain, or they enhance neuronal inhibition on the skeletal muscles.

Centrally Acting Muscle Relaxants

The mechanism of action of centrally acting muscle relaxants is not fully known. Centrally acting muscle relaxants are used in cases of spasticity to suppress hyperactive reflex and for muscle spasms that do not respond to antiinflammatory agents, physical therapy, or other forms of therapy. Table 21.3 presents centrally acting muscle relaxants, and Prototype Drug Chart 21.3 gives the drug data for the centrally acting muscle relaxant cyclobenzaprine.

📄 PROTOTYPE DRUG CHART 21.2

Beta-Interferon

Drug Class	Dosage
Immunomodulators: Interferon beta-1a Interferon beta-1b	*Beta-1a:* A: IM: 30 mcg once/wk A: Subcut: 22 or 44 mcg 3 × wk; give doses at least 48 h apart. *Beta-1b:* A: Subcut: 0.0625 mg every other day; increase by 0.0625 mg q2wk over a 6-wk period up to target of 0.25 mg every other day

Contraindications	Drug Interactions
Albumin hypersensitivity, hamster protein hypersensitivity	Antiretroviral NNRTIs; antiretroviral NRTIs; antiretroviral protease inhibitors; ethanol

Pharmacokinetics	Pharmacodynamics
Absorption: UK Distribution: UK Metabolism: t½: IM, 19 h; subcut: 69 h Excretion: UK Pregnancy category C*	Interferon beta-1a IM/Subcut: Onset: UK Peak 3-15 h; duration: UK Interferon beta-1b Subcut: Onset: Rapid Peak 16 h; duration: UK

Therapeutic Effects/Uses
Interferon beta-1a has been shown to decrease both the number and severity of MS attacks (e.g., relapses) and to significantly slow the progression of physical disability associated with relapsing remitting MS. Mode of Action: Antiviral and immune-regulatory properties are produced by interacting with specific receptor sites on cell surfaces. It is not exactly known how interferon works to treat MS. Beta-interferon is produced by recombinant DNA technology.

Side Effects	Adverse Reactions
Depression, dizziness, fatigue, suicidal ideation, vision problems, dyspnea, chest pain, edema, abdominal pain, autoimmune hepatitis, cystitis, neutropenia, injection site reaction, myalgia, arthralgia, muscle spasm, anaphylaxis, flulike symptoms	Increased myelosuppression may occur with other myelosuppressives including antineoplastics; concurrent use of hepatotoxic agents may increase risk of hepatotoxicity. Avoid concomitant use with immunomodulating natural products such as astragalus, echinacea, and melatonin.

*Pregnancy categories have been revised. See http://www.fda.gov/Drugs/DevelopmentApprovalProcess/DevelopmentResources/Labeling/ucm093307.htm for more information.
A, adult; *h*, hours; *IM*, intramuscular; *MS*, multiple sclerosis; *NNRTI*, nonnucleoside reverse transcriptase inhibitor; *NRTI*, nucleoside reverse transcriptase inhibitor; *q*, every; *subcut*, subcutaneous; *t½*, half-life; *UK*, unknown; *wk*, weeks.

Spasticity

Skeletal muscle spasticity is muscular hyperactivity that causes contraction of the muscles, resulting in pain and limited mobility. Centrally acting muscle relaxants act on the spinal cord. Examples of centrally acting muscle relaxants used to treat spasticity are baclofen, dantrolene, and tizanidine. Diazepam, a benzodiazepine, has also been effective for treating spasticity (Complementary and Alternative Therapies 21.1).

🌿 COMPLEMENTARY AND ALTERNATIVE THERAPIES 21.1

Diazepam

Kava and valerian may potentiate central nervous system depression.

⚡ PATIENT SAFETY

Do not confuse...

- **Baclofen,** a skeletal muscle relaxant, with **Bactroban,** a topical antibacterial, or **Beclovent,** a corticosteroid inhalant.

Muscle Spasms

Various centrally acting muscle relaxants are used for muscle spasm to decrease pain and increase range of motion. They have a sedative effect and should not be taken concurrently with CNS depressants such as barbiturates, narcotics, and alcohol. These agents, with the exception of cyclobenzaprine, can cause drug dependence. In addition, dizziness and drowsiness are common side effects. Examples of this group of centrally acting muscle relaxants are carisoprodol, chlorzoxazone, cyclobenzaprine, metaxalone, methocarbamol, and orphenadrine citrate (see Table 21.3).

Pharmacokinetics Cyclobenzaprine is well absorbed from the GI tract, and its half-life is moderate. Cyclobenzaprine is metabolized in the liver and excreted in urine (see Prototype Drug Chart 21.3).

Pharmacodynamics Cyclobenzaprine alleviates muscle spasm associated with acute painful musculoskeletal conditions. When cyclobenzaprine is taken with alcohol, kava, valerian, sedative-hypnotics, barbiturates, or tricyclic antidepressants (TCAs), increased CNS depression occurs. The onset of action, peak concentration time, and duration of action for cyclobenzaprine are short.

TABLE 21.2   Drugs for Multiple Sclerosis

Drugs	Route and Dosage	Uses and Considerations
IMMUNOMODULATORS		
Beta-Interferon Interferon beta-1a Interferon beta-1b	See Prototype Drug Chart 21.2.	
Glatiramer acetate	A: Subcut: 20 mg/mL once daily Subcut: 40 mg/mL 3 × wk	Treatment of relapsing remitting MS Distribution: Enters lymphatic and systemic circulation Onset/Peak/Duration: UK PB: UK; t½: UK Pregnancy category B*
Teriflunomide	A: PO: 7-14 mg once daily	Treatment of relapsing remitting MS Absorption: Well absorbed Distribution: UK PB: >99%; t½: 18-19 d Pregnancy category X*
IMMUNOSUPPRESSANTS		
Mitoxantrone	A: IV: 12 mg/m² q3mo	Treatment of secondary (chronic) progressive, progressive relapsing, or worsening relapsing remitting MS Absorption: Complete bioavailability Distribution: Widely distributed PB: UK; t½: 5-8 d Pregnancy category D*
Dimethyl fumarate	A: PO: 120 mg bid for 1 wk, then 240 mg bid	Treatment of relapsing forms of MS Absorption: Converted to active metabolite (MMF) by enzymes in the GI tract, blood, and tissue Distribution: UK PB: MMF 27%-45%; t½: MMF 1 h Pregnancy category C*
SPHINGOSINE 1–PHOSPHATE RECEPTOR MODULATORS		
Fingolimod	A: PO: 0.5 mg once daily	Treatment of relapsing forms of MS Absorption: 93% following oral administration Distribution: 86% of drug into RBCs PB: >99.7%; t½: 6-9 h Pregnancy category C*
MONOCLONAL ANTIBODY		
Alemtuzumab	A: IV: 12 mg/1.2 mL on 5 consecutive days (total dose of 60 mg) for first treatment course; follow 12 mo later with 12 mg IV for 3 consecutive days (total dose of 36 mg) for second treatment.	Onset: UK Peak: UK PB: UK; t½: 12 d Pregnancy category C*
Natalizumab	A: IV: 300 mg q4wk	Treatment to reduce frequency of exacerbations of relapsing MS Absorption: Complete bioavailability when given by IV route Distribution: UK PB: 99.7%; t½: 7-15 d Pregnancy category C*

*Pregnancy categories have been revised. See http://www.fda.gov/Drugs/DevelopmentApprovalProcess/DevelopmentResources/Labeling/ucm093307.htm for more information.
>, Greater than; *A*, adult; *bid*, twice daily; *d*, day; *GI*, gastrointestinal; *h*, hour; *IV*, intravenous; *MMF*, metabolite monomethyl fumarate; *mo*, months; *MS*, multiple sclerosis; *PB*, protein binding; *PO*, by mouth; *q*, every; *RBC*, red blood cell; *subcut*, subcutaneous; *t½*, half-life; *UK*, unknown; *wk*, weeks.

Side Effects and Adverse Reactions

The side effects from centrally acting muscle relaxants include drowsiness, dizziness, lightheadedness, headaches, and occasional GI sensitivity (e.g., nausea, vomiting, abdominal distress). Cyclobenzaprine and orphenadrine have anticholinergic effects (Complementary and Alternative Therapies 21.2).

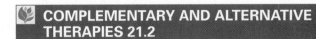

COMPLEMENTARY AND ALTERNATIVE THERAPIES 21.2

Orphenadrine Citrate

Valerian and kava kava potentiate sedation.

TABLE 21.3   Muscle Relaxants

Drugs	Route and Dosage	Uses and Considerations
ANXIOLYTICS		
Diazepam (CSS C-IV controlled substance; a long-acting benzodiazepam)	A: PO: 2 to 10 mg bid/qid Older adults: PO: 2 to 2.5 mg qd/bid A: IV/IM 2-10 mg, may repeat in 3-4 h C >6 mo: PO: 1 to 2.5 mg tid/qid Seizures: C: IM/IV: 0.05-0.3 mg/kg over 3-5 min q15-30min C >5 y: Max 10 mg q2-4h C <5 y: Max 5 mg q2-4h	Diazepam has many uses, one of which is to relieve muscle spasms associated with paraplegia, MS, MG, and cerebral palsy. It is also used for status epilepticus and acute seizure activity. Contraindication: Narrow-angle glaucoma PB: 98%; t½: A: 20 to 50 h (up to 100 h for metabolites) Pregnancy category D*
MUSCLE RELAXANTS		
Centrally Acting Muscle Relaxants (for Spasticity)		
Baclofen	A: PO: Initially 5 mg tid; increase gradually by 5 mg q3d; *max:* 80 mg/d divided over 4 doses	For muscle spasms caused by MS and spinal cord injury. Overdose may cause CNS depression. Drowsiness, dizziness, nausea, and hypotension may occur. PB: 30%; t½: 2.5 to 4 h; Pregnancy category C*
Tizanidine	A: PO: 4 mg q6-8h PRN; *max:* 36 mg/d	To manage spasticity, especially for spinal cord injury and MS. PB: 30%; t½: 2.5 h Pregnancy category C*
Spasticity (Direct Acting)		
Dantrolene sodium	A: PO: Initially 25 mg/d; increase gradually; *maint:* 100 mg bid/qid C >5 y: PO: Initially 0.5 mg/kg/d; increase dose gradually by 0.5 mg/kg tid/qid/d; *max:* 100 mg qid	For chronic neurologic disorders that cause spasms: SCI, cerebral palsy, stroke, and MS. Start with low doses (25 mg/d) and increase q4-7d. Avoid taking with alcohol or CNS depressants. PB: 95%; t½: 8 h Max dose depends on route of administration and indication. Pregnancy category C*
Centrally Acting Muscle Relaxants		
Carisoprodol	A: PO: 250-350 mg qid/daily	For relaxation of skeletal muscles. Has CNS depressant effects. Avoid taking with alcohol or CNS depressants. Should only be used on a short-term basis (2 to 3 wk). PB: UK; t½: 8 h; Pregnancy category C*; increased risk for addiction
Chlorzoxazone	A: PO: 250 to 500 mg tid/qid; *max:* 3 g/d	For relief of acute or severe muscle spasms. Not effective for cerebral palsy. Take with food to decrease GI upset. PB: UK; t½: 1.1 h; Pregnancy category C*
Methocarbamol	A: PO: Initially 1.5 g qid for 2-3/d; *maint:* 4 to 4.5 g/d in 3 to 6 divided doses; *max:* 8 g/d A: IM/IV 1-3 g/d q8h up to 3 d; repeat course after a 48-h rest.	For relief of acute muscle spasms; used for treatment of tetanus. Has CNS depressant effects (sedation). Avoid taking with alcohol or CNS depressants. Urine may turn green, brown, or black. Drowsiness may occur but usually decreases with continued drug use. PB: UK; t½: 1 to 2 h; Pregnancy category C*
Metaxalone	A: PO: Initially 400-800 mg tid/qid; *max:* 3200 mg/d	Relief of acute painful muscle spasticity PB: UK; t½: 2-3 h; Pregnancy category UK*
Orphenadrine	A: PO: 100 mg bid; *max:* 200 mg/d A: IM/IV: 60 mg q12h; *max:* 120 mg/d	For relief of acute muscle spasm. Can be toxic with a mild overdose. Used in combination with aspirin and caffeine. Contraindication: MG PB: <20%; t½: 14 h; Pregnancy category C*
Depolarizing Skeletal Muscle Relaxant (Adjunct to Anesthesia)		
Succinylcholine	A: IV: 0.3-1.1 mg/kg over 10-30 s Short procedure: 1 mg/kg max Long procedure: 10 mg/min max	Used for surgical skeletal muscle relaxation and in endoscopy and intubation PB: UK; t½: UK; Pregnancy category C*
Nondepolarizing Skeletal Muscle Relaxants (Adjunct to Anesthesia) **Neuromuscular blocking agent**		
🚫 Pancuronium bromide	A/C >1 mo: IV: 0.04-0.1 mg/kg; then 0.01 mg/kg at 30- to 60-min intervals	Used in surgery for relaxation of skeletal muscle (e.g., abdominal wall). Does not cause hypotension. May cause respiratory depression. Assess cardio and respiratory status constantly. PB: 30%-87%; t½: 2 h; Pregnancy category C*

TABLE 21.3   Muscle Relaxants—cont'd

Drugs	Route and Dosage	Uses and Considerations
Vecuronium bromide ⊘ Must be administered only by qualified clinicians	A/C >10 y: IV: 0.08-0.1 mg/kg initially, then after 25-40 min, give 0.01-0.15 mg/kg q12-15min or as a continuous infusion 0.001 mg/kg/min	For surgical skeletal muscle relaxation. Can be used for patients with asthma, renal disease, or limited cardiac reserve. Given after general anesthesia has been started. PB: 60%-90%; t½: 30-80 min Pregnancy category C*

*Pregnancy categories have been revised. See http://www.fda.gov/Drugs/DevelopmentApprovalProcess/DevelopmentResources/Labeling/ucm093307.htm for more information.
>, Greater than; <, less than; A, adult; bid, twice a day; C, child; cardio, cardiovascular; CNS, central nervous system; CSS, Controlled Substances Schedule; d, day; GI, gastrointestinal; h, hour; IM, intramuscular; IV, intravenous; maint, maintenance; max, maximum; MG, myasthenia gravis; min, minutes; mo, months; MS, multiple sclerosis; PB, protein binding; PO, by mouth; PRN, as needed; q, every; qid, four times a day; s, seconds; SCI, spinal cord injury; t½, half-life; tid, three times a day; UK, unknown; wk, weeks; y, year.

PROTOTYPE DRUG CHART 21.3

Cyclobenzaprine

Drug Class	Dosage
Centrally acting muscle relaxants	A: PO: 5-10 mg tid; max: 30 mg/d tid; treatment beyond 2-3 wk is not recommended. A: PO: ER cap 15 mg/d; max: 30 mg/d

Contraindications	Drug-Lab-Food Interactions
AV block, acute MI, bradycardia, bundle-branch block, cardiac arrhythmias, children, cerebral palsy, diabetes mellitus, heart failure, hyperthyroidism, hypertension, hypokalemia, paralytic ileus, concurrent use of MAOI therapy, QT prolongation, SCI Caution: Seizure disorder, alcohol, CNS depressants, glaucoma, prostatic hypertrophy, urinary retention, hepatic disease, breastfeeding, driving or operating machinery, morbidity in geriatric patients, sunlight UV exposure	Drug: Increased CNS depression with alcohol, kava (Piper methysticum), valerian, barbiturates, TCAs, and other CNS depressants. Check resource book for multiple interactions. Take with food or milk to decrease GI upset.

Pharmacokinetics	Pharmacodynamics
Absorption: PO: Well absorbed Distribution: PB: 93% Metabolism: t½: 1-3 days Excretion: In urine	PO: Onset: 1 h Peak: 3-8 h Duration: 12-24 h Pregnancy category B*; PB: 93%

Therapeutic Effects/Uses
For short-term treatment of muscle spasms Mode of Action: Relieves muscle spasms through a central action, possibly at the brainstem level

Side Effects	Adverse Reactions
Anticholinergic effects (blurred vision, constipation, dry mouth, tachycardia, urinary retention); arrhythmias, confusion, drowsiness, dizziness, headache, nausea, nervousness, unpleasant taste, urinary retention	Allergic reactions, angioedema, MI, seizures, ileus

*Pregnancy categories have been revised. See http://www.fda.gov/Drugs/DevelopmentApprovalProcess/DevelopmentResources/Labeling/ucm093307.htm for more information.
A, Adult; AV, atrioventricular; cap, capsule; CNS, central nervous system; d, day; ER, extended release; GI, gastrointestinal; h, hour; MAOI, monoamine oxidase inhibitor; max, maximum; MI, myocardial infarction; PB, protein binding; PO, by mouth; SCI, spinal cord injury; t½, half-life; TCA, tricyclic antidepressant; tid, three times a day; UV, ultraviolet; wk, week.

NURSING PROCESS

Patient-Centered Collaborative Care

Muscle Relaxant: Cyclobenzaprine

Assessment

- Obtain a medical history. Cyclobenzaprine is contraindicated if the patient has cardiovascular disorders, hyperthyroidism, or hepatic impairment or is taking concurrent monoamine oxidase inhibitors (MAOIs).
- Obtain baseline vital signs.
- Assess the patient's health history to identify the cause of muscle spasm and determine whether it is acute or chronic.

- Observe the patient's drug history for possible drug interactions.
- Note whether the patient has a history of narrow-angle glaucoma or MG. Cyclobenzaprine and orphenadrine are contraindicated with these health problems.

Nursing Diagnoses

- Physical Mobility, Impaired related to dizziness and hyperactive reflexes
- Activity Intolerance related to drowsiness and hyperactive reflexes

Planning

- The patient will be free of muscular pain within 1 week.

Nursing Interventions

- Monitor serum liver enzyme levels of patients taking dantrolene and carisoprodol. Report to the health care provider elevated levels of liver enzymes such as alkaline phosphatase (ALP), aspartate aminotransferase (AST), alanine aminotransferase (ALT), and gamma-glutamyl transferase (GGT).
- Record vital signs. Report abnormal results.
- Observe for CNS side effects (e.g., dizziness).

Patient Teaching
General

- Teach patients that the muscle relaxant should not be abruptly stopped. The drug should be tapered over 1 week to avoid rebound spasms.
- Advise patients not to drive, operate dangerous machinery, or make important life-changing decisions when taking muscle relaxants. These drugs have a sedative effect and can cause drowsiness.
- Inform patients that most of the centrally acting muscle relaxants for acute spasms are usually taken for no longer than 3 weeks.
- Teach patients to avoid alcohol and CNS depressants. If muscle relaxants are taken with these drugs, CNS depression may be intensified.

- Advise patients that these drugs must be used cautiously when pregnant or nursing.
- Patients should always check with the health care provider prior to stopping medications.

Side Effects
- Encourage patients to report side effects of the muscle relaxant: nausea, vomiting, dizziness, fainting, headache, and diplopia can occur. Dizziness and fainting are most likely caused by orthostatic (postural) hypotension.

Diet
- Advise patients to take muscle relaxants with food to decrease GI upset.

Cultural Considerations
- Use both hands to show respect when offering a prescription, instructions, or pamphlets to Asians and Pacific Islanders.
- Demonstrate respect by addressing patients formally until told otherwise, and do not ask private questions in public.

Evaluation
- Evaluate the effectiveness of the muscle relaxant, and determine whether the patient's muscular pain or spasms have decreased or disappeared.

CRITICAL THINKING CASE STUDY

FR, a 29-year-old woman, was diagnosed with myasthenia gravis (MG) 2 years ago. She is receiving pyridostigmine 120 mg three times daily. Last evening, FR was involved in an automobile accident. She was taken to the emergency department unconscious and missed two evening doses of pyridostigmine.

1. How does pyridostigmine alleviate the symptoms of MG?
2. What are the potential side effects and adverse effects of pyridostigmine?
3. What problems are likely to develop following delayed pyridostigmine dosing?

FR is scheduled for surgery to repair a fractured right femur suffered in the accident. During surgery, FR develops bradycardia.

4. What medications may lead to drug interactions with pyridostigmine?
5. What problems may develop from pyridostigmine overdosing?
6. What are the similarities between myasthenic crisis and cholinergic crisis?

NCLEX STUDY QUESTIONS

1. When the nurse explains the pathophysiology of myasthenia gravis to a patient, which is the best explanation?
   a. Degeneration of cholinergic neurons and a deficit in acetylcholine lead to neuritic plaques and neurofibrillary tangles.
   b. A decreased amount of acetylcholine to cholinergic receptors produces weak muscles and reduced nerve impulses.
   c. Myelin sheaths of nerve fibers in the brain and spinal cord develop lesions or plaques.
   d. An imbalance of dopamine and acetylcholine leads to degeneration of neurons in midbrain and extrapyramidal motor tracts.

2. The nurse is teaching a patient recently diagnosed with multiple sclerosis about the disease. Which statement is *not* correct concerning multiple sclerosis?
   a. The disease has periods of exacerbations and remissions.
   b. Goals of treatment are to decrease the inflammation in the nervous system.
   c. Patients experience muscle weakness, vision problems, and fatigue.
   d. Multiple sclerosis is an autoimmune disorder that causes plaque to develop in the spinal cord.

3. A patient has spasticity following a spinal cord injury. The nurse anticipates that which drug will be prescribed to treat the patient's spasticity?
   a. Neostigmine
   b. Ropinirole
   c. Cyclobenzaprine
   d. Pyridostigmine

4. The nurse anticipates that the health care provider will prescribe which medication to treat a patient with relapsing remitting multiple sclerosis?
   a. Ambenonium
   b. Pyridostigmine
   c. Mitoxantrone
   d. Glatiramer acetate

5. The nurse is providing medication instructions to a patient with acute muscle spasms who has been prescribed cyclobenzaprine. Which statement indicates to the nurse that the patient understands the instructions?
   a. I plan to take this medication with a glass of milk.
   b. Cyclobenzaprine should be taken once daily at bedtime.
   c. I will only drink one glass of wine per day.
   d. I will be able to take this drug with grapefruit juice.

6. Which instructions will the nurse include in the teaching plan for a patient who is taking pyridostigmine? (Select all that apply.)
   a. Pyridostigmine must be taken on time.
   b. Take the prescribed dose every other week.
   c. Underdosing can result in myasthenic crisis.
   d. Overdosing can result in cholinergic crisis.
   e. Report the adverse effect of tachycardia to the health care provider.

7. A patient is beginning to take cyclobenzaprine for treatment of acute back spasms. Which interventions will the nurse include in the care of this patient? (Select all that apply.)
   a. Advise the patient to take this drug on an empty stomach.
   b. Inform the patient not to abruptly stop taking the muscle relaxant. The dose should be tapered down.
   c. Tell the patient to report dizziness and double vision to the health care provider.
   d. Advise the patient to avoid alcohol.
   e. Taking narcotics at the same time can cause serious side effects.

8. The nurse is reviewing a patient's medication history for a patient who has just been prescribed cyclobenzaprine for treatment of back spasms. The nurse plans to contact the health care provider if the patient is taking which of these?
   a. Atorvastatin
   b. Conjugated estrogen
   c. Valerian
   d. Penicillin G procaine

9. The nurse is caring for a patient who has been diagnosed with myasthenia gravis. The patient is experiencing muscle weakness, dyspnea, bradycardia, and diaphoresis. The nurse anticipates that the health care provider will order which medication to distinguish between myasthenic crisis and cholinergic crisis?
   a. Adrenocorticotropic hormone
   b. Diazepam
   c. Edrophonium
   d. Mitoxantrone

Answers: 1, b; 2, b; 3, c; 4, d; 5, a; 6, a, c, d; 7, b, c, d, e; 8, c; 9, c.

Mental and Behavioral Health Drugs

From moods and emotions flow the various thoughts and actions of individuals, which are communicated throughout the central nervous system (CNS) by chemical neurotransmitters. An impulse is communicated by traveling through the presynaptic neuron across the synaptic cleft and binding to a receptor on the postsynaptic neuron, as illustrated in Fig. VI.I.

Neurotransmitters are synthesized in the cytoplasm in the presynaptic neuron and are stored in vesicles, which safeguard neurotransmitters from being destroyed by enzymes. When an impulse arrives by way of an action potential at a presynaptic neuron, vesicles are triggered to move to the cell membrane wall and release the transmitter into the synaptic cleft.

Neurotransmitters function with the help of receptors, which are embedded in the membrane of the postsynaptic neuron. Receptors are configured in size and shape to interlock with specific transmitters. Immediately upon connection of neurotransmitters to receptors, an action is exerted and the transmitter is removed. Once released, transmitters can be broken down into inactive substances by enzymes, diffused away from the synapse into intracellular fluid, or returned to the presynaptic neuron in a process called *reuptake*.

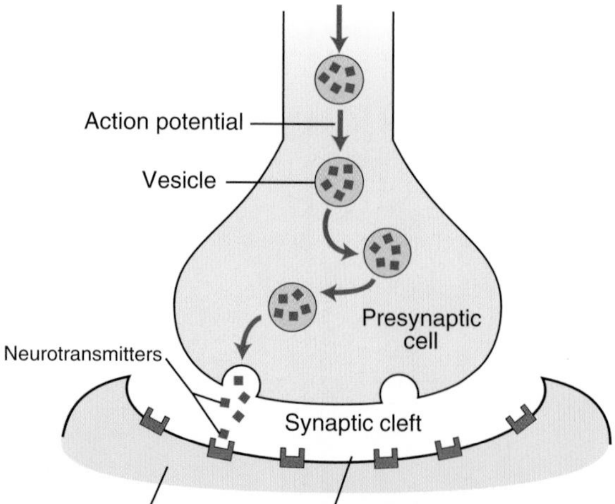

The major neurotransmitters that affect psychopathology include gamma-aminobutyric acid (GABA), serotonin, dopamine, norepinephrine, and acetylcholine. The GABA neurotransmitter is associated with the regulation of anxiety. When the level of GABA neurotransmitters is reduced, anxiety disorders may result. Benzodiazepines (antianxiety drugs) act by binding to a GABA receptor site, making the postsynaptic receptor more sensitive to GABA and its neurotransmission. This connection decreases the signs and symptoms of anxiety.

Serotonin neurotransmission is associated with arousal and general activity levels of the CNS. Serotonin functions to regulate sleep, wakefulness, and mood as well as the delusions, hallucinations, and withdrawal of schizophrenia. Antidepressants block the reuptake of serotonin into the presynaptic neuron. A structurally specific drug is more likely to affect only the specific receptors for which it is intended and not the receptors specific for other neurochemicals, which would produce unintended effects. Selective serotonin reuptake inhibitor (SSRI) drugs are specific and generally produce fewer side effects in the treatment of depression than older antidepressants such as monoamine oxidase inhibitors (MAOIs).

Dopamine-containing neurons are thought to be involved in the regulation of cognition, emotional responses, and motivation, and dopamine neurotransmitters are associated with schizophrenia and other psychoses. Antipsychotic drugs block dopamine receptors in the postsynaptic neuron.

Norepinephrine is associated with control of arousal, attention, vigilance, mood, affect, and anxiety. This neurotransmitter is involved with thinking, planning, and interpreting. Tricyclic antidepressants (TCAs) block the reuptake of norepinephrine into the presynaptic neuron and effectively treat depressive disorders. MAOIs inactivate norepinephrine, dopamine, and serotonin by inhibiting the monoamine oxidase enzyme to relieve signs and symptoms of depression.

FIG. VI.I Chemical Neurotransmitters.

Action potential
Vesicle
Neurotransmitters
Presynaptic cell
Synaptic cleft
Postsynaptic neuron   Stimulus (gated Na⁺ channel)

Faulty release, reuptake, or elimination of neurotransmitters may lead to an imbalance of neurotransmission and subsequent pathology. Disorders can then develop that can affect an individual's thoughts, feelings, and behaviors.

Knowledge of psychopharmacology is essential to psychiatric mental health nursing. A basic understanding of the actions of psychotropic drugs will help nurses rapidly comprehend and apply information and enhance the effectiveness of pharmacologic treatment. Essential responsibilities of the nurse administering psychotropic medications are to assess behavior, monitor for side effects, and educate the patient and family. These actions are crucial to successful psychopharmacologic therapy.

Drugs used to treat psychoses and anxiety are discussed in Chapter 22. Antidepressants and mood stabilizers are discussed in Chapter 23.

Antipsychotics and Anxiolytics

ⓔ http://evolve.elsevier.com/McCuistion/pharmacology

OBJECTIVES

- Differentiate between antipsychotic and anxiolytic drug groups.
- Contrast the action, uses, side effects, and adverse effects of traditional typical and atypical antipsychotics.

- Plan nursing interventions, including patient teaching, for the patient taking antipsychotics and anxiolytics.
- Apply the nursing process to the patient taking an atypical antipsychotic, a typical antipsychotic, and an anxiolytic.

OUTLINE

Psychosis
Antipsychotic Agents
  Pharmacophysiologic Mechanisms of Action
  Adverse Reactions
  Phenothiazines
  Nonphenothiazines
  Antipsychotic Dosage for Older Adults
  Atypical Antipsychotics (Serotonin/Dopamine Antagonists)
  Nursing Process: Patient-Centered Collaborative
    Care—Phenothiazines and Nonphenothiazines

Anxiolytics
  Nonpharmacologic Measures
  Benzodiazepines
  Miscellaneous Anxiolytics
  Nursing Process: Patient-Centered Collaborative
    Care—Benzodiazepines
Critical Thinking Case Study
NCLEX Study Questions

KEY TERMS

Central nervous system (CNS) depressants used to manage symptoms of psychosis and anxiety disorders include antipsychotics and anxiolytics, which may cause psychosis. Antipsychotics are also known as *neuroleptics* or *psychotropics,* but the preferred name for this group is either *antipsychotics* or *neuroleptics.* The term neuroleptic refers to any drug that modifies psychotic behavior and exerts an antipsychotic effect. Anxiolytics are also called *antianxiety drugs* or *sedative-hypnotics.* Certain anxiolytics are used to treat sleep disorders, seizures, and withdrawal symptoms from alcohol or other abuse substances. Some of these drugs are also used for conscious sedation and anesthesia supplementation. However, the anxiolytics described in this chapter are used specifically to treat anxiety and psychotic behaviors.

PSYCHOSIS

Psychosis, or loss of contact with reality, is manifested in a variety of mental or psychiatric disorders. Psychosis is usually characterized by more than one symptom, such as difficulty in processing information, disorganized thoughts, distortion of reality, delusions, hallucinations, incoherence, catatonia, and aggressive or violent behavior. Schizophrenia, a chronic psychotic disorder, is the major category of psychosis in which many of these symptoms are manifested.

The symptoms of schizophrenia usually develop in adolescence or early adulthood and are divided into three groups: (1) cognitive symptoms, (2) positive symptoms, and (3) negative symptoms. *Cognitive symptoms* are characterized by disorganized thinking, memory difficulty, and decreased ability to focus attention. *Positive symptoms* may be characterized by exaggeration of normal function (e.g., agitation), incoherent speech, hallucinations, delusions, and paranoia. *Negative symptoms* are characterized by a decrease or loss in function and motivation. A poverty or simplicity of speech, blunted affect, inertia, poor self-care, and social withdrawal are apparent. Negative symptoms tend to be more chronic and persistent. The typical, conventional, or traditional group of antipsychotics (first-generation antipsychotics) is more helpful for managing positive symptoms. A group of antipsychotics called *atypical* (second-generation antipsychotics) has been found to be the newest treatment for both positive and negative symptoms of schizophrenia.

Antipsychotics compose the largest group of drugs used to treat mental illness. Specifically, these drugs improve the thought processes and behavior of patients with psychotic symptoms, especially those with schizophrenia and other psychotic disorders. They are not used as a primary treatment for anxiety or depression. The theory is that psychotic symptoms result from an imbalance in the neurotransmitter dopamine in the brain. Sometimes these antipsychotics are called *dopamine antagonists*. Antipsychotics block D_2 dopamine receptors in the brain and thus reduce psychotic symptoms. Many antipsychotics block the chemoreceptor trigger zone (CTZ) and vomiting (emetic) center in the brain, producing an antiemetic (prevents or relieves nausea and vomiting) effect. However, when dopamine is blocked, symptoms of extrapyramidal syndrome (EPS) or parkinsonism (a chronic neurologic disorder that affects the extrapyramidal motor tract) such as tremors, masklike facies, rigidity, and shuffling gait may develop. Many patients who take high-potency antipsychotic drugs may require long-term medication for symptoms of parkinsonism.

ANTIPSYCHOTIC AGENTS

Antipsychotics are divided into two major categories: *typical* and *atypical*. The typical antipsychotics, introduced in 1952, are subdivided into phenothiazines and nonphenothiazines. *Nonphenothiazines* include butyrophenones, dibenzoxazepines, dihydroindolones, and thioxanthenes. The butyrophenones block only the neurotransmitter dopamine. The *phenothiazines* and the thioxanthenes block norepinephrine, causing sedative and hypotensive effects early in treatment.

Atypical antipsychotics make up the second category of antipsychotics. Clozapine, discovered in the 1960s and made available in Europe in 1971, was the first atypical antipsychotic agent. It was not marketed in the United States until 1990 because of adverse hematologic reactions. Atypical antipsychotics are effective for treating schizophrenia and other psychotic disorders in patients who do not respond to or are intolerant of typical antipsychotics. Because of their decreased side effects, atypical antipsychotics are often used instead of traditional typical antipsychotics as first-line therapy.

Pharmacophysiologic Mechanisms of Action

Antipsychotics block the actions of dopamine and thus may be classified as dopaminergic antagonists. There are five subtypes of dopamine receptors numbered D_1 through D_5. All antipsychotics block the D_2 (dopaminergic) receptor, which in turn promotes the presence of EPS, resulting in drug-induced pseudoparkinsonism in varying degrees. Atypical antipsychotics have a weak affinity to D_2 receptors and a stronger affinity to D_4 receptors, and they block the serotonin receptor. These agents cause fewer EPS than the typical (phenothiazine) antipsychotic agents, which have a strong affinity to D_2 receptors.

Adverse Reactions
Extrapyramidal Syndrome
Pseudoparkinsonism, which resembles symptoms of parkinsonism, is a major side effect of typical antipsychotic drugs. Symptoms of pseudoparkinsonism or EPS include stooped posture, masklike facies, rigidity, tremors at rest, shuffling gait, pill-rolling motions of the hands, and bradykinesia. When patients take high-potency typical antipsychotic drugs for extended periods, EPS is more pronounced. Patients who take low-strength antipsychotics such as chlorpromazine are not as likely to have symptoms of pseudoparkinsonism as those who take fluphenazine.

During early treatment with typical antipsychotic agents for schizophrenia and other psychotic disorders, two adverse extrapyramidal reactions that may occur are acute dystonia and akathisia. Tardive dyskinesia is a later phase of extrapyramidal reaction to antipsychotics. Use of anticholinergic drugs helps decrease pseudoparkinsonism symptoms, acute dystonia, and akathisia but has little effect on alleviating tardive dyskinesia. Complementary and Alternative Therapies 22.1 details interactions with antipsychotic agents.

COMPLEMENTARY AND ALTERNATIVE THERAPIES 22.1
Antipsychotic Agents

- Kava kava may increase the risk and severity of dystonic reactions when taken with phenothiazines.
- Kava kava may increase the risk and severity of dystonia when taken concurrently with fluphenazine.

The symptoms of acute dystonia usually occur in 5% of patients within days of taking typical antipsychotics. Characteristics of the reaction include muscle spasms of the face, tongue, neck, and back; facial grimacing; abnormal or involuntary upward eye movement; and laryngeal spasms that can impair respiration. This condition is treated with an anticholinergic antiparkinson drug such as benztropine. The benzodiazepine lorazepam may also be prescribed.

Akathisia occurs in approximately 20% of patients who take a typical antipsychotic drug. With this reaction, the patient has trouble standing still, is restless, paces the floor, and is in constant motion (e.g., rocks back and forth). Akathisia is best treated with a benzodiazepine such as lorazepam or a beta blocker such as propranolol.

Tardive dyskinesia is a serious adverse reaction that occurs in approximately 20% to 30% of patients who have taken a typical antipsychotic drug for more than 1 year. The prevalence is higher in cigarette smokers. The likelihood of developing tardive

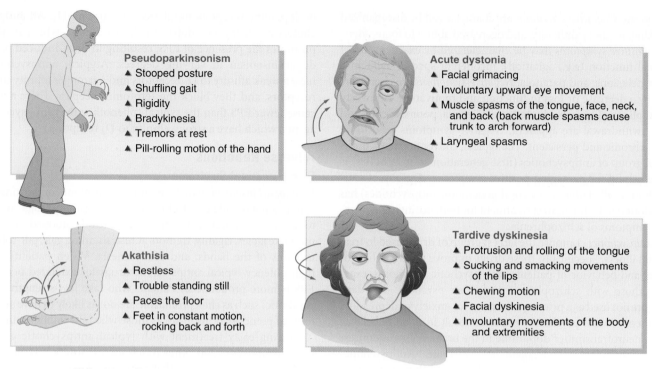

FIG. 22.1 Characteristics of pseudoparkinsonism, acute dystonia, akathisia, and tardive dyskinesia.

dyskinesia depends on the dose and duration of the antipsychotic factor. Characteristics of tardive dyskinesia include protrusion and rolling of the tongue, sucking and smacking movements of the lips, chewing motion, and involuntary movement of the body and extremities. In older adults, these reactions are more frequent and severe. The antipsychotic drug should be stopped in all who experience tardive dyskinesia, and another antipsychotic agent should be substituted. Benzodiazepines, calcium channel blockers, and beta blockers are sometimes helpful in decreasing tardive dyskinesia, although no one agent is effective for all patients. High doses of vitamin E may be helpful, and its use to treat tardive dyskinesia is currently under investigation. Clozapine has also been effective for treating tardive dyskinesia. Tetrabenazine, used to improve symptoms of Huntington disease, seems to be effective in treating tardive dyskinesia. Tetrabenazine reduces dopamine, norepinephrine, and serotonin levels. Amantadine has also been helpful in reducing drug-induced involuntary movements. Fig. 22.1 shows the characteristics of pseudoparkinsonism, acute dystonia, akathisia, and tardive dyskinesia.

Neuroleptic Malignant Syndrome

Neuroleptic malignant syndrome (NMS) is a rare but potentially fatal condition associated with antipsychotic drugs. Predisposing factors include excess agitation, exhaustion, and dehydration. NMS symptoms involve muscle rigidity, hyperthermia, altered mental status, profuse diaphoresis, blood pressure fluctuations, tachycardia, dysrhythmias, seizures, rhabdomyolysis, acute renal failure, respiratory failure, and coma. Treatment of NMS involves immediate withdrawal of antipsychotics, adequate hydration, hypothermic blankets, and administration of antipyretics, benzodiazepines, and muscle relaxants such as dantrolene.

Phenothiazines

Chlorpromazine hydrochloride was the first phenothiazine introduced for treating psychotic behavior in patients in psychiatric hospitals. The phenothiazines are subdivided into three groups: aliphatic, piperazine, and piperidine, which differ mostly in their side effects.

The *aliphatic phenothiazines* produce a strong sedative effect, decreased blood pressure, and may cause moderate EPS (pseudoparkinsonism). Chlorpromazine hydrochloride is in the aliphatic group and may produce pronounced orthostatic hypotension, low blood pressure that occurs when an individual assumes an upright position from a supine position.

The *piperazine phenothiazines* produce more EPS than other phenothiazines. They also cause dry mouth, urinary retention, and agranulocytosis. Examples of piperazine phenothiazines are fluphenazine and perphenazine.

The *piperidine phenothiazines* have a strong sedative effect, cause few EPS, have a low to moderate effect on blood pressure, and have no antiemetic effect. Thioridazine is an example of piperidine phenothiazines. Table 22.1 summarizes the effects of the phenothiazines.

Most antipsychotics can be given orally (tablet or liquid), intramuscularly (IM), or intravenously (IV). For oral use, the liquid form might be preferred because some patients may hide tablets in their cheek or under their tongue to avoid taking them. Mouth checks are necessary for noncompliant patients. In addition, the absorption rate is faster with the liquid form, and a peak serum drug level occurs in 2 to

TABLE 22.1 Effects of Phenothiazines (Varies Within Class)

Group	Sedation	Hypotension	EPS	Antiemetic
aliphatic	+++	+++	++	++
chlorpromazine and triflupromazine				+++
piperazine	++	+	+++	+++
piperidine	+++	+++	+	—
Nonphenothiazines				
haloperidol	+	+	+++	+++
loxapine	++	++	+++	—
molindone	+/++	+	+++	—
thiothixene	+	+	+++	—
Atypical Antipsychotics				
risperidone	+	+	+/0	—

—, No effect; +, mild effect; ++, moderate effect; +++, severe effect; *EPS,* symptoms of extrapyramidal syndrome.

3 hours. The antipsychotics are highly protein bound (>90%), and excretion of the drugs and their metabolites is slow. Phenothiazines are metabolized by liver enzymes into phenothiazine metabolites. Metabolites can be detected in the urine several months after the medication has been discontinued. Phenothiazine metabolites may cause a harmless pinkish to red-brown urine color. The *full* therapeutic effects of oral antipsychotics may not be evident for 3 to 6 weeks following initiation of therapy, but an observable therapeutic response may be apparent after 7 to 10 days.

Noncompliance with antipsychotics is common. Medication teaching in the following areas is of utmost importance: (1) encourage the patient to take the medication as prescribed, (2) explain and emphasize essential information to compensate for the patient's knowledge deficit, and (3) provide an interpreter for patients whose first language is not English.

Prototype Drug Chart 22.1 shows the drug characteristics of fluphenazine, a phenothiazine antipsychotic used to manage psychosis. Box 22.1 shows the symptoms and suggested treatment for overdose of phenothiazines.

Pharmacokinetics Oral absorption of fluphenazine is rapid and unaffected by food. This drug is strongly protein bound and has a long half-life, therefore the drug may accumulate in the body. Fluphenazine is metabolized by the liver, crosses the blood-brain barrier and placenta, and is excreted as metabolites primarily in the urine. With hepatic dysfunction, the phenothiazine dose may need to be decreased. Lack of drug metabolism in the liver will cause an elevation in serum drug level.

Pharmacodynamics Fluphenazine is prescribed primarily for psychotic disorders. This drug has anticholinergic properties and should be cautiously administered to patients with glaucoma, especially narrow-angle glaucoma. Because hypotension is a side effect of these phenothiazines, any antihypertensives simultaneously administered can cause an additive hypotensive effect. Narcotics and sedative-hypnotics administered

PROTOTYPE DRUG CHART 22.1

Fluphenazine

Drug Class
Antipsychotic: Neuroleptic piperazine phenothiazine
Pregnancy category C*

Dosage
A: PO: Initially 2.5-10 mg/d in 2-3 divided doses, increase gradually; maint: 1-5 mg/d; *max:* 40 mg/d
Older adults: PO: 1-2.5 mg/d in 2-3 divided doses; maint: 1-5 mg/d; *max:* 40 mg/d
Immediate release:
A: IM: 1.25 mg single dose; maint: 2.5-10 mg/d in divided doses q6-8h; *max:* 10 mg/d
Fluphenazine decanoate ER:
A/adol/C >12 y: IM/subcut: : 12.5-25 mg q3wk;
max: 100 mg/dose

Contraindications
Hypersensitivity, subcortical brain damage, severe CNS depression, coma
Caution: Dysrhythmias, paralytic ileus, urinary retention, BPH, leukopenia, neutropenia, agranulocytosis, hepatic and renal damage, hypotension, dementia in elderly patients, glaucoma, parkinsonism, seizure disorder

Drug-Lab-Food Interactions
Drug: Increased depressive effects when taken with alcohol or other CNS depressants; MgSO$_4$, lithium, and beta blockers increase effects; antacids and antiparkinsonism drugs decrease effects.
Complementary and alternative therapies: Kava kava may increase dystonia.

Pharmacokinetics
Absorption: Rapidly absorbed
Distribution: PB 91%-99%
Metabolism: t½: HCl, 15 h; decanoate, 14 d
Excretion: In urine

Pharmacodynamics
PO: Onset: HCl, 1 h; decanoate, 24 h
Peak: HCl, 2 h; decanoate, 48-96 h
Duration: HCl, 6-8 h; decanoate, 4 wk

Therapeutic Effects/Uses
To manage symptoms of psychosis including schizophrenia
Mode of Action: Blocks dopamine receptors in the brain and controls psychotic symptoms

Side Effects
Drowsiness, dizziness, headache, dry mouth, blurred vision, excess sweating, weight gain, constipation, urinary retention, peripheral edema, sexual dysfunction

Adverse Reactions
Hypertension, hypotension, tachycardia, ileus, EPS, seizures, psychosis
Life threatening: Agranulocytosis, leukopenia, neutropenia, hepatotoxicity, bronchospasm, dysrhythmias, NMS

*Pregnancy categories have been revised. See http://www.fda.gov/Drugs/Development ApprovalProcess/DevelopmentResources/Labeling/ucm093307.htm for more information.
>, Greater than; *A,* adult; *adol,* adolescent; *BPH,* benign prostatic hyperplasia; *C,* child; *CNS,* central nervous system; *d,* day; *ER,* extended release; *EPS,* symptoms of extrapyramidal syndrome; *h,* hours; *HCl,* hydrochloride; *IM,* intramuscular; *maint,* maintenance; *max,* maximum; *MgSO$_4$,* magnesium sulfate; *NMS,* neuroleptic malignant syndrome; *PB,* protein binding; *PO,* by mouth; *q6-8h,* every 6 to 8 hours; *subcut,* subcutaneous; *t½,* half-life; *wk,* weeks; *y,* years.

simultaneously with these phenothiazines can cause an additive CNS depression. Antacids decrease the absorption rate of both drugs and all phenothiazines, so they should be given 1 hour before or 2 hours after an oral phenothiazine.

BOX 22.1   Symptoms and Suggested Treatment for Overdose of Phenothiazines

Symptoms
- Unable to arouse; blood pressure fluctuations; tachycardia; agitation; delirium; convulsions; dysrhythmias; neuroleptic malignant syndrome; extrapyramidal symptoms; and renal, cardiac, and respiratory failure

Treatment
- Maintain airway, gastric lavage, activated charcoal administration, adequate hydration, anticholinergics, and norepinephrine

The onset of action for fluphenazine hydrochloride is 1 hour, with a duration rate of 6 to 8 hours. Fluphenazine decanoate has delayed absorption, with an onset of action of 24 hours and a duration of 4 weeks.

Nonphenothiazines

The many groups of nonphenothiazine antipsychotics include butyrophenones, dibenzoxazepines, dihydroindolones, and thioxanthenes.

In the *butyrophenone* group, a frequently prescribed nonphenothiazine is haloperidol. Haloperidol's pharmacologic behavior is similar to that of the phenothiazines. It is a potent antipsychotic drug in which the equivalent prescribed dose is smaller than that of drugs of lower potency, such as chlorpromazine. The drug dose for haloperidol is 0.5 to 5 mg, whereas the drug dose for chlorpromazine is 10 to 25 mg. Long-acting preparations of haloperidol decanoate and fluphenazine decanoate are given for slow release via injection every 2 to 4 weeks. Administration precautions should be taken to prevent soreness and inflammation at the injection site. Because the medication is a viscous liquid, a large-gauge needle (e.g., 21 gauge) should be used with the Z-track method for administration in a deep muscle; Chapter 10 provides further explanation of the Z-track method of injection. The injection site should not be massaged, and sites should be rotated. These medications should not remain in a plastic syringe longer than 15 minutes. Prototype Drug Chart 22.2 provides the drug data related to haloperidol.

Pharmacokinetics   Haloperidol is absorbed well through the gastrointestinal (GI) mucosa. It has a long half-life and is highly protein bound, so the drug may accumulate. Haloperidol is metabolized in the liver and is excreted in urine and feces.

Pharmacodynamics   Haloperidol alters the effects of dopamine by blocking dopamine receptors, thus sedation and EPS may occur. The drug is used to control psychosis and to decrease agitation in adults and children. Dosages need to be decreased in older adults because of decreased liver function and potential side effects. Haloperidol may be prescribed for children with hyperactive behavior. Because it has anticholinergic activity, care should be taken when administering it to patients with a history of glaucoma.

Haloperidol has a similar onset of action, peak time of concentration, and duration of action as the phenothiazines. It has strong EPS effects. Skin and sun protection is necessary for prolonged use because of the possible side effect of photosensitivity.

📄 PROTOTYPE DRUG CHART 22.2
Haloperidol and Haloperidol Decanoate

Drug Class	Dosage
Antipsychotic: Neuroleptic (nonphenothiazine) Pregnancy category C*	A/adol: PO: Initially 0.5-5 mg bid/tid; maint: 10-15 mg/d; *max*. 100 mg/d C 3-12 y: PO: Initially 0.25-0.5 mg/d in 2-3 divided doses; *max*. 0.15 mg/kg/d Deconate: A: IM: *max*. 100 mg first dose, 450 mg subsequent monthly doses

Contraindications	Drug-Lab-Food Interactions
Narrow-angle glaucoma; severe hepatic, renal, and cardiovascular diseases; bone marrow depression; parkinsonism; blood dyscrasias; CNS depression; subcortical brain damage; coma *Caution:* Alcoholism, dementia, glaucoma, dehydration, CAD, liver and renal damage, neutropenia, leukopenia	Drug: Increased sedation with alcohol, CNS depressants; increased toxicity with anticholinergics, CNS depressants, lithium; decreased effects with phenobarbital, carbamazepine; decreased effects with caffeine

Pharmacokinetics	Pharmacodynamics
Absorption: PO: 60% absorbed Distribution: PB: 92% Metabolism: t½: 12-22 h Excretion: In urine and feces	PO: Onset: 60-90 min Peak: 4-6 h Duration: 24-72 h IM: Onset: 15-30 min Peak: 20-40 min Duration: 4-8 h IM: Decanoate: Onset: UK Peak: 6 d Duration: 3-4 wk

Therapeutic Effects/Uses
To treat acute psychoses, ADHD, schizophrenia, Tourette syndrome
Mode of Action: Alters the effect of dopamine on the CNS; the mechanism for antipsychotic effects is unknown.

Side Effects	Adverse Reactions
Drowsiness, orthostatic hypotension, headache, lethargy, tremor, dry mouth and eyes, blurred vision, insomnia, agitation, weight gain, sexual dysfunction	Tachycardia, seizures, urinary retention, EPS *Life threatening:* Laryngospasm, bronchospasm, dysrhythmias, NMS, agranulocytosis, leukopenia, neutropenia

*Pregnancy categories have been revised. See http://www.fda.gov/Drugs/DevelopmentApprovalProcess/DevelopmentResources/Labeling/ucm093307.htm for more information.

A, Adult; *ADHD,* attention-deficit/hyperactivity disorder; *adol,* adolescent; *bid,* twice a day; *C,* child; *CAD,* coronary artery disease; *CNS,* central nervous system; *d,* day; *EPS,* symptoms of extrapyramidal syndrome; *h,* hour; *IM,* intramuscularly; *maint,* maintenance; *max,* maximum; *min,* minute; *NMS,* neuroleptic malignant syndrome; *PB,* protein binding; *PO,* by mouth; *t½,* half-life; *tid,* three times a day; *UK,* unknown; *wk,* week; *y,* year.

From the *dibenzoxazepine* group, loxapine is a moderately potent agent. It has moderate sedative and orthostatic hypotensive effects and strong EPS effects.

The typical antipsychotic molindone hydrochloride from the *dihydroindolone* group is a moderately potent agent. It has low sedative and orthostatic hypotensive effects and strong EPS effects.

In the nonphenothiazine group known as *thioxanthenes* is thiothixene, a highly potent typical antipsychotic drug. It has side effects similar to those of molindone with low sedative and orthostatic hypotensive effects and strong EPS effects.

Side Effects and Adverse Reactions

Several side effects are associated with antipsychotics. The most common side effect for all antipsychotics is drowsiness. Many of the antipsychotics have some anticholinergic effects: dry mouth, increased heart rate, urinary retention, and constipation can occur. Blood pressure decreases with the use of antipsychotics; aliphatics and piperidines cause a greater decrease in blood pressure than the others.

EPS can begin within 5 to 30 days after initiation of antipsychotic therapy and are most prevalent with the phenothiazines, butyrophenones, and thioxanthenes. These symptoms include pseudoparkinsonism, akathisia, dystonia (prolonged muscle contractions with twisting, repetitive movements), and tardive dyskinesia. Tardive dyskinesia may develop in 20% of patients taking antipsychotics for long-term therapy. Antiparkinson anticholinergic drugs may be given to control EPS, but they are not always effective in treating tardive dyskinesia.

High dosing or long-term use of some antipsychotics can cause blood dyscrasias (blood cell disorders) such as agranulocytosis. The white blood cell (WBC) count should be closely monitored and reported to the health care provider if an extreme decrease in leukocytes is observed.

Dermatologic side effects seen early in drug therapy are pruritus and marked photosensitivity. Patients are urged to use sunscreen, hats, and protective clothing and to stay out of the sun.

Drug Interactions

Because phenothiazines lower the seizure threshold, dosage adjustment of an anticonvulsant may be necessary. If either aliphatic phenothiazine or the thioxanthene group is administered, a higher dose of anticonvulsant might be necessary to prevent seizures.

Antipsychotics interact with alcohol, hypnotics, sedatives, narcotics, and benzodiazepines to potentiate the sedative effects of antipsychotics. Atropine counteracts EPS and potentiates antipsychotic effects. Use of antihypertensives can cause an additive hypotensive effect.

Antipsychotics should *not* be given with other antipsychotic or antidepressant drugs except to control psychotic behavior for selected individuals who are refractory to drug therapy. Under ordinary circumstances, if one antipsychotic drug is ineffective, a different one is prescribed. Individuals should *not* take alcohol or other CNS depressants (e.g., narcotic analgesics, barbiturates) with antipsychotics because additive depression is likely to occur.

When discontinuing antipsychotics, the drug dosage should be reduced gradually to avoid sudden recurrence of psychotic symptoms and seizures. Table 22.2 lists common antipsychotic drugs—phenothiazines and nonphenothiazines—and their dosages, uses, and considerations, including common side effects and a few serious adverse effects.

Antipsychotic Dosage for Older Adults

Older adults usually require smaller doses of antipsychotics—from 25% to 50% less than young and middle-aged adults. Regular to high doses of antipsychotics increase the risk of severe side effects. Dosage amounts need to be individualized according to the patient's age and physical status. In addition, dosage changes may be necessary during antipsychotic therapy. Antipsychotics have a black box warning that states mortality is increased in elderly patients with dementia-related psychosis.

Atypical Antipsychotics (Serotonin/Dopamine Antagonists)

Atypical antipsychotics differ from typical traditional antipsychotics in that the atypical agents are effective in treating both

TABLE 22.2	**Phenothiazines and Nonphenothiazines**	
Drug	**Route and Dosage**	**Uses and Considerations**
Chlorpromazine hydrochloride	Schizophrenia: A: PO: Initially 10-25 mg 2-4 times/d; maint: 200-400 mg/d; *max:* 1000 mg/d (2000 mg/d for short periods)	For acute psychosis, schizophrenia, intractable hiccups, nausea, and vomiting. May cause psychosis, seizures, weight gain, drowsiness, dry mouth, orthostatic hypotension, constipation, sexual dysfunction, life-threatening dysrhythmias, NMS, and EPS. Pregnancy category: C*; PB: 92%-97%; t½: 23-37 h
Fluphenazine hydrochloride	See Prototype Drug Chart 22.1.	
Perphenazine	Schizophrenia: A: PO: Initially 4-16 mg tid; after obtaining maximum response, gradually reduce dose; *max:* 24 mg/d (64 mg/d for short periods)	For schizophrenia, severe nausea and vomiting. May cause psychosis, seizures, weight gain, dizziness, drowsiness, dry mouth, appetite stimulation, and EPS. Pregnancy category: C*; PB: 91%-99%; t½: 9 h
Thioridazine hydrochloride	A: PO: Initially 50-100 mg tid; maint: 200-800 mg/d; *max:* 800 mg/d for short periods Adol/C >5 y: PO: Initially 0.5 mg/kg/d in divided doses; *max:* 3 mg/kg/d	For schizophrenia. May cause psychosis, seizures, weight gain, dizziness, drowsiness, dry mouth, appetite stimulation, nausea, vomiting, constipation, peripheral edema, hypotension, leukopenia, EPS, and life-threatening dysrhythmias. Pregnancy category: C*; PB: 91%-99%; t½: 5-27 h
Haloperidol	See Prototype Drug Chart 22.2.	

Continued

TABLE 22.2   Phenothiazines and Nonphenothiazines—cont'd

Drug	Route and Dosage	Uses and Considerations
Loxapine	Schizophrenia: A: PO: Initially 10 mg bid (50 mg in severely disturbed patients); maint: 60-100 mg/d; max: 250 mg/d	For schizophrenia and bipolar disorder. May cause seizures, dizziness, drowsiness, dry mouth, dysgeusia, hypotension, tachycardia, bronchospasm, EPS, and NMS. Pregnancy category: C*; PB: 96.6%; t½: 4-12 h
Molindone hydrochloride	A/adol/C >12 y: PO: Initially: 50-75 mg in 3-4 divided doses; max: 225 mg/d	For schizophrenia. May cause seizures, blurred vision, drowsiness, constipation, hypotension, tachycardia, EPS, and NMS. Pregnancy category: C*; PB: UK; t½: 1.5 h
Thiothixene hydrochloride	A/adol/C >12: PO: Initially 2 mg tid; maint: 20-30 mg/d; max: 60 mg/d	For schizophrenia. May cause blurred vision, dry mouth, constipation, weight gain, peripheral edema, hypotension, leukopenia, seizures, NMS, and EPS. Pregnancy category: C*; PB: 90%; t½: 34 h
Clozapine	A: PO: Initially: 12.5 mg/d or bid; gradually increase to maint: 300-450 mg/d in 3 divided doses; max: 900 mg/d	For schizophrenia. May cause dizziness, drowsiness, insomnia, hypersalivation, nausea, vomiting, constipation, hypotension, tachycardia, seizures, agranulocytosis, EPS, and NMS. Monitor white blood cell count. Gradually taper off over 1-2 wk upon discontinuation. Pregnancy category: B*; PB: 97%; t½: 4-12 h
Olanzapine	A: PO: Initially 5-10 mg/d; max: 20 mg/d Older adults: PO: Initially 5 mg/d; max: 20 mg/d Adol: PO: Initially 2.5-5 mg/d; maint: 10 mg/d; max: 20 mg/d	For schizophrenia, bipolar disorder, depression. May cause headache, dizziness, drowsiness, weakness, appetite stimulation, weight gain, hyperglycemia, hypercholesterolemia, hypertriglyceridemia, insomnia, seizures, NMS, and EPS. Pregnancy category: C*; PB: 93%; t½: 21-54 h
Quetiapine	Schizophrenia: Immediate release: A/adol: PO: Initially 25 mg/bid; maint: 300-400 mg/d in divided doses; max: 800 mg/d Extended release: A: PO: 300 mg at bedtime; maint: 400-800 mg/d; max: 800 mg/d Adol/older adults: Initially 50 mg/d, max: 200-800 mg/d	For schizophrenia, bipolar disorder, and depression. May cause dizziness, drowsiness, headache, dry mouth, electrolyte imbalance, psychosis, seizures, nausea, hypercholesterolemia, hypertriglyceridemia, orthostatic hypotension, weight gain, weakness, and EPS. Pregnancy category: C*; PB: 83%; t½: 6 h
Asenapine	Schizophrenia: A: SL: Initially 5 mg bid; may increase after 1 wk, max: 20 mg/d	For schizophrenia and bipolar disorder. May cause dizziness, drowsiness, insomnia, headache, paresthesia, hypertriglyceridemia, seizures, asthenia, and EPS. Pregnancy category: C*; PB: 95%; t½: 24 h
Risperidone	Schizophrenia: A: PO: Initially 2 mg/d; maint: 4-8 mg/d; max: 16 mg/d Older adults: PO: Initially 0.5 mg bid; max: 16 mg/d Adol: PO: Initially 0.5 mg/d; maint: 1-6 mg/d; max: 6 mg/d	For management of schizophrenia and bipolar disorder. May cause dizziness, drowsiness, headache, insomnia, fatigue, appetite stimulation, nausea, vomiting, seizures, dysrhythmias, agranulocytosis, EPS, and NMS. Pregnancy category: C*; PB: 90%; t½: 20 h
Ziprasidone	Schizophrenia: A: PO: 20 mg bid; may increase q2d; max: 80 mg/d A: IM: 10-20 mg; max: 40 mg/d	For schizophrenia and bipolar disorder. Dose should be taken with food; IM dose should not be given for more than 3 consecutive days. May cause dizziness, drowsiness, headache, insomnia, nausea, constipation, psychosis, seizures, weight gain, and EPS. Pregnancy category: C*; PB: 99%; t½: 7 h
Iloperidone	A: PO: Initially 1 mg bid; maint: 6-12 mg bid; max: 24 mg/d	For schizophrenia. May cause dizziness, drowsiness, nausea, dry mouth, weight gain, tachycardia, seizures, and EPS. Pregnancy category: C*; PB: 95%; t½: 23-37 h
Aripiprazole	See Prototype Drug Chart 22.3.	
Cariprazine	Schizophrenia: A: PO: Initially 1.5 mg/d; max: 6 mg/d	For schizophrenia and bipolar disorder. May cause insomnia, dizziness, headache, restlessness, weight gain, nausea, vomiting, constipation, seizures, suicidal ideation, and EPS. Pregnancy category: UK*; PB: 91%-97%; t½: 2 to 4 d
Brexpiprazole	Schizophrenia: A: PO: Initially 1 mg/d; maint: 2-4 mg/d; max: 4 mg/d	For schizophrenia and depression. May cause headache, drowsiness, weight gain, pharyngitis, seizures, suicidal ideation, NMS, and EPS. Pregnancy category: UK*; PB: 99%; t½: 91h
Paliperidone	Extended release tablet: A: PO: Initially 6 mg/d in the morning; may increase dose q5d, max: 12 mg/d A: IM ER: Initially 234 mg, then 1 wk later 156 mg; maint: 5 wk after first dose begin 117 mg/month; max: 234 mg q1month	For schizophrenia. May cause dizziness, drowsiness, headache, agitation, tachycardia, hypertriglyceridemia, weight gain, seizures, NMS, and EPS. Pregnancy category: C*; PB: 74%; t½: 23 h

*Pregnancy categories have been revised. See http://www.fda.gov/Drugs/DevelopmentApprovalProcess/DevelopmentResources/Labeling/ucm093307.htm for more information.

>, Greater than; *A*, adult; *adol*, adolescent; *bid*, twice a day; *C*, child; *d*, day; *EPS*, symptoms of extrapyramidal syndrome; *ER*, extended release; *h*, hour; *IM*, intramuscular; *maint*, maintenance; *max*, maximum; *NMS*, neuroleptic malignant syndrome; *PB*, protein binding; *PO*, by mouth; *q2d*, every 2 days; *SL*, sublingual; *t½*, half-life; *tid*, three times a day; *UK*, unknown; *wk*, weeks; *y*, years.

positive and negative symptoms of schizophrenia. The typical antipsychotics have not been effective in the treatment of negative symptoms. Two advantages of the atypical agents are that they are effective in treating negative symptoms and that they are unlikely to cause symptoms of EPS, including tardive dyskinesia. Atypical drugs available include clozapine, risperidone, olanzapine, ziprasidone, and aripiprazole. These agents have a greater affinity for blocking serotonin and dopaminergic D_4 receptors than primarily blocking the dopaminergic D_2 receptor responsible for mild and severe EPS. Weight gain, drowsiness, unsteady gait, headache, insomnia, depression, diabetes mellitus, and dyslipidemia are common side effects of atypical antipsychotics.

Clozapine was the first atypical antipsychotic agent used to treat schizophrenia and other psychoses. It is not as likely to cause symptoms of EPS, although they may occur. Tremors and occasional rigidity have been reported. Serious adverse reactions of clozapine are seizures and agranulocytosis, a decrease in the production of granulocytes that involves the body's immune defenses. Currently, clozapine is only indicated for the treatment of severely ill schizophrenic patients who have not responded to traditional antipsychotic drugs. The WBC (leukocyte) count needs to be closely monitored for leukopenia; if the level falls below 3000 mm^3, clozapine should be discontinued. Seizures have been reported in 3% of patients taking the drug. Dizziness, sedation, tachycardia, orthostatic hypotension, and constipation are common side effects.

Another atypical agent used to treat the positive and negative symptoms of schizophrenia is risperidone. Its action is similar to that of clozapine, and the occurrence of EPS and tardive dyskinesia is low. It does not cause agranulocytosis. Paliperidone is the major active metabolite of risperidone and is an extended-release tablet with once-a-day dosing. Paliperidone should be swallowed whole and not chewed, divided, or crushed. The most common adverse effects include EPS, insomnia, headache, and akathisia.

Like clozapine and risperidone, the atypical antipsychotic olanzapine is effective for treating the positive and negative symptoms of schizophrenia.

Like all the other atypical antipsychotics, quetiapine is less likely to cause EPS. Severe tardive dyskinesia may occur but it is rare.

For individuals with cardiac dysrhythmias, ziprasidone must be prescribed with caution because its use may lead to a prolonged QT interval; electrocardiograms (ECGs) should be monitored. Ziprasidone is contraindicated in patients with a history of prolonged QT interval or with other concurrent drugs known to prolong QT interval. Patients taking quetiapine, clozapine, risperidone, olanzapine, ziprasidone, and aripiprazole should be monitored for hyperglycemia and other symptoms of diabetes mellitus.

Prototype Drug Chart 22.3 illustrates drug characteristics of aripiprazole, an atypical antipsychotic. When anxiety, hallucinations, agitation, mania, confusion, or depression and other symptoms are noted, the health care provider should check the medications that the patient is taking.

PROTOTYPE DRUG CHART 22.3
Aripiprazole

Drug Class	Dosage
Nonphenothiazine: Atypical antipsychotic Pregnancy category C*	Psychosis: A: PO: 10-15 mg/d, may increase q2wk; maint: 10-30 mg/d; *max:* 30 mg/d Adol >13 y: PO: 2 mg/d, may increase q2d; maint: 10 mg/d; *max:* 30 mg/d Extended release: A: IM: 400 mg/month

Contraindications	Drug-Lab-Food Interactions
Hypersensitivity, dehydration, alcohol intoxication, hypovolemia, agranulocytosis, neutropenia, leukopenia, heart failure, suicidal ideation, myocardial infarction, diabetes mellitus, hyperglycemia, hypotension, seizures, parkinsonism *Caution:* Dysrhythmias, dementia, CNS depression, hyperglycemia, hypotension, parkinsonism, seizures, agranulocytosis, neutropenia, leukopenia	Drug: Antidiabetic agents decrease drug levels and increase risk of hyperglycemia; alpha blockers and antihypertensives increase risk of hypotension; other antipsychotics enhance risk of NMS, EPS, anticholinergic effects, hypotension, and seizures; CNS depressants may increase sedation and orthostatic hypotension; SSRIs may increase risk of serotonin syndrome; calcium channel blockers may increase blood levels Food: Grapefruit juice may increase blood levels Herbal: St. John's wort may decrease blood levels Lab: Increased blood glucose

Pharmacokinetics	Pharmacodynamics
Absorption: Well absorbed, not affected by food Distribution: PB: 99% Metabolism: t½: 75 h; extended release 30-47 d Excretion: In urine and feces	PO: Onset: UK Peak: 3-5 h Duration: 24 h IM: Onset: UK Peak: 1-3 h Duration: 24 h ER: Peak: 5-7 d Duration: 36 d

Therapeutic Effects/Uses

To manage schizophrenia, bipolar disorder, autism, depression, Tourette syndrome

Mode of Action: Interferes with the binding of dopamine to dopamine (D_2) and serotonin 5-hydroxytryptamine (5-HT$_2$) receptors

Side Effects	Adverse Reactions
Drowsiness, memory impairment, weight gain/loss, headaches, fatigue, blurred vision, photosensitivity, peripheral edema, amenorrhea, hyperglycemia, hypoglycemia, insomnia, anxiety, agitation, dizziness, constipation, nausea, vomiting, sexual dysfunction	Orthostatic hypotension, tachycardia, EPS, dysrhythmias, seizures *Life threatening:* Suicidal ideation, NMS, agranulocytosis, leukopenia, laryngospasm

*Pregnancy categories have been revised. See http://www.fda.gov/Drugs/DevelopmentApprovalProcess/DevelopmentResources/Labeling/ucm093307.htm for more information.
>, Greater than; *A,* adult; *adol,* adolescent; *CNS,* central nervous system; *d,* day; *EPS,* symptoms of extrapyramidal syndrome; *ER,* extended release; *h,* hour; *IM,* intramuscularly; *maint,* maintenance; *max,* maximum; *NMS,* neuroleptic malignant syndrome; *PB,* protein binding; *PO,* by mouth; *q2d,* every 2 days; *SSRI,* selective serotonin reuptake inhibitor; *t½,* half-life; *UK,* unknown; *wk,* week.

NURSING PROCESS
Patient-Centered Collaborative Care

Phenothiazines and Nonphenothiazines

Assessment
- Assess baseline vital signs for use in future comparisons.
- Obtain a patient health history that includes present drug therapy. If the patient is taking an anticonvulsant, the drug dose might need to be increased because antipsychotics tend to lower the seizure threshold.
- Assess mental status and cardiac, eye, and respiratory disorders before starting drug therapy, and continue daily assessment.

Nursing Diagnoses
- Relationship, Ineffective related to social withdrawal
- Loneliness, Risk for
- Sleep Pattern, Disturbed related to medication adverse effects
- Activity Intolerance related to sedation
- Confusion, Acute related to psychosis
- Self-Care Deficit, Bathing related to loss of motivation

Planning
- Patient's psychotic behavior will improve with medication, psychotherapy, and adjunct therapies.

Nursing Interventions
- Monitor vital signs. Orthostatic hypotension is likely to occur.
- Remain with patients while medication is taken and swallowed; some patients hide antipsychotics in the mouth to avoid taking them.
- Avoid skin contact with liquid concentrates to prevent contact dermatitis. Liquid must be protected from light and should be diluted with fruit juice.
- Administer oral doses with food or milk to decrease gastric irritation.
- Dilute oral solution of fluphenazine in fruit juice, water, or milk. Avoid apple juice and caffeinated drinks.
- Administer deep into muscle because drug irritates fatty tissue. Do *not* administer intravenously.
- Check blood pressure for marked decrease or increase 30 minutes after drug is injected.
- Do *not* mix in same syringe with heparin, pentobarbital, cimetidine, or dimenhydrinate.
- Chill suppository in refrigerator for 30 minutes before removing foil wrapper.
- Observe for EPS such as acute dystonia, akathisia, pseudoparkinsonism, and tardive dyskinesia (see Fig. 22.1) and report these promptly to the health care provider.
- ⚡ Assess for symptoms of NMS: increased fever, pulse, and blood pressure; muscle rigidity; increased creatine phosphokinase and WBC count; altered mental status; acute renal failure; varying levels of consciousness; pallor; diaphoresis; tachycardia; and dysrhythmias.
- Record urine output; urinary retention may result.
- Monitor serum glucose level.
- Engage patient in interactions with staff, other patients, and attending therapies.

Patient Teaching
General
- Encourage patients to take the drug exactly as ordered. In schizophrenia and other psychotic disorders, antipsychotics do not cure the mental illness but do alleviate symptoms. Many patients on medication can function outside of an institutional setting. Adherence to a drug regimen is extremely important.
- Inform patients that medication may take 6 weeks or longer to achieve full clinical effect.
- ⚡ Caution patients not to consume alcohol or other CNS depressants such as narcotics; these drugs intensify the depressant effect on the body.
- Recommend that patients not abruptly discontinue the drug. Seek advice from a health care provider before making any changes in dosage.
- Encourage patients to read labels on over-the-counter (OTC) preparations. Some are contraindicated when taking antipsychotics.
- Teach smoking cessation because smoking increases the metabolism of some antipsychotics.
- Guide patients to maintain good oral hygiene by frequently brushing and flossing teeth.
- Encourage patients to talk with a health care provider regarding family planning. The effect of antipsychotics on the fetus is not fully known; however, there may be teratogenic effects.
- Explain to the breastfeeding patient that phenothiazine passes into breast milk, possibly causing drowsiness and unusual muscle movement in the infant.
- Warn patients about the importance of routine follow-up examinations.
- ⚡ Encourage patients to obtain laboratory tests on schedule. WBCs are monitored for 3 months, especially during the start of drug therapy. Leukopenia, or decreased WBCs, may occur. Be alert to symptoms of malaise, fever, and sore throat, which may be an indication of agranulocytosis, a serious blood dyscrasia.
- Teach patients, especially those taking clozapine, to report symptoms of infection promptly to the health care provider.
- Advise patients to wear an identification bracelet indicating the medication taken.
- Inform patients that tolerance to the sedative effect develops over a period of days or weeks.

Side Effects
- ⚡ Direct patients to avoid potentially dangerous situations, such as driving, until drug dosing has been stabilized.
- Inform patients about EPS and instruct them to promptly report symptoms to a health care provider.

- Encourage patients to wear sunglasses for photosensitivity, to limit exposure to direct sunlight, and to use sunscreen and protective clothing to prevent a skin rash.
- Warn patients about orthostatic hypotension and possible dizziness.
- Teach patients who are taking aliphatic phenothiazines such as chlorpromazine that the urine might be pink or red-brown; this discoloration is harmless.
- Inform patients that changes may occur related to sexual functioning and menstruation. Women could have irregular menstrual periods or amenorrhea, and men might experience impotence and gynecomastia (enlargement of breast tissue).
- Suggest lozenges or hard candy if mouth dryness occurs. Advise patients to consult a health care provider if dry mouth persists for more than 2 weeks.
- Encourage patients to avoid extremes in environmental temperatures and exercise.
- Advise patients to rise slowly from sitting or lying to standing to prevent a sudden decrease in blood pressure.

🌐 *Cultural Considerations*
- Recognize that some cultural groups may have difficulty in believing and accepting the patient's disorder and the need for medication.

Evaluation
- Evaluate the effectiveness of the drug and whether the patient has acceptably reduced psychotic symptoms at the *lowest* dose possible.
- Ascertain whether the patient can cope with everyday living situations and attend to activities of daily living.
- Determine whether any side effects or adverse reactions to the drug have occurred.

⚡ **PATIENT SAFETY**

Do not confuse
- **Seroquel** with **Serzone**, an antidepressant, or **sertindole** with **Serlect**.

ANXIOLYTICS

Anxiolytics, or *antianxiety drugs,* are primarily used to treat anxiety and insomnia. The major anxiolytic group is benzodiazepines, a minor tranquilizer group. Long before benzodiazepines were prescribed for anxiety and insomnia, barbiturates were used. Benzodiazepines are considered more effective than barbiturates because they enhance the action of gamma-aminobutyric acid (GABA), an inhibitory neurotransmitter within the CNS. Benzodiazepines have fewer side effects and may be less dangerous in overdosing. Long-term use of barbiturates causes drug tolerance and dependence and may cause respiratory distress. Currently, barbiturates are not drugs of choice for treating anxiety. Benzodiazepine-like drugs are used to treat insomnia. Selective serotonin reuptake inhibitors (SSRIs), serotonin norepinephrine reuptake inhibitors

! TABLE 22.3 Approved Uses for Benzodiazepines	
Prescribed Uses	**Drugs**
Anxiety	Alprazolam
	Chlordiazepoxide
	Chlorazepate
	Diazepam
	Lorazepam
Anxiety associated with depression	Alprazolam
	Clonazepam
	Lorazepam
Insomnia, short-term use	Estazolam
	Flurazepam
	Quazepam
	Temazepam
	Triazolam
Seizures and status epilepticus	Clonazepam
	Clorazepate
	Diazepam
	Lorazepam
Alcohol withdrawal	Clorazepate
	Chlordiazepoxide
	Diazepam
	Lorazepam
Skeletal muscle spasms	Diazepam
Preoperative medications	Chlordiazepoxide
	Diazepam
	Lorazepam
	Midazolam

(SNRIs), tricyclic antidepressants (TCAs), and monoamine oxidase inhibitors (MAOIs) are used to treat various anxiety disorders. These drugs are discussed in Chapter 23.

Table 22.3 lists approved uses for benzodiazepines. Drugs used to treat insomnia, including benzodiazepines, are discussed in Chapter 18.

A certain amount of anxiety may make a person more alert and energetic, but when anxiety is excessive, it can be disabling, and anxiolytics may be prescribed. The action of anxiolytics resembles that of the sedative-hypnotics but *not* that of the antipsychotics.

There are two types of anxiety—primary and secondary. *Primary anxiety* is not caused by a medical condition or by drug use; *secondary anxiety* is related to selected drug use or medical or psychiatric disorders. Anxiolytics are not usually given for secondary anxiety unless the medical problem is untreatable, severe, and causes disability. In this case, an anxiolytic could be given for a short period to alleviate any acute anxiety attacks. These agents treat the symptoms but do not cure them. Long-term use of anxiolytics is discouraged because tolerance develops within weeks or months, depending on the agent. Drug tolerance can occur in less than 2 to 3 months in patients who take phenobarbital.

Nonpharmacologic Measures

Some of the symptoms of a severe attack of anxiety, or panic attack, include dyspnea (difficulty in breathing), choking sensation, chest pain, heart palpitations, dizziness, faintness, sweating, trembling and shaking, and fear of losing control. Before giving anxiolytics, nonpharmacologic measures should be used for decreasing anxiety. These measures might include using a relaxation technique, psychotherapy, or support groups.

❶ Benzodiazepines

Benzodiazepines have multiple uses as anticonvulsants, sedative-hypnotics, preoperative drugs, substance abuse withdrawal agents, and anxiolytics. Most of the benzodiazepines are used mainly for severe or prolonged anxiety. Examples include chlordiazepoxide, diazepam, clorazepate dipotassium, lorazepam, and alprazolam. The most frequently prescribed benzodiazepine is lorazepam. Many of the benzodiazepines are used for more than one purpose.

Benzodiazepines are lipid soluble and are absorbed readily from the GI tract. They are highly protein bound (80% to 98%). Benzodiazepines are primarily metabolized by the liver and are excreted in urine, so the drug dosage for patients with liver or renal disease should be lowered accordingly to avoid possible cumulative effects. Traces of benzodiazepine metabolites could be present in the urine for weeks or months after the person has stopped taking the drug. These are Controlled Substance Schedule IV (CSS IV) drugs.

The first benzodiazepine, chlordiazepoxide, became widely used for its sedative effect in 1962. Diazepam was the most frequently prescribed drug in the early 1970s. Lorazepam is the prototype drug of benzodiazepine and is described in Prototype Drug Chart 22.4.

🌿 COMPLEMENTARY AND ALTERNATIVE THERAPIES 22.2
Benzodiazepines

Kava kava should not be combined with benzodiazepines because it increases the sedative effect.

Pharmacokinetics Lorazepam is highly lipid soluble, and the drug is rapidly absorbed from the GI tract. The drug is highly protein bound, and the half-life is 12 hours. Lorazepam is excreted primarily in the urine.

Pharmacodynamics Lorazepam acts on the limbic, thalamic, and hypothalamic levels of the CNS. The onset of action is 15 to 30 minutes for IM administration and 1 to 5 minutes IV. The serum levels of most oral doses of benzodiazepines peak in 2 hours. Oxazepam levels peak in 3 hours. The duration of action varies, but the average is 16 hours when given orally; when given IV, the duration of action is 6 to 8 hours.

It is recommended that benzodiazepines be prescribed for no longer than 3 to 4 months. Beyond 4 months, the effectiveness of the drug lessens. Table 22.4 lists the anxiolytics and their dosages, uses, and considerations, including common side effects and a few serious adverse effects.

Miscellaneous Anxiolytics

The anxiolytic buspirone hydrochloride binds to serotonin and dopamine receptors. It may not be effective until 1 to 2 weeks

PROTOTYPE DRUG CHART 22.4
❶ Lorazepam

Drug Class	Dosage
Anxiolytic: Benzodiazepine Pregnancy category D*	Anxiety: A/C >12 y: PO: initially 2-3 mg in divided doses; increase gradually PRN; maint: 1-10 mg/d in divided doses; max: 10 mg/d Older adults: PO: 1-2 mg/d in divided doses; max: 10 mg/d
Contraindications Hypersensitivity, narrow-angle glaucoma *Caution:* Hepatic or renal dysfunction, alcohol intoxication, depression, seizures, CNS depression, pregnancy, suicidal ideation	**Drug-Lab-Food Interactions** Drug: Increases CNS depression when taken with alcohol, CNS depressants, and anticonvulsants; cimetidine increases lorazepam plasma levels, increases phenytoin levels, decreases levodopa effects; smoking and caffeine decrease antianxiety effects; oral contraceptives decrease effects
Pharmacokinetics Absorption: Rapid from GI tract Distribution: PB: 91% Metabolism: t½: 12 h Excretion: In urine	**Pharmacodynamics** PO: Onset: UK Peak: 2 h Duration: 12-24 h IM: Onset: 15-30 min Peak: 3 h Duration: 6-8 h IV: Onset: 1-5 min Peak: UK Duration: 6-8 h

Therapeutic Effects/Uses
To control anxiety and to treat status epilepticus; for sedation induction; for insomnia
Mode of Action: Potentiates GABA effects by binding to specific benzodiazepine receptors and inhibiting GABA neurotransmission

Side Effects	Adverse Reactions
Drowsiness, dizziness, weakness, confusion, headache, blurred vision, nausea, vomiting, anorexia, restlessness, hallucinations, amnesia, ataxia	Hypertension, hypotension, bradycardia, dependence, seizures *Life threatening:* Suicidal ideation, NMS, respiratory depression

*Pregnancy categories have been revised. See http://www.fda.gov/Drugs/DevelopmentApprovalProcess/DevelopmentResources/Labeling/ucm093307.htm for more information.

>, Greater than; *A,* adult; *C,* child; *CNS,* central nervous system; *d,* day; *GABA,* gamma-aminobutyric acid; *GI,* gastrointestinal; *h,* hour; *IM,* intramuscularly; *IV,* intravenously; *maint,* maintenance; *max,* maximum; *min,* minute; *NMS,* neuroleptic malignant syndrome; *PB,* protein binding; *PO,* by mouth; *PRN,* as needed; *t½,* half-life; *UK,* unknown; *y,* years.

after continuous use. It has fewer of the side effects of sedation and physical and psychological dependency associated with many benzodiazepines. The most common side effects of buspirone include drowsiness, dizziness, headache, nausea, nervousness, and excitement. It is important to note that buspirone has an interaction with grapefruit juice that can lead to toxicity. To avoid this interaction, buspirone users should be advised to limit intake of grapefruit juice to 8 ounces daily or half of a grapefruit.

! TABLE 22.4 Anxiolytics

Drug	Route and Dosage	Uses and Considerations
Benzodiazepines		

Alprazolam
CSS IV
	Immediate release:
	A: PO: Initially 0.25-0.5 mg tid, may increase q3-4d,
	   max: 4 mg/d
	Older A: PO: Initially 0.125 bid/tid, may increase q3-4d;
	   max: 4mg/d
	Extended release:
	A: PO: Initially 0.5-1 mg/d in the morning may increase
	   q3-4d; *max*: 10 mg/d
	Older A: PO: Initially 0.5 mg/d may increase q3-4d;
	   max: 10 mg/d
		For anxiety, panic disorders, and generalized anxiety disorder. May cause dizziness, drowsiness, anxiety, dry mouth, dysarthria, fatigue, confusion, nausea, constipation, tolerance, dependence, withdrawal, weight gain/loss, and tachycardia. Reduce dose gradually upon discontinuation. Pregnancy category: D*; PB: 90%; t½: 11-16 h

Chlordiazepoxide hydrochloride
CSS IV
	Anxiety disorders:
	A: PO: 5-10 mg tid/qid; for severe anxiety: 20-25 mg
	   tid/qid; *max*: 100 mg/d
	Older adult: PO: 5-10 mg/d; maint: 5 mg bid/qid;
	   max: 300 mg/d
	C >6 y: PO: 5 mg bid/qid; *max*: 30 mg/d
	Acute alcohol withdrawal:
	A: PO: 50-100 mg q4-6h until agitation is controlled;
	   max: 300 mg/d
		For anxiety, alcohol withdrawal syndrome (DTs). May cause drowsiness, confusion, dysarthria, constipation, ataxia, tolerance, dependence, withdrawal, and amnesia. Taper off gradually upon discontinuation. Pregnancy category: D*; PB: 96%; t½: 5-30 h

Clorazepate dipotassium
CSS IV
	Anxiety:
	A: PO: 30 mg/d in divided doses; maint: 15-60 mg/d;
	   max: 60 mg/d
	Older adults: 7.5-15 mg/d in divided doses; maint:
	   15-60 mg/d; *max*: 60 mg/d
		For anxiety, alcohol withdrawal syndrome, and partial seizures. May cause drowsiness, dizziness, confusion, blurred vision, hypotension, tolerance, dependence, withdrawal, amnesia, depression, and suicidal ideation. Avoid taking alcohol or CNS depressants with clorazepate. Taper off gradually upon discontinuation. Pregnancy category: D*; PB: 97%; t½: 30-200 h

Diazepam CSS IV	Anxiety: A: PO: 2-10 mg bid/qid; *max*: 40 mg/d Older adults: PO: 2-2.5 mg qd/bid; *max*: 40 mg/d Adol/C >6 months: PO: 1-2.5 mg tid/qid; *max*: 0.6 mg/kg q8h A: IM/IV: 2-5 mg; repeat in 3-4 h PRN	For anxiety, muscle spasms, alcohol withdrawal, seizures, status epilepticus, and sedation induction. May cause drowsiness, confusion, dysarthria, fatigue, paradoxical aggression, dependence, tolerance, and withdrawal. Pregnancy category: D*; PB: 99%; t½: 30-60 h
Lorazepam CSS IV	See Prototype Drug Chart 22.4.	
Oxazepam CSS IV	Anxiety: A/adol: PO: Initially 10-15 mg tid/qid; for severe symptoms, 15-30 mg tid/qid; *max*: A 120 mg/d, adol 60 mg/d Older adults: PO: 10 mg tid; *max*: 60 mg/d	For anxiety and acute alcohol withdrawal. May cause dizziness, drowsiness, blurred vision, amnesia, confusion, dependence, tolerance, and withdrawal. Taper off gradually upon discontinuation. Pregnancy category: D*; PB: 85%-95%; t½: 5-15 h
Azapirones		

Buspirone hydrochloride	A: PO: Initially: 7.5 mg bid; maint: 15-30 mg/d in divided
	   doses; *max*: 60 mg/d
	Older adults: PO: 5 mg bid; maint: 15-30 mg/d in divided
	   doses; *max*: 60 mg/d
		For anxiety and generalized anxiety disorder. Takes several weeks before anxiolytic effects occur. May cause drowsiness, dizziness, headache, nausea, seizures, serotonin syndrome, EPS, and suicidal ideation. Pregnancy category: B*; PB: 86%; t½: 2-4 h

Benzodiazepine Antagonists		

Flumazenil	A: IV: Initially 0.2 mg over 15-30 s; repeat 0.2 mg at 1-min
	   intervals; *max*: 3 mg/h
	C/adol: IV: 0.01 mg/kg over 15 s, repeat at 1-min intervals;
	   max: 0.1 mg/kg/h
		For sedation reversal and benzodiazepine toxicity. Flumenazil should not be used with antipsychotics or antidepressants. May cause dizziness, blurred vision, resedation, ataxia, agitation, insomnia, dry mouth, seizures, and dysrhythmias. Pregnancy category: C*; PB: 50%; t½: 41-79 min

*Pregnancy categories have been revised. See http://www.fda.gov/Drugs/DevelopmentApprovalProcess/DevelopmentResources/Labeling/ucm093 307.htm for more information.

>, Greater than; *A*, adult; *adol*, adolescent; *bid*, twice a day; *C*, child; *CNS*, central nervous system; *CSS*, Controlled Substances Schedule; *d*, day; *DTs*, delirium tremens; *EPS*, symptoms of extrapyramidal symptoms; *h*, hour; *IM*, intramuscularly; *IV*, intravenously; *maint*, maintenance; *max*, maximum; *min*, minute; *PB*, protein binding; *PO*, by mouth; *PRN*, as needed; *q*, every; *q4-6h*, every 4 to 6 hours; *qd*, every day; *qid*, four times a day; *s*, seconds; *t½*, half-life; *tid*, three times a day; *y*, years.

NURSING PROCESS
Patient-Centered Collaborative Care

Benzodiazepines

Assessment
- Assess for suicidal ideation.
- Obtain a history of the patient's anxiety reaction.
- Determine the patient's support system (family, friends, groups).
- Obtain a drug history. Report possible drug-drug interactions.

Nursing Diagnoses
- Anxiety related to situational crisis
- Mobility, Impaired Physical related to drowsiness and weakness
- Noncompliance related to adverse effects of medications.

Planning
- Patient's anxiety and stress will be reduced through non-pharmacologic methods, anxiolytic drugs, or support/group therapy.

Nursing Interventions
- Observe patient for side effects of anxiolytics. Recognize that drug tolerance and physical and psychological dependency can occur with most anxiolytics.
- Recognize that anxiolytic dosages should be lower for older adults, children, and debilitated persons than for middle-aged adults.
- Monitor vital signs, especially blood pressure and pulse; orthostatic hypotension may occur.
- Encourage family to be supportive of the patient.

Patient Teaching
General
- ⚡ Advise patients not to drive a motor vehicle or operate dangerous equipment when taking anxiolytics because sedation is a common side effect.
- ⚡ Warn patients not to consume alcohol or CNS depressants such as narcotics while taking an anxiolytic.
- Teach patients ways to control excess stress and anxiety with relaxation techniques such as long walks.
- Inform patients that an effective response may take 1 to 2 weeks.
- Encourage patients to follow drug regimens and not to abruptly stop taking a drug after prolonged use because withdrawal symptoms can occur. The drug dose is usually tapered when a drug is discontinued.

Side Effects
- Encourage patients to rise slowly from sitting to standing positions to avoid dizziness from orthostatic hypotension.

🌐 *Cultural Considerations*
- Use simple and clear instructions, modifying methods and materials to meet patient and family needs. Ask family members to assist with translation only if an interpreter is not available, and do not ask private questions in public.

Evaluation
- Evaluate the effectiveness of drug therapy by determining whether the patient is less anxious and more able to cope with stresses and anxieties.
- Determine whether the patient is taking the anxiolytic drug as prescribed and is adhering to patient teaching instructions.

Side Effects and Adverse Reactions

The side effects associated with benzodiazepines are sedation, dizziness, headaches, dry mouth, blurred vision, rare urinary incontinence, and constipation. Adverse reactions include leukopenia (decreased WBC count) with symptoms of fever, malaise, and sore throat; tolerance to the drug dosage with continuous use; and physical dependency. Box 22.2 lists guidelines for treating benzodiazepine overdose.

Benzodiazepines should not be abruptly discontinued because withdrawal symptoms are likely to occur. Withdrawal symptoms caused by short-term benzodiazepine use are similar to those from the sedative-hypnotics: agitation, nervousness, insomnia, tremor, anorexia, muscular cramps, and sweating; however, they are slow to develop, taking 2 to 10 days, and can last several weeks, depending on the benzodiazepine's half-life. When discontinuing a benzodiazepine, the drug dosage should be gradually decreased over a period of days, depending on dose or length of time on the drug. Withdrawal symptoms from long-term, high-dose benzodiazepine therapy include paranoia, delirium, panic, hypertension, and status epilepticus. Convulsions during withdrawal may be prevented with simultaneous substitution of an anticonvulsant. Alcohol and other CNS depressants should *not* be taken with benzodiazepines because respiratory depression can result. Tobacco, caffeine, and sympathomimetics decrease the effectiveness of benzodiazepines. Benzodiazepines are contraindicated during pregnancy because of possible teratogenic effects.

BOX 22.2   Suggested Treatment for Overdose of Benzodiazepines

1. Administer an emetic and follow with activated charcoal if the patient is conscious; use gastric lavage if the patient is unconscious.
2. Administer the benzodiazepine antagonist flumazenil intravenously if required.
3. Maintain an airway, give oxygen as needed for decreased respirations, and monitor vital signs.
4. Give intravenous vasopressors for severe hypotension.
5. Request a mental health consultation for the patient.

CRITICAL THINKING CASE STUDY

FS, a 35-year-old woman, is receiving risperidone, 3 mg twice daily, to control a psychotic disorder. She has taken the drug for 6 months but has recently become agitated and is complaining of insomnia.

1. What is the relation between FS's drug dose and her complaints? Explain your answer.

2. What further assessment should be made concerning FS and the drug regimen?

3. How does risperidone compare with other antipsychotics such as chlorpromazine and haloperidol regarding actions and adverse effects?

NCLEX STUDY QUESTIONS

1. The nurse suspects that a patient who is experiencing facial grimacing, involuntary upward eye movement, and muscle spasms of the tongue and face may have which condition?
   a. Akathisia
   b. Acute dystonia
   c. Tardive dyskinesia
   d. Pseudoparkinsonism

2. A patient asks the nurse to explain how antipsychotic drugs work to make him feel better. The nurse understands that antipsychotics act in which way?
   a. Blocking actions of dopamine
   b. Blocking actions of epinephrine
   c. Promoting prostaglandin synthesis
   d. Enhancing the action of gamma-aminobutyric acid

3. An antipsychotic agent, fluphenazine, is ordered for a patient with psychosis. The nurse understands that this agent can lead to symptoms of extrapyramidal syndrome (EPS). What are the symptoms of EPS?
   a. Parkinsonism
   b. Nausea and vomiting
   c. Hyperthermia and dysrhythmias
   d. Tremors, rigidity, and shuffling gait

4. An atypical antipsychotic is prescribed for a patient with psychosis. The nurse understands that this category of medications includes which drugs? (Select all that apply.)
   a. Clozapine
   b. Fluphenazine
   c. Haloperidol
   d. Olanzapine
   e. Aripiprazole

5. A patient is prescribed lorazepam. What does the nurse know to be true regarding lorazepam?
   a. It is used to treat anxiety, status epilepticus, insomnia, and sedation induction
   b. It has a maximum adult dose of 25 mg/day.
   c. It causes plasma levels to be decreased when combined with cimetidine.
   d. It interferes with the binding of dopamine receptors.

6. A patient is receiving aripiprazole. Which nursing intervention(s) will the nurse include in the patient's care plan? (Select all that apply.)
   a. Administer before meals on an empty stomach to facilitate absorption.
   b. Remain with the patient until medication is swallowed.
   c. Monitor vital signs to detect orthostatic hypotension.
   d. Assess the patient for evidence of neuroleptic malignant syndrome.
   e. Observe the patient for acute dystonia, akathisia, and tardive dyskinesia.

7. A patient appears to have had an overdose of phenothiazines. The nurse anticipates that which intervention(s) may be used to treat phenothiazine overdose? (Select all that apply.)
   a. Gastric lavage
   b. Adequate hydration
   c. Maintaining an airway
   d. Fluphenazine
   e. Risperidone
   f. Activated charcoal administration

Answers: 1, b; 2, a; 3, d; 4, a, d, e; 5, a; 6, b, c, d, e; 7, a, b, c, f.

23

Antidepressants and Mood Stabilizers

http://evolve.elsevier.com/McCuistion/pharmacology/

OBJECTIVES

- Contrast the various categories of different antidepressants and give an example of one drug for each category.
- Describe the side effects and adverse reactions of antidepressants.
- Plan nursing interventions, including patient teaching, for antidepressants (tricyclic antidepressants [TCAs], monoamine oxidase inhibitors [MAOIs], selective serotonin
- reuptake inhibitors [SSRIs], serotonin norepinephrine reuptake inhibitors [SNRIs], and atypical antidepressants).
- Explain the uses of lithium and its serum/plasma therapeutic ranges, side effects and adverse reactions, and nursing interventions.
- Apply the nursing process to the patient taking lithium, carbamazepine, and valproic acid.

OUTLINE

KEY TERMS

Antidepressants are used for depressive episodes accompanied by feelings of hopelessness and helplessness. They can be prescribed for 1 month to 12 months or perhaps longer.

Mood-stabilizer agents such as lithium are effective for bipolar disorder. Drug therapy for treating bipolar disorder is discussed in this chapter.

DEPRESSION

Depression is the most common mental illness, affecting approximately 14.8 million Americans. Fewer than 50% of individuals with depression seek treatment despite the fact that about 70% of individuals with depression have a full remission with effective treatment. Women between the ages of 25 and 45 years are two to three times more likely than men to experience major depression. Depression is characterized primarily by mood changes and loss of interest in normal activities and is second only to hypertension as the most common chronic clinical condition.

Contributing causes of depression include genetic predisposition, social and environmental factors, and biologic conditions. Some signs of major depression include loss of interest in most activities, depressed mood, weight loss or gain, insomnia or hypersomnia, loss of energy, fatigue, feelings of despair, decreased ability to think or concentrate, and suicidal thoughts. Approximately 66% of all suicides are related to depression. Depressed men, especially older Causcasian men, are more likely to commit suicide successfully than are depressed women. Antidepressants can mask suicidal ideation.

The three types of depression are (1) *reactive*, (2) *major*, and (3) *bipolar disorder*, previously referred to as *manic depression*. Reactive depression usually has a sudden onset after a precipitating event (e.g., depression resulting from a loss, such as death of a loved one). The patient knows why he or she is depressed and may call this "the blues." Usually, this type of depression lasts for months, and a benzodiazepine agent may be prescribed. *Major depression* is characterized by loss of interest in work and home, inability to concentrate and complete tasks, difficulty sleeping or excessive sleeping, feelings of fatigue and worthlessness, and deep depression, also known as dysphoria. Major depression can be either *primary*, unrelated to other health problems, or *secondary* to a health problem such as a physical or psychiatric disorder or drug use. Antidepressants have been effective in treating major depression. Bipolar disorder involves swings between two moods, the manic (euphoric) and the depressive (dysphoric); lithium was originally the drug of choice for treating this type of disorder. Other mood stabilizers such as carbamazepine; valproic acid, or divalproex; and lamotrigine are also currently first-line drugs of choice for bipolar disorder.

Pathophysiology

Many theories exist as to the cause of major depression. A common one suggests an insufficient amount of brain monoamine neurotransmitters (norepinephrine, serotonin, perhaps dopamine). It is thought that decreased levels of serotonin permit depression to occur, and decreased levels of norepinephrine cause depression. However, there can be other physiologic causes of depression, and social and environmental factors play a role.

Complementary and Alternative Therapy for Depression

St. John's wort and *Gingko biloba* have been suggested for the management of mild depression, but these should not be taken along with prescription antidepression medications. St. John's wort can decrease reuptake of the neurotransmitters serotonin, norepinephrine, and dopamine. The use of these and many complementary and alternative products should be discontinued 1 to 2 weeks before surgery. The patient should check with a health care provider regarding complementary and alternative therapies (Complementary and Alternative Therapies 23.1).

> ### COMPLEMENTARY AND ALTERNATIVE THERAPIES 23.1
> *Selective Serotonin Reuptake Inhibitors*
>
> - Feverfew may interfere with SSRI antidepressants such as fluoxetine.
> - St. John's wort interacts with SSRIs, which may cause serotonin syndrome (dizziness, headache, sweating, and agitation).

ANTIDEPRESSANT AGENTS

Antidepressants are divided into five groups: (1) tricyclic antidepressants (TCAs), or tricyclics; (2) selective serotonin reuptake inhibitors (SSRIs); (3) serotonin norepinephrine reuptake inhibitors (SNRIs); (4) atypical antidepressants that affect various neurotransmitters; and (5) monoamine oxidase inhibitors (MAOIs). TCAs and MAOIs were marketed in the late 1950s, and many of the SSRIs and atypical antidepressants were available in the 1980s. The SSRIs and SNRIs are popular antidepressants because they do not cause sedation, hypotension, anticholinergic effects, or cardiotoxicity as do many of the TCAs. However, users of SSRIs can experience sexual dysfunction, but this can be managed. With unpleasant side effects or lack of improvement, the patient is usually changed to another category of drug.

Tricyclic Antidepressants

Tricyclic antidepressants (TCAs) are used to treat major depression because they are effective and are less expensive than SSRIs and other drugs. Imipramine was the first TCA marketed in the 1950s.

The action of TCAs is to block the uptake of the neurotransmitters norepinephrine and serotonin in the brain. The clinical response of TCAs occurs after 2 to 4 weeks of drug therapy. If there is no improvement after 2 to 4 weeks, the antidepressant is slowly withdrawn and another antidepressant is prescribed. *Polydrug therapy*, the practice of giving several antidepressants or antipsychotics together, should be avoided if possible because of potential serious side effects.

The effectiveness of TCAs in treating major depression is well documented. This group of drugs elevates mood, increases interest in daily living and activity, and decreases insomnia. For agitated depressed persons, amitriptyline, doxepin, or trimipramine may be prescribed because of their highly sedative effect. TCAs are often given at night to minimize problems caused by their sedative action. When discontinuing TCAs, the drugs should be gradually decreased to avoid withdrawal symptoms such as nausea, vomiting, anxiety, and akathisia. Imipramine hydrochloride is used for the treatment of enuresis (involuntary discharge of urine during sleep in children).

The TCA drugs include amitriptyline, imipramine, trimipramine, doxepin, desipramine, nortriptyline, and protriptyline. The TCA drugs desipramine and nortriptyline are major metabolites of imipramine and amitriptyline.

> **Pharmacokinetics** Amitriptyline is strongly protein bound. The half-life is 10 to 50 hours, and a cumulative drug effect may result. Amitriptyline is primarily excreted in urine.
> **Pharmacodynamics** Amitriptyline is well absorbed, but antidepressant effects develop slowly over several weeks. The onset of the antidepressant effect of amitriptyline is 1 to 3 weeks, and the peak concentration is 2 to 5 hours. Drug doses are decreased for older patients to reduce side effects.

Side Effects and Adverse Reactions

The TCAs have many side effects: orthostatic hypotension, sedation, anticholinergic effects, cardiotoxicity, and seizures. Rising from a sitting position too rapidly can cause dizziness and lightheadedness (*orthostatic hypotension*), so the patient should be instructed to rise slowly to an upright position. The TCAs block the histamine receptors, thus sedation is likely to occur initially but decreases with continuous use of the drug. Because TCAs block the cholinergic receptors, they can cause anticholinergic effects such as tachycardia, urinary retention, constipation, dry mouth, and blurred vision. Other side effects of TCAs include allergic reactions (skin rash, pruritus, and petechiae) and sexual dysfunction (erectile dysfunction and amenorrhea). Most TCAs can cause blood dyscrasias (leukopenia, thrombocytopenia, and agranulocytosis) that require close monitoring of blood cell counts. Amitriptyline may lead to symptoms of extrapyramidal syndrome (EPS).

Clomipramine can cause neuroleptic malignant syndrome (NMS). Because the seizure threshold is decreased by TCAs, patients with seizure disorders may need TCA dose adjustment. The most serious adverse reaction to TCAs is cardiotoxicity, such as dysrhythmias that may result from high doses of the drug. The therapeutic serum range of TCAs should be monitored.

Drug Interactions

Alcohol, hypnotics, sedatives, and barbiturates potentiate central nervous system (CNS) depression when taken with TCAs. Concurrent use of MAOIs with amitriptyline may lead to cardiovascular instability and toxic psychosis. Antithyroid medications taken with amitriptyline may increase the risk of dysrhythmias.

Selective Serotonin Reuptake Inhibitors

Selective serotonin reuptake inhibitors (SSRIs) block the reuptake of serotonin into the nerve terminal of the CNS, thereby enhancing its transmission at the serotonergic synapse. These drugs do *not* block the uptake of dopamine or norepinephrine, and they do *not* block cholinergic and alpha$_1$-adrenergic receptors. SSRIs are more commonly used to treat depression than are TCAs, and they have fewer side effects than TCAs.

The primary use of SSRIs is for major depressive disorders. They are also effective for treating anxiety disorders such as obsessive-compulsive disorder (OCD), panic disorders, phobias, posttraumatic stress disorder (PTSD), and other forms of anxiety. Fluvoxamine is useful for treating OCD in children and adults. SSRIs have also been used to treat eating disorders and selected drug abuses. Miscellaneous uses for SSRIs include decreasing premenstrual tension syndrome, preventing migraine headaches, and preventing or minimizing aggressive behavior in patients with borderline personality disorder.

The SSRIs include fluoxetine, fluvoxamine, sertraline, paroxetine, citalopram, and escitalopram. Fluoxetine has been effective in 50% to 60% of patients who fail to respond to TCA therapy (*TCA-refractory depression*). The U.S. Food and Drug Administration (FDA) approved a weekly delayed-release fluoxetine dose of 90 mg. However, before taking the weekly dose, the patient should respond to a daily maintenance dose of 20 mg/day without serious effects.

Many SSRIs have an interaction with grapefruit juice that can lead to possible toxicity. It is recommended that daily intake be limited to 8 ounces of grapefruit juice or one half of a grapefruit.

Prototype Drug Chart 23.1 describes the drug characteristics of the SSRI fluoxetine.

> **Pharmacokinetics** Fluoxetine is strongly protein bound, and the half-life is 4 to 6 days; therefore a cumulative drug effect may result from long-term use. Fluoxetine is metabolized and excreted by the kidneys.
>
> **Pharmacodynamics** Fluoxetine is well absorbed; however, its antidepressant effect develops slowly over several weeks. The onset of fluoxetine's antidepressant effect is between 1 and 12

PROTOTYPE DRUG CHART 23.1

Fluoxetine

Drug Class	Dosage
Antidepressant: Selective serotonin reuptake inhibitor Pregnancy category: C*	Regular release: A: PO: Initially 20 mg/d in the morning; *max:* 80 mg/d Delayed release: A: PO: 90 mg/wk; *max:* 90 mg/wk

Contraindications	Drug-Lab-Food Interactions
Hypersensitivity *Caution:* Myocardial infarction, with MAOIs, dehydration, breastfeeding, suicidal ideation, liver disease, osteoporosis, glaucoma, seizure disorder, diabetes mellitus, malnourished, anticoagulant therapy, diarrhea	Drug: Increased effects of CNS and respiratory depression, hypotensive effect with alcohol and CNS depressants; increased bleeding potential with aspirin, NSAIDs, anticoagulants; MAOIs and SSRIs increase risk of serotonin syndrome. Complementary and alternative therapy: St. John's wort increases risk for serotonin syndrome; increased effect of hypoglycemics

Pharmacokinetics	Pharmacodynamics
Absorption: PO: well absorbed Distribution: PB: 94.5% Metabolism: Fluoxetine: t½: 4-6 d Excretion: Excreted primarily in urine	PO: Onset: 3-4 wk Peak: 6-8 h Duration: UK

Therapeutic Effects/Uses
To treat depression, bipolar disorder, bulimia disorder; obsessive-compulsive disorder; panic disorder; and premenstrual dysphoric disorder Mode of Action: Serotonin is increased in nerve cells because of blockage from nerve fibers.

Side Effects	Adverse Reactions
Headache, dizziness, drowsiness, insomnia, anxiety, asthenia, memory impairment, mydriasis, tremors, dry mouth, akathisia, anorexia, nausea, diarrhea, weight loss, erectile dysfunction	Seizures, angioedema, hyponatremia, hypokalemia, hyperkalemia, hypoglycemia, dehydration, bleeding, osteoporosis *Life threatening:* Stevens-Johnson syndrome, hepatic dysfunction, suicidal ideation

*Pregnancy categories have been revised. See http://www.fda.gov/Drugs/DevelopmentApprovalProcess/DevelopmentResources/Labeling/ucm093307.htm for more information.

A, Adult; *CNS*, central nervous system; *d*, day; *MAOI*, monoamine oxidase inhibitor; *max*, maximum; *NSAID*, nonsteroidal antiinflammatory drug; *PB*, protein binding; *PO*, by mouth; *SSRI*, selective serotonin reuptake inhibitor; *t½*, half-life; *UK*, unknown; *wk*, week.

weeks, and peak concentration with consistent therapy is at 6 to 8 hours after ingestion. The drug dose for older adults should be decreased to reduce side effects.

Side Effects and Adverse Reactions

Fluoxetine produces common side effects such as dry mouth, blurred vision, insomnia, headache, nervousness, anorexia, nausea, diarrhea, and suicidal ideation. Fluoxetine has fewer side effects than amitriptyline.

Some patients may experience sexual dysfunction when taking SSRIs. Men have discontinued taking fluoxetine after

PROTOTYPE DRUG CHART 23.2

Venlafaxine

Drug Class	Dosage
Antidepressant: Serotonin norepinephrine reuptake inhibitor Pregnancy category: C*	Immediate release: A: PO: 75 mg/d in 2-3 divided doses; *max:* 225 mg/d for outpatients, 375 mg/d for inpatients Extended release: A: PO: Initially 37.5-75 mg once daily; *max:* 225 mg/d

Contraindications	Drug-Lab-Food Interactions
Hypersensitivity *Caution:* With MAOIs, CNS depression, SIADH, anticoagulant therapy, pregnancy, breastfeeding, in children, suicidal ideation, renal impairment, hepatic disease, bleeding, narrow-angle glaucoma, seizures, malnourishment, hypovolemia, hypokalemia, hyponatremia, hyperthyroidism, MI, heart failure	Drug: Increased effects of CNS, respiratory depression, and hypotensive effect with alcohol and CNS depressants; drug levels and toxicity increase with cimetidine and haloperidol; bleeding is increased with anticoagulants and aspirin; risk of serotonin syndrome and NMS is increased with other SNRIs, SSRIs, serotonin receptor agonists (triptans), and amphetamines. *Life threatening:* Hypertensive crisis and death may occur with MAOIs; St. John's wort may cause serotonin syndrome (tachycardia, hypertension, confusion, twitching, hyperreflexia, and hyperthermia).

Pharmacokinetics	Pharmacodynamics
Absorption: PO: Well absorbed Distribution: PB: 27% Metabolism: t½: 5 h Excretion: Primarily in urine	Immediate release: PO: Onset: UK Peak: 2-4 h Duration: UK Extended release: PO: UK Peak: 5.5 h Duration: UK

Therapeutic Effects/Uses	
To treat depression, generalized anxiety disorder, social anxiety disorder, panic disorder Mode of Action: Serotonin and norepinephrine are increased in nerve cells because of blockage from nerve fibers.	

Side Effects	Adverse Reactions
Drowsiness, dizziness, insomnia, headache, euphoria, amnesia, blurred vision, mydriasis, dry mouth and eyes, excess sweating, weakness, diarrhea, weight loss, nausea, anorexia, constipation	Tachycardia, seizure, hypertension, serotonin syndrome *Life threatening:* Suicidal ideation, NMS, SIADH, renal failure, Stevens-Johnson syndrome

*Pregnancy categories have been revised. See http://www.fda.gov/Drugs/Development
ApprovalProcess/DevelopmentResources/Labeling/ucm093307.htm for more information.

A, Adult; *CNS,* central nervous system; *d,* day; *h,* hour; *MAOI,* monoamine oxidase inhibitor; *max,* maximum; *MI,* myocardial infarction; *NMS,* neuroleptic malignant syndrome; *PB,* protein binding; *PO,* by mouth; *SIADH,* syndrome of inappropriate antidiuretic hormone secretion; *SNRI,* serotonin norepinephrine reuptake inhibitor; *SSRI,* selective serotonin reuptake inhibitor; *t½,* half-life; *UK,* unknown.

experiencing a decrease in sexual arousal. Some women have become anorgasmic while males reported erectile dysfunction and delayed ejaculation when taking paroxetine HCl. The side effects often decrease or cease over the 1- to 4-week period of waiting for the therapeutic effect to emerge.

Serotonin Norepinephrine Reuptake Inhibitors

Venlafaxine was the first of the serotonin norepinephrine reuptake inhibitors (SNRIs) approved for major depression in 1993. SNRIs inhibit the reuptake of serotonin and norepinephrine, increasing availability in the synapse. SNRIs are used for major depression. Other approved uses are for generalized anxiety disorder and social anxiety disorder. Other SNRIs include duloxetine and desvenlafaxine. The concurrent interaction of venlafaxine and St. John's wort may increase the risk of serotonin syndrome and NMS. Prototype Drug Chart 23.2 describes the drug characteristics of venlafaxine.

> Pharmacokinetics Venlafaxine is well absorbed. The protein-binding capacity is 27%, and the half-life is 5 hours. Venlafaxine is mostly excreted in the urine.
> Pharmacodynamics The onset and duration of venlafaxine are unknown. The peak action is 2 to 4 hours for immediate-release tablets and 5.5 hours for extended-release tablets.

Side Effects and Adverse Effects

Side effects for venlafaxine include drowsiness, dizziness, insomnia, headache, euphoria, amnesia, blurred vision, and ejaculation dysfunction. Adverse effects of this drug are hypertension, tachycardia, angioedema, seizures, and suicidal ideation.

Atypical Antidepressants

Atypical antidepressants, or *second-generation antidepressants*, became available in the 1980s and have been used for major depression, reactive depression, and anxiety. They affect one or two of the three neurotransmitters: serotonin, norepinephrine, and dopamine. One of the first atypical antidepressants marketed was amoxapine; others are maprotiline, nefazodone, and trazodone.

Amoxapine and maprotiline are sometimes considered to be TCAs because of their pharmacologic similarities. Atypical antidepressants should *not* be taken with MAOIs and should not be used within 14 days after discontinuing MAOIs. Trazodone may have a potential drug interaction with ketoconazole, ritonavir, and indinavir that may lead to increased trazodone levels and adverse effects.

Monoamine Oxidase Inhibitors

Another group of antidepressants is the monoamine oxidase inhibitors (MAOIs). The enzyme monoamine oxidase (MAO) inactivates norepinephrine, dopamine, epinephrine, and serotonin. By inhibiting MAO, the levels of these neurotransmitters rise. Two forms of MAO enzyme exist in the body: MAO-A and MAO-B. These enzymes are found primarily in the liver and brain. MAO-A inactivates dopamine in the brain, whereas MAO-B inactivates norepinephrine and serotonin.

The MAOIs are nonselective and inhibit both MAO-A and MAO-B. Inhibition of MAO by MAOIs is thought to relieve the symptoms of depression. Four MAOIs are currently prescribed: (1) tranylcypromine sulfate, (2) isocarboxazid, (3) selegiline HCl, and (4) phenelzine sulfate. These MAOIs are detailed in Table 23.1.

For the treatment of depression, MAOIs are as effective as TCAs; however, because of adverse reactions, such as the risk of hypertensive crisis resulting from food and drug interactions, only 1% of patients who take antidepressants take an MAOI. Currently, MAOIs are not the antidepressants of choice and are usually prescribed when the patient does not respond to TCAs

TABLE 23.1   Antidepressants

Drug	Route and Dosage	Uses and Considerations
Tricyclic Antidepressants (TCAs)		
Amitriptyline hydrochloride	A: PO: 50-100 mg/d; *max:* 300 mg/d for inpatients, 150 mg/d for outpatients Older adults: PO: 10-25 mg at bedtime; *max:* 150 mg/d Therapeutic serum range: 120-150 ng/mL	For depression. May cause drowsiness, dizziness, blurred vision, memory impairment, headache, insomnia, orthostatic hypotension, dysrhythmias, dry mouth, excess sweating, constipation, weight gain/loss, lethargy, tremor, paresthesia, seizures, and suicidal ideation. Pregnancy category: C*; PB: 95%; t½: 10-50 h
Clomipramine hydrochloride	A: PO: Initially 25 mg/d, may increase to 100 mg/d in divided doses with meals; after titration, entire dose may be given at bedtime; *max:* 250 mg/d Adol/C >10 y: PO: Initially 25 mg/d, then 3 mg/kg/d; *max:* 200 mg/d	For depression and OCD. Give initially with meals to decrease GI side effects, later, give at bedtime to reduce daytime sedation. May cause tremor, dizziness, drowsiness, headache, visual impairment, insomnia, fatigue, dry mouth, anorexia, nausea, constipation, weight gain, sexual dysfunction, and pseudoparkinsonism, especially in older adults in high doses. Pregnancy category: C*; PB: 97%; t½: 36 h
Desipramine hydrochloride	A: PO: Initially 50-75 mg/d in 2-4 divided doses, increased gradually; maint: 100-200 mg/d; *max:* 300 mg/d for inpatients, 200 mg/d for outpatients Older adults: Initially 25 mg/d at bedtime; maint: 100 mg/d in divided doses; *max:* 150 mg/d Adol: PO: Initially 25-50 mg/d at bedtime; maint: 100 mg/d; *max:* 150 mg/d Therapeutic serum range: 125-300 ng/mL	For depression. Take with food if GI distress occurs. May administer at bedtime to decrease daytime sedation. May cause dizziness, drowsiness, headache, memory impairment, tremor, paresthesia, dry mouth, urinary retention, orthostatic hypotension, and suicidal ideation. Pregnancy category: C*; PB: 90%; t½: 7-60 h
Doxepin hydrochloride	A: PO: Initially 75 mg/d at bedtime; or in 2-3 divided doses; maint: 75-150 mg/d; *max:* 300 mg/d Adol/C >12 y: PO: Initially 25-50 mg/d; *max:* 100 mg/d Therapeutic serum range: 110-250 ng/mL	For depression and anxiety. May cause dizziness, drowsiness, blurred vision, orthostatic hypotension, dry mouth, sexual dysfunction, sleep-related behaviors, and suicidal ideation. Pregnancy category: C*; PB: 80%; t½: 6-8 h
Imipramine hydrochloride	A: PO: Initially 75-100 mg/d; maint: 150-200 mg/d; *max:* 200 mg/d for outpatients, 300 mg/d for inpatients Adol/older adults: Initially 30-40 mg/d at bedtime; maint: 75-100 mg/d; *max:* Adol 100 mg/d, older adults 200 mg/d for outpatients, 300 mg/d for inpatients Therapeutic serum range: 125-250 ng/mL	For depression. Optimal response may take 1-3 weeks. Can be taken at bedtime to lessen dangers from sedative effect. Take with food if GI distress occurs, and avoid taking with alcohol or CNS depressants. May cause dizziness, drowsiness, fatigue, headache, blurred vision, dry mouth, orthostatic hypotension, tremor, urinary retention, seizures, and suicidal ideation. Pregnancy category: UK*; PB: 85%-95%; t½: 8-16 h
Nortriptyline hydrochloride	A: PO: Initially 25-50 mg tid/qid; *max:* 150 mg/d Adol/older adults: PO: Initially 10-25 mg/d at bedtime; maint: 30-50 mg/d; *max:* 150 mg/d Therapeutic serum range: 50-150 ng/mL	For depression. May cause dizziness, drowsiness, headache, fatigue, orthostatic hypotension, dry mouth, seizures, and suicidal ideation. Pregnancy category: C*; PB: 93%-95%; t½: 16-90 h
Protriptyline hydrochloride	A: PO: Initially 5-10 mg tid/qid; *max:* 60 mg/d Older adults: PO: Initially 5 mg or less tid; *max:* 30 mg/d Therapeutic serum range: 70-250 ng/mL	For depression. Has little sedative effect. May cause dizziness, headache, blurred vision, confusion, insomnia, tremor, dry mouth, nausea, orthostatic hypotension, and suicidal ideation. Gradually taper the dose when discontinuing. Pregnancy category: C*; PB: 90%; t½: 54-92 h
Trimipramine maleate	A: Initially 75 mg/d in divided doses; *max:* 200 mg/d for outpatients, 300 mg/d for inpatients Adol/older adults: Initially 50 mg/d in divided doses; *max:* 100 mg/d	For depression. May cause dizziness, drowsiness, fatigue, tremor, headache, dry mouth, orthostatic hypotension, weight gain, and suicidal ideation. Gradually taper the dose when discontinuing. Pregnancy category: C*; PB: 95%; t½: 20-26 h

TABLE 23.1 Antidepressants—cont'd

Drug	Route and Dosage	Uses and Considerations
Selective Serotonin Reuptake Inhibitors (SSRIs)		
Citalopram	A: PO: Initially 20 mg/d, may increase after 1 wk to 40 mg/d; *max:* 40 mg/d A >60 y: PO: 20 mg/d; *max:* 20 mg/d	For depression. Limit to 20 mg daily if concurrently taking omeprazole. Wait 14 days after stopping MAOIs to avoid serotonin syndrome. May cause drowsiness, insomnia, dry mouth, excess sweating, nausea, ejaculation dysfunction, seizures, prolonged QT, and angioedema. Pregnancy category: C*; PB: 80%; t½: 35 h
Fluoxetine hydrochloride	See Prototype Drug Chart 23.1.	
Paroxetine hydrochloride	Depression: Regular-release tablets: A: PO: Initially 20 mg/d; *max:* 50 mg/d Older adults: PO: Initially 10 mg/d; *max:* 40 mg/d Controlled-release tablets: A: PO: Initially 25 mg/d in the morning; *max:* 62.5 mg/d Older adults: PO: Initially 12.5 mg/d; *max:* 50 mg/d	For depression, general anxiety disorder, social anxiety disorder, PTSD, and OCD. May cause dizziness, drowsiness, insomnia, headache, asthenia, dry mouth, nausea, constipation, diarrhea, tremors, orthostatic hypotension, sexual dysfunction, and suicidal ideation. Pregnancy category: D*; PB: 93%-95%; t½: 15-21 h
Sertraline hydrochloride	Depression: A: PO: 25-50 mg/d; *max:* 200 mg/d	For depression, OCD, PTSD, panic disorder, social anxiety disorder. *Do not* take with MAOIs or TCAs. Take with food if GI distress occurs. May cause dizziness, drowsiness, headache, insomnia, nausea, diarrhea, orthostatic hypotension, and Stevens-Johnson syndrome. Pregnancy category: C*; PB: 98%; t½: 26 h
Fluvoxamine	OCD: Adol/A: PO: Initially 50 mg/d at bedtime; maint: 100-200 mg/d; *max:* 300 mg/d Adol 12-17 y: PO: 25 mg/d at bedtime; *max:* 300 mg/d Extended release: A: PO: 100 mg/d at bedtime; maint: 100-300 mg/d; *max:* 300 mg/d	For OCD and social anxiety disorder. May cause dizziness, drowsiness, headache, insomnia, dry mouth, asthenia, anorexia, nausea, diarrhea, sexual dysfunction, and Stevens-Johnson syndrome. *Caution:* Do not use in patients with hepatic disorders. Pregnancy category: C*; PB: 80%; t½: 15.6 h immediate release, 16.3 h extended release
Escitalopram	Depression: A: PO: 10 mg/d, may increase to 20 mg/d after 1 wk; *max:* 20 mg/d Older adults: PO: 10 mg/d; *max:* 10 mg/d Adol/C >12 y: PO: 10 mg/d; *max:* 20 mg/d	For depression and generalized anxiety disorder. May cause drowsiness, headache, insomnia, nausea, orthostatic hypotension, ejaculation dysfunction, agranulocytosis, and Stevens-Johnson syndrome. Pregnancy category: C*; PB: 56%; t½: 27-32 h
Vilazodone	A: PO: Initially 10 mg/d for 1 wk; maint: 20-40 mg/d with food; *max:* 40 mg/d	For depression. Common side effects include dizziness, headache, dry mouth, insomnia, nausea, diarrhea, serotonin syndrome, and suicidal ideation. Pregnancy category: C*; PB: 96%-99%; t½: 25 h
Nefazodone	A: PO: Initially 100 mg bid; maint: 300-600 mg/d; *max:* 600 mg/d Older adult: Initially 50 mg bid; maint: 300-600 mg/d in 2 divided doses; *max:* 600 mg/d	For depression. May cause headache, drowsiness, dizziness, insomnia, blurred vision, dry mouth, weakness, infection, nausea, diarrhea, constipation, and suicidal ideation. Pregnancy category: C*; PB: 99%; t½: 1.5-2 h
Trazodone hydrochloride	Immediate release: A: PO: Initially 150 mg/d in divided doses; *max:* 400 mg/d for outpatients, 600 mg/d for inpatients Older A: PO: Initially 25-50 mg at bedtime, *maint:* 75-150 mg/d; *max:* 400 mg/d for outpatients, 600 mg/d for inpatients Extended release: A: PO: Initially 150 mg/d at bedtime, *max:* 375 mg/d	For depression. Can be taken at bedtime to lessen dangers from sedative effect. May cause drowsiness, dizziness, blurred vision, headache, insomnia, fatigue, dry mouth, orthostatic hypotension, tachycardia, nausea, vomiting, and suicidal ideation. Take with food to decrease GI distress. Pregnancy category: C*; PB: 85%-95%; t½: 9-13 h
Vortioxetine	A: PO: Initially 10 mg/d; maint: 5-20 mg/d; *max:* 20 mg/d	For depression. May cause dizziness, dry mouth, nausea, diarrhea, sexual dysfunction, and suicidal ideation. Gradually taper off upon discontinuation. Contraindicated within 14 days of an MAOI. Pregnancy category: C*; PB: 98%; t½: 66 h
Atypical (Second-Generation) Antidepressants		
Amoxapine	A/adol >16 y: PO: Initially 50 mg bid/tid; *max:* 400 mg/d for outpatients, 600 mg/d for inpatients Older adults: PO: 25 mg bid/tid; *max:* 300 mg/d	For depression. May cause drowsiness, dizziness, dry mouth, increased appetite, constipation, EPS, and suicidal ideation. Do *not* take with MAOIs or TCAs. Taper off gradually when discontinuing. Pregnancy category: C*; PB: >90%; t½: 6.5-30 h
Maprotiline hydrochloride	A: PO: Initially 25 mg tid or 75 mg at bedtime; *max:* 225 mg/d for inpatients, 150 mg/d for outpatients Older adults: Initially 25 mg at bedtime; maint: 50-75 mg/d; *max:* 225 mg/d for inpatients, 150 mg/d for outpatients	For depression. May cause dizziness, drowsiness, dry mouth, seizures, and suicidal ideation. Gradually taper off when discontinuing. Pregnancy category: B*; PB: 88%; t½: 27-58 h

Continued

TABLE 23.1   Antidepressants—cont'd

Drug	Route and Dosage	Uses and Considerations
Norepinephrine Dopamine Reuptake Inhibitors (NDRIs)		
Bupropion hydrochloride	Depression: Immediate release: A: PO: Initially 100 mg bid; *max:* 450 mg/d, 150 mg/dose Sustained release: A: PO: Initially 150 mg/d in the morning; maint: 200 mg bid; *max:* 400 mg/d, 200 mg single dose Extended release: A: PO: 150 mg/d in the morning; *max:* 450 mg/d	For depression, seasonal affective disorder, and nicotine withdrawal. May cause dizziness, insomnia, lethargy, headache, blurred vision, dry mouth, diaphoresis, agitation, tachycardia, weight loss, and suicidal ideation. Avoid use in patients with a history of seizures. Gradually taper off when discontinuing. Pregnancy category: C*; PB: 84%; t½: 8-24 h immediate release, 20-37 h sustained and extended release
Miscellaneous Antidepressants		
Mirtazapine	A: PO: Initially 15 mg at bedtime; maint: 15-45 mg/d; *max:* 45 mg/d Older adults: PO: Initially 7.5 mg at bedtime, then 15-30 mg/d; *max:* 45 mg/d	For depression. May cause dizziness, drowsiness, restlessness, increased appetite, dry mouth, constipation, weight gain, hypercholesterolemia, and suicidal ideation. Pregnancy category: C*; PB: 85%; t½: 20-40 h
Serotonin Norepinephrine Reuptake Inhibitors (SNRIs)		
Desvenlafaxine	Extended release: A: PO: Initially 50 mg/d; *max:* 400 mg/d	For depression. May cause dizziness, drowsiness, insomnia, dry mouth, nausea, excess sweating, fatigue, withdrawal, and suicidal ideation. Taper off gradually over 2 to 3 weeks. Pregnancy category: C*; PB: 30%; t½: 11 h
Duloxetine	Depression: A: PO: Initially 20 mg/d; maint: 60 mg/d; *max:* 120 mg/d	For major depression, diabetic neuropathy, fibromyalgia, generalized anxiety disorder, musculoskeletal pain, and osteoarthritis. May cause dizziness, drowsiness, headache, insomnia, anxiety, asthenia, dry mouth, anorexia, nausea, constipation, and suicidal ideation. Wait 14 days after stopping MAOIs to use this drug. Gradually taper off when discontinuing. Pregnancy category: C*; PB: 90%; t½: 9.2-19.1 h
Venlafaxine	See Prototype Drug Chart 23.2.	
Levomilnacipran	A: PO: Initially 20 mg/d for 2 d, then 40 mg/d; maint: 40-120 mg/d; *max:* 120 mg/d	For depression. May cause orthostatic hypotension, excess sweating, nausea, constipation, and suicidal ideation. Contraindicated within 14 d of MAOI use. Gradually taper off when discontinuing. Pregnancy category: C*; PB: 22%; t½: 12 h
Monoamine Oxidase Inhibitors (MAOIs)		
Isocarboxazid	A/adol >16 y: PO: Initially 10 mg bid; maint: 40 mg/d in divided doses; *max:* 60 mg/d	For depression. May cause dizziness, headache, dry mouth, weight gain, seizure, withdrawal, and suicidal ideation. Avoid tyramine-rich foods such as cheese, sour cream, wine, beer, figs, cured meat (sausage, salami), soy sauce, anchovies, shrimp, raisins, raspberries, bananas, and chocolate, and avoid drugs such as TCAs. Antidepressant effect may take 1-6 weeks. Taper off gradually when discontinuing. Pregnancy category: C*; PB: UK; t½: 2.5 h
Phenelzine sulfate	A/adol >16 y: PO: Initially 15 mg tid; maint: 60-90 mg/d; *max:* 90 mg/d	For depression. May cause dizziness, drowsiness, headache, blurred vision, nystagmus, edema, ejaculation dysfunction, orthostatic hypotension, hypertensive crisis, and suicidal ideation. Avoid tyramine-rich foods. Gradually taper off when discontinuing. Pregnancy category: UK*; PB: UK; t½: 12 h
Tranylcypromine sulfate	A: PO: Initially 15 mg bid; *max:* 60 mg/d	For depression. May cause dizziness, insomnia, blurred vision, constipation, orthostatic hypotension, peripheral edema, weight gain, erectile dysfunction, withdrawal, and suicidal ideation. Avoid tyramine-rich foods. Pregnancy category: C*; PB: UK; t½: 2.5 h
Selegiline hydrochloride	Depression: A: PO: 7.5 mg/d; *max:* 10 mg/d A: Transdermal: 6 mg/d; *max:* 12 mg/d	For depression and parkinsonism. May cause dizziness, dry mouth, confusion, nausea, orthostatic hypotension, impulse control disorder, and suicidal ideation. Avoid tyramine-rich foods. Taper off gradually when discontinuing. Pregnancy category: C*; PB: 85%; t½: PO 10 h, transdermal 18-25 h

TABLE 23.1 Antidepressants—cont'd

Drug	Route and Dosage	Uses and Considerations
Mood Stabilizers		
Lithium citrate	See Prototype Drug Chart 23.3.	
Carbamazepine	Bipolar disorder: Extended-release capsule: A:PO: Initially 200 mg bid; *max:* 1600 mg/d Therapeutic serum level: 4-12 mcg/mL	For bipolar disorder, seizures, neuropathic pain, trigeminal neuralgia. Contraindicated in bone marrow depression. May cause dizziness, drowsiness, headache, blurred vision, ataxia, pruritus, nausea, vomiting, weakness, anemia, agranulocytosis, and suicidal ideation. Gradually taper off when discontinuing. Pregnancy category: D*; PB: 76%; t½: 25-65 h
Divalproex	Bipolar disorder: Delayed release: A: PO: Initially 750 mg/d in divided doses; *max:* 3000 mg/d or 60 mg/kg/d Extended release: A: PO: Initially 25 mg/kg/d; *max:* 60 mg/kg/d Therapeutic range: 50-100 mcg/mL	For bipolar disorder, seizures, and migraine prophylaxis. May cause dizziness, drowsiness, insomnia, asthenia, blurred vision, nausea, vomiting, diarrhea, thrombocytopenia, and suicidal ideation. Give with food to avoid GI distress. Pregnancy category: C*; PB: 90%; t½: 6-16 h
Lamotrigine	Bipolar disorder: A: PO: Initially 25 mg/d for 2 wk, then 50 mg/d for 2 wk, then 100 mg/d for 1 wk; thereafter give 200 mg/d	For bipolar disorder, seizures, Lennox-Gastaut syndrome. May cause dizziness, drowsiness, blurred vision, pharyngitis, nausea, vomiting, ataxia, and Stevens-Johnson syndrome. Pregnancy category: C*; PB: 55%; t½ 14-59 h
Cariprazine	Bipolar disorder: A: PO: Initially 1.5 mg/d; day 2 give 3 mg/d; maint: 1.5-6 mg/d; *max:* 6 mg/d	For bipolar disorder and schizophrenia. May cause insomnia, dizziness, headache, dry mouth, restlessness, weight gain, nausea, constipation, EPS, and suicidal ideation. Pregnancy category: UK*; PB: 91%-97%; t½: 2-4 d
Aripiprazole	Bipolar disorder: A: PO: Initially 15 mg/d; *max:* 30 mg/d Adol/C >10 y: PO: Initially 2 mg/d; *max:* 30 mg/d	For bipolar disorder, schizophrenia, autism, depression, Tourette syndrome. May cause drowsiness, fatigue, headache, anxiety, agitation, insomnia, EPS, nausea, vomiting, hyperglycemia, and suicidal ideation. Pregnancy category: UK*; PB: 99%; t½: 75 h, extended release 30-47 d

*Pregnancy categories have been revised. See http://www.fda.gov/Drugs/DevelopmentApprovalProcess/DevelopmentResources/Labeling/ucm093307.htm for more information.
>, Greater than; *A*, adult; *adol*, adolescent; *bid*, twice a day; *C*, child; *CNS*, central nervous system; *d*, day; *EPS*, extrapyramidal syndrome symptoms; *GI*, gastrointestinal; *h*, hour; *maint*, maintenance; *MAOI*, monoamine oxidase inhibitor; *max*, maximum; *OCD*, obsessive-compulsive disorder; *PB*, protein binding; *PO*, by mouth; *PTSD*, posttraumatic stress disorder; *qid*, four times a day; *t½*, half-life; *tid*, three times a day; *TCA*, tricyclic antidepressant; *UK*, unknown; *wk*, week(s); *y*, year.

or second-generation antidepressants. However, MAOIs are still used for mild, reactive, and atypical depression (chronic anxiety, hypersomnia, fear). MAOIs and TCAs should not be taken together when treating depression.

Drug and Food Interactions

Certain drug and food interactions with MAOIs can be fatal. Any drugs that are CNS stimulants or sympathomimetics, such as vasoconstrictors and cold medications that contain phenylephrine and pseudoephedrine, can cause a hypertensive crisis when taken with an MAOI. In addition, foods that contain tyramine—aged cheese (cheddar, Swiss, bleu), cream, yogurt, coffee, chocolate, bananas, raisins, Italian green beans, liver, pickled foods, sausage, soy sauce, yeast, beer, and red wines—have sympathomimetic-like effects and can cause a hypertensive crisis. MAOI users *must avoid* these types of food and drugs. Frequent blood pressure monitoring is essential, and patient teaching regarding foods and over-the-counter (OTC) drugs to avoid is an important nursing responsibility. Because of the danger associated with hypertensive crisis, many psychiatrists will not prescribe MAOIs for depression unless other drugs have failed to be effective for the patient. However, this group of drugs is effective for treating depression if taken properly.

In teaching patients about the foods and drugs to avoid when taking MAOIs, some individuals respond better to verbal instructions and education with reinforcement from videos than to printed communications. Complementary and Alternative Therapies 23.2 details complementary and alternative therapy interactions with MAOIs.

Side Effects and Adverse Reactions

Side effects of MAOIs include CNS stimulation (agitation, restlessness, and insomnia), orthostatic hypotension, and anticholinergic effects.

COMPLEMENTARY AND ALTERNATIVE THERAPIES 23.2

Monoamine Oxidase Inhibitors

- Ginseng, ephedra (Ma-huang), and St. John's wort may lead to palpitations, heart attack, and hypertensive crisis when taken with antidepressant MAOIs.
- Ginseng may lead to manic episodes when taken in combination with MAOIs such as tranylcypromine sulfate.
- An excessive dose of anise may interfere with MAOIs.
- An increased use of brewer's yeast with MAOIs can increase blood pressure.

 NURSING PROCESS

Patient-Centered Collaborative Care

Antidepressants

Assessment

- Assess the patient's baseline vital signs and weight for future comparisons. TCAs should be avoided in patients with cardiovascular disease and hypertension and should be used cautiously in patients with seizure disorders.
- Note the patient's hepatic and renal function by assessing urine output (>1500 mL/day), blood urea nitrogen (BUN), and serum creatinine and hepatic enzyme levels.
- Obtain a health history of episodes of depression; assess mental status, and assess for suicidal tendencies.
- Secure a drug history of the current drugs, alcohol, and herbs the patient is taking. CNS depressants can cause an additive effect. Antidepressants that cause anticholinergic-like symptoms are contraindicated if a patient has glaucoma.
- Assess for tardive dyskinesia and NMS, including hyperpyrexia, muscle rigidity, tachycardia, and cardiac dysrhythmias.

Nursing Diagnoses

- Self-Directed Violence, Risk for
- Anxiety related to situational crises
- Social Isolation related to feelings of sadness
- Coping, Ineffective related to negative thought patterns
- Hopelessness related to feelings of despair
- Knowledge, Deficient related to inexperience with medication
- Health Maintenance, Impaired related to lack of interest

Planning

- Patient's depression or bipolar behavior will be decreased.

Nursing Interventions

- Observe patients for signs and symptoms of depression: mood changes, insomnia, apathy, or lack of interest in activities.
- Monitor vital signs. Orthostatic hypotension is common. Check for anticholinergic-like symptoms such as dry mouth, increased heart rate, urinary retention, and constipation. Check weight two to three times per week.

- Monitor patients for suicidal tendencies when marked depression is present.
- Observe patients for seizures when anticonvulsants are taken; antidepressants lower the seizure threshold, and the anticonvulsant dose might need to be increased.
- Monitor for drug-drug and food-drug interactions. Sympathomimetic-like drugs and foods that contain tyramine may cause a hypertensive crisis if taken with MAOIs.
- Check patients for extremely high blood pressure when taking MAOIs.
- Provide patients with a list of foods to avoid when taking MAOIs to avoid hypertensive crisis. These foods include cheese, red wine, beer, liver, bananas, yogurt, and sausage.

Patient Teaching

General

- Teach patients to take the medication as prescribed. Compliance is important.
- Inform patients that full effectiveness of a drug may not be evident until 1 to 2 weeks after the start of therapy.
- Encourage patients to keep medical appointments.
- Caution patients not to consume alcohol or any CNS depressants because of their addictive effect.
- Inform patients that many complementary and alternative therapy products interact with antidepressants, especially MAOIs and SSRIs. Complementary and alternative therapies may need to be discontinued, or the antidepressant drug dosage may need to be modified (see Complementary and Alternative Therapies 23.1 and 23.2).
- Warn patients not to drive or be involved in potentially dangerous mechanical activity until stabilization of the drug dose has been established.
- Advise patients not to abruptly stop taking the drug. The drug dose should be gradually decreased by a health care provider.
- Encourage patients planning pregnancy to consult with a health care provider about possible teratogenic effects of the drug on the fetus.
- Advise patients to take the drug with food if gastrointestinal (GI) distress occurs.

Side Effects

- Advise patients that antidepressants may be taken at bedtime to decrease dangers from the sedative effect, and suggest they check with a health care provider. Transient side effects include nausea, drowsiness, headaches, and nervousness.

 Cultural Considerations

- Explain to Asian patients taking an antipsychotic (such as TCA or lithium) that the dose may need to be decreased. Explain to Hispanic patients that the dose for the antidepressant may be lower than is required for other cultural groups.

Evaluation

- Evaluate the effectiveness of the drug therapy regarding whether a patient's depression is controlled or has ceased.

MOOD STABILIZERS

Mood stabilizers are used to treat bipolar affective disorder. Lithium was the first drug used to manage this disorder. Some refer to lithium as an *antimania drug* effective in controlling manic behavior that arises from underlying bipolar disorder. Lithium has a calming effect but may cause some memory loss and confusion. It controls any evidence of flight of ideas and hyperactivity. If the person stops taking lithium, manic behavior may return. Lithium, carbamazepine, valproic acid or dival-proex, and lamotrigine are currently first-line drugs for bipolar disorder.

Lithium is an inexpensive drug that must be closely monitored, and it has a narrow therapeutic serum range of 0.8 to 1.2 mEq/L. Serum lithium levels greater than 1.5 mEq/L may produce early signs of toxicity. The serum lithium level should be monitored biweekly until the therapeutic level has been obtained, and then it must be monitored at least every 1 to 2 months on the maintenance dose. Serum sodium levels also need to be monitored because lithium tends to deplete sodium. Lithium must be used with caution, if at all, by patients taking diuretics. Prototype Drug Chart 23.3 lists the pharmacologic behavior of lithium.

Pharmacokinetics More than 95% of lithium is absorbed through the GI tract. The half-life of lithium ranges from 18 to 36 hours. Because of its long half-life, cumulative drug action may result. Lithium is metabolized by the liver, and most of the drug is excreted unchanged in the urine.

Pharmacodynamics Lithium is prescribed mostly for the stabilization of bipolar affective disorder. The onset of action is fast, but the patient may not achieve the desired effect for 5 to 6 days. Increased sodium intake increases renal excretion, so the sodium intake needs to be closely monitored. Increased urine output can result in body fluid loss and dehydration, therefore adequate fluid intake of 1 to 2 L should be maintained daily.

Antiseizure drugs such as carbamazepine, lamotrigine, and divalproex/valproic acid have been used in place of lithium for some patients. These agents are further discussed in Chapter 19. The antipsychotic drugs olanzapine, ziprasidone, and aripiprazole are approved to treat acute mania and mixed episodes of bipolar disorder. Antipsychotic drugs are discussed further in Chapter 22.

Side Effects and Adverse Reactions

The many side effects of lithium—dry mouth, thirst, increased urination (loss of water and sodium), weight gain, bloated feeling, metallic taste, and edema of the hands and ankles—can be annoying to the patient. If taken during pregnancy, lithium may have teratogenic effects.

Lithium and nonsteroidal antiinflammatory drugs (NSAIDs) should *not* be given together, as NSAIDs may increase lithium levels. Caffeine and loop diuretics may decrease lithium levels. Lithium should be prescribed with extreme caution for patients who have a cardiovascular disease due to an increased risk of lithium toxicity. Frequent monitoring of lithium levels is necessary. Caution must also be used in patients with thyroid disease, as hypothyroidism may occur.

📄 **PROTOTYPE DRUG CHART 23.3**

Lithium

Drug Class	Dosage
Mood stabilizer	Regular release:
Pregnancy category: D*	A/adol/C >12 y: PO: Initially 600 mg tid;
	maint: 900-1800 mg/d in 3-4 divided doses
	Extended release:
	A/adol/C >12 y: PO: 900 mg bid
	Therapeutic drug range: 0.8 -1.2 mEq/L

Contraindications	Drug-Lab-Food Interactions
Hypersensitivity	Drug: May increase lithium level with thiazide
Caution: Hepatic and renal disease, pregnancy, lactation, breastfeeding, cardiac disease, dehydration, hyponatremia, hypokalemia, children, older adults, hypertension, infection, bradycardia, thyroid disease, seizure disorder, alcoholism	diuretics, methyldopa, haloperidol, NSAIDs, antidepressants, carbamazepine, calcium channel blockers, spironolactone, ACE inhibitors, sodium bicarbonate, phenothiazines; may increase lithium excretion with theophylline, aminophylline; may increase risk of serotonin syndrome with SSRIs and SNRIs; may increase hyperglycemia with antidiabetics; caffeine may decrease lithium levels, and CNS stimulants and direct renin inhibitors may increase risk of mania.
	Lab: Increased urine and blood glucose, protein; decreased serum sodium level
	Food: Increase sodium intake; lithium may cause sodium depletion
	Complementary and alternative therapy: Use of St. John's wort, kava kava, and valerian may lead to neurotoxicity.

Pharmacokinetics	Pharmacodynamics
Absorption: PO: Well absorbed	PO: Onset: UK
	Peak: 0.5-3 h
Distribution: PB: UK	Duration: 24 h
Metabolism: t½: 18-36	Extended release:
Excretion: 98% in urine, mostly unchanged	Onset: UK
	Peak: 4-12 h
	Duration: UK

Therapeutic Effects/Uses
To treat bipolar disorder, manic episodes
Mode of Action: Alteration of ion transport in muscle and nerve cells; increased receptor sensitivity to serotonin

Side Effects	Adverse Reactions
Headache, memory impairment, blurred vision, metallic taste, thirst, dry mouth, dental caries, drowsiness, dizziness, ataxia, tremors, anorexia, nausea, vomiting, diarrhea, polyuria, dehydration, hypotension, abdominal pain, restlessness, erectile dysfunction, weight gain/loss, abnormally dry skin	Urinary and fecal incontinence, hyperglycemia, proteinurea, leukocytosis, nephrotoxicity
	Life threatening: Cardiac dysrhythmias, seizures, angioedema, cardiac arrest, serotonin syndrome, neuroleptic malignant syndrome

*Pregnancy categories have been revised. See http://www.fda.gov/Drugs/DevelopmentApprovalProcess/DevelopmentResources/Labeling/ucm093307.htm for more information.
A, Adult; *ACE*, angiotensin-converting enzyme; *adol*, adolescent; *bid*, twice a day; *C*, child; *CNS*, central nervous system; *d*, day; *h*, hour; *maint*, maintenance; *NSAID*, nonsteroidal antiinflammatory drug; *PB*, protein binding; *PO*, by mouth; *SNRI*, serotonin norepinephrine reuptake inhibitor; *SSRI*, selective serotonin reuptake inhibitor; *t½*, half-life; *tid*, three times a day; *UK*, unknown; *y*, year; *>*, greater than.

NURSING PROCESS
Patient-Centered Collaborative Care

Mood Stabilizer: Lithium

Assessment
- Assess for suicidal ideation.
- Assess baseline vital signs for future comparisons.
- Evaluate neurologic status, including gait, level of consciousness, reflexes, and tremors.
- Note hepatic and renal function by assessing urine output (>600 mL/day) and whether BUN and serum creatinine and liver enzyme levels are within normal range. Assess for toxicity. Draw weekly blood levels initially and then every 1 to 2 months. Therapeutic serum levels for lithium are 0.8 to 1.2 mEq/L. Signs and symptoms of serum levels above 1.5 mEq/L are nausea and vomiting, diarrhea, ataxia, blurred vision, confusion, and tremors. Above 2.5 mEq/L, signs and symptoms of toxicity progress to include seizures, cardiac dysrhythmias, coma, and permanent neurologic impairment. At 3.5 mEq/L or higher, signs of toxicity are potentially lethal. Withhold medication and notify a health care provider immediately if any of these occur.
- Obtain a health history of episodes of depression or manic-depressive behavior.
- Obtain a drug history. Diuretics, tetracyclines, methyldopa, probenecid, and NSAIDs such as ibuprofen decrease renal clearance of lithium, causing drug accumulation.

Nursing Diagnoses
- Injury, Risk for
- Coping, Ineffective related to manic behavior
- Noncompliance related to lack of adequate education regarding lithium

Planning
- The patient's manic-depressive behavior will be decreased.

Nursing Interventions
- Observe patients for signs and symptoms of depression: mood changes, insomnia, apathy, or lack of interest in activities.
- Monitor vital signs. Hypotension is common.
- Draw blood samples for lithium levels immediately before the next dose (8 to 12 hours after the previous dose).
- ⚡ Monitor for signs of lithium toxicity. Report high (>1.5 mEq/L) serum lithium levels immediately to a health care provider.
- ⚡ Monitor patients for suicidal tendencies when marked depression is present.
- Evaluate urine output and body weight. Fluid volume deficit may occur as a result of polyuria.
- Observe patients for fine- and gross-motor tremors and presence of slurred speech, which are signs of adverse reaction.
- Assist patients in conserving energy when in a manic phase.
- Check cardiac status. Loss of fluids and electrolytes may cause cardiac dysrhythmias.
- Monitor serum electrolytes, and report abnormal findings.

Patient Teaching
General
- Teach patients to take lithium as prescribed. Emphasize the importance of adherence to the therapy, laboratory tests, and follow-up visits with a health care provider. If lithium is stopped, manic symptoms will reappear.
- Encourage patients to keep medical appointments. Have patients check with a health care provider before taking OTC preparations.
- Warn patients not to drive a motor vehicle or engage in potentially dangerous mechanical activity until a stable lithium level is established.
- Advise patients to maintain adequate fluid intake (2 to 3 L/day initially and 1 to 2 L/day maintenance). Fluid intake should increase in hot weather.
- Teach patients to take lithium with meals to decrease gastric irritation.
- Inform patients that effectiveness of the drug may not be evident until 1 to 2 weeks after the start of therapy. Compliance in taking the prescribed lithium doses on a daily basis is a major problem with bipolar patients. Sometimes, when a patient has a period of emotional stability, he or she does not believe that the drug is needed and may stop taking the lithium.
- Advise patients planning pregnancy to consult with a health care provider about possible teratogenic effects of the drug on the fetus, especially during the first 3 months.
- Encourage patients to wear or carry an identification tag or bracelet indicating the drug taken.

Diet
- Advise patients to avoid caffeine products (coffee, tea, cola) because they can aggravate the manic phase of bipolar disorder by decreasing lithium levels.
- Advise patients to maintain adequate sodium intake and to avoid crash diets that affect physical and mental health.

Side Effects
- Advise patients to contact a health care provider if they experience symptoms of toxicity. Early symptoms include diarrhea, drowsiness, loss of appetite, muscle weakness, nausea, vomiting, slurred speech, and trembling. Late symptoms include blurred vision, confusion, increased urination, convulsions, severe trembling, and unsteadiness.

🌐 Cultural Considerations
- Obtain an interpreter when necessary; do not rely on family members, who may not fully disclose because of honor, shame, or lack of understanding of medical terminology.

Evaluation
- Evaluate the effectiveness of the drug therapy. Patient is free of bipolar behavior.
- Allow patients to verbalize their understanding of symptoms of toxicity.
- Determine whether the patient demonstrates a subsiding or resolution of symptoms.

CRITICAL THINKING CASE STUDY

ST, a 37-year-old woman, is receiving fluoxetine 20 mg in the evening for depression. ST complains of insomnia and GI upset.
1. What could you suggest to ST to help her avoid insomnia? Explain your answer.
2. How might ST avoid GI upset when taking fluoxetine? What food should be avoided?

ST states that she does not think the fluoxetine is helping. She states that she has heard about complementary and alternative therapies that may be taken for depression. She has also heard that fluoxetine can be taken weekly.
3. Is ST's fluoxetine dose within normal dosage range? Explain your answer.
4. How would you respond to ST about the use of certain complementary and alternative therapies for depression?
5. What would your response be concerning the use of fluoxetine in a weekly dose?

NCLEX STUDY QUESTIONS

1. A patient is admitted with bipolar affective disorder. The nurse acknowledges which medication as one used to treat this disorder for some patients in place of lithium?
   a. Thiopental
   b. *Gingko biloba*
   c. Fluvoxamine
   d. Divalproex
2. The nurse realizes that some complementary and alternative therapies interact with selective serotonin reuptake inhibitors. Which complementary and alternative therapy interaction may cause serotonin syndrome?
   a. Feverfew
   b. Ma-huang
   c. St. John's wort
   d. *Gingko biloba*
3. A selective serotonin reuptake inhibitor is prescribed for a patient. The nurse knows that which drug is a selective serotonin reuptake inhibitor?
   a. Paroxetine
   b. Amitriptyline
   c. Divalproex sodium
   d. Bupropion Hydrochloride
4. A patient is taking tranylcypromine sulfate for depression. What advice should the nurse include in the teaching plan for this medication?
   a. Warn the patient about severe hypotension.
   b. Instruct the patient to avoid beer and cheddar cheese.
   c. Encourage the patient to take ginseng and ephedra.
   d. Encourage the patient to eat fruit such as bananas.

5. Which statement is true concerning lithium?
   a. The maximum dose is 3.4 g/day.
   b. The therapeutic drug range is 2.5 to 3.5 mEq/L.
   c. Lithium increases receptor sensitivity to gamma-aminobutyric acid.
   d. Concurrent nonsteroidal antiinflammatory drugs (NSAIDs) may increase lithium levels.
6. When a patient is taking an antidepressant, what should the nurse do? (Select all that apply.)
   a. Monitor the patient for suicidal tendencies.
   b. Observe the patient for orthostatic hypotension.
   c. Teach the patient to take the drug with food if gastrointestinal distress occurs.
   d. Tell the patient that the drug may not have full effectiveness for 1 to 2 weeks.
   e. Advise the patient to maintain adequate fluid intake of 2 L/day.
7. A patient is taking lithium. The nurse should be aware of the importance of which nursing intervention(s)? (Select all that apply.)
   a. Observe the patient for motor tremors.
   b. Monitor the patient for hypotension.
   c. Draw lithium blood levels immediately after a dose.
   d. Advise the patient to drink 750 mL/day of fluid in hot weather.
   e. Advise the patient to avoid caffeinated foods and beverages.
   f. Teach the patient to take lithium with meals to decrease gastric irritation.

Answers: 1, d; 2, c; 3, a; 4, b; 5, d; 6, a, b, c, d; 7, a, b, e, f.

Pain and Inflammation Management Drugs

Inflammation is a reaction to tissue injury caused by the release of chemical mediators that trigger both a vascular response and the migration of fluid and cells—leukocytes, or white blood cells—to the injured site. The chemical mediators are histamines, kinins, and prostaglandins. *Histamine,* the first mediator in the inflammatory process, causes dilation of the arterioles and increases capillary permeability, allowing fluid to leave the capillaries and flow into the injured area. *Kinins,* such as bradykinin, also increase capillary permeability and the sensation of pain. *Prostaglandins* cause an increase in vasodilation, capillary permeability, pain, and fever. Antiinflammatory agents, such as nonsteroidal antiinflammatory drugs (NSAIDs) and

steroids (cortisone preparations), inhibit chemical mediators and thus decrease the inflammatory process. Fig VII.1 illustrates the process of chemical mediators acting on injured tissues. The five responses to tissue injury are called the *cardinal signs of inflammation:* redness, swelling, pain, heat, and loss of function.

Inflammation may or may not be the result of an infection; only a small percentage of inflammations are caused by infection. Other causes of inflammation include trauma, surgical interventions, extreme heat or cold, and caustic chemical agents. Antiinflammatory drugs reduce fluid migration and pain, lessening loss of function and increasing the patient's mobility and comfort.

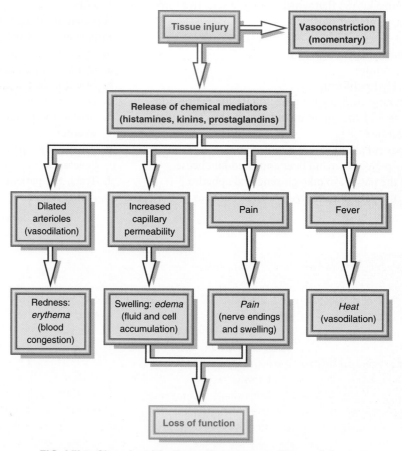

FIG. VII.1 Chemical Mediator Response to Tissue Injury.

24

Antiinflammatories

ⓔ http://evolve.elsevier.com/McCuistion/pharmacology/

OBJECTIVES

- Explain the pathophysiologic basis of the five cardinal signs of inflammation.
- Compare the action of various nonsteroidal antiinflammatory drugs (NSAIDs).
- Explain the use of disease-modifying antirheumatic drugs (DMARDs).

- Differentiate between the side effects and adverse reactions of NSAIDs and DMARDs.
- Correlate the nursing processes associated with NSAIDs and corticosteroids, including patient teaching.
- Apply the nursing process to the patient taking DMARDs.
- Compare the action of various antigout medications.

OUTLINE

KEY TERMS

Inflammation is a response to tissue injury and infection. When the inflammatory process occurs, a vascular reaction takes place in which fluid, elements of blood, leukocytes (white blood cells [WBCs]), and chemical mediators accumulate at the injured tissue or infection site. The process of inflammation is a protective mechanism in which the body attempts to neutralize and destroy harmful agents at the site of injury and to establish conditions for tissue repair.

Although a relationship exists between inflammation and infection, these terms should *not* be used interchangeably. Infection is caused by microorganisms and *results* in inflammation, but not all inflammations are caused by infections.

PATHOPHYSIOLOGY

The five characteristics of inflammation, called *the cardinal signs of inflammation,* are (1) redness, (2) swelling (edema), (3) heat, (4) pain, and (5) loss of function. Table 24.1 gives the description and explanation of the cardinal signs of inflammation. Inflammation also has two phases: the *vascular phase,* which occurs 10 to 15 minutes after an injury, and the *delayed phase.* The vascular phase is associated with vasodilation and increased capillary permeability, during which blood substances and fluid leave the plasma and go to the injured site. The delayed phase occurs when leukocytes infiltrate the inflamed tissue.

TABLE 24.1   Cardinal Signs of Inflammation

Signs	Description and Explanation
Erythema (redness)	Redness occurs in the first phase of inflammation. Blood accumulates in the area of tissue injury because of the release of the body's chemical mediators (kinins, prostaglandins, and histamine). These chemical mediators dilate the arterioles.
Edema (swelling)	Swelling is the second phase of inflammation. Plasma leaks into the interstitial tissue at the injury site. Kinins and histamine increase capillary permeability.
Heat	Heat at the inflammatory site can be caused by increased blood accumulation and may result from pyrogens, substances that produce fever, which interfere with the temperature-regulating center in the hypothalamus.
Pain	Pain is caused by tissue swelling and release of chemical mediators.
Loss of function	Function is lost because of the accumulation of fluid at the tissue injury site and because of pain, which decreases mobility at the affected area.

Various chemical mediators are released during the inflammation process. Among these are **prostaglandins**, chemical mediators that have been isolated from the exudate at inflammatory sites. Prostaglandins have many effects that include vasodilation, relaxation of smooth muscle, increased capillary permeability, and sensitization of nerve cells to pain.

Cyclooxygenase (COX) is the enzyme responsible for converting arachidonic acid into prostaglandins and their products. This synthesis of prostaglandins causes inflammation and pain at a tissue injury site. Cyclooxygenase has two enzyme forms, COX-1 and COX-2. *COX-1* protects the stomach lining and regulates blood platelets, and *COX-2* triggers inflammation and pain.

ANTIINFLAMMATORY AGENTS

Drugs such as aspirin inhibit the biosynthesis of prostaglandin and are therefore called *prostaglandin inhibitors.* Because prostaglandin inhibitors affect the inflammatory process, they are more commonly called *antiinflammatories or antiinflammatory drugs.*

Antiinflammatories also relieve pain (analgesic), reduce elevated body temperature (antipyretic), and inhibit platelet aggregation (anticoagulant). Aspirin is the oldest antiinflammatory drug, but it was first used for its analgesic and antipyretic properties. As a result of searching for a more effective drug with fewer side effects, many other antiinflammatories or prostaglandin inhibitors have been discovered. Although these drugs have potent antiinflammatory effects that mimic the effects of corticosteroids (cortisone), they are *not* chemically related to corticosteroids and therefore are called **nonsteroidal antiinflammatory drugs (NSAIDs).** Most NSAIDs are used to decrease inflammation and pain for patients who have some type of musculoskeletal condition.

NONSTEROIDAL ANTIINFLAMMATORY DRUGS

NSAIDs include aspirin and aspirin-like drugs that inhibit the enzyme COX, which is needed for the biosynthesis of prostaglandins. Chapters 25 and 40 present expanded discussions of NSAIDs in their roles as analgesics and anticoagulants, respectively. These drugs may be called *prostaglandin inhibitors* with varying degrees of analgesic and antipyretic effects, but they are used primarily as antiinflammatories to relieve inflammation and pain. Their antipyretic effect is less than their antiinflammatory effect. With several exceptions, NSAID preparations are not suggested for use in alleviating mild headaches and mildly elevated temperature. Preferred drugs for headaches and fever are aspirin (adults only for fever), acetaminophen, and ibuprofen. NSAIDs are more appropriate for reducing swelling, pain, and stiffness in joints.

Most NSAIDs cost more than aspirin. Other than aspirin, the only NSAIDs that can be purchased over the counter (OTC) are ibuprofen and naproxen. All other NSAIDs require a prescription. Examples of prescription products on the market that contain NSAID contents alone or in combination include celecoxib, meloxicam, oxaprozin, nabumetone, sulindac, and ketorolac. If a patient can take aspirin for the inflammatory process without gastrointestinal (GI) upset, salicylate products are usually recommended.

There are seven groups of NSAIDs:
1. Salicylates
2. *Para*-chlorobenzoic acid derivatives, or indoles
3. Phenylacetic acids
4. Propionic acid derivatives
5. Fenamates
6. Oxicams
7. Selective COX-2 inhibitors

The first six NSAID groups on the list are known as *first-generation NSAIDs,* and the COX-2 inhibitors are called *second-generation NSAIDs.*

Table 24.2 provides dosage information and considerations for use for the most commonly used NSAIDs. The half-lives of NSAIDs differ greatly; some have a short half-life of 2 hours, and others have a moderate to long half-life of 6 to 24 hours. Aspirin should not be taken with an NSAID because of the potentiation of side effects. In addition, combined therapy does not increase effectiveness.

Salicylates

Aspirin comes from the family of salicylates derived from salicylic acid. Aspirin is also called *acetylsalicylic acid (ASA)* after the acetyl group used in its composition. The abbreviation frequently used for aspirin is *ASA.*

Aspirin was developed in 1899 by Adolph Bayer, making it the oldest antiinflammatory agent. It was the most frequently used antiinflammatory agent before the introduction of ibuprofen. Aspirin is a prostaglandin inhibitor that decreases the inflammatory process. It is also considered an antiplatelet drug for patients with cardiac or cerebrovascular disorders; aspirin decreases platelet aggregation, and thus blood clotting is decreased. Because high doses of aspirin are usually needed to relieve inflammation, gastric distress—which includes anorexia,

TABLE 24.2 Antiinflammatory Agents: Nonsteroidal

Drug	Route and Dosage	Uses and Considerations
First-Generation NSAIDs		
Salicylates		
Aspirin	See Prototype Drug Chart 24.1.	
Diflunisal	A/adol: PO: 250-500 mg bid; *max:* 1500 mg/d	For mild to moderate pain, osteoarthritis, and rheumatoid arthritis. Avoid if hypersensitive to aspirin. May cause rash, headache, GI distress, GI bleeding, and elevated hepatic enzymes. Pregnancy category: C*; PB: 99%; t½: 8-12 h
Salicylate Derivatives		
Olsalazine sodium	A: PO: 500 mg q12h; *max:* 3 g/d in divided doses or 1 g/dose	For ulcerative colitis. May cause headache, arthralgia, and GI distress. Pregnancy category: C*; PB: 99%; t½: 1 h
Sulfasalazine	Rheumatoid arthritis: A: PO: Initially 0.5-1 g/d; maint: 2 g/d in 2-3 divided doses; *max:* 3 g/d	For ulcerative colitis and rheumatoid arthritis. Avoid if allergic to sulfonamides or aspirin. May cause dizziness, rash, headache, GI distress, and oligospermia. Pregnancy category: B*; PB: 99%; t½: 5-7 h
Para-Chlorobenzoic Acid (Indoles)		
Indomethacin	Rheumatoid arthritis: Regular release: A: PO: 25 mg bid/tid with food; *max:* 200 mg/d Sustained release: A: PO: 75 mg/d; *max:* 150 mg/d	For mild to severe pain, acute gout, tendinitis, ankylosing spondylitis, and arthritis. May cause dizziness, headache, GI distress, and GI bleeding. Take with food. Avoid if allergic to aspirin. Pregnancy category: C*; PB: 99%; t½: 2.6-11.2 h
Sulindac	Rheumatoid arthritis: A: PO: 150-200 mg bid; *max:* 400 mg/d	For arthritis, bursitis, ankylosing spondylitis, and tendinitis. May cause dizziness, headache, rash, GI distress, elevated hepatic enzymes, and GI bleeding. Take with food or milk. Pregnancy category: C*; PB: 93%; t½: 8 h
Tolmetin	A: PO: Initially: 400 mg tid; maint: 600-1800 mg/d in divided doses; *max:* 1.8 g/d Adol/C >2 y: PO: 20 mg/kg/d in divided doses; *max:* 30 mg/kg/d	For osteoarthritis, rheumatoid arthritis, and juvenile rheumatoid arthritis. May cause dizziness, headache, asthenia, weakness, edema, weight loss/gain, hypertension, GI distress, and stroke. Take with food. Pregnancy category: C, D*; PB: 99%; t½: 1-2 h
Phenylacetic Acid		
Diclofenac sodium	Osteoarthritis: Immediate release: A: PO: 35-50 mg bid/tid; *max:* 150 mg/d Extended release: A: PO: 100 mg/d; *max:* 150 mg/d	For mild to severe pain, rheumatoid arthritis, osteoarthritis, and spondylitis. May cause headache, ocular pain, GI bleeding, and stroke. Take with food. Pregnancy category: C, D*; PB: 99%; t½: 2 h
Etodolac	Arthritis: Regular release: A: PO: Initially 300 mg bid/tid; maint: 600-1200 mg/d; *max:* 1200 mg/d Extended release: A: PO: 400-1000 mg/d; *max:* 1200 mg/d	For mild to moderate pain, rheumatoid arthritis, and osteoarthritis. May cause dizziness, asthenia, GI distress, duodenal ulcers, GI bleeding, and stroke. Take with food. Pregnancy category: C*; PB: 99%; t½: 6-7 h
Ketorolac tromethamine	Short-term pain: A/adol >17 y >50 kg: PO: Initially 20 mg dose, then 10 mg q4-6h; *max:* 40 mg/d Older A/adol >17 y <50 kg: PO: Initially 10 mg dose, then 10 mg q4-6h; *max:* 40 mg/d A/adol >17 y >50 kg: IM/IV: 30 mg q6h; *max:* 120 mg/d Older A/adol >17 y <50 kg: 15 mg q6h; *max:* 60 mg/d Nasal spray: A >50 kg: Intranasal: 1 spray each nostril q6-8h; *max:* 4 doses Older A <50 kg: Intranasal: 1 spray 1 nostril q6-8h; *max:* 4 doses	For short-term moderate to severe pain management of 5 days or less and for ocular inflammation. First injectable NSAID. May cause dizziness, drowsiness, headache, GI distress, edema, GI bleeding/perforation, elevated hepatic enzymes, and ocular inflammation. Pregnancy category: C, D*; PB: 99%; t½: PO, 2.4-9 h; IM, 3.5-9.2 h
Propionic Acid		
Fenoprofen calcium	Rheumatoid arthritis: A: PO: 400-600 mg tid/qid; *max:* 3200 mg/d	For mild to moderate pain, osteoarthritis, and rheumatoid arthritis. Most effective after 2-3 weeks. May cause drowsiness, dizziness, weakness, itching, GI distress, palpitations, and stroke. Take with food. Pregnancy category: C, D*; PB: 99%; t½: 2.5-3 h

Continued

TABLE 24.2   Antiinflammatory Agents: Nonsteroidal—cont'd

Drug	Route and Dosage	Uses and Considerations
Flurbiprofen sodium	A: PO: 200-300 mg/d in 2-4 divided doses; *max:* 300 mg/d	For mild to moderate pain, osteoarthritis, and rheumatoid arthritis. May cause dizziness, blurred vision, GI distress, and GI bleeding. Take with food. Pregnancy category: C, D*; PB: 99%; t½: 3-9 h
Ibuprofen	See Prototype Drug Chart 24.2.	
Ketoprofen	Arthritis: Immediate release: A: PO: Initially 50 mg qid or 75 mg tid (older A, initially 50 mg tid or 75 mg bid); *max:* 300 mg/d Extended release: A: PO: 200 mg/d; *max:* 200 mg/d Older A: PO: 100-150 mg/d; *max:* 200 mg/d	For mild to moderate pain, osteoarthritis, and rheumatoid arthritis. May cause headache, insomnia, dreams, GI distress, elevated hepatic enzymes, and stroke. Take with food or 8 oz of water to avoid GI distress. Pregnancy category: C, D*; PB: 99%; t½: Immediate release, 0.9-3.3 h; Extended release, 5.4 h
Naproxen	A: PO: 250-500 mg bid; *max:* 1500 mg/d C >2 y: PO: 5 mg/kg bid; *max:* 15 mg/kg/d	For mild to moderate pain, osteoarthritis, rheumatoid arthritis, ankylosing spondylitis, gout, bursitis, and dysmenorrhea. May cause drowsiness, dizziness, headache, elevated hepatic enzymes, GI distress, and bleeding. Take with food or with a full glass of water. Pregnancy category: C*; PB: 99%; t½: 12-17 h
Oxaprozin	A: PO: 600-1200 mg/d; *max:* 1800 mg/d	For osteoarthritis and rheumatoid arthritis. May cause rash and GI distress or bleeding. Take with food. Pregnancy category: C, D*; PB: 99%; t½: 41.4 h
Anthranilic Acids (Fenamates)		
Meclofenamate	Arthritis: A/adol >14 y: PO: 200-400 mg/d in 3-4 divided doses; *max:* 400 mg/d	For mild to moderate pain, osteoarthritis, and rheumatoid arthritis. May cause dizziness, headache, rash, severe GI distress/bleeding, and stroke. Take with food. Pregnancy category: C, D*; PB: 99%; t½: 2 h
Mefenamic acid	A/adol >14 y: PO: Initially: 500 mg; then 250 mg q6h PRN; *max:* 1250 mg/d	For mild to moderate pain and dysmenorrhea. May cause dizziness, headache, GI distress (especially diarrhea), elevated hepatic enzymes, angioedema, GI bleeding, renal dysfunction, and stroke. Drug is usually discontinued after 7 days. Pregnancy category: C, D*; PB: 90%; t½: 2 h
Oxicams		
Piroxicam	A: PO: 20 mg/d; *max:* 20 mg/d Older A: PO: 10 mg/d; *max:* 20 mg/d	For osteoarthritis and rheumatoid arthritis. Effective at 2 weeks. May cause edema, dizziness, headache, rash, itching, GI distress, elevated hepatic enzymes, GI bleeding, renal dysfunction, and stroke. Pregnancy category: C, D*; PB: 99%; t½: 50 h
Meloxicam	A: PO: 7.5-15 mg/d; *max:* 15 mg/d	For osteoarthritis and rheumatoid arthritis. Some COX-2 selectivity. May cause dizziness, headache, insomnia, edema, GI distress, and elevated hepatic enzymes. Pregnancy category: C, D*; PB: 99%; t½: 15-20 h
Naphthylalkanones		
Nabumetone	A: PO: 500-1000 mg qd/bid; *max:* 2000 mg/d	For osteoarthritis and rheumatoid arthritis. Inhibits COX-2 more so than COX-1. Causes fewer GI problems but may cause GI distress, dizziness, headache, tinnitus, rash, itching, edema, and stroke. Pregnancy category: C*; PB: 99%; t½: 24 h
COX-2 Inhibitors (Second-Generation NSAIDs)		
Celecoxib	See Prototype Drug Chart 24.3.	

*Pregnancy categories have been revised. See http://www.fda.gov/Drugs/DevelopmentApprovalProcess/DevelopmentResources/Labeling/ucm 093307.htm for more information.

A, Adult; *adol,* adolescent; *bid,* twice a day; *C,* child; *COX,* cyclooxygenase; *d,* day; *GI,* gastrointestinal; *h,* hour; *IM,* intramuscular; *IV,* intravenous; *maint,* maintenance; *max,* maximum; *NSAID,* nonsteroidal antiinflammatory drug; *PB,* protein binding; *PO,* by mouth; *PRN,* as needed; *q12h,* every 12 hours; *qd,* every day; *qid,* four times a day; *t½,* half-life; *tid,* three times a day; *y,* year; *>,* greater than; *<,* less than.

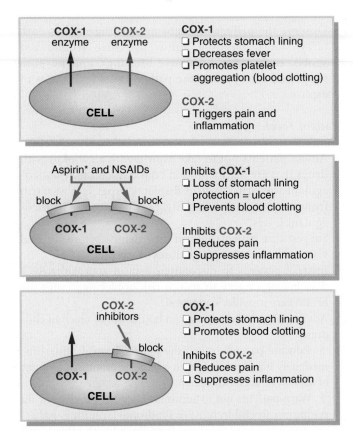

*Aspirin is only one of the NSAIDs.

FIG. 24.1 Uses of COX-1 and COX-2 inhibitors.

PROTOTYPE DRUG CHART 24.1

Aspirin

Drug Class	Dosage
Analgesic: Antiinflammatory drug Pregnancy category: D*	Arthritis: A: PO: 3 g/d in divided doses

Contraindications	Drug-Lab-Food Interactions
Hypersensitivity to salicylates or NSAIDs, flu or virus symptoms in children, GI bleeding *Caution:* Renal or hepatic disorders, gout, alcoholism, anticoagulant therapy, GI bleeding, bone marrow suppression, head trauma, immunosuppression, pregnancy	Drug: Increased risk of bleeding with anticoagulants and other NSAIDs; increased risk of hypoglycemia with oral hypoglycemic drugs; increased ulcerogenic effect with glucocorticoids; decreased effects of ACE inhibitors, loop diuretics, and probenecid; effects are decreased by corticosteroids. Lab: Decreased cholesterol, potassium, T_3, and T_4 levels; increased uric acid, PT, and bleeding time

Pharmacokinetics	Pharmacodynamics
Absorption: PO: 80%-100% Distribution: PB: 90%-95%, crosses placenta Metabolism: t½: Varies with dosage; low doses 15-20 min, high doses 2-18 h Excretion: 50% in urine	PO: Onset: 15-30 min Peak: 1-2 h Duration: 4-6 h

Therapeutic Effects/Uses
To reduce pain and inflammatory symptoms, decrease fever, and inhibit platelet aggregation; for osteoarthritis and rheumatoid arthritis Mode of Action: Inhibition of prostaglandin synthesis, inhibition of hypothalamic heat-regulator center

Side Effects	Adverse Reactions
Dizziness, drowsiness, headache, anorexia, nausea, vomiting, diarrhea, heartburn, abdominal pain, rash	Tinnitus, hearing loss, GI ulceration and bleeding *Life threatening:* Agranulocytosis, hemolytic anemia, leukopenia, bronchospasm, anaphylaxis, thrombocytopenia, Reye syndrome, hepatotoxicity

*Pregnancy categories have been revised. See http://www.fda.gov/Drugs/DevelopmentApprovalProcess/DevelopmentResources/Labeling/ucm093307.htm for more information.
A, Adult; *ACE*, angiotensin-converting enzyme; *d*, day; *GI*, gastrointestinal; *h*, hour; *min*, minute; *NSAID*, nonsteroidal antiinflammatory drug; *PB*, protein binding; *PO*, by mouth; *PT*, prothrombin time; *t½*, half-life; T_3, triiodothyronine; T_4, thyroxine.

dyspepsia, nausea, vomiting, diarrhea, constipation, abdominal pain, heartburn, and flatulence—is a common problem. In such cases, enteric-coated (EC) tablets may be used. Aspirin should *not* be taken with other NSAIDs because it decreases the blood level and effectiveness of NSAIDs.

Aspirin and other NSAIDs relieve pain by inhibiting the COX enzyme, which is needed for the biosynthesis of prostaglandins. As mentioned earlier, the two enzyme forms of cyclooxygenase, COX-1 and COX-2 (Fig. 24.1), serve different purposes: COX-1 protects the stomach lining and regulates blood platelets, promoting blood clotting, whereas COX-2 triggers pain and inflammation at the injured site. NSAIDs usually inhibit or block *both* COX-1 and COX-2. Inhibition of COX-1 produces the desirable effect of decreasing platelet aggregation, but it has the undesirable effect of decreasing protection to the stomach lining; therefore stomach bleeding and ulcers may occur with aspirin and NSAID agents. When COX-2 is inhibited, pain and fever are reduced and inflammation is suppressed, but COX-2 inhibitors do *not* cause gastric ulceration, and they have no effect on platelet function.

Newer NSAIDs, called **COX-2 inhibitors**, block only COX-2 and not COX-1. These drugs leave protection for the stomach lining intact, so no gastric bleeding or ulcers result, but they still deliver relief for pain and inflammation.

A COX-2 inhibitor approved by the U.S. Food and Drug Administration (FDA) is celecoxib. Drugs similar to COX-2 inhibitors include meloxicam and nabumetone, which allow some stomach protection. Patients at risk for stroke or heart attack who take aspirin to prevent blood clotting (decreased platelet aggregation) would not benefit from COX-2 inhibitors. If the COX-1 enzyme was not blocked, increased blood clotting would remain even though the stomach lining is protected.

Many researchers believe that COX-2 inhibitors may prevent some types of cancer, such as colon cancer. Fruits and vegetables block the COX-2 enzyme naturally, protecting the colon from malignant growths.

Pharmacokinetics Aspirin is well absorbed from the GI tract (Prototype Drug Chart 24.1). It can cause GI distress, which includes anorexia, nausea, vomiting, diarrhea, and abdominal pain, so it should be taken with water, milk, or food. The EC or buffered form can decrease gastric distress. EC tablets should not be crushed or broken.

Aspirin has a short half-life. It should not be taken during the last trimester of pregnancy because it could cause premature closure of the ductus arteriosus in the fetus. Aspirin should not be taken by children with flu symptoms because it may cause the potentially fatal Reye syndrome.

Pharmacodynamics Like other NSAIDs, aspirin inhibits prostaglandin synthesis by inhibiting COX-1 and COX-2, thus it decreases inflammation and pain. The onset of action for aspirin is within 30 minutes. It peaks in 1 to 2 hours, and the duration of action is an average of 4 to 6 hours. The action for the rectal preparation of aspirin can be erratic because of blood supply and fecal material in the rectum; it may take a week or longer for a therapeutic antiinflammatory effect.

Hypersensitivity to Salicylate Products

Patients may be hypersensitive to aspirin. Tinnitus (ringing in the ears), vertigo (dizziness), and bronchospasm—especially in asthmatic patients—are symptoms of aspirin overdose or hypersensitivity to aspirin.

Salicylates are present in numerous foods such as prunes, raisins, and licorice and in spices such as curry and paprika.

 NURSING PROCESS
Patient-Centered Collaborative Care

Salicylate: Aspirin

Assessment
• Determine a medical history. Ask the patient about previous gastric distress, gastric bleeding, or liver disease. Aspirin can cause gastric irritation, and it prolongs bleeding time by inhibiting platelet aggregation.
• Obtain a drug history. Report if a drug-drug interaction is probable.

Nursing Diagnoses
• Injury, Risk for
• Pain, Chronic related to tissue swelling of rheumatoid arthritis (RA)

Planning
• The patient's pain will be reduced within 12 to 24 hours.
• The patient's inflammation will be reduced within 1 week.

Nursing Interventions
• Monitor serum salicylate (aspirin) level when a patient takes high doses of aspirin for chronic conditions such as arthritis. The normal therapeutic range is 15 to 30 mg/dL. Mild toxicity occurs at a serum level greater than 30 mg/dL, and severe toxicity occurs above 50 mg/dL.

• Observe the patient for signs of bleeding such as dark tarry stools, bleeding gums, petechiae (round red spots), ecchymosis (excessive bruising), and purpura (large red spots) when the patient takes high doses of aspirin.

Patient Teaching
General
• Advise patients not to take aspirin with alcohol or with drugs that are highly protein bound, such as the anticoagulant warfarin. Aspirin displaces drugs like warfarin from the protein-binding site, causing increased anticoagulant levels.
• Suggest that patients inform their dentist before a dental visit if they are taking high doses of aspirin.
• Instruct patients to discontinue aspirin approximately 7 days before surgery to reduce risk of bleeding (with the health care provider's approval).
• Advise patients to keep aspirin bottles out of reach of children.
• ⚡ Educate parents to call the poison control center immediately if a child has taken a large or unknown amount of aspirin or acetaminophen.
• ⚡ Warn patients not to administer aspirin for virus or flu symptoms in children. Reye syndrome (vomiting, lethargy, delirium, and coma) has been linked with aspirin and viral infections. Acetaminophen is usually prescribed for cold and flu symptoms.
• Inform patients that aspirin tablets can cause GI distress.
• Inform patients with dysmenorrhea to take acetaminophen instead of aspirin 2 days before and during the first 2 days of the menstrual period.
Side Effects
• Direct patients to report side effects such as drowsiness, tinnitus (ringing in the ears), headaches, flushing, dizziness, GI distress, GI bleeding, visual changes, and seizures.
Diet
• Instruct patients to take aspirin and ibuprofen with food, at mealtime, or with plenty of fluids. EC aspirin helps prevent GI distress.

🌐 *Cultural Considerations*
• Provide additional explanation as needed related to the purpose of the drug and its side effects.

Evaluation
• Evaluate the effectiveness of aspirin in relieving pain. If pain persists, another analgesic such as ibuprofen may be prescribed.
• Determine whether the patient shows any of the side effects of aspirin.

Para-Chlorobenzoic Acid

One of the first NSAIDs introduced was indomethacin, a *para*-chlorobenzoic acid. It is used for rheumatoid arthritis (RA), gouty arthritis, and osteoarthritis and is a potent prostaglandin inhibitor. It is highly protein bound (99%) and displaces other protein-bound drugs, resulting in potential toxicity. It has a moderate half-life (2.6 to 11.2 hours). Indomethacin is very irritating to the stomach and should be taken with food.

Two other *para*-chlorobenzoic acid derivatives—sulindac and tolmetin—produce less severe adverse reactions than indomethacin. Tolmetin is not as highly protein bound as indomethacin and sulindac, and it has a short half-life. This group of NSAIDs may cause sodium and water retention and increased blood pressure.

Phenylacetic Acid Derivatives

Diclofenac sodium, a phenylacetic acid derivative, has a plasma half-life of 2 hours. Its analgesic and antiinflammatory effects are similar to those of aspirin, but it has minimal to no antipyretic effects. It is indicated for RA, osteoarthritis, and ankylosing spondylitis. Diclofenac is available in oral, extended-release, and topical 1% gel preparations. Side effects and adverse reactions are similar to those of other NSAIDs, with far less detrimental reactions when using a topical preparation.

Ketorolac, another phenylacetic acid derivative, is the first injectable NSAID. Like other NSAIDs, it inhibits prostaglandin synthesis, but it has greater analgesic properties than other antiinflammatory agents. Ketorolac is recommended for short-term management of pain. For postsurgical pain, it has shown analgesic efficacy equal or superior to that of opioid analgesics. It is administered intramuscularly in doses of 30 to 60 mg every 6 hours for adults. Ketorolac is also available in oral, intravenous (IV), and intranasal preparations.

Propionic Acid Derivatives

The propionic acid group is a relatively new group of NSAIDs. These drugs are aspirin-like but have stronger effects and create less GI irritation. Drugs in this group are highly protein bound, so drug interactions might occur, especially when given with another highly protein-bound drug. Propionic acid derivatives are better tolerated than other NSAIDs. Gastric upset occurs, but it is not as severe as with aspirin and indomethacin. Severe adverse reactions such as blood dyscrasias are not frequently seen. Ibuprofen is the most widely used propionic acid NSAID, and it may be purchased OTC in lower doses (200 mg). Prototype Drug Chart 24.2 details the pharmacologic behavior of ibuprofen. Five other propionic acid agents are fenoprofen calcium, naproxen, ketoprofen, flurbiprofen, and oxaprozin.

Pharmacokinetics Ibuprofens are well absorbed from the GI tract. These drugs have a short half-life but are highly protein bound. If ibuprofen is taken with another highly protein-bound drug, severe side effects may occur. The drug is metabolized in the liver to inactivate metabolites and is excreted as inactive metabolites in the urine.

PROTOTYPE DRUG CHART 24.2

Ibuprofen

Drug Class	Dosage
NSAID: Propionic acid derivative Pregnancy category: C (D third trimester)*	A: PO: 400-800 mg tid/qid; *max:* 3200 mg/d

Contraindications	Drug-Lab-Food Interactions
Hypersensitivity, coronary artery bypass graft surgery *Caution:* Bleeding disorders, pregnancy, lactation, systemic lupus erythematosus, asthma, peptic ulcer, anticoagulant therapy, renal or hepatic disease	Drug: Increased bleeding time with oral anticoagulants; increased effects of phenytoin, sulfonamides, warfarin; decreased effect with aspirin; may increase severe side effects of lithium

Pharmacokinetics	Pharmacodynamics
Absorption: PO: Well absorbed Distribution: PB: 90%-99% Metabolism: t½: 2-4 h Excretion: In urine, mostly as inactive metabolites; some in bile	PO: Onset: 30 min-1 h Peak: 2-4 h Duration: 6-8 h

Therapeutic Effects/Uses
To reduce inflammatory process; to relieve pain; antiinflammatory effect for arthritic conditions; to reduce fever Mode of Action: Inhibition of prostaglandin synthesis, thus relieving pain and inflammation

Side Effects	Adverse Reactions
Headache, dizziness, anorexia, nausea, vomiting, diarrhea, edema, rash, fluid retention	Hearing loss, tinnitus, bleeding *Life threatening:* Anemia, neutropenia, thrombocytopenia, nephrotoxicity, anaphylaxis

*Pregnancy categories have been revised. See http://www.fda.gov/Drugs/DevelopmentApprovalProcess/DevelopmentResources/Labeling/ucm093307.htm for more information.

A, Adult; *d*, day; *h*, hour; *max*, maximum; *min*, minute; *NSAID*, nonsteroidal antiinflammatory drug; *PB*, protein binding; *PO*, by mouth; *qid*, four times a day; *t½*, half-life; *tid*, three times a day.

Pharmacodynamics Ibuprofen inhibits prostaglandin synthesis and are therefore effective in alleviating inflammation and pain. They have a short onset of action, peak concentration time, and duration of action. It may take several days for the antiinflammatory effect to be evident.

Many drug interactions are associated with ibuprofen. Because ibuprofen can increase the effects of warfarin, sulfonamides, many of the cephalosporins, and phenytoin, it should be avoided with these drugs. However, when taken with aspirin, its effect can be decreased. Hypoglycemia may result when ibuprofen is taken with insulin or an oral hypoglycemic drug, and risk of toxicity is high when ibuprofen is taken concurrently with calcium channel blockers.

Fenamates

The fenamate group includes potent NSAIDs used for acute and chronic arthritic conditions. As with most NSAIDs, gastric irritation is a common side effect; patients with a history of peptic ulcer should avoid taking fenamates. Other side effects include edema, dizziness, tinnitus, and pruritus. Two fenamates are meclofenamate sodium monohydrate and mefenamic acid.

Oxicams

Piroxicam and meloxicam, oxicams, are indicated for long-term arthritic conditions such as RA and osteoarthritis. They too can cause gastric problems such as ulceration and epigastric distress, but the incidence is lower than for some other NSAIDs. Oxicams are well tolerated, and their major advantage over other NSAIDs is their long half-life, which allows them to be taken only once daily.

Full clinical response to piroxicam may take 1 to 2 weeks. This drug is also highly protein bound and may interact with another highly protein-bound drug when taken together. Piroxicam should *not* be taken with aspirin or other NSAIDs.

General Side Effects and Adverse Reactions With First-Generation NSAIDs

Most NSAIDs tend to have fewer side effects than aspirin when taken at antiinflammatory doses, but gastric irritation is still a common problem when NSAIDs are taken without food. In addition, sodium and water retention may occur. Alcoholic beverages consumed with NSAIDs may increase gastric irritation and should be avoided.

 NURSING PROCESS
Patient-Centered Collaborative Care
Nonsteroidal Antiinflammatory Drug: Ibuprofen

Assessment
- Check the patient's history for allergy to NSAIDs such as ibuprofen. If an allergy is present, notify the health care provider.
- Obtain a drug and herbal history, and report any possible drug-drug or herb-drug interactions. NSAIDs can increase the effects of phenytoin, sulfonamides, and warfarin. Most NSAIDs are highly protein bound and can displace other highly protein-bound drugs like warfarin.
- Determine the medical history. NSAIDs are contraindicated if a patient has severe renal or liver disease, peptic ulcer, or bleeding disorder.
- Assess for GI distress and peripheral edema, which are common side effects of NSAIDs.

Nursing Diagnoses
- Injury, Risk for
- Activity Intolerance, Risk for

Planning
- The patient's inflammatory process will subside in 1 to 3 weeks.

Nursing Interventions
- Observe the patient for bleeding gums, petechiae, ecchymoses, or black tarry stools. Bleeding time can be prolonged

when NSAIDs are taken, especially with a highly protein-bound drug such as warfarin (anticoagulant).
- Report if a patient has GI discomfort. Administer NSAIDs at mealtime or with food to prevent GI upset.
- Monitor vital signs and check for peripheral edema, especially in the morning.
- Do not give directions such as "take one blue pill" at a specified time. Instead, provide the name and the dosage of medications.

Patient Teaching
General
- ⚡ Advise patients not to take aspirin and acetaminophen with NSAIDs. Taking an NSAID with aspirin could cause GI upset and possibly GI bleeding.
- Advise patients to avoid alcohol when taking NSAIDs. GI distress or gastric ulcer may result.
- Alert patients that many complementary and alternative therapy products may interact with NSAIDs and could cause bleeding. Doses of NSAIDs and/or herbs may need to be modified to avoid possible bleeding (Complementary and Alternative Therapies 24.1).
- Direct patients to inform the dentist or surgeon before a procedure if they are taking ibuprofen or other NSAIDs for a continuous period.
- Warn female patients not to take NSAIDs 1 to 2 days before menstruation to avoid heavy menstrual flow. If discomfort occurs, acetaminophen is usually prescribed.
- ⚡ Advise pregnant patients to avoid NSAIDs. Congenital abnormalities may occur when NSAIDS are taken during early pregnancy, and excess bleeding might occur during delivery.
- Inform patients that it may take several weeks to experience the desired drug effect of some NSAIDs and disease-modifying antirheumatic drugs (DMARDs).

Side Effects
- Educate patients about the common side effects of NSAIDs. GI distress, peripheral edema, purpura or petechiae, and dizziness can occur. Report occurrences of side effects.

Diet
- Advise patients to take NSAIDs with meals or snacks to reduce GI distress.

🌐 *Cultural Considerations*
- Recognize that patients from various cultural backgrounds respond to pain and inflammation in various ways. In some cultures, the use of drugs to alleviate pain and inflammation is not acceptable. Herbal medicine and acupuncture can be used to alleviate pain.
- Be supportive of patients' methods for pain control. Explain the purpose of medications and their actions and side effects.

Evaluation
- Evaluate the effectiveness of the drug therapy, such as a decrease in pain and in swollen joints and an increase in mobility.

Nonsteroidal Antiinflammatory Drugs

Dong quai, feverfew, garlic, ginger, and ginkgo may cause bleeding when
taken with nonsteroidal antiinflammatory drugs (NSAIDs).

Selective COX-2 Inhibitors

Cyclooxygenase-2 (COX-2) inhibitors, second-generation
NSAIDs, became available in the last several years to decrease
inflammation and pain. Most NSAIDs are nonselective inhibitors that inhibit COX-1 and COX-2. By inhibiting COX-1, protection of the stomach lining is decreased, and clotting time is
also decreased, which may benefit the patient with cardiovascular or coronary artery disease (CAD). Selective COX-2 inhibitors are the drugs of choice for patients with severe arthritic
conditions who need high doses of an antiinflammatory drug,
because large doses of NSAIDs may cause peptic ulcer and gastric bleeding.

Currently, only one drug, celecoxib, is classified as a COX-2
inhibitor. Nabumetone is a similar drug that can be used; however, it is not considered a true COX-2 inhibitor, although it
does inhibit COX-2 more than COX-1. Celecoxib is described
in Prototype Drug Chart 24.3.

Use of NSAIDs in Older Adults

Older adults frequently use NSAIDs to treat pain associated with inflammation caused by osteoarthritis, RA, and
neuromuscular-skeletal disorders. As older adults age, the number of drugs taken daily increases; therefore drug interactions
are more common, especially when numerous drugs are taken
with NSAIDs. With the use of NSAIDs, GI distress—including
ulceration—is four times more common in older adults, and
hospitalization is often necessary.

The introduction of COX-2 inhibitors (second-generation
NSAIDs) has decreased the incidence of GI problems associated with NSAID use; however, edema is likely to occur. Renal
function should be evaluated, and older adults should increase
their fluid intake for adequate hydration. To decrease possible
complications, the NSAID dose should be lowered.

CORTICOSTEROIDS

Corticosteroids such as prednisone, prednisolone, and dexamethasone are frequently used as antiinflammatory agents. This
group of drugs controls inflammation by suppressing or preventing many of the components of the inflammatory process
at the injured site. Corticosteroids have been widely prescribed
for arthritic conditions, and although they are not the drug of
choice for arthritis because of their numerous side effects, they
are frequently used to control arthritic flareups.

The half-life of a corticosteroid is long (>24 hours), and it
is administered once a day in a large prescribed dose. When
discontinuing long-term steroid therapy, the dosage should be
tapered over a period of 5 to 10 days. Steroids are discussed in
more detail in Chapter 46.

PROTOTYPE DRUG CHART 24.3

Celecoxib

Drug Class	Dosage
Nonsteroidal antiinflammatory: COX-2 inhibitor Pregnancy category: C, D (third trimester)*	Arthritis: A: PO: 100-200 mg qd/bid; *max:* 800 mg/d
Contraindications	**Drug-Lab-Food Interactions**
Hypersensitivity, coronary artery bypass surgery *Caution:* Renal or hepatic dysfunction, angina, hypertension, dysrhythmias, heart failure, anemia, dehydration, peptic ulcer disease, GI bleeding or perforation, concurrent anticoagulant therapy, steroids, alcoholism, immunosuppression	Drug: Decreased effect of ACE inhibitors, increased INR and GI bleeding with warfarin and SNRIs, may increase toxicity with lithium, fluoroquinolones may increase the risk of seizures; fluconazole and ketoconazole increase celecoxib levels. Complementary and alternative therapies: Ginkgo biloba may increase bleeding risk.
Pharmacokinetics	**Pharmacodynamics**
Absorption: Well absorbed in GI tract Distribution: PB: 97% Metabolism: t½: 11.2 h Excretion: Primarily in feces	PO: Onset: UK Peak: 3 h Duration: UK
Therapeutic Effects/Uses	
To treat osteoarthritis and rheumatoid arthritis, to relieve dysmenorrhea and moderate to severe pain, for ankylosing spondylitis Mode of Action: Inhibits COX-2, which normally promotes prostaglandin synthesis and inflammatory response, but does not inhibit COX-1	
Side Effects	**Adverse Reactions**
Headache, dizziness, sinusitis, abdominal pain, nausea, flatulence, diarrhea, rash	Peripheral edema, bleeding, hypertension *Life threatening:* Stroke

*Pregnancy categories have been revised. See http://www.fda.gov/Drugs/
DevelopmentApprovalProcess/DevelopmentResources/Labeling/ucm093307.htm
for more information.
A, Adult; *ACE,* angiotensin-converting enzyme; *bid,* twice a day; *COX,* cyclooxygenase; *d,* day; *GI,* gastrointestinal; *h,* hour; *INR,* international normalized ratio;
max, maximum; *PB,* protein binding; *PO,* by mouth; *qd,* every day; *SNRI,* serotonin
norepinephrine reuptake inhibitor; *t½,* half-life; *UK,* unknown.

DISEASE-MODIFYING ANTIRHEUMATIC DRUGS

When NSAIDs do not control immune-mediated arthritic
disease sufficiently, other drugs, although more toxic, can be
prescribed to alter the disease process. The disease-modifying
antirheumatic drugs (DMARDs) include immunosuppressive agents, immunomodulators, and antimalarials.
DMARDs help alleviate the symptoms of RA for the 2 million persons in the United States affected by the disorder.
DMARDs are described in Table 24.3. Other indications for
use of DMARDs include osteoarthritis, psoriatic arthritis,
severe psoriasis, ankylosing spondylitis, Crohn disease, and
ulcerative colitis.

Immunosuppressive Agents

Immunosuppressives are used to treat refractory RA, arthritis that does not respond to antiinflammatory drugs. In low doses, selected immunosuppressive agents have been effective in the treatment of RA. Drugs such as azathioprine, cyclophosphamide, and methotrexate—primarily used to suppress cancer growth and proliferation—might be used to suppress the inflammatory process of RA when other treatments fail. In one study of patients receiving cyclophosphamide, few new erosions of joint cartilage were present, suggesting that the disease process was not active.

Immunomodulators

Immunomodulators treat moderate to severe RA by disrupting the inflammatory process and delaying disease progression. Interleukin 1 (IL-1) receptor antagonists and tumor necrosis factor (TNF) blockers are two groups of drugs classified as immunomodulators.

Anakinra, an IL-1 receptor antagonist, blocks activity of IL-1 by inhibiting it from binding to interleukin receptors located in cartilage and bone. IL-1 is a proinflammatory cytokine that contributes to synovial inflammation and joint destruction. Anakinra is administered subcutaneously. The peak is 3 to 7 hours, and the half-life is 4 to 6 hours.

TNF blockers bind to TNF and block it from attaching to TNF receptors on synovial cell surfaces. By neutralizing TNF, a contributor to synovitis, the inflammatory disease process is delayed. Etanercept was the first TNF blocker developed. It is administered subcutaneously, and the half-life ranges from 72 to 132 hours. Signs and symptoms of RA are suppressed rapidly with etanercept therapy but reappear if the drug is discontinued. Other TNF blockers include infliximab, adalimumab, and leflunomide. Infliximab is administered intravenously over at least 2 hours, adalimumab is administered subcutaneously, and leflunomide is administered orally. Infliximab is described in Prototype Drug Chart 24.4.

Both IL-1 receptor antagonists and TNF blockers predispose the patient to severe infections; they are contraindicated in active infection and should be discontinued when an infection occurs. Immunomodulators are usually very expensive.

◎ NURSING PROCESS
Patient-Centered Collaborative Care

Infliximab

Assessment
- Determine a medical history. Ask patient if there is any history of seizures, diabetes mellitus, multiple sclerosis, or kidney or liver disease. Aspirin can cause gastric irritation. It prolongs bleeding time by inhibiting platelet aggregation.
- Obtain baseline complete blood count (CBC) and renal and liver function tests.

Nursing Diagnoses
- Mobility, Impaired Physical related to severe pain
- Pain, Chronic related to tissue swelling from RA

Planning
- The patient's pain will be reduced within 12 to 24 hours.
- The patient's inflammation will be reduced within 1 week.

Nursing Interventions
- Obtain a negative tuberculosis skin test prior to initiating infliximab therapy.
- Monitor patients for signs and symptoms of infection. If a serious infection occurs while a patient is receiving infliximab therapy, antibiotic therapy should be initiated, and infliximab should be discontinued.
- Monitor laboratory tests for blood dyscrasias (CBC) and renal and liver function (blood urea nitrogen [BUN], serum creatinine, alkaline phosphatase [ALP], aspartate aminotransferase [AST], alanine aminotransferase [ALT]).
- Flush IV tubing with normal saline before and after administration. Deliver IV medication through a 1.2-micron or smaller filter.
- Administer each dose over a minimum of 2 hours.
- Discontinue IV dose of infliximab if the patient develops acute infusion reaction (e.g., chest pain, fever, chills, dyspnea, pruritus, urticaria, hypotension, or hypertension).
- Monitor patients up to 2 hours after infusion for acute infusion reaction.

Patient Teaching
General
- Encourage patients to keep medical appointments and to have regularly scheduled laboratory tests that include CBC and renal and liver function tests for early detection of blood dyscrasias and renal and liver damage.
- Advise patients to avoid live vaccines while taking infliximab.
Side Effects
- ⚡ Teach patients to report dizziness, chills, depression, dyspnea, severe infections, seizures, fatigue, or rash immediately.
- Teach patients to report severe infections immediately.

⊕ Cultural Considerations
- Provide additional explanation as needed related to the disease process and the purpose of the drug and its side effects.
- Identify conflicts in values and beliefs.
- Suggest follow-up by a community health nurse to determine patient compliance with the drug regimen and the effectiveness of the prescribed drug therapy.

Evaluation
- Evaluate patient response to the DMARD. If pain persists, the drug regimen may need modification.
- Determine the presence of adverse reactions. Drug therapy for pain may need to be changed.

Antimalarials

Antimalarial drugs may be used to treat RA when other methods of treatment fail. The mechanism of action of antimalarials in suppressing RA is unclear. The effect may take 4 to 12 weeks to become apparent. Antimalarials are usually used in combination with NSAIDs in patients whose arthritis is not under control.

TABLE 24.3 Antiinflammatory Drugs: Disease-Modifying Antirheumatic Drugs

Drug	Route and Dosage	Uses and Considerations
Golimumab	A: Subcut: 50 mg every month	For RA, psoriatic arthritis, ankylosing spondylitis, and ulcerative colitis. May cause injection-site reaction, aplastic anemia, leukopenia, neutropenia, thrombocytopenia, infection, URI, and elevated hepatic enzymes. Pregnancy category: B*; PB: UK; t½: 2 wk
Anakinra	A: Subcut: 100 mg/d; *max:* 100 mg/d	For RA. May cause injection-site reaction, headache, fever, GI distress, arthralgia, nasopharyngitis, infection, and neutropenia. Pregnancy category: B*; PB: UK; t½: 4 to 6 h
Etanercept	A: Subcut: 50 mg 1-2 times/wk; *max:* 100 mg/wk C >2 y: Subcut: 0.8 mg/kg/wk; *max:* 50 mg/wk	For RA, psoriatic arthritis, and ankylosing spondylitis. May cause injection-site reaction, diarrhea, influenza, infection, and URI. Pregnancy category: B*; PB: UK; t½: 72-132 h
Infliximab	See Prototype Drug Chart 24.4.	
Rituximab	Rheumatoid arthritis: A: IV: 1000 mg on day 1 and day 15 with methotrexate, then q24wk Give methylprednisolone 100 mg or equivalent prior to each dose to decrease infusion reactions.	For RA, chronic lymphocytic leukemia, and non-Hodgkin lymphoma. May cause infusion-site reaction, dizziness, headache, insomnia, pain, fever, chills, fatigue, peripheral edema, anemia, hypertension, hypotension, angioedema, GI distress, increased hepatic enzymes, hyperglycemia, cough, rhinitis, epistaxis, neuropathy, weakness, and arthralgia. Pregnancy category: C*; PB: UK; t½: 83.9-407 h
Adalimumab	A: Subcut: 40 mg q2wk	For RA, psoriatic arthritis, Crohn disease, ulcerative colitis, and ankylosing spondylitis. May cause injection-site reaction, headache, nausea, infection, rash, and URI. Pregnancy category: B*; PB: UK; t½: 10 to 20 d
Leflunomide	A: PO: Initially 100 mg/d for 3 d; maint: 20 mg/d	For RA. May cause hypertension, dizziness, headache, alopecia, rash, GI distress, asthenia, elevated hepatic enzymes, infection, and URI. Pregnancy category: X*; PB: 99%; t½: 2 wk
Abatacept	A >100 kg: IV: 1 g over 30 min q2wk for 3 doses, then 1 g q4wk A 60-100 kg: IV: 750 mg over 30 min q2wk for 3 doses, then q4wk	For RA. May cause dizziness, headache, GI distress, infection, URI, hypertension, influenza, and infusion-related reaction. Pregnancy category: C*; PB: UK; t½: 14.3 d
Tofacitinib	A: PO: 5 mg bid; *max:* 5 mg bid	For RA. May cause headache, GI distress, hypertension, elevated hepatic enzymes, hypercholesterolemia, infection, and URI. Pregnancy category: C*; PB: 40%; t½: 3 h
Tocilizumab	A: IV: 4 mg/kg over 1 h q4wk initially; *max:* 800 mg/dose A: Subcut: 162 mg q2wk; *max:* 162 mg/dose	For RA and juvenile idiopathic arthritis. May cause infusion/injection-related reaction, headache, hyperlipidemia, elevated hepatic enzymes, neutropenia, URI, angioedema, and hypertension. Pregnancy category: C*; PB: UK; t½: subcut 5-13 d; IV, 11-13 d
Secukinumab	A: Subcut: 300 mg wks 0-4, followed by 300 mg q4wk; *max:* 300 mg/dose	For psoriasis, psoriatic arthritis, and ankylosing spondylitis. May cause oral ulceration, infection, nasopharyngitis, hypersensitivity, and diarrhea. Pregnancy category: B*; PB: UK; t½: 22-31 d
Apremilast	A: PO: Initially 10 mg in the morning; day 2, 10 mg bid; day 3, 10 mg in morning, and 20 mg in evening; day 4, 20 mg bid; day 5, 20 mg in morning, and 30 mg in evening; maint: 30 mg bid starting on day 6; *max:* 60 mg/d	For psoriatic arthritis and psoriasis. May cause headache, URI, nausea, vomiting, diarrhea, weight loss, infection, and suicidal ideation. Pregnancy category: C*; PB: 68%; t½: 6-9 h
Canakinumab	Adol/C >2 y >7.5 kg: Subcut: 4 mg/kg q4wk; *max:* 4 mg/kg/dose	For systemic juvenile idiopathic arthritis. May cause headache, dizziness, GI distress, injection-site reaction, weight gain, musculoskeletal pain, nasopharyngitis, influenza, infection, leukopenia, and neutropenia. Pregnancy category: C*; PB: UK; t½: 26 d

*Pregnancy categories have been revised. See http://www.fda.gov/Drugs/DevelopmentApprovalProcess/DevelopmentResources/Labeling/ucm093 307.htm for more information.

A, Adult; *adol,* adolescent; *bid,* twice daily; *C,* child; *d,* day; *GI,* gastrointestinal; *h,* hour; *IV,* intravenous; *maint,* maintenance; *max,* maximum; *min,* minute; *PB,* protein binding; *PO,* by mouth; *q2,* every two; *RA,* rheumatoid arthritis; *Subcut,* subcutaneous; *t½,* half-life; *UK,* unknown; *URI,* upper respiratory infection; *wk,* week; *y,* year; >, greater than.

PROTOTYPE DRUG CHART 24.4

Infliximab

Drug Class	Dosage
Immunomodulator: Tumor necrosis factor blocker Pregnancy category: B*	Rheumatoid arthritis: A: IV: Initially 3 mg/kg over 2 h; then 3 mg/kg wks 2 and 6; *max*. 10 mg/kg/dose Crohn disease: A: IV: Initially 5 mg/kg over 2 h and on wks 2 and 6; maint: 5-10 mg/kg q8wk

Contraindications	Drug-Lab-Food Interactions
Hypersensitivity, heart failure *Caution:* Renal or hepatic dysfunction, bone marrow suppression, diabetes mellitus, COPD, immunosuppression, multiple sclerosis, seizures, corticosteroid therapy, with older adults	Drug: May decrease effectiveness of vaccines; concurrent immunosuppressives may increase risk for infection or adverse effects

Pharmacokinetics	Pharmacodynamics
Absorption: UK Distribution: UK Metabolism: t½: 7-12 d Excretion: UK	IV: Onset: 2 wk Peak: UK Duration: UK

Therapeutic Effects/Uses
To treat psoriasis, rheumatoid arthritis, psoriatic arthritis, spondylitis, ulcerative colitis, and Crohn disease Mode of Action: Binds to TNF and blocks it from attaching to TNF receptors on synovial cell surfaces; reduces infiltration of inflammatory cells and delays inflammatory process

Side Effects	Adverse Reactions
Headache, dizziness, cough, fatigue, chills, flushing, fever, anxiety, nausea, vomiting, diarrhea, constipation, flatulence, abdominal pain, weight loss, rash, alopecia, dry skin, pharyngitis	Severe infections, chest pain, hypotension, hypertension, seizures, arthralgia, bone fractures, increased hepatic enzymes, anemia, neutropenia, pancytopenia, Stevens-Johnson syndrome

*Pregnancy categories have been revised. See http://www.fda.gov/Drugs/DevelopmentApprovalProcess/DevelopmentResources/Labeling/ucm093307.htm for more information.

A, Adult; *COPD,* chronic obstructive pulmonary disease; *d,* day; *h,* hour; *IV,* intravenous; *maint,* maintenance; *max,* maximum; *q8,* every 8; *t½,* half-life; *TNF,* tumor necrosis factor; *UK,* unknown; *wk,* week.

ANTIGOUT DRUGS

Gout is an inflammatory condition that attacks joints, tendons, and other tissues. It may be called *gouty arthritis.* The most common site of acute gouty inflammation is at the joint of the big toe. Gout is characterized by a uric acid metabolism disorder and a defect in purine (products of certain proteins) metabolism, which results in an increase in urates (uric acid salts) and an accumulation of uric acid (hyperuricemia) or an ineffective clearance of uric acid by the kidneys. Uric acid solubility is poor in acid urine, and urate crystals may form, causing urate calculi. Gout may appear as bumps, or *tophi,* in the subcutaneous tissue of earlobes, elbows, hands, and at the base of the great

toe. In addition to tophi, the complications of untreated or prolonged periods of gout include gouty arthritis, urinary calculi, and gouty nephropathy.

To promote uric acid excretion and to prevent renal calculi, fluid intake should be increased while taking antigout drugs. Foods high in purine—such as organ meats, sardines, salmon, gravy, herring, liver, and meat soups—and alcohol, especially beer, should be avoided. Alcohol causes both an overproduction and underexcretion of uric acid. To reduce acidity, acetaminophen should be taken for discomfort instead of aspirin (salicylic acid).

Antiinflammatory Gout Drug: Colchicine

The first drug used to treat gout was colchicine, introduced in 1936. This antiinflammatory gout drug inhibits the migration of leukocytes to the inflamed site. It is effective in alleviating acute symptoms of gout, but it is not effective for decreasing inflammation that occurs in other inflammatory disorders. Colchicine does not inhibit uric acid synthesis and does not promote uric acid excretion. It should not be used if the patient has a severe renal, cardiac, or GI problem. Gastric irritation is a common problem, so colchicine should be taken with food. With high doses, nausea, vomiting, diarrhea, or abdominal pain occurs in approximately 75% of patients taking the drug.

Colchicine is well absorbed in the GI tract, and its peak concentration time is within 2 hours. Most of the drug is excreted in the feces, but 10% to 20% is excreted in the urine.

Uric Acid Biosynthesis Inhibitors

Allopurinol, first marketed in 1963, is *not* an antiinflammatory drug; instead, it inhibits the final steps of uric acid biosynthesis and therefore lowers serum uric acid levels, preventing the precipitation of an attack. This drug is frequently used as a prophylactic to prevent gout, and it is a drug of choice for patients with chronic tophaceous gout. Allopurinol is also indicated for gout patients with renal impairment. It is useful for patients who have renal obstructions caused by uric acid stones and for patients with blood disorders such as leukemia and polycythemia vera. It is also given to patients who do not respond well to uricosuric drugs such as probenecid. Increased fluid intake is recommended to promote diuresis and alkalinization of the urine. Prototype Drug Chart 24.5 presents the pharmacologic behavior of febuxostat, another uric acid biosynthesis inhibitor.

Pharmacokinetics Eighty percent of allopurinol is absorbed from the GI tract. Biosynthesis of uric acid occurs in the liver in pure form and as active metabolites. The half-life of the drug itself is 1 to 2 hours, and it is 20 to 24 hours for its active metabolites. The protein-binding percentage is unknown. Approximately 80% to 100% of allopurinol and its metabolites are excreted in urine.

Pharmacodynamics Allopurinol inhibits the production of uric acid by inhibiting the enzyme xanthine oxidase, which is needed in the synthesis of uric acid. Allopurinol also improves the solubility of uric acid. Its onset of action occurs within 30 to 60 minutes; its peak time averages 2 to 4 hours. Allopurinol has a long duration of action.

PROTOTYPE DRUG CHART 24.5

Febuxostat

Drug Class	Dosage
Antigout: Uric acid biosynthesis inhibitor Pregnancy category: C*	A: PO: 40-80 mg/d; *max.* 120 mg/d

Contraindications	Drug-Lab-Food Interactions
Hypersensitivity, severe renal disease *Caution:* Hepatic disorder, cardiac disease	Drug: Increased effect of theophylline, azathioprine, didanosine, mercaptopurine, pegloticase Lab: Increased AST, ALT, BUN

Pharmacokinetics	Pharmacodynamics
Absorption: PO: 49% absorbed Distribution: PB: 99.2% Metabolism: t½: 5-8 h Excretion: 49% in urine	PO: Onset: UK Peak: 1-1.5 h Duration: UK

Therapeutic Effects/Uses
To treat gout and hyperuricemia Mode of Action: Blocks hypoxanthine and xanthine metabolism to reduce uric acid synthesis to decrease uric acid blood and urine concentrations

Side Effects	Adverse Reactions
Dizziness, headache, anorexia, dry mouth, vomiting, diarrhea, flatulence, arthralgia, pruritus, erectile dysfunction	Hepatic impairment, angioedema, bradycardia, gout, hyperglycemia, hyperlipidemia, hypertriglyceridemia *Life threatening:* Thrombocytopenia, neutropenia, leukopenia, pancytopenia, hepatic impairment, dysrhythmias, Steven-Johnson syndrome

*Pregnancy categories have been revised. See http://www.fda.gov/Drugs/DevelopmentApprovalProcess/DevelopmentResources/Labeling/ucm093307.htm for more information.
A, Adult; *ALT,* alanine aminotransferase; *AST,* aspartate aminotransferase; *BUN,* blood urea nitrogen; *d,* day; *h,* hour; *max,* maximum; *PB,* protein binding; *PO,* by mouth; *t½,* half-life; *UK,* unknown.

Alcohol, caffeine, and thiazide diuretics increase the uric acid level. Use of ampicillin or amoxicillin with allopurinol increases the risk of rash formation. Allopurinol can increase the effect of warfarin and oral hypoglycemic drugs.

Uricosurics

Uricosurics increase the rate of uric acid excretion by inhibiting its reabsorption. These drugs are effective in alleviating chronic gout, but they should not be used during acute attacks. Probenecid is a uricosuric that has been available since 1945. It blocks the reabsorption of uric acid and promotes its excretion. Probenecid can be taken with colchicine. To begin initial therapy for relieving symptoms of gout and inhibiting uric acid reabsorption, small doses of colchicine should be given before adding probenecid. If gastric irritation occurs, probenecid should be taken with meals. It has an average half-life of 1.7 to 31.2 hours and is 34% to 44% protein bound.

Another uricosuric is sulfinpyrazone. This drug is a metabolite of phenylbutazone and is more potent than probenecid. Sulfinpyrazone should be taken with meals or with antacids to prevent gastric irritation. Severe blood dyscrasias might occur,

especially in patients with a history of blood dyscrasias. Table 24.4 gives dosages and considerations for the commonly used antigout drugs.

Side Effects and Adverse Reactions

Side effects may include flushed skin, sore gums, and headache. Kidney stones resulting from the uric acid could be prevented by increasing water intake and maintaining a urine pH above 6. Blood dyscrasias occur rarely. Aspirin use should be avoided because it causes uric acid retention.

NURSING PROCESS
Patient-Centered Collaborative Care

Antigout Drug: Allopurinol

Assessment
- Obtain a medical history of any gastric, renal, cardiac, or liver disorders. Antigout drugs are excreted via kidneys, so sufficient renal function is needed. Drug dosage and drug selection might need to be changed.
- Obtain a drug history. Report possible drug-drug interactions.
- Assess serum uric acid value for future comparisons.
- Record urine output. Use initial urine output for future comparisons.
- Check laboratory tests such as BUN, serum creatinine, ALP, AST, ALT, and lactate dehydrogenase [LDH], and compare with future laboratory test results.

Nursing Diagnoses
- Tissue Integrity, Impaired related to inflammation of the great toe
- Pain, Acute related to tissue swelling

Planning
- Patient's pain from gout will be absent or controlled without side effects.

Nursing Interventions
- Report GI symptoms, gastric pain, nausea, vomiting, or diarrhea for patients taking antigout drugs. Administer these drugs with food to alleviate gastric distress.
- Record urine output. Because the drugs and uric acid are excreted through the urine, kidney stones might occur, so both water intake and urine output should be increased.
- ⚡ Monitor laboratory tests for renal and liver function (BUN, serum creatinine, ALP, AST, ALT).

Patient Teaching
General
- ⚡ Encourage patients to keep medical appointments and to have regularly scheduled laboratory tests for renal and liver function and CBC. Some antigout drugs may cause blood dyscrasias, so blood tests should be monitored.

- Instruct patients to increase fluid intake; it will increase drug and uric acid excretion.

Side Effects

- Advise patients to report to a health care provider any side effects of antigout drugs such as anorexia, nausea, vomiting, diarrhea, stomatitis, dizziness, rash, pruritus, and metallic taste.
- Advise patients to have a yearly eye examination because visual changes can result from prolonged use of allopurinol.

Diet

- Warn patients to avoid alcohol and caffeine because they can increase uric acid levels.
- Suggest that patients not take large doses of vitamin C while taking allopurinol; kidney stones may occur.
- Tell patients not to ingest foods high in purine content such as organ meats, salmon, sardines, gravy, and legumes. Foods with purine increase uric acid levels.

- Direct patients to report any gastric distress. Encourage them to take antigout drugs with food or at mealtime.

Cultural Considerations

- Provide additional explanation as needed related to the disease process and the purpose of the drug and its side effects.
- Identify conflicts in values and beliefs.
- Suggest follow-up by a community health nurse to determine patient compliance with the drug regimen and the effectiveness of the prescribed drug therapy.

Evaluation

- Evaluate response to the antigout drug. If pain persists, the drug regimen may need modification.
- Determine the presence of adverse reactions. Drug therapy for gout pain may need to be changed.

TABLE 24.4 Antigout Drugs

Drug	Route and Dosage	Uses and Considerations
Antiinflammatory Gout Drugs		
Colchicine	Acute gout attack: A/adol >16 y: PO: Initially 1.2 mg; then 0.6 mg in 1 h; *max:* 2.4 mg/d Prophylaxis: A/adol >16 y: PO: 0.6 mg qd/bid; *max:* 1.2 mg/d	For gout. Not for patients with renal or gastric disorders. May cause nausea, vomiting, diarrhea, elevated hepatic enzymes, anemia, agranulocytosis, leukopenia, neutropenia, thrombocytopenia, pancytopenia, and rhabdomyolysis. Take with food. Pregnancy category: C*; PB: 34%-44%; t½: 1.7-31.2 h
Uric Acid Biosynthesis Inhibitors		
Allopurinol	Gout: A: PO: Initially 100 mg/d; *max:* 800 mg/d	For gout, hyperuricemia, and renal calculi. May cause nausea, vomiting, diarrhea, anemia, and GI bleeding. Pregnancy category: C*; PB: UK; t½: 1-2 h
Febuxostat	See Prototype Drug Chart 24.5.	
Uricosurics		
Probenecid	A: PO: Initially 250 mg bid for 1 wk; maint: 500 mg bid; *max:* 2 g/d	For hyperuricemia and gout. May cause dizziness, flushing, headache, fever, GI distress, and anemia. Increase fluid intake. Pregnancy category: B*; PB: 75%-95%; t½: 1-2 h, oxypurinol metabolite approximately 24 h

*Pregnancy categories have been revised. See http://www.fda.gov/Drugs/DevelopmentApprovalProcess/DevelopmentResources/Labeling/ucm 093307.htm for more information.

A, Adult; *adol,* adolescent; *bid,* twice a day; *d,* day; *GI,* gastrointestinal; *h,* hour; *maint,* maintenance; *max,* maximum; *PB,* protein binding; *PO,* by mouth; *qd,* every day; *t½,* half-life; *UK,* unknown; *wk,* week; *y,* year; *>,* greater than.

CRITICAL THINKING CASE STUDY

PQ, a 72-year-old woman, had taken 650 mg of aspirin four times a day for 8 months to alleviate her chronic symptoms of pain and inflammation associated with arthritis. Four weeks ago, a peptic ulcer developed.

1. Explain the process by which PQ could have a peptic ulcer. How could this have been prevented?
2. Compare the similarities and differences in the side effects of salicylates with those of acetic acid agents, propionic acid agents, COX-2 inhibitors, and phenylacetic acid.

3. What patient teaching points should PQ receive before and during the time she takes aspirin?
4. How would COX-2 inhibitors prevent the development of a peptic ulcer?
5. Would DMARDs be more helpful in alleviating PQ's symptoms? Explain your answer.
6. Compare the differences in the various types of DMARDs.

NCLEX STUDY QUESTIONS

1. A patient is taking ibuprofen. The nurse understands that COX-1 and COX-2 inhibitors are different in that ibuprofen is more likely than celecoxib to cause which adverse effect?
   a. Fever
   b. Constipation
   c. Peptic ulcer disease
   d. Metallic taste when eating

2. When teaching a patient who is receiving allopurinol, what should the nurse encourage the patient to do?
   a. Eat more meat.
   b. Increase vitamin C intake.
   c. Have annual eye examinations.
   d. Take medication 2 hours before meals.

3. A patient is admitted to the hospital with an acute gout attack. The nurse expects that which medication will be ordered to treat acute gout?
   a. Colchicine
   b. Allopurinol
   c. Probenecid
   d. Sulfinpyrazone

4. A patient is taking aspirin for arthritis. Which adverse reaction should the nurse teach the patient to report to the health care provider?
   a. Tinnitus
   b. Seizures
   c. Sinusitis
   d. Palpitations

5. The nurse is teaching a patient about taking aspirin. Which are important points to include? (Select all that apply.)
   a. Advise the patient to avoid alcohol while taking aspirin.
   b. Instruct the patient to take aspirin before meals on an empty stomach.
   c. Instruct the patient to inform the dentist of the aspirin dosage before having dental work.
   d. Instruct the patient to inform the surgeon of the aspirin dosage before having surgery.
   e. Suggest that aspirin may be given to children for flu symptoms.

6. A patient is taking infliximab and asks the nurse what side effects/adverse reactions to expect from this drug. The nurse lists which side effects? (Select all that apply.)
   a. Fatigue
   b. Headache
   c. Chest pain
   d. Renal damage
   e. Severe infections

Answers: 1, c; 2, c; 3, a; 4, a; 5, a, c, d; 6, a, b, c, e.

25

Analgesics

http://evolve.elsevier.com/McCuistion/pharmacology

OBJECTIVES

- Differentiate between acute and chronic pain.
- Compare indications for nonopioid and opioid analgesics.
- Describe the serum therapeutic ranges of aspirin and acetaminophen.
- Contrast the side effects of aspirin and opioids.
- Explain the methadone treatment program.
- Discuss nursing interventions and patient teaching related to nonopioid and opioid analgesics.
- Formulate a nursing process for a patient with morphine patient-controlled analgesia.

OUTLINE

Pathophysiology
   Undertreatment of Pain
Nonopioid Analgesics
   Nonsteroidal Antiinflammatory Drugs
   Acetaminophen
   Nursing Process: Patient-Centered Collaborative
      Care—Analgesic: Acetaminophen
Opioid Analgesics
   Morphine
   Nursing Process: Patient-Centered Collaborative
      Care—Opioid Analgesic: Morphine Sulfate
   Meperidine
   Hydromorphone
   Combination Drugs
   Patient-Controlled Analgesia

Transdermal Opioid Analgesics
   Analgesic Titration
   Opioid Use in Special Populations
Adjuvant Therapy
Treatment for Opioid-Addicted Individuals
Opioid Agonist-Antagonists
   Nursing Process: Patient-Centered Collaborative
      Care—Opioid Agonist-Antagonist Analgesic: Nalbuphine
Opioid Antagonists
Headaches: Migraine and Cluster
   Pathophysiology
   Treatment of Migraine Headaches
Critical Thinking Case Study
NCLEX Study Questions

KEY TERMS

addiction, p. 326
adjuvant analgesics, p. 333
analgesics, p. 323
cluster headaches, p. 336
endorphins, p. 323
migraine headaches, p. 336
neuropathic pain, p. 323
nociceptors, p. 323
nonopioid analgesics, p. 324

nonsteroidal antiinflammatory drugs (NSAIDs), p. 323
opioid agonist-antagonists, p. 334
opioid agonists, p. 326
opioid antagonist, p. 335
orthostatic hypotension, p. 330
pain threshold, p. 322
pain tolerance, p. 323
patient-controlled analgesia (PCA), p. 332
withdrawal syndrome, p. 330

Pain is an unpleasant sensory and emotional experience related to tissue injury. Due to the subjective nature of pain, the nurse must be knowledgeable and skillful in the assessment and measurement of pain to achieve optimal pain management.

Pain management is regarded as such a significant component of nursing care that pain has become known as the "fifth vital sign." The Joint Commission (TJC) has incorporated the assessment, documentation, and management of pain into its standards, which reflect the importance of this vital sign. The

nurse's role is to assess the patient's pain level, alleviate the patient's pain through nonpharmacologic and pharmacologic treatments, thoroughly document the patient's response to treatment, and teach patients and their significant others to manage pain control when appropriate.

An individual's **pain threshold** reflects the level of stimulus needed to create a painful sensation, and individual genetic makeup contributes to the variations in pain threshold from person to person. The mu (μ) opioid receptor gene controls the number of μ-receptors present. When an individual has a large number of μ-receptors, the pain threshold is high, and pain sensitivity is reduced.

The amount of pain a person can endure without having it interfere with normal functioning is called pain tolerance. This psychological aspect of pain varies greatly in individuals because it is subjective and because pain tolerance is influenced by factors such as age, gender, culture, ethnicity, previous experience, anxiety level, and specific circumstances, such as a traumatic event.

Analgesics, both nonopioid and opioid, are prescribed for the relief of pain. The choice of analgesic depends upon the severity of the pain. Mild to moderate pain is frequently relieved with the use of nonopioid, also known as *nonnarcotic,* analgesics. Moderate to severe pain usually requires an opioid, or *narcotic,* analgesic.

Drugs used for pain relief are presented in this chapter. Many of the same nonopioid analgesics that are taken for pain, such as the nonsteroidal antiinflammatory drugs (NSAIDs), are also taken for antiinflammatory purposes. This application for these drugs is covered in Chapter 24.

The most common classification of pain is by duration. Acute pain can be mild, moderate, or severe and is usually associated with a specific tissue injury. The onset of acute pain is usually sudden and of short duration lasting less than 3 months. Chronic pain usually has a vague origin and gradual onset with a prolonged duration (more than 3 months) of long-lasting discomfort.

Pain may also be classified by its origin. Nociceptors, sensory receptors for pain, are activated by noxious stimuli—mechanical, thermal, and chemical—in peripheral tissues. When tissue damage occurs, injured cells release chemical mediators that affect the exposed nerve endings of the nociceptors. Pain that originates from tissue injury is nociceptor pain, which includes somatic pain—that is, pain from structural tissues such as bones and muscles—and visceral (organ) pain. Neuropathic pain is an unusual sensory disturbance that often involves neural supersensitivity. This pain is due to injury or disease of the peripheral nervous system (PNS) or central nervous system (CNS). The patient with neuropathic pain usually complains of burning, tingling, or electric shock sensations in the affected area, often triggered by light touch. Diabetic neuropathy associated with diabetes mellitus is an example of peripheral neuropathic pain. Severe, intractable pain from a herniated disk or spinal cord injury is evidence of neuropathic pain from the CNS.

PATHOPHYSIOLOGY

The most common pain theory is called the *gate theory,* proposed by Melzack and Wall in 1965. According to this theory, tissue injury activates nociceptors and causes the release of chemical mediators such as substance P, prostaglandins, bradykinin, histamine, serotonin, acetylcholine, glutamate, adenosine triphosphate, leukotrienes, and potassium. These substances initiate an action potential along a sensory nerve fiber and sensitize pain receptors. Nociceptive action potentials are transmitted via afferent nerve fibers. One type of pain fiber that primarily transmits impulses from the periphery is the A-delta (A-δ) fiber. Because A-δ pain fibers are wrapped in a myelin sheath, they transmit impulses rapidly in acute pain. The C-fiber is a type of pain fiber that is small and unmyelinated, and because C-fibers are unmyelinated, they transmit impulses slowly. C-fibers are more often associated with chronic, dull pain.

A pain signal begins at the nociceptors in the periphery and proceeds throughout the CNS. Knowing how and where pharmacologic agents work is essential to controlling pain. The body produces neurohormones called endorphins (peptides) that naturally suppress pain conduction, although the method is not completely understood. Opioids such as morphine activate the same receptors as endorphins to reduce pain. NSAIDs control pain at the peripheral level by blocking the action of cyclooxygenase, a pain-sensitizing chemical, and interfering with the production of prostaglandins. Cortisone decreases pain by blocking the action of phospholipase, reducing the production of both prostaglandins and leukotrienes. In neuropathic pain, anticonvulsant drugs inhibit the transmission of nerve impulses by stabilizing the neuronal membrane and inactivating peripheral sodium channels.

To ascertain severity of pain, the health care provider should ask the patient to rate the degree of pain on a scale of 0 to 10, with 10 being the worst or most severe pain. For example, a patient who indicates a pain level of 9 may verbalize a decrease in pain to a level of 7 within 30 to 45 minutes after receiving pain medication. Many scales and instruments are available to the nurse for assessment and measurement of the patient's pain level. Table 25.1 lists the types of pain and the drug groups that may be effective in relieving each type.

Undertreatment of Pain

Undertreatment of pain is a major issue in health care today. The National Pharmaceutical Council and TJC state that up to 75% of patients have unrelieved pain. Some reasons for undertreatment are sociocultural variables that mediate a patient's willingness to acknowledge being in pain, the patient's inability to describe pain, the patient's fear of addiction, the nurse's inability to measure pain, lack of regular pain-assessment rounds, attitudes of the health care team, an unwillingness to believe the patient's report of pain, inaccurate knowledge on the part of the health care provider concerning addiction and tolerance, and prescription of an inadequate analgesic dose.

Unrelieved pain leads to a multitude of harmful effects that involve almost all organs of the body. As a result of unrelieved pain, the patient may develop increased respiratory and heart rates, hypertension, increased stress response, urinary retention, fluid overload, electrolyte imbalance, glucose intolerance, hyperglycemia, pneumonia, atelectasis, anorexia, paralytic ileus, constipation, weakness, confusion, and infection.

In addition to psychological and physical suffering, inadequate pain management leads to high health care costs. It is estimated that the cost of extended hospital stays, readmissions to the hospital, and outpatient visits due to inadequate pain management exceeds $200 billion per year.

TABLE 25.1   Types of Pain

Type of Pain	Definition	Drug Treatment
Acute	Pain occurs suddenly, is of short duration (less than 3 months), and responds to treatment; it can result from trauma, tissue injury, inflammation, or surgery.	Mild pain: Nonopioid drugs, such as acetaminophen and NSAIDs Moderate pain: Combination of nonopioid and opioid drugs, such as oxycodone and acetaminophen Severe pain: Potent opioids, such as morphine or hydrocodone
Chronic	Pain persists for more than 3 months and is difficult to treat or control.	Nonopioid drugs are suggested. Opioids, if used, should meet these criteria: • Oral or transdermal • Long duration of action • Include adjunct therapy • Cause minimal respiratory depression
Cancer	Pain occurs from pressure on nerves and organs, blockage to blood supply, or metastasis to bone.	NSAIDs and opioid drugs administered PO, transdermally, via IM or IV routes, intrathecally, or with PCA
Somatic	Pain is in skeletal muscle, ligaments, and joints.	Nonopioids: NSAIDs; also act as antiinflammatories and muscle relaxants
Superficial	Pain is from surface areas such as skin and mucous membranes.	Mild pain: Nonopioid Moderate pain: Combination of opioid and nonopioid analgesic drugs
Vascular	Pain occurs from vascular or perivascular tissues contributing to headaches or migraines.	Nonopioid drugs
Visceral	Pain is from smooth muscle and organs.	Opioid drugs

IM, Intramuscular; *IV,* intravenous; *NSAIDs,* nonsteroidal antiinflammatory drugs; *PCA,* patient-controlled analgesia; *PO,* by mouth.

NONOPIOID ANALGESICS

Nonopioid analgesics such as aspirin, acetaminophen, ibuprofen, and naproxen are less potent than opioid analgesics and are used to treat mild to moderate pain. Nonopioids are usually purchased over the counter, but cyclooxygenase 2 (COX-2) inhibitors require a prescription. Nonopioids are effective for the dull, throbbing pain of headaches, dysmenorrhea (menstrual pain), inflammation, minor abrasions, muscular aches and pain, and mild to moderate arthritis. Most analgesics also have an antipyretic effect and will lower an elevated body temperature. Some, such as aspirin, have antiinflammatory and antiplatelet effects as well.

Nonsteroidal Antiinflammatory Drugs

All NSAIDs have an analgesic effect as well as an antipyretic and antiinflammatory action. NSAIDs such as aspirin, ibuprofen, and naproxen can be purchased as over-the-counter (OTC) drugs. Aspirin, a salicylate NSAID, is the oldest nonopioid analgesic drug still in use. Adolf Bayer marketed the original formulation in 1899, and currently aspirin can be purchased under many names and with added ingredients.

The American Academy of Pediatrics, Centers for Disease Control and Prevention (CDC), U.S. Food and Drug Administration (FDA), National Reye's Syndrome Foundation, U.S. Surgeon General, and World Health Organization (WHO) recommend aspirin products not be given to children and adolescents younger than 19 years of age during episodes of fever or viral illnesses because of the danger of Reye syndrome. Reye syndrome is a rare but serious condition associated with viral infections treated with salicylates that causes swelling of the brain and liver. In these circumstances, acetaminophen is recommended instead of aspirin.

In addition to its analgesic, antipyretic, and antiinflammatory properties, aspirin decreases platelet aggregation (clotting). Some health care providers may therefore prescribe one

81-mg, 162-mg, or 325-mg aspirin tablet every day or one 325-mg tablet every other day as a preventive measure against transient ischemic attacks (TIAs, or ministrokes), heart attacks, or any thromboembolic episode. Aspirin is discussed in depth in Chapter 24 along with other NSAIDs.

Aspirin and other NSAIDs relieve pain by inhibiting biosynthesis of prostaglandin by different forms of the COX enzyme. As explained in Chapter 24, NSAIDs inhibit or block both COX-1 and COX-2 enzymes, while COX-2 inhibitors are selective and only inhibit COX-2 enzyme. Inhibition of COX-1 decreases protection of the stomach lining while inhibition of COX-2 decreases inflammation and pain. As a result of an NSAID's inhibition of COX-1, gastric irritation and bleeding may occur. Aspirin is the drug of choice for alleviating pain and inflammation in arthritic conditions, but when given in high doses, severe gastrointestinal (GI) irritation and possible ulceration develop in approximately 20% of patients. Some pharmaceutical companies have developed antiinflammatory and analgesic drugs that inhibit only COX-2. The COX-2 inhibitors were developed to eliminate the GI side effects associated with aspirin and other NSAIDs. COX-2 inhibitors are discussed in depth in Chapter 24.

Side Effects and Adverse Reactions

A common side effect of NSAIDs is gastric distress, including anorexia, nausea, vomiting, and diarrhea. These drugs should be taken with food, at mealtime, or with a full glass of fluid to help reduce this problem. Excessive bleeding might occur as a side effect if an NSAID is taken for dysmenorrhea during the first 2 days of menstruation. Adverse effects of salicylate toxicity includes tinnitus, vertigo, hyperventilation, and potential metabolic acidosis.

Some patients are hypersensitive to aspirin. Dyspnea, bronchospasm, and urticaria are some of the symptoms that indicate

PROTOTYPE DRUG CHART 25.1
Acetaminophen

Drug Class	Dosage
Analgesic Pregnancy category: B, C*	A/adol/C >12 y >60 kg: PO/PR: 325-650 mg q4-6h PRN; *max:* 3000 mg/d; rectal supp: 650 mg qid Adol/C <60 kg: PO/PR: 10-15 mg/kg q4-6h PRN; *max:* 75 mg/kg/d Neonates: PO/PR: 10-15 mg/kg q6-8h PRN; *max:* 60 mg/kg/d TDM: 10-20 mcg/mL
Contraindications Acetaminophen hypersensitivity, severe hepatic disease *Caution:* Renal disease, alcoholism, severe hypovolemia, chronic malnutrition	**Drug-Lab-Food Interactions** Increased effect with caffeine, diflunisal Decreased effect with oral contraceptives, antacids, anticholinergics, cholestyramine, charcoal, barbiturates, carbamazepine, and phenytoin
Pharmacokinetics Absorption: Rapidly absorbed PO; rectal absorption is erratic. Distribution: PB: 10%-25%; crosses the placenta, excreted in breast milk Metabolism: t½: 2-3 h Excretion: In urine as metabolites	**Pharmacodynamics** PO: Onset: 10-30 min Peak: 30-60 min Duration: 3-5 h Rectal: Onset: UK Peak: UK Duration: 4-6 h
Therapeutic Effects/Uses To decrease pain and fever Mode of Action: Inhibition (weak) of prostaglandin synthesis, inhibition of hypothalamic heat-regulator center	
Side Effects Headache, insomnia, anorexia, nausea, vomiting, constipation, rash	**Adverse Reactions** Oliguria, elevated hepatic enzymes *Life threatening:* Hepatotoxicity, hemolytic anemia, agranulocytosis, leukopenia, neutropenia, thrombocytopenia, renal failure

*Pregnancy categories have been revised. See http://www.fda.gov/Drugs/DevelopmentApprovalProcess/DevelopmentResources/Labeling/ucm093307.htm for more information.
A, Adult; *adol*, adolescent; *C*, child; *d*, day; *h*, hour; *max*, maximum dosage; *min*, minute; *PB*, protein binding; *PO*, by mouth; *PR*, per rectum; *PRN*, as needed; *q*, every; *qid*, four times a day; *supp*, suppository; *t½*, half-life; *TDM*, therapeutic drug monitoring; *UK*, unknown; *y*, year; >, greater than; <, less than.

anaphylaxis to salicylate products. Certain foods also contain salicylates: prunes, raisins, paprika, and licorice. Those with a hypersensitivity to aspirin and salicylate products may be sensitive to other NSAIDs. This hypersensitivity may be related to inhibition of the COX enzyme by the salicylate.

Acetaminophen

The analgesic acetaminophen, a para-aminophenol derivative, was first marketed in the mid-1950s as an analgesic and antipyretic drug used for muscular aches and pains and for fever caused by viral infections in infants, children, adults, and older adults. It is a popular nonprescription drug: it constitutes 25% of all OTC drugs sold. Acetaminophen is a nonopioid drug, but it is *not* an NSAID. Because acetaminophen does not have the antiinflammatory properties of aspirin, it is not the drug of choice for any inflammatory process. Acetaminophen is a safe, effective drug when used at therapeutic doses, causes little to no gastric distress, and does not interfere with platelet aggregation. Complementary and Alternative Therapies 25.1 describes the use of these products in pain relief. An intravenous (IV) formulation was approved by the FDA for treating pain and fever. It should be administered undiluted over 15 minutes. There is no link between acetaminophen and Reye syndrome, and unlike aspirin and NSAIDs, it does not increase the potential for excessive bleeding if taken for dysmenorrhea (Prototype Drug Chart 25.1).

Pharmacokinetics Acetaminophen is well absorbed from the GI tract. Rectal absorption may be erratic because of the presence of fecal material or a decrease in blood flow to the colon. Because of acetaminophen's short half-life, it can be administered every 4 hours as needed with a maximum dose of 4 g/day for adults. However, it is suggested that a patient who frequently takes acetaminophen limit the dose to 2000 mg/day (2 g/day) to avoid the possibility of hepatic or renal dysfunction. More than 85% of acetaminophen is metabolized to drug metabolites by the liver.

Large doses or overdoses can be toxic to the hepatic cells, so when large doses are administered over a long period, the serum level of acetaminophen should be monitored. The therapeutic serum range is 10 to 20 mcg/mL. Hepatic enzyme levels (aspartate aminotransferase [AST], alanine aminotransferase [ALT], alkaline phosphatase [ALP]) and serum bilirubin should also be monitored. Ingesting alcohol concurrently with acetaminophen may lead to hepatic injury, hepatic failure, and death. When acetaminophen toxicity occurs, acetylcysteine is the antidote, which reduces liver injury by converting toxic metabolites to a nontoxic form.

Pharmacodynamics Acetaminophen weakly inhibits prostaglandin synthesis, which decreases pain sensation. It is effective in eliminating mild to moderate pain and headaches and is useful for its antipyretic effect. Acetaminophen does not possess antiinflammatory action. When given orally, its onset of action is within 10 to 30 minutes, and the duration of action is 3 to 5 hours. Severe adverse reactions may occur with an overdose, so acetaminophen in liquid or chewable form should be kept out of children's reach.

Side Effects and Adverse Reactions

An overdose of acetaminophen can be extremely toxic to liver cells; death could occur in 1 to 4 days from hepatic necrosis. If a child or adult ingests excessive amounts of acetaminophen tablets or liquid, a poison control center should be contacted immediately, and the child or adult should be taken to the emergency department. Early symptoms of hepatic damage include nausea, vomiting, diarrhea, and abdominal pain.

Table 25.2 lists the commonly used nonopioid analgesics and their dosages, uses, and considerations.

NURSING PROCESS
Patient-Centered Collaborative Care

Analgesic: Acetaminophen

Assessment
- Obtain a medical history of liver dysfunction. Overdosing or extremely high doses of acetaminophen can cause hepatotoxicity, hepatic failure, and death.
- Ascertain the severity of pain. Nonopioid NSAIDs, such as ibuprofen, or an opioid may be necessary to relieve pain.

Nursing Diagnoses
- Injury, Risk for
- Pain, Acute related to edema from the surgical incision

Planning
- The patient's pain will be relieved or diminished.

Nursing Interventions
- Check hepatic enzyme tests such as ALT, ALP, gamma-glutamyl transferase (GGT), 5'-nucleotidase, and bilirubin for elevations in patients who take high doses of acetaminophen or overdoses.

Patient Teaching
General
- Teach patients to keep acetaminophen out of children's reach. Acetaminophen for children is available in flavored tablets and liquid, and high doses can cause hepatotoxicity, hepatic failure, and death.
- Advise patients not to self-medicate with acetaminophen for more than 10 days. Teach adult caregivers not to medicate children for more than 5 days without a health care provider's approval.
- ⚡ Direct parents to call a poison control center immediately if a child has taken a large or unknown amount of acetaminophen.
- ⚡ Teach patients to check acetaminophen dosages on the label of OTC drugs. Do not exceed the recommended

dosage. The suggested safe maximum adult acetaminophen dosage is 4 g/day to avoid hepatic damage (see Prototype Drug Chart 25.1).
- Teach patient to avoid alcohol ingestion while taking acetaminophen.

Side Effects
- Encourage patients to report side effects. Overdosing can cause severe hepatic damage, hepatic failure, and death.
- ⚡ Check the serum acetaminophen level if toxicity is suspected. The therapeutic serum level is 10 to 20 mcg/mL; the toxic level is greater than 200 mcg/mL 4 hours after ingestion and is usually associated with hepatotoxicity. The antidote for acetaminophen is acetylcysteine. Dosage is based on the serum acetaminophen level.

Cultural Considerations
- Involving the extended family may be important for teaching health strategies and providing support.

Evaluation
- Evaluate the effectiveness of acetaminophen in relieving pain using consistent pain scale. If pain persists, another analgesic may be needed.
- Determine whether the patient is taking the recommended dosage. Observe and report any side effects.

COMPLEMENTARY AND ALTERNATIVE THERAPIES 25.1

Capsaicin

Capsaicin, which is found naturally in cayenne pepper, is selective for C-fiber nociceptors and relieves some arthritis pain in topical cream or gel form.

❶ OPIOID ANALGESICS

Opioid analgesics, called opioid agonists, are prescribed for moderate and severe pain. In the United States, the Harrison Opioid Act of 1914 required that all forms of opium be sold with a prescription and that it no longer be used as a nonprescription drug. The Controlled Substances Act of 1970 classified drugs with high abuse potential, opioids among them, in five schedule categories according to their potential for drug abuse (see Chapter 7). Addiction is defined as a psychological and physical dependence upon a substance beyond normal voluntary control, usually after prolonged use of a substance.

Morphine, a prototype opioid, is obtained from the sap of seed pods of the opium poppy plant. Codeine is another drug obtained from opium. In the past decades, many synthetic and semisynthetic opioids have been developed, for example, meperidine.

Although nonopioid analgesics act on the PNS at the pain receptor sites, opioid analgesics act mostly on the CNS. Opioids act primarily by activating the μ-receptors, but they also exert a weak activation of the kappa (κ) receptors. Analgesia, respiratory depression, euphoria, and sedation are effects of μ-receptor activation. Activation of κ-receptors leads to analgesia and sedation but has no effect on respiratory depression and euphoria.

TABLE 25.2   Analgesics

Generic	Route and Dosage	Uses and Considerations
PARA-AMINOPHENOL		
Acetaminophen	See Prototype Drug Chart 25.1.	
NONSTEROIDAL ANTIINFLAMMATORY DRUGS (NSAIDS)		
Aspirin	Pain: A: PO/PR: 325 to 650 mg, q4h PRN; *max:* 4 g/d	For relief of headaches, pain, inflammation, fever, and mild anticoagulant to prevent thromboembolism. May cause GI distress, dizziness, drowsiness, tinnitus, hearing loss (reversible), and bleeding. Aspirin should be taken with food. Avoid with alcohol. Avoid in children and teenagers younger than 19 years during episodes of fever or viral illnesses. Pregnancy category: D*; PB: 90%-95%; t½: 15-20 min
Diflunisal	Pain: A/adol >50 kg: PO: Initially 1000 mg; maint: 500 mg q8-12h; *max:* 1500 mg/d Older A/adol <50 kg: PO: Initially 500 mg; maint: 250 mg q8-12h; *max:* 1500 mg/d	For mild to moderate pain, osteoarthritis, and RA. May cause headache, dizziness, insomnia, fatigue, rash, GI distress and bleeding, and elevated hepatic enzymes. Pregnancy category: C*; PB: 99%, t½: 8-12 h
PROPIONIC ACID		
Ibuprofen	Pain: A: PO: 400 mg q4-6h; *max:* 3200 mg/d A/adol >17 y: IV: 400-800 mg over 30 min q6h; *max:* 3200 mg/d	For reducing fever, mild to severe pain, osteoarthritis, and RA. May cause GI distress, tinnitus, hearing loss, fluid retention, nephrotoxicity, edema, anemia, thrombocytopenia, and neutropenia. Should be taken with food, at mealtime, or with plenty of fluids. Pregnancy category: C*; PB: 90%-99%; t½: 2-4 h
Naproxen	Pain: A: PO: Initially 500 mg, then 250 mg q6-8h; *max:* 1250 mg/d	For mild to moderate pain, osteoarthritis, RA, bursitis, ankylosing spondylitis, gout, and dysmenorrhea. May cause drowsiness, dizziness, headache, rash, skin eruptions, elevated hepatic enzymes, GI distress, and bleeding. Pregnancy category: C*; PB: 99%; t½: 12-17 h
Ketorolac	A/adol >17 y >50 kg: PO: Initially 20 mg, maint: 10 mg q4-6h PRN; *max:* 40 mg/d Older A/adol >17 y <50 kg: PO: 10 mg q4-6h PRN; *max:* 40 mg/d A/adol >17 y >50 kg: IM/IV: 30 mg q6h PRN; *max:* 120 mg/d Older A/adol >17 y <50 kg: IM/IV: 15 mg q6h PRN; *max:* 60 mg/d	For short-term pain management (5 days or less). May cause dizziness, drowsiness, edema, headache, GI distress, GI bleeding and perforation, elevated hepatic enzymes, and ocular inflammation. Pregnancy category: C*; PB: 99%; t½: PO, 2.4-9 h; IM, 3.5-9.2 h
OXICAMS		
Meloxicam	A: PO: 7.5-15 mg/d; *max:* 15 mg/d	For pain from osteoarthritis and RA. May cause dizziness, headache, insomnia, edema, GI distress, and elevated hepatic enzymes. Pregnancy category: C, D*; PB: 99%; t½: 15-20 h
NAPHTHYLALKANONES		
Nabumetone	A: PO: 1000 mg/d or 500 mg bid; *max:* 2000 mg/d	For pain from osteoarthritis and RA. May cause dizziness, headache, tinnitus, rash, itching, GI distress, edema, and cardiovascular thrombotic events. Pregnancy category: C*; PB: 99%; t½: 24 h
CYCLOOXYGENASE 2 (COX-2) INHIBITORS		
Celecoxib	Pain: A >18 y: PO: initially 400 mg followed by additional 200 mg on day 1 as needed; maint: 200 mg bid; *max:* 800 mg/d	For moderate to severe pain, osteoarthritis, and RA. May cause dizziness, headache, hypertension, edema, bleeding, and cardiovascular thrombotic events. Use caution in patients with severe renal or liver disorders and for those allergic to salicylates or sulfonamides. Pregnancy category: C, D*; PB: 97%; t½: 11.2 h
MISCELLANEOUS		
Tramadol	Immediate release: A/adol >17 y: PO: Initially: 25 mg/d; maint: 50-100 mg q4-6h PRN; *max:* 400 mg/d, 300 mg/d for A >75 y Extended release: A: PO: 100 mg/d; *max:* 300 mg/d	For moderate to severe pain. Contraindicated in severe alcoholism or with use of opioids and CNS depressants. May cause nausea, vomiting, drowsiness, dizziness, weakness, constipation, headache, anxiety, and agitation. Pregnancy category: C*; PB: 20%; t½: 6.3 h for immediate release, 7.9 h for extended release

Continued

TABLE 25.2   Analgesics—cont'd

Generic	Route and Dosage	Uses and Considerations
MISCELLANEOUS		
Indomethacin	Pain: Regular release: A: PO: 75-150 mg/d in 3-4 divided doses with food for 7-14 d; *max:* 200 mg/d Extended release: A: PO: 75 mg daily/bid with food for 7-14 d; *max:* 150 mg/d	For mild to severe pain, gout, tendinitis, osteoarthritis, RA, and ankylosing spondylitis. May cause dizziness, headache, GI distress, and GI bleeding. Take with food. Avoid if allergic to aspirin. Pregnancy category: C*; PB: 99%; t½: 2.6-11.2 h

*Pregnancy categories have been revised. See http://www.fda.gov/Drugs/DevelopmentApprovalProcess/DevelopmentResources/Labeling/ucm093307.htm for more information.
A, Adult; *adol,* adolescent; *bid,* twice a day; *CNS,* central nervous system; *d,* day; *GI,* gastrointestinal; *h,* hour; *IM,* intramuscular; *IV,* intravenous; *maint,* maintenance; *max,* maximum dosage; *min,* minute; *PB,* protein binding; *PO,* by mouth; *PR,* per rectum; *PRN,* as needed; *q,* every; *RA,* rheumatoid arthritis; *t½,* half-life; *y,* year; >, greater than; <, less than.

 COMPLEMENTARY AND ALTERNATIVE THERAPIES 25.2

Sedatives

Opioids taken with kava, valerian, and St. John's wort may increase sedation.

Opioids not only suppress pain impulses but also suppress respiration and coughing by acting on the respiratory and cough centers in the medulla of the brainstem. One example of such an opioid is morphine, a potent analgesic that can readily depress respirations. Codeine is not as potent as morphine (1/15 to 1/20 as potent), but it also relieves mild to moderate pain and suppresses cough, which allows it also to be classified as an antitussive. Most opioids, with the exception of meperidine, have an antitussive (cough suppression) effect. The opioids have two isomers, levo and dextro. The levo-isomers of opioids produce an analgesic effect only; however, both levo- and dextro-isomers possess an antitussive response. The dextro-isomers do not cause physical dependence, but the

levo-isomers do. Synthetic cough suppressants are discussed in Chapter 35.

In addition to pain relief and antitussive effects, many opioids possess antidiarrheal effects. Common side effects with high doses of most opioids include nausea and vomiting, particularly in ambulatory patients; constipation; a moderate decrease in blood pressure; and orthostatic hypotension. High doses of opioids may also cause respiratory depression; urinary retention, usually in older adults; and antitussive effects. See Complementary and Alternative Therapies 25.2 for interactions with opioids.

Morphine

Morphine, an extraction from opium, is a potent opioid analgesic (Prototype Drug Chart 25.2). Morphine is effective against acute pain resulting from acute myocardial infarction (AMI) and cancer, relieves dyspnea resulting from pulmonary edema, and may be used as a preoperative medication to relieve anxiety. Although it is effective in relieving severe pain, it can cause

PROTOTYPE DRUG CHART 25.2

❶ Morphine Sulfate

Drug Class	Dosage
Opioid CSS II Pregnancy category: C*	Regular release: A: PO: Initially 10-30 mg q4h PRN Extended release: A: PO: 15 mg q8-12h PRN or 30 mg/d A: IV/IM/subcut: 2-10 mg/70 kg q3-4h PRN Adol/C/Infants >6 mo: IV/IM/subcut: 0.05-0.2 mg/kg q2-4h PRN
Contraindications Hypersensitivity, CNS or respiratory depression, status asthmaticus, increased intracranial pressure, shock, alcoholism, ileus, hypovolemia *Caution:* Respiratory insufficiency, renal or hepatic diseases; urinary retention; sleep apnea; older adults	**Drug-Lab-Food Interactions** Drug: Increased effects of alcohol, sedative-hypnotics, antipsychotic drugs, muscle relaxants Complementary and Alternative Therapies: St. John's wort may decrease drug effect (see Complementary and Alternative Therapies 25.2). Lab: Increased AST, ALT
Pharmacokinetics Absorption: PO, varies; IV, rapid Distribution: PB: 30%-35%; crosses placenta, excreted in breast milk Metabolism: t½: 1.5-2 h Excretion: 90% in urine	**Pharmacodynamics** PO: Onset: Variable Peak: 1 h Duration: 4-5 h; SR, 8-12 h Subcut/IM: Onset: 15-30 min Peak: 50-90 min Duration: UK IV: Onset: Rapid Peak: 20 min Duration: 3-5 h

PROTOTYPE DRUG CHART 25.2—cont'd

❶ *Morphine Sulfate*

Therapeutic Effects/Uses	
To relieve moderate to severe pain	
Mode of Action: Depression of the CNS; depression of pain impulses by binding with opiate receptors in the CNS	

Side Effects	Adverse Reactions
Anorexia, nausea, vomiting, abdominal pain, diarrhea, constipation, flatulence, fever, drowsiness, dizziness, agitation, anxiety, sedation, confusion, depression, urinary retention, rash, blurred vision, miosis, weakness, flushing, euphoria, pruritus	Hypotension, urticaria, seizures, ileus, psychological dependence *Life threatening:* Respiratory depression

*Pregnancy categories have been revised. See http://www.fda.gov/Drugs/DevelopmentApprovalProcess/DevelopmentResources/Labeling/ucm093307.htm for more information.
A, Adult; *adol,* adolescent; *ALT,* alanine aminotransferase; *AST,* aspartate aminotransferase; *C,* child; *CNS,* central nervous system; *CSS,* Controlled Substances Schedule; *d,* day; *h,* hour; *IM,* intramuscular; *IV,* intravenous; *min,* minute; *mo,* month; *PB,* protein binding; *PO,* by mouth; *PRN,* as necessary; *q,* every; *subcut,* subcutaneous; *SR,* sustained release; *t½,* half-life; *UK,* unknown.

respiratory depression, orthostatic hypotension, miosis, urinary retention, constipation resulting from reduced bowel motility, and cough suppression. An antidote for morphine excess or overdose is the opioid antagonist naloxone.

Pharmacokinetics Morphine may be taken orally, although GI absorption can be somewhat erratic. For quick relief of severe pain, such as with AMI, or for fast relief of anxiety and to reduce hypertension, it is given intravenously. Morphine is 30% to 35% protein bound and may also be administered rectally and epidurally. Oral morphine undergoes first-pass hepatic metabolism, meaning the liver metabolizes the drug before morphine is available to the rest of the body. Only a small amount of morphine crosses the blood-brain barrier to produce an analgesic effect. It has a short half-life of 1.5 to 2 hours, and 90% is excreted in the urine. Morphine crosses the placenta and is excreted in breast milk.

Pharmacodynamics Morphine binds with the opiate receptor in the CNS. Parenterally, the onset of action is rapid, especially

◎ NURSING PROCESS
Patient-Centered Collaborative Care
❶ *Opioid Analgesic: Morphine Sulfate*

Assessment

- Obtain a medical history. Contraindications for morphine include severe respiratory disorders, increased intracranial pressure, and severe renal disease. Morphine may cause seizures.
- Determine a drug history and check for drug allergies. Report if a drug-drug interaction is probable. Morphine increases the effects of alcohol, sedatives and hypnotics, antipsychotic drugs, and muscle relaxants, and it can cause respiratory depression.
- Assess vital signs, noting the rate and depth of respirations, as well as pupil size for future comparisons; opioids commonly decrease respirations and systolic blood pressure and may cause miosis.
- Monitor urinary output; morphine can cause urinary retention.
- Assess the type of pain, location, and duration before giving opioids.

Nursing Diagnoses

- Pain, Acute related to surgical tissue injury
- Breathing Pattern, Ineffective related to excess morphine dosage
- Falls, Risk for
- Constipation related to morphine

Planning

- The patient's pain will be reduced or alleviated.

Nursing Interventions

- Administer morphine before pain reaches its peak to maximize effectiveness of the drug.
- ⚡ Monitor vital signs at frequent intervals to detect respiratory changes. Fewer than 10 respirations per minute can indicate respiratory distress.
- Record the patient's urine output because urinary retention is a side effect of morphine. Urine output should be at least 600 mL/day.
- Check bowel sounds for decreased peristalsis; constipation is a side effect of morphine. A dietary change or mild laxative might be needed.
- ⚡ Check for pupil changes and reaction. Pinpoint pupils can indicate morphine overdose.
- ⚡ Have naloxone available as an antidote to reverse respiratory depression if morphine overdose occurs.
- Validate the dose of morphine before administration. Check older adults for alertness and orientation because confusion is a side effect of morphine. Use side rails and take other safety precautions as necessary.

Patient Teaching
General

- Encourage patients not to use alcohol or CNS depressants with any opioid analgesics such as morphine. Respiratory depression can result, as well as dizziness and the potential fall risk.
- Suggest nonpharmacologic measures to relieve pain as the patient recuperates from surgery. As recovery progresses, a nonopioid analgesic may be prescribed.

Side Effects

- Alert patients that with continuous use, opioids such as morphine can become addicting. If addiction occurs, inform patients about methadone treatment programs and other resources in the area.
- Encourage patients to report dizziness while taking morphine. Dizziness could be due to orthostatic hypotension. Advise patients to ambulate with caution or only with assistance.
- ⚡ Teach patients to report difficulty in breathing, blurred vision, and headaches.

🌐 *Cultural Considerations*

- Identify conflicts in values and beliefs about pain and pain management.
- Respect cultural and religious differences concerning refusal of opioid analgesics.
- Incorporate traditional practices into Western medicine whenever possible.

Evaluation

- Evaluate the effectiveness of morphine in lessening or alleviating pain using a consistent pain scale. If pain persists after several days, the dose should be increased or the opioid should be changed.
- Determine the stability of vital signs. Any decrease in respiration or blood pressure should be reported.

when administered intravenously. Onset of action is slower for subcutaneous (subcut) and intramuscular (IM) injections. The duration of action with most types of drug administration is 3 to 5 hours; with controlled-release morphine sulfate tablets, duration is 8 to 12 hours.

Meperidine

One of the first synthetic opioids, meperidine became available in the mid-1950s. It is classified as a Schedule II drug according to the Controlled Substances Act. Meperidine has a shorter duration of action than morphine, and its potency varies according to the dosage. Meperidine can be given orally or via IM and IV routes, and it is primarily effective in GI procedures. It does not have the antitussive property of opium preparations.

During pregnancy, meperidine is preferred to morphine because it does not diminish uterine contractions and causes less neonatal respiratory depression. Meperidine causes less constipation and urinary retention than morphine. Meperidine is not indicated for patients with chronic pain, severe liver dysfunction, sickle cell disease, a history of seizures, severe coronary artery disease (CAD), or cardiac dysrhythmias. When older adults and patients with advanced cancer receive large doses of meperidine, neurotoxicity (e.g., nervousness, tremors, agitation, irritability, seizures) are reported. Meperidine should *not* be prescribed for long-term use; the dosage is frequently limited to 150 mg/dose for a period no longer than 48 to 72 hours.

Meperidine is metabolized in the liver to an active metabolite, therefore the dose should be decreased for patients with hepatic or renal insufficiency. It is excreted in the urine in a metabolite form called *normeperidine*. Meperidine should not be taken with alcohol or sedative-hypnotics because combination of these drugs causes an additive CNS depression. A major side effect of meperidine is a decrease in blood pressure, which should be monitored, especially if the patient is an older adult.

Table 25.3 lists opioids and their dosages, uses, and considerations.

⚡ **PATIENT SAFETY**

Do not confuse...
- **Meperidine** (opioid analgesic) with **morphine** (opioid analgesic), **meprobamate** (antianxiety), or **hydromorphone** (opioid analgesic).
- **Demerol** (opioid analgesic) with **Desyrel** (antidepressant) **or Dilaudid** (opioid analgesic).

Hydromorphone

Hydromorphone is a semisynthetic opioid similar to morphine. The analgesic effect is approximately six times more potent than that of morphine with fewer hypnotic effects and less GI distress. This opioid has a faster onset and shorter duration of action than morphine. Hydromorphone is classified as a Schedule II drug according to the Controlled Substances Act. Tolerance to hydromorphone increases gradually.

This drug is given orally, rectally, or via subcut, IM, and IV routes for the relief of moderate to severe pain. When given intravenously, dilution of each dose with 5 mL of sterile water or normal saline is preferred. Direct IV administration of 2 mg or less should be given over 2 to 3 minutes. Hydromorphone is readily absorbed in the body and is excreted in the urine. Respirations should be monitored closely, and adequate hydration should be provided.

Side Effects and Adverse Reactions

Many side effects are known to accompany the use of opioids. Of particular importance are signs of respiratory depression (respiration <10/min). Other side effects include orthostatic hypotension (decrease in blood pressure when rising from a sitting or lying position), drowsiness, dizziness, weakness, confusion, constipation, and urinary retention. In addition, pupillary constriction (a sign of toxicity), tolerance, and psychological and physical dependence may occur with prolonged use.

Increased metabolism of opioids contributes to tolerance, which causes an increased need for higher doses of the opioid. If chronic use of the opioid is discontinued, symptoms of withdrawal that result from cessation of drug administration usually occur within 24 to 48 hours after the last opioid dose. Withdrawal syndrome is caused by physical dependence. Symptoms of withdrawal syndrome include irritability, diaphoresis (sweating), restlessness, muscle twitching, tachycardia, and increased blood pressure. Withdrawal symptoms from opioids are unpleasant but not as severe or life threatening as those that accompany withdrawal from sedative-hypnotics, a process that may lead to seizures.

! TABLE 25.3 Opioids: Opium and Synthetics

Generic	Route and Dosage	Uses and Considerations
Codeine sulfate, codeine phosphate CSS II	A: PO/subcut/IM: 15-60 mg q4h PRN; *max:* 360 mg/d Adol <17 y/C >6 y: PO/subcut/IM: 0.5-1 mg/kg q4-6h PRN; *max:* 60 mg/dose	For mild to moderate pain and as an antitussive. May cause drowsiness, dizziness, headache, anxiety, insomnia, euphoria, miosis, fatigue, confusion, respiratory depression, GI distress, constipation, tolerance, and dependence. Pregnancy category: C*; PB: 7%, t½: 3-4 h
Hydrocodone bitartrate CSS II	Pain: A: PO: Initially 2.5-10 mg hydrocodone/300-660 mg acetaminophen q4-6h PRN	For moderate to severe pain. May cause dizziness, drowsiness, confusion, euphoria, headache, miosis, GI distress, constipation, dependence, tolerance, and respiratory depression. Do not abruptly discontinue. Taper off upon discontinuation. Pregnancy category: C*; PB: 36%; t½: 7-9 h
Hydromorphone hydrochloride CSS II	A: PO: Initially 2.5-10 mg q4-6h PRN A: IM/subcut: 1-2 mg q2-3h PRN A: IV: 0.2-1 mg over 2-3 min q2-3h PRN Rectal: 3 mg q6-8h PRN	For moderate to severe pain. May cause dizziness, drowsiness, headache, miosis, euphoria, fatigue, insomnia, dry mouth, GI distress, constipation, weakness, orthostatic hypotension, urinary reten-tion, tolerance, dependence, and respiratory depression. Pregnancy category: C*; PB: 8%-19%; t½: Immediate release, 2-3 h; extended release, 11 h
Meperidine CSS II	Pain: A: PO/subcut/IM/IV: 50-150 mg q3-4h PRN, give IV over 4-5 min; *max:* 150 mg/dose C: PO/subcut/IM/IV: 1-1.8 mg/kg q3-4h PRN; *max:* 150 mg/dose as a single dose	For moderate to severe pain and sedation induction and maintenance. May cause dizziness, drowsiness, flushing, headache, euphoria, miosis, fatigue, GI distress, constipation, hypotension, tolerance, dependence, and respiratory depression. Pregnancy category: C, D*; PB: 65%-75%; t½: 3-5 h
Morphine sulfate CSS II	See Prototype Drug Chart 25.2.	
Oxycodone hydrochloride CSS II	Immediate release: A: PO: Initially 5-15 mg q4-6h PRN Extended release: A: PO: 10 mg q12h PRN	For moderate to severe pain. Avoid taking drug over an extended period of time. May cause dizziness, drowsiness, confusion, headache, miosis, dry mouth, GI distress, constipation, weakness, and itching. Take with food to avoid GI distress. Pregnancy category: B*; PB: 45%; t½: Immediate release, 3-5 h; extended release, 4.5 h
Oxycodone with acetaminophen and oxycodone with aspirin CSS II	Immediate release: A: PO: 1-2 tabs (2.5-10 mg oxycodone/325 mg acet-aminophen) q6h PRN Extended release: A: PO: 2 tabs q12h With aspirin: A: PO: 1 tab (2.25 mg oxycodone/325 mg aspirin) q6h PRN; max: 12 tabs/d	For moderate to severe pain. May cause dizziness, drowsiness, head-ache, euphoria, miosis, hypotension, itching, dry mouth, GI distress, constipation, dependence, tolerance, elevated hepatic enzymes, and weakness. Take with food or liquid. Pregnancy category: C*; PB: 45%-99%; t½: 2-4 h
Fentanyl CSS II	Pain: A: IM/IV: 2-20 mcg/kg (slow IV over 1-2 min) Chronic severe pain: Transdermal patch: Initially 25 mcg/h patch A: Transmucosal: Initially 200 mcg sucked (not chewed) over 15 min	For moderate to severe pain and anesthesia induction and maintenance. May cause drowsiness, dizziness, euphoria, miosis, headache, confu-sion, weakness, bradycardia, hypokalemia, edema, GI distress, consti-pation, dry mouth, tolerance, dependence, and respiratory depression. Pregnancy category: C*; PB: 80%-85%; t½: IV, 2-4 h; transdermal, 20-27 h; transmucosal, 3-14 h
Methadone CSS II	Pain: A: PO/subcut/IM: Initially 2.5 mg q8-12h PRN	For moderate to severe pain, opiate agonist dependence and with-drawal. Similar to morphine but longer duration of action. Used in drug abuse programs. Helps alleviate craving for opioids. May cause dizziness, drowsiness, blurred vision, agitation, confusion, eupho-ria, hallucinations, seizure, headache, bradycardia, dysrhythmias, hypotension, edema, diaphoresis, dry mouth, GI distress, weakness, urinary retention, tolerance, dependence, and respiratory depression. Pregnancy category: C*; PB: 85%-90%; t½: 2-3 h

*Pregnancy categories have been revised. See http://www.fda.gov/Drugs/DevelopmentApprovalProcess/DevelopmentResources/Labeling/ucm093307.htm for more information.
A, Adult; *Adol,* adolescent; *C,* child; *CSS,* Controlled Substances Schedule; *d,* day; *ER,* extended release; *GI,* gastrointestinal; *h,* hour; *IM,* intramuscular; *IV,* intravenous; *max,* maximum; *min,* minute; *PB,* protein binding; *PO,* by mouth; *PRN,* as necessary; *q,* every; *subcut,* subcutaneous; *t½,* half-life; *tab,* tablet; *y,* year.

Contraindications

Use of opioid analgesics is contraindicated for patients with head injuries. Opioids decrease respiration, which promotes carbon dioxide (CO_2) retention leading to increased intracranial pressure.

Opioid analgesics given to a patient with a respiratory disorder only intensify the respiratory distress. In a patient with asthma, opiates decrease respiratory drive while simultaneously increasing airway resistance.

Opioids may cause hypotension and are not indicated for patients in shock or for those who have very low blood pressure. If an opioid is necessary, the dosage needs to be adjusted accordingly; otherwise, the hypotensive state may worsen. For an older adult or a person who is debilitated, the opioid dose usually needs to be decreased.

Morphine is the opioid analgesic prototype; all other opioids are measured in comparison to morphine.

Combination Drugs

To treat moderate to severe pain, combination drugs that comprise an NSAID and an opioid analgesic may be used. Examples are ibuprofen and hydrocodone, a combination of an NSAID and an opioid. Another combination for the treatment of mild to moderate pain is acetaminophen and codeine. When using a combination of drugs, smaller doses of each drug are required, thereby decreasing side effects. Also, using a combination of drugs for pain helps to decrease drug dependency that may result from possible long-term use of an opioid agent.

Patient-Controlled Analgesia

Patient-controlled analgesia (PCA) is an alternative route for opioid administration for self-administered pain relief as needed. Usually a loading dose (e.g., 2 to 10 mg of morphine) is given initially to achieve pain relief. Within predetermined safety limits, the patient controls administration of the opioid analgesic based on the amount of pain. To receive the opioid, the patient pushes a button on the PCA device, which releases a specific dose of analgesic (e.g., 1 mg morphine) into the IV line. The nurse sets the PCA pump with the opioid analgesic dose prescribed by the health care provider by regulating the time intervals (every several minutes) at which the drug can be received. A lockout mechanism on the electronically controlled infusion pump prevents the patient from constantly pushing the button and causing a drug overdose. The PCA device maintains a near-constant analgesic level, avoiding episodes of severe pain or oversedation. It is imperative that the patient, not the family or the nurse, control the PCA device to avoid overdosing. Morphine is used most often for PCA, but fentanyl and hydromorphone may also be given.

Transdermal Opioid Analgesics

Transdermal opioid analgesics provide continuous, around-the-clock pain control that is helpful to patients who suffer from chronic pain. The transdermal method is not useful for acute or postoperative pain. An example of a transdermal opioid analgesic is fentanyl, which is administered via a transdermal patch. This patch comes in various strengths—12.5, 25, 50, 75, and 100 mcg/h. Maximum serum fentanyl levels occur within 24 hours of when the patch is first applied. Fentanyl is also available for IM and IV use. Fentanyl is more potent than morphine. For older adults, the use of a lower fentanyl transdermal dose is usually suggested. The health care provider must exercise caution when prescribing fentanyl for patients who weigh less than 110 pounds.

Analgesic Titration

Analgesics may be titrated to increase or decrease the dosage. Usually postoperative pain will decrease over time, and analgesics will be titrated downward. However, the patient with cancer-related pain usually has a continual increase in pain and will require an upward titration. Titration can be accomplished by changing the dose, the interval between doses, the route of administration, or the drug. When titrating analgesics, the dosage is decided after assessing the patient's respiratory rate and pain level.

Opioid Use in Special Populations
Children

Pain management in children is complex because it is more difficult to assess their pain. Some children will not verbalize discomfort when they are in severe pain, and some are fearful of treatments like injections that relieve pain. Nurses should use age-appropriate communication skills to ascertain a child's need for pain relief. The "ouch scale" illustrated in Fig. 25.1 can be helpful in determining a child's level of pain. Also, the parent may help identify the presence and degree of the child's pain. Crying and whining may be indicators of a need for pain relief or may represent other needs.

A child, like an adult, should be given medication before the pain becomes severe. The use of oral liquid medication for pain relief, if appropriate, is generally more acceptable to the child. The nurse may alleviate the child's fear and help with drug compliance by using drawings and pictures related to areas of pain in the body and pain relief with smiling faces.

Older Adults

Usually, adults who are 65 years of age or older require adjustment to drug doses to avoid severe side effects. Merely decreasing the usual adult dosage of opioid analgesic is not always the answer for older adults. Many take an array of medications for their health problems, increasing the possibility of drug interactions and drug side effects. In older adults, side effects from the use of opioids are more pronounced; therefore the nurse must closely monitor for adverse reactions in older adults who take opioid analgesics. As a person ages, liver and renal functions decrease, causing the rate of metabolism and excretion of the drug to decrease. As a result, drug accumulation may occur.

Older adults tend to have different beliefs and fears than younger generations regarding opioids. They may believe that pain is inevitable due to aging, or they may fear addiction. Older adults may not want to report pain because they do not want to be a burden. The nurse must perform pain assessment with a supportive approach in an unhurried manner and should give the patient accurate drug information.

Pain assessment may be more difficult with older adults due to the decrease in cognitive and sensory-perceptual abilities. Dementia or hearing and visual deficits may interfere

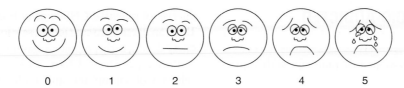

1. Explain to the child that each face is for a person who feels happy because he has no pain (hurt, or whatever word the child uses) or feels sad because he has some or a lot of pain.

2. Point to the appropriate face and state, "This face is ..."
   0-"very happy because he doesn't hurt at all."
   1-"hurts just a little bit."
   2-"hurts a little more."
   3-"hurts even more."
   4-"hurts a whole lot."
   5-"hurts as much as you can imagine, although you don't have to be crying to feel this bad."

3. Ask the child to choose the face that best describes how he feels. Be specific about which pain (e.g., "shot" or incision) and what time (e.g., now? earlier? before lunch?).

FIG. 25.1 A scale used to rate the intensity of pain in children. From Hockenberry, M. (2013). *Wong's essentials of pediatric nursing* (9th ed.). St. Louis: Mosby.

with communication. The nurse may need to rely on a more thorough physical assessment to discover the presence of pain, because self-reporting may not be reliable.

In the presence of decreased renal and hepatic function, drugs that tend to be more toxic in older adults include meperidine, pentazocine, and propoxyphene. Analgesics are usually metabolized in the liver and are excreted in the urine. Usual doses of analgesics in older adults may result in excessive sedation and prolonged duration of action. Chronologic age is one of several factors that influence medication use and dosage. Comorbidity must also be considered.

Cognitively Impaired Individuals

Any cognitively impaired individual may be unable to report pain adequately. The nurse should use a measurement scale that is appropriate for the patient. Some physical signs of pain include moans, grimacing, clenched teeth, noisy respirations, and restlessness.

Oncology Patients

Cancer pain is managed according to three levels of analgesia based on the WHO "ladder" as follows:
Step 1—Mild Pain: Nonopioids with or without an adjuvant medication
Step 2—Moderate Pain: Nonopioids and mild opioids with or without an adjuvant medication
Step 3—Severe Pain: Stronger opioids at higher dosage levels with or without an adjuvant medication

Opioids are titrated for oncology patients until pain relief is achieved or the side effects become intolerable. For effective pain management in patients with cancer, extremely high doses may be required. There are no set dosage limits for oncology patients.

Individuals With a History of Substance Use Disorder

Often patients with a history of substance use disorder require pain medication. A thorough pain assessment is necessary to find out the cause of pain. The nurse needs to know that opioids are effective and safe in this population, even though larger doses in greater frequency may be required. Studies have shown that withholding opioids in this population has not increased recovery from addiction. However, opioid agonist-antagonists such as pentazocine should be avoided in chemically dependent patients because these drugs may precipitate withdrawal syndrome.

ADJUVANT THERAPY

Medications used as **adjuvant analgesics** have been developed for other purposes and were later found to be effective for pain relief in neuropathy. Adjuvant therapy is usually used along with a nonopioid and opioid analgesic. Examples of adjuvant analgesics include anticonvulsants, antidepressants, corticosteroids, antidysrhythmics, and local anesthetics.

Antiseizure medications such as gabapentin act on the peripheral nerves and CNS by inhibiting spontaneous neuronal firing. They are used for neuropathic pain and for prevention of migraine headaches. Tricyclic antidepressants (TCAs) such as amitriptyline prevent the reuptake of serotonin and norepinephrine in the cells. Lower doses of TCAs than those usually prescribed for depression are effective in treating peripheral neuropathy. Corticosteroids serve as effective analgesics by reducing nociceptive stimuli. Antidysrhythmics such as mexiletine block sodium channels to reduce pain. Local anesthetics—for example, a lidocaine patch—can provide effective analgesia by interrupting the transmission of pain signals to the brain.

Adjuvant medications potentiate opioid analgesia for severe persistent pain in diabetic neuropathy, cancer, migraine headaches, and rheumatoid arthritis. When any of the adjuvant medications are used in conjunction with an NSAID and an opioid, dosages may be kept lower to reduce adverse effects.

TREATMENT FOR OPIOID-ADDICTED INDIVIDUALS

Refer to Chapter 7 for a discussion of therapies for addiction.

OPIOID AGONIST-ANTAGONISTS

Opioid agonist-antagonists, medications in which an opioid antagonist is added to an opioid agonist, may be used to decrease opioid abuse. Pentazocine, an opioid agonist-antagonist analgesic, can be given orally as a tablet or by injection (subcut, IM, and IV). Pentazocine is classified as a Schedule IV drug. Butorphanol tartrate, buprenorphine, and nalbuphine hydrochloride are examples of other opioid agonist-antagonist analgesics. Reports say that pentazocine and butorphanol can cause dependence. Opioid agonist-antagonist drugs are not given for cancer pain because of

the risk of potential CNS toxicity from the high doses required. These analgesics are considered safe for use during labor, but their safety during early pregnancy has not been established.

Prototype Drug Chart 25.3 details the pharmacologic behavior of nalbuphine, and Table 25.4 lists the various opioid agonist-antagonists.

Pharmacokinetics Nalbuphine can be administered orally or via IM, subcut, or IV routes. It is rapidly absorbed parenterally. Nalbuphine has a short half-life. It is metabolized in the liver and excreted in the urine.

Pharmacodynamics Nalbuphine is effective in alleviating moderate to severe pain. The onset of action is rapid, and peak time occurs within 30 minutes with IV administration. The duration of action is the same for all routes of administration: approximately 5 hours.

PROTOTYPE DRUG CHART 25.3
Nalbuphine

Drug Class	Dosage
Opioid agonist-antagonist Pregnancy category: B*	A: IV/IM/subcut: 10 mg q3-6h; *max:* 20 mg/dose, 160 mg/d
Contraindications	**Drug-Lab-Food Interactions**
Hypersensitivity *Caution:* History of alcohol or drug abuse, respiratory insufficiency, head injury, increased ICP, biliary tract disease, renal or hepatic dysfunction	Drug: CNS depression is potentiated with alcohol or other CNS depressants.
Pharmacokinetics	**Pharmacodynamics**
Absorption: Readily occurs parenterally Distribution: PB: <30%; crosses placenta, excreted in breast milk Metabolism: t½: 3-6 h Excretion: In urine, bile, and feces	Onset: 2-3 min IV; <15 min IM/subcut Peak: 30 min IV; 30 min IM Duration: 3-4 h IV; 3-6 h IM/subcut
Therapeutic Effects/Uses	
To relieve moderate to severe pain and for anesthesia induction and maintenance Mode of Action: Inhibits pain impulses transmitted in the CNS by binding with opiate receptors and increasing pain threshold	
Side Effects	**Adverse Reactions**
Dizziness, drowsiness, headache, dry mouth, nausea, vomiting, diaphoresis	Bradycardia, tachycardia, hypotension, hypertension, dyspnea *Life threatening:* Respiratory depression

*Pregnancy categories have been revised. See http://www.fda.gov/Drugs/DevelopmentApprovalProcess/DevelopmentResources/Labeling/ucm093307.htm for more information.
A, Adult; *CNS,* central nervous system; *d,* day; *h,* hour; *ICP,* intracranial pressure; *IM,* intramuscular; *IV,* intravenous; *max,* maximum; *min,* minute; *PB,* protein binding; *q,* every; *subcut,* subcutaneous; *t½,* half-life; <, less than.

TABLE 25.4 Opioid Agonist-Antagonists

Generic	Route and Dosage	Uses and Considerations
Buprenorphine hydrochloride CSS V	Pain: A: IM/IV: Initially, 0.3 mg (older adults 0.15 mg); may repeat in 30-60 min, then q6-8h PRN; *max:* 0.6 mg/dose IM, 0.3 mg/dose IV	For moderate to severe pain, opiate dependence, and withdrawal. Avoid alcohol and CNS depressants. May cause dizziness, drowsiness, miosis, headache, anxiety, insomnia, euphoria, flushing, diaphoresis, GI distress, weakness, hypotension, and respiratory depression. Pregnancy category: C*; PB: 96%; t½: IV 1.2-7.2 h, transdermal 26 h, sublingual 37 h
Butorphanol tartrate CSS IV	A: IM: 2 mg q3-4h PRN Older A: IM: 1 mg q6h PRN A: IV: 1 mg q3-4h PRN Older A: IV: 0.5 mg q6h PRN A: Nasal spray: 1 mg (1 spray into 1 nostril), may apply additional spray in 60-90 min as needed q3-4h PRN	For moderate to severe pain and anesthesia induction and maintenance. May cause dizziness, drowsiness, insomnia, anxiety, confusion, euphoria, headache, tinnitus, paresthesia, GI distress, nasal congestion, palpitations, dependence, tolerance, and respiratory depression. Pregnancy category: C*; PB: 80%; t½: 4.8-5.8 h

TABLE 25.4 Opioid Agonist-Antagonists—cont'd

Generic	Route and Dosage	Uses and Considerations
Nalbuphine hydrochloride CSS IV	See Prototype Drug Chart 25.3.	
Pentazocine lactate CSS IV	A/adol >17 y: Subcut/IM/IV: 30 mg q3-4 h PRN; *max:* 360 mg/d	For moderate to severe pain and anesthesia induction and maintenance. May cause miosis, dizziness, drowsiness, euphoria, headache, confusion, insomnia, irritability, nightmares, GI distress, flushing, hypotension, blurred vision, tachycardia, tolerance, and dependence. Pregnancy category: C*; PB: UK; t½: 1.5-10 h

*Pregnancy categories have been revised. See http://www.fda.gov/Drugs/DevelopmentApprovalProcess/DevelopmentResources/Labeling/ucm093307.htm for more information.
A, Adult; *adol,* adolescent; *CNS,* central nervous system; *CSS,* Controlled Substances Schedule; *d,* day; *GI,* gastrointestinal; *h,* hour; *IM,* intramuscular; *IV,* intravenous; *max,* maximum; *min,* minutes; *PB,* protein binding; *PRN,* as needed; *q,* every; *subcut,* subcutaneous; *t½,* half-life; *UK,* unknown; *>,* greater than.

⚡ PATIENT SAFETY

Do not confuse...
- **Nubain,** a narcotic agonist-antagonist analgesic for moderate to severe pain, with **Nebcin,** an aminoglycoside antibiotic, or **Nuprin,** an OTC analgesic, antipyretic NSAID.

◎ NURSING PROCESS
Patient-Centered Collaborative Care
Opioid Agonist-Antagonist Analgesic: Nalbuphine

Assessment
- Obtain a drug history from the patient. Report if a drug-drug interaction is probable. When taken with nalbuphine, CNS depressants can cause respiratory depression.
- Note baseline vital signs for future comparisons.
- Assess the type of pain, duration, and location before giving the drug.

Nursing Diagnosis
- Pain, Acute related to trauma
- Knowledge Deficit related to lack of familiarity with a drug

Planning
- The intensity of the patient's pain will be lessened.

Nursing Interventions
- Monitor vital signs. Note any changes in respirations.
- Check bowel sounds and the date of the last bowel movement to identify constipation. Decreased peristalsis may result in constipation. A mild laxative may be necessary.
- Determine urine output. Report if urine output is less than 30 mL/h or less than 600 mL/day.
- Administer IV nalbuphine undiluted. Do not mix with barbiturates.

Patient Teaching
General
- ⚡ Warn patients not to use alcohol or CNS depressants while taking nalbuphine. Respiratory depression can occur.

- Suggest nonpharmacologic methods for lessening pain, such as changing position or ambulation.

Side Effects
- Advise patients to report side effects of nalbuphine: dizziness, headaches, constipation, dysuria, rash, or blurred vision. Hallucinations, tachycardia, and respiratory depression are adverse reactions that might occur.

 Cultural Considerations
- Accept various cultural groups' use of alternative methods for relief of pain.

Evaluation
- Evaluate the effectiveness of nalbuphine in relieving pain. If ineffective, another opioid analgesic may need to be ordered.
- Determine stability of vital signs. Note whether a change in respirations, pulse rate, or blood pressure occurs. Report abnormal findings.

OPIOID ANTAGONISTS

Opioid antagonists are antidotes for drug toxicity of natural and synthetic opioid analgesics. The opioid antagonists have a higher affinity to the opiate receptor site than the opioid being taken. An opioid antagonist blocks the receptor and displaces any opioid that would normally be at the receptor, which inhibits the opioid action. Indications for opioid antagonists include reversal of postoperative opioid depression and opioid overdose.

Naloxone is administered via an IM or IV route, and naltrexone hydrochloride is administered orally by tablet or liquid. These drugs are perfect examples of pharmacologic antagonists because they reverse the respiratory and CNS depression (sedation and hypotension) caused by opioids. Table 25.5 lists the opioid antagonists.

When receiving opioid antagonists, the patient should be monitored continuously. The opioid action may exceed that of opioid antagonists, and further analgesia may be needed. For example, fentanyl and a combination of drugs given during surgery may lead to excessive respiratory depression. Naloxone may be given as an opioid antidote. The patient's respiratory and CNS status should be monitored closely for indications of

TABLE 25.5   Opioid Antagonists

Generic	Route and Dosage	Uses and Considerations
Naloxone hydrochloride	Opiate agonist overdose: A: IV/IM/Subcut: 0.4-2 mg; may repeat q2-3 min; *max:* 2 mg/dose or 10 mg total Adol/C >5 y >20 kg: IV: 2 mg q2-3min; *max:* 2 mg/dose C <5 y <20 kg: IV: 0.1 mg/kg; may repeat q2-3min; *max:* 0.1 mg/dose	For opioid overdose and opioid-induced respiratory depression. Dose often needs repeating as the half-life is shorter than opioids and the opioid effects may reoccur. May cause flushing, agitation, hypotension or hypertension, tachycardia, hyperhidrosis, nausea, vomiting, and dyspnea. Pregnancy category: C*; PB: UK; t½: 30-81 min
Naltrexone hydrochloride	A: PO: 50 mg/d with food for 12 wk; *max:* 150 mg/d A: IM: 380 mg/dose q4wk; *max:* 380 mg/dose	For opioid agonist and alcohol dependence. Decreases but does not prevent craving for opioids. Patient must be opioid free for 7-10 days prior. May cause dizziness, headache, insomnia, anxiety, GI distress, arthralgia, myalgia, weakness, injection site reaction, elevated hepatic enzymes, and suicidal ideation. Pregnancy category: C*; PB: 21%-28%; t½: PO, 4 h; IM, 5-10 d

*Pregnancy categories have been revised. See http://www.fda.gov/Drugs/DevelopmentApprovalProcess/DevelopmentResources/Labeling/ucm093307.htm for more information.
A, Adult; *adol,* adolescent; *C,* child; *d,* day; *GI,* gastrointestinal; *IM,* intramuscular; *IV,* intravenous; *max,* maximum; *min,* minute; *PB,* protein binding; *PO,* by mouth; *q,* every; *subcut,* subcutaneous; *t½,* half-life; *UK,* unknown; *wk,* weeks; *y,* years; >, greater than; <, less than.

analgesic reversal (tachycardia, nausea, vomiting, and sweating) and the possible need for further analgesia. The patient receiving naloxone should also be observed for bleeding because this drug may cause an elevated partial thromboplastin time.

HEADACHES: MIGRAINE AND CLUSTER

Migraine headaches are characterized by a unilateral throbbing head pain accompanied by nausea, vomiting, and photophobia. These symptoms frequently persist for 4 to 24 hours and for several days in some cases. Two thirds of migraine headaches are experienced by women in their twenties and thirties. Symptoms usually decrease or are absent during pregnancy and menopause. The intensity of migraine pain can disrupt daily activities.

Pathophysiology

The exact etiology of migraine headaches are unknown, although many theories exist. A common theory suggests a series of neurovascular events initiates a migraine headache. Neuronal hyperexcitability occurs in the cerebral cortex, especially in the occipital cortex. Specific factors that trigger a migraine headache include foods, monosodium glutamate, aspartame, fatigue, stress, too much or too little sleep, missed meals, odors, light, hormone changes, drugs, and weather. Foods such as cheese, chocolate, and red wine can trigger an attack.

The two types of migraine are *migraines associated with an aura,* which occurs minutes to 1 hour before onset, and *migraines without aura.*

Cluster headaches are characterized by a severe, unilateral, nonthrobbing pain usually located around the eye. They occur in a series of cluster attacks in which one or more attacks occur every day for several weeks. Cluster headaches are not associated with an aura and do not cause nausea and vomiting. Men are more commonly affected by cluster headaches than women are.

Treatment of Migraine Headaches

Preventive treatment for migraines includes (1) beta-adrenergic blockers, such as propranolol and atenolol; (2) anticonvulsants, such as valproic acid and gabapentin; and (3) TCAs, such as amitriptyline and imipramine.

Treatment of a migraine attack depends on the intensity of pain. Drugs used to treat migraines include analgesics, opioid analgesics, ergot alkaloids, and selective serotonin (5-HT) receptor agonists, also known as *triptans.* For mild migraine attacks, aspirin, acetaminophen, or NSAIDs such as ibuprofen or naproxen may be prescribed. Aspirin may be used in combination with caffeine. Meperidine and butorphanol nasal spray are opioid analgesics that are occasionally used.

Antimigraine medication should be taken early during a migraine attack. Nausea and vomiting might occur, and antiemetics decrease these symptoms. Dihydroergotamine, an ergot alkaloid, can be administered subcutaneously, intramuscularly, intravenously, and by means of a nasal spray.

The triptans, 5-HT receptor agonists, are the most recently developed group of drugs for the treatment of migraine headaches. Sumatriptan, a selective serotonin receptor agonist with a short duration of action, was the first triptan drug. It is considered more effective than ergot alkaloids in treating acute migraine attacks. Table 25.6 lists the ergot alkaloids and the selective serotonin (5-HT) receptor agonists and their dosages, uses, and considerations.

⚡ PATIENT SAFETY

Do not confuse...
- **Sumatriptan** with **zolmitriptan.** Both drugs are triptans but have different dosages.
- **Amerge,** a triptan used for migraines, with **Amaryl,** a sulfonylurea used for diabetes mellitus, or **Altace,** an angiotensin-converting enzyme (ACE) inhibitor used for hypertension and heart failure.

Prototype Drug Chart 25.4 provides further information on the pharmacology of sumatriptan.

TABLE 25.6   Drugs Used to Treat Severe Migraine Headaches

Drug	Route and Dosage	Uses and Considerations
ERGOT ALKALOIDS		
Dihydroergotamine mesylate	A: Intranasal: 1 spray (0.5 mg) in each nostril; may repeat in 15 min; *max:* 4 sprays (2 mg total dose), 3 mg/d, 4 mg/wk A: IM/subcut/IV: 1 mg; may repeat q1h until resolved; *max:* Subcut/IM, 3 mg/dose; IV, 2 mg/dose, 6 mg/wk	For migraine and cluster headaches. May cause rhinitis, dysgeusia, and GI distress. Pregnancy category: X*; PB: 90%-93%; t½: 9-10 h
SELECTIVE SEROTININ RECEPTOR AGONISTS (TRIPTANS)		
Sumatriptan	See Prototype Drug Chart 25.4.	
Naratriptan	A: PO: 1-2.5 mg; may repeat in 4 h; *max:* 5 mg/d	For migraines. Avoid if a patient has uncontrolled hypertension, IHD, or prior MI. May cause dizziness, drowsiness, blurred vision, GI distress, and bradycardia. Pregnancy category: C*; PB: 28%-31%; t½: 6 h
Rizatriptan benzoate	A: PO: 5-10 mg; may repeat q2h; *max:* 30 mg/d	For migraines. Avoid if a patient has uncontrolled hypertension, CAD, or acute MI. May cause dizziness, drowsiness, dry mouth, nausea, weakness, paresthesia, and fatigue. Pregnancy category: C*; PB: 14%; t½: 2-3 h
Zolmitriptan	A: PO: 1.25-2.5 mg; may repeat in 2 h; *max:* 5 mg/dose; 10 mg/d Oral disintegrating tab: 2.5 mg; *max:* 5 mg/dose, 10 mg/d Nasal inhalation: A/adol/C >12 y: 2.5-5 mg in 1 nostril; may repeat in 2 h; *max:* 10 mg/d	For migraines. Avoid in uncontrolled hypertension, IHD, and prior MI. May cause dizziness, drowsiness, dysgeusia, dry mouth, nausea, paresthesia, hyperesthesia, and weakness. Pregnancy category: C*; PB: 25%; t½: 3 h
Almotriptan	A/C >12 y: PO: 6.25-12.5 mg; may repeat in 2 h; *max:* 25 mg/d	For migraines. May cause drowsiness, dizziness, paresthesia, and GI distress. Pregnancy category: C*; PB: 35%; t½: 3-4 h
Frovatriptan	A: PO: 2.5 mg; may repeat in 2 h; *max:* 7.5 mg/d	For migraines. May cause dizziness, dysgeusia, dry mouth, GI distress, paresthesia, and fatigue. Pregnancy category: C*; PB: 15%; t½: 26 h
Eletriptan	A: PO: 20-40 mg; may repeat in 2 h; *max:* 40 mg/dose, 80 mg/d	For migraines. May cause dizziness, drowsiness, hyperhidrosis, dry mouth, nausea, weakness, and paresthesia. Pregnancy category: C*; PB: 85%; t½: 4-5 h

*Pregnancy categories have been revised. See http://www.fda.gov/Drugs/DevelopmentApprovalProcess/DevelopmentResources/Labeling/ucm093307.htm for more information.
A, Adult; *adol*, adolescent; *C*, child; *CAD*, coronary artery disease; *d*, day; *GI*, gastrointestinal; *h*, hour; *IHD*, ischemic heart disease; *IM*, intramuscular; *IV*, intravenous; *max*, maximum; *MI*, myocardial infarction; *min*, minute; *PB*, protein binding; *PO*, by mouth; *q*, every; *subcut*, subcutaneous; *t½*, half-life; *tab*, tablet; *wk*, week; *y*, years; >, greater than.

PROTOTYPE DRUG CHART 25.4

Sumatriptan

Drug Class	Dosage
5-HT receptor agonist: Antimigraine Pregnancy category: C*	A: PO: 25-100 mg for 1 dose, may repeat in 2 h; *max:* 100 mg/dose, 200 mg/d A: Subcut: 6 mg, may repeat with 6 mg after 1 h; *max:* 6 mg/dose, 12 mg/d A: Intranasal: 5-20 mg in 1 nostril, may repeat after 2 h; *max:* 40 mg/d
Contraindications	**Drug-Lab-Food Interactions**
Hypersensitivity, CAD, peripheral vascular disease, hypertension, cerebrovascular disease *Caution:* Renal or hepatic dysfunction, obesity, DM, smoking, seizures, older adults	Drug: Risk of vasospasm and blood pressure elevation with dihydroergotamine and other ergot alkaloids; increased levels and toxicity within 2 weeks of MAOIs; increased risk of serotonin syndrome or neuroleptic malignant syndrome with SSRIs
Pharmacokinetics	**Pharmacodynamics**
Absorption: Rapidly absorbed following subcut injection Distribution: PB: 14%-21% Metabolism: t½: 1.9 h Excretion: Urine and feces	PO: Onset: 60 min Peak: 2-4 h; duration: 24-48 h Subcut: Onset: 10 min Peak: 5-20 min; duration: 24-48 h Intranasal: Onset: 15 min Peak: 1-1.5 h; duration: 24-48 h

Continued

PROTOTYPE DRUG CHART 25.4—cont'd
Sumatriptan

Therapeutic Effects/Uses	
To treat migraine and cluster headaches	
Mode of Action: Causes vasoconstriction of cranial arteries to relieve migraine attacks	

Side Effects	Adverse Reactions
Dizziness, vertigo, headache, paresthesia, fatigue, flushing, drowsiness, dysgeusia, nausea, vomiting, injection site reaction, pruritis	Hypotension, hypertension, AV block, angina, dysrhythmias, bradycardia, elevated hepatic enzymes, thromboembolism, seizures
	Life threatening: Coronary artery vasospasm, MI, cardiac arrest, suicidal ideation

*Pregnancy categories have been revised. See http://www.fda.gov/Drugs/DevelopmentApprovalProcess/DevelopmentResources/Labeling/ucm093307.htm for more information.
5-HT, Serotonin; *A,* adult; *AV,* atrioventricular; *CAD,* coronary artery disease; *d,* day; *DM,* diabetes mellitus; *h,* hour; *MAOI,* monoamine oxidase inhibitor; *max,* maximum; *MI,* myocardial infarction; *min,* minute; *PB,* protein binding; *PO,* by mouth; *SSRI,* selective serotonin reuptake inhibitor; *subcut,* subcutaneous; *t½,* half-life.

CRITICAL THINKING CASE STUDY

RJ, a 79-year-old man, underwent abdominal surgery for resection of his colon. After the surgery, his physician prescribed morphine 10 mg every 3 to 4 hours as needed. RJ did not ask for pain medication because he worried he might become addicted. A day after the surgery, RJ's nurse noted that he was restless and grimaced whenever he moved in bed. He refused to breathe deeply or cough when instructed to do so. The nurse compared RJ's vital signs to his baseline findings and noted an increased pulse rate and a drop in systolic blood pressure of 6 mm Hg.

1. Should the nurse give morphine? Explain your answer.
2. What would your reaction be to RJ in regard to his restlessness, grimacing, and refusal to breathe deeply and cough?

3. What is the significance of the change in vital signs?
4. What classic side effects of opioid analgesics should the nurse assess?
5. What are some possible nonpharmacologic measures that might be helpful in alleviating RJ's pain?

The second postoperative day, RJ began asking for morphine every 3 hours. On the fifth day, the physician discontinued RJ's morphine and prescribed acetaminophen with codeine.

6. Why was the opioid analgesic order changed?
7. RJ does not want to ambulate. What is an appropriate nursing response?

NCLEX STUDY QUESTIONS

1. A patient requires a nonopioid medication. The nurse knows that which medication will cause the least gastrointestinal distress?
   a. Aspirin
   b. Ketorolac
   c. Celecoxib
   d. Ibuprofen
2. A patient states during a medical history that he takes several acetaminophen tablets throughout the day for acute pain. The nurse teaches the patient that the dosage should not exceed which amount?
   a. 1 g/day
   b. 3 g/day
   c. 4 g/day
   d. 6 g/day

3. For the patient receiving periodic morphine via intravenous push, which of the following findings would be of utmost concern to the nurse?
   a. Increased temperature
   b. Decreased bowel sounds
   c. Decreased respirations
   d. Increased red blood cell count
4. A patient is admitted to the emergency department with signs of respiratory depression following self-injection with hydromorphone. The admitting nurse knows that which drug will reverse respiratory depression caused by opioid overdose?
   a. Fentanyl
   b. Naloxone
   c. Butorphanol
   d. Sufenta

5. Assessing a patient following intravenous morphine administration, the nurse notes cold, clammy skin; a pulse of 40 beats/min; respirations of 10 breaths/min; and constricted pupils. Which medication will the patient likely need next?
   a. Naloxone
   b. Meloxicam
   c. Pentazocine
   d. Propoxyphene
6. For the patient who is taking acetaminophen, what should the nurse do? (Select all that apply.)
   a. Monitor routine liver enzyme tests.
   b. Encourage the patient to check package labels of over-the-counter drugs to avoid overdosing.
   c. Report side effects immediately, as toxicity can cause severe hepatic damage.
   d. Teach the female patient that oral contraceptives can increase the effect of acetaminophen.
   e. Teach the patient that caffeine decreases the effects of acetaminophen.
7. For the patient who is taking nalbuphine, what should the nurse do? (Select all that apply.)
   a. Monitor any changes in respirations.
   b. Instruct the patient to report bradycardia.
   c. Administer intravenous nalbuphine undiluted.
   d. Explain to the patient to expect an excessive amount of urine output.
   e. Instruct the patient to avoid alcohol when taking nalbuphine to avoid respiratory depression.
8. A patient is having a migraine attack. The nurse should know that which drugs are used to treat migraine attacks?
   a. Triptans
   b. Anticonvulsants
   c. Tricyclic antidepressants
   d. Beta-adrenergic blockers

Answers: 1. c; 2, b; 3, c; 4, b; 5, a; 6, a, b, c; 7, a, c, e; 8, a.

Antimicrobial Drugs

Disease-producing microorganisms may be gram-positive or gram-negative bacteria, viruses, protozoans, or fungi. The degree to which they are pathogenic depends on the microorganism and its virulence. This unit discusses drugs prescribed to combat disease-producing microorganisms.

Bacteria are single-celled organisms that lack a true nucleus and nuclear membrane. Most bacteria have a rigid cell wall, and the structure of the cell wall determines the shape of the bacteria. One classification of bacteria involves the appearance or shape under a microscope. A bacillus is a rod-shaped organism, whereas cocci are spherical. When cocci appear in clusters, they are called *staphylococci*; when cocci are arranged in chains, they are called *streptococci*. Bacteria reproduce by cell division about every 20 minutes. Chapter 26, Antibacterials, discusses substances that inhibit bacterial growth or that kill bacteria and other microorganisms.

Tuberculosis (TB) is caused by the acid-fast bacillus *Mycobacterium tuberculosis*. Antitubercular drugs treat persons with active TB and those exposed to active TB. Antifungals treat infection caused by a fungus. A fungal infection may be superficial or systemic. Fungi known as *dermatophytes* can cause superficial fungal infections that involve the integumentary system, which includes mucous membranes, hair, nails, and moist skin areas. Systemic fungal infections may involve the lungs, central nervous system (CNS), or abdomen. With the exception of human immunodeficiency virus (HIV), viruses are self-limiting illnesses that usually do not require treatment with specific antivirals. Current antivirals target influenza, herpes, and hepatitis. Viruses enter healthy cells and use their deoxyribonucleic acid (DNA) and ribonucleic acid (RNA) to generate more viruses. The growth cycle of viruses depends on the host cell enzymes and cell substrates for viral replication. Three categories of drugs are covered in Chapter 27: Antituberculars, Antifungals, and Antivirals. Although these differ from one other significantly, each category contains drugs that inhibit or kill organisms that cause disease.

Malaria is a life-threatening disease caused by protozoan parasites of several species of the genus *Plasmodium* that are carried by infected *Anopheles* mosquitoes. Malaria remains one of the most prevalent protozoan diseases, although antimalarial drugs provide treatment and prophylaxis. Helminths are large parasitic worms that live and lay eggs in warm, moist soil where sanitation and hygiene are poor. Transmission occurs from infected soil to a person, and the helminth then feeds on host tissues. The most common site for helminthiasis is the intestine. Other sites for parasitic infestation are the lymphatic system, blood vessels, and liver. Antimicrobial peptides are broad-spectrum antimicrobials with activity against bacteria, viruses, and fungi. Peptides are derived from cultures of *Bacillus subtilis*, and this group appears to interfere with bacterial cell membrane function. Chapter 28—Antimalarials, Anthelmintics, and Peptides—discusses these antimicrobial drugs.

26

Antibacterials

http://evolve.elsevier.com/McCuistion/pharmacology/

OBJECTIVES

- Explain the mechanisms of action of antibacterial drugs.
- Differentiate between bacteria that are naturally resistant and those that have acquired resistance to an antibiotic.
- Summarize the three general adverse effects associated with antibacterial drugs.
- Differentiate between narrow-spectrum and broad-spectrum antibiotics.
- Compare the effects of the natural, broad-spectrum (extended), penicillinase-resistant, and antipseudomonal penicillins.
- Contrast the effects of first-, second-, third-, fourth-, and fifth-generation cephalosporins.
- Apply the nursing process for patients receiving penicillins and cephalosporins.
- Describe the pharmacokinetics and pharmacodynamics of erythromycin.
- Apply the nursing process for tetracyclines, including patient teaching.

- Summarize the nurse's role in detecting ototoxicity and nephrotoxicity associated with the administration of aminoglycosides.
- Explain the importance for ordering peak and trough concentration levels for aminoglycosides.
- Develop a teaching plan for a patient prescribed a fluoroquinolone (quinolone).
- Contrast the nursing interventions for each of the drug categories: macrolides, tetracyclines, aminoglycosides, and fluoroquinolones.
- Differentiate between short-acting and intermediate-acting sulfonamides.
- Compare the similarities and differences between the sulfonamides and sulfadiazine.
- Explain the pharmacokinetics of the sulfonamides.
- Apply the nursing process to the patient taking trimethoprim-sulfamethoxazole.
- Develop a teaching plan for a patient prescribed metronidazole.

OUTLINE

Pathophysiology
Antibacterial Drugs
    Antibacterials/Antibiotics

SECTION 26A: PENICILLINS AND CEPHALOSPORINS

Penicillins
    Broad-Spectrum Penicillins (Aminopenicillins)
    Penicillinase-Resistant Penicillins (Antistaphylococcal Penicillins)
    Extended-Spectrum Penicillins (Antipseudomonal Penicillins)
    Beta-Lactamase Inhibitors
    Geriatrics
    Side Effects and Adverse Reactions
    Drug Interactions
Other Beta-Lactam Antibacterials
    Side Effects and Adverse Reactions

Nursing Process: Patient-Centered Collaborative Care—
    Antibacterials: Penicillins
Cephalosporins
First-, Second-, Third-, Fourth-, and Fifth-Generation Cephalosporins
Side Effects and Adverse Reactions
Drug Interactions
Nursing Process: Patient-Centered Collaborative Care—
    Antibacterials: Cephalosporins

SECTION 26B: MACROLIDES, OXAZOLIDINONES, LINCOSAMIDES, GLYCOPEPTIDES, KETOLIDES, TETRACYCLINES, AND GLYCYLCYCLINES

Macrolides
    Side Effects and Adverse Reactions
    Drug Interactions
    Extended Macrolide Group

Nursing Process: Patient-Centered Collaborative Care—
    Antibacterials: Macrolides
Oxazolidinones
    Side Effects and Adverse Reactions

SECTION 26C: AMINOGLYCOSIDES, FLUOROQUINOLONES, AND LIPOPEPTIDES

SECTION 26D: SULFONAMIDES AND NITROIMIDAZOLES

KEY TERMS

This chapter discusses the antibacterials and their effects and includes mechanisms of antibacterial action, body defenses, resistance to antibacterials, use of antibacterial combinations, general adverse reactions to antibacterials, and narrow- and broad-spectrum antibiotics.

The groups of antibacterials discussed in this chapter include penicillins, cephalosporins, macrolides (erythromycin, clarithromycin, and azithromycin), lincosamides, glycopeptides, ketolides, tetracyclines, glycylcyclines, aminoglycosides, fluoroquinolones (quinolones), lipopeptides, sulfonamides, and nitroimidazoles.

The penicillins, macrolides, lincosamides, tetracyclines, and sulfonamides are primarily bacteriostatic drugs, those that inhibit bacterial growth, but they may also be bactericidal (bacteria killing), depending on the drug dose, serum level, and the pathogen (the disease-producing microorganism). Cephalosporins, glycopeptides, aminoglycosides, and fluoroquinolones are bactericidal drugs.

Macrolides, lincosamides, glycopeptides, and ketolides are discussed together because they have spectrums of antibiotic effectiveness similar to that of penicillin, although they differ in structure. Drugs from these groups are used as penicillin substitutes, especially in individuals who are allergic to penicillin. Erythromycin is the drug frequently prescribed if the patient has a hypersensitivity to penicillin.

Sulfonamides are one of the oldest antibacterial agents used to combat infection. When penicillin was initially marketed, the sulfonamide drugs were not widely prescribed because penicillin was considered a "miracle drug." However, use of sulfonamides has increased as a result of newer sulfonamides and drugs that combine a sulfonamide with an antibacterial agent in preparations such as trimethoprim-sulfamethoxazole.

PATHOPHYSIOLOGY

Bacteria, known as *prokaryotes,* are single-celled organisms that lack a true nucleus and nuclear membrane. Most bacteria have a rigid cell wall, and the structure of the cell wall determines the shape of the bacteria. One classification of bacteria involves the appearance or shape under a microscope. A *bacillus* is a rod-shaped organism, and *cocci* are spherical. When cocci appear in clusters, they are called *staphylococci;* when they are arranged in chains, they are called *streptococci.* Bacteria reproduce by cell division ranging from 12 minutes to 24 hours.

Another classification of bacteria involves staining properties of the cell. The Gram-staining method was devised in 1882 by Hans Christian Gram, a Danish bacteriologist. Gram staining determines the ability of the bacterial cell wall to retain a purple stain by a basic dye. Crystal violet is normally used in the staining process but may be substituted with methylene blue. If bacteria retain a purple stain, they are classified as gram-positive microorganisms. Those bacteria not stained are known as gram-negative microorganisms. Examples of gram-positive bacteria include *Staphylococcus aureus, Streptococcus pneumoniae,* group B *Streptococcus* (GBS), and *Clostridium perfringens.* Examples of gram-negative bacteria include *Neisseria meningitides, Escherichia coli,* and *Haemophilus influenzae.*

Bacteria produce toxins that cause cell lysis (cell breakdown). Many bacteria produce the enzyme beta-lactamase, which destroys beta-lactam antibiotics such as penicillins and cephalosporins.

ANTIBACTERIAL DRUGS

Antibacterials/Antibiotics

Although the terms *antibacterial, antimicrobial,* and *antibiotic* are frequently used interchangeably, there are some subtle differences in meaning. Antibacterials and antimicrobials are substances that inhibit bacterial growth or kill bacteria and other microorganisms—microscopic organisms that include viruses, fungi, protozoa, and rickettsiae. Technically, the term *antibiotic* refers to chemicals produced by one kind of microorganism that inhibit the growth of or kill another. For practical purposes, however, these terms may be used interchangeably. Several drugs, including antiinfective and chemotherapeutic agents, have actions similar to those of antibacterial and antimicrobial agents. Antibacterial drugs do not act alone in destroying bacteria. Natural body defenses, surgical procedures to excise infected tissues, and dressing changes may be needed along with antibacterial drugs to eliminate the infecting bacteria.

Antibacterial drugs are either obtained from natural sources or are manufactured. The use of moldy bread on wounds to fight infection dates back 3500 years. In 1928, British bacteriologist Alexander Fleming noted that a mold that

had contaminated his bacterial cultures was inhibiting bacterial growth. The mold was *Penicillium notatum,* thus Fleming called the substance *penicillin.* Sulfonamide, a synthetic antibacterial, was introduced in 1935. In 1939, Howard Florey expanded on Fleming's findings and purified penicillin so it could be used commercially. Penicillin was used during World War II and was marketed in 1945.

For drugs with a narrow therapeutic index, such as the aminoglycosides, peaks and troughs of serum antibiotic levels are monitored to determine whether the drug is within the therapeutic range for its desired effect. If the serum *peak* level is too high, drug toxicity could occur. If the serum *trough* level (drawn minutes before administration of the next drug dose) is below the therapeutic range, the patient is not receiving an adequate antibiotic dose to kill the targeted microorganism.

Mechanisms of Antibacterial Action

Five mechanisms of antibacterial action are responsible for the inhibition of growth or destruction of microorganisms: (1) inhibition of bacterial cell-wall synthesis, (2) alteration of membrane permeability, (3) inhibition of protein synthesis, (4) inhibition of the synthesis of bacterial ribonucleic acid (RNA) and deoxyribonucleic acid (DNA), and (5) interference with metabolism within the cell (Table 26.1).

Pharmacokinetics Antibacterial drugs must not only penetrate the bacterial cell wall in sufficient concentrations but also have an affinity for (attraction to) the binding sites on the bacterial cell. The length of time the drug remains at the binding sites increases the effect of the antibacterial action. This time factor is controlled by the pharmacokinetics—the distribution, half-life, and elimination—of the drug.

TABLE 26.1 Mechanisms of Action of Antibacterial Drugs

Action	Effect	Drugs
Inhibition of cell-wall synthesis	Bactericidal effect Enzyme breakdown of cell wall Inhibition of enzyme in synthesis of cell wall	Penicillin Cephalosporins Bacitracin Vancomycin
Alteration of membrane permeability	Bacteriostatic or bactericidal effect Increases membrane permeability Cell lysis caused by loss of cellular substances	Amphotericin B Nystatin Polymyxin Colistin
Inhibition of protein synthesis	Bacteriostatic or bactericidal effect Interferes with protein synthesis without affecting normal cell Inhibits steps of protein synthesis	Aminoglycosides Tetracyclines Erythromycin Lincomycin
Inhibition of synthesis of bacterial RNA and DNA	Inhibits synthesis of RNA and DNA in bacteria Binds to nucleic acid and enzymes needed for nucleic acid synthesis	Fluoroquinolones
Interference with cellular metabolism	Bacteriostatic effect Interferes with steps of metabolism within cells	Sulfonamides Trimethoprim Isoniazid Nalidixic acid Rifampin

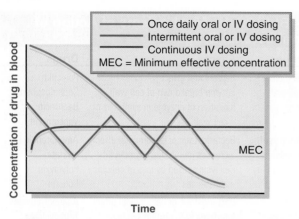

FIG. 26.1 Effects of Concentrated Drug Dosing.

Antibacterials that have a longer half-life usually maintain a greater concentration at the binding site, therefore frequent dosing is not required. Most antibacterials are not highly protein bound, with a few exceptions (e.g., oxacillin, ceftriaxone, cefprozil, cloxacillin, nafcillin, clindamycin). Protein binding does not have a major influence on the effectiveness of most antibacterial drugs. The steady state of the antibacterial drug occurs after the fourth to fifth half-lives, and after the seventh half-life, the drug is eliminated from the body, mainly through urine.

Pharmacodynamics The drug concentration at the site and the exposure time for the drug play important roles in bacterial eradication. Antibacterial drugs are used to achieve the minimum effective concentration (MEC) necessary to halt the growth of a microorganism. Many antibacterials have a bactericidal effect against the pathogen when the drug concentration remains constantly above the MEC during the dosing interval. Duration of use of the antibacterial varies according to the type of pathogen, site of infection, and immunocompetence of the host. With some severe infections, a continuous infusion regimen is more effective than intermittent dosing because of constant drug concentration and time exposure. Once-daily antibacterial dosing—such as with aminoglycosides, macrolides, and fluoroquinolones—has been effective in eradicating pathogens and has not caused severe adverse reactions (ototoxicity, nephrotoxicity) in most cases. The ease of compliance with once- or twice-daily drug dosing also increases the patient's adherence to the drug regimen.

Fig. 26.1 illustrates the effect of three methods of drug dosing. The drug dose is effective when it remains above the MEC.

Body Defenses

Body defenses and antibacterial drugs work together to stop the infectious process. The effect that antibacterial drugs have on an infection depends not only on the drug but also on the host's defense mechanisms. Factors such as age, nutrition, immunoglobulins, white blood cells (WBCs), organ function, and circulation influence the body's ability to fight infection. Older adults and undernourished individuals have less resistance to infection than younger, well-nourished populations. If the host's natural body defense mechanisms are inadequate, drug therapy might not be as effective. As a result, drug therapy may need to be closely monitored or revised. When circulation is impeded, an antibacterial drug may not be distributed properly to the infected area.

In addition, **immunoglobulins**—antibody proteins such as IgG and IgM—and other elements of the immune response system, such as WBCs needed to combat infections, may be depleted in individuals with poor nutritional status.

Resistance to Antibacterials

Bacteria can be either sensitive or resistant to certain antibacterials. When bacteria are *sensitive* to a drug, the pathogen is inhibited or destroyed; however, if bacteria are *resistant*, the pathogen continues to grow despite administration of that antibacterial drug.

Bacterial resistance can result naturally, called **inherent resistance**, or it may be acquired. A natural, or inherent, resistance occurs without previous exposure to the antibacterial drug. For example, the gram-negative bacterium *Pseudomonas aeruginosa* is inherently resistant to penicillin G. An **acquired resistance** is caused by prior exposure to the antibacterial. Although *S. aureus* was once sensitive to penicillin G, repeated exposures have caused this organism to evolve and become resistant to that drug. Penicillinase, an enzyme produced by the microorganism, is responsible for causing its penicillin resistance. Penicillinase metabolizes penicillin G, causing the drug to be ineffective; however, penicillinase-resistant penicillins that are effective against *S. aureus* are now available.

Antibiotic resistance is a major problem. In the early 1980s, pharmaceutical companies thought that enough antibiotics were on the market, so they concentrated on developing antiviral and antifungal drugs. As a result, fewer new antibiotics were developed during the 1980s. Now pharmaceutical companies have developed many new antibiotics, but antibiotic resistance continues to develop, especially when antibiotics are used frequently. As bacteria reproduce, some mutation occurs, and eventually the mutant bacteria survive the effects of the drug. One explanation is that the mutant bacterial strain may have grown a thicker cell wall.

In large health care institutions, there is a tendency toward drug resistance in bacteria. Mutant strains of organisms have developed, thus increasing their resistance to antibiotics that were once effective against them. Infections acquired while patients are hospitalized are called **health care acquired infections** (previously known as nosocomial infections). Many of these infections are caused by drug-resistant bacteria, and this can prolong hospitalization, which is costly to both the patient and third-party health care insurers.

Another problem related to antibiotic resistance is that bacteria can transfer their genetic instructions to another bacterial species, and the other bacterial species then becomes resistant to that antibiotic as well. Bacteria can also pass along high resistance to a more virulent and aggressive bacterium (e.g., *S. aureus,* enterococci).

Methicillin was the first penicillinase-resistant penicillin; it was developed in 1959 in response to the resistance of *S. aureus*. In 1968, strains of *S. aureus* were beginning to become resistant to methicillin. Highly resistant bacteria, so-called methicillin-resistant *S. aureus* (MRSA), became resistant not only to methicillin but to all penicillins and cephalosporins as well. Resistance that was once found only in hospitals began to emerge in 1981 in the community. Methicillin is now off the market, and the treatment of choice for MRSA is vancomycin. Other effective drugs used to treat MRSA include linezolid, tedizolid, daptomycin, trimethoprim-sulfamethoxazole, doxycycline, clindamycin, *and* televancin, a glycopeptide antiinfective.

Many enterococcal strains are resistant to penicillin, ampicillin, gentamicin, streptomycin, and vancomycin. Another big resistance problem is vancomycin-resistant *Enterococcus faecium* (VREF), which can cause death in persons with weakened immune systems. The incidence of VREF in hospitals has increased, and a strain of MRSA has also been reported to be resistant to vancomycin (vancomycin-resistant *S. aureus,* or VRSA). One antibiotic after another is ineffective against new resistant strains of bacteria, and major medical problems result. As new drugs are developed, drug resistance will probably also develop.

Pharmaceutical companies and biotech firms are working on new classes of drugs to overcome the problem of bacterial resistance to antibiotics. A class of antibiotics known as *oxazolidinones* was discovered by a pharmaceutical company in 1988, but the company could not overcome the toxicity problems with this class of drug; however, another pharmaceutical company has taken the compound and made it less toxic. This antibiotic, linezolid, is effective against MRSA, VREF, and penicillin-resistant streptococci. Quinupristin-dalfopristin, which consists of two streptogramin antibacterials, is marketed in a 30:70 combination for intravenous (IV) use against life-threatening infection caused by VREF and for treatment of bacteremia, *S. aureus,* and *Streptococcus pyogenes.*

Another way to attack antimicrobial resistance is to develop drugs that disable the antibiotic-resistant mechanism in the bacteria. Patients would take the antibiotic-resistance disabler along with the antibiotic already on the market, making the drug effective again. Developing a bacterial vaccine is another way to combat bacteria and lessen the need for antibiotics. The bacterial vaccine against pneumococcus has been effective in decreasing the occurrence of pneumonia and meningitis among various age groups.

Antibiotic misuse, a major problem today, increases antibiotic resistance. Studies reveal that 23% to 37.8% of patients in hospitals receive antibiotics, and 50% of this population is receiving antibiotics inappropriately. When antibiotics are taken unnecessarily—such as for viral infections, when no bacterial infection is present—or incorrectly (e.g., skipping doses, not taking the full antibiotic regimen), resistance to antibacterials may develop. Consumer education is important because many patients *demand* antibiotics for viral conditions, even though antibiotics are ineffective against viruses; however, viral infections that persist could compromise the body's immune system and thus promote a secondary bacterial infection. The nurse should teach patients about the proper use of antibiotics to prevent situations that promote drug resistance to bacteria.

Cross-resistance can also occur among antibacterial drugs that have similar actions, such as the penicillins and cephalosporins. To ascertain the effect antibacterial drugs have on a specific microorganism, culture and sensitivity (C&S) or antibiotic susceptibility laboratory testing is performed. C&S can detect the infective microorganism present in a sample (e.g., blood, sputum, swab) and the best drug to kill it. The organism causing the infection is determined by culture, and antibiotics the organism is sensitive to are determined by sensitivity. The susceptibility or resistance of one microorganism to several antibacterials can be determined by the C&S test. Multiantibiotic therapy, or daily use of several antibacterials, delays the development of microorganism resistance.

Use of Antibiotic Combinations

Combination antibiotics should not be routinely prescribed or administered except for specific uncontrollable infections. Usually a single antibiotic will successfully treat a bacterial infection; however, when severe infection persists and is of an unknown origin or has been unsuccessfully treated with several single antibiotics, a combination of two or three antibiotics may be suggested. Before beginning antibiotic therapy, a culture or cultures should be taken to identify the bacteria.

When two antibiotics are combined, the result may be additive, potentiative, or antagonistic. The *additive* effect is equal to the sum of the effects of two antibiotics. The *potentiative* effect occurs when one antibiotic potentiates the effect of the second antibiotic, *increasing* its effectiveness. The *antagonistic* result is achieved with combination of a drug that is bactericidal, such as penicillin, and a drug that is bacteriostatic, such as tetracycline; when these two drugs are used together, the desired effect may be greatly *reduced*.

General Adverse Reactions to Antibacterials

Three major adverse reactions associated with the administration of antibacterial drugs are (1) allergic (hypersensitivity, anaphylaxis) reactions, (2) superinfection, and (3) organ toxicity. Table 26.2 describes these adverse reactions, all of which require close monitoring of the patient.

Narrow-Spectrum and Broad-Spectrum Antibiotics

Antibacterial drugs can be classified as either narrow spectrum or broad spectrum. The narrow-spectrum antibiotics are primarily effective against one type of organism. For example, penicillin and erythromycin are used to treat infections caused by gram-positive bacteria. Certain broad-spectrum antibiotics, such as tetracycline and cephalosporins, can be effective against both gram-positive and gram-negative organisms. Because narrow-spectrum antibiotics are selective, they are more active against those single organisms than the broad-spectrum antibiotics. Broad-spectrum antibiotics are frequently used to treat infections when the offending microorganism has not been identified by the C&S test.

TABLE 26.2   General Adverse Reactions to Antibacterial Drugs

Type	Considerations
Allergy or hypersensitivity	Allergic reactions to drugs may be mild or severe. Examples of mild reactions are rash, pruritus, and hives. An example of a severe response is anaphylactic shock, which results in vascular collapse, laryngeal edema, bronchospasm, and cardiac arrest. Severe allergic reaction generally occurs within 20 minutes, and shortness of breath is often the first symptom of anaphylaxis. Mild allergic reaction is treated with an antihistamine, whereas anaphylaxis requires treatment with epinephrine, bronchodilators, and antihistamines.
Superinfection	Superinfection is a secondary infection that occurs when the normal microbial flora of the body are disturbed during antibiotic therapy. Superinfections can occur in the mouth, respiratory tract, intestine, genitourinary tract, and skin. Fungal infections frequently result in superinfections, although bacterial organisms (e.g., *Proteus*, *Pseudomonas*, *Staphylococcus*) may be the offending microorganisms. Superinfections rarely develop when drug is administered for less than 1 week, and they occur more commonly with the use of broad-spectrum antibiotics. For fungal infection of the mouth, nystatin is frequently used.
Organ toxicity	The liver and kidneys are involved in drug metabolism and excretion, and antibacterials may result in damage to these organs. For example, aminoglycosides can be nephrotoxic and ototoxic.

SECTION 26A: Penicillins and Cephalosporins

PENICILLINS

Penicillin, a natural antibacterial agent obtained from the mold genus *Penicillium,* was introduced to the military during World War II and is considered to have saved many soldiers' lives. It became widely used in 1945 and was considered a "miracle drug." With the advent of penicillin, many patients survived who would have normally died from wound and severe respiratory infections.

Penicillin's beta-lactam ring structure interferes with bacterial cell-wall synthesis by inhibiting the bacterial enzyme that is necessary for cell division and cellular synthesis. The bacteria die of cell lysis (cell breakdown). The penicillins can be both bacteriostatic and bactericidal, depending on the drug and dosage. Penicillin G is primarily bactericidal.

Penicillins are mainly referred to as *beta-lactam antibiotics.* Bacteria can produce a variety of enzymes, such as beta-lactamases, that can inactivate penicillin and other beta-lactam antibiotics such as the cephalosporins. The beta-lactamases, which attack penicillins, are called *penicillinases.*

Penicillin G was the first penicillin administered orally and by injection. With oral administration, only about one third of the dose is absorbed. Because of its poor absorption, penicillin G given by injection (IV and intramuscular [IM]) is more effective in achieving a therapeutic serum penicillin level. Because it is an aqueous drug solution, aqueous penicillin G has a short duration of action, and the IM injection is very painful. As a result, a longer-acting form of penicillin, procaine penicillin (milky color), was produced to extend the activity of the drug. Procaine (an anesthetic) in the penicillin decreases the pain related to injection.

Penicillin V was the next type of penicillin produced. Although two thirds of the oral dose is absorbed by the gastrointestinal (GI) tract, it is a less potent antibacterial drug than penicillin G. Penicillin V is effective against mild to moderate infections, including anthrax as a weapon of bioterrorism.

Initially, penicillin was overused. It was first introduced for the treatment of staphylococcal infections, but after a few years, mutant strains of *Staphylococcus* developed that were resistant to penicillins G and V because of the bacterial enzyme penicillinase, which destroys penicillin. This led

to the development of new broad-spectrum antibiotics with structures similar to penicillin to combat infections resistant to penicillins G and V.

Food in the stomach does not significantly alter absorption of penicillin V, so it should be taken after meals. Amoxicillins are penicillins that are unaffected by food.

Broad-Spectrum Penicillins (Aminopenicillins)

Broad-spectrum penicillins are used to treat both gram-positive and gram-negative bacteria. They are not, however, as broadly effective against all microorganisms as they were once considered to be. This group of drugs is costlier than penicillin and therefore should not be used when ordinary penicillins, such as penicillin G, are effective. The broad-spectrum penicillins are effective against some gram-negative organisms such as *E. coli, H. influenzae, Shigella dysenteriae, Proteus mirabilis,* and *Salmonella* species. However, these drugs are not penicillinase resistant; because they are readily inactivated by beta-lactamases, they are ineffective against *S. aureus.* Examples of this group are ampicillin and amoxicillin (Table 26.3). Amoxicillin is the most prescribed penicillin derivative for adults and children.

Penicillinase-Resistant Penicillins (Antistaphylococcal Penicillins)

Penicillinase-resistant penicillins (antistaphylococcal penicillins) are used to treat penicillinase-producing *S. aureus.* Dicloxacillin is an oral preparation of these antibiotics, whereas nafcillin and oxacillin are IM and IV preparations. This group of drugs is *not* effective against gram-negative organisms and is less effective than penicillin G against gram-positive organisms. See Prototype Drug Chart 26.1 and Table 26.3 to compare the similarities and differences in the broad-spectrum penicillin amoxicillin and the penicillinase-resistant penicillin dicloxacillin.

Extended-Spectrum Penicillins (Antipseudomonal Penicillins)

The antipseudomonal penicillins are a group of broad-spectrum antibiotics effective against *P. aeruginosa,* a gram-negative

TABLE 26.3 Antibacterials: Penicillins

Generic	Route and Dosage	Uses and Considerations
BASIC PENICILLINS		
Penicillin G procaine	Severe pneumococcal pneumonia: A/adol/C >27 kg: IM: 600,000-1.2 million units/d for at least 10 d Infants/C <27 kg: IM: 300,000 units/d for at least 10 d	For treating anthrax, diphtheria, endocarditis, syphilis, and skin and respiratory infections. May cause anaphylaxis, angioedema, headache, GI distress, superinfection, CDAD, and tongue discoloration. Pregnancy category: B*; PB: 60%; t½: UK
Penicillin G benzathine	Upper respiratory infection: A: IM: 1.2 million units as a single dose Adol/C >27 kg: IM: 900,000 units as a single dose C/infants <27 kg: IM: 600,000 units as a single dose	For treating syphilis and respiratory infections and for rheumatic fever prophylaxis. May cause anaphylaxis, angioedema, GI distress, tongue discoloration, headache, superinfection, and CDAD. Pregnancy category: B*; PB: 60%; t½: UK
Penicillin G sodium	Streptococcal infection: A: IM/IV: 5-24 million units/d in divided doses q4-6h; *max:* 80 million units/d Infants/C/adol: IM/IV: 200,000-300,000 units/kg/d in divided doses q4-6h; *max:* 300,000 units/kg/d	For treating septicemia, gas gangrene, tetanus, anthrax, STIs, meningitis, diphtheria, pericarditis, endocarditis, and respiratory infections. May cause anaphylaxis, angioedema, GI distress, tongue discoloration, superinfection, and CDAD. Pregnancy category: B*; PB: 45%-68%; t½: 20-30 min
Penicillin VK	Upper respiratory infection: A/adol/C >12 y: PO: 250-500 mg q6h; *max:* 2 g/d	For treating ulcerative gingivitis, otitis media, and respiratory and skin infections and for endocarditis prophylaxis. May cause anaphylaxis, angioedema, rash, GI distress, oral candidiasis, tongue discoloration, superinfection, and CDAD. Not recommended in renal failure. Pregnancy category: B*; PB: 75%-89%; t½: UK
BROAD-SPECTRUM PENICILLINS		
Amoxicillin	See Prototype Drug Chart 26.1.	
Amoxicillin-clavulanate	Lower respiratory infection: Immediate release: A/adol/C >40 kg: PO: 500 mg amoxicillin and 125 mg clavulanate q8h Extended release: A/adol/C >40 kg: PO: 2000 mg amoxicillin and 125 mg clavulanate q12h	For treating otitis media, sinusitis, and respiratory, skin, and urinary tract infections. May cause anaphylaxis, angioedema, GI distress, tongue discoloration, superinfection, and CDAD. Pregnancy category: B*; PB: 18%-25%; t½: 1-1.3 h
Ampicillin	Respiratory infection: A/adol/C >20 kg: PO: 250 mg four times daily Adol/C/infants <20 kg: PO: 50 mg/kg/d in four divided doses A/adol/C >40 kg: IM/IV: 250-500 mg q6h A/adol/C/infants <40 kg: IM/IV: 25-50 mg/kg/d IV in divided doses q6-8h or 150-200 mg/kg/d IM/IV in divided doses q6h	For meningitis, endocarditis, septicemia, gastroenteritis, and skin, respiratory, and urinary tract infections. May cause anaphylaxis, angioedema, rash, stomatitis, tongue discoloration, GI distress, superinfection, and CDAD. Pregnancy category: B*; PB: 20%; t½: 1-1.5 h
Ampicillin sulbactam	Skin infections: A: IM/IV: 1 g ampicillin/0.5 g sulbactam q6h Adol/C >40 kg: IV: 1 g ampicillin/0.5 g sulbactam q6h Adol/C <40 kg: IV: 200 mg/kg/d ampicillin/100 mg/kg/d sulbactam in divided doses q6h	For treating skin, respiratory, intraabdominal, and gynecologic infections. May cause anaphylaxis, angioedema, phlebitis, rash, GI distress, tongue discoloration, CDAD, and superinfection. Pregnancy category: B*; PB: 15%-25%; t½: 1-1.5 h
PENICILLINASE-RESISTANT PENICILLINS		
Dicloxacillin sodium	A/adol/C >40 kg: PO: 125-500 mg q6h; *max:* 4 g/d Adol/C/infants <40 kg: PO: 12.5-50 mg/kg/d in divided doses q6h	For treating bacteremia, endocarditis, and bone/joint, skin structure, and respiratory infections. May cause anaphylaxis, angioedema, myalgia, rash, GI distress, tongue discoloration, CDAD, superinfection, and renal dysfunction. Pregnancy category: B*; PB: 95%-99%; t½: 30-42 min
Nafcillin	A: IM/IV: 500 mg-2 g q4h; *max:* 6 g/d	For treating endocarditis, meningitis, bacteremia, and skin, respiratory, and bone/joint infections. May cause anaphylaxis, angioedema, tongue discoloration, GI distress, CDAD, superinfection, phlebitis, and injection site reaction. Pregnancy category: B*; PB: 70%-90%; t½: 0.5-1.5 h
Oxacillin sodium	Mild/moderate infection: A/adol/C >40 kg: IM/IV: 250 mg-500 mg q4-6h; *max:* 6 g/d Adol/C/infants <40 kg: IM/IV: 50-100 mg/kg/d in divided doses q4-6h	For treating endocarditis, meningitis, bacteremia, and skin, respiratory, and bone/joint infections. May cause anaphylaxis, angioedema, rash, GI distress, tongue discoloration, CDAD, superinfection, and injection site reaction. Pregnancy category: B*; PB: 89%-94%; t½: 0.5 h

Continued

TABLE 26.3 Antibacterials: Penicillins—cont'd

Generic	Route and Dosage	Uses and Considerations
EXTENDED-SPECTRUM PENICILLINS		
Piperacillin tazobactam	Moderate/severe respiratory infection: A: IV: 3 g piperacillin/3.375 g tazobactam over 30 min q6h for 7-10 d; *max:* 16 g piperacillin/2 g tazobactam/d	For treating PID and skin, intraabdominal, and respiratory infections. May cause anaphylaxis, angioedema, GI distress, CDAD, rash, and superinfection. Pregnancy category: B*; PB: 30%; t½: 0.7-1.5 h

*Pregnancy categories have been revised. See http://www.fda.gov/Drugs/DevelopmentApprovalProcess/DevelopmentResources/Labeling/ucm093 307.htm for more information.

A, Adult; *adol,* adolescent; *C,* child; *CDAD, Clostridium difficile*–associated diarrhea; *d,* day; *GI,* gastrointestinal; *h,* hour; *IM,* intramuscular; *IV,* intravenous; *max,* maximum; *min,* minutes; *PB,* protein binding; *PID,* pelvic inflammatory disease; *PO,* by mouth; *q,* every; *STI,* sexually transmitted infection; *t½,* half-life; *UK,* unknown; *y,* year; *>,* greater than; *<,* less than.

📄 PROTOTYPE DRUG CHART 26.1

Amoxicillin

Drug Class	Dosage
Amoxicillin: Broad-spectrum penicillin Pregnancy category: B*	Respiratory infection: Immediate release: A: PO: 250-875 mg q8-12h; *max:* 1750 mg/d Adol/C/infants >3 mo: PO: 20-40 mg/kg/d in divided doses; *max:* 500 mg/dose Neonates/infants <3 mo: PO: 30 mg/kg/d in divided doses q12h
Contraindications	**Drug-Lab-Food Interactions**
Allergy to penicillin, hypersensitivity, asthma, inflammatory bowel disease, pseudomembranous colitis, ulcerative colitis Amoxicillin: Mononucleosis *Caution:* Hypersensitivity to cephalosporins Amoxicillin: Renal impairment	Drug: Increased effect with aspirin, allopurinol, probenecid; increased bleeding with oral anticoagulants; increased effect of methotrexate; decreased effect with tetracycline, erythromycin Lab: Increased serum AST, ALT, BUN, and creatinine; increased PT, INR Food: Decreased effect with acidic fruits and juices
Pharmacokinetics	**Pharmacodynamics**
Absorption: PO: >80% in the GI tract Distribution: PB: 20% Metabolism: t½: 1-1.5 h Excretion: 70% in urine	PO: Onset, duration: UK Peak: 1-2 h
Therapeutic Effects/Uses	
For rheumatic fever prophylaxis and to treat otitis media, tonsillitis, sinusitis, and gastric/duodenal ulcers, and skin, respiratory, and urinary tract infections. Amoxicillin is effective against *Helicobacter pylori* and *Escherichia coli* and species of *Haemophilus, Enterococcus, Proteus, Staphylococci,* and *Streptococci.* Mode of Action: Amoxicillin inhibits the enzyme in cell-wall synthesis and has a bactericidal effect.	
Side Effects	**Adverse Reactions**
Nausea, vomiting, diarrhea, abdominal pain, rash, stomatitis, dysgeusia, tongue and tooth discoloration, headache, dizziness, anxiety, confusion, edema, insomnia, crystalluria, dermatitis	Superinfection (vaginitis) *Life threatening:* Anaphylaxis, angioedema, hemolytic anemia, eosinophilia, leukopenia, thrombocytopenia, CDAD, Stevens-Johnson syndrome, hepatic damage, seizures

*Pregnancy categories have been revised. See http://www.fda.gov/Drugs/DevelopmentApprovalProcess/DevelopmentResources/Labeling/ucm093307.htm for more information.

A, Adult; *Adol,* adolescent; *ALT,* alanine aminotransferase; *AST,* aspartate aminotransferase; *BUN,* blood urea nitrogen; *C,* child; *CDAD, Clostridium difficile*–associated diarrhea; *d,* day; *GI,* gastrointestinal; *h,* hour; *INR,* international normalized ratio; *max,* maximum dosage; *mo,* months; *PB,* protein binding; *PO,* by mouth; *PT,* prothrombin time; *q,* every; *t½,* half-life; *UK,* unknown; *>,* greater than; *<,* less than.

bacillus that is difficult to eradicate. These drugs are also useful against many gram-negative organisms such as *Proteus, Serratia, Enterobacter,* and *Acinetobacter* species and also *Klebsiella pneumoniae.* The antipseudomonal penicillins are *not* penicillinase resistant. Their pharmacologic action is similar to that of aminoglycosides, but they are less toxic.

Table 26.3 lists the drugs in the four categories of penicillin-type antibacterials. The administration routes (oral, IM, or IV) of various types of penicillins, along with the cephalosporins, are available on the Evolve website.

Beta-Lactamase Inhibitors

When a broad-spectrum antibiotic such as amoxicillin is combined with a beta-lactamase enzyme inhibitor such as clavulanic acid, the resulting antibiotic combination inhibits the bacterial beta-lactamases, making the antibiotic effective and extending its antimicrobial effect. There are three beta-lactamase inhibitors: (1) clavulanic acid, (2) sulbactam, and (3) tazobactam. These inhibitors are not given alone but are combined with a penicillinase-sensitive penicillin such as amoxicillin, ampicillin, or piperacillin. The combination drugs currently marketed include amoxicillin-clavulanic acid (for oral use) and ampicillin-sulbactam and piperacillin-tazobactam (for use parenterally).

Pharmacokinetics Amoxicillin is well absorbed from the GI tract, whereas dicloxacillin is only partially absorbed. Protein-binding power differs between the two drugs—amoxicillin is 20% protein bound, but dicloxacillin is highly protein bound (95%). Drug toxicity may result when other highly protein-bound drugs are used with dicloxacillin. Both drugs have short half-lives. Sixty percent of amoxicillin is excreted in the urine; dicloxacillin is excreted in bile and urine.

Pharmacodynamics Both amoxicillin and dicloxacillin are penicillin derivatives and are bactericidal. These drugs interfere with bacterial cell-wall synthesis, causing cell lysis. Amoxicillin may be produced with or without clavulanic acid, an agent that prevents the breakdown of amoxicillin by decreasing resistance to the antibacterial drug. The addition of clavulanic acid intensifies the effect of amoxicillin. The amoxicillin–clavulanic acid preparation and amoxicillin trihydrate have similar pharmacokinetics and pharmacodynamics as well as similar side effects and adverse reactions. When probenecid is taken with amoxicillin or dicloxacillin, the serum antibacterial levels may be increased. The effects of amoxicillin are decreased when taken with erythromycin and tetracycline. The onset of action, serum peak concentration time, and duration of action for amoxicillin and dicloxacillin are very similar.

Geriatrics

Most beta-lactam antibiotics are excreted via the kidneys. With older adults, assessment of renal function is most important. Serum blood urea nitrogen (BUN) and serum creatinine should be monitored. With a decrease in renal function, the antibiotic dose should be decreased.

Side Effects and Adverse Reactions

Common adverse reactions to penicillin administration are hypersensitivity and superinfection, the occurrence of a secondary infection when the flora of the body are disturbed (see Table 26.2). Anorexia, nausea, vomiting, and diarrhea are common GI disturbances, often referred to as GI distress. This may be alleviated some by taking penicillin with food. Rash is an indicator of a mild to moderate allergic reaction; severe allergic reaction leads to anaphylactic shock. Clinical manifestations of a severe allergic reaction include laryngeal edema, severe bronchoconstriction with stridor, and hypotension. Allergic effects occur in 5% to 10% of persons receiving penicillin compounds, therefore close monitoring during the first and subsequent doses of penicillin is essential.

Drug Interactions

The broad-spectrum penicillins, amoxicillin and ampicillin, may decrease the effectiveness of oral contraceptives. Potassium supplements can increase serum potassium levels when taken with potassium penicillin G or V. When penicillin is mixed with an aminoglycoside in IV solution, the actions of both drugs are inactivated.

OTHER BETA-LACTAM ANTIBACTERIALS

Like penicillins, these beta-lactam antibacterials preferentially bind to specific penicillin-binding proteins located inside the bacterial cell wall and are bactericidal. This group includes aztrenam, imipenem/cilastatin, and meropenem. Aztrenam's effectiveness is limited to aerobic gram-positive infections. Imipenem/cilastatin and meropenem are effective against a broader spectrum of activity than many other beta-lactam antibacterials. These three antibacterials are less nephrotoxic than many other antibacterials. Table 26.4 describes these other beta-lactam antibacterials and their dosages, uses, and considerations.

Side Effects and Adverse Reactions

Side effects and adverse reactions to aztrenam, imipenem/cilastatin, and meropenem include headache, nausea, vomiting, diarrhea, anemia, eosinophilia, and neutropenia. Rash may also occur. Severe adverse reactions include anaphylaxis, angioedema, seizures, and *Clostridium difficile*–associated diarrhea.

 NURSING PROCESS
Patient-Centered Collaborative Care
Antibacterials: Penicillins

Assessment
- Assess for allergy to penicillin or cephalosporins. The patient who is hypersensitive to amoxicillin should not take *any* type of penicillin products because severe allergic reaction could occur. A small percentage of patients who are allergic to penicillin could also be allergic to a cephalosporin product.
- Evaluate laboratory results, especially liver enzymes. Report elevated alkaline phosphatase (ALP), alanine aminotransferase (ALT), and aspartate aminotransferase (AST).
- Record urine output. If amount is inadequate (<30 mL/h or <600 mL/day), the drug or drug dosage may need to be changed.

Nursing Diagnoses
- Infection, Risk for
- Skin Integrity, Risk for Impaired
- Noncompliance with drug regimen related to decreased finances
- Nutrition, Imbalanced: Less than Body Requirements related to nausea and vomiting

Planning
- The patient's infection will be controlled and ultimately eliminated.

Nursing Interventions
- Obtain a sample (e.g., swab, blood, sputum) for laboratory culture and antibiotic sensitivity testing (C&S test) to discern the infective organism before antibiotic therapy is started.
- Monitor for signs and symptoms of superinfection, especially in patients taking high doses of an antibiotic for a

TABLE 26.4 Other Beta-Lactam Antibiotics

Generic	Route and Dosage	Uses and Considerations
Aztreonam	Severe infections: A: IM/IV: 1-2 g q8-12h; *max:* 8 g/d	For treating septicemia and intraabdominal, skin, respiratory, and urinary tract infections. May cause anaphylaxis, angioedema, fever, rash, nasal congestion, cough, wheezing, GI distress, CDAD, neutropenia, injection site reaction, and superinfection. Pregnancy category: B*; PB: 56%-65%; t½: 1.7-2.1h
Ertapenem	Skin infections: A/adol: IM/IV: 1 g/d for 7-14 d; *max:* 1 g/d for 7-14 d C/infants >3 mo: IM/IV: 15 mg/kg; *max:* 1 g/d for 7-14 d	For bacteremia, community-acquired pneumonia, complicated UTI, skin, pelvic, and intraabdominal infections. May cause anaphylaxis, diarrhea, vomiting, abdominal pain, constipation, headache, drowsiness, fever, elevated hepatic enzymes, injection site reaction, superinfection, and anemia. Pregnancy category B*; PB: 95%; t½: 4.5 h
Imipenem and cilastatin	Urinary tract infection: A: IV: 250-500 mg q6h; *max:* 4 g/d Adol/C/infants >3 mo: IV: 15-25 mg/kg/dose q6h; *max:* Adol/C - 4 g/d; Infants - 100 mg/kg/d	For treating septicemia, endocarditis, and gynecologic, intraabdominal, respiratory, urinary tract, skin, and bone/joint infection. May cause anaphylaxis, angioedema, rash, GI distress, tongue discoloration, dysgeusia, CDAD, seizures, eosinophilia, thrombocytosis, elevated hepatic enzymes, and superinfection. Pregnancy category: C*; PB: 20%-40%; t½: 1 h
Meropenem	Skin infections: A/adol/C >50 kg: IV: 500 mg-1 g q8h; *max:* 1 g q8h Adol/C/infants >3 mo, <50 kg: IV: 10-20 mg/kg q8h; *max:* 40 mg/kg/dose	For treating meningitis and intraabdominal, respiratory, and skin infections. May cause anaphylaxis, angioedema, headache, rash, GI distress, glossitis, constipation, CDAD, anemia, seizure, and superinfection. Pregnancy category: B*; PB: 2%: t½: 1.2 h

*Pregnancy categories have been revised. See http://www.fda.gov/Drugs/DevelopmentApprovalProcess/DevelopmentResources/Labeling/ucm093307.htm for more information.

A, Adult; *adol,* adolescent; *C,* child; *CDAD, Clostridium difficile*–associated diarrhea; *d,* day; *GI,* gastrointestinal; *h,* hour; *IM,* intramuscular; *IV,* intravenous; *max,* maximum; *mo, months;* *PB,* protein binding; *PO,* by mouth; *q,* every; *t½,* half-life; *>,* greater than.

prolonged time. Signs and symptoms include stomatitis (mouth ulcers), genital discharge (vaginitis), and anal or genital itching.

- ⚡ Examine the patient for allergic reaction to the penicillin product, especially after the first and second doses. This may be a mild reaction, such as a rash, or a severe reaction, such as respiratory distress or anaphylaxis.
- ⚡ Have epinephrine available to counteract a severe allergic reaction.
- Do not mix aminoglycosides with a high-dose or extended-spectrum penicillin G because this combination may inactivate the aminoglycoside.
- Assess the patient for bleeding if high doses of penicillin are being given; a decrease in platelet aggregation (clotting) may result.
- Monitor body temperature and the infected area.
- Dilute antibiotic for IV use in an appropriate amount of solution as indicated in the package insert.

Patient Teaching
General
- Teach patients to always take the *entire* prescribed penicillin product, such as amoxicillin, until the bottle is empty. If only a portion of the penicillin is taken, drug resistance to that antibacterial agent may develop in the future.
- Advise patients allergic to penicillin to wear a medical alert bracelet or necklace and to carry a card that indicates the allergy. Patients should notify their health care providers of any allergy to penicillin when reporting their health history.

- Keep drugs out of reach of small children. Request child-proof containers.
- Tell patients to report any side effects or adverse reactions that may occur while taking the drug.
- Encourage patients to increase fluid intake; fluids can aid in regulating body temperature and in excreting the drug.
- Warn patients or the parents of children taking antibiotics that chewable tablets must be chewed or crushed before swallowing.
- Advise female patients of childbearing years to use an additional form of birth control while taking penicillins.

Diet
- Advise patients to take medication with food to avoid gastric irritation.

🌐 Cultural Considerations
- Recognize that patients and family members from various cultural backgrounds may have alternative practices for alleviating infections. Accept adjunctive alternative methods if these are not harmful to the patient.
- Request a translator to obtain a history of symptoms related to infection and any allergies to antibiotics if the patient does not speak English.

Evaluation
- Evaluate the effectiveness of antibacterial agents by determining whether the infection has resolved and whether any side effects, including superinfection, have occurred.

TABLE 26.5 Activity of the Five Generations of Cephalosporins

Generation	Activity
First	Effective mostly against gram-positive bacteria (streptococci and most staphylococci) and some gram-negative bacteria (*Escherichia coli* and species of *Klebsiella, Proteus, Salmonella,* and *Shigella*)
Second	Same effectiveness as first generation but with a broader spectrum against other gram-negative bacteria such as *Haemophilus influenzae, Neisseria gonorrhoeae* and *N. meningitidis, Enterobacter* species, and several anaerobic organisms
Third	Same effectiveness as first and second generations and also effective against gram-negative bacteria (*Pseudomonas aeruginosa* and *Serratia* and *Acinetobacter* species) but with increased resistance to destruction by beta-lactamases
Fourth	Similar to third-generation drugs and highly resistant to most beta-lactamase bacteria with broad-spectrum antibacterial activity and good penetration to cerebrospinal fluid; effective against *E. coli, P. aeruginosa,* and *Klebsiella, Proteus,* and *Streptococcus* species and certain staphylococci
Fifth	Similar characteristics of third and fourth generations, also broad spectrum, and the only cephalosporins effective against methicillin-resistant *Staphylococcus aureus* (MRSA)

Cephalosporins

In 1948, a fungus called *Emericellopsis minimum* (*Cephalosporium acremonium*) was discovered in seawater at a sewer outlet off the coast of Sardinia. This fungus was found to be active against gram-positive and gram-negative bacteria and resistant to beta-lactamase, an enzyme that acts against the beta-lactam structure of penicillin. In the early 1960s, cephalosporins were used with clinical effectiveness. For cephalosporins to be effective against numerous organisms, their molecules were chemically altered, and semisynthetic cephalosporins were produced. Like penicillin, the cephalosporins have a beta-lactam structure and act by inhibiting the bacterial enzyme necessary for cell-wall synthesis. Lysis to the cell occurs, and the bacterial cell dies.

First-, Second-, Third-, Fourth-, and Fifth-Generation Cephalosporins

Cephalosporins are a major antibiotic group used in hospitals and in health care offices. These drugs are bactericidal with actions similar to penicillin. For antibacterial activity, the beta-lactam ring of cephalosporins is necessary.

Five groups of cephalosporins have been developed, identified as *generations*. Each generation is effective against a broader spectrum of bacteria, an increased resistance to destruction by beta-lactamases, and an increased ability to reach cerebrospinal fluid (Table 26.5).

Not all cephalosporins are affected by the beta-lactamases. First-generation cephalosporins are effective against most gram-positive bacteria and are destroyed by beta-lactamases, but not all second-generation cephalosporins are affected by beta-lactamases. Second-generation cephalosporins are effective against gram-positive and some gram-negative bacteria. Third-generation cephalosporins are resistant to beta-lactamases. They have broad-spectrum antibacterial activity and are effective against *P. aeruginosa*. The fourth-generation cephalosporin, cefepime, has broad-spectrum activity, is highly resistant to beta-lactamases, and has good penetration to cerebrospinal fluid. The fifth-generation cephalosporins are broad-spectrum drugs effective against MRSA.

Approximately 10% of persons allergic to penicillin are also allergic to cephalosporins because both groups of antibacterials have similar molecular structures. If a patient is allergic to penicillin and taking a cephalosporin, the nurse should watch for a possible allergic reaction to the cephalosporin, although the likelihood of a reaction is small.

Only a few cephalosporins are administered orally. These include cephalexin, cefadroxil, cefaclor, cefuroxime, cefdinir, cefprozil, cefixime, cefpodoxime, cefditoren, and ceftibuten. The rest of the cephalosporins are administered IM and IV. Prototype Drug Chart 26.2 describes the drug data related to ceftriaxone.

Pharmacokinetics Cefazolin is administered IM and IV, and cefaclor is given orally. The protein-binding power of cefazolin is greater than that of cefaclor. The half-life of each drug is short, and the drugs are excreted 60% to 80% unchanged in the urine.

Pharmacodynamics Cefazolin and cefaclor inhibit bacterial cell-wall synthesis and produce a bactericidal action. For IM and IV use of cefazolin, the onset of action is almost immediate, and peak concentration time is 5 to 15 minutes with IV use. The peak concentration time for an oral dose of cefaclor is 30 to 60 minutes.

When probenecid is administered with either of these drugs, urine excretion of cefazolin and cefaclor is decreased, which increases the action of the drug. The effects of cefazolin and cefaclor can be decreased if the drug is given with tetracyclines or erythromycin. These drugs can cause false-positive laboratory results for proteinuria and glucosuria, especially when they are taken in large doses.

Table 26.6 lists the cephalosporins by their designated generation and also gives dosages, uses, and considerations.

Side Effects and Adverse Reactions

The side effects and adverse reactions to cephalosporins include GI disturbances (nausea, vomiting, diarrhea), alteration in blood clotting time (increased bleeding) with administration of large doses, and nephrotoxicity (toxicity to the kidney) in individuals with a preexisting renal disorder.

Drug Interactions

Drug interactions can occur with certain cephalosporins and alcohol. For example, alcohol consumption may cause a disulfiram-like reaction (flushing, dizziness, headache, nausea, vomiting, and muscular cramps) while taking cefotetan. Uricosuric drugs increase the excretion rate of uric acid by inhibiting its reabsorption. Taking uricosurics concurrently can decrease the excretion of cephalosporins, thereby greatly increasing serum levels.

PROTOTYPE DRUG CHART 26.2

Ceftriaxone

Drug Class	Dosage
Ceftriaxone: Third-generation cephalosporin Pregnancy category: B*	Intraabdominal, skin, and bone/joint infections: A: IM/IV: 1-2 g q12-24h; *max:* 4 g/d Adol/C/infants: IM/IV: 50-75 mg/kg/d in divided doses q12-24h; *max:* 100 mg/kg/d
Contraindications	**Drug-Lab-Food Interactions**
Hypersensitivity to cephalosporins, gallbladder disease, pseudomembranous colitis, renal impairment *Caution:* Bleeding, receiving calcium IVs, hypersensitivity to penicillins, vitamin K deficiency, anticoagulants, diabetes mellitus, hepatic dysfunction	Drug: Increased nephrotoxicity with loop diuretics, aminoglycosides, calcium salts, and vancomycin; increased bleeding with anticoagulants Lab: May increase AST, ALT, ALP, LDH, PT, and INR
Pharmacokinetics	**Pharmacodynamics**
Absorption: IM, IV Distribution: PB: 85%-95% Metabolism: t½: 6-9 h Excretion: In urine	IM: Onset, duration: UK Peak: 1.5-4 h IV: Onset: Immediate; duration: UK Peak: 30 min
Therapeutic Effects/Uses	
For treating otitis media, meningitis, appendicitis, gonorrhea, septicemia, and surgical infection prophylaxis, and skin, respiratory, bone/joint, gynecologic, and urinary tract infections. Ceftriaxone is effective against *Klebsiella, Haemophilus, Clostridium, Citrobacter, Bacteroides, Acinetobacter, Neisseria, Proteus, Salmonella, Serratia, Shigella, Staphylococci, Staphylococci,* and *Escherichia coli.* Mode of Action: Inhibits bacterial cell-wall synthesis causing cell lysis; bactericidal effect	
Side Effects	**Adverse Reactions**
Anorexia, nausea, dyspepsia, dysgeusia, stomatitis, glossitis, vomiting, diarrhea, abdominal cramps, flatulence, rash, flushing, diaphoresis, fever, pruritus, headaches, dizziness, edema, injection site reaction	Superinfection, bleeding, epistaxis, angioedema, palpitations, biliary obstruction, cholelithiasis, elevated hepatic enzymes, jaundice, hematuria *Life threatening:* Seizures, anaphylaxis, agranulocytosis, aplastic anemia, hemolytic anemia, leukopenia, thrombocytopenia, neutropenia, eosinophilia, renal failure, CDAD, Stevens-Johnson syndrome

*Pregnancy categories have been revised. See http://www.fda.gov/Drugs/DevelopmentApprovalProcess/DevelopmentResources/Labeling/ucm093307.htm for more information.
A, Adult; *Adol,* adolescent; *ALP,* alkaline phosphatase; *ALT,* alanine aminotransferase; *AST,* aspartate aminotransferase; *C,* child; *CDAD, Clostridium difficile–*associated diarrhea; *d,* day; *h,* hour; *IM,* intramuscular; *INR,* international normalized ratio; *IV,* intravenous; *LDH,* lactic dehydrogenase; *max,* maximum; *min,* minute; *PB,* protein binding; *PT,* prothrombin time; *q,* every; *t½,* half-life; *UK,* unknown.

 NURSING PROCESS
Patient-Centered Collaborative Care

Antibacterials: Cephalosporins

Assessment
- Assess for allergy to cephalosporins or penicillins. If a patient is allergic to one type or class of cephalosporin, that patient should not receive any other type of cephalosporin or penicillin.
- Record vital signs and urine output. Report abnormal findings, which may include elevated temperature or decreased urine output.
- Evaluate laboratory results, especially those that indicate renal and liver function (BUN, serum creatinine, AST, ALT, ALP, and bilirubin). Use these laboratory results for baseline values, and report any abnormal findings.

Nursing Diagnoses
- Skin Integrity, Risk for Impaired
- Infection, Risk for
- Noncompliance with the drug regimen related to lack of knowledge relevant to regimen behavior

- Nutrition, Imbalanced: Less than Body Requirements related to nausea and vomiting

Planning
- The patient's infection will be controlled and ultimately eliminated.

Nursing Interventions
- Culture the infected area before cephalosporin therapy is started. The organism causing the infection can be determined by culture, and the antibiotics the organism is sensitive to are determined by sensitivity. If antibiotic therapy is started before culture result is reported, the antibiotic may need to be changed after C&S test results are received.

Patient Teaching
General
- Keep drugs out of reach of children. Request childproof containers.
- Tell patients to report signs of superinfection, such as mouth ulcers or discharge from the anal or genital area.
- Advise patients to ingest buttermilk, yogurt, or an acidophilus supplement to prevent superinfection of the intestinal flora.

TABLE 26.6   Antibacterials: Cephalosporins

Generic	Route and Dosage	Uses and Considerations
FIRST GENERATION		
Cefadroxil	UTI: A: PO: 1-2 g/d in 1-2 divided doses for 3-7 d; *max:* 2 g/d Adol/C/infants: PO: 30 mg/kg/d in 2 divided doses; *max:* 30 mg/kg/d	For treating pharyngitis, tonsillitis, and urinary tract and skin infections. May cause anaphylaxis, angioedema, fever, rash, arthralgia, GI distress, CDAD, elevated hepatic enzymes, nephritis, superinfection, and Stevens-Johnson syndrome. Well absorbed by the GI tract and not affected by food. Pregnancy category: B*; PB: UK; t½: 1-2 h
Cefazolin sodium	URI and UTI: A: IM/IV: 250 mg-1 g q8h; *max:* 12 g/d Adol/C/infants >1 mo: IM/IV: 25-100 mg/kg/d in 3 divided doses; *max:* 6 g/d	For treating endocarditis, septicemia, and skin, bone/joint, biliary, respiratory, and urinary tract infections. May cause anaphylaxis, angioedema, rash, GI distress, CDAD, superinfection, seizures, injection site reaction, Stevens-Johnson syndrome, and elevated hepatic enzymes. Pregnancy category: B*; PB: 75%-85%; t½: 1-2 h
Cephalexin	URI: A: PO: 250-500 mg q6-12h; *max:* 4 g/d Adol/C: PO: 25-100 mg/kg/d in 2-4 divided doses; *max:* 4 g/d	For treating otitis media and skin, bone/joint, respiratory, and urinary tract infections. May cause anaphylaxis, nephritis, GI distress, CDAD, rash, elevated hepatic enzymes, eosinophilia, superinfection, and Stevens-Johnson syndrome. Pregnancy category: B*; PB: 10%-15%; t½: 1 h
SECOND GENERATION		
Cefaclor	URI: Immediate release: A/adol: PO: 250-500 mg q8h; *max:* 1.5 g/d C/infants >1 mo: PO: 20-40 mg/kg/d divided q8h; *max:* 1 g/d Extended release: A/adol >16 y: PO: 375 mg q12h for 10 d; *max:* 1 g/d	For pharyngitis, tonsillitis, otitis media, and skin, skin structures, respiratory, and urinary tract infections. May cause anaphylaxis, headache, rhinitis, rash, GI distress, CDAD, seizure, Stevens-Johnson syndrome, and superinfection. Pregnancy category: B*; PB: 25%; t½: 1 h
Cefotetan	UTI: A: IM/IV: 500 mg-2 g q12-24h; *max:* 6 g/d	For treating PID and gynecologic, intraabdominal, respiratory, urinary tract, skin, and bone/joint infections. May cause anaphylaxis, angioedema, GI distress CDAD, seizures, bleeding, hypoprothrombinemia, anemia, superinfection, and Stevens-Johnson syndrome. Pregnancy category: B*; PB: 75%-90%; t½: 3-4.5 h
Cefoxitin sodium	Respiratory infection: A: IM/IV: 1-2 g q6-8h; *max:* 12 g/d Adol/C/infants >3 mo: IM/IV: 80-100 mg/kg/d in divided doses q6-8h; *max:* 12 g/d	For treating septicemia and intraabdominal, gynecologic, skin, respiratory, bone/joint, and urinary tract infections. May cause anaphylaxis, GI distress, anemia, seizure, renal dysfunction, Stevens-Johnson syndrome, and superinfection. Pregnancy category: B*; PB: 73%; t½: 40-60 min
Cefprozil monohydrate	Skin infection: A: PO: 250-500 mg/d or q12h for 10 d; *max:* 1 g/d C 2-12 y: PO: 20 mg/kg q12h for 10 d; *max:* 30 mg/kg/d	For treating otitis media and respiratory and skin infections. May cause anaphylaxis, angioedema, GI distress, CDAD, elevated hepatic enzymes, Stevens-Johnson syndrome, and superinfection. Pregnancy category: B*; PB: 36%; t½: 1.3 h
Cefuroxime	Respiratory infection: A/adol: PO: 250-500 mg q12h for 5-10 d A: IM/IV: 750 mg-1.5 g q8h Adol/C/infants >3 mo: IM/IV: 50-100 mg/kg/d in divided doses q6-8h	For treating meningitis, Lyme disease, otitis media, gonorrhea, septicemia, and skin, respiratory, urinary tract, and bone/joint infections. May cause anaphylaxis, rash, GI distress, CDAD, elevated hepatic enzymes, seizure, Stevens-Johnson syndrome, and superinfection. Pregnancy category: B*; PB: 33%-50%; t½: 1-2 h
THIRD GENERATION		
Cefdinir	Skin infection: A/adol: PO: 300 mg q12h for 10 d; *max:* 600 mg/d	For treating otitis media, acute sinusitis, tonsillitis, and respiratory, and skin infections. May cause anaphylaxis, headache, rash, GI distress, CDAD, superinfection, and Stevens-Johnson syndrome. Pregnancy category: B*; PB: 60%-70%; t½: 1.7 h
Cefixime	Respiratory infection: A/adol/C >45 kg: PO: 400 mg/d in divided doses q12-24h; *max:* 400 mg/d Infant >6 mo/C <45 kg: PO: 8 mg/kg/d in divided doses q12-24h; *max:* 8 mg/kg/d	For treating otitis media, tonsillitis, gonorrhea, and respiratory and urinary tract infections. May cause anaphylaxis, headache, dizziness, GI distress, CDAD, superinfection, and Stevens-Johnson syndrome. Pregnancy category: B*; PB: 65%-70%; t½: 3-4 h
Cefotaxime	A/adol/C >50 kg: IM/IV: 1-2 g q6-12h; *max:* 12 g/d Adol/C/infants <50 kg: IM/IV: 50-225 mg/kg/d in divided doses q4-8h; *max:* 225 mg/kg/d	For treating bacteremia, septicemia, meningitis, typhoid fever and gynecologic, skin, bone/joint, intraabdominal, respiratory, and urinary tract infections. May cause anaphylaxis, rash, pruritus, GI distress, CDAD, nephritis, eosinophilia, injection site reaction, superinfection, and Stevens-Johnson syndrome. Pregnancy category: B*; PB: 13%-38%; t½: 1-2 h

Continued

TABLE 26.6   Antibacterials: Cephalosporins—cont'd

Generic	Route and Dosage	Uses and Considerations
THIRD GENERATION		
Cefpodoxime	Respiratory infection: A/adol/C >12 y: PO: 200 mg q12h for 14 d; *max:* 800 mg/d	For treating otitis media, tonsillitis, sinusitis, gonorrhea, proctitis, and skin, respiratory, and urinary tract infections. May cause anaphylaxis, headache, rash, GI distress, CDAD, superinfection, and nephritis. Food enhances drug absorption. Pregnancy category: B*; PB: 22%-33%; t½: 3 h
Ceftazidime	Intraabdominal infection: A: IM/IV: 1-2 g q8-12h; *max:* 6 g/d C/infants >1 mo: IV: 30-50 mg/kg q8h; *max:* 150 mg/kg/d	For treating bacteremia, meningitis and gynecologic, intraabdominal, skin, respiratory, bone/joint, and urinary tract infections. May cause anaphylaxis, angioedema, dizziness, injection site reaction, GI distress, CDAD, eosinophilia, superinfection, and Stevens-Johnson syndrome. Pregnancy category: B*; PB: 10%; t½: 1.5-2 h
Ceftriaxone	See Prototype Drug Chart 26.2.	
Ceftibuten	Bronchitis: A/adol/C >12 y: PO: 400 mg/d for 10 d; *max:* 400 mg/d	For treating otitis media, tonsillitis, and respiratory infections. May cause anaphylaxis, rash, fever, dysgeusia, GI distress, CDAD, superinfection, eosinophilia, and Stevens-Johnson syndrome. Pregnancy category: B*; PB: 65%; t½: 2-2.5 h
Cefditoren	A/adol/C >12 y: PO: 200-400 mg bid for 10-14 d; *max:* 800 mg/d	For treating tonsillitis and respiratory and skin infections. May cause anaphylaxis, dizziness, headache, GI distress, CDAD, hematuria, hyperglycemia, superinfection, and Stevens-Johnson syndrome. Avoid in patients with milk-protein hypersensitivity. Pregnancy category: B*; PB: 88%; t½: 1.6 h
Ceftazi-dime and avibactam	Urinary tract infection: A: IV: 2 g ceftazidime/0.5 g avibactam over 2 h q8h for 7-14 d; *max:* 6 g ceftazidime/1.5 g avibactam/d	For treating intraabdominal and urinary tract infections. May cause anxiety, headache, dizziness, rash, dysgeusia, GI distress, constipation, CDAD, elevated hepatic enzymes, hypokalemia, superinfection, and renal dysfunction. Pregnancy category: B*; PB: 5%-10%; t½: 1.5-2 h
FOURTH GENERATION		
Cefepime	Moderate to severe pneumonia: A/adol >16 y: IV: 1-2 g q12h for 10 d; *max:* 6 g/d Adol <16 y/C/infants >2 mo: IV: 50 mg/kg q12h for 10 d; *max:* 150 mg/kg/dose	For treating bacteremia and respiratory, skin, intraabdominal, and urinary tract infections. May cause anaphylaxis, headache, confusion, fever, rash, GI distress, CDAD, hallucinations, seizure, superinfection, and Stevens-Johnson syndrome. Pregnancy category: B*; PB: 16%-19%; t½: 2-2.3 h
FIFTH GENERATION		
Ceftaroline fosamil	A/adol >33 kg: IV: 600 mg q12h for 5-14 d; *max:* 1200 mg/d	For treating skin and respiratory infections. May cause anaphylaxis, headache, fever, rash, GI distress, and CDAD. Pregnancy category: B*; PB: 20%; t½: 1.6-2.6 h
Ceftolo-zane and tazobactam	Intraabdominal infection: A: IV: 1 g ceftolozane/0.5 g tazobactam q8h for 4-14 d; *max:* 3 g ceftolozane/1.5 g tazobactam/d	For treating intraabdominal and urinary tract infections. May cause headache, insomnia, GI distress, constipation, CDAD, fever, and hypokalemia. Pregnancy category: B*; PB: 16%-30%; t½: 0.91-3.12 h

*Pregnancy categories have been revised. See http://www.fda.gov/Drugs/DevelopmentApprovalProcess/DevelopmentResources/Labeling/ucm093 307.htm for more information.

A, Adult; *adol,* adolescent; *bid,* two times a day; *C,* child; *CDAD, Clostridium difficile*–associated diarrhea; *d,* day; *GI,* gastrointestinal; *h,* hour; *IM,* intramuscularly; *IV,* intravenously; *max,* maximum; *min,* minutes; *mo,* month; *PB,* protein binding; *PID,* pelvic inflammatory disease; *PO,* by mouth; *q,* every; *t½,* half-life; *UK,* unknown; *URI,* upper respiratory infection; *UTI,* urinary tract infection; *y,* years; <, less than; >, greater than.

- Instruct patients to take the complete course of medication, even when symptoms of infection have ceased.
- Infuse all IV cephalosporins over 30 minutes or as ordered to prevent pain and irritation.
- ⚡ Observe for hypersensitivity reactions.

Side Effects
- Warn patients to report any side effects from use of oral cephalosporin drugs; these may include anorexia, nausea, vomiting, headache, dizziness, itching, and rash.

Diet
- Advise patients to take medication with food if gastric irritation occurs.
- Encourage patients to take an adequate amount of fluids to avoid dehydration from diarrhea.

🌐 Cultural Considerations
- Allow adequate time for information processing for patients whose first language is not English. Failing to do so may result in an inaccurate response or no response.
- Provide time for patients to respond to questions, especially when there is a language barrier.
- Speak clearly and slowly, giving time for translation. Obtain an interpreter if necessary.

Evaluation
- Evaluate the effectiveness of the cephalosporin by determining whether the infection has ceased and that no side effects, including superinfection, have occurred.

SECTION 26B: Macrolides, Oxazolidinones, Lincosamides, Glycopeptides, Ketolides, Tetracyclines, and Glycylcyclines

MACROLIDES

Macrolide antibiotics—which include azithromycin, clarithromycin, and erythromycin—are called *broad-spectrum antibiotics*. Erythromycin, the first macrolide, was derived from the funguslike bacteria *Streptomyces erythreus* and was first introduced in the early 1950s. Macrolides bind to the 50S ribosomal subunits and inhibit protein synthesis. At low to moderate drug doses, macrolides have a bacteriostatic effect, and with high drug doses, their effect is bactericidal. Macrolides can be administered orally or by IV but not intramuscularly because it is too painful. IV macrolides should be infused slowly to avoid unnecessary pain (phlebitis).

Gastric acid destroys erythromycin in the stomach, therefore acid-resistant salts are added (e.g., ethylsuccinate, stearate, estolate) to decrease breakdown into small particles (dissolution) in the stomach. This allows the drug to be absorbed in the intestine. Normally, food does not hamper the absorption of acid-resistant macrolides. Table 26.7 lists the dosages, uses, and considerations of macrolides.

Macrolides are active against most gram-positive bacteria and are moderately active against some gram-negative bacteria, although resistant organisms may emerge during treatment. Macrolides are used to treat mild to moderate infections of the respiratory tract, sinuses, GI tract, and skin and soft tissue in addition to treating diphtheria, impetigo contagiosa, and sexually transmitted infections (STIs).

Erythromycin is the drug of choice for the treatment of mycoplasmal pneumonia and Legionnaires' disease. Clarithromycin is also available in a once-a-day extended-release tablet to be taken for 7 days. Azithromycin is frequently prescribed for upper and lower respiratory infections, STIs, and uncomplicated skin infections. Table 26.7 lists the drugs developed from the derivatives of erythromycin, and Prototype Drug Chart 26.3 details the pharmacologic behavior of azithromycin.

Pharmacokinetics Clarithromycin and erythromycin are readily absorbed from the GI tract, mainly by the duodenum. Azithromycin is incompletely absorbed from the GI tract, and only 37% reaches systemic circulation. Azithromycin and erythromycin can be administered intravenously, but intermittent infusions should be diluted in normal saline (NS) or in 5% dextrose in water (D_5W) to prevent phlebitis or burning sensations at the injection site. Azithromycin 500 mg should be diluted in 250 to 500 mL of fluid, and erythromycin lactobionate 1 g should be diluted in 200 to 1000 mL. Macrolides are excreted in bile, feces, and urine. Because only a small amount is excreted in urine, renal insufficiency is not a contraindication for macrolide use.

Pharmacodynamics Macrolides suppress bacterial protein synthesis. The onset of action of oral preparations of erythromycin is 1 hour, peak concentration time is 4 hours, and duration of action is 6 hours. Newer macrolides have a longer half-life and are administered less frequently. Clarithromycin is administered twice a day for immediate release, and the extended-release formulation is administered once a day. Azithromycin has up to a 40- to 68-hour half-life and is prescribed to be taken only once a day for 5 days.

Side Effects and Adverse Reactions

Side effects and adverse reactions to macrolides include GI disturbances such as nausea, vomiting, diarrhea, and abdominal cramping. Severe diarrhea occurs when antibacterials kill normal flora, allowing an overgrowth of *Clostridium difficile*. This superinfection is called *Clostridium difficile*–associated diarrhea (CDAD),

Generic	Route and Dosage	Uses and Considerations
TABLE 26.7 Antibacterials: Macrolides, Oxazolidinones, Lincosamides, Glycopeptides, Ketolides, and Lipopeptides		
MACROLIDES		
Azithromycin	See Prototype Drug Chart 26.3.	
Clarithromycin	Skin infections: Immediate release: A: PO: 250 mg q12h for 7-14 d; *max:* 1 g/d Adol/C/infants >6 mo: PO: 7.5 mg/kg q12h for 10 d; *max:* 15 mg/kg/d	For treating otitis media, tonsillitis, duodenal ulcer due to *Helicobacter pylori*, and skin, respiratory, and soft-tissue infections. May cause anaphylaxis, headache, insomnia, rash, dysgeusia, tooth discoloration, GI distress, CDAD, superinfection, myasthenia, seizures, Stevens-Johnson syndrome, and renal failure. Pregnancy category: C*; PB: 42%-70%; t½: 3-7 h
Erythromycin base	Respiratory infections: A: PO: 250-500 mg q6h; *max:* 4 g/d Adol/C/infants: PO: 30-50 mg/kg/d in divided doses; *max:* 2 g/d A/adol/C/infants: IV: 15-20 mg/kg/d in divided doses q6h; *max:* 4 g/d	For treating acne, impetigo, tonsillitis, urethritis, STIs, Legionnaires' disease, PID, diphtheria, and respiratory and skin infections. May cause skin irritation, reversible hearing loss, superinfection, dysrhythmias, GI distress, CDAD, seizures, elevated hepatic enzymes, and Stevens-Johnson syndrome. Pregnancy category: B*; PB: 73%-81%; t½: 1.5-2 h
Fidaxomicin	A: PO: 200 mg bid for 10 d; *max:* 400 mg/d	For treating CDAD. May cause anaphylaxis, angioedema, anemia, neutropenia, GI distress and bleeding, and elevated hepatic enzymes. Pregnancy category: B*; PB: UK; t½: 6.9-16.5 h

Continued

TABLE 26.7   Antibacterials: Macrolides, Oxazolidinones, Lincosamides, Glycopeptides, Ketolides, and Lipopeptides—cont'd

Generic	Route and Dosage	Uses and Considerations
OXAZOLIDINONES		
Linezolid	Respiratory infection: A/adol/C >12 y: PO/IV: 600 mg q12h for 10-14 d; *max:* 1200 mg/d C <12 y/infants/neonates: PO/IV: 10 mg/kg q8h for 10-14 d; *max:* 10 mg/kg q8h	For treating bacteremia, sepsis, MRSA, VREF, and respiratory and skin infections. May cause anaphylaxis, headache, rash, seizure, tongue/tooth discoloration, GI distress, dizziness, thrombocytopenia, anemia, peripheral neuropathy, CDAD, and Stevens-Johnson syndrome. Pregnancy category: C*; PB: 31%; t½: 4.26-5.4 h
Tidezolid	A: PO/IV: 200 mg/d for 6 d; *max:* 200 mg/d	For treating skin infections. May cause headache, GI distress, CDAD, anemia, neutropenia, thrombocytopenia, peripheral neuropathy, and serotonin syndrome. Pregnancy category: C*; PB: 70%-90%; t½: 12 h
LINCOSAMIDES		
Clindamycin hydrochloride	Lower respiratory infection: A: PO: 150-450 mg q6h for 7-21 days Adol/C: PO: 8-20 mg/kg/d divided doses q6-8h A/adol >16y: IM/IV: 300 mg q6-12h; *max:* 2700 mg/d Adol <16y/C/infants: IM/IV: 20-40 mg/kg/d in divided doses q6-8h	For treating PID, acne, bacteremia, septicemia, MRSA, and respiratory, intraabdominal, skin, gynecologic, and bone/joint infections. May cause anaphylaxis, xerosis, dysgeusia, GI distress, CDAD, erythema, pruritus, elevated hepatic enzymes, superinfection, and Stevens-Johnson syndrome. Should be taken with full glass of water. Pregnancy category: B*; PB: 92%-94%; t½: 2-3 h
Lincomycin	A: IM: 600 mg q12-24h Adol/C/Infants >1 mo: IM: 10 mg/kg q12-24h A: IV: 600 mg-1 g q8-12h; *max:* 8 g/d Adol/C/Infants >1 mo: IV: 10-20 mg/kg/d in divided doses q8-12h; *max:* 20 mg/kg/d	For treating bacteremia, septicemia, and intraabdominal, respiratory, bone/joint, and skin infections. May cause anaphylaxis, angioedema, glossitis, stomatitis, GI distress, CDAD, pancytopenia, Stevens-Johnson syndrome, superinfection, injection site reaction, and hypotension if given by too-rapid IV infusion. Pregnancy category: B*; PB: 72%; t½: 2-11.5 h
GLYCOPEPTIDES		
Vancomycin hydrochloride	*Clostridium difficile* infection: A: PO: 125 mg four times daily for 10 d; *max:* 2 g/d Therapeutic range: Trough: 10-20 mcg/mL	For treating bacteremia, septicemia, endocarditis, MRSA, CDAD, and respiratory, skin, and bone/joint infections. May cause anaphylaxis, hypotension, fever, headache, flushing, GI distress, peripheral edema, hypokalemia, neutropenia, ototoxicity, nephrotoxicity, disulfiram-like reaction to alcohol, red man syndrome, superinfection, and Stevens-Johnson syndrome. Pregnancy category: B*; PB: 55%; t½: 4-6 h
Oritavancin	Skin infection: A: IV: 1200 mg as a single dose over 3 h; *max:* 1200 mg	For treating skin infections, MRSA, and cellulitis. May cause angioedema, wheezing, bronchospasm, dizziness, headache, phlebitis, peripheral edema, elevated hepatic enzymes, GI distress, and CDAD. Pregnancy category: C*; PB: 85%; t½: 245 h
Telavancin	A: IV: 10 mg/kg/d over 60 min for 7-21 d; *max:* 10 mg/kg/d	For treating MRSA and respiratory and skin infections. May cause anaphylaxis, headache, insomnia, chills, dizziness, pruritus, rash, dysgeusia, GI distress, CDAD, red man syndrome, nephrotoxicity, and superinfection. Pregnancy category: C*; PB: 93%; t½: 8-9 h
KETOLIDES		
Telithromycin	A: PO: 800 mg/d for 7-10 d; *max:* 800 mg/d	For treating MRSA and community-acquired pneumonia. May cause anaphylaxis, dizziness, dysgeusia, GI distress, CDAD, hepatotoxicity, dysrhythmias, and myasthenia. Pregnancy category: C*; PB: 60%-70%; t½: 10 h
LIPOPEPTIDES		
Daptomycin	Skin infection: A: IV: 4 mg/kg/d for 7-14 d; *max:* 6 mg/kg/d	For treating MRSA, endocarditis, bacteremia, and skin infections. May cause anaphylaxis, rash, pruritis, anemia, insomnia, GI distress, edema, chest pain, hypertension, headache, hyperhidrosis, and Stevens-Johnson syndrome. Pregnancy category: B*; PB: 90%-93%; t½: 7.7-8.3 h

*Pregnancy categories have been revised. See http://www.fda.gov/Drugs/DevelopmentApprovalProcess/DevelopmentResources/Labeling/ucm093 307.htm for more information.

A, Adult; *Adol,* adolescent; *bid,* twice daily; *C,* child; *CDAD, Clostridium difficile*–associated diarrhea; *d,* day; *GI,* gastrointestinal; *h,* hour; *IM,* intramuscular; *IV,* intravenous; *max,* maximum; *min,* minutes; *mo,* month; *MRSA,* methicillin-resistant *Staphylococcus aureus; PB,* protein binding; *PID,* pelvic inflammatory disease; *PO,* by mouth; *q,* every; *STI,* sexually transmitted infection; *t½,* half-life; *UK,* unknown; *VREF,* vancomycin-resistant *Enterococcus faecium; wk,* weeks; *y,* years; <, less than; >, greater than.

PROTOTYPE DRUG CHART 26.3

Azithromycin

Drug Class	Dosage
Antibacterial macrolide Pregnancy category: B*	Upper respiratory infection: A: PO: 500 mg on day 1, then follow with 250 mg/d for 4 days
Contraindications	**Drug-Lab-Food Interactions**
Hypersensitivity, hepatic dysfunction *Caution:* Bradycardia, hypokalemia, hypomagnesemia, dysrhythmias, renal dysfunction	Drug: Increases effects of digoxin, cyclosporine, and warfarin; decreases effects of penicillins and clindamycin
Pharmacokinetics	**Pharmacodynamics**
Absorption: PO: 38% absorbed Distribution: PB: 51% Metabolism: t½: 68 h Excretion: In bile, a small amount in urine	PO: Onset, duration: UK Peak: 2-3 h Extended release: Peak: 5 h IV: Onset, duration, peak: UK
Therapeutic Effects/Uses	
For treating bacterial conjunctivitis, otitis media, tonsillitis, sinusitis, PID, STIs, and skin and respiratory infections. For patients who are allergic to penicillin. Azithromycin is effective against species of *Clostridium, Haemophilus, Chlamydia, Mycobacterium, Neisseria, Staphyloccus,* and *Streptococcus.* Mode of Action: Inhibits the steps of protein synthesis; bacteriostatic or bactericidal effect	
Side Effects	**Adverse Reactions**
Blurred vision, ocular irritation, photosensitivity, headache, tinnitus, drowsiness, dizziness, fever, fatigue, tongue discoloration, dysgeusia, anorexia, nausea, vomiting, diarrhea, abdominal cramps, pruritus, rash, injection site reaction, weakness	Superinfection, hearing loss, angioedema, seizures, elevated hepatic enzymes, hyperbilirubinemia *Life threatening:* Hepatotoxicity, anaphylaxis, bronchospasm, CDAD, leukopenia, anemia, Stevens-Johnson syndrome

*Pregnancy categories have been revised. See http://www.fda.gov/Drugs/DevelopmentApprovalProcess/DevelopmentResources/Labeling/ucm093307.htm for more information.
A, Adult; *CDAD, Clostridium difficile*–associated diarrhea; *d,* day; *h,* hour; *IV,* intravenous; *max,* maximum; *PB,* protein binding; *PID,* pelvic inflammatory disease; *PO,* by mouth; *STI,* sexually transmitted infection; *t½,* half-life; *UK,* unknown.

also known as pseudomembraneous colitis. A release of bacterial toxins causes injury, inflammation, and bleeding in the colon lining. This condition causes abdominal cramping, 5 to 10 watery diarrheal stools per day, and bloody stools. Frequency of stools may increase to 20 per day in severe cases. Conjunctivitis may develop as a side effect of azithromycin, and the patient should avoid wearing contact lenses if this occurs. Allergic reactions to erythromycin are rare. Hepatotoxicity (liver toxicity) can occur when erythromycin and azithromycin are taken in high doses with other hepatotoxic drugs, such as acetaminophen (high doses), phenothiazines, and sulfonamides. Liver damage is usually reversible when the drug is discontinued. Erythromycin should not be taken with clindamycin or lincomycin because they compete for receptor sites.

Drug Interactions

Macrolides can increase serum levels of theophylline (a bronchodilator), carbamazepine (an anticonvulsant), and warfarin (an anticoagulant). If these drugs are given with macrolides, their drug serum levels should be closely monitored. To avoid severe toxic effects, erythromycin should not be used with other macrolides. Antacids may reduce azithromycin peak levels when taken at the same time.

Extended Macrolide Group

Derivatives of erythromycin have been effective in the treatment of numerous organisms. Like erythromycin, they also inhibit protein synthesis. Many of these macrolides have a longer half-life and are administered once a day. After the introduction of erythromycin, the first extended macrolide drug developed was clarithromycin, which has been effective against

many bacterial infections. Clarithromycin is administered twice a day for immediate-release form, and the extended-release formulation is given once a day. Another extended macrolide is azithromycin. This drug has a long half-life of 40 to up to 68 hours, therefore it is only prescribed once a day for 5 days.

Elimination of these drugs is via bile and feces. Azithromycin is frequently prescribed for upper and lower respiratory tract infections, STIs, and uncomplicated skin infections.

When erythromycin is given concurrently with verapamil, diltiazem, clarithromycin, fluconazole, ketoconazole, and itraconazole, erythromycin blood concentration and the risk of sudden cardiac death increase. Table 26.7 lists the drugs developed from the derivatives of erythromycin.

Common side effects of clarithromycin are nausea, diarrhea, and abdominal discomfort. With azithromycin, the side effects of nausea, diarrhea, and abdominal pain are common.

 NURSING PROCESS
Patient-Centered Collaborative Care

Antibacterials: Macrolides

Assessment
- Assess vital signs and urine output. Report abnormal findings.
- Check laboratory tests (liver enzyme values) to determine liver function. Order liver enzyme tests periodically for patients taking large doses of azithromycin for a continuous period.
- Obtain a history of drugs the patient currently takes. The peak level of azithromycin may be decreased by antacids.

Nursing Diagnoses
- Infection, Risk for
- Tissue Integrity, Risk for Impaired

Planning
- The patient's infection will be controlled and ultimately eliminated.

Nursing Interventions
- Obtain a sample from the infected area and send it to the laboratory for C&S testing before starting azithromycin therapy. Antibiotic therapy can be initiated after obtaining the culture sample.
- Monitor vital signs, urine output, and laboratory values, especially liver enzymes (ALP, ALT, AST, and bilirubin).
- Monitor the patient for liver damage resulting from prolonged use and high dosage of macrolides such as azithromycin. Signs of liver dysfunction include elevated liver enzyme levels and jaundice.
- Administer oral azithromycin 1 hour before or 2 hours after meals. Give with a full glass of water, *not* fruit juice. Give the drug with food if GI upset occurs. Chewable tablets should be chewed, *not* swallowed whole.
- Dilute in an appropriate amount of solution as indicated in the drug circular for IV azithromycin.
- Administer antacids either 2 hours before or 2 hours after azithromycin.

Patient Teaching
General
- Instruct patients to take the full course of the antibacterial agent as prescribed. Drug compliance is most important for all antibacterials (antibiotics).
Side Effects
- Encourage patients to report side effects, including adverse reactions (nausea, vomiting, diarrhea, abdominal cramps, itching).
- Teach patients to report any evidence of superinfection, secondary infection resulting from drug therapy; for some patients, stomatitis or vaginitis may occur.
- ⚡ Tell patients to report the onset of loose stools or diarrhea. CDAD should be ruled out.

🌐 *Cultural Considerations*
- Recognize that patients and family members from various cultural backgrounds may need a written schedule that shows when the drug should be taken. Have instructions available in the language the patient speaks or reads most easily, and emphasize reporting possible side effects to the health care provider.

Evaluation
- Evaluate the effectiveness of azithromycin by determining whether the infection has been controlled or has ceased and that no side effects, including superinfection, have occurred.

OXAZOLIDINONES

Like macrolides, oxazolidinones inhibit protein synthesis on the 50S ribosomal subunit of bacteria. This action prevents formation of 70S initiation complex which is necessary for bacterial reproduction. Linezolid and tidezolid are examples of oxazolidinones. Drugs in this antibacterial classification are bacteriostatic or bactericidal and are effective against gram-positive infections. Table 26.7 lists the oxazolidinones.

Side Effects and Adverse Reactions

Side effects and adverse reactions to linezolid and tidezolid include headache, nausea, vomiting, diarrhea, anemia, and thrombocytopenia. Rash may also occur. Severe adverse reactions include CDAD and serotonin syndrome.

LINCOSAMIDES

Like erythromycin, lincosamides inhibit bacterial protein synthesis and have both bacteriostatic and bactericidal actions, depending on drug dosage. Clindamycin and lincomycin are examples of lincosamides. Clindamycin is more widely prescribed than lincomycin because it is active against most gram-positive organisms, including *S. aureus* and anaerobic organisms. It is not effective against gram-negative bacteria (e.g., *E. coli* and *Proteus* and *Pseudomonas* species). Clindamycin is absorbed better than lincomycin through the GI tract and maintains a higher serum drug concentration. Clindamycin is considered more effective than lincomycin and has fewer toxic effects. Table 26.7 lists the lincosamides.

Side Effects and Adverse Reactions

Side effects and adverse reactions to clindamycin and lincomycin include GI irritation, which may manifest as nausea, vomiting, and stomatitis. Rash may also occur. Severe adverse reactions include colitis and anaphylactic shock.

Drug Interactions

Clindamycin and lincomycin are incompatible with aminophylline, phenytoin, barbiturates, and ampicillin.

GLYCOPEPTIDES

Vancomycin, a glycopeptide bactericidal antibiotic, was widely used in the 1950s to treat staphylococcal infections. Vancomycin is used against drug-resistant *S. aureus* and in cardiac surgical prophylaxis for individuals with penicillin allergies. Serum vancomycin levels should be monitored.

Vancomycin has become ineffective for treating enterococci. Quinupristin-dalfopristin is a combined antibacterial used to treat life-threatening VREF infections. Antibiotic-resistant enterococci can cause staphylococcal endocarditis.

Telavancin, a glycopeptide, treats selected gram-positive bacteria and skin infections. This drug is a semisynthetic derivative of vancomycin with bactericidal action against MRSA. Telavancin has an advantage of once-daily dosing. Oritavancin has the further advantage of being administered in a single dose.

Pharmacokinetics Vancomycin is given orally for treatment of staphylococcal enterocolitis and antibiotic-associated pseudomembranous colitis due to *C. difficile*. When vancomycin is given orally, it is not absorbed systemically and is excreted in the feces. Vancomycin is also given intravenously for septicemia, for severe infections due to MRSA, and for bone, skin, and lower respiratory tract infections that do not respond or are resistant to other antibiotics. Intermittent vancomycin doses should be diluted in 100 mL for 500 mg and 200 mL for 1 g of D₅W, NS, or Lactated Ringer's (LR) and should be administered over 60 to 90 minutes. Vancomycin is excreted in the urine when given by IV route. It is 55% protein bound, and the half-life is 4 to 6 hours.

Pharmacodynamics Vancomycin inhibits bacterial cell-wall synthesis and is active against several gram-positive microorganisms. The peak action is 30 minutes after the end of the infusion.

Side Effects and Adverse Reactions

Vancomycin may cause nephrotoxicity and ototoxicity. Ototoxicity results in damage to the auditory or vestibular branch of cranial nerve VIII. Such damage can result in permanent hearing loss (auditory branch) or temporary or permanent loss of balance (vestibular branch). Side effects may include chills, dizziness, fever, rashes, nausea, vomiting, and thrombophlebitis at the injection site. Too-rapid injection of IV vancomycin can cause a condition known as *red man syndrome* or *red neck syndrome*. Characterized by red blotching of the face, neck, and chest, this is a toxic effect rather than an allergic reaction. Other adverse effects include eosinophilia, neutropenia, and Stevens-Johnson syndrome. Severe hypotension, tachycardia, generalized tingling, and, rarely, cardiac arrest are also known adverse reactions.

Drug Interactions

Dimenhydrinate can mask ototoxicity when taken with vancomycin. The risk of nephrotoxicity and ototoxicity may be potentiated when vancomycin is taken with furosemide, aminoglycosides, amphotericin B, colistin, cisplatin, and cyclosporine. Vancomycin may inhibit methotrexate excretion and can increase methotrexate toxicity. The absorption of oral vancomycin may be decreased when given with cholestyramine and colestipol.

KETOLIDES

Ketolides are structurally related to macrolides. The first drug in this class, telithromycin, is used for adults 18 years of age and older to treat mild to moderate community-acquired pneumonia. This disorder is usually caused by *S. pneumoniae* and *H. influenzae*.

Pharmacokinetics Telithromycin is given orally and is well absorbed by the GI tract; it is unaffected by food intake. Telithromycin is excreted in the feces and urine. It is 60% to 70% protein bound, and the half-life is 10 hours.

Pharmacodynamics Telithromycin inhibits protein synthesis in microorganisms by binding to the bacterial ribosomal RNA site of the 50S subunit, resulting in bacterial cell death. The peak action is 1 hour.

Side Effects and Adverse Reactions

Side effects and adverse reactions to telithromycin include visual disturbances (blurred vision and diplopia), headache, dizziness, altered taste, nausea, vomiting, diarrhea, and liver failure. Telithromycin may also lead to an exacerbation of myasthenia gravis.

Drug Interactions

Telithromycin levels are increased when taken concurrently with antilipidemics (simvastatin, lovastatin, and atorvastatin), itraconazole, ketoconazole, and benzodiazepines. Class 1A or class III antidysrhythmics may lead to life-threatening dysrhythmias. Blood levels of telithromycin are decreased when taken with rifampin, phenytoin, carbamazepine, or phenobarbital, producing a subtherapeutic drug level. Telithromycin can increase levels of cisapride and pimozide, which can lead to toxicity; these two drugs are therefore contraindicated for the patient taking telithromycin. Digoxin, metoprolol, midazolam, ritonavir, sirolimus, and tacrolimus levels are increased when taken concurrently with telithromycin. Concurrent use of telithromycin with ergot alkaloid derivatives leads to ergot toxicity (severe peripheral vasospasm and impaired sensation).

TETRACYCLINES

Tetracyclines, isolated from *Streptomyces aureofaciens* in 1948, were the first broad-spectrum antibiotics effective against gram-positive and gram-negative bacteria and many other organisms—mycobacteria, rickettsiae, spirochetes, and chlamydiae, to name a few. Tetracyclines act by inhibiting bacterial protein synthesis and have a bacteriostatic effect.

Tetracyclines are not effective against *S. aureus* (except for the newer tetracyclines), nor are they effective against *Pseudomonas* or *Proteus* species, but they can be used against *Mycoplasma pneumoniae*. Tetracycline in combination with metronidazole and bismuth subsalicylate is useful in treating *Helicobacter pylori*, a bacterium in the stomach that can cause peptic ulcer. For years, oral and topical tetracyclines have been used to treat severe acne vulgaris, and low doses are usually prescribed to minimize the toxic effect of the drug.

The tetracyclines are frequently prescribed for oral use, although they are also available for IV use to treat severe infections (Prototype Drug Chart 26.4). The newer oral preparations of tetracyclines (i.e., doxycycline, minocycline) are more rapidly and completely absorbed. Tetracyclines should not be taken with magnesium and aluminum antacid preparations, milk products containing calcium, or iron-containing drugs because these substances bind with tetracycline and prevent absorption of the drug. It is suggested that tetracyclines, except for doxycycline and minocycline, be taken on an empty stomach 1 hour before or 2 hours after mealtime; the absorption of doxycycline and minocycline is improved with food ingestion. Table 26.8 describes the tetracycline preparations and their dosages, uses, and considerations. The tetracyclines are listed according to whether they are short-, intermediate-, or long-acting drugs.

Although tetracyclines are widely used, they have numerous side effects, adverse reactions, toxicities, and drug interactions.

Side Effects and Adverse Reactions

GI disturbances such as nausea, vomiting, and diarrhea are side effects of tetracyclines. Photosensitivity (sunburn reaction) may occur in persons taking tetracyclines, especially demeclocycline.

Doxycycline

Drug Class	Dosage
Antibacterial: Tetracycline Pregnancy category: D*	Urinary track infection: A/adol/C >8 y, >45 kg: PO: 100 mg q12h on day 1, then 100 mg/d C >8 y, <45 kg: PO: 2.2 mg/kg q12h on day 1, then 2.2 mg/kg/d A/adol/C >8 y, >45 kg: IV: 200 mg on day 1, then 100-200 mg/d C >8 y, <45 kg: IV: 4.4 mg/kg on day 1, then 2.2-4.4 mg/kg/d in 1-2 divided doses
Contraindications	**Drug-Lab-Food Interactions**
Hypersensitivity, sulfite hypersensitivity *Caution:* Renal and hepatic dysfunction, photosensitivity, hyperpigmentation	Drug: May increase effects of digoxin and warfarin; doxycycline absorption decreases with sucralfate, antacids, iron, calcium, magnesium, zinc, barbiturates, phenytoin, quinapril, and rifampin; decreases effects of oral contraceptives, ciprofloxacin, and penicillin; may alter lithium levels Lab: Decreases serum potassium level Food: Dairy products decrease effect.
Pharmacokinetics	**Pharmacodynamics**
Absorption: PO: 100% absorbed Distribution: PB: 23%-93% Metabolism: t½: 14-24 h Excretion: Urine and feces	PO: Onset, duration: UK Peak: 1.5-4 h IV: Onset: Rapid Peak, duration: UK

Therapeutic Effects/Uses

For treating acne, anthrax, amebiasis, gingivitis, plague, STIs, rickettsia, and respiratory, urinary tract, and skin infections. Doxycycline is effective against *Escherichia coli* and MRSA, and species of *Clostridium, Haemophilus, Enterococcus, Chlamydia, Neisseria, Klebsiella, Staphylococcus, Streptococcus,* and *Shigella.*

Mode of Action: Inhibits the steps of protein synthesis; bacteriostatic or bactericidal

Side Effects	Adverse Reactions
Abdominal pain, glossitis, dry mouth, tooth/nail discoloration, nausea, vomiting, diarrhea, headache, vision changes, diplopia, photosensitivity, rash, pruritus, injection site reaction	Superinfection, angioedema, hypertension, renal dysfunction *Life threatening:* Anaphylaxis, anemia, eosinophilia, thrombocytopenia, hepatotoxicity, increased intracranial pressure, CDAD, Stevens-Johnson syndrome

*Pregnancy categories have been revised. See http://www.fda.gov/Drugs/DevelopmentApprovalProcess/DevelopmentResources/Labeling/ucm093307.htm for more information.
A, Adult; *adol,* adolescent; *C,* child; *CDAD, Clostridium difficile*–associated diarrhea; *d,* day; *h,* hour; *IV,* intravenous; *MRSA,* methicillin-resistant *Staphylococcus aureus; PB,* protein binding; *PO,* by mouth; *q,* every; *STI,* sexually transmitted infection; *t½,* half life; *UK,* unknown; *UTI,* urinary tract infection; *y,* year; <, less than; >, greater than.

TABLE 26.8 Antibacterials: Tetracyclines and Glycylcyclines

Generic	Route and Dosage	Uses and Considerations
SHORT-ACTING TETRACYCLINE		
Tetracycline	URI: A: PO: 1-2 g/d in 2-4 divided doses; *max:* 4 g/d Adol/C >8 y: PO: 25-50 mg/kg/d in 4 divided doses	For treating anthrax, plague, gingivitis, *Helicobacter pylori,* cholera, MRSA, STIs, and skin, urinary tract, and respiratory infections. May cause anaphylaxis, headache, diplopia, dermatitis, glossitis, tooth/tongue/nail discoloration, GI distress, CDAD, photosensitivity, nephrotoxicity, hepatotoxicity, and superinfection. Pregnancy category: D*; PB: 65%; t½: 6-12 h
INTERMEDIATE-ACTING TETRACYCLINE		
Demeclocycline Hydrochloride	Respiratory infection: A: PO: 150 mg q6h or 300 mg q12h; *max:* 1.2 g/d Adol/C >8 y: PO: 7-13 mg/kg/d in 2-4 divided doses	For treating acne, gingivitis, anthrax, cholera, plague, STIs, and skin, respiratory, and urinary tract infections. May cause anaphylaxis, angioedema, headache, photosensitivity, tooth discoloration, glossitis, GI distress, CDAD, elevated hepatic enzymes, Stevens-Johnson syndrome, and superinfection. Pregnancy category: D*; PB: 65%-90%; t½: 10-17 h
LONG-ACTING TETRACYCLINES		
Doxycycline hyclate	See Prototype Drug Chart 26.4.	
Minocycline Hydrochloride	Respiratory infection: A: PO/IV: Initially: 200 mg; maint: 100 mg q12h; *max:* 200 mg/d PO; 400 mg/d IV Adol/C >8 y: PO/IV: Initially: 4 mg/kg/d, followed by 2 mg/kg q12h	For treating anthrax, cholera, plague, meningitis, gingivitis, MRSA, STIs, acne, and respiratory, urinary tract, and skin infections. May cause anaphylaxis, dizziness, fatigue, headache, stomatitis, tongue/tooth discoloration, dental caries and pain, GI distress, CDAD, photosensitivity, hepatotoxicity, superinfection, pancytopenia, and Stevens-Johnson syndrome. Take drug with food. Pregnancy category: D*; PB: 76%; t½: 11-24 h
GLYCYLCYCLINES		
Tigecycline	A: IV: Initially: 100 mg over 30-90 min; maint: 50 mg q12h for 7-14 d; *max:* 100 mg/d	For treating community-acquired pneumonia, MRSA, and skin and intraabdominal infections. May cause anaphylaxis, dizziness, photosensitivity, headache, weakness, anemia, superinfection, GI distress, CDAD, and Stevens-Johnson syndrome. Pregnancy category: D*; PB: 71%-89%; t½: 27-42 h

*Pregnancy categories have been revised. See http://www.fda.gov/Drugs/DevelopmentApprovalProcess/DevelopmentResources/Labeling/ucm093 307.htm for more information.
A, Adult; *Adol,* adolescent; *C,* child; *CDAD, Clostridium difficile*–associated diarrhea; *d,* day; *GI,* gastrointestinal; *h,* hour; *IV,* intravenous; *maint,* maintenance; *max,* maximum; *min,* minutes; *MRSA,* methicillin-resistant *Staphylococcus aureus; PB,* protein binding; *PO,* by mouth; *q,* every; *STI,* sexually transmitted infection; *t½,* half-life; *URI,* upper respiratory infection; *y,* year; >, greater than.

Pregnant patients should *not* take tetracycline during the first trimester of pregnancy because of possible teratogenic effects. Women in the last trimester of pregnancy and children younger than 8 years of age should also *not* take tetracycline because it irreversibly discolors the permanent teeth. Minocycline can cause damage to the vestibular part of the inner ear, which may result in difficulty maintaining balance. Outdated tetracyclines should always be discarded, because the drug breaks down into a toxic by-product. Nephrotoxicity (kidney toxicity) results when tetracycline is given in high doses with other nephrotoxic drugs. Because tetracycline can disrupt the microbial flora of the body, superinfection (secondary infection resulting from drug therapy) is another adverse reaction that might result.

Drug Interactions

Antacids and iron-containing drugs can prevent absorption of tetracycline from the GI tract. Milk and foods high in calcium can inhibit tetracycline absorption. To avoid drug interaction, these should be taken at least 2 hours apart from tetracycline. Be aware that lipid-soluble tetracyclines, such as doxycycline and minocycline, are actually better absorbed from the GI tract when taken *with* milk products and food.

The desired action of oral contraceptives can be lessened when taken with tetracyclines. The activity of penicillins given with a tetracycline can be decreased because the tetracyclines could cause a bacterial resistance to the action of penicillin. Administering tetracycline with an aminoglycoside may increase the risk of nephrotoxicity.

◎ NURSING PROCESS
Patient-Centered Collaborative Care

Antibacterials: Tetracyclines

Assessment
- Assess vital signs and urine output. Report abnormal findings.
- Check laboratory results, especially those that indicate renal and liver function (BUN, serum creatinine, AST, ALT, bilirubin).
- Obtain a history of dietary intake and drugs the patient currently takes. Dairy products, antacids, iron, calcium, and magnesium decrease drug absorption. Digoxin absorption is increased, which may lead to digitalis toxicity.

Nursing Diagnoses
- Infection, Risk for
- Noncompliance with drug regimen related to denial of illness
- Skin Integrity, Risk for Impaired
- Nutrition, Imbalanced: Less than Body Requirements related to nausea and vomiting

Planning
- The patient's infection will be controlled and ultimately eliminated.

Nursing Interventions
- Obtain a sample for culture from the infected area and send it to the laboratory for C&S. Antibiotic therapy can be started after the culture sample has been taken.
- Administer tetracycline 1 hour before or 2 hours after meals for optimum absorption.
- Monitor laboratory values to assess liver and kidney function (in particular, liver enzymes, BUN, and serum creatinine).
- Record vital signs and urine output.

Patient Teaching
General
- Instruct patients to store tetracycline away from light and extreme heat. Tetracycline decomposes in light and heat and causes the drug to become toxic.
- Advise patients to check expiration dates on bottles of tetracycline; out-of-date tetracycline can be toxic.
- ⚡ Inform female patients who are contemplating pregnancy to avoid taking tetracycline because of possible teratogenic effects.
- Warn parents that children younger than 8 years of age should not take tetracycline because it can cause discoloration of permanent teeth.
- Encourage patients to take the complete course of tetracycline as prescribed.

Side Effects
- Advise patients to use a sun block and protective clothing during sun exposure. Photosensitivity is associated with tetracycline.
- Encourage patients to report signs of a superinfection (mouth ulcers, anal or genital discharge).
- Advise patients to use additional contraceptive techniques and *not* to rely on oral contraceptives when taking the drug because contraceptive effectiveness may decrease.
- Teach patients to use effective oral hygiene several times a day to prevent or alleviate mouth ulcers (stomatitis).

Diet
- Educate patients to avoid milk products, iron, and antacids. Tetracycline should be taken 1 hour before or 2 hours after meals with a full glass of water. If GI upset occurs, the drug can be taken with nondairy foods.

🌐 *Cultural Considerations*
- Recognize that patients and family members from various cultural backgrounds may need a written schedule that shows when the drug should be taken. Explain how dairy products should not be taken with specific tetracyclines but that food helps with the absorption of minocycline and doxycycline.
- Provide a detailed explanation orally or in written form of the possible side effects that should be reported to the health care provider.

Evaluation
- Evaluate the effectiveness of tetracycline by determining whether the infection has been controlled or has ceased and that there are no side effects.

GLYCYLCYCLINES

Tigecycline is an antibiotic in a category called *glycylcyclines*, synthetic analogues of the tetracyclines (see Table 26.8). Tigecycline acts by blocking protein synthesis in bacterial cells, resulting in a bacteriostatic action. Indications for use are complicated skin infections and intraabdominal infections, including *S. aureus, E. coli, S. pyogenes, K. pneumoniae,* and *C. perfringens.*

Pharmacokinetics Tigecycline is administered IV at an initial loading dose of 100 mg over 30 to 90 minutes, followed by 50 mg every 12 hours. The protein-binding capacity of tigecycline ranges from 71% to 89%, and the half-life is 27 to 42 hours. The drug is eliminated from the body in bile, feces, and urine, but biliary excretion is the primary route.

Pharmacodynamics Tigecycline binds to the 30S ribosomal subunit and causes cell death. It has broad-spectrum activity against gram-positive and gram-negative bacterial pathogens.

Side Effects and Adverse Reactions

Because of their related structural formulas, many side effects of tigecycline are similar to those of tetracycline. The most common side effects of tigecycline involve the GI tract and include nausea, vomiting, abdominal pain, and diarrhea. Pseudomembranous colitis may occur but is rare. Other side effects are photosensitivity, headache, dizziness, insomnia, hypertension, hypotension, anemia, leukocytosis, and thrombocythemia. Hyperglycemia, hypokalemia, elevated BUN, and elevated liver enzymes may also occur.

Drug Interactions

Oral contraceptives may be less effective when given concurrently with tigecycline. Warfarin levels may be increased and may lead to bleeding when taken with tigecycline.

SECTION 26C: Aminoglycosides, Fluoroquinolones, and Lipopeptides

AMINOGLYCOSIDES

Aminoglycosides act by inhibiting bacterial protein synthesis. The aminoglycoside antibiotics are used against gram-negative bacteria such as *E. coli* and *Proteus* and *Pseudomonas* species. Some gram-positive cocci are resistant to aminoglycosides, so penicillins or cephalosporins may be used.

Streptomycin sulfate, derived from the bacterium *Streptomyces griseus* in 1944, was the first aminoglycoside available for clinical use and was used to treat tuberculosis. Because of its ototoxicity and the bacterial resistance that can develop, it is infrequently used today. Despite its toxicity, streptomycin is the drug of choice to treat tularemia and plague.

Aminoglycosides are for serious infections, and they cannot be absorbed from the GI tract, nor can they cross into the cerebrospinal fluid; they cross the blood-brain barrier in children but not in adults. These agents are primarily administered IM and IV, except for a few aminoglycosides (e.g., neomycin) that may be given orally to decrease bacteria and other organisms in the bowel. Neomycin is frequently used as a preoperative bowel antiseptic.

The aminoglycosides currently used to treat *P. aeruginosa* infection include gentamicin, tobramycin, and amikacin. *P. aeruginosa* is sensitive to gentamicin. Amikacin may be used when there is bacterial resistance to gentamicin and tobramycin. Prototype Drug Chart 26.5 lists the drug data related to the aminoglycoside gentamicin.

Pharmacokinetics Gentamicin is administered IM and IV. This drug has a short half-life, and the drug dose can be given three to four times a day. Excretion of this drug is primarily unchanged in the urine.

Pharmacodynamics Gentamicin inhibits bacterial protein synthesis, has a bactericidal effect, and was previously designated pregnancy category D by the manufacturer and C by some experts. The onset of action is rapid or immediate, and the peak action for gentamicin is 30 minutes to 1 hour for IM and 30 minutes for IV administration.

To ensure a desired blood level, aminoglycosides are usually administered IV. The patient's blood levels are drawn periodically to determine the drug's peak (highest concentration) and trough (lowest concentration) blood levels. A therapeutic drug level can be maintained by monitoring the trough level, and peak levels are useful to monitor for toxicity. Many other antibiotics should be monitored as well to maintain effective blood levels.

IV aminoglycosides can be given concurrently with penicillins and cephalosporins but should not be mixed together in the same container. When combinations of antibiotics are given by IV, the IV line is flushed after each antibiotic has been administered to ensure that the antibiotic was completely delivered.

Side Effects and Adverse Reactions

Serious adverse reactions to aminoglycosides include ototoxicity and nephrotoxicity. Renal function, drug dose, and age are all factors that determine whether a patient will develop nephrotoxicity from aminoglycoside therapy. Careful drug dosing is especially important with younger and older patients. The nurse must assess changes in patients' hearing, balance, and urinary output. Prolonged use of aminoglycosides could result in a superinfection, and specific serum aminoglycoside levels should be closely monitored to avoid adverse reactions. Table 26.9 lists the aminoglycosides and their dosages, uses, and considerations.

Drug Interactions

When aminoglycosides are administered concurrently with penicillins, the desired effects of the aminoglycosides are greatly decreased; preferably, these drugs should be given several hours apart. The drug action of oral anticoagulants such as warfarin can increase when taken simultaneously with aminoglycoside administration, and the risk of ototoxicity increases when ethacrynic acid and an aminoglycoside are given.

Gentamicin Sulfate

Drug Class	Dosage
Antibacterial: Aminoglycoside Pregnancy category: D*	Respiratory infection: A: IM/IV: 3-5 mg/kg/d in 3-4 divided doses Adol/C: IM/IV: 2-2.5 mg/kg q8h TDM: Peak: 5-8 mcg/mL Trough: <1-2 mcg/mL
Contraindications	**Drug-Lab-Food Interactions**
Hypersensitivity *Caution:* Renal disease, pseudomembranous colitis, neuromuscular disorders (myasthenia gravis, parkinsonism), hypocalcemia, dehydration, hearing impairment	Drug: Increases risk of ototoxicity with loop diuretics and methoxyflurane; increases risk of nephrotoxicity with NSAIDs, amphotericin B, cephalosporins, cisplatin, furosemide, and vancomycin Lab: Increases BUN, serum AST, ALT, LDH, bilirubin, and creatinine; decreases serum potassium and magnesium
Pharmacokinetics	**Pharmacodynamics**
Absorption: IM, IV Distribution: PB: 0%-30% Metabolism: t½: 2 h Excretion: Unchanged in urine	IM/IV: Onset: rapid Peak: IM 30-60 min, IV 30 min Duration: UK

Therapeutic Effects/Uses

For treating endocarditis, meningitis, bacteremia, septicemia, and respiratory, intraabdominal, bone/joint, skin, and urinary tract infections. Gentamicin is effective against MRSA, *Pseudomonas aeruginosa, Escherichia coli, and* species of *Proteus, Enterococcus, Haemophilus, Klebsiella, Salmonella, Serratia, Staphylococcus,* and *Streptococcus.*

Mode of Action: Inhibits bacterial protein synthesis; bactericidal effect

Side Effects	Adverse Reactions
Anorexia, stomatitis, nausea, vomiting, alopecia, rash, pruritus, skin/ocular irritation, visual disturbances, photosensitivity, headache, dizziness, confusion, depression, tinnitus, weakness, arthralgia	Superinfection, peripheral neuropathy, laryngeal edema, hearing loss, hypokalemia, hypomagnesemia, hyponatremia *Life threatening:* Anaphylaxis, nephrotoxicity, thrombocytopenia, anemia, agranulocytosis, hepatic dysfunction, increased intracranial pressure

*Pregnancy categories have been revised. See http://www.fda.gov/Drugs/DevelopmentApprovalProcess/DevelopmentResources/Labeling/ucm093307.htm for more information.

A, Adult; *Adol,* adolescent; *ALT,* alanine aminotransferase; *AST,* aspartate aminotransferase; *BUN,* blood urea nitrogen; *C,* child; *d,* day; *h,* hour; *IM,* intramuscular; *IV,* intravenous; *LDH,* lactic dehydrogenase; *min,* minutes; *MRSA,* methicillin-resistant *Staphylococcus aureus; NSAID,* nonsteroidal antiinflammatory drug; *PB,* protein binding; *q,* every; *t½,* half-life; *TDM,* therapeutic drug monitoring; *UK,* unknown; <, less than.

TABLE 26.9 Antibacterials: Aminoglycosides

Generic	Route and Dosage	Uses and Considerations
Amikacin sulfate	Respiratory infections: A: IM/IV: 15 mg/kg/d in divided doses; *max:* 1.5 g/d Adol/C/infants: IM/IV: 15 mg/kg/d divided q8-12h; *max:* 1.5 g/d TDM: Peak: 25-35 mcg/mL; trough: <5 mg/mL	For treating meningitis, septicemia, bacteremia, and respiratory, urinary, bone/joint, skin, and intraabdominal infections. May cause GI distress, CDAD, anemia, ototoxicity, seizures, nephrotoxicity, and superinfection. Pregnancy category: C/D*; PB: 0%-11%; t½: 2 h
Gentamicin sulfate	See Prototype Drug Chart 26.5.	
Neomycin sulfate	Skin infections: A/adol/C: Topical: Apply a thin film of 0.5% cream or ointment to infected area up to four times daily. Hepatic coma: A: PO: 1-3 g q6h for 5-6 d; *max:* 12 g/d	For treating hepatic encephalopathy, skin infections, and bowel preparation. May cause stomatitis, rash, GI distress, eosinophilia, seizures, superinfection, neurotoxicity, nephrotoxicity, and ototoxicity. Pregnancy category: D*; PB: 0%-30%; t½: UK
Streptomycin sulfate	Respiratory infection: A: IM: 1-2 g/d in divided doses q6-12h; *max:* 4 g/d Adol/C/infants: IM: 20-40 mg/kg/d in divided doses q6-12h; *max:* 2 g/d TDM: Peak: 40-50 mcg/mL; trough: <5 mcg/mL	For treating meningitis, endocarditis, bacteremia, tuberculosis, plague, and respiratory and urinary tract infections. May cause anaphylaxis, angioedema, rash, headache, dizziness, GI distress, weakness, pancytopenia, ototoxicity, nephrotoxicity, and neurotoxicity. Pregnancy category: D*; PB: 35%; t½: 2-3 h
Tobramycin sulfate	Bone/joint infection: A: IM/IV: 3-5 mg/kg/d in divided doses; give IV over 30-60 min; *max:* 5 mg/d Adol/C/infants: IM/IV: 2.5 mg/kg/dose q8h; *max:* 6-7.5 mg/kg/d in 3-4 divided doses	For treating bacteremia, septicemia, PID, meningitis, and respiratory, urinary tract, intraabdominal, skin, and bone/joint infections. May cause anaphylaxis, headache, dizziness, dysgeusia, GI distress, CDAD, dysphonia, weakness, chest pain, superinfection, neurotoxicity, ototoxicity, nephrotoxicity, and Stevens-Johnson syndrome. Pregnancy category: D*; PB: 30%; t½: 2-3 h

*Pregnancy categories have been revised. See http://www.fda.gov/Drugs/DevelopmentApprovalProcess/DevelopmentResources/Labeling/ucm093307.htm for more information.

A, Adult; *Adol,* adolescent; *C,* child; *CDAD, Clostridium difficile*–associated diarrhea; *d,* day; *GI,* gastrointestinal; *h,* hour; *IM,* intramuscular; *IV,* intravenous; *max,* maximum; *min,* minutes; *PB,* protein binding; *PID,* pelvic inflammatory disease; *PO,* by mouth; *q,* every; *t½,* half-life; *TDM,* therapeutic drug monitoring; *UK,* unknown; <, less than.

NURSING PROCESS
Patient-Centered Collaborative Care
Antibacterials: Aminoglycosides

Assessment
- Record vital signs and urine output. Compare these results with future vital signs and urine output. Nephrotoxicity is an adverse reaction to most aminoglycosides.
- Assess laboratory results to determine renal and liver function, including BUN, serum creatinine, ALP, ALT, AST, and bilirubin. Serum electrolytes should also be checked. Aminoglycosides may decrease serum potassium and magnesium levels.
- Obtain a medical history related to renal or hearing disorders. Large doses of aminoglycosides could cause nephrotoxicity or ototoxicity.

Nursing Diagnoses
- Infection, Risk for
- Tissue Integrity, Risk for Impaired
- Nutrition, Imbalanced: Less than Body Requirements related to an inability to ingest food
- Tissue Perfusion, Risk for Ineffective Peripheral

Planning
- The patient's infection will be controlled and ultimately eliminated.

Nursing Interventions
- Send a sample from the infected area to the laboratory for culture to determine the organism and its antibiotic sensitivity before the aminoglycoside is started.
- Monitor intake and output. Urine output should be at least 600 mL/day. Immediately report any decrease in urine output. Urinalysis may be ordered daily, and results should be checked for proteinuria, casts, blood cells, and appearance.
- ⚡ Check for hearing loss. Aminoglycosides can cause ototoxicity.
- Evaluate laboratory results and compare with baseline values. Report abnormal results.
- Monitor vital signs. Note whether body temperature has decreased.
- Dilute gentamicin in 50 to 200 mL of NS or D₅W solution and administer IV over 30 to 60 minutes.
- ⚡ Check that therapeutic drug monitoring (TDM) has been ordered for peak and trough drug levels. Blood should be drawn 45 to 60 minutes after drug has been administered for peak levels and minutes before next drug dosing for trough levels. Gentamicin peak values should be 5 to 8 mcg/mL, and trough values should be less than 1 to 2 mcg/mL.
- Monitor for signs and symptoms of superinfection; these include stomatitis (mouth ulcers), genital discharge (vaginitis), and anal or genital itching.

Patient Teaching
General
- Encourage patients to increase fluid intake unless fluids are restricted.
Side Effects
- Advise patients to report aminoglycoside side effects that include nausea, vomiting, tremors, tinnitus, pruritus, and muscle cramps.
- Direct patients to use a sun block and protective clothing during sun exposure because aminoglycosides can cause photosensitivity.

🌐 Cultural Considerations
- Do not give directions such as "take one blue pill" at a specified time. Instead, provide the name and dosage of the medication in the language the patient speaks and reads most easily.

Evaluation
- Evaluate the effectiveness of the aminoglycoside by determining whether the infection has ceased and whether any side effects have occurred.

FLUOROQUINOLONES (QUINOLONES)

The mechanism of action of fluoroquinolones is to interfere with the enzyme DNA gyrase, which is needed to synthesize bacterial DNA. Their antibacterial spectrum includes bactericidal action on both gram-positive and gram-negative organisms. The fluoroquinolones are effective against some gram-positive organisms, such as *S. pneumoniae,* and also against *H. influenzae, P. aeruginosa,* and *Salmonella* and *Shigella* species. This group of antibiotics is useful in the treatment of urinary tract, bone, and joint infections; bronchitis; pneumonia; gastroenteritis; and gonorrhea. Table 26.10 lists the various fluoroquinolones.

Ciprofloxacin is a synthetic antibacterial related to nalidixic acid. This fluoroquinolone has a broad spectrum of action on gram-positive and gram-negative organisms, including *P. aeruginosa*. Ciprofloxacin is approved for use for urinary tract and lower respiratory tract infections and for skin, soft tissue, bone, and joint infections.

The use of fluoroquinolones as urinary antibiotics is discussed in Chapter 48. Prototype Drug Chart 26.6 lists the drug data related to levofloxacin. Levofloxacin is used primarily to treat respiratory problems such as community-acquired pneumonia, chronic bronchitis, acute sinusitis, and uncomplicated skin infections in addition to urinary tract infections.

Moxifloxacin is available for once-a-day oral and parenteral dosing. This drug is prescribed to treat the same infections other fluoroquinolones are effective against. Moxifloxacin is more active than levofloxacin against *S. pneumoniae.* It is also effective against some strains of *S. aureus* and enterococci but is not effective against VREF. The fluoroquinolones are included in Table 26.10.

TABLE 26.10   Antibacterials: Fluoroquinolones (Quinolones) and Unclassified Drugs

Generic	Route and Dosage	Uses and Considerations
FLUOROQUINOLONES		
Ciprofloxacin Hydrochloride	UTI: Immediate release: A: PO: 250 mg q12h for 3 d; *max:* 1.5 g/d C: PO: 10-20 mg/kg q12h for 7-14 d; *max:* 40 mg/kg/d Extended release: A: PO: 500 mg for 3 d; *max:* 1 g/d A: IV: 200-400 mg q12h for 7-14 d; *max:* 1.2 g/d C: IV: 6-10 mg/kg/dose q8h for 10-21 d; *max:* 30 mg/kg/d	For treating STIs, anthrax, otitis media, and intraabdominal, gynecologic, bone/joint, skin, respiratory, and urinary tract infections. May cause anaphylaxis, dizziness, irritability, headache, retinal detachment, corneal deposits, ocular pruritus, tendon rupture, injection site reaction, dysgeusia, GI distress, CDAD, superinfection, and Stevens-Johnson syndrome. Pregnancy category: C*; PB: 20%-40%; t½: 4 h
Levofloxacin	See Prototype Drug Chart 26.6.	
Moxifloxacin	Sinusitis: A: PO/IV: 400 mg/d for 10 d; *max:* 400 mg/d	For treating sinusitis, PID, plague, and respiratory, intraabdominal, and skin infections. May cause anaphylaxis, visual impairment, ocular irritation/bleeding, conjunctivitis, retinal detachment, keratitis, hyperemia, headache, GI distress, CDAD, superinfection, nephrotoxicity, and Stevens-Johnson syndrome. Pregnancy category: C*; PB: 30%-50%; t½: 12 h
Ofloxacin	UTI: A: PO: 200 mg q12h for 3-10 d; *max:* 800 mg/d	For treating otitis media, PID, STIs, prostatitis, and respiratory, urinary tract, and skin infections. May cause anaphylaxis, headache, dizziness, dysgeusia, insomnia, GI distress, CDAD, pruritus, photosensitivity, visual disturbances, superinfection, tendon rupture, and Stevens-Johnson syndrome. Pregnancy category: C*; PB: 20%-40%; t½: 4-8 h
UNCLASSIFIED DRUGS		
Chloramphenicol	Septicemia: A/adol/C/infants: IV: 50-100 mg/kg/d in 4 divided doses; *max:* 100 mg/kg/d TDM: Meningitis Peak: 15-25 mcg/mL Trough: 5-15 mcg/mL All other infections, Peak: 10-20 mcg/mL Trough: 5-10 mcg/mL	For treating bacteremia, septicemia, typhoid fever, and meningitis. May cause anaphylaxis, angioedema, optic neuritis, headache, glossitis, stomatitis, GI distress, nephritis, neurotoxicity, anemia, and pancytopenia. Pregnancy category: C*; PB: 60%; t½: 4.1 h
Quinupristin-dalfopristin	Skin infections: A/C >12 y: IV: 7.5 mg/kg given over 1 h, q12h for at least 7 d; *max:* 15 mg/kg/d	For treating skin infections and VREF. May cause anaphylaxis, angioedema, infusion site reaction, arthralgia, myalgia, GI distress, CDAD, hyperbilirubinemia, edema, dysrhythmias, and superinfection. Pregnancy category: B*; PB: 11%-19%; t½: 0.7-0.85 h
Obiltoxaximab	A >40 kg: IV: 16 mg/kg as single dose A/adol/C/Infants <40 kg: IV: 24 mg/kg as single dose	For prophylaxis and treatment of anthrax. May cause anaphylaxis, headache, URI, cough, rash, pruritus, and injection site reaction. Pregnancy category: B*; PB: UK; t½: UK

*Pregnancy categories have been revised. See http://www.fda.gov/Drugs/DevelopmentApprovalProcess/DevelopmentResources/Labeling/ucm093307.htm for more information.

A, Adult; *adol*, adolescent; *C*, child; *CDAD, Clostridium difficile*–associated diarrhea; *d*, day; *GI*, gastrointestinal; *h*, hour; *IV*, intravenous; *max*, maximum; *PB*, protein binding; *PID*, pelvic inflammatory disease; *PO*, by mouth; *q*, every; *STI*, sexually transmitted infection; *t½*, half-life; *TDM*, therapeutic drug monitoring; *UK*, unknown; *URI*, upper respiratory infection; *UTI*, urinary tract infection; *VREF*, vancomycin-resistant *Enterococcus faecium*; *y*, year; >, greater than; <, less than.

⚡ PATIENT SAFETY

Fluoroquinolones, especially levaquin, should be reserved for patients who have no other alternative treatment options for uncomplicated UTI, acute bacterial exacerbation of chronic bronchitis, or acute bacterial sinusitis due to disabling and potentially irreversible serious adverse reactions. These adverse reactions include tendon rupture, tendinitis, peripheral neuropathy, CNS effects, and exacerbation of myasthenia gravis. (Black Box Warning.)

Pharmacokinetics Levofloxacin is well absorbed from the GI tract. It has a low protein-binding effect of 50% and a moderately short half-life of 6 to 8 hours. Levofloxacin is excreted unchanged in the urine.

Pharmacodynamics Levofloxacin inhibits bacterial DNA synthesis by inhibiting the enzyme DNA gyrase. The drug has a high tissue distribution. If possible, it should be taken before meals because food slows the absorption rate; antacids also decrease the absorption rate. Levofloxacin increases the effect of oral hypoglycemics, theophylline, and caffeine.

Levofloxacin has an average onset of action of 30 minutes to 1 hour, and the peak concentration time is 1 to 2 hours. The duration of action is unknown.

PROTOTYPE DRUG CHART 26.6
Levofloxacin

Drug Class	Dosage
Antibacterials: Quinolone, fluoroquinolone Pregnancy category: C*	Sinusitis: A: PO/IV: 500 mg/d for 10 d or 750 mg/d for 5 d
Contraindications	**Drug-Lab-Food Interactions**
Severe renal disease, hypersensitivity to other quinolones, seizures, myasthenia gravis *Caution:* Renal and hepatic dysfunction, children and older adults, theophylline therapy, dehydration, rheumatoid arthritis, cardiac dysrhythmias	Drug: Increases effects of oral hypoglycemics, theophylline, and caffeine; increases levels of levofloxacin with corticosteroids, NSAIDs, and probenecid; decreases drug absorption with antacids, iron, and calcium; may increase warfarin effects Lab: Increased AST, ALT, prolonged bleeding time
Pharmacokinetics	**Pharmacodynamics**
Absorption: PO: well absorbed Distribution: PB: 24%-38% Metabolism: t½: 6-8 h Excretion: Unchanged in urine	PO: Onset: 0.5-1 h Peak: 1-2 h Duration: UK
Therapeutic Effects/Uses	
For treating sinusitis, cellulitis, impetigo, plague, anthrax, and respiratory, urinary tract, and skin infections. Levofloxacin is effective against *Escherichia coli*, *Clostridium perfringens*, and species of *Enterobacter*, *Haemophilus*, *Klebsiella*, *Neisseria*, *Proteus*, *Pseudomonas*, *Serratia*, *Staphylococcus*, and *Streptococcus*. Mode of Action: Interferes with the enzyme DNA gyrase, which is needed for bacterial DNA synthesis; bactericidal effect	
Side Effects	**Adverse Reactions**
Anorexia, dysgeusia, stomatitis, nausea, vomiting, diarrhea, abdominal cramps, flatulence, constipation, headache, blurred vision, dizziness, restlessness, confusion, depression, insomnia, weakness, nightmares, tremor, rash, injection site reaction, tinnitus, ocular irritation/pain, photosensitivity, weakness, tendon rupture (rare)	Palpitations, superinfection, edema, hypotension, peripheral neuropathy, crystalluria, myasthenia, hypoglycemia/hyperglycemia, retinal detachment *Life threatening:* Anaphylaxis, angioedema, anemia, leukopenia, agranulocytosis, thrombocytopenia, increased intracranial pressure, Stevens-Johnson syndrome, hepatotoxicity, nephrotoxicity, seizures, CDAD, dysrhythmias, suicidal ideation

*Pregnancy categories have been revised. See http://www.fda.gov/Drugs/DevelopmentApprovalProcess/DevelopmentResources/Labeling/ucm093307.htm for more information.
A, Adult; ALT, alanine aminotransferase; AST, aspartate aminotransferase; CDAD, Clostridium difficile–associated diarrhea; d, day; DNA, deoxyribonucleic acid; h, hour; IV, intravenous; NSAID, nonsteroidal antiinflammatory drug; PB, protein binding; PO, by mouth; t½, half-life; UK, unknown.

NURSING PROCESS
Patient-Centered Collaborative Care
Antibacterials: Fluoroquinolones

Assessment
- Record vital signs along with intake and urine output. Compare these results with future vital signs and urine output. Fluid intake should be at least 2000 mL/day.
- Assess laboratory results (BUN and serum creatinine) to determine renal function.
- Obtain a drug and diet history. Antacids and iron preparations decrease absorption of fluoroquinolones such as levofloxacin, and levofloxacin can increase the effects of theophylline and caffeine and can also increase the effects of oral hypoglycemics. When levofloxacin is taken with nonsteroidal antiinflammatory drugs (NSAIDs), central nervous system (CNS) reactions may occur, which includes seizures.

Nursing Diagnoses
- Infection, Risk for
- Tissue Integrity, Risk for Impaired
- Noncompliance with drug regimen related to lack of understanding of importance of drug regimen

Planning
- The patient's infection will be controlled and ultimately eliminated.

Nursing Interventions
- Obtain a specimen from the infected site, and send it to the laboratory for C&S before initiating antibacterial drug therapy.
- Monitor intake and output. Urine output should be at least 750 mL per day. The patient should be well hydrated, and fluid intake should be greater than 2000 mL daily to prevent crystalluria (crystals in the urine). Urine pH should be below 6.7.
- Record vital signs and report any abnormal findings.
- Check laboratory results, especially BUN and serum creatinine. Elevated values may indicate renal dysfunction.
- Administer levofloxacin 2 hours before or after antacids and iron products for best absorption. Give with a full glass of water. If GI distress occurs, the drug may be taken with food.
- Dilute IV levofloxacin in an appropriate amount of solution (250 mg in 50 mL, 500 mg in 100 mL, 750 mg in 150 mL. NS, D₅W, D₅NS, D₅LR). Infuse over 60 minutes.
- Check for signs and symptoms of superinfection: stomatitis (mouth ulcers), furry black tongue, and anal or genital discharge or itching.
- ⚡ Monitor serum theophylline levels when taken concurrently with levofloxacin, which can increase theophylline levels. Check for symptoms of CNS stimulation such as nervousness, insomnia, anxiety, and tachycardia.
- ⚡ Monitor blood glucose. Levofloxacin can increase the effects of oral hypoglycemics.

General

- Teach patients to drink at least 6 to 8 glasses (8 oz) of fluid daily.
- Encourage patients to avoid caffeinated products.

Side Effects

- Direct patients to avoid operating motor vehicles or hazardous machinery while taking the drug, at least until drug stability has occurred, because of possible drug-related dizziness.
- Inform patients that photosensitivity is a side effect of most fluoroquinolones. Patients should wear sunglasses, sun block, and protective clothing when in the sun.
- Encourage patients to report side effects such as dizziness, nausea, vomiting, diarrhea, flatulence, abdominal cramps, tinnitus, rash, and tendon rupture (very rare). Older adults are more likely to develop side effects.

 🌐 *Cultural Considerations*

- Demonstrate an interest in the patient's family and other personal matters to establish trust among some Hispanic and Appalachian patients.
- Solicit the patient's opinions and advice.

Evaluation

- Evaluate the effectiveness of the fluoroquinolone by determining whether the infection has ceased and the body temperature has returned within normal range.

LIPOPEPTIDES

Daptomycin is a U.S. Food and Drug Administration (FDA)-approved antibiotic in the category of *lipopeptides*. Daptomycin acts by binding to the bacterial membrane and causing rapid depolarization of its membrane potential, inhibiting protein, DNA, and RNA synthesis. This action results in bacterial cell death.

Indications for daptomycin include complicated skin infections due to gram-positive microorganisms, septicemia due to *S. aureus* infection, and infective endocarditis due to MRSA infection.

Pharmacokinetics Daptomycin is administered by IV at a dose of 4 mg/kg daily. Each 500-mg vial of the medication is diluted in 10 mL of NS 0.9% and allowed to stand for 10 minutes. After gentle rotation of the vial to ensure dilution, further dilute in 50 to 100 mL of NS and administer over 30 minutes. Drug should *not* be mixed with dextrose-containing diluents.

The protein-binding capacity is 90% to 93%, and half-life averages 8 hours. Daptomycin is primarily excreted by the kidneys.

Pharmacodynamics Daptomycin binds to the bacterial membrane and causes cell death. An effective trough concentration of 5.9 mcg/mL is usually achieved by the third dose.

Side Effects and Adverse Reactions

Side effects that may occur when taking daptomycin include hypertension, hypotension, anemia, numbness, tingling, dizziness, insomnia, pain or burning on urination, nausea, vomiting, diarrhea, constipation, and pallor. More serious adverse effects that have occurred with daptomycin are chest pain, hypokalemia, hyperkalemia, hyperglycemia, hypoglycemia, bleeding, rhabdomyolysis, and pleural effusion.

Drug Interactions

When daptomycin is given with 3-hydroxy-3-methylglutaryl coenzyme A (HMG-CoA) reductase inhibitors (statins, such as simvastatin, atorvastatin), the risk of rhabdomyolysis and elevated levels of creatine phosphokinase (CPK) is increased. Daptomycin toxicity may be increased when given concurrently with tobramycin, and warfarin may lead to increased bleeding when taken with daptomycin.

UNCLASSIFIED ANTIBACTERIAL DRUGS

Several antibacterials, such as chloramphenicol and quinupristin-dalfopristin, do not belong to any major drug group. Chloramphenicol was discovered in 1947 and exerts its bacteriostatic action by inhibiting bacterial protein synthesis. Because of the toxic effects of chloramphenicol, including blood dyscrasias related to bone marrow suppression, it is used only to treat serious infections. It is effective against gram-negative and gram-positive bacteria and many other microorganisms, such as rickettsiae, *Mycoplasma*, and *H. influenzae*.

Quinupristin-dalfopristin is effective for treating VREF bacteremia and skin infected by *S. aureus* and *S. pyogenes*. It acts by disrupting the protein synthesis of the organism. When administering the drug through a peripheral IV line, pain, edema, and phlebitis may occur.

Obiltoxaximab was FDA approved in 2016 for prophylaxis and treatment of anthrax. It prevents the lethal factor of anthrax from intracellular entry by inhibiting the binding of the protective antigen of *Bacillus anthracis* toxin to cellular receptors. This drug is administered IV as a single dose over 1 hour and 10 minutes.

SECTION 26D: Sulfonamides and Nitroimidazoles

SULFONAMIDES

Sulfonamides were first isolated from a coal tar derivative compound in the early 1900s and were produced for clinical use against coccal infections in 1935. Sulfonamides were the first group of drugs used against bacteria, although they are not classified as antibiotics because they were not obtained from biologic substances. The sulfonamides are bacteriostatic because they inhibit bacterial synthesis of folic acid, which is essential for bacterial growth. Humans do not synthesize folic acid, rather they acquire

TABLE 26.11   Antibacterials: Sulfonamides

Generic	Route and Dosage	Uses and Considerations
SHORT-ACTING		
Sulfadiazine	Urinary tract infection: A: PO: Initially 2-4 g, then 2-4 g/d in 3-6 divided doses; *max:* 4 g/d Adol/C/infants >2 mo: PO: Initially 75 mg/kg, then 150 mg/kg/d in 4-6 divided doses; *max:* 6 g/d	For treating otitis media, meningitis, malaria, and UTIs and for rheumatic fever prophylaxis. May cause anaphylaxis, photosensitivity, headache, insomnia, seizure, crystalluria, stomatitis, GI distress, peripheral neuropathy, and Stevens-Johnson syndrome. Increase fluid intake to >2000 mL/d. Pregnancy category: C*; PB: 38%-48%; t½: 17 h
INTERMEDIATE-ACTING		
Sulfasalazine	Ulcerative colitis: Uncoated tablets: A: PO: Initially 1 g q6-8h; maint: 500 mg q6h; *max:* 4 g/d Adol/C >6 y: PO: Initially 40-60 mg/kg/d in divided doses; maint: 30 mg/kg/d in divided doses; *max:* 2 g/d	For treating ulcerative colitis and rheumatoid arthritis. May cause anaphylaxis, headache, dizziness, stomatitis, GI distress, skin/urine discoloration, peripheral neuropathy, crystalluria, oligospermia, nephritis, hepatotoxicity, rash, hematuria, anemia, and Stevens-Johnson syndrome. Take drug after eating. Pregnancy category: B*; PB: 99%; t½: 5.7-7.6 h
Trimethoprim-sulfa-methoxazole	See Prototype Drug Chart 26.7.	

*Pregnancy categories have been revised. See http://www.fda.gov/Drugs/DevelopmentApprovalProcess/DevelopmentResources/Labeling/ucm093307.htm for more information.

A, Adult; *Adol,* adolescent; *C,* child; *d,* day; *GI,* gastrointestinal; *h,* hour; *IV,* intravenous; *maint,* maintenance; *max,* maximum; *mo,* month; *PB,* protein binding; *PO,* by mouth; *q,* every; *t½,* half-life; *UTI,* urinary tract infection; *y,* year; *>,* greater than.

it through the diet, therefore sulfonamides selectively inhibit bacterial growth without affecting normal cells. Folic acid (folate) is required by cells for biosynthesis of RNA, DNA, and proteins.

The clinical usefulness of sulfonamides alone, not in combination, has decreased for several reasons. The availability and effectiveness of penicillin and other antibiotics has increased, and bacterial resistance to some sulfonamides can develop. Sulfonamides may be used as an alternative drug for patients who are allergic to penicillin. They are still used to treat urinary tract and ear infections and may be used for newborn eye prophylaxis. Sulfonamides are approximately 90% effective against *E. coli,* therefore they are frequently a preferred treatment for urinary tract infections, which are often caused by *E. coli.* They are also useful in the treatment of meningococcal meningitis and against *Chlamydia* species and *Toxoplasma gondii.* Sulfonamides are *not* effective against viruses and fungi.

Pharmacokinetics Sulfonamide drugs are well absorbed by the GI tract and are well distributed to body tissues and the brain. The liver metabolizes the sulfonamide drug, and the kidneys excrete it.

Pharmacodynamics Many sulfonamides are for oral administration because they are absorbed readily by the GI tract. They are also available in solution and as ointments for ophthalmic use and in cream form (silver sulfadiazine and mafenide acetate) for burns. Most of the early sulfonamides were highly protein bound and displaced other drugs by competing for protein sites. The two categories of sulfonamides, classified according to their duration of action, are *short-acting sulfonamides* that have a rapid absorption and excretion rate and *intermediate-acting sulfonamides* with moderate to slow absorption and a slow excretion rate.

Sulfadiazine is useful in prophylactic treatment of streptococcal infections in patients with rheumatic fever who are hypersensitive to penicillin. Older sulfonamides such as sulfadiazine are poorly soluble in urine and can cause crystallization, which

could damage the kidneys if fluid and water intake are insufficient; however, newer sulfonamides have greater water solubility, therefore crystal formations in the urine and renal damage are unlikely. Table 26.11 describes the sulfonamides.

Side Effects and Adverse Reactions

Side effects of sulfonamides may include an allergic response such as skin rash and itching. Anaphylaxis is uncommon. Blood disorders such as hemolytic anemia, aplastic anemia, and low WBC and platelet counts could result from prolonged use and high dosages. GI disturbances such as anorexia, nausea, and vomiting may also occur. The early sulfonamides were insoluble in acid urine, and crystalluria (crystals in the urine) and hematuria (blood in the urine) were common problems. Increasing fluid intake dilutes the drug, which helps prevent crystalluria. Photosensitivity, an excessive reaction to direct sunlight or ultraviolet (UV) light that leads to redness and burning of the skin, can also occur; therefore the patient should avoid sunbathing and excess ultraviolet light. Cross-sensitivity, a sensitivity or allergy to one sulfonamide that leads to sensitivity to another sulfonamide, might occur with the different sulfonamides but does not occur with other antibacterial drugs. Sulfonamides should be avoided during pregnancy to avoid congenital malformations, neural tube defects, and kernicterus.

⚡ PATIENT SAFETY

Preventing Medication Errors

Do not confuse...
- **Septra**, an antibacterial sulfonamide, with **Sectral**, a beta-adrenergic antagonist used to manage dysrhythmias.
- **Sulfadiazine**, a short-acting antibacterial sulfonamide, with **sulfasalazine**, an intermediate-acting antibacterial sulfonamide.

Trimethoprim-Sulfamethoxazole

Trimethoprim-sulfamethoxazole (TMP-SMZ) contains one part trimethoprim and five parts sulfamethoxazole to produce a synergistic effect that increases the desired drug response. Trimethoprim is an antibacterial agent that interferes with bacterial folic acid synthesis just as sulfonamides do; it is classified as a urinary tract antiinfective that may be used alone for uncomplicated urinary tract infections, and it is also effective against the gram-negative bacteria *E. coli* and also *Proteus* and *Klebsiella* species. In the 1970s, trimethoprim was combined with sulfamethoxazole, an intermediate-acting sulfonamide, to prevent bacterial resistance to sulfonamide drugs and to obtain a better response against many organisms. Giving both drugs together in one compounded form causes bacterial resistance to develop much more slowly than if only one of the drugs were to be used alone.

TMP-SMZ is effective in treating urinary, intestinal, lower respiratory tract, and middle ear (otitis media) infections; prostatitis; and gonorrhea. It is also used to prevent *Pneumocystis carinii* in patients with acquired immunodeficiency syndrome (AIDS). Increased fluid intake is strongly recommended to avoid complications such as crystalluria. Prototype Drug Chart 26.7 describes the pharmacologic behavior of TMP-SMZ.

Pharmacokinetics TMP-SMZ is well absorbed from the GI tract and is moderately protein bound. Its half-life is 8 to 12 hours, thus it is administered twice a day. It is excreted as unchanged metabolites in the urine.

Pharmacodynamics Trimethoprim, a nonsulfonamide antibiotic, enhances the activity of the drug combination. TMP-SMZ blocks steps in the bacterial synthesis of protein and nucleic acid, producing a bactericidal effect.

TMP-SMZ can be administered orally or by IV. Orally the drug has a moderately rapid onset of action; drug action is immediate via the IV route. Serum peak concentration time for oral use is 1 to 4 hours and 30 minutes to 1 hour for IV use. TMP-SMZ increases the hypoglycemic response when taken with sulfonylureas (oral hypoglycemic agents). It can also increase the activity of oral anticoagulants.

Side Effects and Adverse Reactions

Side effects of TMP-SMZ may include mild to moderate rashes, anorexia, nausea, vomiting, diarrhea, stomatitis, crystalluria, and photosensitivity. Serious adverse reactions are rare; however, agranulocytosis, aplastic anemia, and myocarditis have been reported as possible life-threatening conditions.

Topical and Ophthalmic Sulfonamides

Sulfonamides can be administered for topical and ophthalmic uses, but because topical use of sulfonamides can

---

PROTOTYPE DRUG CHART 26.7

Trimethoprim-Sulfamethoxazole (TMP-SMZ)

Drug Class	Dosage
Antibacterial: Sulfonamide Pregnancy category: D*	Chronic bronchitis: A: PO: TMP 160 mg, SMZ 800 mg q12h for 14 d

Contraindications	Drug-Lab-Food Interactions
Severe renal or hepatic disease, hypersensitivity to sulfonamides, megaloblastic or folate-deficiency anemia, pregnancy, breastfeeding, infants *Caution:* Diabetes mellitus, hypothyroidism, advanced age	Drug: Increased anticoagulant effect with warfarin; increased hypoglycemic effect with oral hypoglycemic drugs, increased potassium levels with ACE inhibitors and spironolactone, increased digoxin and sulfonylurea levels, increased phenytoin and methotrexate toxicity Lab: May increase BUN, serum creatinine, AST, ALT, and ALP

Pharmacokinetics	Pharmacodynamics
Absorption: PO: Well absorbed Distribution: PB: 44% for TMP; 70% for SMZ; crosses placenta Metabolism: t½: 8-10 h for TMP, 6-12 h for SMZ Excretion: In urine as metabolites	PO: Onset: UK Peak: 1-4 h Duration: UK IV: Onset: Immediate Peak: UK Duration: UK

Therapeutic Effects/Uses	
For treating otitis media, gastroenteritis, MRSA, and respiratory and urinary tract infections. TMP-SMZ is effective against *Escherichia coli,* MRSA, and species of *Enterobacter, Haemophilus, Pneumocystis, Streptococcus, Klebsiella, Proteus,* and *Shigella.* Mode of Action: Inhibits folic acid synthesis and protein synthesis of nucleic acids; bactericidal effect	

Side Effects	Adverse Reactions
Anorexia, stomatitis, nausea, vomiting, diarrhea, abdominal pain, weakness, rash, depression, headache, vertigo, insomnia, photosensitivity, tinnitus, arthralgia, myalgia	*Life threatening:* Anaphylaxis, angioedema, seizures, myocarditis, leukopenia, thrombocytopenia, hemolytic anemia, aplastic anemia, agranulocytosis, eosinophilia, neutropenia, hyperkalemia, hyponatremia, hypoglycemia, crystalluria, CDAD, Stevens-Johnson syndrome, renal failure

*Pregnancy categories have been revised. See http://www.fda.gov/Drugs/DevelopmentApprovalProcess/DevelopmentResources/Labeling/ucm093307.htm for more information.

A, Adult; *ACE,* angiotensin-converting enzyme; *ALP,* alkaline phosphatase; *ALT,* alanine aminotransferase; *AST,* aspartate aminotransferase; *BUN,* blood urea nitrogen; *CDAD,* Clostridium difficile–associated diarrhea; *d,* day; *h,* hour; *IV,* intravenous; *MRSA,* methicillin-resistant *Staphylococcus aureus;* *PB,* protein binding; *PO,* by mouth; *q,* every; *SMZ,* sulfamethoxazole; *TMP,* trimethoprim; *t½,* half-life; *UK,* unknown.

cause hypersensitivity reactions, they are used infrequently. Mafenide acetate is a sulfonamide derivative prescribed to prevent sepsis in cases of second- and third-degree burns. Silver sulfadiazine is another topical sulfonamide used to treat burns. Both of these drugs are discussed in more detail in Chapter 45.

Sulfacetamide sodium is a sulfonamide for ophthalmic and topical uses. In ophthalmic preparations (liquid drops and ointments), sulfacetamide sodium is used to treat ocular infections. It is often used as prophylactic treatment after an eye injury or after removal of a foreign body. Do *not* use ointment for the eye unless it has *ophthalmic* printed on the drug label. Sulfacetamide sodium is discussed in more detail in Chapter 44.

Topical sulfacetamide sodium *for the skin* is a cream, gel, lotion, or cleanser and is used to treat seborrheic dermatitis and acne. This dermatologic form is *not* used for the eye.

◎ NURSING PROCESS
Patient-Centered Collaborative Care

Antibacterials: Sulfonamides

Assessment
- Assess the patient's renal function by checking urinary output (>600 mL/day), BUN (normal, 8 to 25 mg/dL), and serum creatinine (normal, 0.5 to 1.5 mg/dL).
- Obtain a medical history from the patient. Sulfonamides such as TMP-SMZ are contraindicated for patients with severe renal or liver disease.
- Determine whether the patient is hypersensitive to sulfonamides. An allergic reaction can include rash, skin eruptions, and itching. A severe hypersensitivity reaction includes erythema multiforme—an erythematous macular, papular, or vesicular eruption that can cover the entire body—or exfoliative dermatitis, characterized by desquamation, scaling, and itching of the skin.
- Obtain a history of drugs the patient currently takes. Oral antidiabetic drugs (sulfonylureas) given with sulfonamides increase the hypoglycemic effect; use of warfarin with sulfonamides increases the anticoagulant effect.
- Assess baseline laboratory results, especially complete blood count (CBC). Blood dyscrasias may occur as a result of high doses of sulfonamides over a continuous period, causing life-threatening conditions.

Nursing Diagnoses
- Infection, Risk for
- Protection, Ineffective as evidenced by photosensitivity related to sulfonamides
- Elimination, Impaired Urinary related to prolonged high doses of sulfonamides

Planning
- The patient's infection will be controlled and ultimately alleviated.

Nursing Interventions
- Administer sulfonamides with a full glass of water. Extra fluid intake can prevent crystalluria and kidney stone formation.
- Record intake and output. To decrease the risk of crystalluria, fluid intake should be at least 2000 mL/day, and urine output should be at least 1200 mL/day. The sulfonamide sulfadiazine is more likely to cause crystalluria than combination drugs.
- Monitor vital signs. Note whether the patient's temperature has gone down.
- Observe the patient for hematologic reactions that may lead to life-threatening anemias. Early signs are sore throat, purpura, and decreasing WBC and platelet counts. Check CBC, and compare values with baseline findings.
- Check for signs and symptoms of superinfection. Symptoms include stomatitis (mouth ulcers), furry black tongue, anal or genital discharge, and itching.

Patient Teaching
General
- Encourage patients to drink several quarts of fluid daily while taking sulfonamides to avoid crystalluria.
- Advise pregnant patients to avoid sulfonamides during the last 3 months of pregnancy.
- Counsel patients not to take antacids with sulfonamides because antacids decrease the absorption rate of sulfonamide drugs.
- ⚡ Warn patients with an allergy to one sulfonamide that all sulfonamide preparations should be avoided, with health care provider's approval, because of the possibility of cross-sensitivity. Observe the patient for rash or any skin eruptions.

Self-Administration
- Teach patients to take sulfonamides 1 hour before or 2 hours after meals with a full glass of water.

Side Effects
- ⚡ Direct patients to report bruising or bleeding that could be a result of a drug-induced blood disorder. Advise patients to have their blood cell count monitored on a regular basis.
- Warn patients to wear sunglasses, avoid direct sunlight, and use sun block and protective clothing to decrease the risk of photosensitive reactions.

🌐 *Cultural Considerations*
- Respect cultural beliefs and values regarding alternative methods for treating infections. Explain the purpose of the drug therapy and how often the drug should be taken.
- Communicate that patients should increase fluid intake to 10 to 12 glasses per day. Written instructions in the patient's preferred language may be necessary if the patient's cultural background prevents understanding of the health problem and drug regimen.

Evaluation
- Evaluate the effectiveness of sulfonamide therapy by determining whether the infection has been alleviated and the blood cell count is within normal range.

TABLE 26.12 Antibacterials: Nitroimidazoles

Generic	Route and Dosage	Uses and Considerations
Metronidazole	**CDAD:** A: PO/IV: 500 mg q8h for 10-14 d; *max:* 4 g/d Adol/C: PO/IV: 30 mg/kg/d in 4 divided doses for 10 d; *max:* 2 g/d	For treating acne, amebiasis, bacterial vaginosis, endocarditis, meningitis, giardiasis, septicemia, trichomoniasis, CDAD, and bone/joint, *Helicobacter pylori*, gynecologic, skin, intraabdominal, and respiratory infection, and surgical infection prophylaxis. May cause headache, insomnia, dizziness, weakness, seizure, dry mouth, dysgeusia, GI distress, tongue/urine discoloration, peripheral neuropathy, superinfection, leukopenia, disulfiram-like reaction with alcohol, and Stevens-Johnson syndrome. Pregnancy category: B*; PB: 10%; t½: 8 h
Tinidazole	**Intestinal amebiasis:** A: PO: 2 g with food for 3 d; *max:* 2 g/d Adol/C >3 y: 50 mg/kg/d with food for 3-5 days; *max:* 2 g/d	For treating amebiasis, giardiasis, trichomoniasis, bacterial vaginosis, and anaerobic bacterial infections. May cause headache, dizziness, insomnia, dysgeusia, GI distress, tongue/urine discoloration, peripheral neuropathy, weakness, superinfection, seizures, leukpenia, angioedema, and Stevens-Johnson syndrome. Pregnancy category: C*; PB: 12%; t½: 12-14 h

*Pregnancy categories have been revised. See http://www.fda.gov/Drugs/DevelopmentApprovalProcess/DevelopmentResources/Labeling/ucm093 307.htm for more information.

A, Adult; *Adol*, adolescent; *C*, child; *CDAD*, *Clostridium difficile*–associated diarrhea; *d*, day; *GI*, gastrointestinal; *h*, hour; *IV*, intravenous; *max*, maximum; *PB*, protein binding; *PO*, by mouth; *q*, every; *t½*, half- life; *y*, year; *>*, greater than.

NITROIMIDAZOLES

Nitroimidazoles act by disrupting DNA and protein synthesis in susceptible bacteria and protozoa. The nitroimidazoles are effective against *H. pylori* and bacterial species (such as *Bacteroides*, *Clostridium*, *Gardnerella*, *Prevotella*, *Peptococcus*, *Giardia*), and protozoa (such as *Trichomones vaginalis*). Nitroimidazoles are used for prophylaxis for surgical infections and to treat CDAD, anaerobic infections, amebiasis, giardiasis, trichomoniasis, bacterial vaginosis, and acne rosacea. Metronidazole and tinidazole are two of the most effective drugs available to treat anaerobic bacterial infections. Both nitroimidazoles are used with other agents to treat *H. pylori* infections associated with peptic and duodenal ulcers. Metronidazole was FDA approved in 1963 and tinidazole was approved in 2004.

Nitroimidazoles are primarily administered orally, parenterally, and topically. When metronidazole is given IV intermittently, it should be administered slowly over 30 to 60 minutes. Avoid contact with the eyes when using topical product. Table 26.12 lists nitroimidazoles and their dosages, uses, and considerations.

Pharmacokinetics Both metronidazole and tinidazole are well absorbed from the GI tract and are usually not given parenterally unless the patient cannot tolerate oral medications. The protein-binding capacity of nitroimidazoles range from 10% to 12% and the half-life is 8 to 14 hours. These drugs are eliminated from the body via urine and feces.

Pharmacodynamics Nitroimidazoles disrupt DNA and protein synthesis becoming bactericidal, amebicidal, and trichomonacidal. It is recommended that tinidazole be taken with food, but metronidazole can be given without regard to food. When metronidazole is used in the extended release form, it should be taken on an empty stomach. The topical form is only minimally absorbed. The peak action for both of these agents is 1 to 3 hours.

Side Effects and Adverse Reactions

Common side effects that may occur when taking nitroimidazoles include headache, dizziness, insomnia, weakness, dry mouth, dysgeusia, anorexia, nausea, vomiting, diarrhea, tongue/urine discoloration, and superinfection. More serious adverse reactions that have occurred with metronidazole and tinidazole are leukopenia, peripheral neuropathy, seizures, and Stevens-Johnson syndrome. A disulfiram-like reaction may occur when metronidazole is taken with excessive amounts of alcohol. Symptoms of disulfiram-like reaction include flushing, throbbing headache, visual disturbance, confusion, dyspnea, nausea, vomiting, tachycardia, syncope, and circulatory collapse.

■ CRITICAL THINKING CASE STUDY

JN, a 46-year-old woman, has a wound infection. The culture report states that the infection is due to *Pseudomonas aeruginosa*, and JN's temperature has risen to 104°F (40°C). Amikacin sulfate is to be administered intravenously in 100 mL of 5% dextrose in water (D₅W solution) over 45 minutes every 8 hours. The dosage is 15 mg/kg/day in three divided doses. JN weighs 165 pounds.

1. What is the drug classification of amikacin? How many milligrams of amikacin should JN receive every 8 hours?

2. What type of intravenous (IV) infusion should be used? What would be the IV flow rate?

3. When would a wound culture be obtained to determine the appropriate antibacterial agent? Explain your answer.

4. What are the similarities of amikacin to other aminoglycosides such as gentamicin? Would one aminoglycoside be preferred over another? Explain your answer.

The nurse assesses JN for hearing and urinary function before and during amikacin therapy.

5. Why should a hearing assessment be included?
6. JN's urine output in the last 8 hours was 125 mL. Explain the possible cause for the amount of urine output. What nursing action should be taken?

7. What laboratory tests monitor renal function?
8. The health care provider requests peak and trough serum amikacin levels. When should the blood samples to determine peak serum level and trough serum level be drawn?

NCLEX STUDY QUESTIONS

1. Amoxicillin is prescribed for a patient who has a respiratory infection. The nurse is teaching the patient about this medication and realizes that more teaching is needed when the patient makes which statement?
   a. This medication should not be taken with food.
   b. I will take my entire prescription of medication.
   c. I should report to the physician any genital itching.
   d. If I experience any excess bleeding, I will contact the health care provider.

2. A patient is taking a cephalosporin. The nurse anticipates which appropriate nursing intervention(s) for this medication? (Select all that apply.)
   a. Monitoring renal function studies
   b. Monitoring liver function studies
   c. Infusing intravenous medication over 30 minutes
   d. Monitoring the patient for mouth ulcers
   e. Advising the patient to stop the medication when he or she feels better

3. Penicillin G has been prescribed for a patient. Which nursing intervention(s) should the nurse perform for this patient? (Select all that apply.)
   a. Collect culture and sensitivity before the first dose.
   b. Monitor the patient for mouth ulcers.
   c. Instruct the patient to limit fluid intake to 1000 mL/day.
   d. Have epinephrine on hand for a potential severe allergic reaction.
   e. No particular interventions are required for this patient.

4. A patient is prescribed daptomycin. Which action(s) should the nurse implement? (Select all that apply.)
   a. Monitor blood values for toxicity.
   b. Dilute in 50 to100 mL of normal saline and administer intravenously over 30 minutes.
   c. Monitor the patient for allergic reactions such as rhabdomyolysis.
   d. Advise the patient to take the medication on an empty stomach, even if gastrointestinal distress occurs.
   e. Culture the infected area before administering the first dose.

5. A patient is taking azithromycin. Which nursing intervention(s) would the nurse plan to implement for this patient? (Select all that apply.)
   a. Monitor periodic liver function tests.
   b. Dilute with 50 mL of 5% dextrose in water for intravenous administration.
   c. Instruct the patient to report any loose stools or diarrhea.
   d. Instruct the patient to report evidence of superinfection.
   e. Teach the patient to take oral drug 1 hour before or 2 hours after meals.
   f. Advise the patient to avoid antacids from 2 hours prior to 2 hours after administration.

6. For which serious adverse effect should the nurse closely monitor a patient who is taking lincosamides?
   a. Seizures
   b. Ototoxicity
   c. Hepatotoxicity
   d. *Clostridium difficile*–associated diarrhea

7. The nurse enters a patient's room to find that his heart rate is 120, his blood pressure is 70/50, and he has red blotching of his face and neck. Vancomycin is running intravenous piggyback. The nurse believes that this patient is experiencing a severe adverse effect called *red man syndrome*. What action will the nurse take?
   a. Stop the infusion and call the health care provider.
   b. Reduce the infusion to 10 mg/minute.
   c. Encourage the patient to drink more fluids, up to 2 L/day.
   d. Report onset of Stevens-Johnson syndrome to the health care provider.

8. A patient is receiving tetracycline. Which advice should the nurse include when teaching this patient about tetracycline?
   a. Take sunscreen precautions when at the beach.
   b. Take an antacid with the drug to prevent severe gastrointestinal distress.
   c. Obtain frequent hearing tests for early detection of hearing loss.
   d. Obtain frequent eye checkups for early detection of retinal damage.

9. A patient is taking levofloxacin. What does the nurse know to be true regarding this drug?
   a. It is administered by intravenous only.
   b. Levofloxacin may cause hypertension.
   c. This drug is classified as an aminoglycoside.
   d. An adverse effect is dysrhythmia.

10. Which instruction(s) will the nurse include when teaching patients about gentamicin? (Select all that apply.)
    a. Patients should report any hearing loss.
    b. Patients should use sunscreen when taking gentamicin.
    c. Intravenous gentamicin will be given over 20 minutes.
    d. Patients are monitored for mouth ulcers and vaginitis.
    e. Peak levels will be drawn 30 minutes before the intravenous dose.
    f. Patients should increase fluid intake.

11. Which nursing intervention(s) should the nurse consider for the patient taking ciprofloxacin? (Select all that apply.)
    a. Obtain culture before drug administration.
    b. Tell the patient to avoid taking ciprofloxacin with antacids.
    c. Monitor the patient for tinnitus.
    d. Encourage fluids to prevent crystalluria.
    e. Infuse intravenous ciprofloxacin over 60 minutes.
    f. Monitor blood glucose because ciprofloxacin can decrease effects of oral hypoglycemics.

12. A patient is taking sulfasalazine. What should the nurse teach the patient to do?
    a. Drink at least 10 glasses of fluid per day.
    b. Monitor blood glucose carefully to avoid hyperglycemia.
    c. Avoid operating a motor vehicle because this drug may cause drowsiness.
    d. Take this drug with an antacid to decrease the risk of gastrointestinal distress.

13. The nurse is teaching a patient about trimethoprim-sulfamethoxazole. Which instructions will the nurse plan to include? (Select all that apply.)
    a. Report any bruising or bleeding.
    b. Report any diarrhea or bloody stools.
    c. Report any fever, rash, or sore throat.
    d. Avoid unprotected exposure to sunlight.
    e. Report thirst and polyuria.

Answers: 1, a; 2, a, b, c, d; 3, a, b, d; 4, a, b, c, e; 5, a, c, d, e; 6, d, f; 7, a; 8, a; 9, d; 10, a, b, d, f; 11, a, b, c, d, e; 12, a; 13, a, b, c, d.

27

Antituberculars, Antifungals, and Antivirals

http://evolve.elsevier.com/McCuistion/pharmacology/

OBJECTIVES

- Compare first-line and second-line antitubercular drugs and give examples of each.
- Differentiate between the groups of antifungal drugs.
- Explain the uses of polyenes.
- Differentiate the adverse reactions of antitubercular, antifungal, and antiviral drugs.
- Apply the nursing process for patients taking antitubercular, antifungal, and antiviral drugs.

OUTLINE

Tuberculosis
Pathophysiology
Antitubercular Drugs
Side Effects and Adverse Reactions
Special Populations
Pregnancy and Tuberculosis
Tuberculosis and HIV Coinfection
Pediatric Tuberculosis
Nursing Process: Patient-Centered Collaborative Care—Antitubercular Drugs
Fungus
Pathophysiology
Antifungal Drugs
Polyenes
Azole Antifungals

Antimetabolites
Echinocandins
Nursing Process: Patient-Centered Collaborative Care—Antifungals
Viruses
Pathophysiology
Non-HIV Antivirals
Influenza Antivirals
Herpes Antivirals
Cytomegalovirus Antivirals
Nursing Process: Patient-Centered Collaborative Care—Antiviral: Acyclovir
Hepatitis Antivirals
Critical Thinking Case Study
NCLEX Study Questions

KEY TERMS

This chapter covers antituberculars, antifungals, and antivirals. Although these drug categories differ from one another, they each contain drugs that inhibit or kill organisms that cause disease.

TUBERCULOSIS

Tuberculosis (TB) is caused by the acid-fast bacillus *Mycobacterium tuberculosis*. The number of TB cases had declined until the mid-1980s, when the number of cases started to increase. The increase in cases of TB was attributed to multiple factors, such as human immunodeficiency virus (HIV), increased immigration, and the spread of multidrug-resistant TB (MDR TB). According to the U.S. Department of Health and Human Services (DHHS), tuberculosis is one of the world's leading causes of death due to infectious diseases in persons older than 5 years of age. Each year, about 9 million people develop TB, and 2 million die because of it. With increased funding, prompt identification of persons with TB, appropriate initial treatment, and completion of treatments, the number of TB cases started declining again in the mid-1990s. However, MDR TB continues to be a serious health concern. Patients started on therapy for TB who do not finish the prescribed therapy can develop and spread resistant strains of *M. tuberculosis*.

Pathophysiology

TB is transmitted from one person to another by droplets dispersed in the air through coughing, sneezing, and speaking. TB microorganisms can be inhaled into the lungs, therefore persons in close contact with the infected patient are at highest risk of becoming infected. Others at high risk for contracting the disease include the immunocompromised (e.g., patients with HIV, diabetes, and renal failure and those taking certain medications, such as cortisol), people living or working in high-risk residential settings (e.g., nursing homes, shelters, correctional facilities), those who inject illegal drugs, and health care workers who serve high-risk patients.

Not everyone infected with TB will develop clinical manifestations, rather some will harbor the microorganisms and will have what is called latent tuberculosis infection; these persons are at risk of developing TB disease later, and only those with TB disease can infect others. Symptoms of TB disease include anorexia, cough with sputum production or blood, chest pain, fever, night sweats, weight loss, and positive acid-fast bacilli in the sputum. Isolating infectious persons and initiating treatment for TB disease as soon as possible is the best way to decrease transmission.

Nurses should be aware that persons coming to the United States from high-risk countries where TB disease is common may have been vaccinated with bacille Calmette-Guérin (BCG) as a child. This vaccine is seldom used in the United States. Previous vaccination with BCG may cause a positive reaction to skin testing; however, it does not affect interferon-gamma release assay (IGRA) blood testing.

ANTITUBERCULAR DRUGS

Antitubercular drugs (Table 27.1), which include antimycobacterials, treat persons with TB disease and those exposed to TB disease. Streptomycin was the first drug used in the treatment of TB disease in 1943. However, it was noted that patients began to deteriorate after 3 months of therapy due to drug resistance. In 1952, isoniazid (INH) began to see widespread use in the treatment of TB disease and was felt to be a "wonder drug." To this day, INH remains the first-line treatment for TB disease. INH

TABLE 27.1 Antitubercular Drugs

Generic	Route and Dosage	Uses and Considerations
FIRST-LINE TREATMENT FOR TUBERCULOSIS DISEASE		
Ethambutol hydrochloride	A: PO: Based on lean body weight: 15-25 mg/kg/d	Used in combination with other antitubercular drugs. A common adverse effect is eye damage that causes blurred or changed vision, including color vision. Pregnancy category: B*; PB: 20%-30%; t½: 3-4 h
Isoniazid (INH)	See Prototype Drug Chart 27.1.	
Pyrazinamide	A/C: PO: 15-30 mg/kg/d or 50-70 mg/kg 2 ×/wk; *max:* 30 mg/kg/d	Used in combination with other antitubercular drugs. Can be given without regard to meals; promote fluid intake to decrease renal complications. Common adverse effects include hepatitis with patients exhibiting abdominal pain, abnormal hepatic transaminases, fatigue, anorexia, nausea or vomiting, jaundice, and icteric, dark urine. May also cause photosensitivity, angioedema, hepatic failure, and thrombocytopenia. Monitor LFTs and serum uric acid. Pregnancy category: C*; PB: 50%; t½: 9-10 h
Rifabutin	A: PO: 300 mg/d; *max:* 600 mg/d	May divide dose to 150 mg twice daily with GI concerns (e.g., nausea, vomiting). Pregnancy category: B*; PB: 85%; t½: Average 45 h
Rifampin†	A: PO: 10 mg/kg/d; *max:* 600 mg/d C: PO: 10-20 mg/kg/d; *max:* 600 mg/d	Used in combination with other antitubercular drugs. Best taken on an empty stomach. Contents of capsules may be mixed with applesauce or jelly. Pregnancy category: C*; PB: 80%; t½: 3-5 h
Rifapentine	Active: A/C ≥12 y: PO: 600 mg twice weekly Latent: A/C ≥2 y: Single weight-based dose weekly × 12 wk; *max:* 900 mg/wk	Rifapentine *must* be used in combination with other antitubercular drugs in patients with TB disease who are HIV negative or for latent TB infection to prevent progression to TB disease. Rifapentine has a longer half-life than rifampin; the interval between doses should be at least 72 h. Monitor for toxicity if drug is taken with an anticoagulant or anticonvulsant or with digoxin. Monitor for thrombocytopenia, ecchymosis, and indigestion. Do not use concurrently with oral contraceptives. Pregnancy category: C*; PB: 98%; t½: 13 h
DRUGS FOR MULTIDRUG-RESISTANT TUBERCULOSIS		
(Used in combination with first-line drugs based on sensitivity)		
Aminosalicylate sodium	A: PO: 8-12 g/d in 2-3 divided doses C: PO: 200-300 mg/kg/d in 2-4 divided doses taken with food; *max:* 10 g/d	Used in combination with other antitubercular drugs as a second-line therapy. Administer as a suspension mixed in acidic liquid (e.g., applesauce, yogurt, or tomato or orange juice) without chewing. Nonacidic foods will dissolve the acid-resistant coating of the granules. GI disturbances (e.g., nausea, vomiting, diarrhea, abdominal pain) are the most common complaints. Pregnancy category: C*; PB: 50%-60%; t½: 26 min
Capreomycin	A ≤59 y: IV/IM: 15 mg/kg/d; *max:* 1 g/d A >59 y: IV/IM: 10 mg/kg/d; *max:* 750 mg/d	Used in combination with other antitubercular drugs. Inject into a large muscle mass. Because of possible nephrotoxicity, use caution when administering to patients with renal impairment. Other toxicity includes ototoxicity. Pregnancy category: C*; PB: UK; t½: 5.2-6.8 h

Continued

TABLE 27.1   Antitubercular Drugs—cont'd

Generic	Route and Dosage	Uses and Considerations
DRUGS FOR MULTIDRUG-RESISTANT TUBERCULOSIS		
Cycloserine	A: PO: 500-1000 mg/d in divided doses	Used in combination with other antitubercular drugs. May be taken without regard to food. Pyridoxine taken concurrently can relieve or prevent neurotoxic effects. Contraindicated in patients with a history of ETOH abuse, severe anxiety, major depression, psychosis, severe renal disease, and seizure disorders. Monitor cycloserine concentrations. Pregnancy category: C*; PB: UK; t½: 10 h
Ethionamide	A/C >12 y: PO: 15-20 mg/kg/d as a single dose or in 2-3 divided doses; *max:* 1 g/d	Used in combination with other antitubercular drugs. Contraindicated in severe hepatic impairment. An ophthalmologic exam should be done and blood glucose and hepatic function should be monitored before and periodically during treatment. Drug may be taken without regard to food. Pregnancy category: C*; PB: 30%; t½: 2 h
Streptomycin sulfate	A: IM: 15 mg/kg/d; *max:* 1 g/d C: IM: 20-40 mg/kg/d	Used in combination with other antitubercular drugs. Inject into a large muscle mass. Contraindicated in people with aminoglycoside hypersensitivity. Monitor for ototoxicity, nephrotoxicity, and neurotoxicity. Pregnancy category: D*; PB: 35%; t½: 2-3 h

*Pregnancy categories have been revised. See http://www.fda.gov/Drugs/DevelopmentApprovalProcess/DevelopmentResources/Labeling/ucm093 307.htm for more information.
†Rifampin is the preferred agent from the class of rifamycins (rifabutin, rifampin, and rifapentine).
A, Adult; *C,* child; *d,* day; *ETOH,* ethanol (alcohol); *GI,* gastrointestinal; *h,* hour; *HIV,* human immunodeficiency virus; *IM,* intramuscular; *IV,* intravenous; *LFT,* liver function test; *max,* maximum; *min,* minutes; *PB,* protein binding; *PO,* by mouth; *t½,* half-life; *TB,* tuberculosis; *UK,* unknown; *wk,* week; *y,* year; >, greater than; ≥, greater than or equal to; ≤, less than or equal to.

PROTOTYPE DRUG CHART 27.1

Isoniazid

Drug Class	**Dosage**
Antimycobacterial (antitubercular) Pregnancy category: C*	Latent TB infection: A: PO/IM: 300 mg/d *or* 900 mg/d 2 ×/wk with pyridoxine *or* 15 mg/kg with rifapentine 1 ×/wk C: PO/IM: 10-15 mg/kg/d *or* 20-30 mg/kg/d 2 ×/wk with pyridoxine *or* 15 mg/kg with rifapentine 1 ×/wk; *max:* 900 mg/d Do not give rifapentine to children under 2 y. TB disease: A: PO/IM: 5 mg/kg/d or 5 d/wk or 15 mg/kg once, twice, or thrice weekly; *max:* 900 mg/d Adol: PO/IM: 5-15 mg/kg/d or 5 d/wk *or* 15-40 mg/kg twice or thrice weekly C: PO/IM: 10-15 mg/kg once daily or 5 ×/wk *or* 20-40 mg/kg 2-3 ×/wk See the CDC website at www.cdc.gov for complete dosing regimens.
Contraindications	**Drug-Lab-Food Interactions**
Severe renal or hepatic disease, alcoholism, diabetic retinopathy; severe hypersensitivity to pyrazinamide or ethionamide; concurrent use with MAOI therapy	Drug: Potent inhibitor of CYP450 enzyme system; many drug-drug interactions can occur (see the package insert for a complete list). Increased effect with alcohol, rifampin, and cycloserine; decreased GI absorption while taking aluminum antacids; inhibits the metabolism of benzodiazepines, phenytoin, fosphenytoin, SSRIs, SNRIs, and valproic acid. MAOIs could potentiate the effects of INH. Food: Food decreases the rate and extent of drug absorption. Foods rich in histamine (e.g., aged cheese, tuna), tyramine (e.g., aged cheese, bananas, avocadoes, overripe fruit, fava beans, smoked meats and fish, soy sauce, yeast), and caffeine can increase the effects of INH. Herb: Green tea, guarana, and ginseng could potentiate the effects of INH. Lab: Increases AST, ALT, bilirubin
Pharmacokinetics	**Pharmacodynamics**
Absorption: Rapidly absorbed in the GI tract when given PO Distribution: PB: Nonsignificant Metabolism: t½: 1-4 h Excretion: 75% in urine; remainder in feces, saliva, and sputum	PO/IM: Onset: UK Peak: 1-2 h Duration: UK
Therapeutic Effects/Uses	

To treat active tuberculosis and as a prophylactic measure against tuberculosis

Mode of Action: Bactericidal or bacteriostatic, depending on the drug concentration; inhibits bacterial cell-wall synthesis and MAO without affecting mitochondrial MAO, which interferes with the metabolism of tyramine and histamine. No cross-resistance with other antitubercular drugs occurs except with ethionamide. Pyridoxine supplementation reduces neurotoxic side effects.

PROTOTYPE DRUG CHART 27.1—cont'd

Isoniazid

Side Effects	Adverse Reactions
Drowsiness, tremors, rash, blurred vision, photosensitivity, tinnitus, dizziness, nausea, vomiting, dry mouth, constipation, diarrhea with oral solution, injection site reaction with IM administration	Psychotic behavior, peripheral neuropathy, vitamin B6 deficiency, hyperglycemia, metabolic acidosis, optic neuritis *Life threatening:* Blood dyscrasias, seizures, thrombocytopenia, agranulocytosis, hepatotoxicity, exfoliative dermatitis

*Pregnancy categories have been revised. See http://www.fda.gov/Drugs/DevelopmentApprovalProcess/DevelopmentResources/Labeling/ucm093 307.htm for more information.

A, adult; *Adol*, adolescent; *ALT*, alanine aminotransferase; *AST*, aspartate aminotransferase; *C*, child; *CDC*, Centers for Disease Control and Prevention; *CYP450*, cytochrome P450; *d*, day; *GI*, gastrointestinal; *h*, hour; *IM*, intramuscular; *INH*, isoniazid; *MAO*, monoamine oxidase; *MAOI*, monoamine oxidase inhibitor; *max*, maximum; *PB*, protein binding; *PO*, by mouth; *SNRI*, serotonin norepinephrine reuptake inhibitor; *SSRI*, selective serotonin reuptake inhibitor; *t½*, half-life; *TB*, tuberculosis; *UK*, unknown; *wk*, week; *y*, year.

BOX 27.1   Determining When to Treat Latent Tuberculosis Infection

People with a positive tuberculin skin test (TST) reaction of ≥5 mm if they are:
- HIV positive
- Recent contacts of someone with active tuberculosis (TB disease)
- Persons with fibrotic changes on chest radiography consistent with old TB
- Organ transplant recipients
- Persons who are immunosuppressed for other reasons (e.g., those taking the equivalent of >15 mg/day of prednisone for 1 month or longer, those taking tumor necrosis factor alpha [TNF-α] antagonists)

People with a positive TST reaction of ≥10 mm if they are:
- Recent immigrants (<5 years) from high-prevalence countries
- Injection drug users
- Residents and employees of high-risk congregate settings (e.g., correctional facilities, nursing homes, homeless shelters, hospitals, and other health care facilities)
- Mycobacteriology laboratory personnel
- Children under 4 years of age or children or adolescents exposed to adults in high-risk categories

From http://www.cdc.gov/tb/topic/treatment/decideltbi.htm

---

is a bactericidal drug that inhibits tubercle cell-wall synthesis and blocks pyridoxine (vitamin B6), which is used for intracellular enzyme production. When INH is prescribed, pyridoxine may also be prescribed to avoid vitamin B deficiency and to minimize peripheral neuropathy. INH is administered orally. Prototype Drug Chart 27.1 lists the data for INH.

Prophylactic antituberculars are drugs to prevent TB disease in individuals with latent TB infection. Prophylaxis is recommended for those who have a clinically significant result on tuberculin skin testing (≥5 mm for immunocompromised individuals or ≥10 mm for high-risk groups; Box 27.1) or a positive IGRA result. Patients who have converted from a negative to a positive TB skin test (TST) or from a negative to positive IGRA should be considered candidates for prophylactic therapy as well. Prototype Drug Chart 27.1 shows guidelines for latent TB infection treatment with INH.

Prophylactic therapy is contraindicated for persons with liver disease because INH is the primary antitubercular drug used, and it may cause INH-induced liver damage. Other antitubercular drugs may also cause liver damage if given in high doses over an extended period.

Single-drug therapy is ineffective in the treatment of TB disease due to drug resistance. Using a combination of antitubercular drugs has been shown to decrease bacterial resistance. Additionally, using combination therapy has decreased the duration of treatment from 2 years to 6 to 9 months. Different combinations of drugs can be used with INH, rifampin, ethambutol, and pyrazinamide.

Antitubercular drugs are divided into two categories: first-line drugs that form the core of treatment regimens and drugs used in the treatment of drug-resistant TB. **First-line drugs**—those drugs chosen first, such as INH, rifampin, pyrazinamide, and ethambutol—are considered more effective and less toxic than drugs used in the treatment of drug-resistant TB. Drugs used in the treatment of drug-resistant TB, in which *M. tuberculosis* is resistant to at least one first-line drug, or MDR TB, in which *M. tuberculosis* is resistant to INH and rifampin plus one other first-line drug, are used in combination with first-line drugs to treat drug-resistant *M. tuberculosis*. See Table 27.1 for drugs used in the treatment of drug-resistant TB.

Combination therapy against TB disease is more effective in eradicating infection than any single drug. The treatment regimen is divided into two phases: the initial phase lasts 2 months, and the continuation phase consists of the next 4 or 7 months. The total treatment plan can be up to 9 months or longer, depending on response to drug therapy. If drug resistance develops, other antibacterial drugs such as aminoglycosides (streptomycin, kanamycin, amikacin) or fluoroquinolones (levofloxacin, ciprofloxacin, or ofloxacin) may be given as part of combination therapy. Combination therapy for drug-resistant TB disease consists of a minimum of three drugs, but preferably four to five drugs, administered as part of directly observed therapy to ensure adherence. Drug therapy should be managed by an expert in the disease, and susceptibility testing to determine drug resistance should be performed before drug therapy; however, treatment with first-line therapy should not be delayed if TB disease is suspected. Aminoglycoside antibiotics should not be taken if kidney dysfunction is present. When antibacterial agents are used continuously or at high doses, serum drug levels should be closely monitored to avoid drug toxicity.

Many drug-drug interactions and side effects occur with antituberculars. To increase adherence to drug therapy, direct observation therapy (DOT) is recommended.

Side Effects and Adverse Reactions

Side effects and adverse reactions to antituberculars differ according to the drug prescribed. For INH, peripheral neuropathy can be a problem, especially for those who are malnourished, have diabetes mellitus, or are alcoholics. This condition can be prevented if pyridoxine (vitamin B6) is administered. Hepatotoxicity (liver toxicity) is an adverse reaction to many antituberculars. Patients with moderate to severe liver dysfunction should *not* take these drugs. Patients with liver disease should have hepatic transaminases monitored closely. Patients may also develop headaches, blood dyscrasias, paresthesias, gastrointestinal (GI) distress (e.g., nausea, vomiting, diarrhea, dyspepsia), and ocular toxicity. An ophthalmic exam before and during treatment is warranted. INH may cause hyperglycemia, hyperkalemia, hypophosphatemia, and hypocalcemia. Rifampin turns body fluids orange, and soft contact lenses may be permanently discolored. It may also cause thrombocytopenia and GI intolerance. The patient taking ethambutol may develop dizziness, confusion, hallucinations, and joint pain. Streptomycin may lead to many adverse effects such as ototoxicity, optic nerve toxicity, encephalopathy, angioedema, central nervous system (CNS) and respiratory depression, nephrotoxicity, and hepatotoxicity.

⚡ PATIENT SAFETY

Do not confuse...
- *Rifampin* with other antituberculars such as *rifabutin* and *rifapentine*.

SPECIAL POPULATIONS

Pregnancy and Tuberculosis

The benefits of treating a pregnant woman with TB disease outweigh the risks of treatment. Women with untreated TB disease are at risk for passing the disease to their fetus and delivering an infant with low birthweight. The drugs used in initial treatment of TB disease do cross the placenta but do not appear to harm the fetus.

Treatment of latent TB infection in the pregnant woman includes INH daily or twice weekly for 9 months with pyridoxine supplementation. Three-month combination therapy of INH with rifapentinem, *referred to as 3HP,* is not recommended for pregnant women or those planning to become pregnant within 3 months.

The pregnant woman with TB disease should be treated with INH, rifampin, and ethambutol daily for 2 months followed by INH and rifampin daily or twice weekly for 7 months for a total of 9 months. Streptomycin should *not* be used due to potential harmful effects on the fetus. Pyrazinamide is also *not* recommended due to unknown effects on the fetus.

Tuberculosis and HIV Coinfection

HIV is a risk factor for the development of TB, and TB disease is one of the leading causes of death for people living with HIV. Left untreated, latent TB infection can quickly develop into TB disease. The recommended treatment for an adult with latent TB infection and HIV is INH daily for 9 months.

Adults with HIV and TB disease should be treated for 6 months with INH, rifabutin, pyrazinamide, and ethambutol during the initial phase. The 4-month continuation phase should consist of INH and rifabutin.

A pregnant woman with HIV and TB disease should be treated the same as a nonpregnant woman but with concern for the fetus when choosing drug therapy.

Pediatric Tuberculosis

Children are more likely than adults to be sickened more quickly by TB. Because of this, children with latent TB infection should be treated to prevent development of TB disease. The recommended treatment is INH for 9 months. Treatment of TB disease should be managed by a pediatric TB expert in conjunction with drug susceptibility studies. It is very important for the nurse to make sure parents understand that if a child stops taking the drugs before therapy is finished, the child can become sick again. Additionally, nurses should stress to parents that if drugs are not taken correctly, the bacteria may become drug resistant. Drug-resistant TB is harder and more expensive to treat.

◎ NURSING PROCESS
Patient-Centered Collaborative Care
Antitubercular Drugs

Assessment
- Determine any past instances of TB in the patient's health history—including the last purified protein derivative (PPD) tuberculin test and the reaction or the serum IGRA result, the last chest radiograph and result, and the last ophthalmic exam—along with any allergies.
- Obtain a general medical history from the patient. Most antitubercular drugs are contraindicated if the patient has severe hepatic disease.
- Check laboratory results for liver function studies, bilirubin, blood urea nitrogen (BUN), and serum creatinine. These baseline values can be compared with future laboratory test results.
- Evaluate the patient for signs and symptoms of paresthesia (tingling, numbness, or burning).
- Assess for hearing changes if the antitubercular drug regimen includes streptomycin. Drug-induced ototoxicity is the major irreversible toxicity of aminoglycosides.

Nursing Diagnoses
- Nonadherence, Risk for
- Infection, Risk for
- Knowledge, Deficient related to unfamiliarity with medications

Planning
- The patient's sputum test for acid-fast bacilli will be negative 2 to 3 months after the prescribed antitubercular therapy.

Nursing Interventions
- If INH is ordered, administer the drug 1 hour before or 2 hours after meals because food decreases the absorption rate. Other antitubercular drugs are given without regard to meals.

- Give pyridoxine (vitamin B6) as prescribed with INH to prevent peripheral neuropathy.
- Monitor serum liver enzyme levels. Elevated levels may indicate liver toxicity.
- Collect sputum specimens for acid-fast bacilli early in the morning. Usually three consecutive morning sputum specimens are sent to the laboratory.
- Encourage eye examinations for patients taking INH and ethambutol because these antitubercular drugs may cause visual disturbances.
- Emphasize the importance of complying with the drug regimen.

Patient Teaching
- Tell patients who take INH to take the drug 1 hour before meals or 2 hours after meals for better absorption.
- ⚡ Direct patients to take antitubercular drugs as prescribed. Ineffective treatment and development of drug resistance might occur if drugs are taken intermittently or discontinued when symptoms are decreased or when the patient is feeling better. *Adherence to the drug regimen is essential to prevent the spread of drug-resistant M. tuberculosis.*
- Instruct patients not to take antacids while taking antitubercular drugs because they decrease drug absorption. Patients should also avoid alcohol because it increases the risk of hepatotoxicity.
- Advise patients to keep medical appointments and to participate in sputum testing, which is important in evaluating the effectiveness of drug regimens.
- Warn patients contemplating pregnancy to first check with their health care provider about taking the antitubercular drugs ethambutol and rifampin.
- Guide patients to report any numbness, tingling, or burning of hands and feet. Peripheral neuropathy is a common side effect of INH. Vitamin B6 prevents peripheral neuropathy.
- Encourage patients to avoid direct sunlight to decrease the risk of photosensitivity. Patients should use a sunscreen with a minimum sun protection factor (SPF) of 30 and ultraviolet A and B (UVA/UVB) protection while in the sun.
- Inform patients taking rifampin that urine, feces, saliva, sputum, sweat, and tears may turn a harmless red-orange color. Soft contact lenses may be permanently stained.
- Alert patients receiving ethambutol to take daily single doses to avoid visual problems. Divided doses of ethambutol may cause visual disturbances.
- Increase access to health care. Community involvement and culturally sensitive patient education are important. Explain to patients who have active TB that family members should get a TB skin test and may receive a prophylactic drug for 6 months to 1 year. Emphasize the importance of family members seeking medical care.
- Provide a written sheet for drug and treatment regimens in the language the patient speaks or reads most easily.

- Explain the importance of good hygiene (e.g., discarding tissues that contain sputum, separating dishes, using a dishwasher to clean dishes if possible).
- Understand the significance of community if multiple individuals in the same community are treated for latent TB infection. Make all attempts to place community members on a treatment plan to increase compliance through social support.

Evaluation
- Evaluate the effectiveness of the antitubercular drugs. Sputum specimens for acid-fast bacilli should be negative after taking antitubercular drugs for several weeks or months.

FUNGUS

Pathophysiology

An infection caused by a fungus may also be called *mycosis*, *tinea*, or *candidiasis*. A fungal infection may be local or systemic. Local fungal infections can be acquired by contact with an infected person. Fungi known as *dermatophytes* can cause local fungal infections involving the integumentary system, which includes mucous membranes, hair, nails, and moist skin areas. When *Candida albicans* affects the mouth, it is called *oral candidiasis* or *thrush*. Vaginal candidiasis is common in women who are pregnant, diabetic, immunocompromised, or taking certain medications (e.g., antibiotics, oral contraceptives, and dapagliflozin). Systemic fungal infections may involve the lungs, CNS, or abdomen and are usually transmitted to an individual through inhalation into the lungs. Fungal infections may be mild, such as tinea pedis (athlete's foot), or severe, such as fungal disease of the lungs or fungal meningitis.

Fungal infections are also classified as *opportunistic* or *primary*. Opportunistic infections usually occur in the immunocompromised or debilitated population (e.g., patients who have cancer or AIDS) or in those taking antibiotics, corticosteroids, chemotherapy, or other immunosuppressives. Fungi such as *Candida* species (yeast) are part of the normal flora of the mouth, skin, intestine, and vagina. An opportunistic infection, such as systemic candidiasis, may occur when the body's defense mechanisms are impaired such that they allow overgrowth of the fungus. Other opportunistic infections are aspergillosis, mucormycosis, *Pneumocystis* pneumonia, and fusariosis. Primary infections typically occur in immunocompetent persons and result from inhaled spores. Primary infections include coccidioidomycosis, blastomycosis, paracoccidioidomycosis, cryptococcosis, and histoplasmosis, including progressive disseminated histoplasmosis.

ANTIFUNGAL DRUGS

Antifungal drugs, also called antimycotic drugs, are used to treat fungal infections. Typically, antifungals are fungistatic or fungicidal depending upon the susceptibility of the fungus and the dosage. The antifungal drugs are classified into the following groups (Table 27.2):
- Polyenes (amphotericin B, nystatin)
- Azoles (fluconazole)

TABLE 27.2 Antifungal Drugs

Generic	Route and Dosage	Uses and Considerations
POLYENES		
Amphotericin B deoxycholate	A: IV: 0.25-1.5 mg/kg/d; *max:* 1.5 mg/kg/d	For a variety of systemic fungal infections. May require pretreatment with an analgesic, antihistamine, antipyretic, and corticosteroid for pain, fever, chills, or rigor. Electrolyte loss and nephrotoxicity can occur. Protect drug against light and infuse slowly via an in-line filter. Pregnancy category: B*; PB: 90%-95%; t½: 24 h
Nystatin	See Prototype Drug Chart 27.2.	
AZOLE ANTIFUNGALS		
Fluconazole	See Prototype Drug Chart 27.3.	
Itraconazole	A: PO: 200-400 mg/d Other dosing regimens are available for severe infection or for patients who are immunocompromised.	For a variety of fungal infections. Targets CYP450 enzymatic pathway. Avoid concurrent use with PPIs, H₂ blockers, or antacids. Take on an empty stomach. Pregnancy category: C*; contraindicated in pregnancy and in those contemplating pregnancy; PB: 99%; t½: 34-42 h
Ketoconazole	Systemic: A: PO: 200-400 mg/d as a single dose C ≥2 y: PO: 3.3-6.6 mg/kg/d as a single dose Topical: A: Apply a sufficient amount to affected and surrounding areas once daily for 2 wk.	For a variety of fungal infections. Treatment may last 1 to 6 months for systemic infections. Take with food to avoid GI discomfort. Higher doses can inhibit adrenal cortisol synthesis. Pregnancy category: C*; PB: 84%-99%; t½: 2-8 h
Posaconazole	Oral candidiasis: A: PO: 100 mg/d up to 200 mg tid for 14-21 d Prophylactic: A: PO: 200-300 mg bid/tid A: IV: 300 mg bid initially, then 300 mg/d	For oral candidiasis and prophylactic treatment of invasive *Aspergillus* and *Candida* infections in immunosuppressed patients. Different formulations are not interchangeable. Ensure proper dosage formulation, strength, and frequency. Do not chew, divide, or crush delayed-release tablets. Administer with food or as an IV infusion via a central line with an in-line filter. Pregnancy category: UK* (avoid use during pregnancy); PB: >98%; t½: 20-66 h depending on formulation
Voriconazole	A/C: PO: Weight-based dosing: 200-400 mg q12h A/C: IV: 6 mg/kg q12h on day 1, then 3-4 mg/kg q12h	For aspergillosis, candidiasis, fusariosis, and scedosporiosis. Patients with HIV coinfection may need a higher dose. Grapefruit juice should be avoided. Take PO dose on an empty stomach. Pregnancy category: D*; PB: 58%; t½: 6 h to 6 d, depending on the dose
ANTIMETABOLITES		
Flucytosine	A: PO: 50-150 mg/kg/d in divided doses q6h for 7-10 d; *max:* 150 mg/kg/d TDM: 50-150 mcg/mL	Usually given in conjunction with amphotericin B to decrease the development of resistance to flucytosine. Fungal resistance occurs if drug is given alone. Fungal cells convert flucytosine to trace amounts of fluorouracil intracellularly. Monitor flucytosine concentrations, liver transaminases, and renal function. Pregnancy category: C*; PB: 2%-4%; t½: 2.5-6 h
ECHINOCANDINS		
Anidulafungin	A: IV: 100-200 mg loading dose on day 1, then 50-100 mg/d	For *Candida* infections. Infusion time is dose dependent. Monitor liver function tests. Pregnancy category: C*; PB: 99%; t½: 30-60 min
Caspofungin	A: IV: 70 mg on day 1, then 50 mg/d C ≥3 mo: IV: 70 mg/m² on day 1, then 50-70 mg/m²; *max:* 70 mg/d	For *Aspergillus* and *Candida* infections. Give IV as an infusion over 1 h. Monitor CBC and liver transaminases. Pregnancy category: C*; PB: 97%; t½: 9-50 h
Micafungin	A: IV: 100-150 mg/d C ≥4 mo: IV: 2-4 mg/kg/d; *max:* 100 mg/d	For *Candida* infection. Patients with HIV coinfection may require a higher dose. Does not have significant effect on the CYP450 enzyme system. To minimize excessive foaming, do not vigorously shake the vial. Infuse slowly over 1 h. Rapid infusion can cause histamine-mediated reactions. Pregnancy category: C*; PB: 99%; t½: 13-17 h

Generic	Route and Dosage	Uses and Considerations
MISCELLANEOUS ANTIFUNGALS		
Griseofulvin	A: PO: 300-750 mg/d; can be given in 2-4 divided doses/d; *max:* 1000 mg/d C >2 y: PO: 5-20 mg/kg/d; *max:* 1000 mg/d	For tinea infection, including onychomycosis. Available in microsize and ultramicrosize; dosage depends on formulation. Give with a fatty meal to increase absorption. Tablets can be crushed and mixed with food; swallow without chewing. Pregnancy category: X*; PB: UK; t½: 9-24 h

TABLE 27.2 **Antifungal Drugs—cont'd**

*Pregnancy categories have been revised. See http://www.fda.gov/Drugs/DevelopmentApprovalProcess/DevelopmentResources/Labeling/ucm093307.htm for more information.

A, Adult; *bid,* twice daily; *C,* child; *CBC,* complete blood count; *CYP450,* cytochrome P450; *d,* day; *GI,* gastrointestinal; *h,* hour; *H₂,* histamine 2; *HIV,* human immunodeficiency virus; *IV,* intravenous; *max,* maximum; *min,* minute; *mo,* month; *PB,* protein binding; *PO,* by mouth; *PPI,* proton pump inhibitor; *q,* every; *t½,* half-life; *TDM,* therapeutic drug monitoring; *tid,* three times daily; *UK,* unknown; *wk,* weeks; *y,* year; *>,* greater than; *≥,* greater than or equal to.

- Antimetabolites (flucytosine)
- Echinocandins (caspofungin)
- Miscellaneous antifungals (griseofulvin)

Polyenes
Amphotericin B
The polyene antifungal drug of choice for severe systemic infection is amphotericin B, which is effective against numerous fungal diseases that include histoplasmosis, cryptococcosis, coccidioidomycosis, aspergillosis, blastomycosis, and systemic candidiasis. Polyene antifungals act by binding to the fungal cell membrane to form open channels that increase cell permeability and leakage of intracellular components, especially potassium. Because of its toxicity, amphotericin B is administered with close supervision.

Pharmacokinetics Amphotericin B is highly protein bound and has a long half-life. Only 5% of the drug is excreted in the urine. Renal disease does not affect the excretion of amphotericin B.

Pharmacodynamics Amphotericin B is not absorbed from the GI tract, therefore it is administered intravenously in low doses for treating systemic fungal infections. Peak effect occurs 1 to 2 hours after intravenous (IV) infusion, and the duration is 24 hours.

Side Effects and Adverse Reactions. Side effects and adverse reactions for amphotericin B include fever, shaking, chills, flushing, loss of appetite, dizziness, nausea, vomiting, headache, shortness of breath, and tachypnea. These symptoms may occur 1 to 3 hours after the infusion has started. Pretreatment with acetaminophen, diphenhydramine, or hydrocortisone administered 30 to 60 minutes prior to infusion may alleviate these symptoms. Additionally, patients may experience hypotension, paresthesia, and thrombophlebitis. Amphotericin B is *highly toxic* and can cause nephrotoxicity and electrolyte imbalance, especially hypokalemia and hypomagnesemia (low serum potassium and magnesium levels). Urinary output, BUN, and serum creatinine levels must be closely monitored. Amphotericin B is also toxic to bone marrow, therefore complete blood counts should be monitored periodically.

Nystatin
Nystatin is another polyene antifungal drug that is administered orally or topically to treat *Candida* infection. It is available in suspension, cream, and ointment forms. Nystatin is poorly absorbed by the GI tract. The more common use of nystatin is as an oral suspension for *Candida* infection in the mouth (oral thrush). The suspension is swished in the mouth for several minutes to ensure contact with the mucous membranes and then is either spit out or swallowed. If the throat area is involved, the patient should also gargle with nystatin prior to swishing and swallowing or spitting. Prototype Drug Chart 27.2 lists the data for nystatin.

Azole Antifungals
The azole group is effective against candidiasis (local and systemic), coccidioidomycosis, cryptococcosis, histoplasmosis, and paracoccidioidomycosis. Ketoconazole was the first effective antifungal drug that was orally absorbed. Fluconazole, itraconazole, posaconazole, and voriconazole are other azole drugs used to treat systemic fungal infections. These antifungals can be taken orally, unlike amphotericin B and caspofungin, which are administered by the IV route only. Fluconazole, a systemic azole antifungal agent, is described in Prototype Drug Chart 27.3.

Azoles inhibit cytochrome P450 (CYP450) in fungal cells, interfering with the formation of ergosterol. Because ergosterol is a major sterol in the fungal cell membrane, cell permeability and leakage are increased. Numerous azoles are used in topical preparations (e.g., creams, ointments, powders, shampoos, sprays, and solutions) to treat candidiasis and tinea infections. Azoles and other topical antifungal agents are presented in Table 27.2.

Antimetabolites
The antimetabolite flucytosine acts by selectively penetrating the fungal cell, which converts the drug into fluorouracil, an antimetabolite that disrupts fungal DNA and RNA synthesis. Flucytosine is well absorbed from the GI tract, and it is used in combination with other antifungal drugs, such as amphotericin B. Antimetabolites are discussed further in Chapter 32.

PROTOTYPE DRUG CHART 27.2

Nystatin

Drug Class	Dosage
Antifungal antibiotic Pregnancy category: C*	A/C: PO susp: 4-6 mL swished in the mouth 4 ×/d for 7-14 d Infants: PO susp: 1-2 mL in each side of the mouth 4 ×/d for at least 48 h A/C: Top: Apply to affected area bid until healed. A: PO cap: 500,000 to 1 million units tid for at least 48 h
Contraindications	**Drug-Lab-Food Interactions**
Caution: Pregnancy, diabetes mellitus, paraben hypersensitivity, breastfeeding	Drug: Azole antifungals inhibit the synthesis of the fungal sterol ergosterol, which decreases the effectiveness of nystatin.
Pharmacokinetics	**Pharmacodynamics**
Absorption: Poorly absorbed in the GI the tract when given PO Absorption: Susp/top: Not absorbed from intact skin or mucous membranes Distribution: PB: UK Metabolism: t½: UK Excretion: PO: In feces	PO: Onset: 24-72 h; peak and duration: UK Susp/top: Onset, peak, and duration: UK
Therapeutic Effects/Uses	
To treat candidiasis Mode of Action: Binds to sterols (ergosterol) causing the loss of intracellular potassium and other cellular contents	
Side Effects	**Adverse Reactions**
PO: Diarrhea, nausea, vomiting, dyspepsia Top: Skin irritation	Top/susp: Pruritus, urticaria, rash, hyperglycemia *Life threatening:* PO/top/susp: Angioedema, bronchospasm, sinus tachycardia, Stevens-Johnson syndrome

*Pregnancy categories have been revised. See http://www.fda.gov/Drugs/DevelopmentApprovalProcess/DevelopmentResources/Labeling/ucm093307.htm for more information.

A, Adult; *bid,* twice daily; *C,* child; *cap,* capsule; *d,* day; *GI,* gastrointestinal; *h,* hour; *PB,* protein binding; *PO,* by mouth; *susp,* suspension; *t½,* half-life; *tid,* three times daily; *Top,* topical; *UK,* unknown.

PROTOTYPE DRUG CHART 27.3

Fluconazole

Drug Class	Dosage
Azole antifungal Pregnancy category: C/D*	Cryptococcal meningitis: A: PO/IV: 400 mg on day 1, then 200-400 mg/d C: PO/IV: 12 mg/kg on day 1, then 10-12 mg/kg/d Systemic candidiasis (candidemia): A: PO/IV: 800 mg on day 1, then 400 mg/kg/d C: PO/IV: 6-12 mg/kg/d Candiduria (UTI due to candidiasis): A: PO/IV: 200-400 mg/d Most other candidiasis: A: PO/IV: 200 mg on day 1, then 100 mg/d Other treatment regimens are available.
Contraindications	**Drug-Lab-Food Interactions**
Caution: Azole antifungal hypersensitivity, pregnancy, cardiac disease, renal or hepatic disease	Drug: Because this drug inhibits the CYP450 isoenzyme, many drug-drug interactions are possible. See package insert for complete detail. Increases PT in patients taking warfarin; increases hypoglycemia when taken with oral sulfonylureas; increases phenytoin, cyclosporine, and haloperidol levels; decreases fluconazole level with cimetidine and rifampin; decreases the effect of clopidogrel; increases incidences of QT prolongation with cisapride, terfenadine, thioridazine, ondansetron, and other CYP3A4 substrates Food: May be administered without regard to food Herb: Increases serum caffeine (e.g., with coffee, green tea, soft drinks, and guarana)
Pharmacokinetics	**Pharmacodynamics**
Absorption: PO: Rapid and essentially complete Distribution: PB: 11%-12% Metabolism: t½: 20-50 h; does not undergo first-pass metabolism Excretion: 60%-80% in urine unchanged, 11% as metabolites	PO: Onset: Rapid Peak: 1-2 h Duration: UK IV: Onset, peak, and duration: UK

PROTOTYPE DRUG CHART 27.3—cont'd

Fluconazole

Therapeutic Effects/Uses	
To treat *Candida* infections and cryptococcal meningitis; as prophylaxis for patients undergoing BMT or radiation therapy	
Mode of Action: Increases permeability of the fungal cell membrane by inhibiting ergosterol synthesis	
Side Effects	**Adverse Reactions**
PO: GI upset (e.g., nausea, vomiting, diarrhea, abdominal pain, dysgeusia, dyspepsia), rash, headache, hypokalemia	Elevated liver transaminases, hepatic failure, renal failure, fatal cardiac arrhythmias, toxic epidermal necrolysis

*Pregnancy categories have been revised. See http://www.fda.gov/Drugs/DevelopmentApprovalProcess/DevelopmentResources/Labeling/ucm 093307.htm for more information.

A, Adult; *BMT,* bone marrow transplant; *C,* child; *CYP,* cytochrome P; *d,* day; *GI,* gastrointestinal; *h,* hour; *IV,* intravenous; *PB,* protein binding; *PO,* by mouth; *PT,* prothrombin time; *t½,* half-life; *UK,* unknown; *UTI,* urinary tract infection.

Echinocandins

Echinocandins are the newest class of antifungals. Three echinocandins are available in the United States: anidulafungin, caspofungin, and micafungin. The action of echinocandins is to inhibit biosynthesis of essential components of the fungal cell wall, which interferes with growth and reproduction of *Candida* and *Aspergillus* species. Echinocandins are administered intravenously because they are not absorbed in the GI tract. Phlebitis at the IV site and increased aspartate aminotransferase (AST) and alanine aminotransferase (ALT) are common adverse effects. Rapid infusion can cause histamine-mediated reactions.

⚡ PATIENT SAFETY

Amphotericin B
The two formulations of amphotericin B are amphotericin B deoxycholate and liposomal amphotericin B. Dosing for each formulation is different, therefore caution is advised.

◎ NURSING PROCESS
Patient-Centered Collaborative Care

Antifungals

Assessment
- Obtain a medical history that includes any serious renal or hepatic disorders. Antifungal agents such as amphotericin B, fluconazole, flucytosine, and ketoconazole are contraindicated if the patient has a serious renal or liver disease.
- Check laboratory tests for liver function (alkaline phosphatase [ALP], ALT, AST, gamma-glutamyl transferase [GGT]), BUN, bilirubin, and serum creatinine because elevated levels can indicate liver or renal dysfunction. Use these test results for future comparisons.
- Assess any prior use of antifungals.
- Record baseline vital signs for future comparisons.

Nursing Diagnoses
- Knowledge, Deficient related to the treatment regimen
- Infection, Risk for
- Injury, Risk for

Planning
- The patient's fungal infection will be resolved without life-threatening adverse reactions.

Nursing Interventions
- Obtain a culture to determine the fungus type (e.g., *Candida*).
- Monitor the patient's urinary output; many antifungal drugs can cause nephrotoxicity.
- Check laboratory results for BUN, serum creatinine, ALP, ALT, AST, bilirubin, and electrolytes and compare these with baseline findings. Certain antifungals can cause hepatotoxicity and nephrotoxicity when high doses are taken for an extended period.
- Record vital signs and compare these with baseline findings.
- Observe for side effects and adverse reactions to antifungal drugs, which may include nausea, vomiting, headache, phlebitis, and signs and symptoms of electrolyte imbalance.

Patient Teaching
- Advise patients to take drugs as prescribed. Compliance is of the utmost importance because discontinuing a drug too soon may result in relapse.
- Instruct patients to keep appointments to monitor laboratory testing of serum liver enzymes, BUN, creatinine, and electrolytes.
- Advise patients not to consume alcohol.
- Educate patients on proper administration of topical preparations.
- Teach patients to avoid operating hazardous equipment or motor vehicles when taking antifungals that may cause visual changes, sleepiness, dizziness, or lethargy (e.g., amphotericin B, ketoconazole, or flucytosine).
- Encourage patients to report side effects such as nausea, vomiting, diarrhea, dermatitis, rash, dizziness, tinnitus, edema, and flatulence. These symptoms may occur when taking certain antifungal drugs.
- Respect the patient's apprehension and fear concerning the use of topical antifungal drugs and the desire to use alternative methods. Evaluate the patient's method of topical administration in regard to safe practice. If the method is considered unsafe, explain why and suggest modifications. If appropriate, involve other persons for clarification.

Evaluation
- Evaluate the effectiveness of the antifungal drug by noting the diminishing or absence of the fungal infection.

VIRUSES

A **virus** is an obligate intracellular organism that must reside within a living host cell to survive and reproduce. Viruses enter healthy cells, live and reproduce within living cells, and use their DNA and RNA to generate more viruses. The growth cycle of viruses depends on host cell enzymes and cell substrates for viral replication. With the exception of HIV and certain kinds of viral hepatitis, viruses are self-limiting illnesses that usually do *not* require treatment with a specific antiviral. Current antivirals target influenza, herpes, and hepatitis.

Pathophysiology

Influenza, commonly called *the flu,* is a highly contagious viral infection that causes mild to severe illness that can result in hospitalization or even death. Influenza is usually seasonal and is more prevalent from fall to spring. There are three main types of influenza: A, B, and C. *Influenza A* causes a moderate to severe infection. There are two subtypes found in humans, designated by the hemagglutinin (H) and neuraminidase (N) proteins, H1N1 and H3N2, found on the viral surface. *Influenza B* usually causes mild illness in children. Two strains are currently found in humans: B/Yamagata and B/Victoria. *Influenza C* infection is a mild respiratory illness not thought to cause epidemics. Influenza is transmitted easily via contaminated droplets during coughing, sneezing, or talking. Droplets enter into the respiratory tract of the unaffected person and begin replication 24 hours before the appearance of symptoms. Usually influenza has an abrupt onset with the first symptoms being high fever, headache, fatigue, and myalgia (muscle aches). Chills, sore throat, nonproductive cough, watery nasal discharge, weakness, red watery eyes, and photophobia can also occur.

Herpesviruses are large viruses that cause infections. Among the most familiar are herpes simplex virus type 1 (HSV-1) and type 2 (HSV-2); varicella-zoster viruses (HSV-3, or VZV), more commonly known as *chickenpox* and *shingles*; Epstein-Barr virus (EBV, or human herpesvirus 4 [HHV-4]); and cytomegalovirus (CMV, or human herpesvirus 5 [HHV-5]). HSV-1 is usually associated with cold sores (vesicular lesions) and is capable of **latency**, the establishment and maintenance of latent infection in nerve cell ganglia proximal to the site of infection. HSV-2 is usually associated with vesicular lesions and small ulcerations on the genitalia (genital herpes). The HSV-2 virus remains dormant by traveling through the peripheral nerves to the sacral dorsal nerve root ganglia. The reactivation and replication of latent HSV always occurs in the area supplied by the ganglia in which latency was established. Reactivation can be induced by various factors that include fever, trauma, emotional stress, sunlight, and menstruation. Both HSV-1 and HSV-2 are capable of causing recurrent infections, and both can replicate in the mucous membranes and skin of the oropharynx or genitalia. Virus is transmitted by contact with infectious lesions or secretions. Signs and symptoms usually include eruption of small pustules and vesicles; fever; headache; malaise; myalgia; and tingling, itching, and pain in the affected area.

The varicella-zoster virus (VZV, or HSV-3) causes chickenpox and shingles. Chickenpox is a highly contagious viral infection that causes generalized pruritic vesicles and fever. Serious illness, hospitalizations, and deaths from VZV have decreased by 90% since vaccination began in 1995; however, some outbreaks still occur. When a person who has previously been infected with chickenpox becomes older or develops a weakened immune system, VZV that has lain dormant in nerve root ganglia can reactivate. The reactivation, called **shingles,** is a painful vesicular rash along the region of skin innervated by the nerve root ganglia, or **dermatome,** where the virus had lain dormant. In addition to the rash, the patient may also develop fever, malaise, myalgia, and pain along the involved dermatome.

Epstein-Barr virus (EBV, or HHV-4) most commonly causes infectious mononucleosis, a condition manifested by fever, tonsillitis, and enlarged lymph nodes in the neck. EBV resides in lymphocytes, epithelial cells, and muscle cells and has a latency period.

Cytomegalovirus (CMV, or HHV-5) is a common viral infection that affects people of all ages. Most people infected with CMV do not exhibit symptoms and are unaware they have the virus. However, people with weakened immune systems—such as those with HIV, transplant recipients, and those taking immunosuppressant drugs—along with pregnant women, unborn babies, and neonates are at risk for developing signs and symptoms (e.g., lymphadenopathy and splenomegaly). In susceptible individuals, CMV infection can lead to blindness (CMV retinitis) or fatal pneumonia.

Viral hepatitis infections, such as with hepatitis B and C viruses (HBV and HCV, respectively), are serious liver infections. Many people with HBV and HCV are unaware they have the virus. These viruses can persist undetected for years, increasing the likelihood of transmitting the disease to others. HBV and HCV are **blood-borne pathogens** spread through blood and body fluids. They are leading causes of hepatic cancer and the most common reason for hepatic failure and subsequent liver transplant. Signs and symptoms of viral hepatitis include fatigue, jaundice, abdominal pain, malaise, and nausea.

NON-HIV ANTIVIRALS

Antiviral drugs are used to prevent or delay the spread of viral infections. They inhibit viral replication by interfering with viral nucleic acid synthesis in the cell. Some groups of antiviral drugs are effective against various viruses, such as influenzas A and B, herpesviruses, HBV and HCV, and HIV. The non-HIV antiviral drugs are listed in Table 27.3. Interferon alfa-2a and -2b used to treat HBV and HCV are discussed in Chapter 34. Drugs for HIV are discussed in Chapter 29.

Influenza Antivirals

Current recommendations for the treatment of influenza type A and B are oseltamivir or zanamivir. These are neuraminidase inhibitors, a group of drugs that decrease the release of the virus from infected cells by inhibiting the activity of neuraminidase, a viral glycoprotein, thus decreasing viral spread and shortening the duration of flu symptoms. Zanamivir and oseltamivir should be taken within 48 hours of flu symptoms, but they are *not* substitutes for the influenza vaccines.

TABLE 27.3 Non-HIV Antivirals

Generic	Route and Dosage	Uses and Considerations
ANTIVIRALS: INFLUENZA		
Amantadine hydrochloride	Influenza A: A <65 y/C >9 y: PO: 200 mg/d in 1-2 divided doses Older adults >65 y: 100 mg/d C 1-8 y: PO: 4.4-8.8 mg/kg/d in 2 divided doses; *max.* 150 mg/d	Primary use is as prophylaxis against influenza A. Because of resistance in circulating influenza A, amantadine is no longer recommended; influenza A is sensitive to oseltamivir and zanamivir. If used, amantadine should be started within 24-48 h of onset of signs/symptoms and continued for 24-48 h after resolution. Avoid aspirin-containing products in children with influenza virus. Can be taken without regard to food. Pregnancy category: C*; PB: 67%; t½: 11-15 h
Cidofovir	A: IV: 5 mg/kg every other week	For CMV retinitis in HIV-infected patients. Give concomitantly with hydration and probenecid to minimize renal toxicity. Use chemotherapeutic precautions, including preparing the drug under laminar flow and using protective gloves and gowns. *Contraindications:* Sulfonamide hypersensitivity, renal impairment Pregnancy category: C*; PB: <6%; t½: 6-48 h
Foscarnet	Acyclovir-resistant herpesvirus: A: IV: 40-80 mg/kg q8h CMV retinitis: A: IV: 90 mg/kg q12h or 60 mg/kg/d q8h	For CMV retinitis and acyclovir-resistant mucocutaneous HSV. Administer via slow IV infusion. Patient must be hydrated to minimize renal toxicity. Monitor renal function. Pregnancy category: C*; PB: 14%-17%; t½: 3-7 h
Oseltamivir phosphate	A/C >40 kg: PO: 75 mg bid for 5 d C 15-40 kg: PO: 30-60 mg bid for 5 d Infants ≥14 d: PO: 3 mg/kg bid for 5 d	Blocks the function of viral neuraminidase protein by stopping the release of viruses from infected cells. Effective against influenzas A and B. Treatment should begin within 48 h of flu symptoms. Also used as prophylaxis for influenza A within 48 h of exposure; treat for 10 d. Dose is based on weights. May be taken without regard to food. Monitor renal function. Pregnancy category: C*; PB: 3%, t½: 1-3 h
Rimantadine hydrochloride	A/C >10 y: PO: 100 mg bid; *max:* 200 mg/d Older adults: PO: 100 mg/d; *max:* 100 mg/d	Formerly used for prophylaxis and treatment against influenza A virus. If used, monitor renal and hepatic functions; dosing may need to be adjusted. Because of resistance in circulating influenza A, amantadines (e.g., amantadine, rimantadine) are *not* recommended; influenza A is sensitive to oseltamivir and zanamivir. Avoid aspirin-containing products in children with influenza. Pregnancy category: C*; PB: 40%; t½: 13-65 h
Zanamivir	Inhaler: A/C ≥7 y: 2 oral inhalations bid for 5 d Prophylaxis: A/C ≥5 y: 2 oral inhalations once daily for 10 or 28 d	Effective against influenzas A and B. Blocks the function of viral neuraminidase protein by stopping the release of viruses from infected cells. Treatment should begin within 48 h of flu symptoms. Take bronchodilators before zanamivir. Pregnancy category: C*; PB: <10%; t½: 2.5-5 h
ANTIVIRALS: HERPES SPECIES		
Acyclovir	See Prototype Drug Chart 27.4.	Also available as a topical
Famciclovir	Herpes zoster: A: PO: 500 mg q8h for 7 d Herpes simplex: A: PO: 250 mg tid for 7-10 d Herpes genitalis: A: PO: 1000 mg bid for 1 d Herpes labialis: A: PO: 1500 mg single dose	For herpes zoster, herpes genitalis, herpes labialis, and HSV. Start treatment within 48 h of rash onset. Dose adjustment is necessary in patients coinfected with HIV. Monitor renal function; dose adjustment may be necessary with impaired renal function. Can be taken without regard to food. Pregnancy category: B*; PB: <20%; t½: 2-3 h
Ganciclovir sodium	A/C: IV: 5 mg/kg for 7-14 d; then 5 m/kg/dose once daily for 7 d A/C ≥2 y: Ophthal: 1 drop to each affected eye 5 ×/d until healed, then 1 drop tid for 7 d	For CMV infection in immunocompromised patients and for herpes simplex keratitis. Monitor for hematologic toxicity. Handle drugs according to guidelines for chemotherapeutics. *Contraindicated in patients with severe thrombocytopenia.* Monitor renal function; dose may need to be adjusted. Pregnancy category: C*; PB: 1%-2%; t½: 2-6 h
Penciclovir	A/C ≥12 y: Topical: Apply q2h while awake for 4 d	For recurrent herpes labialis (cold sores). Start within 1 h of onset of symptoms. Do not administer to mucous membranes. Pregnancy category: B*; PB: UK; t½: UK
Trifluridine	A/C ≥6 y: Ophthal: 1 gtt q2h to each affected eye while awake; *max:* 9 gtt/d	Used primarily for keratoconjunctivitis due to HSV. Remove contact lenses prior to use. If more than one ophthalmic drug is used, separate instillations by at least 5-10 min. Pregnancy category: C*; PB: UK; t½: 12 min

Continued

TABLE 27.3   Non-HIV Antivirals—cont'd

Generic	Route and Dosage	Uses and Considerations
ANTIVIRALS: HERPES SPECIES		
Valacyclovir hydrochloride	HSV: A/C ≥12 y: PO: 2 g q12h × 2 doses Herpes zoster: A: PO: 1 g tid for 7 d Varicella: C ≥2 y: 20 mg/kg tid for 5 d	Effective against varicella and HSV. May be taken without regard to food. Monitor kidney function. Half-life is increased in patients with ESRD. Pregnancy category: B*; PB: 14%-18%; t½: 2.5-3.3 h
Valganciclovir	CMV retinitis: A: PO: 900 mg bid CMV prophylaxis: A: PO: 900 mg once daily C ≥4 mo: PO: Dose is based on BSA: 7 × BSA × CrCl as a single dose; round the dose to the nearest 10-mg increment; *max.* 900 mg/d	For CMV disease prophylaxis and CMV retinitis in AIDS patients. As with ganciclovir, monitor renal function. May cause hematologic toxicity. Monitor CBC. Do not crush or break tablets. Oral solution is not recommended for adults and should not be mixed with other liquids. Pregnancy category: C*; PB: 1%-2% as ganciclovir; t½: 18 h
ANTIVIRALS: HEPATITIS		
Adefovir dipivoxil (nucleotide analogue)	A/C ≥12 y: PO: 10 mg/d	For chronic HBV, used in combination with lamivudine. Can be taken without regard to food. Monitor renal function. Renal impairment may require dose adjustment. Monitor HBV DNA. Pregnancy category: C*; PB: <4%; t½: 7.5 h
Daclatasvir	A: PO: 30-90 mg once daily	For HCV with or without other comorbidities (e.g., liver transplant, decompensated cirrhosis, HIV). Must be given with sofosbuvir. Dose amount and duration depends on genotype. Monitor liver function and HCV RNA concentration. Monitor HIV RNA if patient has HIV. May be taken without regard to food. Pregnancy category: UK*; PB: 99%; t½: 12-15 h
Convenience drug pack with ombitasvir/ paritaprevir/ ritonavir and dasabuvir	A: PO: 1-day convenience pack with fixed dosage: ombitasvir 12.5 mg, paritaprevir 75 mg, ritonavir 50 mg × 2 tabs and dasabuvir 250 mg × 2 tabs	For HCV with or without cirrhosis. Monitor liver function and HCV RNA concentration. May take with food. Duration of treatment depends on genotype. Pregnancy category: B*; PB: 99.5%; t½: 5.5-6 h
Entecavir	A/C >30 kg: PO: 0.5-1 mg/d C <30 kg: PO: 0.15-0.9 mg/d; weight based	Nucleoside analogue for chronic HBV. Take on an empty stomach. Monitor liver function and HBV DNA viral load. Patients with renal impairment may need dose adjustment. Pregnancy category: C*; PB: 13%; t½: 128-149 h
Lamivudine	See Chapter 29.	Synthetic nucleoside analogue for HBV and HIV
Ledipasvir/ sofosbuvir	A: PO: ledipasvir 90 mg/sofosbuvir 400 mg fixed dose tab; 1 tab daily	For chronic HCV; includes patients with other comorbid conditions (e.g., decompensated liver disease, HIV, liver transplant) as combination therapy with sofosbuvir. Monitor liver function, HCV RNA concentration, and renal function. Must be taken with food if coadministering with ribavirin. Duration of treatment depends on genotype; dependent on genotype, ribavirin may be added. Pregnancy category: X*; PB: 99.8%; t½: 47 h
Ombitasvir, paritaprevir, ritonavir	A: PO: Ombitasvir 12.5 mg/paritaprevir 75 mg/ritonavir 50 mg fixed-dose tab; 2 tabs per day	For HCV without hepatic scarring or cirrhosis. Recommendation to administer with ribavirin for genotype 4. Monitor liver function and HCV RNA concentration. Take with food. Pregnancy category: B*; PB: 97%-99%; t½: 21-25 h (ombitasvir), 5.5 h (paritaprevir), 4 h (ritonavir)
Peginterferon alfa-2a	HBV: A: Subcut or IM: 30-35 million units/wk in divided doses × 16 wk C: Subcut: 3 million units/m² 3 ×/wk for 1 wk then increase to 6 million units HCV: A/C ≥3 y >61 kg: Subcut or IM: 3 million units 3 ×/wk C ≥3 y <61 kg: Subcut: 3 million units/m² 3 ×/wk	For HBV and HCV with compensated liver disease. See Chapter 34 for other uses and considerations. If severe reactions occur, reduce dose. For HCV, may be used in combination with ribavirin. Duration of treatment depends on HCV genotype.

TABLE 27.3 Non-HIV Antivirals—cont'd

Generic	Route and Dosage	Uses and Considerations
ANTIVIRALS: HEPATITIS		
Ribavirin	RSV: C: Aerosol inhalation: 20 mg over 12-18 h/d for 3-7 d Hepatitis C, in combination therapy: A ≥75 kg: PO: 1200 mg/d in 2 divided doses A <75 kg: PO: 1000 mg/d in 2 divided doses C: PO: 15 mg/kg/d Other dosing regimens are available.	Effective for HCV when used as combination therapy with other antivirals. Aerosolized ribavirin therapy requires an experienced clinician. Health care workers should protect eyes when administering aerosol to prevent ocular irritation. Contraindicated during pregnancy. Dosage and duration, as well as coadministration of peginterferon alfa-2a or -2b dependent on genotype. Pregnancy category: X*; PB: NA; t½: 43-298 h
Simeprevir	A: PO: 150 mg once daily	For chronic HCV as combination therapy with sofosbuvir or peginterferon alfa and ribavirin. Duration dependent on genotype and presence of cirrhosis. Monitor liver transaminases, bilirubin, and HCV RNA concentrations. Take with food, and swallow capsules whole. Pregnancy category: C*; PB: 99.9%; t½: 10-13 h
Sofosbuvir	A: PO: 400 mg once daily	For chronic HCV as combination therapy with daclatasvir, ledipasvir, ribavirin, or peginterferon alfa/ribavirin. Drug combination and treatment duration are dependent upon genotype. Monitor HCV RNA concentration and renal function. May be taken without regard to food. Pregnancy category: B*; PB: 61%-65%; t½: 0.4 h (sofosbuvir) and 27 h (metabolite GS-41203)
Tenofovir disoproxil	A: PO: 300 mg once daily. Available as an oral powder in a 40 mg/scoop given with food	Nucleoside analogue for chronic HBV and HIV. Has an additive or synergistic activity when combined with other antiretroviral agents.

*Pregnancy categories have been revised. See http://www.fda.gov/Drugs/DevelopmentApprovalProcess/DevelopmentResources/Labeling/ucm093307.htm for more information.

A, Adult; *AIDS*, acquired immunodeficiency syndrome; *bid*, twice daily; *BSA*, body surface area; *C*, child; *CBC*, complete blood count; *CMV*, cytomegalovirus; *CrCl*, creatinine clearance; *d*, day; *ESRD*, end-stage renal disease; *gtt*, drops; *h*, hour; *HBV*, hepatitis B virus; *HCV*, hepatitis C virus; *HIV*, human immunodeficiency virus; *HSV*, herpes simplex virus; *IM*, intramuscular; *IV*, intravenous; *max*, maximum; *min*, minutes; *mo*, month; *NA*, not applicable; *Ophthal*, ophthalmic solution; *PB*, protein binding; *PO*, by mouth; *q*, every; *RSV*, respiratory syncytial virus; *subcut*, subcutaneous; *t½*, half-life; *tab*, tablet; *tid*, three times daily; *UK*, unknown; *wk*, weeks; *y*, year; *>*, greater than; *≥*, greater than or equal to; *<*, less than.

Side Effects and Adverse Reactions

The side effects and adverse reactions of these two neuraminidase inhibitors include dizziness, headache, insomnia, vertigo, fatigue, and GI disturbances such as nausea, vomiting, and diarrhea. ⚡ Nurses must be aware of a Food and Drug Administration (FDA) advisory that persons receiving oral oseltamivir should be monitored closely for abnormal behavior. Incidence of self-injury and delirium have been reported in postmarketing surveillance.

Herpes Antivirals

The synthetic purine nucleoside antiviral group is effective in interfering with the steps of viral nucleic acid (DNA) synthesis. Drugs in this group of nucleoside analogues include ribavirin, acyclovir, famciclovir, ganciclovir sodium, valacyclovir, and valganciclovir. These drugs are effective in managing herpes simplex viruses (HSV-1, HSV-2), and VZV (chickenpox and shingles).

Acyclovir, famciclovir, and valacyclovir appear equally effective in the treatment of initial episodes and recurrent episodes of genital herpes, but famciclovir appears somewhat less effective for suppression of viral shedding. Topical antivirals for herpes simplex viruses include acyclovir, penciclovir, and trifluridine.

Cytomegalovirus Antivirals

Four antivirals are effective in treating CMV retinitis in persons with **acquired immunodeficiency syndrome (AIDS)**:

ganciclovir, valganciclovir, cidofovir, and foscarnet. Ganciclovir and valganciclovir are synthetic purine nucleoside analogues. Ganciclovir was the first drug approved for treatment of CMV retinitis. Cidofovir is a nucleotide analogue that suppresses viral replication by inhibiting DNA polymerase. Foscarnet selectively inhibits viral-specific DNA polymerases and reverse transcriptases. Due to the emergence of drug resistance, many times it is necessary to use a combination of agents to effectively manage CMV retinitis (Prototype Drug Chart 27.4).

Side Effects and Adverse Reactions

A limiting factor in all antiviral therapy is hematologic toxicity. All patients should be closely monitored for signs of bone marrow suppression and toxicity, including thrombocytopenia, granulocytopenia, and leukopenia. Additionally, all antivirals should be dose adjusted in the setting of kidney dysfunction. Kidney function should be closely monitored during drug therapy because acute kidney failure can occur.

Side effects and adverse reactions to antiviral drugs include nausea, vomiting and diarrhea, headache, dizziness, rash and pruritus, and hematuria. Additionally, when antiviral drugs are administered IV, extravasation may lead to sloughing of the skin. Topical preparations can cause local irritations, and contact lenses should be removed prior to instilling ophthalmic antivirals.

PROTOTYPE DRUG CHART 27.4
Acyclovir Sodium

Drug Class	Dosage
Antiviral Pregnancy category: B*	Neonatal HSV: Neo/Inf <3 mo: IV: 20 mg/kg q8h for 10-21 d based on progression of disease HSV: A: PO: 200-400 mg for 7-10 days; amount, frequency, and duration depend on disease A: IV: 5-10 mg/kg q8h; amount, frequency, and duration depend on disease Herpes zoster virus, immunocompetent: A/C ≥12 y: PO: 800 mg q4h 5 ×/d Herpes zoster virus, immunocompromised and immunocompetent children: A/C ≥12 y: IV: 10 mg/kg q8h C <12 y: 10 mg/kg Herpes simplex encephalitis: A: IV: 5-10 mg/kg q8h until clinical resolution Inf/C ≥3 mo: IV: 10-15 mg/kg q8h for 14-21 d Inf <3 mo: 20 mg/kg q8h for 21 d Also available as a topical preparation for superficial candidiasis
Contraindications	**Drug-Lab-Food Interactions**

Known hypersensitivity to acyclovir and its components, milk protein
  hypersensitivity
Caution: Renal impairment, electrolyte imbalance, dehydration, seizure disorder,
  nursing mothers, young children
	Drug: Increased nephrotoxicity and neurotoxicity with aminoglycosides, probenecid,
	  interferon, and ibuprofen; decreases effect of phenytoin; increases serum
	  concentrations of other antivirals (e.g., tenofovir, entecavir)
	Lab: May increase AST, ALT, serum creatinine, BUN
	Food: Food does not affect absorption.

Pharmacokinetics	**Pharmacodynamics**
Absorption: PO: Poorly absorbed, 15%-30% Distribution: PB: 9%-33% Metabolism: t½: PO: 2.5-3.3 h Excretion: Mostly in urine	PO: Onset: UK; peak: 1.5-2 h; duration: UK IV: Onset: UK; peak: 1 h; duration: UK
Therapeutic Effects/Uses	
To treat herpes simplex and varicella-zoster viruses Mode of Action: Inhibits viral DNA synthesis and inhibits viral DNA polymerase and viral DNA chain; inactivates viral DNA polymerase	
Side Effects	**Adverse Reactions**

Nausea, anorexia, vomiting, diarrhea, headache, tremors, agitation,
  lethargy, rash, pruritus, increased bleeding time, phlebitis at IV site
	Urticaria, anemia, paresthesias
	Life threatening: Crystalluria, neuropathy, seizures, nephrotoxicity (large doses), blood
	  dyscrasias

*Pregnancy categories have been revised. See http://www.fda.gov/Drugs/DevelopmentApprovalProcess/DevelopmentResources/Labeling/ucm
093307.htm for more information.

A, Adult; *ALT,* alanine aminotransferase; *AST,* aspartate aminotransferase; *BUN,* blood urea nitrogen; *C,* child; *d,* day; *h,* hour; *HSV,* herpes simplex
virus; *IV,* intravenous; *mo,* months; *Neo/Inf,* neonate/infant; *PB,* protein binding; *PO,* by mouth; *q,* every; *t½,* half-life; *UK,* unknown; *y,* year; <, less
than; ≥, greater than or equal to.

NURSING PROCESS
Patient-Centered Collaborative Care

Antiviral: Acyclovir

Assessment
- Obtain a medical history from the patient that includes any serious renal or hepatic diseases.
- Determine baseline vital signs and obtain a complete blood count (CBC). Use these findings for comparisons with future results.
- Assess baseline laboratory results, particularly BUN, serum creatinine, liver function studies, bilirubin, and electrolytes. Use these results for future comparisons.
- Evaluate baseline vital signs and urine output. Report abnormal findings.

Nursing Diagnoses
- Infection, Risk for
- Injury, Risk for
- Knowledge, Deficient related to inexperience with antiviral medications

Planning
- Patient's symptoms of viral infections will be eliminated or diminished.

Nursing Interventions
- Check the patient's CBC. Report abnormal results (leukopenia, thrombocytopenia, low hemoglobin and hematocrit).
- Monitor other laboratory tests (BUN, serum creatinine, liver function studies); compare with baseline values.

- Record the patient's urinary output. An antiviral drug such as acyclovir can affect renal function.
- Monitor vital signs, especially blood pressure. Acyclovir and amantadine may cause orthostatic hypotension.
- Observe for signs and symptoms of side effects. Most antiviral drugs have many side effects.
- Check for superimposed infection (superinfection) caused by high doses and prolonged use of an antiviral drug such as acyclovir.
- Administer oral acyclovir as prescribed. Oral doses can be taken at mealtime.
- Dilute the antiviral drug in an appropriate amount of solution as indicated in the drug circular when giving intravenously. Administer IV drug over 60 minutes. Never give acyclovir as a bolus (IV push).

Patient Teaching

- Advise patients to maintain adequate fluid intake to ensure sufficient hydration for drug therapy and to increase urine output.
- Instruct patients with genital herpes to avoid spreading infection by practicing sexual abstinence or by using condoms correctly and consistently. Patients must be aware that while condoms reduce the transmission of disease, they may not eliminate it. Advise women with genital herpes to have a Pap test done as indicated by their health care provider. Cervical cancer is more prevalent in women with genital herpes simplex.
- Guide patients to report adverse reactions, including a decrease in urine output and CNS changes such as dizziness, anxiety, or confusion.
- Warn patients with dizziness resulting from orthostatic hypotension to arise slowly from a sitting to a standing position.
- Tell patients to report any side effects associated with the antiviral drug; this may include nausea and vomiting, diarrhea, increased bleeding time, rash, urticaria, and menstrual abnormalities.
- Teach non–English-speaking patients and family members how to properly use antivirals by providing materials in the patient's first language. Pictures may be helpful.

Evaluation

- Evaluate the effectiveness of the antiviral drug in eliminating the virus or in decreasing symptoms.
- Determine whether any side effects are present.

Hepatitis Antivirals

Viral hepatitis can be caused by at least five distinct viruses that affect the liver: hepatitis A virus (HAV), HBV, HCV, hepatitis D (delta hepatitis, HDV), and hepatitis E. Hepatitis A and E are self-limiting illnesses and do not usually require antiviral therapy. HBV and HCV can develop into chronic hepatitis; those with HBV can be coinfected with HDV. The Centers for Disease Control and Prevention (CDC) and the World Health Organization (WHO) have developed guidelines for screening, treatment, and surveillance of persons with HBV and HCV. Currently, HAV and HBV are vaccine preventable. Vaccines are discussed in Chapter 31.

No specific therapy exists for people with acute HBV. Instead, treatment is mostly supportive. Antivirals are given for people with chronic HBV and signs of liver disease progression to attempt to suppress viral replication and potentially halt liver disease and liver-related deaths. Treatment with antivirals is recommended for all people with chronic HBV who are at high risk of disease progression regardless of age. Currently, five antiviral drugs are approved for this indication: lamivudine, adefovir, entecavir, tenofovir, and peginterferon alfa-2a. Except for peginterferon alfa-2a, all of these are nucleoside analogues, and all have been shown to delay the progression of liver disease (e.g., cirrhosis, hepatic carcinoma). Adefovir inhibits reverse transcription, entecavir inhibits several major stages of viral replication, and lamivudine and tenofovir inhibit the synthesis of viral DNA; however, no antiviral therapy cures HBV. Lamivudine and adefovir are no longer the preferred agents in the treatment of HBV.

Hepatitis C is more prevalent among people who inject drugs. HCV is an RNA virus, whereas HBV is a DNA virus. As with HBV, HCV can cause chronic infection that leads to liver cirrhosis, liver failure, and hepatic carcinoma. No vaccine against HCV is currently available. In addition to peginterferon alfa-2a and -2b, ribavirin, protease inhibitors (e.g., simeprevir and paritaprevir), NS5A inhibitors (e.g., daclatasvir, ledipasvir, ombitasvir), and polymerase inhibitors (e.g., dasabuvir, sofosbuvir) can treat HCV. Many of these antivirals are prepackaged as combination therapy.

Persons with HCV should have genotype testing; HCV has 6 genotypes and more than 50 subtypes, and genotyping can help predict treatment response and duration of treatment. For example, genotypes 2 and 3 respond better to peginterferon alfa-2a or a combination of peginterferon alfa-2a and ribavirin than does genotype 1. Genotypes 2 and 3 only need 24 months of treatment, whereas genotype 1 requires 48 months. Genotype 1 is the most common genotype in the United States. The Infectious Diseases Society of America (IDSA) and the American Association for the Study of Liver Diseases (AASLD) have published treatment guidelines based on genotype (see http://www.hcvguidelines.org/node/72).

Table 27.3 lists the antivirals, uses, and considerations for viral hepatitis. Chapter 29 further illustrates nucleoside analogues.

Side Effects and Adverse Effects

Side effects range from mild to life threatening. Transient exacerbations of viral hepatitis can occur if antivirals are suddenly stopped. HBV and HCV can become resistant to antivirals, therefore routine monitoring of renal and hepatic functions are warranted in addition to monitoring viral load. Nucleoside analogues can cause hepatotoxicity or lactic acidosis, and dose adjustments are recommended in patients with renal impairment. Side effects for peginterferon include depression, fatigue, flulike symptoms, pancytopenia, alopecia, arthralgia, myalgia, anorexia, dysgeusia, thyroid dysfunction, and infection. Ophthalmic dysfunction can also occur (e.g., papilledema, vasculature obstruction). Ribavirin is teratogenic and can also cause hemolytic anemia, and protease inhibitors can cause skin reactions, dysgeusia, and photosensitivity.

CRITICAL THINKING CASE STUDY

CJ, a 41-year-old homeless man, has had a constant cough and night sweats for several months. He consumes about a fifth of liquor over 2 days. Acid-fast bacilli (AFB) smear on the sputum is positive. The health care provider orders a 6- to 9-month antitubercular drug regimen, with the time of therapy to be determined according to sputum and radiograph test results. For 2 months, CJ takes isoniazid (INH), rifampin, and pyrazinamide daily. For the next 4 to 7 months, CJ takes INH and rifampin biweekly.

1. What are some of CJ's risk factors for contracting tuberculosis (TB)? Give other risk factors for contracting TB.
2. CJ received first-line antitubercular drugs for treatment of TB. How can the health professional determine whether the drugs are effective in eradicating the bacillus *Mycobacterium tuberculosis*? Explain your answer.
3. What is the nurse's role in patient teaching concerning the drug regimen?
4. Name at least two serious adverse reactions that can occur when antitubercular drugs are given over an extended period.
5. What laboratory tests should be monitored while CJ takes isoniazid and rifampin? Why?
6. The health care provider orders pyridoxine to be given daily. Give the rationale for the use of pyridoxine.

NCLEX STUDY QUESTIONS

1. A patient is beginning isoniazid and rifampin treatment for tuberculosis. The nurse gives the patient which instruction?
   a. Do not skip doses.
   b. Take both drugs three times daily with food.
   c. Take an antacid with the drugs to decrease gastrointestinal distress.
   d. Take rifampin initially, and begin isoniazid after 2 months.
2. A patient taking isoniazid is worried about the side effects. Which of the following does the nurse realize is an adverse effect of the drug?
   a. Ototoxicity
   b. Hepatotoxicity
   c. Nephrotoxicity
   d. Optic nerve toxicity
3. The nurse teaches a patient taking amphotericin B to report which signs and symptoms to the health care provider?
   a. Change in sight
   b. Decrease in hearing
   c. Decrease in urine
   d. Painful red rash and blisters
4. A patient has been diagnosed with tuberculosis and is to begin antitubercular therapy with isoniazid, rifampin, and ethambutol. What should the nurse do? (Select all that apply.)
   a. Encourage periodic eye examinations.
   b. Instruct the patient to take medications with meals.
   c. Suggest that the patient take antacids with medications to prevent gastrointestinal distress.
   d. Advise the patient to report numbness and tingling of the hands or feet.
   e. Alert the patient that body fluids may develop a red-orange color.
   f. Teach the patient to avoid direct sunlight and to use sunblock.

5. Zanamivir is ordered for a patient. What does the nurse know about use of this drug?
   a. It is a treatment for herpes simplex virus type 2.
   b. Oral administration is for treatment of herpes simplex virus type 1.
   c. It treats varicella-zoster virus.
   d. Administration must be within 48 hours of onset of symptoms to be effective.
6. Acyclovir has been ordered for a patient with genital herpes. Which nursing interventions are appropriate for this patient? (Select all that apply.)
   a. Monitor the patient's blood urea nitrogen and creatinine.
   b. Monitor the patient's blood pressure for hypertension.
   c. Administer intravenous acyclovir over 30 minutes.
   d. Advise maintenance of adequate fluid intake.
   e. Monitor complete blood count for blood dyscrasias.
7. A mother of two children was just diagnosed with hepatitis C virus. Which of the following is *incorrect* about hepatitis C virus?
   a. A vaccine is available.
   b. Hepatitis C virus can be transmitted by blood and body fluids.
   c. Hepatitis C virus can cause hepatic carcinoma.
   d. Persons with hepatitis C virus can become chronic carriers.

Answers: 1, a; 2, b; 3, c; 4, a, d, e, f; 5, d; 6, a, d, e; 7, a.

28

Antimalarials, Anthelmintics, and Peptides

http://evolve.elsevier.com/McCuistion/pharmacology/

OBJECTIVES

- Explain the action of antimalarial drugs.
- Identify side effects and adverse reactions of antimalarial drugs.
- Correlate transmission with prevention in people with malaria.
- Apply the nursing process for people receiving antimalarial drugs.
- Explain the action of anthelmintic drugs.
- Identify adverse reactions of anthelmintic drugs.

- Correlate transmission with prevention in people with helminthic infections.
- Apply the nursing process for people receiving anthelmintic drugs.
- Explain the use of peptides as an antibacterial.
- Summarize the side effects and adverse reactions possible with peptides.
- Apply the nursing process for people taking antibacterials.

OUTLINE

Antimalarial Drugs
    Side Effects and Adverse Reactions
    Nursing Process: Patient-Centered Collaborative Care
        —Antimalarials
Anthelmintic Drugs
    Side Effects and Adverse Reactions
    Nursing Process: Patient-Centered Collaborative Care
        —Anthelmintics

Peptides
    Colistimethate
    Polymyxins
    Bacitracin
    Metronidazole
    Nursing Process: Patient-Centered Collaborative Care
        —Antiinfectives: Peptides
Critical Thinking Case Study
NCLEX Study Questions

KEY TERMS

anthelmintics, p. 395
antibiotic resistance, p. 397
antimalarial drugs, p. 392
drug-resistant infection, p. 397
erythrocytic phase, p. 391
helminthiasis, p. 395
helminths, p. 395

peptides, p. 397
prophylaxis, p. 392
superinfection, p. 400
tissue phase, p. 391
trichinosis, p. 395
World Health Organization (WHO), p. 391

ANTIMALARIAL DRUGS

Malaria is a life-threatening disease that was eliminated from the U.S. in the early 1950s. Since that time, 1500 to 2000 cases of malaria have been reported mostly by recent travelers. The World Health Organization (WHO) is an agency of the United Nations with the purpose of monitoring communicable and noncommunicable disease outbreaks globally. WHO reported an estimated 214 million new cases of malaria in 2015. Sub-Saharan Africa has the highest rate, at 88%. Malaria

is caused by multiple species of protozoan parasites of the genus *Plasmodium* that are carried by infected *Anopheles* mosquitoes, and it remains one of the most prevalent protozoan diseases. After the mosquito infects the human, the protozoan parasite passes through two phases: the tissue phase and the erythrocytic phase. The tissue phase (invasion of body tissue) produces no clinical symptoms in the human, but the erythrocytic phase (invasion of the red blood cells) causes symptoms of chills, fever, and sweating. The incubation period is 10 to 35 days, followed by flulike symptoms. Preventing transmission of malaria can be done by controlling the mosquito firstly through insecticide-treated mosquito nets and secondly with spraying.

There are approximately 50 species of *Plasmodium,* four of which cause malaria: *P. malariae, P. ovale, P. vivax,* and *P. falciparum. P. vivax* is the most prevalent, whereas *P. falciparum* is the most severe. In spite of having over 200 million cases of malaria globally, in the United States malaria is confined mainly to persons who enter the country after having traveled abroad. The incidence of malaria has increased since 1960, primarily because of travel to regions in the world where malaria is endemic and drug-resistant malaria parasites have evolved.

Treatment of malaria depends on the type of *Plasmodium* and the organism's life cycle. Quinine was the only antimalarial drug available from 1820 until the early 1940s. Antimalarial drugs provide treatment and prophylaxis, and synthetic antimalarial drugs have since been developed that are as effective as quinine and cause fewer toxic effects. When drug-resistant

malaria occurs, combinations of antimalarials are used to facilitate effective treatment. Chloroquine is a commonly prescribed drug for malaria. If drug resistance to chloroquine occurs, another antimalarial such as mefloquine hydrochloride (HCl) or combinations of antimalarials with or without antibiotics (e.g., tetracycline, doxycycline, clindamycin) may be prescribed.

Three methods used to eradicate malaria are prophylaxis (prevention), treatment for the acute attack, and prevention of relapse. Many synthetic antimalarials, chloroquine and primaquine among them, are used prophylactically. Chloroquine and mefloquine are frequently used to treat an acute malarial attack. Mefloquine HCl and the combination drug atovaquone-proguanil are used to treat chloroquine-resistant *P. falciparum.* Chloroquine and hydroxychloroquine can be toxic to children and may even cause death, therefore the drug dose should be closely monitored. Prototype Drug Chart 28.1 lists the drug data for chloroquine phosphate.

PROTOTYPE DRUG CHART 28.1
Chloroquine Phosphate

Drug Class	Dosage
Antimalarial Pregnancy category: C*	Acute malaria: 500 mg chloroquine phosphate (salt) = 300 mg chloroquine base; doses expressed as chloroquine base A: PO: 600 mg base (=1000 mg salt) x 1, then 300 mg base (=500 mg salt) x 1 in 6 h, then 300 mg base (=500 mg salt) x 1 at 24 h and 48 h C: PO: 10 mg base/kg x 1, then 5 mg base/kg x 1 at 6 h, 24 h, and 48 h Prophylaxis: 1-2 wk before exposure; discontinue 4 wk after exposure A: PO: 300 mg base (=500 mg salt) every 6 h x 2 doses, then 300 mg base (=500 mg salt) every week C: PO: 5 mg base/kg every 6 h x 2 doses before exposure, then 5 mg base/kg every week discontinuing 4 wk after exposure
Contraindications Chloroquine hypersensitivity, renal disease, psoriasis, ocular disease *Caution:* Alcoholism, liver dysfunction, G-6-PD deficiency, and with GI, neurologic (seizures, hearing impairment), and hematologic disorders; breastfeeding.	**Drug-Lab-Food Interactions** Drug: Increases effects of digoxin, neuromuscular blockers; decreased absorption with antacids and laxatives Lab: Elevated liver enzymes; decreased RBC count, hemoglobin, hematocrit; monitor ophthalmic exams.
Pharmacokinetics Absorption: Well absorbed from GI tract Distribution: Widely distributed into body tissue PB: 50%-65% Metabolism: Partially in the liver Half-life: 1-2 months Excretion: Excreted slowly in urine	**Pharmacodynamics** Onset: Rapid Peak: 1-2 h Duration: Days to weeks
Therapeutic Effects/Uses To treat acute malaria, as prophylaxis for malaria Mode of Action: Increased pH in the malaria parasite inhibits parasitic growth.	
Side Effects Anorexia, nausea, vomiting, diarrhea, abdominal cramps, fatigue, pruritus, headache, nervousness, visual impairment, insomnia, photosensitivity, hair discoloration	**Adverse Reactions** ECG changes, hypotension, psychosis, seizures; may cause dizziness, so use caution driving a vehicle; avoid sun exposure. *Life threatening:* Agranulocytosis, aplastic anemia, corneal opacity, macular degeneration, thrombocytopenia, ototoxicity, cardiovascular collapse

*Pregnancy categories have been revised. See http://www.fda.gov/Drugs/DevelopmentApprovalProcess/DevelopmentResources/Labeling/ucm093307.htm for more information.
A, Adult; *C,* child; *ECG,* electrocardiogram; *G-6-PD,* glucose-6-phosphate dehydrogenase; *GI,* gastrointestinal; *h,* hour; *PB,* protein binding; *PO,* by mouth; *RBC,* red blood cell; *wk,* week.

Pharmacokinetics Chloroquine phosphate is well absorbed from the gastrointestinal (GI) tract. It is moderately protein binding, and the drug has a long half-life. The first two doses have a loading dose effect. Because of the drug's long half-life, the next dose is given in 6 hours, the third and fourth doses are given at 24 and 48 hours. Chloroquine is metabolized in the liver to active metabolites and is excreted in the urine. Antimalarial drugs concentrate first in the liver; if the patient drinks large amounts of alcohol or has a liver disorder, the liver enzymes will require closer monitoring. Renal impairment may also occur as an adverse effect of antimalarials.

Pharmacodynamics Chloroquine phosphate inhibits the malaria parasite's growth by interfering with its protein synthesis. Whether the drug is given orally or intramuscularly (IM), the onset of action is rapid. The peak effect is slower when given orally. The duration of effect of the drug is very long, from days to weeks.

Side Effects and Adverse Reactions

General side effects and adverse reactions to antimalarials include GI upset, cranial nerve VIII involvement (quinine and chloroquine), renal impairment (quinine), and cardiovascular effects (quinine).

Table 28.1 lists commonly ordered antimalarial drugs and their dosage, uses, and considerations. Note that *quinine* is an antimalarial drug, and *quinidine* is an antidysrhythmic drug. A medication guideline developed by the U.S. Food and Drug Administration (FDA) accompanies mefloquine each time it is dispensed. This type of guideline is used only for drugs that require monitoring for serious adverse effects. Adverse effects of mefloquine include severe anxiety, restlessness, disorientation, depression, hallucinations, paranoia, and suicidal thoughts, which may continue after the drug is discontinued.

> ⚡ **PATIENT SAFETY**
>
> **Do not confuse...**
> - *Quinine* (antimalarial) with *quinidine* (antidysrhythmic)
> - *Hydroxychloroquine* (antimalarial drug) and *hydroxyurea* (chemotherapy drug)

TABLE 28.1	Antimalarials	
Generic	**Route and Dosage**	**Uses and Considerations**
Chloroquine phosphate	See Prototype Drug Chart 28.1.	
Hydroxychloroquine sulfate	Acute malaria: A: PO: 800 mg, then 400 mg at 6, 18, 24, and 36 h Prophylaxis: A: 400 mg once every day for 7 d; begin 2 wk before exposure, continue after leaving endemic area, then continue for 8 wk. C: PO: 13 mg/kg/dose, then 6.4 mg/kg once every day for 7 d; begin 2 wk before exposure and continue for 8 wk after leaving endemic area.	Alternative to chloroquine. Dosage varies for treating malaria. Can be used adjunctively with primaquine. Give with meals to reduce GI distress. Administration requires an experienced clinician. *Caution:* During pregnancy, in patients with psoriasis or retinal disturbances, and with history of alcoholism or hepatic impairment Pregnancy category: C*; PB: 45%; t½: 32-50 d
Mefloquine hydrochloride	Treatment of mild/moderate disease: A: PO: Single dose: 1250 mg Malaria prophylaxis: A: PO: 250 mg/wk for 1-2 wk before travel and 4 wk after; take with plenty of water.	For prophylaxis and treatment of acute malaria. Contraindicated in people with cardiac conditions, seizures, psychosis, and alcoholism. Use with caution with hepatic impairment. Safety and efficacy have not been established for infants and children under 20 kg. Is secreted in breast milk. Pregnancy category: C*; PB: 98%; t½: 10-21 d
Primaquine phosphate	Malaria treatment: (26.3 mg primaquine phosphate = 15 mg primaquine base; doses are given as primaquine base) A: PO: 30 mg base/d for 14 d C: PO: 0.8 mg/kg for 14 d Malaria prophylaxis: A: PO: 30 mg base/d for 14 d; continue during stay in the endemic area and for 7 d after returning.	For malaria caused by *Plasmodium vivax, P. ovale,* and *P. falciparum* as well as for *Pneumocystis carinii* pneumonia. Can affect WBC production (granulocytopenia) and can cause acute hemolytic anemia in patients with G-6-PD deficiency. Pregnancy category: C*; PB: UK; t½: 6 h
Quinine	Acute malaria: A/Adol >16 y: PO: 648 mg q8h for 3-7 d C <16 y: 10 mg/kg/dose every 3-7 h for 7 d; *max:* 648 mg	Used in combination drug therapy (with tetracycline, clindamycin, or doxycycline) or for chloroquine-resistant malaria. Quinine may be used as step-down therapy from IV quinidine. Avoid in patients with hepatic or cardiac impairment, hypersensitivity to quinine drugs, hypoglycemia (it stimulates insulin; blood glucose levels should be monitored), and thrombocytopenia (monitor platelet count). Pregnancy category: C*; PB: 70%; t½: 8-21 h

Continued

TABLE 28.1 Antimalarials—cont'd

Generic	Route and Dosage	Uses and Considerations
COMBINATION ANTIMALARIAL DRUGS		
Atovaquone-proguanil combination tablet	A/C >40 kg: PO: 4 adult tabs of atovaquone 250 mg/proguanil 100 mg in a single dose (for a total of atovaquone 1000 mg/proguanil 400 mg) for 3 d C 31-40 kg: PO: 3 tabs atovaquone 250 mg/proguanil 100 mg in a single dose (for a total of atovaquone 750 mg/proguanil 300 mg) for 3 d C 21-30 kg: PO: 2 tabs atovaquone 250 mg/proguanil 100 mg in a single dose (for a total of atovaquone 500 mg/proguanil 200 mg) for 3 d C 11-20 kg: PO: 1 tab atovaquone 250 mg/proguanil 100 mg each day for 3 d	For acute and uncomplicated prophylaxis and treatment of malaria; effective for chloroquine-resistant strains. *Caution:* Renal and hepatic impairment Pregnancy category: C*; PB: 75%-99%; t½: 2-3 d/12-20 h
Artemether-lumefantrine combination tablet	A/C >35 kg: PO: 4 tabs of artemether 20 mg/lumefantrine 120 mg twice daily for 3 d, for a total of 6 doses C 25-35 kg: PO: 3 tabs artemether 20 mg/lumefantrine 120 mg twice daily for 3 d, for a total of 6 doses C 15-25 kg: PO: 2 tabs artemether 20 mg/lumefantrine 120 mg twice daily for 3 d, for a total of 6 doses C 5-15 kg: PO: 1 tab artemether 20 mg/lumefantrine 120 mg twice daily for 3 d for a total of 6 doses	For malaria infections that are both drug-sensitive and drug-resistant *P. falciparum.* Acts by inhibiting nucleic acid and protein synthesis. Rapid onset allows drug to control fever quickly. Has a cure rate >40%. Adverse effects include nystagmus, wheezing, hypokalemia, blood dyscrasias, and hepatomegaly. Pregnancy category: C*; PB: 95%-99%; t½: 2-3 h/3-6 d

*Pregnancy categories have been revised. See http://www.fda.gov/Drugs/DevelopmentApprovalProcess/DevelopmentResources/Labeling/ucm093 307.htm for more information.

A, Adult; *Adol,* adolescent; *C,* child; *d,* day; *G-6-PD,* glucose-6-phosphate dehydrogenase; *GI,* gastrointestinal; *h,* hour; *IV,* intravenous; *max,* maximum; *PB,* protein binding; *PO,* by mouth; *q,* every; *t½,* half-life; *tabs,* tablets; *UK,* unknown; *WBC,* white blood cell; *wk,* week; *y,* year; *>,* greater than; *<,* less than.

◎ NURSING PROCESS
Patient-Centered Collaborative Care
Antimalarials

Assessment
- Assess patient's hearing, especially if receiving quinine or chloroquine. These drugs may affect cranial nerve VIII.
- Assess patient for visual changes; this is especially important if a patient is taking chloroquine and hydroxychloroquine.
- Assess the patient's level of consciousness.
- Assess whether the patient has traveled out of the country to a malaria-endemic area.
- Obtain a patient history of malaria and whether antimalarial drugs were taken.
- Assess baseline urinary output.
- Assess whether the patient has allergies to any drugs.

Nursing Diagnoses
- Infection, Risk for
- Knowledge, Readiness for Enhanced
- Skin Integrity, Risk for Impaired
- Nutrition, Imbalanced: Less than Body Requirements

Planning
- The patient will exhibit vital signs at baseline level showing absence of malarial symptoms.
- The patient will take antimalarial drugs at the times and dosages prescribed.
- The patient will utilize preventive measures when in the outside environment.

Nursing Interventions
- ⚡ Monitor renal and liver function by checking urine output (>600 mL/d) and liver enzymes.
- ⚡ Report if the patient's serum liver enzymes are elevated or if renal function tests are abnormal.
- Monitor the patient for impaired consciousness, headache, or seizures.

Patient Teaching
- Advise patients traveling to malaria-endemic countries to receive prophylactic doses of an antimalarial drug before leaving, during the visit, and upon their return.
- Teach patients to take oral antimalarial drugs with food or at mealtime if GI upset occurs.
- Monitor patients returning from malaria-endemic areas for malarial symptoms.
- Inform patients who take chloroquine or hydroxychloroquine to report vision changes immediately.
- Advise patients to avoid consuming large quantities of alcohol.

Side Effects
- Direct patients to report signs and symptoms of anorexia, nausea, vomiting, diarrhea, abdominal cramps, pruritus, visual disturbances, and dizziness.

Cultural Considerations
- Advise patients returning from malaria-endemic areas to be tested for malaria if they experience chills, high fever, and profuse sweating.
- Provide patient education in clear, understandable language about any prescribed antimalarial drug.

Evaluation
- Evaluate the effectiveness of the antimalarial drug by determining that the patient is free of symptoms.
- Evaluate the patient's understanding of the medication regimen.

ANTHELMINTIC DRUGS

Helminths are large parasitic worms that live and lay eggs in warm, moist soil where sanitation and hygiene are poor (Centers for Disease Control and Prevention [CDC], 2013). Transmission occurs from infected soil to the person, whereupon the helminth then feeds on host tissue. The most common site for helminthiasis (worm infection) is the intestine. Other sites for parasitic infection are the lymphatic system, blood vessels, and liver. These parasites cause disability and developmental delays in children and adolescents.

Groups of helminths include (1) cestodes (tapeworms), (2) trematodes (flukes), (3) intestinal nematodes (roundworms), and (4) tissue-invading nematodes (tissue roundworms and filariae). They enter the human host via contaminated food, bites of carrier insects, or direct penetration of the skin. The cestodes (tapeworms) are segmented and enter the intestine via contaminated food. There are four species of cestodes: *Taenia solium* (pork tapeworm), *T. saginata* (beef tapeworm), *Diphyllobothrium latum* (fish tapeworm), and *Hymenolepis nana* (dwarf tapeworm). The segmented cestodes have heads and hooks or suckers that attach to the tissue.

The trematodes (flukes) are flat, nonsegmented parasites that feed on the host. Four types of trematodes exist: *Fasciola hepatica* (liver fluke), *Fasciolopsis buski* (intestinal fluke), *Paragonimus westermani* (lung fluke), and *Schistosoma* species (blood flukes).

Five types of nematodes may feed on intestinal tissue: *Ascaris lumbricoides* (giant roundworm), *Necator americanus* (hookworm), *Enterobius vermicularis* (pinworm), *Strongyloides stercoralis* (threadworm), and *Trichuris trichiura* (whipworm).

Two types of nematodes are tissue-invading: *Trichinella spiralis* (pork roundworm) and *Wuchereria bancrofti* (filariae). The pork roundworm *T. spiralis* can cause trichinosis, a disease caused by ingestion of raw or inadequately cooked pork that contains larvae of the *T. spiralis* parasite, which can be diagnosed by muscle biopsy. By thoroughly cooking pork, the roundworm is destroyed.

Side Effects and Adverse Reactions

The common side effects of anthelmintics (agents that destroy worms) include various manifestations of GI distress, such as anorexia, nausea, vomiting, and occasionally diarrhea and stomach cramps. The neurologic problems associated with anthelmintics are dizziness, weakness, headache, and drowsiness. Adverse reactions do not occur frequently because the drugs usually are given for a short period (1 to 3 days). Prototype Drug Chart 28.2 lists dosages and drug data for ivermectin, and Table 28.2 lists anthelmintic drugs prescribed to treat various types of parasitic worms.

PROTOTYPE DRUG CHART 28.2

Ivermectin

Drug Class	Dosage
Synthetic anthelmintic Pregnancy category: C*	Topically (for head lice only): Apply to affected area. Avoid contact with eyes and mouth. Onchocerciasis: A/C >15 kg: PO: 0.15 mg/kg single dose with retreatment in 3-12 months Strongyloidiasis: A/C >15 kg: PO: 0.2 mg/kg single dose followed with stool exam
Contraindications	**Drug-Lab-Food Interactions**
Pediatric dosage safety and efficacy have not been established. Contraindicated for those hypersensitive to the drug's components. *Caution:* Asthma, hepatic impairment; not recommended with breastfeeding	Take on an empty stomach with water. Monitor ophthalmic exams, and follow up with stool exams.
Pharmacokinetics	**Pharmacodynamics**
Absorption: Well absorbed Distribution: Widely distributed within the body; does not cross blood-brain barrier Mode of Action: Binds with chloride ions, increases cell permeability, and kills the parasite PB: 93% Half-life: 18 h Metabolism: Liver Excretion: In feces (over 12 d) and urine (<1%)	Peak: 4 h
Therapeutic Effects/Uses	
Drug of choice for strongyloidiasis and onchocerciasis Follow up and retreat as necessary.	
Side Effects	**Adverse Reactions**
Dizziness, nausea, pruritus	Lymph node swelling, abdominal pain, ocular effects and opacity, tachycardia, and increased liver enzymes (AST, ALT)

*Pregnancy categories have been revised. See http://www.fda.gov/Drugs/DevelopmentApprovalProcess/DevelopmentResources/Labeling/ucm093307.htm for more information.
A/C, Adult/child; *ALT,* alanine aminotransferase; *AST,* aspartate aminotransferase; *d,* day; *h,* hour; *PB,* protein binding; *PO,* by mouth; <, less than; >, greater than.

TABLE 28.2 Anthelmintics

Generic	Route and Dosage	Uses and Considerations
Bithionol	A: PO: 30-50 mg/kg in 2 daily doses given every other day with food for 10-15 doses	Effective against flukes. For *Paragonimus* or *Fasciola* species when a patient cannot receive praziquantel due to resistance or adverse effect.
Ivermectin	See Prototype Drug Chart 28.2.	
Praziquantel	A/C >4 y: PO: 20-25 mg/kg tid for 1-2 d	Anthelmintic/antiparasitic for treatment of beef, pork, and fish tapeworms; blood flukes; and liver, lung, and intestinal flukes. *Caution:* Dizziness can occur; caution patient to avoid driving and operating machinery; use with caution in patients with cardiac or hepatic impairment, seizures Pregnancy category: B*; PB: 80%-85%; t½: 0.8-1.5 h
Pyrantel pamoate	A/C >2 y: PO: Roundworm: 11 mg/kg, single dose Pinworm: 11 mg/kg every 2 wk x 2 doses Hookworm: 11 mg/kg daily x 3 doses *max:* 1 g	For giant roundworm, hookworm, and pinworm. Pregnancy category: C*; PB: UK; t½: UK

*Pregnancy categories have been revised. See http://www.fda.gov/Drugs/DevelopmentApprovalProcess/DevelopmentResources/Labeling/ucm093307.htm for more information.
A, Adult; *C,* child; *d,* day; *h,* hour; *max,* maximum; *PB,* protein binding; *PO,* by mouth; *t½,* half-life; *tid,* three times a day; *UK,* unknown; *wk,* week; *y,* year; *>,* greater than; *<,* less than.

◎ NURSING PROCESS
Patient-Centered Collaborative Care
Anthelmintics

Assessment
- Assess whether the patient has traveled to other countries.
- Assess the patient's health behavior when at home; also assess handwashing facilities, disposal of waste, access to safe drinking water, and whether the patient walks barefoot in soil.
- Obtain a history of foods the patient has eaten and how the food was prepared.
- Document whether any other person in the household has been checked for helminths (worms).
- Assess the patient for complaints of anal itching and abdominal discomfort.
- Assess baseline vital signs, and collect a stool specimen.

Nursing Diagnoses
- Coping, Defensive
- Activity Intolerance, Risk for
- Nutrition, Imbalanced: Less than Body Requirements
- Body Image, Disturbed
- Knowledge, Deficient
- Gastrointestinal Motility, Risk for Dysfunctional

Planning
- The patient will demonstrate handwashing before eating.
- The patient will explain how to prepare foods properly to avoid recurrence.
- The patient will identify changes needed at home to ensure sanitation in food preparation.
- The patient will describe methods of infection control within the home.

Nursing Interventions
- ⚡ Discuss benefits of handwashing before eating and after working in the soil or with animals.
- Monitor intake and output.
- Collect the stool specimen in a clean container. Avoid having stool come in contact with water, urine, or chemicals, which could destroy parasitic worms.
- ⚡ Administer the prescribed anthelmintic after meals to prevent or minimize occurrence of GI distress.
- ⚡ Monitor adverse reactions, which can include wheezing, abdominal pain, and high fever.
- Check laboratory values of iron, iodine, and vitamin A to monitor nutritional status.

Patient Teaching
- Explain to the patient the importance of handwashing before meals and after going to the toilet. The parasite can be transferred within the family if proper hygiene is not used.
- Advise the patient to take daily showers and not baths.
- Encourage the patient to change sheets, bedclothes, towels, and underwear daily.
- Advise the patient that a second course of anthelmintic may be necessary if helminthiasis persists after therapy.
- Emphasize the importance of taking the prescribed drug at the designated times and keeping health care appointments.
- Teach the patient to read all directions regarding over-the-counter (OTC) drugs before use.
- Warn the patient that drowsiness may occur and that operating a car or machinery should be avoided if this should happen.
- Teach the patient to report any side effects or adverse reactions to the health care provider.

- Recognize that community involvement may be needed if an area is at high risk for poor sanitation.
- Obtain an interpreter when necessary; do not rely on family members, who may not fully disclose because of honor or shame or because of lack of understanding of medical terminology.

Evaluation
- Evaluate effectiveness of anthelmintic therapy and absence of side effects.
- Determine whether the patient is using proper hygiene to avoid the spread of parasitic worms.
- Evaluate the patient's knowledge of preventative measures for helminthiasis.

PEPTIDES

The Center for Communicable Disease, a governmental health agency that prevents and reduces communicable diseases in the United States and globally, has launched an initiative for health care providers and patients to prevent drug-resistant infection. Antibiotic therapy is challenged by increasing occurrence of drug-resistant infections such as methicillin-resistant *Staphylococcus aureus* (MRSA) and carbapenem-resistant *Enterobacteriaceae* (CRE). Antimicrobial peptides provide a broad spectrum and bactericidal ability to kill a range of parasites and viruses. There is ongoing research in combining antibiotics as multidrug regimens, which in turn can reduce antibiotic resistance.

Peptides classifications include antiviral, antimicrobial, antifungal, and antiparasitic. The two groups of peptides used as antibiotics are the polymyxins and bacitracin. Peptides are derived from cultures of *Bacillus subtilis,* and this group appears to interfere with bacterial cell membrane function.

Colistimethate

Colistimethate is a polypeptide antibiotic that targets aerobic gram-negative bacteria. It is used to treat *Pseudomonas aeruginosa,* CRE, and *Klebsiella* and *Shigella* species. This antibiotic has the capacity to penetrate and disrupt the bacterial cell. Colistimethate is available in forms administrated IM, intravenously (IV), and by inhalation. Common reactions include dyspepsia, tingling, slurred speech, dizziness, paresthesia, pruritus, rash and fever. Serious reactions include nephrotoxicity, neurotoxicity, neuromuscular blockade, respiratory distress, apnea, superinfection and *C. difficile*–associated diarrhea. Acute respiratory distress syndrome can occur when the antibiotic is administered by inhalation.

Polymyxins

Polymyxins were one of the early groups of antimicrobials, but many of the early drugs were discontinued because of severe toxic reactions such as neurotoxicity and nephrotoxicity. Polymyxins are polypeptide antibiotics that consist of five different chemical compounds, polymyxins A through E. Currently, polymyxin B and polymyxin E (also known as colistin) are used in clinical practice. Polymyxins produce a bactericidal effect by interfering with the cell membrane of the bacterium, thereby causing cell death. They affect most gram-negative bacteria, such as *P. aeruginosa, Escherichia coli,* and *Klebsiella* and *Shigella* species.

The polymyxins are not absorbed through the oral route except for colistin, which exerts action on the colon and is excreted in the feces. Intramuscular injection of polymyxins produces intense pain at the injection site. Consequently, parenteral polymyxins are administered at a slow IV infusion rate. Table 28.3 lists antiinfective peptides with dosage and uses.

Severe Adverse Effects

High serum levels of polymyxins can cause nephrotoxicity and neurotoxicity. In nephrotoxicity, the blood urea nitrogen (BUN) and serum creatinine levels are elevated, but when the serum drug level decreases, renal toxicity is usually reversed. Signs and symptoms of neurotoxicity (toxicity of the nerves) include paresthesias—abnormal sensations such as numbness, tingling, burning, and prickling—and dizziness. Neurotoxicity is usually reversible when the drug is discontinued.

Bacitracin

Bacitracin has a polypeptide structure and acts by inhibiting bacterial cell-wall synthesis and damaging the cell-wall membrane, which results in death of the cell. The drug action can be bacteriostatic or bactericidal. Bacitracin is not absorbed by the GI tract; if given orally, it is excreted in the feces. Bacitracin is effective against most gram-positive bacteria and some gram-negative bacteria. OTC bacitracin ointment is available for application to the skin. The side effects of bacitracin include skin redness and rash, nausea, and vomiting. Severe adverse reactions are renal damage and ototoxicity, and mild to severe allergic reactions that range from hives to anaphylaxis may occur.

Metronidazole

Metronidazole is a synthetic antibiotic and antiprotozoal (nitroimidazole class) that works by disrupting the bacterial DNA and inhibiting cell synthesis, which causes cell death. Metronidazole as a protozoal treats *Trichomonas vaginalis,* amebiasis, and giardiasis; as an antibiotic, it is used for anaerobic bacteria, including *Helicobacter pylori,* a pathogen in GI infections. Additionally, this drug has immunosuppressive and antiinfective properties that treat rosacea. This drug can be added to multidrug regimens in order to reduce antibiotic resistance, which occurs when the bacteria are not sensitive to the antibiotic. Metronidazole can be administered orally, parenterally, topically, and intravaginally. Toxic reactions include neurologic disturbances such as seizures and peripheral neuropathies. Prototype Drug Chart 28.3 provides information on metronidazole.

⚡ PATIENT SAFETY

To avoid antibiotic resistance, counsel patients to:
- Ask their health care provider if they can be treated without antibiotics.
- Take antibiotics as prescribed.
- Never skip doses and complete all of the antibiotic, even if they feel better.
- Never take someone else's antibiotic.

TABLE 28.3   Antiinfectives

Generic	Route and Dosage	Uses and Considerations
PEPTIDES		
Bacitracin	A/C: Topical: Apply a thin layer two or three times daily. A/C: Ophthalmic ointment: Apply a thin film to the affected eye q3-4h for 7-10 d.	Topical ointment is for skin infections; ophthalmic ointment is for eye infections. Pregnancy category: C*; PB: <20%; t½: UK
Colistimethate sodium	A/C: IM/IV: 2.5-5 mg/kg/d in divided doses; *max.* 5 mg/kg/d NEB: 75 mg every 12 h	For *Pseudomonas aeruginosa, Escherichia coli,* and *Klebsiella* and *Shigella* species; can be used for CRE infection. Pregnancy category: C*; PB: UK: t½: 2-3 h Treats multidrug-resistant strains of serious gram-negative infections (e.g. UTI, septicemia, bacteremia, meningitis, skin infections) when other antibiotics are ineffective or contraindicated. Side effects include GI discomfort, headache, and depression. Adverse reactions include respiratory failure, neurotoxicity, and nephrotoxicity. *Prolonged use may result in fungal or bacterial superinfection.* Use with caution in renal patients and in pregnancy. Pregnancy category: B*; PB: 10%; t½: 6-8 h
ADDITIONAL ANTIINFECTIVE AGENTS		
Metronidazole	See Prototype Drug Chart 28.3	
Polymyxin B	A/C: Ophthalmic: 25,000 U/kg/d A/C: Topical: 0.1%-0.25% A/C: IM: 25,000-30,000 U/kg in divided doses q4-6h	Routine IM administration is not recommended. Commonly used as an ophthalmic, otic, and topical treatment. Also combined with neomycin for urinary tract irrigation. *Caution:* In pregnancy and while breastfeeding; with IM administration, renal disease, hypersensitivity to the drug A polypeptide antibiotic for gram-negative bacteria including *P. aeruginosa, E. coli, Haemophilus influenzae, Enterobacter aerogenes,* and *Klebsiella* spp. Rarely used via the IM route because of toxic reactions (nephrotoxicity, neurotoxicity) and pain at the injection site. *Adverse reactions:* Facial swelling, difficulty breathing, paresthesias

*Pregnancy categories have been revised. See http://www.fda.gov/Drugs/DevelopmentApprovalProcess/DevelopmentResources/Labeling/ucm093307.htm for more information.

A, Adult; *bid,* twice daily; *C,* child; *CNS,* central nervous system; *CRE,* carbapenem-resistant *Enterobacteriaceae; d,* day; *GI,* gastrointestinal; *h,* hour; *IM,* intramuscular; *IV,* intravenous; *max,* maximum; *NEB,* nebulizer; *PB,* protein binding; *PO,* by mouth; *q,* every; *t½,* half-life; *UK,* unknown; *UTI,* urinary tract infection; <, less than; ≥, greater than or equal to.

PROTOTYPE DRUG CHART 28.3

Metronidazole

Drug Class	Dosage
Antibacterial peptide, amebicide Systemic and topical Pregnancy category: B*	Topical: Apply a thin layer to the affected area. Systemic for anaerobic infections: A: IV: 15 mg/kg x 1, then 7.5 mg/kg q6h C: IV: 30 mg/kg/d in divided doses q6h (*max.* 4 g/d) Trichomoniasis: A and C >45 kg: PO: 2 g x 1 or 500 mg bid for 7 d C <45 kg: 15 mg/kg/day PO, divided doses q8h x 7 d Giardiasis: A: 250 mg q8h for 5-7 d Amebiasis: A: PO: 750 mg q8h for 5-10 d C: PO: 35-50 mg/kg divided dose q8h for 10-14 d *Clostridium difficile*–associated diarrhea: A: PO: 500 mg tid for 10-14 d C: PO: 30 mg/kg/d divided doses q6h x 7-10 d Bacterial vaginosis: A and C >45 kg: PO: 500 mg q12h x 7 d C <45 kg: PO: 15 mg/kg/d divided doses q12h x 7 d (*max.* 1 g/d)
Contraindications	**Drug-Lab-Food Interactions**
Hypersensitivity to drug components, first trimester of pregnancy; breastfeeding should be withheld. *Caution:* Liver impairment and cardiac conditions, neoplastic disease	Alcohol is contraindicated. Take immediate-release tablet with food; take extended-release tablet on an empty stomach.
Pharmacokinetics	**Pharmacodynamics**
Absorption: Well absorbed orally; does not cross the blood-brain barrier Distribution: Bile, seminal fluid, bone, liver, lung, vagina Metabolism: PB: 10% Excretion: In urine (60%-80%) and feces (6%-15%) Half-life: 8 h	Oral: Peak: 1-3 h immediate-release tablet Peak: 5 h extended-release tablet

Therapeutic Effects/Uses

Bactericidal in anaerobic infections such as *Helicobacter pylori*; antiprotozoal agent used for *Trichomonas vaginalis* vaginosis, giardiasis, *Clostridium difficile* infection, and amebiasis. Anaerobic infections include skin, intraabdominal, CNS, and lower respiratory infections and endocarditis. Can be applied topically twice daily for rosacea (0.75%).

Mode of Action: Interacts with DNA to inhibit cell nucleic acid synthesis resulting in cell death

Side Effects	Adverse Reactions
Headaches, nausea, flushing, dizziness, superinfection (*Candida* overgrowth) resulting in oral and vaginal candidiasis	Seizures, diarrhea, optic and peripheral neuropathy, hypersensitivity, pruritus, urticaria

*Pregnancy categories have been revised. See http://www.fda.gov/Drugs/DevelopmentApprovalProcess/DevelopmentResources/Labeling/ucm093307.htm for more information.

A, Adult; *bid*, twice daily; *C*, child; *CNS*, central nervous system; *d*, day; *h*, hour; *IV*, intravenous; *max*, maximum; *PO*, by mouth; *q*, every; *tid*, three times daily ; <, less than; >, greater than.

NURSING PROCESS
Patient-Centered Collaborative Care

Antiinfectives: Peptides

Assessment
- Assess whether the patient has any allergies to medications.
- Assess the patient's prior use of antimalarial drugs.
- Assess the patient's level of consciousness.
- Assess renal function and urinary output.
- Assess skin integrity and evaluate for skin rash and pruritus.

Nursing Diagnosis
- Allergy Response, Risk for
- Infection, Risk for
- Injury, Risk for
- Tissue Integrity, Risk for Impaired

Planning
- The patient will show liver and kidney laboratory values at baseline level.
- The patient's skin will be intact without pruritus, swelling, or rash.
- The patient will be able to explain how to properly take the prescribed drug.
- The patient will describe the side effects and adverse reactions that require notification of a health care provider.

Nursing Interventions
- ⚡ Monitor lab values, including liver function tests (aspartate aminotransferase [AST], alanine aminotransferase [ALT]) and evaluation of renal function (BUN, creatinine clearance [CrCl]) and blood serum (platelet count, hemoglobin, hematocrit).
- ⚡ Check urinary function by monitoring intake and output.
- ⚡ Monitor the patient for an altered level of consciousness.

Patient Teaching
- Teach patients to read all instructions prior to taking medications.
- Inform patients to take all prescribed medication.
- Discuss possible side effects that can occur as a reaction to the drug.
- Instruct patients to check for signs of superinfection, such as white patches on the tongue.
- Advise patients to report all adverse reactions to a health care provider, including fever, diarrhea, trouble breathing, and decreased urination.
- Describe urinary signs that indicate impairment, such as decreased urinary flow.
- Advise patients to avoid alcohol.

Side Effects
- Direct patients to report all side effects and adverse reactions.

 Cultural Considerations
- Provide patient information in a clear, concise manner using understandable terms about the action, dose, and precautions of antiinfectives.
- With the patient's approval, include family members to participate in teaching sessions.

Evaluation
- Evaluate effectiveness of treatment by absence of manifestations.
- Evaluate patient understanding of the medication regimen by encouraging patient feedback and questions.

CRITICAL THINKING CASE STUDY

SM is a 40-year-old male who has returned from working in a missionary health clinic in sub-Saharan Africa. He is experiencing fever, headache, and chills. SM states he took his antimalarial pills but stopped when he got to the clinic in Africa. Chloroquine is ordered.

1. Which key factors should be assessed in SM's history?
2. What is the significance of monitoring lab enzymes and hemoglobin?
3. Describe the correct method of preventive prophylaxis when taking antimalarial drugs.

NCLEX STUDY QUESTIONS

1. A patient is diagnosed with malaria and is prescribed mefloquine hydrochloride. The nurse anticipates that which lab test will be ordered?
   a. Liver enzymes
   b. Blood glucose
   c. Sputum culture and sensitivity
   d. White blood cell count

2. A patient is admitted to the hospital with multidrug-resistant urinary tract infection. Lab tests show *Pseudomonas aeruginosa*. Colistimethate sodium is ordered by intramuscular injection. The nurse understands that which of the following is the purpose for this drug?
   a. This drug prevents toxic adverse reactions.
   b. This drug treats aerobic gram-negative bacteria.
   c. This drug is safe for patients with renal impairments.
   d. This drug prevents antibiotic resistance.

3. A patient with a history of malaria who is being treated with chloroquine is in the clinic for a follow-up visit. What should the nurse advise the patient to do?
   a. Get frequent hearing checks.
   b. Take antimalarials before meals.
   c. Get frequent testing of stool specimens.
   d. Check your heart rate before taking this medication.
4. A patient is taking thiabendazole for trichinosis. What does the nurse realize about this condition and its treatment?
   a. The medication is given for 7 days.
   b. The medication should be avoided if the patient has renal disease.
   c. Family members should be checked for the same disease.
   d. Proper hygiene must be taught to avoid the spread of disease.

5. A 50-year-old woman is being discharged from the hospital after treatment for malaria. Which teaching topic would best inform the patient about adverse reactions?
   a. The occurrence of headaches
   b. Experiencing dizziness
   c. Developing mild pruritus
   d. Respiratory distress
6. A 30-year-old woman presents with a recurrence of *Trichomonas vaginalis* infection, and metronidazole is ordered. The patient's history reveals which of the following contraindications?
   a. A recent pregnancy test is negative.
   b. She previously took metronidazole and had no side effects.
   c. She drinks an occasional glass of wine.
   d. She takes an oral contraceptive.

Answers: 1, a; 2, b; 3, a; 4, d; 5, d; 6, c.

Immunologic Drugs

Immunity comprises those functions that protect people from the effects of invasion of the body by microscopic organisms such as bacteria, viruses, molds, spores, pollens, protozoa, and cells from other persons or animals. A person remains in harmony with these organisms as long as the organisms do not enter the body's internal environment. The body has various defenses (e.g., skin) that prevent microorganisms from gaining access to its internal environment. However, these defenses are not infallible, and invasion of the body's internal environment by microorganisms occurs often. A properly functioning immune system neutralizes, eliminates, or destroys the invading microorganisms. To do this without harming the body, immune system cells use defensive actions against only nonself proteins and cells. This means that immune system cells can differentiate between the body's own healthy cells and other nonself proteins and cells.

Nonself proteins and cells include (1) all foreign cells and microorganisms, (2) infected or debilitated body cells, and (3) self cells that have undergone malignant transformation into cancer cells. This ability to recognize self versus nonself, which is necessary to prevent healthy body cells from being destroyed along with the invaders, is called *self-tolerance.* Immune system cells are the only body cells capable of recognizing self from nonself.

Unique proteins on the surface of all body cells of each individual serve as a personal identification code for that person. The cell-surface proteins of one person are recognized as foreign by the immune system of another person. These are antigens—proteins capable of stimulating an immune response.

Immune function is generally most efficient when people are in their twenties and thirties; it slowly declines with increasing age. Older adults have marginal immune function, causing increased susceptibility to a variety of pathologic conditions.

IMMUNE SYSTEM STRUCTURE

The immune system is not confined to any one organ or body area. Instead, immune system cells originate in the bone marrow. Some of these cells mature in the bone marrow; others leave the bone marrow

and mature in different body sites. After maturation, most immune system cells are released into the blood, where they circulate throughout the body and exert specific effects.

IMMUNE SYSTEM FUNCTION

The three processes necessary for immunity, together with the cells involved in these responses, can be categorized as inflammation, antibody-mediated immunity (humoral immunity), and cell-mediated immunity. Inflammation is discussed in the introduction to Unit VII. Full immunity, or *immunocompetence,* requires the adequate function and interaction of all three processes, although some functions of each overlap. Long-lasting immune actions are those generated by antibody-mediated immunity and cell-mediated immunity.

Antibody-Mediated Immunity

Antibody-mediated immunity (AMI), also called *humoral immunity,* involves antigen-antibody interactions that neutralize, eliminate, or destroy foreign proteins. Antibodies for these interactions are produced by populations of B lymphocytes.

Antigen-Antibody Interactions

Antigen-antibody interactions occur in the body's internal environment. To make an antibody that can exert its effects on a specific antigen, the body must first be exposed to that antigen to the degree that the antigen enters the body. Even when exposure includes penetration, not all exposures result in the stimulation of antibody production. Invasion by the antigen must occur in such large numbers that some of the antigen either evades detection by the normal nonspecific defenses or overwhelms the abilities of the inflammatory response to neutralize, eliminate, or destroy the invader.

Acquiring Antibody-Mediated Immunity

The two broad categories of immunity are *innate immunity* and *acquired immunity.* Innate immunity is a genetically determined characteristic of an individual, group, or species. A person either has or does not have innate immunity. For example, humans have many innate immunities to viruses and other microorganisms that cause specific diseases in animals. As a result, humans are not susceptible to diseases such as mange, distemper, hog cholera, or any of a variety of animal afflictions. This type of immunity cannot be developed or transferred from one person to another and is not an adaptive response to exposure or invasion by foreign proteins.

Acquired immunity is the immunity that every person's body makes, or can receive, as an adaptive response to invasion by foreign proteins. *Antibody-mediated immunity* is an acquired immunity that occurs either naturally or artificially and can be either active or passive. Active immunity occurs when antigens enter the body and the body responds by making specific antibodies against the antigen. This type of immunity is active because the body takes an active part in making the antibodies. *Active immunity* can occur under conditions that are either natural or artificial. Natural active immunity occurs when an antigen enters the body without human assistance, and the body responds by actively making antibodies against that antigen (e.g., chickenpox virus). Most of the time, the first invasion of the body by this antigen results in the person manifesting signs and symptoms of the disease. However, processes that occur in the body at the same time allow the person to acquire immunity to that antigen so that a second exposure to the same antigen will not cause illness. This type of immunity is the most effective and the longest lasting.

Artificial active immunity is a type of protection developed against illnesses that produce such serious side effects that total avoidance of the disease is most desirable. Small amounts of specific antigens are deliberately placed in the body via vaccination so that the body responds by actively making antibodies against the antigen. Because antigens used for this procedure have been specially processed to make them less likely to proliferate within the body, this exposure does not in itself cause the disease.

Examples of diseases for which artificially acquired active immunity can be obtained include tetanus, diphtheria, measles, smallpox, mumps, and rubella. This type of immunity lasts many years, although repeated but smaller doses of the original antigen are periodically required as a "booster" to maintain complete protection against the antigen.

Passive immunity occurs when antibodies against a specific antigen are in a person's body, but the person did not actively generate these antibodies. Instead, these antibodies are made in the body of another person or animal and are then transferred to the body of a specific individual. Because these antibodies are foreign to the individual, the body recognizes the antibodies as nonself and takes steps to eliminate them relatively quickly. For this reason, passive immunity can provide only immediate, short-term protection against a specific antigen.

Cell-Mediated Immunity

Cell-mediated immunity (CMI), or *cellular immunity,* involves many leukocyte actions, reactions, and interactions that range from the simple to the complex. This type of immunity is provided by committed lymphocyte stem cells that mature in the secondary lymphoid tissues of the thymus and pericortical areas of lymph nodes. Certain CMI responses influence and regulate the activities of antibody-mediated immunity and inflammation by producing and releasing cytokines, therefore total immunocompetence relies on optimal CMI function.

The leukocytes that play the most important roles in CMI include several specific T-lymphocyte subsets along with a special population of cells known as *natural killer cells* (NK cells). T lymphocytes further differentiate into a variety of subsets, each of which has a specific function. The three T-lymphocyte subsets crucial to the development and continuation of CMI are helper/inducer T cells, suppressor T cells, and cytotoxic/cytolytic T cells.

Protection Provided by Cell-Mediated Immunity

Specific components of CMI assist in providing protection to the body by their highly developed abilities to differentiate self from nonself. The nonself cells most easily recognized by CMI are self cells that are infected by organisms that live within host cells and self cells that are mutated at the DNA level and are thus abnormal. CMI provides a surveillance system that rids the body of self cells that might potentially harm the body. CMI is critically important in preventing development of cancer and metastasis after exposure to carcinogens.

In this unit, Chapter 29 discusses drugs related to HIV and AIDS; Chapter 30 reviews drugs used in solid organ transplantation; and Chapter 31 covers vaccines.

29

HIV- and AIDS-Related Drugs

http://evolve.elsevier.com/McCuistion/pharmacology/

OBJECTIVES

- Describe the life cycle of the human immunodeficiency virus (HIV) and relate it to the actions of pharmacologic drugs used in the treatment of HIV disease.
- Identify the common risk factors for HIV transmission.
- Describe the six classifications of antiretroviral therapy, and give examples of medications in each group.
- Explain specific issues of medication adherence to antiretroviral agents.

- Discuss the nurse's role in medication management and issues of adherence.
- Discuss medical management for preventing mother-to-child transmission of HIV infection during pregnancy.
- Discuss health care workers' exposure risks and relate the risk and type of exposure to recommendations.
- Apply the nursing process, including teaching, to the care of patients with HIV infection.

OUTLINE

KEY TERMS

Since the acquired immunodeficiency syndrome (AIDS) epidemic began in the United States in the early 1980s, advancement of antiretroviral therapy (ART) has dramatically improved human immunodeficiency virus (HIV)-related morbidity and mortality and has reduced perinatal and behaviorally associated HIV transmission. The Centers for Disease Control and Prevention (CDC) reports that more than 1.2 million people in the United States are infected with HIV; between 10% and 15% of persons living with HIV do not know they have it. Approximately 50,000 new cases of HIV infection occur annually. Improvement of health, prolonging lives, reducing transmission risk, and suppression of HIV necessitates the use of combination treatments with antiretroviral drugs. Current clinical guidelines recommend ART for all persons infected with HIV-1, regardless of their viral load (CD4+ cell count). Prophylactic treatment of HIV-negative partners minimizes their risk of contracting HIV. It is critical that nurses educate patients regarding ART and, in partnership with the patient, develop strategies to optimize adherence.

Although strides have been made in the treatment of HIV/AIDS, challenges remain. One important aspect is increased drug resistance to current therapies. The makeup of the HIV DNA strands allows the virus to mutate from a drug-sensitive to a drug-resistant form. To minimize resistant strains, clinical and nonclinical providers and health departments need to strive for the highest possible adherence to ART. At each health care visit, persons with HIV and their partners should receive ongoing counseling to reinforce HIV prevention measures, screening for high-risk behaviors, diagnosis and treatment of sexually transmitted infections (STIs), and reinforcement of the importance of medication adherence. Open communication between the health care provider and patient should be fostered.

The goals for initiating ART are to (1) reduce HIV-associated morbidity and mortality, (2) prolong the duration and quality of life, (3) restore and preserve immunologic function, (4) maximally and durably suppress plasma HIV viral load, and (5) prevent HIV transmission.

HIV INFECTION: PATHOPHYSIOLOGY

HIV is an RNA retrovirus. It is unable to survive and replicate unless it is inside a living human cell. HIV destroys CD4+ T cells, also called *helper T cells* or *CD4+ T lymphocytes*; these play a critical role in the human immune response through recognition of infectious and neoplastic processes. The destruction of CD4+ cells by HIV results in immune deficiency, so the CD4+ cell count is an indicator for immune function in those with HIV.

Normal CD4+ counts range from 500 to 1200 cells/mm^3. After initial infection, rapid viral replication occurs, resulting in a high level of HIV in circulation (high viral load); the virus then attacks and destroys CD4+ cells. There is a corresponding drop in CD4+ cells, which triggers an immune response that results in CD4+ cell replacement and HIV antibody production. HIV uses the CD4+ cell's apparatus to replicate itself and spread throughout the body. The CD4+ cells continue to drop as HIV viral load increases, which further weakens the person's natural

immune system such that it cannot fight off infection and disease (e.g., cancer). Symptoms of HIV infection range from mild to severe and include fever, fatigue, pharyngitis, myalgia or arthralgia, lymphadenopathy, headache, and night sweats in those recently infected; these symptoms can be experienced 2 to 12 weeks after HIV exposure. This period is called *acute retroviral syndrome, acute seroconversion syndrome,* or *primary HIV infection.* At this stage, people are highly infectious and symptoms can often be mistaken, by both patient and health care provider, for a transient flulike illness. Consequently, few people are diagnosed during this time. Additionally, the time delay from infection to a positive HIV test result—the so-called window period—averages 10 to 14 days, but some do not seroconvert for 3 to 4 weeks. Almost all patients seroconvert within 6 months. For this reason, patients who are at risk for HIV infection and test negative should be counseled to have the test repeated in 3 months (the close of the window period). If HIV is strongly suspected, an HIV RNA quantitative test can be done. A viral load of 10,000 copies/mL usually indicates the virus is adequately suppressed.

HIV LIFE CYCLE

The phases of the HIV life cycle (Fig. 29.1) are binding, fusion, reverse transcription, integration, replication, assembly, and budding. HIV begins its life cycle when it *binds* to CD4+ receptors on the surface of a CD4+ T lymphocyte. The virus then *fuses* with the host cell, allowing entrance into the CD4+ cell.

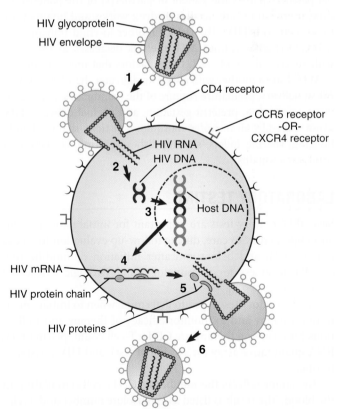

FIG. 29.1 The Life Cycle of the Human Immunodeficiency Virus (HIV). (Courtesy National Institutes of Health)

After fusion, the virus releases RNA, its genetic material, into the host cell to be converted into HIV DNA. This *reverse transcription* (RT) lets the virus enter into the host cell's nucleus and *integrate* (combine) with the cell's DNA. The integrated HIV DNA, a provirus, creates copies of the HIV genomic material (*replication*) and shorter strands of RNA called *messenger RNA* (mRNA). The mRNA is used as a blueprint to make long chains of HIV proteins. The new HIV proteins and HIV RNA *assemble* into an immature, noninfectious HIV, which then pushes out of the host cell (*budding*). Finally, these immature HIV cells release HIV enzymes (proteases) that disassemble the long protein chains of immature HIV virus. The now individual proteins can combine to make copies of mature HIV and can then move on to infect other cells.

HIV TRANSMISSION

HIV is spread via intimate contact with blood, semen, vaginal fluids, and breast milk. Transmission of the virus occurs primarily by (1) sexual contact, which includes oral, vaginal, and anal sex; (2) direct blood contact including intravenous (IV) drug use with shared needles or shared drug works, shared contaminated personal care items such as razors, and blood transfusions (now extremely rare in the United States); and (3) mother-to-child contact through shared maternal-fetal blood circulation, direct blood contact during delivery, or breast milk. Included in these modes are accidental needle injury, artificial insemination with donated semen, and organ transplant. Those at highest risk include persons who engage in unprotected sex, those with multiple sexual partners (either the patient or partner[s] of the patient), IV drug users who share needles or drug works, and infants born to women with HIV. The risk of mother-to-child transmission (MTCT) is 25% without ART; the risk decreases to 1% to 2% with successful use of ART. Other factors that increase the risk of MTCT are a mother with a viral load greater than 1000 copies/mL at delivery, premature rupture of the membranes, hepatitis C virus coinfection, preterm gestation, and vaginal delivery. HIV is not spread by air or water, mosquitoes or ticks, shaking hands, hugging, sharing toilets, sharing dishes or drinking glasses, or drinking fountains.

LABORATORY TESTING

Several laboratory tests are important for initial patient evaluation upon entry to care, during follow-up evaluation for those not on ART, and before and after initiation or modification of ART to assess for immunologic and virologic efficacy of treatment.

The laboratory tests used to determine when to initiate medication therapy and to monitor efficacy of therapy and indications for changing therapy are CD4+ T-cell count, plasma HIV RNA quantitative assay (or viral load test), and HIV resistance testing.

The count reflects the number of CD4+ cells circulating in the blood. The result is listed as an absolute number and a relative percentage. The absolute count can vary in the same patient depending on the laboratory used, the time of day laboratory

blood work is drawn, or acute illness. The CD4+ percentage is a more stable reflection of the immune system and is used in conjunction with the absolute count to monitor health status and response to medication therapy. The patient should be encouraged to use the same laboratory at approximately the same time of day to promote consistency of results. The nurse should monitor the laboratory used because lab value references vary from laboratory to laboratory. The HIV viral load is indicative of the level of virus circulating in the blood and is the best determinant of treatment efficacy. A key goal of therapy is to achieve and maintain a viral load below the limits of detection (<20 to 40 copies/mL, depending on the assay used). This goal should be achieved in 16 to 24 weeks of therapy. Resistance to ART leads to treatment failure and the risk of transmitting drug-resistant virus. Determination of the presence of a drug-resistant strain of HIV is important to prevent ineffective treatment. Individuals who experience failure of ART should have drug-resistance testing, assessment of drug adherence, and a review of possible drug-drug and drug-food interactions and drug intolerability, treatment history, and HIV RNA and CD4+ cell counts.

CLASSIFICATION

HIV disease staging and classification systems are important tools for tracking and monitoring the HIV epidemic and for providing the clinician and patient with information about HIV disease stage and clinical management. The two major classification systems are the CDC staging system (revised in 2014) and the World Health Organization (WHO) system (revised in 2015).

The CDC system assesses the severity of HIV disease by CD4+ cell counts and by presence of specific HIV-related conditions; the system is based on the lowest documented CD4+ cell count (*nadir CD4+*) and on previously diagnosed HIV-related conditions. The WHO system is useful in resource-constrained settings without access to CD4+ cell measurements and classifies HIV disease based on clinical manifestations that clinicians and those with varying levels of HIV expertise and training can recognize in diverse settings.

INDICATIONS FOR ANTIRETROVIRAL THERAPY

ART has dramatically reduced HIV-associated morbidity and mortality. However, the CDC reported that in the United States, fewer than one-third of HIV-infected individuals have adequate viral suppression. Many individuals with HIV infection are undiagnosed or they are not retained within the health care system for routine monitoring.

A set of guidelines was developed by the U.S. Department of Health and Human Services Expert Panel on Antiretroviral Guidelines for Adults and Adolescents (the Panel). The Panel last updated the guidelines in 2016 and recommends ART for all HIV-infected individuals regardless of CD4+ count to reduce HIV-related morbidity and mortality and to prevent HIV transmission. The Panel also seeks to educate patients on the benefits and considerations for ART, especially the importance of adherence. The current guidelines for treatment-naïve persons with HIV include initial therapy with two nucleoside reverse transcriptase inhibitors (NRTIs) in combination with a third active antiretroviral (ARV) drug from one of three drug classes: an integrase strand transfer inhibitor (INSTI), a nonnucleoside reverse transcriptase inhibitor (NNRTI), or a protease inhibitor (PI) with a pharmacokinetic (PK) enhancer (booster) (cobicistat or ritonavir). All HIV-infected persons diagnosed with active tuberculosis (TB) should be started on antiretroviral and TB therapy. Rifamycin (rifabutin, rifampin) should be included in the TB regimen despite drug interactions. Chapter 27 further discusses antituberculars.

Suppression of HIV with ART may decrease inflammation and immune activation that is thought to contribute to higher rates of cardiovascular, kidney, and liver disease; neurologic complications; and malignancy in HIV-infected cohorts. If therapy is to be initiated, medications are selected based on results of genotypic resistance testing where applicable; comorbidities (e.g., liver disease, renal dysfunction, depression); potential drug-drug interactions; pregnancy status; and assessment of the patient's willingness and readiness to start therapy. Evaluation of medication readiness should include dosage regimen, pill burden, dosing frequency, food restrictions, side effects, and the patient's daily routine. Tools for promoting medication adherence (e.g., alarms, pill planners) and plans for management of potential medication side effects should be reviewed before medication initiation. The patient should be instructed in the need for a better than 95% medication adherence, the potential for development of medication resistance with less than optimal adherence, and the clinical implications of resistance.

ANTIRETROVIRAL DRUGS

NRTIs, NNRTIs, PIs, fusion (entry) inhibitors, CCR5 antagonists, and INSTIs make up the drugs used as ART. Table 29.1 lists dosages, uses, and considerations for several ARVs. More than 25 different ARVs have received U.S. Food and Drug Administration (FDA) approval, and various agents are available in fixed-dose combinations that contain two or more HIV medications from one or more drug classes. In addition to the above classes of antiretrovirals, PK enhancers are approved to be taken with some ARVs (e.g., PIs and certain INSTIs).

Since the 1980s, when zidovudine monotherapy showed survival benefits in advanced HIV patients, much progress has been made. Newer agents have improved adherence (e.g., fewer pills for more convenient dosing, formulation changes that reduce dosing frequency or pill burden, combination dosage forms with two or three drugs in one pill). Other improvements include increased potency, improved side-effect profile (e.g., decreased gastrointestinal [GI] effects), and PI enhancers.

ART is the standard of care in the treatment of HIV infection. Currently, there are six recommended regimens for treatment-naïve patients, five of which are INSTI based and one that is ritonavir-boosted–PI based. For treatment-naïve patients, ART generally consists of two NRTIs plus an INSTI, NNRTI, or PK-enhanced PI. Treatment-experienced patients who encounter drug resistance should begin a new regimen that includes two to three fully active drugs. Adding a single

ARV is not recommended because of the increased risk of drug resistance to all ARVs. Furthermore, drug interruption is not recommended due to a risk of rapid increase of HIV RNA viral load and a decrease in CD4+ cell count.

The Panel reports that nevirapine (NVP) should not be given to ARV-naïve women whose CD4+ count is greater than 250 cells/mm^3 or to men with CD4+ greater than 400 cells/mm^3 due to a high incidence of hepatotoxicity; however, if no other ARV option is available, NVP can be administered, but patients should be closely monitored. On the other hand, the Panel reports no exceptions to stavudine plus zidovudine (antagonistic effect) and unboosted darunavir, saquinavir, or tipranavir (inadequate bioavailability).

INSTI-based regimens include the following:
- Dolutegravir-abacavir-lamivudine (DTG-ABC-3TC), but only for human leukocyte antigen (HLA)-B*5701–negative patients (presence of the HLA-B*5701 allele increases the risk of hypersensitivity to abacavir and is not recommended to individuals positive for the gene)
- Dolutegravir plus tenofovir disoproxil fumarate–emtricitabine (DTG plus TDF-FTC)
- Elvitegravir–cobicistat–tenofovir alafenamide–emtricitabine (EVG-c-TAF-FTC), but only for patients with pretreatment creatinine clearance (CrCl) greater than or equal to 30 mL/min
- Elvitegravir–cobicistat–tenofovir disoproxil fumarate–emtricitabine (EVG/c/TDF/FTC), but only for patients with pretreatment CrCl greater than or equal to 70 mL/min
- Raltegravir plus tenofovir disoproxil fumarate–emtricitabine (RAL plus TDF/FTC)

PI-based regimens include ritonavir-boosted darunavir plus tenofovir disoproxil fumarate–emtricitabine (DRV/r plus TDF/FTC).

Nucleoside/Nucleotide Reverse Transcriptase Inhibitors

Of the antiretroviral drugs, NRTIs were the first type of drug to treat HIV. NRTIs act by interfering with HIV viral RNA-dependent DNA polymerase, resulting in inhibition of viral replication. Seven NRTIs, also known as "nukes," are approved for use in the United States: zidovudine, didanosine, stavudine, lamivudine, abacavir, tenofovir, and emtricitabine. All but didanosine and stavudine are available in a fixed-dose combination with other classes of ARV drugs.

All NRTIs except didanosine can be taken without regard to food. Didanosine should be taken 30 minutes before or 2 hours after meals for optimal absorption. Fifty percent or more of NRTIs are excreted by the kidneys, therefore NRTIs require dosage adjustment in persons with renal insufficiency. With abacavir, dosage adjustment is recommended in individuals with hepatic insufficiency.

As a class, NRTIs are associated with changes in the body's metabolism secondary to mitochondrial toxicity. GI side effects such as nausea, diarrhea, and abdominal pain are transient and improve within the first 2 weeks of therapy. Rash is a common hypersensitivity reaction. Complications include peripheral neuropathy, myopathy, pancreatitis, and lipoatrophy. Lipoatrophy—or wasting of fat on the extremities, face, and buttocks—is

TABLE 29.1 Antiretroviral Agents

Generic	Route and Dosage	Uses and Considerations
NUCLEOSIDE/NUCLEOTIDE REVERSE TRANSCRIPTASE INHIBITORS (NRTIs)		
Abacavir (ABC) Also available as a component of fixed-dose combinations	Tablets: A/C ≥25 kg: PO: 300 mg bid or 600 mg once daily Solution: A: PO: 300 mg bid or 600 mg once daily C ≥3 mo: PO: 8 mg/kg/dose bid or 16 mg/kg/dose once daily	Used in combination with other ARVs. Screen for HLA-B*5701 before initiation. Hypersensitivity reactions are highest in patients who test positive for HLA-B*5701. Avoid in persons with cardiovascular risk factors. A black-box warning exists for hepatotoxicity or lactic acidosis. May be administered without regard to meals. Metabolized by alcohol dehydrogenase and glucuronyl transferase; ethanol decreases elimination of ABC. A reduced dose is recommended in persons with hepatic impairment. Pregnancy category: C*
Didanosine (DDI)	Extended-release capsule: A/C ≥60 kg: PO: 400 mg once daily A/C <60 kg: PO: 250 mg once daily C ≥6 y and 20-24 kg: 200 mg once daily Powder for oral solution: A ≥60 kg: PO: 400 mg once daily A <60 kg: PO: 250 mg once daily C: Dosage is based on age and weight. *Dosages are decreased if administered with TDF.*	DDI is not recommended for initial therapy due to inferior virologic efficacy. Used in combination with other ARVs. Metabolized by the liver. A black-box warning exists for hepatotoxicity or lactic acidosis and pancreatitis. Take on an empty stomach. ER capsules must be swallowed whole. Reduce the dose in persons with renal impairment. Pregnancy category: B*
Emtricitabine (FTC) Also available as a component of fixed-dose combinations	Capsule: A: PO: 200 mg once daily Solution: A: PO: 240 mg once daily C ≥3 mo: PO: 3 mg/kg/d	Used in combination with other ARVs. Metabolized by oxidation. A black-box warning exists for acute severe exacerbation of hepatitis B upon discontinuation of FTC and hepatitis or lactic acidosis. Otherwise, minimal toxicity is noted with FTC. Take without regard to meals. Reduce dose in patients with renal impairment. Pregnancy category: B*
Lamivudine (3TC) Also available as a component of fixed-dose combinations	HIV: Tablet: A/C ≥25 kg: PO: 300 mg once daily or 150 mg bid C <25 kg: Dosage is based on age and weight. Solution: A: PO: 300 mg once daily or 150 mg bid C ≥3 mo/Adol: PO: 8 mg/kg/dose once daily or 4 mg/kg/dose bid	Used in combination with other ARVs for treating HIV. Minimal toxicity with 3TC; a black-box warning exists for acute severe exacerbation of hepatitis B upon discontinuation of 3TC and hepatitis or lactic acidosis. Take without regard to meals. Adjust dosage in patients with renal insufficiency. Pregnancy category: C*
Stavudine (d4T)	A/C ≥60 kg: PO: 40 mg q12h A/C <60 kg: PO: 30 mg q12h	Used in combination with other ARVs for treating HIV. Crosses the blood-brain barrier. A black-box warning exists for hepatotoxicity or lactic acidosis and pancreatitis. Take without regard to meals. Adjust dosage in patients with renal insufficiency Pregnancy category: C*
Tenofovir (TDF)	See Prototype Drug Chart 29.2.	
Zidovudine (ZDV) Also available as a component of fixed-dose combinations	See Prototype Drug Chart 29.1.	
NONNUCLEOSIDE REVERSE TRANSCRIPTASE INHIBITORS (NNRTIs)		
Delavirdine (DLV)	A/C ≥16 y: PO: 400 mg tid	Used in combination with NRTIs. Take without regard to meals. Acidic food improves absorption, and 100-mg tablets may be dispersed in liquid prior to administration. DLV is metabolized extensively by the CYP450 isoenzymes. Pregnancy category: C*
Efavirenz (EFV) Also available as a component of fixed-dose combinations	See Prototype Drug Chart 29.3.	

TABLE 29.1   Antiretroviral Agents—cont'd

Generic	Route and Dosage	Uses and Considerations
NONNUCLEOSIDE REVERSE TRANSCRIPTASE INHIBITORS (NNRTIs)		
Etravirine (ETR)	A/C ≥6 y and ≥30 kg: PO: 200 mg bid C ≥6 y but <30 kg: PO: 16-19 kg: 100 mg bid 20-24 kg: 125 mg bid 25-29 kg: 150 mg bid	Used in combination with NRTIs. However, patients with virologic failure on NNRTIs should not receive ETR solely with NRTIs. Administer after meals to enhance absorption. Tablets may be dispensed in water. Do not use grapefruit juice, carbonated beverages, or warm liquids. Do not add ETR to juice or milk without first adding it to water. Add more fluids to the glass to ensure the full dose is consumed. Metabolized by CYP450 enzymes; numerous drug-drug interactions exist. No dosage adjustment is needed in patients with renal insufficiency. Hypersensitivity reactions include rash, including Stevens-Johnson syndrome, and hepatitis that includes hepatic necrosis. Pregnancy category: B*
Nevirapine (NVP)	Immediate release: A: PO: 200 mg/d for 14 d, then 200 mg bid C: Dosage is based on age and weight. Extended release: A: PO: Initial dosing with IR as above for 14 d, then 400 mg ER once daily C ≥6 y: PO: 150 mg/m²/dose for 14 d, then 200-400 mg ER based on BSA	NVP should not be used as an initial treatment option for treatment-naïve patients because fatal toxicities can occur. Used in combination with other ARVs (NRTIs, NNRTIs, PIs). A black-box warning exists for females whose CD4+ counts are >250/mm³ because risk of hepatotoxicity is increased. Take without regard to meals. Do not crush or chew ER tablets. Metabolized by CYP450. NVP is contraindicated in persons with hepatic impairment because of increased risk for hepatotoxicity. Numerous drug-drug interactions exist. Discontinue with hepatotoxicity or rash, including Stevens-Johnson syndrome. Pregnancy category: B*
Rilpivirine (RPL) Also available as a component of fixed-dose combinations	A/C ≥12 y and ≥35 kg: PO: 25 mg once daily	Must be administered in combination with other ARVs. Take with a meal. Primarily metabolized by the liver. Numerous drug-drug interactions exist, and hepatotoxicity can occur. Monitor for depression, insomnia, cephalgia. Pregnancy category: C*
PROTEASE INHIBITORS (PIs)		
Atazanavir (ATV) Also available as a component of fixed-dose combinations	See Prototype Drug Chart 29.4.	
Darunavir (DRV) Also available as a component of fixed-dose combinations	A: PO: 600-800 mg bid C: Dosage is based on age and weight.	Used in combination with other ARVs. Must be administered with PK enhancer (cobicistat or low-dose ritonavir). Administer with food. DRV is metabolized by CYP450 isoenzymes. Adjust dosage in patients with hepatic insufficiency. Caution in patients with sulfa hypersensitivity. Monitor closely for rash, including Stevens-Johnson syndrome, toxic epidermal necrolysis, acute generalized exanthematous pustulosis, and erythema multiforme. Hepatotoxicity, DKA, and pancreatitis can occur. Other adverse effects include lipodystrophy, elevated transaminases, nausea, and diarrhea. Pregnancy category: C*
Fosamprenavir (FPV)	A: PO: 700 mg bid with ritonavir 100 mg PO bid C: PO: ≥6 mo: <11 kg: 45 mg/kg PO bid w/ritonavir 7 mg/kg PO bid 11-14 kg: 30 mg/kg PO bid w/ritonavir 3 mg/kg PO bid 15-19 kg: 23 mg/kg PO bid w/ritonavir 3 mg/kg PO bid >20 kg: 18 mg/kg up to 700 mg PO bid w/ritonavir 3 mg/kg up to 100 mg PO bid	Used in combination with other ARVs. A PK enhancer with low-dose ritonavir and twice-daily dosing are recommended. Monitor in patients with sulfa hypersensitivity; cross-reaction can occur. Metabolized by CYP450 isoenzymes and drug transporters. Dose adjustment is required in patients with hepatic impairment. Tablets can be taken without regard to meals. Oral suspension is taken on an empty stomach in adults and with food in children. Can readminister dose if emesis occurs within 30 min of administration. Adverse effects include rash, diarrhea, nausea, vomiting, headache, hyperlipidemia, elevated transaminase levels, hyperglycemia, fat maldistribution, and possible increased bleeding in patients with hemophilia. Pregnancy category: C*

Continued

TABLE 29.1	Antiretroviral Agents—cont'd	
Generic	**Route and Dosage**	**Uses and Considerations**
	PROTEASE INHIBITORS (PIs)	
Indinavir (IDV)	A: PO: 800 mg q12h	Used in combination with other ARVs and PK enhancers (e.g., ritonavir). CYP450 3A4 inhibitor and substrate. Adjust dosage in patients with hepatic insufficiency. For optimal absorption, take on an empty stomach. Hydrate with at least 1.5 L of fluid during a 24-h period. Adverse effects include nephrolithiasis, GI intolerance, nausea, indirect hyperbilirubinemia, headache, asthenia, blurred vision, dizziness, rash, metallic taste, thrombocytopenia, alopecia, hemolytic anemia, hyperlipidemia, elevated transaminase levels, hyperglycemia, fat maldistribution, and risk of increased bleeding in patients with hemophilia. Pregnancy category: C*
Lopinavir–ritonavir (LPV/r)	A: PO: 400/100 mg bid *or* 800/200 mg once daily C/Adol: PO: Dosage is based on weight.	Used in combination with other ARVs. CYP450 3A4 inhibitor and substrate. May take tablet with or without food; take oral solution with food. Adverse effects include GI intolerance, asthenia, PR interval prolongation, pancreatitis, hyperlipidemia, elevated transaminase levels, hyperglycemia, fat maldistribution, and risk of increased bleeding in patients with hemophilia. Pregnancy category: C*
Nelfinavir (NFV)	A/Adol: PO: 1250 mg bid or 750 mg tid C 2-13 y: PO: 45-55 mg/kg bid or 25-35 mg/kg tid	Used in combination with other ARVs. Not recommended in treatment-naïve patients as initial therapy. CYP450 3A4 inhibitor and substrate. Take with food; do not mix with acidic food or juice. Tablets can be dispersed in a small amount of water prior to mixing with food or juice. Nelfinavir oral powder may be added to water, milk, formula, soymilk, or dietary supplements. Do not mix nelfinavir oral powder with acidic food or juice (orange juice, apple juice, or applesauce). Do not mix nelfinavir with water in the original container. Adverse effects include diarrhea, hyperlipidemia, elevated transaminase levels, hyperglycemia, fat maldistribution, and risk of increased bleeding in patients with hemophilia. ⚡ Persons with phenylketonuria should not take nelfinavir powder as it contains phenylalanine. Pregnancy category: B*
Ritonavir (RTV)	Other ARVs: A: PO: 600 mg bid C/Adol: Dosage is based on weight. Booster: A: PO: 100-400 mg in 1-2 divided doses C/Adol: Dosage is based on concomitant PI.	Used in combination with other ARVs and as a PK enhancer (booster) of other PIs. Dosage depends on use of RTV. CYP450 3A4 potent inhibitor; use extreme caution when administering other drugs, especially antihistamines, sedative hypnotics, antiarrhythmics, and ergot alkaloids. If coadministering with didanosine, separate drugs by 2 h. Take with food. Swallow tablets and capsules whole. Refrigerate capsules; RTV oral solution should not be refrigerated, but left at room temperature for up to 30 days. Adverse effects include GI intolerance, paresthesias, hepatitis, asthenia, hyperlipidemia, hyperglycemia, fat maldistribution, and risk of increased bleeding in patients with hemophilia. Titrating the dosage may help to reduce side effects. ⚡ RTV oral solution contains significant amounts of ethanol (43.2%) and propylene glycol (26.57%). Accidental ingestion by small children may lead to deadly ethanol or propylene glycol toxicity. Pregnancy category: B*
Saquinavir (SQV)	A: PO: 1000 mg bid	*Must* be dosed concurrently with low-dose ritonavir. SQV is not recommended for treatment-naïve adults due to its serious adverse effects. CYP450 3A4 inhibitor and substrate. Take with food. Adverse effects include nausea, diarrhea, headache, hyperlipidemia, elevated transaminase levels, hyperglycemia, PR and QT interval prolongation, fat maldistribution, and risk of increased bleeding in patients with hemophilia. Contraindicated in patients with PR or QT prolongation, hypokalemia, or hypomagnesemia. Pregnancy category: B*

TABLE 29.1 Antiretroviral Agents—cont'd

Generic	Route and Dosage	Uses and Considerations
PROTEASE INHIBITORS (PIs)		
Tipranavir (TPV)	A: PO: 500 mg bid C ≥2 y/Adol: PO: Dosage is based on weight.	Used in combination with other ARVs; *must* be coadministered with ritonavir. TPV has a black-box warning for hepatotoxicity and intracranial bleeding. CYP450 3A4 inducer and substrate. Take with food if coadministered with RTV tablets; if administered with RTV capsules or solutions, TPV can be taken regardless of food. Adverse effects include hepatotoxicity, rash hyperlipidemia, hyperglycemia, fat maldistribution, and risk of increased bleeding in patients with hemophilia. Use with caution in patients with sulfa hypersensitivity. Pregnancy category: C*
FUSION (ENTRY) INHIBITOR (FI)		
Enfuvirtide (T20)	A/Adol >16 y: subcut: 90 mg bid C ≤16 y: subcut: Dosage is weight based and ranges from 27 to 90 mg bid.	Used in treatment-experienced patients in combination with other ARVs. Administer via subcut, and rotate site. Store vial at room temperature; once reconstituted, refrigerate and use within 24 h. Adverse effects include local injection site reaction (pain, erythema, induration, nodules, cysts, pruritus, ecchymosis), increased rate of bacterial pneumonia, hypersensitivity reaction (rash, fever, nausea, vomiting, chills, rigors, hypotension, elevated transaminases), fatigue. To minimize local reactions, apply ice or heat after injection or gently massage the site to better disperse the drug. Pregnancy category: B*
CCR5 ANTAGONISTS		
Maraviroc (MRV)	A: PO: 150-600 mg bid	Used in combination with other ARVs. MRV is administered *only* to patients with CCR5-tropic HIV infection. Dosing depends on other drugs taken concomitantly. CYP3A substrate; drugs that inhibit or induce the enzymes will alter the pharmacokinetics of MRV. May take without regard to food. Concentration may increase in kidney dysfunction (CrCl <30), therefore caution is advised when used in renal-compromised patients; it is contraindicated in patients with CrCl <30 who are taking strong inhibitors and/or inducers of CYP3A. May need to adjust dose with concomitant CYP3A inhibitors or inducers (because of interactions) or with postural hypotension. Adverse effects include fever, upper respiratory tract infection, flatulence, orthostatic hypotension, hepatotoxicity, rash, cough, abdominal pain, and dizziness. Pregnancy category: B*
INTEGRASE STRAND TRANSFER INHIBITORS (INSTIs)		
Dolutegravir (DTG) Also available as a component of fixed-dose combinations	A/C ≥12 y and ≥40 kg: PO: 50 mg once daily	Used in treatment-naïve or -experienced patients in combination with other ARVs. Metabolized by CYP3A4 enzyme. Can be taken without regard to meals. Take polyvalent cation products (e.g., Mg^{++}, Fe, and Ca^{++} salts); ASA on an empty stomach can reduce bioavailability of DTG. Adverse effects include headache, insomnia, rash, and liver injury. Pregnancy category: B*
Elvitegravir (EVG) Also available as a component of fixed-dose combinations	A: PO: 85-150 mg once daily depending on ritonavir and other ARVs taken concurrently	Used in treatment-naïve or -experienced patients in combination with other ARVs; unboosted EVG is not recommended. EVG is metabolized by CYP3A. Take with food. Adverse effects are rare, but nausea and vomiting can occur; suicide ideation, albeit rare, can also occur, especially in those with a history of psychiatric illness. Pregnancy category: B*
Raltegravir (RAV)	A: PO: 400 mg bid C/Adol: PO: Dosage is weight based.	Used in treatment-naïve or -experienced patients in combination with other ARVs. Does not affect the CYP450 isoenzymes, nor is it a substrate of CYP450 enzymes. Can be taken without regard to meals. Coated tablets are not bioequivalent with chewable tablets or powder for oral suspension; swallow coated tablets whole. Adverse effects include GI symptoms, headache, pyrexia, increased total cholesterol, fatigue, rhabdomyolysis, insomnia, and rash that includes Stevens-Johnson syndrome and epidermal necrolysis. Pregnancy category: C*

*Pregnancy categories have been revised. See http://www.fda.gov/Drugs/DevelopmentApprovalProcess/DevelopmentResources/Labeling/ucm093307.htm for more information.

A, Adult; *Adol*, adolescent; *ARV*, antiretroviral; *ASA*, acetylsalicylic acid (aspirin); *bid*, twice a day; *BSA*, body surface area; *C*, child; *Ca++*, calcium; *CrCl*, creatinine clearance; *CYP450*, cytochrome P450; *d*, day; *DKA*, diabetic ketoacidosis; *ER*, extended-release; *Fe*, iron; *GI*, gastrointestinal; *h*, hour; *HIV*, human immunodeficiency virus; *HLA*, human leukocyte antigen; *IR*, immediate release; *Mg++*, magnesium; *min*, minute; *mo*, months; *PI*, protease inhibitor; *PK*, pharmacokinetic; *PO*, by mouth; *q*, every; *subcut*, subcutaneous; *tid*, three times a day; *y*, years; *>*, greater than; *<*, less than; *≥*, greater than or equal to; *≤*, less than or equal to.

associated with chronic NRTI administration. Rare fatalities have occurred due to lactic acidosis and hepatic steatosis associated with NRTIs. Persons coinfected with hepatitis B virus (HBV) are at risk for severe acute exacerbation of their HBV upon discontinuation of emtricitabine, lamivudine, or tenofovir disoproxil fumarate.

Drug interactions are minimal with NRTIs because these drugs are not metabolized by the cytochrome P450 (CYP450) isoenzymes. However, drug interactions can still occur: for example, ribavirin inhibiting phosphorylation of zidovudine can cause hematologic toxicities; and coadministration of ribavirin with didanosine is contraindicated because fatal hepatic failure can occur; didanosine coadministered with stavudine can worsen lactic acidosis and pancreatitis; allopurinol is contraindicated in individuals taking didanosine; and PIs can increase serum concentration of tenofovir disoproxil fumarate.

Prototype Drug Chart 29.1 gives pharmacologic data for zidovudine, and Prototype Drug Chart 29.2 shows the data for tenofovir.

Nonnucleoside Reverse Transcriptase Inhibitors

Five NNRTIs are used in the United States: delavirdine, efavirenz, etravirine, nevirapine, and rilpivirine. NNRTIs ("non-nukes") do not require intracellular metabolism; they directly bind to the reverse transcriptase (RT) enzymes and block DNA polymerization. The primary advantage of using NNRTIs is to reserve a PI-based therapy for future use. In general, an NNRTI regimen has a lower pill burden compared with most PI-based regimens. Major disadvantages are the prevalence of NNRTI-resistant viral strains and the low genetic barrier of NNRTIs for development of resistance. (Resistance testing is recommended for treatment-naïve patients before starting therapy.)

📄 PROTOTYPE DRUG CHART 29.1

Zidovudine (ZDV)

Drug Class	Dosage
Nucleoside/nucleotide reverse transcriptase inhibitor (NRTI) Pregnancy category: C* Also available as a component of fixed-dose combinations	Prevention of maternal-fetal HIV transmission for HIV RNA >400 copies/mL: Intrapartum: IV: 2 mg/kg LD over 30-60 min followed by continuous infusion of 1 mg/kg/h until cord is clamped. For scheduled cesarean delivery, begin IV 3 h before surgery Neonates ≥35 wk: IV: 3 mg/kg q12h; increase to 9 mg/kg q12h after 4 wk of age Neonates ≥35 wk: PO: 4 mg/kg q12h; increase to 12 mg/kg q12h after 4 wk of age Treatment in combination with other ARV: A: PO: 200 mg q8h or 300 mg q12h A: IV: 1 mg/kg over 1 h q4h (total daily dose: 6 mg/kg/d). Initiate oral therapy as soon as possible. C ≥30 kg: PO: 300 mg bid; 9-29 kg: 9 mg/kg/dose bid; 4-8 kg: 12 mg/kg/dose bid
Contraindications	**Drug-Lab-Food Interactions**
Life-threatening allergies to ZDV or components of the preparation *Black Box Warning:* Hepatotoxicity, lactic acidosis, myopathy, bone marrow suppression *Caution:* Severe anemia (interruption of therapy or reduction in daily dose should be considered); renal impairment/failure; viral hepatitis	*Drug:* Ganciclovir, probenecid, valproic acid may increase concentration/adverse effects. Rifampin, interferon, and ritonavir may decrease concentration/effects. May potentiate hematologic toxicity with other drugs (e.g., interferon alfa, ganciclovir, primaquine, etc.), causing myelosuppression; interferon beta can increase ZDV levels leading to drug toxicity. Can be taken without regard to food. *Lab:* May increase ALT, AST
Pharmacokinetics	**Pharmacodynamics**
Absorption: PO: 66%-70% Distribution: PB: <38%, crosses blood-brain barrier, crosses placenta, excreted in breast milk Metabolism: t½: 0.5-3 h; extensive first-pass effect in liver to GZDV (metabolite) Excretion: 63%-95% in urine as GZDV (metabolite)	Route: PO/IV Onset: UK Peak: 30-90 min; can be taken without regard to meals Duration: UK
Therapeutic Effects/Uses	
Management of patients with HIV infection, prevention of maternal-fetal HIV transmission Mode of Action: Inhibits viral enzyme reverse transcriptase and thymidine kinase, enzymes necessary for viral HIV replication.	
Side Effects	**Adverse Reactions**
Headache, malaise, nausea, anorexia, vomiting, asthenia (abnormal weakness and loss of energy), constipation, abdominal cramps/pain, arthralgia, rigors, dyspepsia, fatigue, insomnia, musculoskeletal pain, myalgia, neuropathy, elevated liver enzymes, anemia, fever, cough, hepatomegaly, rash, diarrhea, lipodystrophy, and stomatitis.	Severe anemia, lactic acidosis, pancreatitis, neutropenia, pancytopenia, seizures, congestive heart failure, myelosuppression, rhabdomyolysis, anaphylaxis, hyperlipidemia, insulin resistance, Stevens-Johnson syndrome, and toxic epidermal necrolysis.

*Pregnancy categories have been revised. See http://www.fda.gov/Drugs/DevelopmentApprovalProcess/DevelopmentResources/Labeling/ucm093307.htm for more information.
A, Adult; *ALT,* alanine aminotransferase; *ARV,* antiretroviral; *AST,* aspartate aminotransferase; *bid,* twice a day; *C,* child; *d,* day; *GZDV,* 5'-glucuronyl zidovudine; *h,* hour; *HIV,* human immunodeficiency virus; *IV,* intravenously; *LD,* loading dose; *min,* minute; *PB,* protein binding; *PO,* by mouth; *q,* every; *t½,* half-life; *UK,* unknown; *wk,* weeks; *>,* greater than; *≥,* greater than or equal to; *<,* less than.

Efavirenz (EFV) and rilpivirine are available as components of fixed-dose regimens. EFV should be taken on an empty stomach; delavirdine and nevirapine (NVP) can be taken without regard to food; all other NNRTIs should to be taken with food to enhance absorption. Except for NVP, all NNRTIs are metabolized by the liver and excreted in feces, whereas NVP is mostly excreted in urine.

EFV is the first-choice drug within the NNRTI class, and it is the only NNRTI that penetrates the cerebrospinal fluid (CSF). It should be used with caution in pregnancy because neural tube defects have been reported after early human gestational exposure. Because of CSF involvement, neuropsychiatric symptoms such as dizziness, sedation, nightmares, euphoria, or loss of concentration can occur. Common complications among all the NNRTIs are rashes, which includes Stevens-Johnson syndrome. Elevated liver transaminases and hepatotoxicity, including hepatic failure, can also occur.

Drug-drug interactions are many because of the extensive metabolizing effects by cytochrome P3A4 (CYP3A4). Acid reducers (e.g., antacids, H2-receptor antagonists, proton pump inhibitors [PPIs]) can decrease the bioavailability of rilpivirine, therefore coadministration of rilpivirine with PPIs is contraindicated; all other acid reducers can be taken at least 2 hours before or 4 hours after rilpivirine. Coadministration with drugs that induce or inhibit any of the CYP isoenzymes can alter the therapeutic effects of other drugs (e.g., anticonvulsants, antidepressants, anticoagulants, antiplatelets, antifungals, antimycobacterials, statins, and calcium channel blockers [CCBs]). Other drugs used concomitantly can alter NNRTI serum levels (e.g., corticosteroids, hepatitis antivirals, and St. John's wort). NNRTIs can decrease the efficacy of hormonal contraceptives, therefore individuals should use alternative means of contraception or additional contraceptive methods.

Prototype Drug Chart 29.3 presents the pharmacologic data for efavirenz.

Protease Inhibitors

PI-based regimens (one or two PIs plus two NRTIs) have revolutionized the treatment of HIV infection, especially with PK enhancement (boosters such as cobicstat and ritonavir); this has led to sustained viral suppression, improved immunologic function, and prolonged patient survival. PIs that have been approved by the FDA include atazanavir (ATV), atazanavir/cobicistat (ATV/c), darunavir (DRV), darunavir/cobicistat (DRV/c), fosamprenavir (FPV), indinavir (IDV), lopinavir/ritonavir (LPV/r), nelfinavir (NFV), saquinavir (SQV), ritonavir (RTV),

PROTOTYPE DRUG CHART 29.2
Tenofovir Disoproxil Fumarate (TDF)

Drug Class	Dosage
Nucleoside/nucleotide reverse transcriptase inhibitor (NRTI) Pregnancy category: B* Also available as a component of fixed-dose combinations	HIV treatment: A/C ≥35 kg: PO: 300 mg once daily C ≥2 y and 28-34 kg: PO: 250 mg once daily C ≥2 y and 22-27 kg: PO: 100 mg once daily C ≥2 y and 17-21 kg: PO: 150 mg once daily Hepatitis B treatment: A/C ≥12 y and ≥35 kg: PO: 300 mg once daily
Contraindications *Black Box Warning:* Hepatitis B exacerbation, hepatotoxicity, lactic acidosis *Caution:* Renal and hepatic dysfunction	**Drug-Lab-Food Interactions** *Drug:* Concomitant use with streptozocin is contraindicated because it can increase risk of nephrotoxicity and ototoxicity. Tenofovir can decrease levels of some drugs (e.g., dabigatran, edoxaban) and increase levels of other drugs (e.g., adefovir, bacitracin, diltiazem, metformin); acyclovir, amikacin, cisplatin, ganciclovir, and gentamicin may increase levels and adverse effects of TDF. *Lab:* May increase triglycerides, AST, ALT, ALP
Pharmacokinetics Absorption: PO: 25%-40% Distribution: PB: 7.2% Metabolism: t½: 17 h; is not metabolized by CYP450 isoenzymes; converted intracellularly by hydrolysis and phosphorylated to active tenofovir diphosphate Excretion: 70%-80% primarily in urine as unchanged drug	**Pharmacodynamics** Route: PO Onset: UK Peak: 1 h (fasting), 2 h (food) Duration: UK
Therapeutic Effects/Uses Management of patients with HIV infection, treatment of chronic hepatitis B Mode of Action: Inhibits viral enzyme reverse transcriptase, an enzyme necessary for viral HIV replication, by competing with AMP as substrate	
Side Effects Diarrhea, nausea, vomiting, flatulence, insomnia, dizziness, depression, fever, hyperlipidemia, elevated transaminases, chest pain	**Adverse Reactions** Lactic acidosis, hepatomegaly, bone fractures, renal insufficiency, Fanconi syndrome

*Pregnancy categories have been revised. See http://www.fda.gov/Drugs/DevelopmentApprovalProcess/DevelopmentResources/Labeling/ucm093307.htm for more information.
A, Adult; *ALP*, alkaline phosphatase; *ALT*, alanine aminotransferase; *AMP*, adenosine monosphosphate; *AST*, aspartate aminotransferase; *C*, child; *CYP*, cytochrome P; *h*, hour; *HIV*, human immunodeficiency virus; *PB*, protein binding; *PO*, by mouth; *t½*, half-life; *UK*, unknown; *y*, years; ≥, greater than or equal to.

PROTOTYPE DRUG CHART 29.3

Efavirenz (EFV)

Drug Class	Dosage
Nonnucleoside reverse transcriptase inhibitor (NNRTI) Pregnancy category: D* Also available as a component of fixed-dose combination.	Note: Take dose at bedtime to minimize CNS adverse effects; take on an empty stomach to reduce adverse reactions. A/C ≥40 kg: PO: 600 mg at bedtime C 32.5-40 kg: PO: 400 mg at bedtime C 25-32.5 kg: PO: 350 mg at bedtime C 20-25 kg: PO: 300 mg at bedtime C 15-20 kg: PO: 250 mg at bedtime C 10-15 kg: PO: 200 mg at bedtime Alternate dosing for children: 367 mg/m^2/d Do not crush tablets. Capsules may be opened and sprinkled into a small amount of age-appropriate soft food or formula; administer within 30 min of mixing; no additional food for 2 h after dosing.
Contraindications	**Drug-Lab-Food Interactions**
Life-threatening allergies to EFV or components of the preparation; concurrent use with rifapentine, St. John's wort, dasabuvir, ombitasvir, paritaprevir, simeprevir, triazolam Caution: Patients with history of mental illness or drug abuse; liver impairment; seizure disorder	Drug: EFV can increase or decrease levels of warfarin, carbamazepine, nevirapine, phenobarbital, bupropion, sertraline, phenytoin, rifampin, CCBs, hormonal contraceptives, HMG-CoA reductase inhibitors; EFV can increase the levels of triazolam. Drugs that can increase or decrease EFV include dexamethasone, boceprevir, St. John's wort. Food: Avoid alcohol because of liver/CNS adverse effects; high-fat meals increase absorption. Lab: May cause a false-positive result for cannabinoid and benzodiazepine screening assays.
Pharmacokinetics	**Pharmacodynamics**
Absorption: PO: Increased following high-fat meal Distribution: PB: >99%, widely distributed (found in CSF) Metabolism: t½: 40-76 h; metabolized in liver; CYP3A4 inducer/inhibitor Excretion: 16%-61% in feces, primarily as unchanged drug; 14%-34% in urine, primarily as metabolite	Route: PO Onset: UK Peak: 3-5 h Duration: UK
Therapeutic Effects/Uses	
Treatment of HIV-1 infections Mode of Action: Binds directly to reverse transcriptase, blocking RNA- and DNA-dependent DNA polymerase activities, including HIV-1 replication	
Side Effects	**Adverse Reactions**
Rash, nausea, diarrhea, CNS effects (dizziness, insomnia, abnormal dreams/thinking, impaired concentration, amnesia, agitation, hallucinations, euphoria, anxiety)	Aggressive reaction, allergic reaction, convulsion, liver failure, neuropathy, suicide, abnormal vision, hyperlipidemia

*Pregnancy categories have been revised. See http://www.fda.gov/Drugs/DevelopmentApprovalProcess/DevelopmentResources/Labeling/ucm093307.htm for more information.
A, Adult; C, child; CCB, calcium channel blocker; CNS, central nervous system; CSF, cerebrospinal fluid; CYP3A4, cytochrome P450 3A4; d, day; h, hour; HMG-CoA, hydroxymethylglutaryl coenzyme A; min, minutes; PB, protein binding; PO, by mouth; t½, half-life; UK, unknown; ≥, greater than or equal to; >, greater than.

and tipranavir (TPV). RTV as the sole PI is not recommended; instead, it should be used as a boosting agent with other PIs. TPV is only approved for ARV-experienced patients. Unlike NRTIs and NNRTIs, PIs act at the end of the HIV life cycle to target viral assembly by inhibiting the activity of protease, an enzyme used to cleave nascent proteins for final assembly of new virions, resulting in formation and release of immature, defective, and noninfectious virus particles. Each PI has unique characteristics based on clinical efficacy, side-effect profile, and pharmacokinetic properties. PIs are highly protein bound, metabolized by the liver, and primarily eliminated in feces.

The Panel's recommended PI regimen is DRV/r plus two NRTIs (tenofovir disoproxil fumarate/emtricitabine [TDF/FTC]). RTV boosting is a relatively new concept and one of the mainstays of PI therapy. The potent inhibitory effect of RTV on the cytochrome P450 3A4 isoenzyme (CYP3A4) allows the addition of 100 mg to 400 mg of RTV to other PIs as a PK booster. This helps reduce dietary restrictions, increase drug exposure, inhibit metabolism, and maximize blood levels of the coadministered PI, thus reducing dosing frequency and pill burden and overcoming viral resistance. Because "boosted" regimens may be less complex, patients may be able to follow and tolerate them better.

Selection of a PI-based regimen should consider dosing frequency, food and fluid requirements, pill burden, drug interaction potential, and side-effect profile. PIs result in numerous metabolic abnormalities that include dyslipidemia and insulin resistance; PK enhancers can alter these adverse effects. Some

PROTOTYPE DRUG CHART 29.4

Atazanavir (ATV)

Drug Class	Dosage
Protease inhibitor Pregnancy category: B*	Also available as a component of fixed-dose combinations. Note: HIV guidelines recommend administering concurrently with a PK enhancer (cobicistat or RTV). Capsules and powder packets are not interchangeable. Capsules: A/C 6 y and ≥40 kg: PO: 300 mg plus RTV 100 mg once daily C 20-40 kg: PO: 200 mg with RTV 100 mg once daily C 15-20 kg: PO: 150 mg with RTV 100 mg once daily Powder: C 15-25 kg: PO: 250 mg (5 pk) plus 80 mg once daily C 5-15 kg: PO: 200 mg (4 pk) plus RTV 80 mg once daily Capsules must be swallowed whole. Powder may be mixed with age-appropriate food; use oral dosing syringe in persons unable to drink from a cup.
Contraindications	**Drug-Lab-Food Interactions**
Hypersensitivity to ATV or any component, concurrent use with alfuzosin, ergot derivatives, lovastatin, midazolam (oral), rifampin, simvastatin, St. John's wort *Caution:* Patients with preexisting conduction abnormalities (may prolong PR interval), hepatitis B or C, hepatic impairment, hemophilia A or B	*Drug:* Drug-drug interactions are numerous. Some known interactions include drugs that can decrease or decrease ATV; acid reducers, including H2-receptor antagonists and PPIs, carbamazepine, phenytoin, phenobarbital, itraconazole, rifampin, boceprevir, and St. John's wort. ATV can increase or decrease levels of dabigatran, warfarin, buspirone, rifabutin, amiodarone, BBs, CCBs, digoxin, corticosteroids, hormonal contraceptives, lovastatin, and simvastatin. *Lab:* May increase liver function tests, cholesterol, triglycerides, glucose *Food:* Bioavailability increases when taken with food.
Pharmacokinetics	**Pharmacodynamics**
Absorption: PO: Rapidly, increased with food Distribution: PB: 86% Metabolism: t½: 7-8 h (9-18 h when boosted with RTV). Metabolized in the liver; inhibitor of CYP450 isoenzymes Excretion: Primarily in feces (79%) but also in urine (13%)	Route: PO Onset: UK Peak: 2-3 h Duration: UK
Therapeutic Effects/Uses	
Treatment of HIV-1 infection Mode of Action: Inhibits HIV protease, rendering enzyme incapable of processing polyprotease precursors, thus rendering immature HIV particles noninfectious	
Side Effects	**Adverse Reactions**
Rash, nausea, vomiting, diarrhea, cough, fever	Atrioventricular block, hyperglycemia, diabetes mellitus, jaundice, hyperlipidemia, lipodystrophy, cholelithiasis, nephrolithiasis, elevated liver transaminases

*Pregnancy categories have been revised. See http://www.fda.gov/Drugs/DevelopmentApprovalProcess/DevelopmentResources/Labeling/ucm093307.htm for more information.

A, Adult; *BB*, beta blocker; *C*, child; *CCB*, calcium channel blocker; *CYP450*, cytochrome P450; *h*, hour; *H2*, histamine 2; *HIV*, human immunodeficiency virus; *PB*, protein binding; *PK*, pharmacokinetic; *pk*, pack; *PO*, by mouth; *PPI*, proton pump inhibitor; *RTV*, ritonavir; *t½*, half-life; *UK*, unknown; *y*, year; ≥, greater than or equal to.

PIs come with a risk factor for causing myocardial infarction (MI). When initiating therapy with PIs, GI side effects (nausea, vomiting, and diarrhea) can be bothersome and may negatively affect adherence. Skin reactions such as rash, which includes Stevens-Johnson syndrome, can occur with PIs. Other adverse effects include hemolytic anemia, electrocardiogram (ECG) changes, and MI.

In patients with hepatic impairment, dosing adjustment may be necessary. All PIs inhibit the CYP450 system, which can lead to many drug-drug interactions. Drugs such as H2-receptor antagonists (e.g., cimetidine, famotidine, or ranitidine) should be given 10 or more hours before PIs. PPIs are not recommended in PI-experienced patients, and concomitant use with anticoagulants/antiplatelets should also be avoided. Ritonavir-boosted PIs can decrease warfarin levels. Anticonvulsants (e.g., carbamazepine, phenobarbital, phenytoin) are contraindicated with certain PIs, whereas some antidepressants (e.g., bupropion,

selective serotonin reuptake inhibitors [SSRIs]) may need dose adjustments. Trazodone is contraindicated with saquinavir/ritonavir, and antimycobacterials and cardiac drugs can worsen cardiac toxicities. Many PIs without the ritonavir boost can increase drug levels of hormonal contraceptives, whereas boosted PIs can decrease the levels. It is important that nurses instruct patients to use an alternative contraceptive method when taking boosted PIs. Rifampin and rifapentine are contraindicated with PIs, as are many other classes of drugs (e.g., antiarrhythmics, antivirals for viral hepatitis, St. John's wort, hydroxymethylglutaryl coenzyme A [HMG-CoA] reductase inhibitors, and some hypnotics) due to a decrease in PI drug levels and toxic drug levels in the other classes of drugs. Benefits of corticosteroid use should outweigh the risks with concomitant administration with corticosteroids.

Prototype Drug Chart 29.4 presents the pharmacologic data for atazanavir.

Fusion (Entry) Inhibitors

Enfuvirtide (T20) is the only agent approved in this class. T20 acts by a mechanism that inhibits the fusion of the virus to healthy cell membranes, thus preventing HIV entry into healthy cells. T20 is indicated only in combination with other ARVs for patients with limited treatment options who require salvage therapy. It is not indicated for HIV-2. Before initiating a fusion (entry) inhibitor, immunoassay and subsequent testing for HIV-1/HIV-2 is recommended.

Enfuvirtide does not require dosage adjustment in patients with renal failure or hepatic impairment. It is not metabolized by CYP enzymes and is not associated with any CYP-mediated drug-drug interactions. Injection-site reactions (e.g., subcutaneous nodules, redness) occur in up to 98% of patients. Other side effects reported include rash and diarrhea. Serious allergic reactions—including anaphylaxis, fever, and hypotension—have occurred in less than 1% of patients.

Chemokine (CCR5) Coreceptor Antagonists

Maraviroc (MVC), the only agent in this class, blocks the CCR5 coreceptor needed for CCR5-tropic HIV entry into immune cells, thus preventing viral replication. MVC is indicated in combination with other ARVs for treatment-experienced adult patients with evidence of viral replication and HIV-1 strains resistant to multiple antiretroviral therapy. The most common side effects are cough, pyrexia, upper respiratory tract infection, rash, abdominal pain, and dizziness. Because MVC is metabolized by the liver, drug-drug interactions exist.

Maraviroc is metabolized by the CYP3A substrate. Coadministration with St. John's wort or rifampin or other CYP3A inducers is not recommended due to reduced effectiveness of maraviroc. Rifapentine and some NRTI fixed-drug combinations are contraindicated with CCR5 coreceptor antagonists. Possible drug-induced hepatotoxicity with allergy-type features has been reported. Use caution in patients with liver or heart disease or a history of orthostatic hypotension and in those on medication that lowers blood pressure. Other adverse reactions include rash, musculoskeletal symptoms, upper respiratory infections, and pyrexia.

Integrase Strand Transfer Inhibitors

Integrase strand transfer inhibitors (INSTIs) such as dolutegravir (DTG), elvitegravir (EVG), and raltegravir (RTG) exert their action by interfering with integrase, the enzyme that HIV needs to multiply and divide, thus limiting the ability of the virus to replicate and infect new cells. INSTIs are used for the treatment of HIV-1 infections with at least two or three other ARVs in both treatment-naïve (recommended initial agent) and treatment-experienced patients. DTG and EVG are also available in fixed-dose combinations. INSTIs distribute into the CSF. DTG and RTG are metabolized by the UDP-glucuronosyltransferases (UGTs) 1A1-mediated glucuronidation pathway; EVG is metabolized by the CYP450 enzymes. Strong inducers (e.g., efavirenz, rifampin, rifabutin) or inhibitors (e.g., tenofovir, atazanavir) of UGT1A1 can significantly alter the concentration of RTG. DTG distributes into the CSF. Common side effects include rash, nausea, headache,

insomnia, diarrhea, and pyrexia; liver injury can also occur. Caution is advised in patients at increased risk for muscle problems (e.g., myopathy, rhabdomyolysis), which includes patients who take medications that can cause these adverse effects, such as statins.

IMMUNE RECONSTITUTION INFLAMMATORY SYNDROME

Immune reconstitution inflammatory syndrome (IRIS) is related to a disease- or pathogen-specific inflammatory response in patients with ART being initiated or changed. IRIS comprises two distinct entities: *paradoxical IRIS* is an exacerbation of treated (successful or partial) opportunistic infection (OI), whereas *unmasking IRIS* is a response to undiagnosed or subclinical OI. Diagnosis is a challenge because there are no laboratory markers; it is a condition of exclusion. For example, new OI or concurrent illness must be excluded before IRIS can be diagnosed. CD4+ cells usually increase in patients with IRIS because of the acute inflammatory response. IRIS may occur in response to many diseases and pathogens, such as Kaposi sarcoma or infection with mycobacteria, viruses, bacteria, or fungi.

Risk factors for developing IRIS include a low CD4+ cell count when ART is initiated and a high baseline HIV RNA. Starting ART soon after initiation of treatment for recognized OI also increases risk for IRIS. Severity of IRIS ranges from mild to life threatening. Treatment varies according to the specific pathogen and clinical situation but typically includes continuing ART if possible, treating the OI as indicated, and adding antiinflammatory therapy (including corticosteroids) as needed.

THE NURSE'S ROLE IN ANTIRETROVIRAL THERAPY

Thorough assessment of the patient's physiologic and psychosocial health needs and literacy levels is required initially and for the duration of care. Follow-up assessment after ART initiation should include drug side effects, adherence to the therapy regimen, and issues that affect medication adherence. Patients may confuse drug side effects with new onset of symptoms. Careful follow-up assessment can detect the need for additional medical care or drug management.

Adherence challenges are common with any drug therapy, but ART presents a greater challenge because patients are asked to achieve an adherence of 95% or greater. Nonadherence can result in HIV viral replication and can potentiate drug resistance. Multiple strategies for adherence are available and should be discussed with patients. Drug organizers, alarms on cell phones or mobile devices, medication "maps" with pictures, and drug diaries are available tools to improve adherence. Friends, family members, and personal support systems can also assist patients with adherence. Nurses can facilitate adherence by allowing sufficient time to educate patients about drugs, developing a trusting relationship, and building a partnership with the patient.

Nursing assessment for adherence should include asking the reasons for missing drug dosages. Reasons commonly include stigma, forgetting, feeling ill, side effects, not having the medicine when doses are due, pill fatigue (nonadherence due to the stress and monotony of constant pill swallowing), drug costs, loss of health insurance, and lack of transportation to the pharmacy. If barriers to adherence are identified, individualized plans should be addressed with the patient and the prescriber.

Patient education should include the purpose of each drug, the dosage schedule, food and fluid restrictions, recommended food choices, and storage of drugs. Additional suggestions include taking drugs during a daily routine, such as brushing teeth, or using a drug calendar to track drugs taken. The nurse should assess whether scheduled appointments to assist the patient with filling a drug organizer would be helpful until the patient is comfortable with completing this task. Discussion of anticipated drug side effects and management of drug side effects is necessary.

 NURSING PROCESS
Patient-Centered Collaborative Care

Antiretroviral Therapy

Assessment
- Obtain an in-depth patient history and assess physiologic and psychosocial needs.
- Assess for signs and symptoms related to clinical progression of HIV disease, and refer to medical care and psychological support as indicated.
- Perform a drug reconciliation that includes all prescription, over-the-counter (OTC), and herbal products. Assess for use of illegal and other nonprescription drugs. Report potential drug-drug or drug-herb interactions.
- Obtain a nutritional history to assess for nutritional deficits and for potential drug-food interactions. Assess for the potential need for therapeutic lifestyle change.
- Assess readiness to learn and discern the preferred method of instruction (written, verbal, pictorial).
- With each patient visit, conduct a pill count to determine treatment adherence.

Nursing Diagnoses
- Health Maintenance, Ineffective related to knowledge deficit about HIV/AIDS and the drug regimen.
- Health Management, Ineffective related to complex drug management
- Fear related to perceived stigma of HIV diagnosis
- Coping, Ineffective (patient) and/or Coping, Compromised Family (significant other) related to HIV diagnosis
- Infection, Risk for

Planning
- The patient will adhere to the drug regimen and will report any difficulties related to adherence.
- The patient will participate in medical treatment and in the spiritual and psychological support that best fits the patient's needs and belief system; the patient will verbalize fears.
- The patient will verbalize ways of maintaining self-health management such as a daily calendar and reminders.

- The patient will verbalize ways to cope with side effects of the drug regimen.
- The patient will verbalize signs and symptoms of potential infection and can reiterate when to notify the health care provider.
- The patient's viral load will become and remain undetectable.
- The patient will not experience secondary or opportunistic infections.

Nursing Interventions
- Provide information on the necessity of adhering to the drug regimen and regular health care. Inconsistent dosing can promote drug resistance. Effectiveness and side effects of ART need to be monitored and/or treated.
- Provide information on various methods of remembering to take drugs. Inconsistent dosing can increase the risk of drug resistance.
- Refer the patient for health care maintenance and appropriate health screening examinations, including Pap tests, ophthalmologic and dental examinations, and age- or risk-related colonoscopies. Side effects and adverse reactions are common in patients receiving ART.
- Refer the patient for spiritual support and for mental health or substance use counseling as needed.
- Provide opportunities for the patient and/or support persons to verbalize feelings.
- Encourage strategies to cope with the side effects of medications.
- Monitor laboratory reports for indications of decreasing CD4+ counts and/or rising viral load; inform the HIV health care provider.
- Refer the patient for nutritional counseling as needed.

Patient Teaching
General
- Educate patients about adherence to the therapeutic regimen by providing information on drugs and a timetable of dosing in patients' preferred method of learning.
- Explain how HIV can damage the immune system and promote infection.
- Explain common emotional responses.
- To decrease risk for exposure to infection, emphasize protective precautions as necessary, such as frequent hand washing, avoiding crowds, and receiving influenza vaccines.
- For patients of childbearing age, explain how HIV transmission to the unborn baby can occur.
- Teach about safe sex practices and other ways to prevent transmission of HIV.
- Inform patients that certain drugs—including OTC medications—and foods and herbal products may interact with antiretrovirals.

Self-Administration
- Assist patients in developing a system for taking the correct dose of the correct drugs at the correct time.

- Counsel patients about the importance of having an adequate supply of drugs to avoid interruption in the dosing schedule. Omission of drugs may result in deterioration of the patient's condition.
- For pediatric patients unable to swallow drugs, teach swallowing techniques.

🌐 Cultural Considerations

- Some members of certain cultural groups may distrust health care providers and may refuse treatment regimens that include research.
- Be aware that some cultures pressure women to reproduce regardless of health status.
- Remember that HIV remains a highly stigmatized disease in many cultures.
- Know that some religions prohibit the use of contraception.

Evaluation

- The patient will have at least a 95% drug adherence.
- Viral load will decrease or become undetectable.
- The patient and/or the significant other will openly discuss any fears or concerns related to HIV and ART.
- The patient will verbalize safe sex practices and methods to reduce HIV transmission.

In addition to patient assessment, education, and advocacy, nurses should identify problems that require additional investigation and research. Because of individual needs, research on strategies to promote adherence is needed. Whenever drug regimens change, nurses should contribute to the ongoing evaluation of the drug regimen, any side effects, and adverse event reporting. See Box 29.1 for HIV resources.

OPPORTUNISTIC INFECTIONS

As HIV advances, patients are more vulnerable to malignancies and opportunistic infections (OIs). Since the introduction of ART, there has been a dramatic reduction in the incidence of OIs among HIV-positive patients receiving ARVs. Although hospitalizations and deaths have decreased, OIs continue to be a leading cause of morbidity and mortality among patients with HIV. Prevention and treatment of OIs remain essential. The most common HIV-related OIs include pulmonary tuberculosis

---

BOX 29.1   HIV Resources

AIDS Info
The website www.aidsinfo.nih.gov provides information on HIV/AIDS clinical research, treatment, and prevention.

National HIV/AIDS Clinicians' Consultation Center
The website www.nccc.ucsf.edu provides up-to-date HIV/AIDS information to pharmacists, physicians, and nurses and is staffed by pharmacists, physicians, and nurse practitioners.

(TB), pneumococcal pneumonia, *Cryptosporidium*, fungal infections, Kaposi sarcoma, toxoplasmosis, histoplasmosis, and cytomegalovirus (CMV), among others.

Tuberculosis infection predominantly affects the lungs but can affect other organs, such as the bowel, brain, and lining of the heart, lungs, central nervous system (CNS), or integument. The CD4+ cell count is not a reliable predictor of increased risk for TB disease. Treatment for TB is discussed in Chapter 27.

Kaposi sarcoma causes dark blue lesions that can occur in a variety of locations, including the skin, mucous membranes, GI tract, lungs, or lymph nodes; they usually appear early in the course of HIV infection. Treatment depends on the symptoms and location, but chemotherapy is the preferred treatment for severe widespread disease.

Pneumocystis jiroveci **pneumonia (PJP)** is caused by a fungus that shares biologic characteristics with protozoa that infect the lungs. Symptoms include fever, dry cough, chest pain, and dyspnea. Even though PJP is classified as a fungal infection, it does not respond to antifungals. Trimethoprim-sulfamethoxazole (TMP-SMX), dapsone plus trimethoprim, pentamidine, or atovaquone are recommended treatment for persons with HIV and PJP.

Toxoplasmosis encephalitis caused by a protozoan can be found in uncooked meat and cat feces. Infection in the brain can cause headache, confusion, motor weakness, and fever. If left untreated, the disease progression results in seizures, stupor, and coma. Treatment includes pyrimethamine, sulfadiazine, and clindamycin. Leucovorin is added to decrease hematologic toxicities associated with pyrimethamine therapy.

Cryptosporidiosis is an infection caused by the protozoan parasite *Cryptosporidium,* usually in the bowel mucosa; in persons with low CD4+ counts, *Cryptosporidium* may involve the biliary tract or respiratory tract. GI symptoms include profuse, nonbloody, watery diarrhea, often with nausea, vomiting, and lower abdominal cramping. In addition to symptomatic therapy, treatment includes nitazoxanide or paromomycin combined with azithromycin. Treatment may be only partially effective in the setting of a low CD4+ count.

Diseases common with a CD4+ count below 50 cells/mL include:

Mycobacterium avium **complex (MAC)** is a blood infection caused by bacteria related to *M. tuberculosis,* the pathogen in TB. MAC generally affects multiple organs with symptoms that include fever, night sweats, weight loss, fatigue, diarrhea, and abdominal pain. Localized syndromes include pneumonitis, osteomyelitis, skin or soft-tissue abscesses, or CNS infections. Treatment includes clarithromycin, azithromycin, ethambutol, amikacin, moxifloxacin, rifabutin, or rifampin.

Cytomegalovirus (CMV) infection is caused by a virus that infects the entire body, but it most commonly appears as retinitis, causing blurred vision that can lead to blindness. CMV can also affect other organs and can cause fever, diarrhea, nausea, pneumonia-like symptoms, and dementia. Treatment includes ganciclovir, valganciclovir, foscarnet, or cidofovir.

ANTIRETROVIRAL THERAPY IN PREGNANCY

Optimal drug therapy should be used for women of reproductive age and for those who are pregnant. When initiating ART for women of reproductive age, the criteria for starting therapy and the goals of treatment are identical to those for other adults and adolescents. Because of considerations related to the prevention of HIV transmission to the fetus during pregnancy, the timing of initiation of treatment and the selection of regimens for pregnant patients may differ from those nonpregnant adults or adolescents. Women of childbearing potential should undergo a pregnancy test prior to initiation of efavirenz (EFV). If the patient expresses interest in becoming pregnant, and EFV is considered as part of the ARV regimen, a risk-benefit discussion must take place regarding the risk of neural tube defects related to EFV use in the first 5 to 6 weeks of pregnancy. EFV can be continued in pregnant patients receiving an efavirenz-based regimen who present for antenatal care in the first trimester, provided the regimen produces virologic suppression.

A patient infected with HIV can transmit the virus during pregnancy, labor, and delivery and through breastfeeding. To prevent mother-to-child transmission of HIV, ART is recommended in all pregnant patients who test positive for HIV infection, regardless of virologic, immunologic, or clinical parameters. Combination drug therapy is considered the standard of care for both treatment of maternal HIV infection and prophylaxis to reduce the risk for perinatal HIV transmission. The goal of ART is to achieve maximal and sustained viral suppression during pregnancy to prevent perinatal transmission of HIV. If viral load is greater than or equal to 400 copies/mL, IV zidovudine is recommended regardless of current ART. Prototype Drug Chart 29.1 presents the pharmacologic data for zidovudine.

OCCUPATIONAL HIV EXPOSURE AND POSTEXPOSURE PROPHYLAXIS

Treatment regimens after percutaneous exposure to HIV are called postexposure prophylaxis (PEP) regimens. Many PEP regimens are available, with varying degrees of tolerability and probability of patients completing 4 weeks of treatment. PEP management of potential HIV exposure should be initiated within 72 hours of the event and should be continued for 4 weeks. Health care workers who take PEP have reported adverse reactions, with the most common being nausea, malaise, and fatigue. More information from the Panel on the treatment of HIV/AIDS can be found at https://aidsinfo.nih.gov.

CRITICAL THINKING CASE STUDY

JP is a 35-year-old patient recently diagnosed with HIV. Other than a recent "case of the flu" approximately 1 month ago, she has been healthy. She has been divorced for 2 years and has a 3-year-old child from her previous marriage. JP tested HIV negative in the first trimester of her pregnancy and was not retested during the third trimester. She reports that the relationship with her husband was monogamous and that they did not use condoms. JP began a relationship with a new partner 1 year after her divorce. He claimed to be HIV negative, and they did not use condoms (JP takes oral contraceptives for pregnancy prevention). JP denies a history of intravenous drug use and other high-risk behaviors. Her baseline labs include a CD4+ count of 450 cells/mm³ and a viral load of 75,000 copies/mL. Her genotypic resistance assay shows no baseline resistance. Her preference is for a once-a-day regimen. She may want to have another child but is not certain.

1. JP asks the nurse when she may have become infected with HIV. What are some of the responses that the nurse should include in a discussion with the patient? What else should the nurse discuss with the patient about HIV transmission?
2. Considering JP's preference for a daily antiretroviral regimen and in view of her history, which medication regimens could be considered? What, if any, risk-benefit discussion should occur with regard to choices?
3. JP is told she will begin therapy with a fixed-dose combination regimen containing three different ARVs. JP asks why she needs to be on more than one drug. What should be the explanation by the nurse for the multidrug regimen?
4. At her next routine visit, JP says that she missed two doses of her medications because she had an unplanned overnight stay during a trip. What counseling and interventions should the nurse include in her discussion with the patient?

NCLEX STUDY QUESTIONS

1. During routine prenatal testing, a patient is diagnosed with human immunodeficiency virus infection. To help prevent perinatal transmission of human immunodeficiency virus to the fetus, what is the nurse's best action?
   a. Provide the patient with contact information for an acquired immunodeficiency syndrome support group.
   b. Educate the patient about the risks of human immunodeficiency virus disease to the fetus.
   c. Notify the Centers for Disease Control and Prevention of the patient's diagnosis.
   d. Provide written and oral education about the use of antiretroviral therapy during pregnancy.

2. When a patient does not appear for a routine clinic visit, the nurse calls to ask about the missed visit. The patient says, "I don't need to come any longer. I'm so glad I no longer have human immunodeficiency virus." The nurse learns that recent laboratory results indicated an "undetectable" human immunodeficiency virus viral load and that the patient stopped his medication several weeks earlier. What is the nurse's best response?
   a. Inform the patient that he must be seen immediately because the undetectable viral load indicates that his medication stopped working.
   b. Have the patient reschedule his clinic visit.
   c. Congratulate the patient on his treatment success.
   d. Educate the patient about the continued need for his medications and ongoing laboratory monitoring.

3. The nurse advises human immunodeficiency virus–positive patients about blood draws to obtain a CD4+ count. What is the correct information to give them about when and how this laboratory blood work should be done?
   a. At the same laboratory at approximately the same time of day whenever possible
   b. After a 10-hour fast
   c. Approximately 1 hour after taking antiretroviral medications
   d. At any laboratory at any time of day

4. In collaboration with a patient on antiretroviral therapy, the nurse formulates a plan of care. Which items are appropriate to include in planning? (Select all that apply.)
   a. The patient's viral load will become and remain undetectable.
   b. The patient will not experience secondary infection.
   c. The patient will promptly report new onset of symptoms and side effects.
   d. Laboratory blood work will be within normal limits.
   e. The patient will adhere to the medication regimen and will report any difficulties related to adherence.

5. A patient is to start on efavirenz. Which points are important for the nurse to include in health teaching for this patient? (Select all that apply.)
   a. The dose is given at bedtime to minimize central nervous system adverse effects.
   b. Alcohol should be avoided because of adverse effects to the liver.
   c. The dose should be taken after breakfast to minimize central nervous system adverse effects.
   d. High-fat meals can increase absorption of the medication.
   e. Hyperglycemia, jaundice, and diabetes mellitus are side effects.

Answers: 1, d; 2, d; 3, a; 4, a, b, c, e; 5, a, b, d.

30

Transplant Drugs

http://evolve.elsevier.com/McCuistion/pharmacology/

OBJECTIVES

- Describe the mechanism of action of the six maintenance therapy drugs and relate the processes to the principles of immunosuppression.
- Differentiate the three drugs used in the treatment of transplant rejection.
- Calculate the absolute neutrophil count of a patient on immunosuppressive drugs and relate it to neutropenic precautions.

- Describe the issues surrounding nonadherence in transplant recipients.
- Describe the nurse's role in promoting adherence to the therapeutic drug regimen.

OUTLINE

KEY TERMS

ORGAN TRANSPLANTATION

Organ transplantation is a life-saving procedure. In cadaveric transplantation, a healthy organ donated at the time of a person's death is transplanted into the body of a patient with end-stage organ failure. In living-donor transplantation, a kidney or a portion of liver donated by a living person is transplanted into the body of a patient with end-stage kidney or liver disease. Organ transplant is an acceptable treatment option when organs fail (e.g., kidney, heart, liver, and lung). More than 122,000 people are currently waiting for an organ transplant. Every 10 minutes, another person is added to the wait list, and over 8000 people die each year while waiting for a donor organ.

Principles of Immunosuppression

The immune system remains the biggest barrier to transplantation as a routine medical treatment because it has effective mechanisms to fight off foreign organisms. These same mechanisms are involved in the rejection of transplanted organs, which are recognized as foreign by the recipient's immune system. The underlying premise of immunosuppression is to use multiple drugs that alter different aspects of the immune system (Fig. 30.1), thereby reducing the chances of transplant rejection

and enabling the use of lower doses of individual drugs, which reduces the likelihood of drug toxicity. Transplantation has revolutionized care for patients with end-stage organ failure, yet significant problems remain with treatments designed to promote transplant survival and prevent rejection. Immunosuppressant drugs are not always effective; in addition, they are expensive and must be taken daily, and they are associated with toxic effects.

Immunosuppressant Drugs

Induction Therapy

Induction therapy provides intense immunosuppression with drugs designed to diminish antigen presentation and T-cell response, thus reducing the risk for acute rejection during the initial transplant period.

Basiliximab is a monoclonal antibody that inhibits interleukin 2 (IL-2)–mediated activation of lymphocytes, a critical component of the cellular immune response involved in transplant rejection. By inhibiting activation of lymphocytes, it prevents the body from mounting an immune response against the transplanted organ. Basiliximab has been approved for induction therapy in kidney transplants. Complete pharmacokinetic data are not available, but drug half-life is known to be 7.2 days in adults and 9.5 days in children.

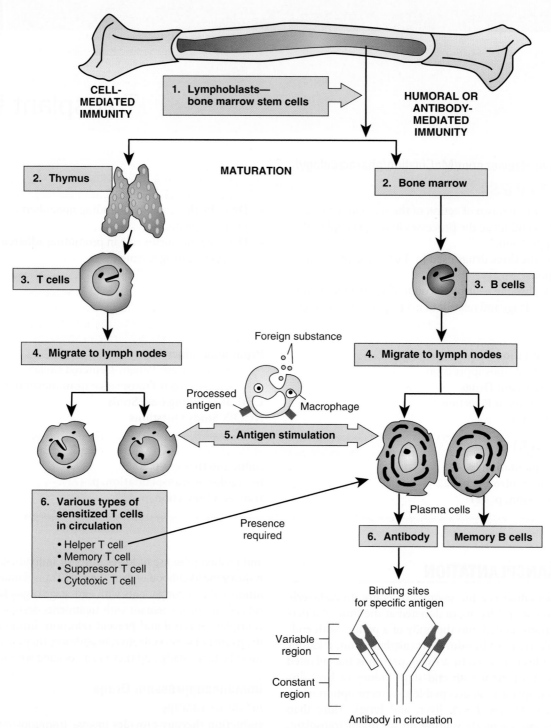

FIG. 30.1 The Immune Response. From Gould, B., & Dyer, R. (2011). *Pathophysiology for the health professions* (4th ed.). St Louis: Saunders.

Basiliximab is administered intravenously (IV), 20 mg within 2 hours before transplant surgery, followed by a second 20-mg dose 4 days after transplantation. The second dose should be withheld if complications occur (including severe hypersensitivity reactions or loss of the transplanted organ). Children under 35 kg should receive 10 mg IV within 2 hours before transplant surgery, followed by a second 10-mg dose 4 days after transplantation; the second dose should be withheld if complications occur (including severe hypersensitivity

reactions or loss of the transplanted organ); children over 35 kg should receive the adult dose.

Side effects of basiliximab include abdominal and back pain, coughing, dizziness, fever or chills, fatigue, weakness, dysuria, dyspnea, sore throat, edema, tremor, nausea and vomiting, and anemia. Serious reactions include sepsis, opportunistic infections, malignancy, lymphoproliferative disorders, thrombocytopenia, leukopenia, diabetes mellitus, anaphylaxis, capillary leak syndrome, and cytokine release syndrome (Box 30.1).

BOX 30.1 Cytokine Release Syndrome

Cytokine release syndrome is a symptom complex associated with the use of anti-T–cell antibody infusions, such as antithymocyte globulin (rabbit) and muromonab-CD3. Commonly referred to as an *infusion reaction*, cytokine release syndrome results from the release of cytokines from cells targeted by the antibody. When cytokines are released into the circulation, systemic symptoms such as fever, nausea, chills, hypotension, tachycardia, asthenia, headache, rash, scratchy throat, and dyspnea can result. In most patients, the symptoms are mild to moderate in severity and are managed easily. Premedication with corticosteroids or acetaminophen plus an antihistamine have been reported to be effective in reducing the severity of symptoms caused by cytokine release. Other management measures include reduction of the infusion rate. However, some patients may experience life-threatening reactions, therefore nurses must closely monitor patients receiving anti-T–cell antibody infusions. Patients with asthma, autoimmune disease, history of drug allergies, and previous exposure to the drug are at increased risk of developing cytokine release syndrome. During infusions, nurses must assess the patient frequently, monitoring vital signs and watching for any signs or symptoms of a reaction. Reactions are most likely to occur in the first hour, but a reaction could occur at any time. Any delay in recognition of the signs of anaphylaxis can compromise the patient's outcome.

From Vogel, W. H. (2010). Infusion reactions: Diagnosis, assessment and management. *Clinical Journal of Oncology Nursing, 14*(2), E10-E21. Retrieved from http://chemotherapy.vc.ons.org/file_depot/0-10000000/0-10000/3365/folder/87592/Infusion+Reactions+(Vogel+2010).pdf

Transplant recipients who receive basiliximab should not receive live vaccines because they may produce an inadequate immune response and are at risk for disseminated infection resulting from the live virus. Caution is advised when basiliximab is administered with other drugs that lower the immune response because of the increased risk of serious infection.

Basiliximab was designated pregnancy category B; no adequate and well-controlled studies have been done on the drug's use in pregnant women, therefore women of childbearing potential should use effective contraceptive measures before beginning treatment, during treatment, and for 4 months after completion of therapy. It is not known whether basiliximab is excreted in breast milk. Because of the potential for adverse drug reactions, a decision should be made whether to discontinue nursing or to discontinue the drug, taking into account the importance of the drug to the mother.

Maintenance Therapy

Calcineurin Inhibitors. The calcineurin inhibitors (CNIs) suppress the immune system by binding to cytoplasmic proteins that inhibit calcineurin phosphatase, resulting in a reduction in cytokine synthesis and inhibition of T-lymphocyte proliferation. There are two CNIs, cyclosporine and tacrolimus; the prototype CNI is cyclosporine. The drug became available in 1983 and was modified to improve bioavailability in 1994. ⚡ Cyclosporine oral solution USP modified and cyclosporine oral solution USP *are not* bioequivalent and *cannot* be used interchangeably.

After oral administration, absorption of cyclosporine is incomplete and varies widely from patient to patient. Drug distribution is concentration dependent; cyclosporine is 90% protein bound. The drug is extensively metabolized by the cytochrome P450 (CYP450) 3A enzyme system in the liver. Elimination is primarily biliary with only 6% excreted in urine. The average drug half-life is 8.4 hours.

Initial dosing of cyclosporine is 7 to 9 mg/kg orally per day in two divided doses; the first dose is given 4 to 12 hours before the transplant or postoperatively in both adult and pediatric patients. Adjustments to drug dosing are based on therapeutic drug monitoring (TDM), with the desired level between 100 and 500 ng/mL, depending on the organ transplanted and the length of time posttransplant.

The daily dose of cyclosporine oral solution USP *modified* should *always* be given in two divided doses and on a consistent schedule with regard to time of day and relation to meals. Grapefruit and grapefruit juice affect drug metabolism, increasing blood concentration of cyclosporine; for this reason, grapefruit should be avoided. To make cyclosporine oral solution USP modified more palatable, it should be diluted with room-temperature orange or apple juice; patients should avoid switching diluents frequently. When mixed with juice, the cyclosporine solution may appear cloudy. Cyclosporine is also available as immediate-release capsules (25 mg and 100 mg) and as an IV solution (250 mg/5 mL).

Common side effects of cyclosporine include elevated blood urea nitrogen (BUN) and creatinine, hypertension, hirsutism, infection, tremor, gingival hyperplasia, headache, hypertriglyceridemia, nausea and vomiting, diarrhea, hyperuricemia, hyperglycemia, arthralgia, edema, acne, hypomagnesemia, and hyperkalemia. Serious reactions include opportunistic infections, nephropathy and nephrotoxicity, diabetes mellitus, leukopenia, thrombocytopenia, hemolytic anemia, malignancy, and seizures.

Transplant recipients taking cyclosporine should not receive live vaccines because they may have inadequate immune response and are at risk for disseminated infection resulting from the live virus.

Multiple antibiotics, melphalan (an antineoplastic drug), antifungals, antiinflammatory drugs, cimetidine and ranitidine (histamine 2–receptor blockers), tacrolimus (an immunosuppressant), fibric acid derivatives, and methotrexate may potentiate kidney dysfunction when administered with cyclosporine. Calcium channel blockers, azole antifungals, macrolide antibiotics, and glucocorticoids can increase cyclosporine concentrations, as can allopurinol, amiodarone, bromocriptine, colchicine, danazol, imatinib, metoclopramide, nefazodone, and oral contraceptives. Other drugs—nafcillin, rifampin, anticonvulsants, bosentan, octreotide, orlistat, sulfinpyrazone, terbinafine, ticlopidine—and St. John's wort can decrease cyclosporine concentrations.

Concomitant administration of cyclosporine with 3-hydroxy-3-methylglutaryl-coenzyme A (HMG-CoA) reductase inhibitors (e.g., lovastatin, simvastatin, pravastatin, fluvastatin, and atorvastatin) may increase the risk for rhabdomyolysis. The dosage of HMG-CoA reductase inhibitors should be reduced.

In addition to TDM (drug levels should be drawn just prior to the dose), patients taking cyclosporine should have frequent monitoring of BUN, creatinine, potassium, and magnesium levels in addition to liver function tests (LFTs) and lipid profiles.

Cyclosporine was designated pregnancy category C; it does not appear to be a major human teratogen; however, it may be associated with increased rates of prematurity. Cyclosporine is present in breast milk. Because of the potential for serious adverse drug reactions in nursing infants, a decision should be made whether to discontinue nursing or to discontinue the drug, taking into account the importance of the drug to the mother.

Tacrolimus. Approved by the FDA in 1994, tacrolimus is the second calcineurin inhibitor approved for prophylaxis of rejection in heart, liver and kidney transplants. It carries a boxed warning for malignancies and serious infections. Patients taking this drug are at increased risk for developing lymphoma and other malignancies. Additionally, patients taking tacrolimus are at risk for developing bacterial, viral, fungal, and protozoal infections.

Dosing for heart transplant recipients begins no sooner than 6 hours posttransplant with a continuous infusion at 0.01 mg/kg/day IV. When oral dosing begins, it should be at a dose of 0.075 mg/kg/day orally divided every 12 hours. For patients with a liver transplant, tacrolimus is administered with a continuous infusion at 0.03 to 0.05 mg/kg/day IV. When oral dosing begins, it should be dosed 0.1 to 0.15mg/kg/day orally divided every two hours. Kidney transplant recipients should begin tacrolimus within 24 hours of receiving the transplanted organ. Dosing ranges from 0.1 to 0.2 mg/kg/day orally divided every 12 hours, and may vary based on drugs used for induction.

For all transplant recipients, dosing is adjusted based on serum drug levels with trough levels ranging between 5 and 20 ng/mL, depending on organ transplanted and length of time since transplant.

The drug is highly nephrotoxic and should be administered at the lowest recommended dose for those with renal impairment. For those with postoperative oliguria, use of tacrolimus may be delayed until kidney function is adequate. All patients on tacrolimus should have their kidney function monitored periodically during therapy.

Tacrolimus may prolong the QT/QTc interval and may cause Torsade de Pointes. Avoid Tacrolimus in patients with congenital long QT syndrome. In patients with congestive heart failure, bradyarrhythmias, those taking certain antiarrhythmic medications or other medicinal products that lead to QT prolongation, and those with electrolyte disturbances such as hypokalemia, hypocalcemia, or hypomagnesemia, consider obtaining electrocardiograms and monitoring electrolytes (magnesium, potassium, calcium) periodically during treatment.

Tacrolimus is slowly absorbed in the GI tract. Bioavailability averages 25% and peak serum concentration is reached in 3 hours. Food, especially food high in fat, slows absorption and reduces bioavailability. It is metabolized extensively in the liver and is over 90% excreted in the feces, with the remaining excreted in the urine. Genetic variations in activity of the CYP3A5 protein can affect serum concentrations of tacrolimus. Its half-life is variable depending on organ transplanted (3.5 to 40.6 hours).

Tacrolimus has multiple common side effects, including tremor, diarrhea, headache, hypertension, nephrotoxicity, infection, insomnia, electrolyte, metabolic and lipid abnormalities, constipation, edema, fever, anemia, hyperglycemia, hepatotoxicity, anorexia, dyspepsia, dyspnea, pruritus, dizziness, cough, leukopenia, and photosensitivity. Serious reactions include malignancy, posttransplant lymphoproliferative disorder, severe infections, Stevens-Johnson syndrome, toxic epidermal necrolysis, anaphylaxis, neurotoxicity, seizures, myocardial hypertrophy, QT prolongation, torsades de pointes, pericardial effusion, diabetes, myelosuppression, DIC, thrombocytopenic purpura, and hemolytic anemia.

Persons receiving tracrolimus have absolute contraindication for live vaccines, mifepristone, pimozide, quinidine, saquinavir, streptozocin, talimogene laherparepvec (a genetically modified oncolytic viral therapy used in patients with recurrent melanoma), and ziprasidone. Multiple other drugs should be used with caution. Protease inhibitors may increase serum drug levels, as can antifungal agents, calcium channel blockers, gastric acid suppressors/antacids, and antibacterials. Anticonvulsants can decrease serum drug levels, as can St. John's wort. Patients receiving tacrolimus should avoid grapefruit juice, as it too, may increase serum drug levels.

Costimulation Blockers. Belatacept is a first-in-class selective T-cell costimulation blocking agent indicated for use in combination with basiliximab induction, mycophenolate mofetil, and corticosteroids to prevent kidney transplant rejection. It inhibits T-cell CD28 activation and proliferation by binding costimulatory ligands (CD80, CD86) of antigen-presenting cells, thereby inhibiting T-lymphocyte proliferation and the production of the cytokines IL-2 and IL-4, interferon-alfa, and tumor necrosis factor alpha (TNF-α), which are involved in systemic inflammation. Metabolism and excretion of belatacept are unknown, but half-life is 8.2 to 9.8 days.

The prescribed dose must be divisible by 12.5 to accurately prepare the dose from the reconstituted solution. Initial dosing is 10 mg/kg IV prior to surgery on the day of transplant; the dose is repeated on day 5 and at the end of weeks 2, 4, 8, and 12 after transplantation. Maintenance dosing is 5 mg/kg IV at the end of week 16 after transplantation and then every 4 weeks thereafter. Belatacept is not approved for pediatric use.

⚡ This drug carries a boxed warning for increased risk of developing posttransplant lymphoproliferative disorder (PTLD), predominantly involving the central nervous system (CNS). Additionally, recipients without immunity to EBV are at a particularly increased risk, therefore belatacept is for use in EBV-seropositive patients only.

Common side effects of belatacept include infection, anemia, diarrhea, peripheral edema, hypertension, constipation, fever, cough, nausea and vomiting, altered potassium levels, headache, leukopenia, abdominal pain, dyslipidemia, hypophosphatemia, arthralgia, hyperglycemia, proteinuria, increased creatinine, insomnia, hypocalcemia, back pain, dysuria, and anxiety. Serious reactions include PTLD, malignancy, serious infections, progressive multifocal leukoencephalopathy (PML), neutropenia, acute renal failure, nephropathy, and diabetes mellitus.

Transplant recipients receiving belatacept should not receive live vaccines because their immune response may be inadequate, and they are at risk for disseminated infection resulting from the live virus. Caution is advised when belatacept is administered with other drugs that lower the immune response because of the increased risk of serious infection.

Belatacept was designated pregnancy category C, and adverse events have been observed in animal studies. According to the manufacturer, belatacept should not be used in pregnancy unless the potential benefit to the mother outweighs the potential risk to the fetus. ⚡ A pregnancy registry has been established to monitor outcomes of women exposed to belatacept during pregnancy (1-877-955-6877). Safety during breastfeeding is unknown, therefore a decision should be made whether to discontinue nursing or to discontinue the drug, taking into account the importance of the drug to the mother.

Mammalian Target of Rapamycin Inhibitors. There are two mammalian target of rapamycin (mTOR) inhibitors approved for the prevention of organ rejection in kidney transplant recipients aged 13 years and older: sirolimus and everolimus. Sirolimus is the prototype drug: it inhibits T-lymphocyte activation and proliferation and inhibits antibody production by binding to the FK binding protein, thereby inhibiting IL-2–mediated signal transduction. This results in cell-cycle arrest in the G1-S phase (growth phase and DNA replication), blocking T- and B-cell activation by cytokines. Time to peak concentration is 1 to 3 hours for sirolimus solution and 1 to 6 hours for tablets. Systemic bioavailability is 14% for solution and 47% for tablets. Sirolimus is extensively protein bound (92%) and is extensively metabolized in the intestine and liver. Excretion is 91% in the feces and 2.2% in the urine, and drug half-life is 2.5 days.

⚡ There are two boxed warnings for sirolimus: use of sirolimus increases susceptibility to infection and the possible development of lymphoma and other malignancies, and the safety and efficacy has not been established in liver or lung transplant patients, therefore use is not advised in liver or lung transplant patients due to increased morbidity and mortality.

For patients who weigh less than 40 kg, the loading dose should be 3 mg/m^2 once orally as soon as possible after transplantation; maintenance dosing should be adjusted based on body surface area (BSA) to 1 mg/m^2 per day orally. In patients who weigh more than 40 kg, the loading dose is 6 mg once orally as soon as possible after transplantation, and maintenance dosing is 2 mg/day orally.

It is recommended that the maintenance dose of sirolimus tablets be reduced by approximately one third in patients with mild or moderate hepatic impairment and by half in patients with severe hepatic impairment. Dosing should not exceed 40 mg/day.

TDM is recommended for all patients. Target whole-blood trough levels should range between 16 and 24 ng/mL for the first year following transplantation; thereafter, trough levels should range between 12 and 20 ng/mL. Sirolimus tablets are to be administered orally once daily, consistently with or without food. Tablets should not be crushed, chewed, or split. It is recommended that sirolimus tablets be taken 4 hours after administration of cyclosporine.

The most common side effects of sirolimus are peripheral edema, hypertriglyceridemia, hypertension, hypercholesterolemia, increased creatinine, constipation, abdominal pain, diarrhea, headache, fever, urinary tract infection, anemia, nausea, arthralgia, pain, and thrombocytopenia. Serious reactions include malignancy, lymphoma, severe infection, PML, nephropathy, hemolytic uremic syndrome, thrombotic microangiopathy, venous thromboembolism, myelosuppression, exfoliative dermatitis, pericardial effusion, ascites, interstitial lung disease, hepatotoxicity, and osteonecrosis.

Concurrent administration of sirolimus with ketoconazole, mifepristone, or voriconazole is contraindicated due to increased serum drug levels secondary to reduced metabolism of sirolimus.

Transplant recipients taking sirolimus should not receive live vaccines because their immune response may be inadequate, and they are at risk for disseminated infection resulting from the live virus. Caution is advised when sirolimus is administered with other drugs that lower the immune response because of the increased risk of serious infection.

Sirolimus was designated pregnancy category C; no adequate and well-controlled studies have been done in pregnant women, therefore effective contraception must be initiated before sirolimus therapy, and it should continue during sirolimus therapy and for 12 weeks after therapy has been stopped. Sirolimus should be used during pregnancy only if the potential benefit outweighs the potential risk. Whether sirolimus is excreted in breast milk is unknown, therefore a decision should be made whether to discontinue nursing or to discontinue the drug, taking into account the importance of the drug to the mother.

Purine Antimetabolites. Azathioprine, a purine antimetabolite, is converted into 6-mercaptopurine in the body, where it blocks purine metabolism and DNA synthesis, thereby suppressing T- and B-lymphocyte proliferation. It is indicated for the prevention of kidney transplant rejection. Azathioprine is well absorbed following oral administration. Both azathioprine and the metabolite 6-mercaptopurine are moderately bound to serum proteins (30%) and undergo extensive metabolism in the liver; both are primarily excreted in bile, and drug half-life is 5 hours.

⚡ Azathioprine has a boxed warning that chronic immunosuppression with azathioprine increases risk of malignancy in humans.

Dosing ranges from 1 to 3 mg/kg per day orally (an IV form is not currently available in the United States). In the setting of kidney dysfunction, the dose should be reduced by 25% for a creatinine clearance (CrCl) between 10 and 50 mL/min; if CrCl is less than 10 mL/min, the dose should be reduced by 50%.

Common side effects include leukopenia, thrombocytopenia, anemia, infection, nausea and vomiting, anorexia, diarrhea, elevated LFTs, malaise, myalgia, fever, and rash. Serious side effects include myelosuppression, PML, pancreatitis, hepatotoxicity, lymphomas, and other malignancies.

Transplant recipients taking azathioprine should not receive live vaccines because their immune response may be inadequate, and they are at risk for disseminated infection resulting from the live virus. Caution is advised when azathioprine is administered with other drugs that lower the immune response because of an increased risk of serious infection. Combining azathioprine with antihypertensive drugs increases the risk of leukopenia.

Patients who receive azathioprine should have a complete blood count (CBC), including a platelet count, taken weekly during the first month, twice monthly for the second and third months of treatment, then monthly. Creatinine and LFTs should be monitored.

Azathioprine was designated pregnancy category D because it can cause fetal harm when given to pregnant women and should be avoided; however, maternal benefit may outweigh fetal risk in serious or life-threatening situations. Azathioprine is found in breast milk and is possibly unsafe during breastfeeding, therefore a decision should be made whether to discontinue nursing or to discontinue the drug, taking into account the importance of the drug to the mother.

Inosine Monophosphate Dehydrogenase Inhibitors. Mycophenolate mofetil blocks synthesis of purine nucleotides by inhibition of the enzyme inosine monophosphate dehydrogenase (IMPDH), thereby preventing the proliferation of T cells and lymphocytes and preventing the formation of antibodies from B cells; it also may inhibit recruitment of leukocytes to inflammatory sites. Mycophenolate mofetil is rapidly absorbed following oral administration with 94% bioavailability, and it is 98% protein bound. It is a prodrug that is metabolized in the liver to mycophenolic acid (MPA); it is excreted in the urine (93%) and in feces (6%). Drug half-life for the oral formulation is 17.9 hours; the half-life for the IV formulation is 16.6 hours.

Recommended dosing for kidney transplant recipients is 1 g orally twice daily; for heart and liver transplant recipients, the dosage is 1.5 g orally twice daily. Kidney function should be monitored; for a CrCl less than 25 mL/min, the maximum dosage is 1 g twice daily. In pediatric transplant recipients, the recommended dose of mycophenolate mofetil oral suspension is 600 mg/m^2 twice daily, up to a maximum of 1 g twice daily.

The dose of mycophenolate mofetil should be reduced or interrupted for an absolute neutrophil count (ANC) of less than 1300. To calculate the ANC, the following formula is used (*WBC* is white blood cell count):

$$WBC \times total\ neutrophils\ (segmented\ neutrophils\ \% + segmented\ bands\ \%) \times 10 = ANC$$

A normal ANC is over 1500. An ANC of 500 to 1500 is considered neutropenic, and an ANC less than 500 indicates severe neutropenia and significantly increases a person's risk for infection (Box 30.2).

Common side effects of mycophenolate mofetil include hypertension, infection, diarrhea, edema, anemia, abdominal pain, constipation, headache, nausea and vomiting, dyspnea and cough, hypercholesterolemia, tremor, hypokalemia, acne, and insomnia. Serious reactions include thrombocytopenia, leukopenia, neutropenia, severe infection, viral reactivation, nephropathy, PML, lymphoma, lymphoproliferative disorders, malignancy, gastrointestinal (GI) bleeding, acute renal failure, and interstitial lung disease.

Transplant recipients taking mycophenolate mofetil should not receive live vaccines because their immune response may be inadequate, and they are at risk for disseminated infection resulting from the live virus. Caution is advised when mycophenolate mofetil is administered with other drugs that lower the immune response because of the increased risk of serious infection. Combining mycophenolate mofetil with nonsteroidal anti-inflammatory drugs (NSAIDs) increases the risk of GI bleeding.

BOX 30.2 Neutropenic Precautions

In addition to receiving treatment from your doctor, the following suggestions can help prevent infections:

- Clean your hands frequently.
- Try to avoid crowded places and contact with people who are sick.
- Do not share food, drink cups, utensils, or other personal items, such as toothbrushes.
- Shower or bathe daily and use an unscented lotion to prevent your skin from becoming dry and cracked.
- Cook meat and eggs all the way through to kill any germs.
- Carefully wash raw fruits and vegetables.
- Protect your skin from direct contact with pet bodily waste (urine or feces) by wearing vinyl or household cleaning gloves when cleaning up after your pet. Wash your hands immediately afterwards.
- Use gloves for gardening.
- Clean your teeth and gums with a soft toothbrush, and if your doctor or nurse recommends one, use a mouthwash to prevent mouth sores.
- Try and keep all your household surfaces clean.
- Get the seasonal flu shot as soon as it is available.
- If you go to the emergency room, you should not sit in the waiting room for a long time; when you check in, tell them right away you are receiving immunosuppressant drugs.
- Know the signs and symptoms of an infection:
  - Fever that is 100.4°F (38°C) or higher for more than one hour, or a one-time temperature of 101°F or higher.
  - Chills and sweats.
  - Change in cough or new cough.
  - Sore throat or new mouth sore.
  - Shortness of breath.
  - Nasal congestion.
  - Stiff neck.
  - Burning or pain with urination.
  - Unusual vaginal discharge or irritation.
  - Increased urination.
  - Redness, soreness, or swelling in any area, including surgical wounds.
  - Diarrhea.
  - Vomiting.
  - Pain in the abdomen or rectum.
  - New onset of pain.
  - Changes in skin, urination, or mental status.

From: Retrieved 12/23/16 from https://www.cdc.gov/cancer/preventinfections/pdf/neutropenia.pdf

---

Patients taking mycophenolate mofetil should have a baseline creatinine level drawn and should have CBCs done weekly during the first month, twice monthly for the second and third months of treatment, then monthly throughout the first year.

Mycophenolate mofetil was designated pregnancy category D; it is associated with an increased risk of first-trimester pregnancy loss and an increased risk of congenital malformations. ⚡ Females of reproductive potential must be made aware of the increased risk of first-trimester pregnancy loss and congenital malformations and must be counseled regarding pregnancy prevention and planning. It is unknown whether mycophenolate mofetil is found in breast milk, therefore a decision should be made whether to discontinue breastfeeding or to discontinue the drug, taking into account the importance of the drug to the mother.

Corticosteroids. Prednisone, a corticosteroid, is a glucocorticoid receptor agonist. It decreases inflammation by suppression of migration of polymorphonuclear leukocytes and reversal of increased capillary permeability; it suppresses the immune system by reducing the activity and volume of the lymphatic system; prednisone suppresses adrenal function at high doses and is readily absorbed from the GI tract (up to 90%). Plasma protein binding is less than 50% but is concentration dependent. Prednisone is metabolized by the liver to its active metabolite, prednisolone. It is excreted in the urine as sulfate and glucuronide conjugates. Prednisone has a plasma half-life of 2 to 4 hours and should be administered after meals or with food or milk to decrease GI upset.

In addition to their use in maintenance therapy, corticosteroids are used in high doses for the treatment of acute transplant rejection. The drug, methylprednisolone sodium succinate, is administered IV in doses that range from 250 mg to 500 mg daily for 3 to 5 days.

Common side effects of corticosteroid use include sodium retention, edema, hypokalemia, hypertension, diaphoresis, muscle atrophy, nausea and vomiting, dyspepsia, petechiae and ecchymosis, facial erythema, acne, rash, headache, dizziness and vertigo, insomnia, emotional lability, depression, anxiety, glucose intolerance, menstrual irregularities, hirsutism, appetite changes, and weight gain. Serious reactions include anaphylaxis, adrenal insufficiency, steroid psychosis, infection, diabetes mellitus, seizures, heart failure, peptic ulcer disease and GI bleeding, osteonecrosis, and tendon rupture. Long-term use may lead to impaired wound healing, skin atrophy, Cushing syndrome, glaucoma and cataracts, Kaposi sarcoma, and growth suppression in children. Cessation of corticosteroids may lead to withdrawal symptoms with high doses or long-term use.

Transplant recipients taking corticosteroids should not receive live vaccines because their immune response may be inadequate, and they are at risk for disseminated infection resulting from the live virus. Caution is advised when corticosteroids are administered with other drugs that lower the immune response because of the increased risk of serious infection. Combining corticosteroids with certain antibiotics increases the risk of QT prolongation and arrhythmias; combining corticosteroids with diuretics increases the risk of hypokalemia.

Transplant recipients taking corticosteroids should have periodic monitoring of their electrolytes, blood pressure, weight, and glucose levels. Pediatric patients should have their height monitored. Chest x-rays and ophthalmic examinations are indicated with long-term use.

Caution is advised during pregnancy, especially in the first trimester or with long-term use, because of the possible risk of low birthweight and premature birth. Corticosteroids are probably safe during breastfeeding.

Drugs for Transplant Rejection

Transplant rejection occurs when the immune system of the transplant recipient attacks the transplanted organ. This happens because the immune system recognizes foreign tissues and attempts to destroy them, just as it attempts to destroy infecting organisms, such as bacteria and viruses. Treatment of rejection with an anti–T-cell antibody is used when corticosteroids have failed to reverse rejection or for treatment of a recurrent rejection.

Antithymocyte globulin (rabbit), or *ATG rabbit*, is a polyclonal (depleting) antibody that blocks T-cell membrane proteins CD2, CD3, and CD45; this causes altered T-cell function and lysis and prolonged T-cell depletion, which begins within 24 hours. Complete pharmacokinetic data are not available, but drug half-life is 2 to 3 days.

Dosing is 1.5 mg/kg IV each day for 7 to 14 days in adults. This drug is not approved for use in children. Dosage should be decreased by 50% if the white blood cell (WBC) count decreases to 2000 to 3000 or the platelet count is 50,000 to 75,000. Treatments should be discontinued if the WBC count falls to less than 2000 or the platelet count falls to less than 50,000.

Common side effects of ATG rabbit include high fever, chills, nausea and vomiting, headache, diarrhea, malaise, shortness of breath, leukopenia, thrombocytopenia, peripheral edema, and increased risk for infection. Serious side effects include anaphylaxis, severe infusion reaction, cytokine release syndrome, serum sickness, sepsis, cytomegalovirus (CMV), malignancy, and lymphoproliferative disorders. Premedication with corticosteroids and antihistamines decreases the incidence and severity of adverse reactions. ⚡ Close supervision of the patient is required during and after IV infusion, to include frequent vital signs and assessment of the site for signs of extravasation.

Transplant recipients receiving ATG rabbit should not receive live vaccines because their immune response may be inadequate, and they are at risk for disseminated infection resulting from the live virus. Caution is advised when ATG rabbit is administered with other drugs that lower the immune response because of the increased risk of serious infection.

Patients should have WBC and platelets monitored frequently during treatment. ATG rabbit was designated pregnancy category C, and there are no adequate and well-controlled studies in pregnant women. Inadequate information is available to assess the risk of ATG rabbit when breastfeeding, therefore a decision should be made whether to discontinue nursing or to discontinue the drug, taking into account the importance of the drug to the mother.

Muromonab-CD3 is a monoclonal antibody that binds specifically to the CD3 complex on the surface of T lymphocytes; the CD3 complex is involved in antigen recognition and cell stimulation. Immediately after administration, CD3-positive T lymphocytes are abruptly removed from circulation. Complete pharmacokinetic data are not available, but drug half-life is 18 hours.

Dosing is 5 mg IV push daily for 10 to 14 days in adults. In pediatric patients under 30 kg, dosage is 2.5 mg IV push daily for 10 to 14 days; pediatric patients over 30 kg are dosed the same as adults.

⚡ Muromonab-CD3 carries a boxed warning for the risk of anaphylactic reactions occurring with any dose and life-threatening or lethal systemic, cardiovascular, and CNS reactions.

Common side effects of muromonab-CD3 include fever, chills, nausea and vomiting, diarrhea, headache, tachycardia, hypotension, dyspnea, tremor, rash, edema, fatigue, diaphoresis, dyspepsia, arthralgia, pruritus, leukopenia, and increased risk of infection. Serious reactions include anaphylaxis, Stevens-Johnson syndrome, cytokine release syndrome, cardiorespiratory arrest, seizures, encephalopathy, aseptic meningitis, opportunistic infection, malignancy, lymphoproliferative disorders, thrombosis, thrombocytopenia, anemia, neutropenia, and leukopenia.

Transplant recipients receiving muromonab-CD3 should not receive live vaccines because their immune response may be inadequate, and they are at risk for disseminated infection resulting from the live virus. Caution is advised when muromonab-CD3 is administered with other drugs that lower the immune response because of the increased risk of serious infection.

Transplant recipients receiving muromonab-CD3 should have BUN, creatinine, LFTs, and a CBC with differential drawn at baseline.

Muromonab-CD3 was designated pregnancy category C, and there are no adequate and well-controlled studies in pregnant women; however, potential benefits may warrant use of the drug in pregnant women despite potential risks. The drug is unsafe during breastfeeding.

Drugs for Infection
Bacterial

Pneumocystis jiroveci pneumonia (PJP) is a life-threatening illness in immunocompromised patients. Routine prophylaxis with trimethoprim-sulfamethoxazole (TMP-SMZ) has significantly reduced the morbidity and mortality of PJP following transplantation. TMP-SMZ is dosed once every morning or one tablet three times a week (Monday, Wednesday, and Friday). TMP-SMZ can make the skin more sensitive to sunlight, therefore patients should be instructed to use a lotion with a minimum sun protection factor (SPF) of 25 when in the sun. See Chapter 26 for further information regarding antibacterial drugs.

Fungal

Transplant recipients use nystatin to prevent or treat thrush in the mouth and esophagus. This is usually given when the patient is on a high-dose immunosuppression regimen and is stopped when the steroid dose is reduced below 20 mg per day. Nurses must instruct the transplant recipient in proper administration of nystatin liquid:
- Shake the preparation well before measuring the dose.
- Swish the dose around in the mouth for at least 2 minutes before swallowing.
- Allow the nystatin to coat the mouth for as long as possible.
- Do not eat or drink anything for 30 minutes after taking the medication.
  See Chapter 27 for further information regarding antifungal drugs.

Viral

One common virus that patients develop after transplantation is CMV. It may present as a viral syndrome or as invasive disease, and it plays a role in organ rejection. Transplant recipients receive antiviral prophylaxis with oral ganciclovir or valganciclovir for 3 to 6 months following surgery. If untreated, CMV can cause serious complications, particularly in the liver,

intestine, kidneys, heart, lungs and eyes. See Chapter 27 for further information regarding antiviral drugs.

PROMOTING ADHERENCE

On discharge from the hospital, transplant recipients begin a lifelong journey of close medical supervision that includes frequent visits to their health care provider, monitoring of blood work, and maintenance of a complex drug regimen. The 1-year survival rates are over 80% for liver transplants and over 90% for kidney transplants; most recipients experience an improved quality of life. However, long-term adherence is a problem, with reports of nonadherence ranging from a low of 2% to as high as 68%. Nonadherence to the posttransplant regimen (e.g., drug regimen, exercise and health promotion) is one of the top three reasons for transplant failure. Factors that affect adherence include episodes of rejection, comorbid illness and disease, side effects of drugs, and health care costs. Nurses play a key role in promoting adherence by incorporating education, motivational strategies, and coping skills into an individually tailored posttransplant plan of care.

NURSING PROCESS
Patient-Centered Collaborative Care
Organ Transplants: Immunosuppression

Assessment
- Assess for clinical signs of rejection including malaise, fever, edema, pain over the transplant site, and increased weight.
- Assess for presence of risk factors for infection, including drugs, travel, and exposure to individuals with active infections.
- Assess for signs and symptoms of infection, including redness, swelling, pain, and elevated temperature.
- Assess immunization status.
- Assess nutritional status, including weight and history of weight loss.

Nursing Diagnosis
- Protection, Ineffective related to the possibility of transplant rejection
- Infection, Risk for

Planning
- Infection is recognized early to allow prompt treatment.
- The transplant recipient and family members will verbalize understanding of early signs and symptoms of rejection.
- The transplant recipient will remain free of infection.

Nursing Interventions
- Instruct the transplant recipient on the benefits of a balanced and healthy diet accompanied by exercise.
- Instruct the transplant recipient on proper adherence to the drug regimen.

- Patients should be instructed to avoid anyone with an active infection and to be careful not to injure themselves, which may increase the chance of acquiring a wound infection. They should stay away from anyone who has a cold, mumps, measles, chickenpox, or other communicable diseases.
- Promote health education with patients and families in order to recognize and minimize the risk of complications and rejection and to facilitate optimum quality of life.
- Teach the transplant recipient the signs and symptoms of rejection and infection, and instruct them on when to call their health care provider.

- Teach the transplant recipient to self-monitor vital signs, daily weights, and blood glucose (if appropriate); ensure the recipient knows when to call the health care provider.
- Transplant recipients and their families should be taught to wash hands properly, especially after toileting, before meals, and before administering drugs.

Evaluation
- Evaluate effectiveness of the plan, including adherence to the immunosuppressive drug regimen and freedom from infection and transplant rejection.

CRITICAL THINKING CASE STUDY

EM is a 24-year-old female kidney transplant recipient 6 months out from surgery. She is experiencing an episode of acute rejection. In addition to cyclosporine oral solution, mycophenolate mofetil, and prednisone, she is now receiving antithymocyte globulin (rabbit), having failed high-dose steroid treatment for the rejection. EM has had a CBC with differential drawn and her WBC counts are $2.0 \times 10^3/\mu L$, segmented neutrophils are 14.8%, and the segmented bands are 5%.
1. What would be your primary nursing diagnosis? Why?

2. Why is EM prescribed multiple immunosuppressant drugs?
3. When questioning EM about her drug regimen, she states she mixes her cyclosporine in orange juice. She has also been drinking a small glass of grapefruit juice at night because she's heard it helps to lower lipid levels, and she knows cyclosporine can cause elevated lipids. How would you respond to EM?
4. Calculate the ANC. What precautions are necessary if the ANC is less than 500?

NCLEX STUDY QUESTIONS

1. All transplant drugs have the same advisory, to use caution when administering them with another immunosuppressant drug because of the increased risk for:
   a. Nausea and vomiting
   b. Edema
   c. Anemia
   d. Infection
2. Which virus has been associated with posttransplant lymphoproliferative disorder?
   a. Cytomegalovirus
   b. Herpes simplex virus
   c. Epstein-Barr virus
   d. Human immunodeficiency virus
3. Nurses are key to promoting adherence in transplant recipients. What factors influence whether a recipient adheres to a drug regimen? (Select all that apply.)
   a. Drug side effects
   b. Episodes of rejection
   c. Cost
   d. Other health care issues

4. Your patient is receiving basiliximab and develops cytokine release syndrome. You would expect to see:
   a. Coughing
   b. Chills
   c. Tremors
   d. Weakness
5. Your patient taking belatacept becomes pregnant. After discussion with her partner, you, and her health care provider, she decides the best thing to do is continue taking the drug while pregnant. In addition to making this informed decision, what else should she do?
   a. Discontinue all other drugs
   b. Contact the pregnancy registry
   c. Ensure her blood level stays between 16 and 24 ng/mL
   d. Decrease her dose by 50%

Answers: 1, d; 2, c; 3, a, b, c, d; 4, b; 5, b.

31

Vaccines

http://evolve.elsevier.com/McCuistion/pharmacology/

OBJECTIVES

- Describe active and passive immunity as both relate to the action of vaccines used in immunizations.
- Differentiate between active natural and active acquired immunity as it relates to the human immune system.
- Identify the diseases that can be prevented with vaccines.
- Review the recommended immunization schedule for children and teens.

- Correlate the manifestations and administration routes for adult vaccines.
- Discuss contraindications to the administration of recommended immunizations.
- Apply the nursing process to include teaching for patients receiving vaccines.

OUTLINE

KEY TERMS

Over the years, immunizations have prevented global epidemics, such as smallpox in 1977 and the eradication of polio in the United States in 1979. The U.S. National Immunization Survey (NIS; www.cdc.gov/vaccines) tracks vaccination coverage of children 19 to 35 months and teens 13 to 17 years. In 2014, vaccine coverage was high (at 90%) for 19- to 35-month-old children who received the recommended doses of diphtheria, tetanus, acellular pertussis (DTaP; for children <7 years old); *Haemophilus influenzae* type B (Hib); measles, mumps, and rubella (MMR); polio; hepatitis B (HepB); pneumococcal conjugate vaccine (PCV); varicella; rotavirus (RV); and hepatitis A (HepA). The survey also estimated that 0.8% of children below

the federal poverty level had lower coverage for all vaccinations compared with children at or above the poverty level.

The 2014 national coverage also indicated that the Healthy People 2020 target goal of 90% was met for children aged 19 to 35 months who received the recommended doses of DTaP, polio, MMR, Hib, HepB, PCV, and varicella vaccines.

The NIS estimated that from 2013 to 2014, vaccination coverage among teens aged 13 to 17 years increased from 84.7% to 87.6% for tetanus, diphtheria, and acellular pertussis (Tdap; for individuals >11 years old), and from 76.6% to 79.3% for meningococcus 4-valent conjugate (MenACWY). Although human papillomavirus (HPV) vaccination increased for females (from 56.7% to 60%) and males (from 33.6% to 41.7%), vaccination coverage remained low. These results indicate an increase in all vaccinations for teens, with a need to improve HPV coverage.

IMMUNITY

Active Immunity

The body can obtain immunity in different ways. Active immunity occurs when the body's immune response is stimulated by an antigen or when a pathogen enters the body. The body recognizes this pathogen as a foreign substance and produces antibodies, also called *immunoglobulins,* which defend the body against pathogens. The immune response is slow, taking several days or weeks to develop immunity. Yet the immunity is often long lasting. During this process, the immune system retains memory of the pathogen then produces antibodies to defend against the disease. Natural acquired active immunity occurs from exposure to a pathogen or disease. Active acquired artificial immunity occurs when a weakened antigen or immunoglobulin (Ig) is injected into an individual as a vaccination, which then stimulates an immune response.

Passive Immunity

When an individual is unable to make antibodies and memory cells, antibodies are given from another source to provide passive immunity. These antibodies may be produced using recombinant deoxyribonucleic acid (DNA) technology or pooled antigens from several human or animal sources that have been exposed to disease-causing pathogens.

Passive immunity can be natural, in which case the body produces its own antibodies, or it can be acquired—that is, the body receives antibodies from an outside source. Either way the immunity is immediate and short lived, lasting no more than several weeks to a few months; the recipient does not induce his or her own immune response. One example of natural immunity passively acquired is in infants, who are unable to protect against disease because of immature immune systems but instead require antibodies from an outside source, such as the mother's placenta and breast milk. Another example is receiving an Ig to provide antibodies against a specific disease. Passive acquired immunity is essential when (1) time does not permit active vaccination alone, (2) the exposed individual is at high risk for complications of the disease, or (3) the individual suffers from an immune system deficiency that renders that person unable to produce an effective immune response.

Community Immunity

Community immunity, also known as *herd immunity,* occurs when most of the community is immunized against contagious diseases, allowing protection of those not immunized. In contrast, when most of the community is *not* immunized, there is an increased risk for the spread of contagious disease within the community (Fig. 31.1). For more information, see www.vaccines.gov/basics/protection/.

VACCINES

Vaccination involves the administration of a small amount of antigen, which although capable of stimulating an immune response does not typically produce the disease. Different types of vaccines are available, but the type used in vaccinations depends on the person's immune response. The antigen in vaccines may be produced in several ways. Traditional vaccines contain the whole or components of an inactivated (killed) microorganism. Other vaccines are attenuated viruses composed of live, attenuated (weakened) microorganisms. Persons who are immunocompromised because of illness or who take medication that causes immunosuppression should avoid live vaccines. Toxoids are inactivated toxins that can no longer produce harmful diseases but do stimulate formation of antitoxins, which produces active immunity (e.g., tetanus toxoid).

Newer vaccines, called conjugate vaccines, require a protein or toxoid from an unrelated organism to link to the outer coating of the disease-causing microorganism. This linkage creates a substance that can be recognized by the immature immune system of young infants. One example is *H. influenzae* type B.

Recombinant subunit vaccines involve the insertion of some of the genetic material (e.g., DNA) of a pathogen into another cell or organism, where the antigen is then produced in massive quantities. These antigens are then used as a vaccine in

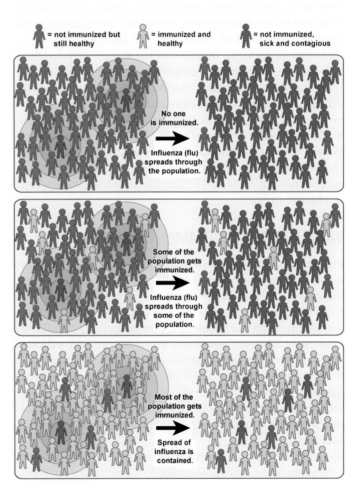

FIG. 31.1 Community immunity. Courtesy National Institute of Allergy and Infectious Diseases.

place of the whole pathogen. The HepB vaccine is an example of this type of vaccine.

An **adjuvant**—often an aluminum salt such as aluminum hydroxide, aluminum phosphate, or aluminum potassium sulfate—is a substance added to a vaccine to increase the body's immune response to the vaccine. One value of adding adjuvant to a vaccine is to reduce the amount of antigen needed to produce a dose of vaccine. Vaccines with adjuvants are rigorously tested for safety before being licensed. In the United States, vaccines against measles, mumps, rubella, chickenpox, rotavirus, polio, and seasonal influenza do *not* contain adjuvants.

Regardless of the composition of the vaccine, each vaccine is designed to stimulate an immune response against a specific pathogen. Some vaccines require booster doses to maintain sufficient immunity. The immune system's memory responds rapidly to prevent disease when exposed to a booster, which provides an active albeit artificially acquired immunity.

VACCINE-PREVENTABLE DISEASES

Vaccinations maintain health by preventing disease. In the United States, more than 20 infectious diseases may be prevented by active vaccination. Many of these vaccines are routinely administered to healthy children and adults. Others are reserved for special populations such as health care providers, military personnel, immigrants, adults with special health needs, the chronically ill, and travelers to certain foreign countries. Table 31.1 provides an overview of the disease manifestations and vaccine information, including route of administration and storage temperature. Vaccine-preventable diseases for children, adolescents, and adults include—but are not limited to—anthrax, diphtheria, *H. influenzae* type B, hepatitis A and B, human papillomavirus, influenza (flu), Japanese encephalitis, measles, meningococcal disease, mumps, pertussis, pneumococcal disease, poliomyelitis, rabies, rotavirus, rubella, smallpox, tetanus, tuberculosis (TB), typhoid, varicella, yellow fever, and herpes zoster.

VACCINATION RECOMMENDATIONS

Immunization schedules are approved by the Advisory Committee on Immunizations (ACIP). Each schedule identifies recommended vaccinations, ages to vaccinate, dosage, and route for children, adolescents, and adults. For the most current information on childhood immunizations, consult the Centers for Disease Control and Prevention (CDC) website at www.cdc.gov/vaccines. A vaccine information statement (VIS) is also produced by the CDC for each vaccine, and provides information on the (1) route of administration, (2) schedule for routine vaccine administration, (3) minimum dosing intervals, (4) contraindications, and (5) standing orders for administering vaccines.

The childhood immunization schedule from birth to 6 years recommends HepB, RV, DTaP, Hib, PCV, inactivated polio virus (IPV), MMR, varicella, and HepA. Before immunizations are administered, screen for medical conditions that put the child

at risk, use of prescription and over-the-counter (OTC) drugs to include herbal preparations, and any food or drug allergies (Complementary and Alternative Therapies 31.1).

The adolescent immunization schedule from ages 7 to 18 years recommends Tdap, influenza, HPV, and meningococcal vaccinations. Adolescents may also need to catch up on any vaccines missed, such as MMR, HepA, HepB, IPV, and varicella (chickenpox).

A catch-up immunization schedule is available for those up to 18 years of age who fall behind or start late with immunizations. Childhood and adolescent immunization schedules are also available as a combined schedule (birth to 18 years).

Adult (19 years and older) vaccination rates remain low, which indicates a need to improve. One way is to increase awareness that routine vaccines for adults are important for well-being, to provide information on how vaccines protect from diseases, and to assess immunization status during clinical visits. Adult vaccines are based on factors such as age and health status and include Tdap, tetanus-diphtheria (Td) booster, influenza, pneumococcal polysaccharide vaccine (PPSV23), HPV, MMR, varicella vaccine (chickenpox), and zoster vaccine (shingles). In certain situations, adults may also be immunized with certain additional vaccines, including HepA, HepB, smallpox (2016 update: routine for lab personnel handling vaccine cultures), and meningococcal vaccine. Current recommendations for adult immunization can be found at www.cdc.gov/vaccines/schedules/.

🌿 COMPLEMENTARY AND ALTERNATIVE THERAPIES 31.1

Vaccines

Although patients should always be asked about their use of prescription drugs, OTC drugs, and complementary and alternative therapies, there are no known interactions between vaccinations and herbal preparations.

⚡ PATIENT SAFETY

Do not confuse...

- Hepatitis A, inactivated/hepatitis B (recombinant) vaccine provides active immunity against both hepititis A virus (HAV) and hepititis B virus (HBV) for adults >18 years of age who are at high risk for HAV and HBV.
- There are different types of **meningococcal vaccine**: MCV4 or MenACWY (conjugate; administered to pre-teens 11 to 12 years old), MenB (serogroup B; administered to teens and young adults ages 16 to 23), and MPSV4 (polysaccharide; for adults ≥56 who require a single dose [traveling or at risk due to community outbreak]).
- HepA and HepB vaccines are *dosed differently* for children, adolescents, and adults.
- Do not confuse HepB *vaccine* and HepB *immunoglobulin*.
- **Zoster vaccine,** a vaccine administered to adults to prevent shingles, and **varicella vaccine,** which prevents chickenpox and is approved for use in susceptible children and adults.
- ❶ **DTaP,** for active immunization in children 6 weeks to 6 years, and **Tdap,** the active booster for those aged 10 years and older; antigens in both are the same, but the amount of antigen component varies.

TABLE 31.1 Vaccine-Preventable Diseases

Disease, Route of Administration, Storage, Pregnancy Category	Manifestations	Vaccine
Anthrax, subcut 2°-8°C Do not freeze Pregnancy category: D*	*Cutaneous:* An itchy sore that may blister and form a black ulcer (eschar). The sore is usually painless but may have surrounding edema. *Gastrointestinal:* Abdominal pain, vomiting, mouth sores, bloody diarrhea, toxemia, shock, and possibly death *Inhaled,* wool sorter's disease or associated with the use of biologic warfare: Fever, malaise, headache, cough, shortness of breath, and chest pain (due to bleeding and swelling in chest cavity) are often followed by shock within 36 hours of symptom onset due to bacteremia.	Routine vaccinations are not recommended but are administered to specific groups: laboratory workers who work with anthrax; people who handle animals or animal products, such as some veterinarians; some members of the U.S. military. These persons sould receive 5 shots over 18 months with annual boosters. When used as postexposure prophylaxis, the vaccine is given as a three-dose series, administered at 0, 2, and 4 weeks after exposure, along with 60 days of antibiotic therapy (ciprofloxacin and doxycycline).
Diphtheria, IM (diphtheria toxoids) 35°-46°F (2°-8°C) Do not freeze Pregnancy category: C*	Respiratory infection, blocked airway, myocardial damage, nerve damage, sore throat, weakness, swollen glands	Toxoid A single-antigen toxoid is not available. Currently combined as DTaP, Tdap, DT, and Td. DTaP is used for active immunity in those 6 wk to 6 y. Tdap (active booster) is given as a single dose for those 10 years and older.
Haemophilus influenzae type B (Hib), IM 35°-46°F (2°-8°C) Do not freeze Pregnancy category: C*	Sepsis, arthritis, skin and throat infections, meningitis, intellectual disability, epiglottitis, pneumonia, and death Increased severity is seen in those younger than 5 y and older than 65 y.	Bacterial conjugate is contained in Hib vaccine. There are different types of influenza; Hib is specific to influenza B. Not all influenza bacteria have vaccines.
Hepatitis A virus (HAV), IM 36°-46°F (2°-8°C) Do not freeze Pregnancy category: C*	Fever; can cause liver damage or failure, malaise, jaundice, anorexia, nausea, arthralgia, kidney, pancreatic, and blood disorders This acute, self-limited illness is highly contagious.	Inactivated viral antigen is available as HepA vaccine and in HepA/HepB. Routinely administered to children 12-23 mo, high-risk populations, close contacts to persons with HAV, and persons traveling to certain countries. Because it is inactivated, the vaccine can be given to immunocompromised persons.
Hepatitis B virus (HBV), IM 35°-46°F (2°-8°C) Do not freeze Pregnancy category: C*	Fever, headache, malaise, anorexia, arthralgia, arthritis, jaundice Chronic infection can occur, leading to liver cirrhosis, liver cancer, and death.	Recombinant viral antigen is available as HepB and HepA/HepB vaccines. Vaccines are recommended for at-risk infants, health care personnel, those who share injectable/IV drug needles and equipment, men who have sex with men, those whose sex partners are HBV positive, and those not in a monogamous relationship. HepB vaccine is available as a single dose and as a combined vaccine. Administer monovalent HepB to all infants at birth. Combination HepA-HepB is recommended only for those 18 y and older and for at-risk infants.
Human papillomavirus (HPV; various disease strains), IM 35°-46°F (2°-8°C) Protect from light, and shake well before administering Pregnancy: Administer only if needed	Sexually transmitted and seen as cervical, vaginal, anal, and oropharyngeal cancers and genital warts	The HPV vaccine is recommended for preteen boys and girls at age 11 or 12 so they are protected before ever being exposed to the virus. Women and men can receive the HPV vaccine through age 26.
Influenza, IM/ID/IN Inactivated influenza vaccine (IIV) 35°-46°F (2°-8°C): Administer IM/ID Live attenuated influenza vaccine (LAIV) ≤5°F (−15°C): Administer IN Pregnancy category: C*	Fever, chills, headaches, malaise, myalgias, nasal congestion, and cough Can cause pneumonia.	*Trivalent flu vaccine* (influenza A [H1N1 and an H3N2] and influenza B). *Quadravalent flu vaccine* (2 influenza A and 2 influenza B). Everyone 6 months and older should have the flu vaccine annually, particularly those at high risk. Those who should NOT receive the flu shot include infants <6 months old, those with allergies to the flu vaccine or any of its components, those with allergies to eggs, and those with or who have recovered from Guillain-Barré syndrome. The IN flu vaccine should not be administered to children <2 y or adults >50 y, or children >2 or <17 y receiving aspirin-containing therapy or with asthma.
Japanese encephalitis, subcut Keep at 35°-46°F (2°-8°C) before and after reconstitution Pregnancy category: B*	Headache, vomiting, fever, myalgias, confusion, encephalitis, and possible death	Inactivated virus is given to travelers going to some Asian locations.

Continued

TABLE 31.1   Vaccine-Preventable Diseases—cont'd

Disease, Route of Administration, Storage, Pregnancy Category	Manifestations	Vaccine
Measles, subcut (rubeola) 35°-46°F (2°-8°C) or colder; may be frozen Protect from light, and discard after 8 hours Pregnancy category: C*	Rash, fever, cough, nasal congestion, conjunctivitis, pneumonia Occasionally results in encephalitis	Live virus is contained in measles, MMR and MMRV vaccines. ❶ Contraindicated in pregnancy
Meningococcal disease, subcut/IM 35°-46°F (2°-8°C) Groups A, C, W, Y Meningococcal Haemophilus influenzae type b conjugate vaccine Pregnancy category: C*	Fever, sepsis, rash, meningitis	Meningococcal conjugate vaccines MenACWY: quadrivalent (protects against serogroups A, C, W, and Y). Recommended for children 2 mo to 10 y who are at increased risk and children/adolescents 11-18 y. First dose is recommended between 11 and 12 y with booster at 16 y. Also for adults following splenectomy, persons working with the pathogen, college freshmen, and military recruits. Meningococcal polysaccharide vaccine (MPSV4): quadrivalent (protects against serogroups A, C, W, and Y) meningococcal vaccine. For adults following splenectomy, persons working with the pathogen, college freshmen, and military recruits. Serogroup B meningococcal vaccine (MenB): monovalent (protects against serogroup B) meningococcal vaccine. Recommended for children/adolescents 10-18 y who are at increased risk.
Mumps, subcut 35°-46°F (2°-8°C), but may be frozen Pregnancy category: C*	Swelling of salivary glands, fever, headache, fatigue, and myalgia Can cause meningitis, encephalitis, inflammation of testicles or ovaries, deafness	Live attenuated virus is contained in MMR and MMRV. ❶ Contraindicated in pregnancy
Pertussis ("whooping cough"), IM 35°-46°F (2°-8°C) Pregnancy category: C*	Highly contagious Severe coughing spasms; can cause pneumonia, seizures, encephalitis, and death Symptoms are more severe in infants and young children.	Antigenic components of inactivated bacteria (acellular) are contained in the two vaccines that are available, DTap and Tdap.
Pneumococcal disease, IM/subcut 35°-46°F (2°-8°C) Pregnancy category: B*	Ear infections, sinus infections, pneumonia; can cause sepsis, meningitis, and death	Pneumococcal polysaccharide vaccine (PPSV23) protects against 23 types of pneumococcal bacteria (IM/subcut). PPSV23 is recommended for all adults ≥65 y. Immunocompromised patients ≥2 but ≤64 y should also receive PPSV23. Pneumococcal conjugate vaccine (PCV13) protects against 13 types of pneumococcal bacteria (IM). PCV13 is recommended for all children <5 y as a series of 4 injections starting at 2 mo, then 4 mo, 6 mo, and between 12 and 15 mo; adults ≥65 y, and people ≥6 y with certain chronic illnesses should also receive the vaccine.
Poliomyelitis, subcut/IM 35°-46°F (2°-8°C) Pregnancy category: C*	Invades brain and spinal cord; the milder form causes fever, sore throat, nausea, and headaches; the severe form causes paralysis and death.	Children should receive a series of 4 inactive polio vaccine (IPV) injections starting at 2 mo, then at 4 mo, 6-18 mo, and a booster at 4-6 y.
Rabies, IM 35°-46°F (2°-8°C) Pregnancy category: C*	Anxiety, difficulty swallowing, seizures; almost always progresses to death	Administer killed virus to high-risk groups (e.g., veterinarians, animal handlers) and to persons traveling to areas where rabies is common. The pre-exposure schedule for rabies vaccination is three doses, given on the following schedule: 1st dose: prior to potential exposure 2nd dose: 7 days after the first dose 3rd dose: 21 days or 28 days after the second dose
Rotavirus, PO 35°-46°F (2°-8°C) Pregnancy category: C*	Acute gastroenteritis; contagious and may be particularly severe in infants and young children but mild in adults	Two vaccines are available: RV5 is given in 3 doses at ages 2 mo, 4 mo, and 6 mo RV1 is given in 2 doses at ages 2 mo and 4 mo ❶ Due to the small increase in cases of intussusception from rotavirus vaccination, health care providers should weigh the potential risks and benefits of administering rotavirus vaccine to infants with a previous history of intussusception.

TABLE 31.1 Vaccine-Preventable Diseases—cont'd

Disease, Route of Administration, Storage, Pregnancy Category	Manifestations	Vaccine
Rubella ("German measles"), subcut 35°-46°F (2°-8°C) May be frozen Pregnancy category: C*	Rash, fever, swollen lymph nodes Birth defects occur if rubella is acquired by a pregnant patient.	The rubella vaccine is a live attenuated virus. Recommended vaccination schedule: 1st dose: 12 through 15 mo 2nd dose: 4 through 6 y ❗ Contraindicated in pregnancy
Smallpox, percutaneous skin prick of 15 jabs using a steel bifurcated needle 35°-46°F (2°-8°C) Protect from light and use within 6-8 hours after reconstitution, then discard Pregnancy category: C*	High fever, severe headache, backache, abdominal pain, and lethargy that lasts 2-5 days; then an extensive rash develops that begins as macules and progresses to papules; then firm vesicles form; and finally, deep-seated, hard pustules form that cause significant scarring.	Smallpox vaccine (live vaccinia virus) is stockpiled in case of an outbreak and emergency. Immunization program for at-risk lab personnel and health care providers, emergency personnel, military personnel Vaccinate only if exposed to smallpox. ❗ Contraindicated in pregnancy; can cause stillbirth. Can cause myocarditis and pericarditis.
Tetanus ("lockjaw"), IM 35°-46°F (2°-8°C) Pregnancy category: C*	Stiffness in neck and abdominal muscles, difficulty swallowing, muscle spasms, fever; can cause broken bones, breathing difficulty, and death	Toxoid conjugate contained in tetanus, DTaP, DT, Tdap, and Td vaccines. Children should receive a series of 5 doses of DTaP vaccine, beginning at 2 mo; then at 4 and 6 mo; then between 15 and 18 mo; and between 4 and 6 y. The Td booster should be given every 10 y.
Tuberculosis (TB), ID (preferred)/ subcut 35°-46°F (2°-8°C) Pregnancy category: C*	Highly contagious respiratory infection Symptoms include cough lasting 3 wk or longer, pleuritic chest pain, coughing up blood or sputum, weakness or fatigue, weight loss, anorexia, fever and night sweats. May also cause meningitis and bone, joint, and skin infections	Live attenuated bacteria Called bacille Calmette-Guérin (BCG) Not routinely administered in the United States, it prevents severe disease but does not prevent infection with the bacterium. Should only be considered for children who have a negative tuberculin skin test and who are continually exposed, or for select health care workers.
Typhoid, subcut/PO 35°-46°F (2°-8°C) Pregnancy category: C*	Sustained high fever, headache, anorexia, abdominal pain, enlarged liver and spleen, constipation, and later, diarrhea	Vaccine given in exposure to *Salmonella paratyphi* and *S. typhi B* is available as live attenuated bacteria (Ty21a; PO) or inactivated components of the typhoid bacterial capsule (Vi; subcut). Routine vaccinations are not required in the United States but are recommended for travelers to certain foreign countries.
Varicella (chickenpox), subcut ≤5°F (−15°C) Contraindicated in pregnancy	Fever and rash, consisting of a few to hundreds of itchy, blisterlike lesions; symptoms are more severe in older children and adults. Complications may include encephalitis, bacterial skin infections, pneumonia, Reye syndrome, and death.	Varicella vaccine, live, is recommended as a two-dose series, first at 12-15 mo, then again between 4 and 6 y. ❗ Contraindicated in pregnancy
Yellow fever, subcut 35°-46°F (2°-8°C) Pregnancy category: C*	Fever, jaundice, and gastrointestinal hemorrhage	Yellow fever vaccine, live A single primary dose is recommended for persons ≥9 mo traveling to, or living in, areas at risk for yellow fever virus transmission (e.g., South America and Africa). The vaccine is required by international regulations for travel to and from certain countries.
Herpes zoster (shingles), subcut ≤5°F (−15°C) Contraindicated in pregnancy	A painful, blisterlike rash in a dermatomal distribution occurs due to reactivation of varicella virus. Following resolution of the rash, prolonged severe pain (postherpetic neuralgia) may occur.	Herpes zoster vaccine approved by the FDA for people ≥50 y.

*Pregnancy categories have been revised. See http://www.fda.gov/Drugs/DevelopmentApprovalProcess/DevelopmentResources/Labeling/ucm093307.htm for more information.

DT, Diphtheria-tetanus; *DTaP*, Diphtheria-tetanus–acellular pertussis; FDA, U.S. Food and Drug Administration; *HepA*, hepatitis A; *HepB*, hepatitis B; *ID*, intradermal; *IM*, intramuscular; *IN*, intranasal; *IV*, intravenous; *MMR*, measles-mumps-rubella; *MMRV*, measles-mumps-rubella-varicella; *mo*, months; *PO*, by mouth; *subcut*, subcutaneous; *Td*, tetanus-diphtheria; *Tdap*, tetanus-diphtheria–acellular pertussis; *wk*, weeks; *y*, years; >, greater than; ≥, greater than or equal to; <, less than; ≤, less than or equal to.

IMMUNIZATION BEFORE INTERNATIONAL TRAVEL

International travel warrants the updating of routine vaccines based on age and immunization history, and travelers to some areas should consider additional vaccines. For example, the CDC currently recommends U.S. travelers 6 months and older to have an updated MMR vaccine based on the travel destination.

Travelers may need to consider vaccination against typhoid and yellow fever. Typhoid fever is caused by a bacterium, *Salmonella typhi,* which is generally spread via contaminated food and water (see Table 31.1). Risk of contracting this infection is greatest for travelers to India, Pakistan, Mexico, Bangladesh, the Philippines, and Haiti. Even stays of less than 2 weeks pose significant risk. Two forms of typhoid vaccine are available for use in the United States. Typhoid vaccine live oral contains the Ty21a strain of *S. typhi*, and is a live attenuated vaccine, which can be administered to persons 6 years of age and older and consists of four capsules, one taken every 48 hours, with the series completed 1 week before potential exposure. A booster dose consisting of the same four-capsule regimen is recommended every 5 years. The other vaccine, parenteral typhoid Vi polysaccharide vaccine, is an inactivated vaccine that contains purified cell surface polysaccharide antigens extracted from *S. typhi* of the Ty2 strain, and may be administered to travelers 2 years of age and older. It is administered at least 2 weeks before expected exposure as a single, intramuscular (IM) injection. A booster dose is recommended every 2 years for those who remain at risk.

Yellow fever is a mosquito-borne viral illness endemic to sub-Saharan Africa and tropical South America. The vaccine is administered as a single injection for persons older than 9 months. Boosters are no longer recommended (ACIP and World Health Organization [WHO], 2016) except for persons at risk. In the United States, the vaccine is administered only at authorized vaccine centers throughout the country. Other vaccines needed for travel may include those for meningococcus, rabies, hepatitis A and B, and Japanese encephalitis. Current vaccine recommendations and related travel information, such as with the Zika virus and cholera, are available from the CDC at 1-800-CDC-INFO or www.cdc.gov/travel.

VACCINE SAFETY: REPORTING DISEASES AND ADVERSE REACTIONS

Vaccines are generally safe, although mild reactions include swelling at the injection site and low-grade fever. Awareness of the contraindications for use of vaccines decreases the incidence of serious adverse reactions. Contraindications include moderate or severe illness or anaphylaxis, a serious, life-threatening allergic reaction to a specific vaccine or vaccine component. Therefore it is important to review vaccine-specific contraindications prior to administering any vaccine. In general, vaccines may be given in cases of mild acute illness or the convalescent phase of illness, antimicrobial therapy, exposure to infectious disease, or premature birth.

Health care providers are responsible for reporting cases of vaccine-preventable diseases and adverse reactions following immunizations. These data identify whether an outbreak is occurring and assess the impact of immunization policies and procedures. Providers must report adverse reactions to the Vaccine Adverse Events Reporting System (VAERS). Information and forms are available at http://vaers.hhs.gov/index. VAERS is a surveillance system that receives and acts on reports of adverse events. The National Childhood Vaccine Injury Act of 1986 initiated the National Vaccine Injury Compensation Program (NVICP), which provides compensation for injury or death caused by a vaccination. More information is available at www.hrsa.gov/vaccinecompensation. To provide safety through communication, the NVICP requires providers to distribute a VIS before vaccines are administered. Federal law requires health care providers to provide information to those receiving vaccines. These information statements include indications, age recommendations, schedule of doses, side effects, special circumstances, and resources to notify if an adverse reaction occurs. For more information, visit www.cdc.gov/vaccines/hcp/vis.

VARICELLA VACCINE

Prior to the development of the varicella vaccine in 1995, about 4 million people came down with varicella zoster virus (VZV), resulting in 10,600 hospitalizations and close to 150 deaths per year. Since implementation of the varicella vaccine, cases of VZV have declined over 75%, hospitalizations have declined over 90%, and deaths from VZV have been reduced by 85% or more.

Prototype Drug Chart 31.1 provides the pharmacologic data for varicella vaccine.

> **Pharmacokinetics** Biologic products such as vaccines do not undergo the pharmacokinetic processes associated with other drug therapy.
>
> **Pharmacodynamics** Seroconversion is the acquisition of detectable levels of antibodies in the bloodstream. In the case of varicella vaccine, seroconversion occurs in more than 98% of 12-month-old to 12-year-old recipients approximately 6 weeks after receiving a single dose of vaccine. Susceptible persons 13 years of age and older who receive two doses of varicella vaccine 4 to 8 weeks apart show a seroconversion rate of approximately 75% 4 weeks after the first dose and 99% 4 weeks after the second dose. Despite the high rate of initial seroconversion among children 12 months to 12 years of age, clinical trials have shown that over a 10-year period, the vaccine's effectiveness in preventing disease was 94% for children who received one dose of vaccine and 98% for those who received two doses. Therefore, beginning in 2007, a second dose of varicella vaccine was recommended for all susceptible individuals, including children.

Contraindications

Varicella vaccine should be avoided in patients with a history of previous anaphylaxis to this vaccine or to any of its components, including gelatin and neomycin. It is also contraindicated in the presence of moderate to severe acute illness or active untreated tuberculosis.

PROTOTYPE DRUG CHART 31.1

Varicella Vaccine

Drug Class	Dosage
Vaccine Pregnancy category: C*	0.5 mL subcut × 2 doses First dose: 12-15 mo; second dose: 4-6 y Catch-up initiated any time after 12-15 mo <13 y, space doses at least 3 mo apart ≥13 y, space doses 4-8 wk apart *For varicella prophylaxis for outbreak control of local epidemics of wild-type varicella virus in susceptible persons following varicella exposure,* consult the current recommendations of the CDC (www.cdc.gov/chickenpox/outbreaks.html)
Contraindications	**Drug-Lab-Food Interactions**
Previous anaphylaxis to this vaccine or to any of its components; pregnancy or possibility of pregnancy within 1 mo; immunocompromised vaccine recipient; presence of moderate to severe acute illness; active untreated tuberculosis	Drug: Separate from other live virus vaccines (e.g., MMR, intranasal flu) by 4 wk if not given on the same day; delay VV for up to 11 mo after blood transfusion or Ig; delay Ig for 2 mo after VV, high-dose immunosuppressant medications; avoid salicylates for 6 wk after VV.
Pharmacokinetics	**Pharmacodynamics**
Not applicable	Seroconversion rates: 12 mo-12 y: >98% at 4-6 wk after vaccination ≥13 y: ~75% 4 wk after first dose and 99% 4 wk after second dose
Therapeutic Effects/Uses	
For prevention of chickenpox; when administered to susceptible individuals, vaccine results in complete protection from chickenpox for the majority of persons. For the minority in whom breakthrough chickenpox develops after vaccination, the disease is typically very mild. The vaccine may also provide prophylaxis protection if administered within 3-5 d of exposure to chickenpox. Mode of Action: Stimulates active immunity against natural disease	
Side Effects	**Adverse Reactions**
Pain and redness at injection site, fever, chickenpox-like rash (generalized or confined to area surrounding injection site)	Anaphylaxis, thrombocytopenia, encephalitis, Stevens-Johnson syndrome

*Pregnancy categories have been revised. See http://www.fda.gov/Drugs/DevelopmentApprovalProcess/DevelopmentResources/Labeling/ucm093307.htm for more information.
CDC, Centers for Disease Control and Prevention; *d,* day; *Ig,* immunoglobulin; *MMR,* measles-mumps-rubella; *mo,* month; *subcut,* subcutaneous; *VV,* varicella vaccine; *wk,* week; *y,* year; <, less than; >, greater than; ≥, greater than or equal to; ~, approximately.

Although varicella infection can cause fetal harm, the possible effects of the vaccine on fetal development are currently unknown. Therefore varicella vaccine is contraindicated during pregnancy. Pregnancy should also be avoided for at least 1 month after each dose of the vaccine. It is important to note that this recommendation differs from the product package insert, which suggests a 3-month delay in pregnancy.

Patients who are immunocompromised because of malignancies, high-dose systemic steroids, or other immunosuppressive therapy should avoid varicella vaccine. Likewise, the vaccine is generally contraindicated in the presence of primary or acquired immunodeficiencies. However, vaccination may be considered in children with certain classes of human immunodeficiency virus (HIV) infection.

Drug Interactions

Frequently a patient is eligible for several immunizations at a visit. A patient receiving varicella vaccine may receive all other vaccines concurrently as long as each is administered at a separate site. If the MMR or other live virus vaccine is not given the same day as the varicella vaccine, administration of the two vaccines should be separated by at least 4 weeks.

If a patient has received a transfusion of blood or blood products, including Ig, administration of the varicella vaccine will need to be deferred for as long as 11 months. Likewise, such blood products should be avoided for at least 2 months after vaccination if possible. Blood products and Ig interfere with the body's production of antibodies specific to chickenpox, thereby decreasing the likelihood that active immunity will develop.

Reye syndrome has occasionally occurred in children following natural chickenpox infection. The majority of these children were also receiving salicylate medications (e.g., aspirin). Therefore, it is generally recommended that patients avoid salicylates for 6 weeks after vaccination.

FUTURE DEVELOPMENTS IN VACCINES

A small outbreak of anthrax cases in the United States in 2001 increased the level of awareness of the anthrax vaccine. Anthrax is caused by the bacteria *Bacillus anthracis.* A serious disease, cutaneous anthrax is the most common form (95% of cases). Anthrax can also occur in the gastrointestinal (GI) tract and lungs. As a biologic weapon, anthrax is highly lethal. It is easily produced, stored, and spread over large areas. Proper vaccination is an essential part of protection against this disease. Approved by the Food and Drug Administration (FDA) in 1970, anthrax vaccine adsorbed (AVA) has been routinely and safely administered to laboratory and military personnel, livestock farmers, and veterinarians. The vaccine requires 5 injections over 18 months with annual boosters. No serious side effects have been reported, but the vaccination is contraindicated during pregnancy. In the event of a bioterrorism attack, persons exposed to anthrax should receive 3 doses of vaccine over 4 weeks and be given ciprofloxacin and doxycycline for 60 days to prevent anthrax. Additional information is available at www.cdc.gov/anthrax/medical-care/prevention.html.

Smallpox, caused by the variola virus, is transmitted through human body fluids or contaminated materials. Smallpox was eradicated in the United States by 1972 and worldwide by 1977; therefore the United States discontinued routine childhood immunization against smallpox in 1972. The vaccine is no longer in use, except in persons who have a high risk of exposure. When the vaccine is administered, most people usually have a mild reaction, such as a sore arm, fever, and body aches. However, persons with a weakened immune system may experience more serious side effects, including death. Since the events of September 2001, concern has arisen that smallpox could be used as a bioterrorist weapon. A smallpox immunization response plan is available for outbreaks or emergencies (http://emergency.cdc.gov/agent/smallpox/vaccination/index.asp).

It has long been known that immunity to pertussis, or "whooping cough," weakens over time and that adolescents and adults are often responsible for transmitting this infection to vulnerable, incompletely immunized infants and young children. Although a relatively benign illness in the older population, pertussis in infants is associated with significant morbidity and mortality. Tdap contains tetanus and diphtheria toxoids along with acellular pertussis; these are licensed for use in older children and adults. Tdap may be used as an active booster for people 11 to 64 years of age, and DTaP is approved for use in children 6 weeks to 6 years. Each vaccine contains the same antigens, but the quantities of diphtheria and acellular pertussis vary. It is recommended that for booster immunization, adolescents and adults receive a one-time dose of Tdap in lieu of the Td vaccine.

Herpes zoster, commonly known as *shingles* or *zoster*, occurs as the result of reactivation of the varicella virus. Following a primary varicella infection (chickenpox), the virus persists but becomes dormant in the body, usually settling in a dorsal root ganglion. Zoster often occurs decades after the primary varicella infection. It appears that development of zoster may be related to a decline in immunity to the VZV. Zoster is characterized by a painful rash that presents in a dermatomal distribution. Especially in older adults, resolution of the rash may be followed by a chronic, severe, sometimes debilitating pain, referred to as *postherpetic neuralgia*. A live attenuated vaccine (zoster vaccine, live) is licensed for use as a one-time injection in adults 50 years of age and older. The vaccine has been shown to boost VZV immunity among vaccine recipients. In clinical trials, zoster vaccine prevented zoster in about 50% of people who received the vaccine. Effectiveness appears to decrease with increasing age of the vaccine recipient. In those who received the vaccine yet went on to develop zoster, the duration of pain was reduced.

Rotavirus is a leading cause of severe acute gastroenteritis in infants and young children. Rotavirus vaccine, live oral, containing five strains of rotavirus, is effective in protecting against severe gastroenteritis and significantly reduces the need for hospitalization among infected children. The vaccine is administered as a three-dose series at 2, 4, and 6 months of age. It is recommended that the third dose be administered before 8 months.

HPV is a sexually transmitted virus that causes cancer of the cervix, vagina, vulva, and penis and can cause genital warts. It also causes anal and oropharyngeal cancers in both men and women. There are over 100 different types of this disease. Two vaccines are approved as routine prophylaxis to prevent HPV disease: human papillomavirus quadrivalent vaccine (recombinant) and human papillomavirus 9-valent vaccine (recombinant). HPV quadrivalent vaccine prevents cervical, vulvar vaginal, and anal cancer caused by HPV types 16 and 18; genital warts caused by HPV types 6 and 11; and precancerous/dysplastic lesions of the cervix, vagina, vulva, and anus caused by HPV types 6, 11, 16, and 18.

HPV 9-valent vaccine (recombinant) is used for prevention of cervical, vaginal, vulvar, and anal cancer caused by HPV types 16, 18, 31, 33, 45, 52 and 58; genital warts caused by HPV types 6 and 11, and precancerous/dysplastic lesions of the cervix, vagina, vulva, and anus caused by HPV types 6, 11, 16, 18, 31, 33, 45, 52, and 58.

Both HPV vaccines are administered as a three-dose series to 9- to 26-year-old males and females. The HPV vaccine is contraindicated in pregnancy. The FDA denied Merck's request for expanded use in women 27 to 45 years of age. Because HPV is sexually transmitted, the vaccine is most effective if administered before initiation of sexual intercourse.

The pneumococcal vaccine provides protection against multiple strains of *Streptococcus pneumoniae* (pneumococcus). Pneumococcal disease includes serious infections of the blood, brain, and lungs. Each year in the United States, around 22,000 persons (both children and adults) die from this vaccine-preventable disease. Two forms of the vaccine are available: pneumococcal 23-valent polysaccharide vaccine (PPV) targeting 23 of the most common serotypes, and pneumococcal 13-valent conjugate vaccine (PCV13) targeting 13 serotypes. PPV is indicated in high-risk persons between the ages of 2 and 65 years (e.g., those undergoing splenectomy, cochlear implant, or immunosuppression) and in all persons older than 65 years. PPV should be repeated after 5 years. PCV13 is recommended for all high-risk persons and for all persons older than 65 years. Since initiation of pneumococcal vaccination, the incidence of antibiotic-resistant disease has dropped significantly.

Bacterial meningitis is a potentially life-threatening infection. Annually, over 1000 cases occur in the United States; 10% to 15% of patients die and 1 out of 5 who live have permanent disability, including brain damage, hearing loss, amputations, or loss of kidney function. ACIP recommends routine vaccination to prevent meningococcal infection for those aged 2 to 55 years. The quadrivalent meningococcal conjugate vaccine (MCV4) and meningococcal polysaccharide vaccine (MPSV4) are approved in the United States. MCV4 is preferred for those between the ages of 2 and 55 years; MPSV4 should be used for those over 55 years of age. For those receiving MCV4, the first dose should be given at 11 or 12 years, with a booster at 16 years. For those who receive the first dose between 13 and 15 years, a one-time booster should be given between 16 and 18 years. If the first dose of MCV4 is given after 16 years, a booster is not needed unless the individual remains at high risk (e.g., microbiologists exposed to *Neisseria meningitidis*, military recruits, those traveling outside the U.S., or those with asplenia).

◎ NURSING PROCESS
Patient-Centered Collaborative Care
Vaccines

Assessment
- Identify benefits and barriers to timely and complete immunization (e.g., beliefs that vaccine-preventable diseases no longer exist, misunderstanding of true contraindications to immunization, concerns regarding vaccine safety and efficacy, fear of multiple injections, cost).
- Obtain a medical history, including history of malignancy or other immune deficiency.
- Determine history of pregnancy or possible pregnancy within the next month. Many vaccines are contraindicated during pregnancy.
- Obtain a drug history that includes high-dose immunosuppressants, blood transfusions, and Ig.
- Obtain a list of complementary and alternative therapies used, and in the case of a breastfed infant, include herbal products used by the mother.
- Determine a complete allergy history that includes drugs, vaccines, food, and environmental allergies.
- Assess for adverse reactions (other than allergic) to previous doses of vaccine or any vaccine component.
- Assess for symptoms of moderate to severe acute illness with or without fever.
- Screen for unvaccinated or immunocompromised household contacts at every visit.
- Obtain an immunization history and a history of vaccine-preventable diseases to determine current vaccine needs. For example, a person with a reliable history of chickenpox or herpes zoster (shingles) does not need the varicella vaccine; natural immunity is assumed.

Nursing Diagnoses
- Knowledge, Deficient about vaccination risks and benefits
- Health Maintenance, Ineffective in adhering to the recommended immunization schedule
- Injury, Risk for due to adverse reactions to immunizations
- Knowledge, Readiness for Enhanced regarding immunization information

Planning
- The patient or the patient's parent or guardian will possess knowledge of vaccine-preventable diseases and risks and benefits of vaccination.
- The patient or the patient's parent or guardian will adhere to the recommended immunization schedule for vaccine-preventable diseases unless contraindications exist.
- The patient will be free of adverse reactions.

Nursing Interventions
- Strictly adhere to individual vaccine storage requirements to ensure potency of the product.
- Upon preparation, including reconstitution of a given vaccine, administer within the time limits stated in the package insert to ensure potency.
- ⚡ Administer at separate sites all vaccines for which a patient is eligible at the time of the visit. Do *not* mix vaccines in the same syringe.
- ⚡ Document in a patient's record the vaccination date, route, and site of administration; the vaccine type, manufacturer, lot number, and expiration date; and the name, business address, and title of the person administering the vaccine.
- ⚡ Observe the patient for signs and symptoms of adverse reactions to vaccines.
- Keep epinephrine readily available for immediate use in case of an anaphylactic reaction.
- Provide the patient with a record of immunizations administered.

Patient Teaching
General
- Discuss vaccine-preventable diseases with the patient and/or the patient's family, including manifestations and risk of contracting the disease.
- Answer all questions regarding vaccine safety, effectiveness, and risk factors in clear, understandable language.
- Advise female patients of childbearing age to avoid pregnancy for 1 month, depending on the vaccines administered.
- Advise patients to avoid contact with immunocompromised persons, depending on the vaccines to be administered.
- Provide the patient or the patient's family with a current VIS, available from the CDC, for each vaccine before its administration as required by federal law.
- Remind the patient or the patient's family to maintain a vaccine immunization record and to bring it to all visits.
- Provide the patient or the patient's family with a return date for the next vaccination(s) based on assessment of the immunization history.

Side Effects
- Discuss common side effects of vaccines, such as injection site soreness, fever, and side effects specific to individual vaccines.
- Offer suggestions for management of common side effects (e.g., cold compresses for injection site soreness, acetaminophen for soreness or fever).
- Advise the patient or the patient's family to contact the health care provider if signs of a serious reaction are noted.

Cultural Considerations
- Modify communications to meet the cultural needs of the patient and the patient's family.
- Use a professional interpreter when necessary.
- Provide the patient and the patient's family with a VIS in the patient's preferred language (available at www.immunize.org).

Evaluation
- Evaluate patient and family understanding of rationale for immunizations.
- Evaluate patient adherence to the recommended immunization schedule.
- Evaluate whether the patient is free from adverse reactions.

PATIENT SAFETY

❶ Don't Wait! Vaccinate!
Use the SHARE method (see https://www.cdc.gov/vaccines/hcp/adults/downloads/standards-immz-practice-recommendation.pdf):
Share reasons why the vaccine is right for the patient.
Highlight positive experiences.
Address the patient's questions about the vaccine.
Remind the patient that vaccines protect against diseases.
Explain the costs and consequences of getting the disease.

CRITICAL THINKING CASE STUDY

RR, a 22-year-old college student, is in the wellness clinic with her 3-month-old daughter and her 13-year-old sister. They live with RR's grandmother, who is 68 years old. RR requests immunizations for her daughter and asks if there are any immunizations she and her sister need.

1. RR says her daughter needs her "regular shots." The infant received her first hepatitis B vaccine while in the newborn nursery but has not had any shots since coming home. Against what vaccine-preventable illnesses should the nurse plan to vaccinate this infant today?
2. RR is worried that she will need to start her immunizations over because "she's so far behind." How should the nurse respond to her concern? When would her infant be due for another series of immunizations?
3. Which vaccines is RR's daughter due for today?
4. RR reports she is afraid the baby will have a reaction. Compare the mild side effects with the more severe allergic reactions. What is the best way of allaying RR's fears?
5. The nurse asks RR about her vaccine history. RR says she had her "baby shots" a long time ago but did not keep her personal vaccine record; however, she remembers receiving a flu shot 2 years ago. What immunizations will she need at this point? How can she best keep track of her immunizations?
6. RR informs the nurse that she is a college freshman and just received an email informing her that there is a campus-wide meningitis outbreak. She doesn't live on campus and asks the nurse if she needs a meningitis shot anyway. Identify the manifestations of this vaccine-preventable disease.
7. After administering RR's meningitis vaccine, RR's 13-year-old sister mentions that she heard that high school students should get a vaccination for human papillomavirus (HPV). She wants to know if she should get one or if it is too late. Who is eligible to receive the HPV vaccine, and what assessment questions would the nurse ask? What type and dosage of vaccine would the nurse administer?
8. RR appears relaxed and comfortable during the visit. However, she states that she is worried about her grandmother's health because her grandmother has diabetes and high blood pressure. RR wants to know if her grandmother should get any immunizations or if those would just make her sick. Identify which vaccine-preventable diseases and vaccines should be given.
9. After the visit, how does the nurse ensure that the vaccines were safely administered?

NCLEX STUDY QUESTIONS

1. The father of a 4-month-old infant calls in to the clinic reporting that his child is having a reaction to immunizations. What is the most important piece of information the nurse should elicit?
   a. The time the immunization was received
   b. Whether the father has given the infant any acetaminophen
   c. The signs and symptoms the infant is experiencing
   d. The sites used to administer the immunizations
2. The nurse is preparing to administer varicella vaccine to a young woman. Which of the following findings has the greatest implication for this young woman's care?
   a. The patient tells the nurse she is "deathly afraid of needles."
   b. The medical record indicates that the patient is allergic to eggs.
   c. The medical history indicates that the patient had leukemia as a young child.
   d. The patient appears to be pregnant.
3. A 38-year-old migrant farm worker is seen in the clinic with a cut to his arm from an old metal drum. The patient has sutures placed, and a tetanus, diphtheria, and acellular pertussis vaccine is given. What is the nurse's most important action after the vaccine has been administered?
   a. The nurse provides the patient with a vaccine information statement about the tetanus, diphtheria, and acellular pertussis vaccine in the patient's primary language.
   b. The nurse determines the exact date of the patient's last tetanus booster.
   c. The nurse documents that the patient did not experience any side effects immediately following immunization.
   d. The nurse provides the patient with a record of the immunization administered at the visit.

4. The nurse is preparing to administer routine, recommended immunizations to an immunocompromised 1-year-old child. What is the most important information to know prior to administering a vaccination?
   a. The type of vaccine to be administered to the child
   b. The child presents with a temperature of 99.8°F.
   c. The child's vaccine report shows immunizations were received on time.
   d. The child did not experience adverse reactions to prior immunizations.

5. A 14-year-old girl requests a vaccination for human papillomavirus. After the nurse administers the first dose, which of the following is important to include in the patient's teaching?
   a. Human papillomavirus prevents all sexually transmitted diseases.
   b. Pap smears are no longer needed after the human papillomavirus vaccination.
   c. The patient needs to notify the health care provider about pain at the injection site.
   d. The date the patient needs to return to the clinic for the next human papillomavirus dose

6. An 18-month-old child is accompanied to the clinic by her grandmother, the child's legal guardian. The grandmother reports that the child is due for her fourth diphtheria, tetanus, and acellular pertussis vaccination. The nurse determines that the child should *not* receive the diphtheria, tetanus, and acellular pertussis vaccine that day for which reason?
   a. The child received a varicella vaccine 2 weeks ago.
   b. The grandmother is receiving chemotherapy.
   c. The third diphtheria, tetanus, and acellular pertussis dose was administered 4 months ago.
   d. The nurse sees that the child has a runny nose during the visit.

7. Which of the following patients would be eligible to receive the influenza vaccine?
   a. The patient who is taking care of her son with human immunodeficiency virus
   b. The patient who is pregnant
   c. The patient with an egg allergy
   d. The child who is 18 months old

8. With the help of an interpreter, the nurse has just immunized a 35-year-old woman with the tetanus, diphtheria, and acellular pertussis vaccine and the vaccine against measles, mumps, and rubella. It is essential that the nurse proceed with which action(s)? (Select all that apply.)
   a. Provide a vaccine information statement in the patient's preferred language for each vaccine received.
   b. Document in the patient's record the date; site and route of administration; vaccine type, manufacturer, lot number, and expiration date; and the name, business address, and title of the person administering the vaccine.
   c. Administer a dose of ibuprofen to prevent postimmunization fever.
   d. Instruct the patient to call about any injection site soreness.

Answers: 1, c; 2, d; 3, a; 4, a; 5, d; 6, c; 7, d; 8, a, b.

Antineoplastics and Biologic Response Modifiers

The development of cancer is a multistep process that is influenced by the environment (e.g., chemicals, radiation); genetics (e.g., genetic mutations); lifestyle factors (e.g., smoking, alcohol use); diet (e.g., high fat); infection (e.g., Epstein-Barr virus, *Helicobacter pylori*, human papillomavirus [HPV]); and the immune system (e.g., human immunodeficiency virus [HIV] infection, immunosuppressive drugs). It must be remembered that *tumor* and *cancer* are not synonyms. Tumors are a collection of unstructured new cells and are benign—that is, they have no known physiologic function—and they will not invade other unrelated tissues or organs. Cancer, or malignant cells, has the potential to invade or spread to other parts of the body (metastasis); and is further characterized by unregulated growth and poor differentiation.

THE CELL CYCLE

All cells progress through a distinct cycle that consists of five phases, four of which are directed toward cell replication and a fifth phase in which the cell stops dividing. The first phase of the cell cycle is called *gap 1* (G_1), and it is the presynthesis phase that produces ribonucleic acid (RNA), protein, and the enzymes necessary to synthesize deoxyribonucleic acid (DNA). The second phase is the *synthesis* (S) phase, in which DNA synthesis and replication occur. Next is the *gap 2* (G_2), the postsynthesis phase, in which the cell continues to grow and prepares for mitosis. Cell division (cytokinesis) of daughter cells occurs in the fourth, or *mitosis* (M), phase. The last phase, *gap 0* (G_0), is a dormant phase.

Most cells in the human body are in the G_0 stage. Exceptions include metabolically active cells (e.g., granulocytes) and epithelial cells. As each cell moves through the cell cycle, it must pass a number of checkpoints before it can progress to the next phase. At these **checkpoints**, cells deemed defective undergo **apoptosis** (self-destruction). The cell cycle is illustrated in Fig. X.1. The cell cycles of normal cells are similar to those of cancer cells with the exception that cancer cells ignore signals at the various checkpoints of the cell cycle to stop dividing, to specialize, or to undergo apoptosis.

GROWTH RATE

Growth rate, also called *doubling time,* is defined as the time it takes for a tumor to double in size. **Growth fraction,** the percent of actively dividing cells, decreases as the tumor enlarges, and doubling time increases. Growth rate depends on several factors, including the cell-cycle activity of the proliferating cells in the tumor mass, the number of cells proliferating within the tumor (*growth fraction*), and the rate of cell loss from the tumor. In general, anticancer drugs are more effective against cancer cells that have a high growth fraction. Anticancer drugs interfere with cell replication and thereby interfere with the growth of cancer cells. Malignant tumors that have prolonged cell cycles and a slower growth rate are more likely to be locally confined and therefore are more amenable to surgical excision.

ANTICANCER THERAPY

Chemotherapy is the use of chemicals to kill cancer cells. Research has led to the use of new anticancer drugs and to the development of standard treatment protocols (drug, dose, and schedule) to guide therapy. Nurses play a vital role in managing the treatment of patients with cancer. This includes the administration of chemotherapy in health care facilities (inpatient treatment) and in the homes of clients (outpatient treatment). To provide the best possible care, nurses should understand the chemotherapy regimen, contraindications, drug interactions, therapeutic effects, side effects, and adverse reactions of the chemotherapy that clients receive.

Chapter 32 provides information on selected anticancer drugs and how they inhibit cellular replication or prevent cellular reproduction. The anticancer drugs are divided into major classes that include alkylating drugs, antimetabolites, antitumor

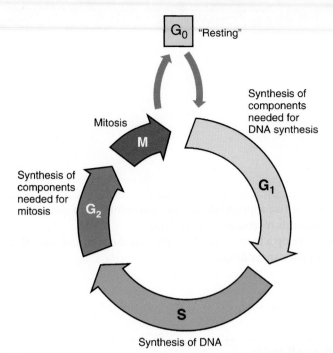

FIG. X.1 Cell cycle G_1 *phase* (postmitotic gap): Production of RNA, protein, and enzymes for DNA synthesis; the G_1 phase lasts 15 to 18 hours. *S phase* (synthesis): All the components of DNA are synthesized, and the cells have doubled; the S phase lasts 10 to 20 hours. *G_2 phase* (premitotic gap): The cell continues to grow and ensures it is not defective; the G_2 phase lasts approximately 3 hours. *M phase* (mitosis): Cell growth has stopped, and the cell divides into two identical (daughter) cells; the M phase lasts approximately 1 hour. *G_0 phase* (resting): Cells remain in this phase and leave the cell cycle or return to the cell cycle for cell replication. Cells in this phase are not as sensitive to many antineoplastic drugs. The cells must pass through a series of checkpoints to continue through the cycle. Defective cells undergo apoptosis (self-destruction). From Burcham, J., & Rosenthal, L. (2016). *Lehne's pharmacology for nursing care* (9th ed.). St Louis: Elsevier.

antibiotics, plant alkaloids, immunomodulators, liposomal drugs, and hormonal drugs.

Some chemotherapy agents negatively affect cancer cells when they are actively dividing. These are called *cell cycle–specific (CCS)* drugs. *Cell cycle–nonspecific (CCNS)* drugs work in any phase of the cell cycle, including in the G_0 (resting) phase. Chemotherapy usually targets RNA or DNA in cancer cells to prevent mitosis or to induce apoptosis. The specific drugs are selected based on the cancer cell type, the rate at which cancer cells divide, and the point in the cell cycle at which the drugs will be most effective. In general, chemotherapy is most effective in destroying cells that are rapidly dividing.

Chapter 33 explores targeted therapies to treat cancer. This modality targets malignant cells, and targeted therapies work by interfering with cancer cell growth and division in different ways and at various points in its development, growth, and spread.

Chapter 34 describes the evolving state of biologic response modifiers (BRMs) that work to (1) enhance host immunologic function, (2) destroy or interfere with tumor activities, and (3) promote differentiation of stem cells.

32

Anticancer Drugs

http://evolve.elsevier.com/McCuistion/pharmacology/

OBJECTIVES

- Discuss ways the nurse can avoid exposure to anticancer drugs.
- Differentiate between cell cycle–specific and cell cycle–nonspecific anticancer drugs.
- Compare the uses and considerations for alkylating compounds, antimetabolites, antitumor antibiotics, hormones, and biotherapy agents.
- Prioritize appropriate nursing interventions to use while patients receive anticancer drugs.
- Develop a focused teaching plan on the uses and side effects of anticancer drugs.

OUTLINE

KEY TERMS

Cancer-related deaths rank second only to heart disease in the United States. Even though cancer-related mortality has decreased since the early 1990s, approximately 1 in 3 women and 1 in 2 men are projected to develop cancer over their lifetime. Excluding basal and squamous cell skin cancers, the highest incidence rates in men are prostate, lung, and colorectal cancer. In women, breast, lung, and colorectal cancers occur with the highest frequency. Lung cancer remains the leading cause of cancer-related death regardless of gender.

The incidences and mortality rates of cancer differ by ethnicity. Non-Hispanic blacks (henceforth "African Americans") have higher incidences (except breast cancer) and higher death rates from cancer (except breast and lung) than any racial or ethnic group. African American women have lower incidences of breast cancer but higher mortality rates than Caucasian women do. Hispanics have the lowest incidences and mortality rates of lung cancer. Incidences and mortality rates for liver and stomach cancers due to hepatitis B virus (HBV) and *Helicobacter pylori* (*H. pylori*) are the highest among Asians and Pacific Islanders. Incidences of cancer increase among all immigrants as they adopt a more westernized lifestyle.

Cancer is a group of diseases in which abnormal cells grow out of control and can spread to other areas of the body. DNA is the genetic substance in the body cells that transfers information necessary for the production of enzymes and protein synthesis. In most cases, cancer is caused by damage to the DNA within the cell. Although some cancers are inherited, most develop when genes in a normal cell become damaged or lost. More than one mutation is required before a malignancy can develop, therefore the development of cancer is a multistep process that may take years to complete.

Pharmaceuticals are often used to destroy cancer cells and are called by different names, including *anticancer drugs, cancer chemotherapeutic agents,* antineoplastic drugs, or cytotoxic therapy. In the 1970s, combination chemotherapy—the use of two or more chemotherapy agents to treat cancer—was adopted and led to improved response rates and increased survival times. Chemotherapy may be used as the only treatment of cancer, or it may be used in conjunction with other modalities such as radiation, surgery, and biologic response modifiers. Combination chemotherapy increases the chance for months to years of cancer remission. If cancer can no longer be controlled, palliative treatment with chemotherapy may be used to relieve disease-related symptoms and improve quality of life.

GENETIC, INFLAMMATORY, INFECTIVE, ENVIRONMENTAL, AND DIETARY INFLUENCES

Cancer can be influenced by genetic mutations, inflammation, infectious organisms, environment, and an unhealthy diet.

Box 32.1 gives examples of environmental substances, viruses, and foods that have a carcinogenic effect in humans. Genes provide the instructions for the production and function of cellular proteins essential for normal cellular activities. Genetic defects may occur in a variety of ways, including deletion, translocation, duplication, inversion, or insertion of genetic material. When defects cannot be effectively repaired, cells exhibit abnormal characteristics and unregulated growth. More than 2000 genes have been causally implicated in the formation of cancer. Cancers with a proven genetic influence include breast, ovarian, prostate, endometrial, colon, pancreatic, and lung cancers; retinoblastoma; and malignant melanoma, to name a few. Many more genetic influences are expected to be found as cancer research continues.

Genes can cause cells to become cancerous in several ways. Proto-oncogenes are normal genes involved in cell differentiation and division, and they regulate cell death, also known as apoptosis. These processes are necessary for healthy tissues and organs. An oncogene is a mutation in a proto-oncogene that affects cellular growth-control proteins and triggers unregulated cell division. Some genes, called antioncogenes, protect others. One such gene is the tumor-suppressor (TS) genes that signal a cell to cease multiplying and stop the action of oncogenes. Uncontrollable cell growth can occur if TS genes become lost or dysfunctional. Other genes repair damage to DNA. If these DNA-repair genes are damaged, mutations are not corrected and are subsequently passed on to the next generation of daughter cells. These and other gene mutations can take place over a long time before cancer develops. As a result, cancers more commonly occur in older individuals.

Inflammation is a normal physiologic process to heal injured tissues. Chronic inflammation, such as chronic inflammatory bowel disease, is an ongoing inflammatory process. The continued inflammation can lead to DNA damage and can result in cancer.

A number of viruses are associated with the development of cancer. The human papillomavirus (HPV) has been found in most women with invasive cervical cancer. Individuals with human immunodeficiency virus (HIV) may develop lymphomas and rectal or genital cancers. The Epstein-Barr virus (EBV) is found in almost all people with Burkitt lymphoma in central Africa and has been implicated in the development of nasopharyngeal cancer. Hepatocellular carcinoma (liver cancer) is linked to hepatitis B and C viruses. Other viruses linked to cancer include human T-cell lymphotropic virus (HTLV) and Kaposi sarcoma–associated herpesvirus.

Bacteria can play a role in the development of cancer. The presence of *H. pylori* in the stomach is associated with an increased risk of gastric cancer. Some reports have indicated a link between certain bacteria and cancer of the gallbladder, colon, and lung. However, no clear evidence supports a link between bacterial infection and other cancers.

BOX 32.1   Environmental, Infective, and Dietary Influences on Cancer Development

Environmental

Tobacco
Gastric cancers and cancer of the bladder, cervix, colon, esophagus, head and neck, kidney and ureter, liver, lung, pancreas, trachea and bronchus, and acute myeloid leukemia

Asbestos
Lung cancer

Benzene
Acute myelogenous leukemia

Formaldehyde
Cancer of the nose, throat, and trachea

Vinyl Chloride
Sarcoma, leukemia

Arsenic
Cancer of the lung and skin, sarcoma

Ionizing Radiation
Leukemia; cancer of the thyroid, breast

Ultraviolet Rays
Skin cancer

Aflatoxin
Liver cancer

Infective

Herpes Simplex 2 Virus (Genital Herpes)
Cervical and penile cancer

Hepatitis B and C Viruses
Cancer of the liver

Epstein-Barr Virus
Non-Hodgkin lymphoma, Hodgkin disease, nasopharyngeal cancers

Human Papillomavirus (HPV)
Cancer of the cervix, vulva, vagina, anus, penis, head and neck

Human Immunodeficiency Virus (HIV)
Kaposi sarcoma, non-Hodgkin lymphoma, cervical cancer

Human T-Cell Lymphotropic Virus
T-cell leukemia

Helicobacter pylori
Cancer of the stomach, gastric mucosa-associated lymphoid tissue (MALT) lymphoma

Diet
Animal Fat
Cancer of the colon, rectum, breast, uterus, prostate, ovary

Heterocyclic Amines (found in some smoked meats)
Cancer of the stomach, colon, rectum, pancreas, breast

Alcohol
Cancer of the mouth, throat, esophagus, liver, breast

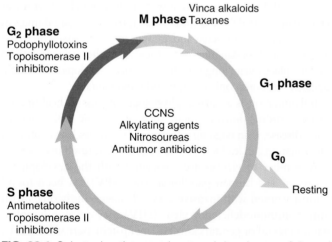

FIG. 32.1 Selected anticancer drugs and the phases of the cell cycle in which they are most effective. *CCNS,* cell cycle non-specific.

Environmental factors associated with the development of cancer include tobacco use, poor diet, decreased physical activity, chemicals, and excessive sun and radiation exposures. According to the Centers for Disease Control and Prevention (CDC), 90% of lung cancers in men and 80% in women occur due to smoking. Other cancer-causing environmental agents include alcohol consumption on a regular basis, which raises the risk of mouth, larynx, and throat cancers; being overweight or obese, which

increases the risk of uterine, breast, prostate, and colorectal cancers; and excessive exposure to sun and other forms of ultraviolet (UV) rays, which promotes skin cancers. Many of these cancers can be prevented. According to the American Cancer Society (ACS), about 43,840 people were expected to succumb to cancer during the year 2015.

CELL CYCLE–NONSPECIFIC AND CELL CYCLE–SPECIFIC ANTICANCER DRUGS

The cell cycle for normal and cancer cells and the growth fraction and doubling time are discussed in the opening pages for Unit X (see Fig. 32.1).

Anticancer drugs stop or slow the growth of cancer cells by interfering with cell replication and are classified according to their action. **Cell cycle–nonspecific (CCNS) drugs** act during any phase of the cell cycle, including the G_0 phase. CCNS drugs include most alkylating drugs, antitumor antibiotics, and hormones. **Cell cycle–specific (CCS) drugs** exert their influence during a specific phase of the cell cycle and are most effective against rapidly growing cancer cells. The CCS drugs include antimetabolites, some alkylating agents, and vinca alkaloids. Fig. 32.1 shows selected categories of anticancer drugs and the phase of the cell cycle in which they are most effective.

Growth fraction and **doubling time** are two factors that play a major role in how the cancer cells respond to anticancer drugs. Anticancer drugs are more effective against neoplastic cells that have a high growth fraction. Leukemia and some lymphomas have high growth fractions and thus respond well to anticancer drug therapy.

Solid tumors have a large percentage of their cell mass in the G_0 phase, thus they generally have a low growth fraction and are less sensitive to anticancer drugs. As the tumor grows, the blood supply decreases, thereby slowing the growth rate. High-dose chemotherapy results in better tumor-killing (tumoricidal) effects. Depending on the type of cancer, malignant cell growth is usually faster in the earlier stages of tumor development. Adequate vascularization is needed for the anticancer drugs to be effective. Anticancer drugs are more effective against small, fast-growing tumors with sufficient blood supply. The vascularization in solid tumors can be inconsistent. Some areas of tumor may have an adequate blood supply, whereas other areas are poorly perfused. This characteristic may make some large tumors resistant to anticancer drugs and therefore difficult to treat.

CANCER CHEMOTHERAPY

Anticancer drugs do not affect just cancer cells; instead, the drugs affect both cancer and normal cells. The side effects of chemotherapy are largely related to the toxic effects on normal cells. Normal cells are able to repair themselves and continue to grow, thus the side effects of chemotherapeutic agents are often temporary. Chemotherapy is usually administered systemically for cancer that has spread to other parts of the body, for cancers in multiple sites, or for cancers too large to be removed by other means (e.g., surgery). The most common route of chemotherapy administration is through intravenous (IV) infusion, although other routes may be used and include oral, intramuscular, subcutaneous, intraperitoneal, intraventricular (intrathecal), intrapleural, intravesicular, intraarterial, and topical routes.

Some types of cancer can be cured with chemotherapy (e.g., Hodgkin disease, Burkitt lymphoma, and testicular cancer). Other types of cancer (e.g., breast and colon cancer) may be treated with surgery first, followed by chemotherapy to eliminate any residual cancer cells (microscopic metastases) that may remain in the body. This is referred to as adjuvant therapy. Sometimes neoadjuvant chemotherapy may be given first to help shrink a large tumor, so that it can be surgically removed. Palliative chemotherapy, used to relieve symptoms associated with advanced disease (e.g., pain and shortness of breath), can improve quality of life.

Chemotherapy administration is guided by specific protocols based on the results of controlled research studies. The length of treatment is determined by the type and extent of the malignancy, the type of chemotherapy given, expected side effects of the drugs, and the amount of time that normal cells need to recover. Chemotherapy is usually given in cycles to improve the likelihood that cancer cells will be destroyed and that normal cells can recover. The duration, frequency, and number of chemotherapy cycles are based on the cancer type and size, the spread of the disease to other areas of the body (metastasis), and the condition of the patient. Chemotherapy treatment may consist of one drug or a combination of drugs. Combination chemotherapy may be administered in one day or may be spread out over several days. The duration of treatment is based on the protocol being followed; it can vary from minutes to days and may be repeated weekly, biweekly, or monthly. Selected anticancer drugs are listed in Box 32.2 according to classification.

Combination Chemotherapy

Single-agent drug therapy is not usually used to treat cancer because combination therapy with two or more anticancer drugs has demonstrated more effective tumoricidal activity.

BOX 32.2   Anticancer Drugs by Classification*

Alkylating Agents
Nitrogen Mustard Gas Derivatives
Bendamustine
Chlorambucil
Cyclophosphamide
Estramustine
Ifosfamide
Mechlorethamine hydrochloride
Melphalan

Nitrosoureas
Carmustine (bis-chloroethylnitrosourea [BCNU])
Lomustine (1-[2-chloroethyl]-3-cyclohexyl-1-nitrosourea [CCNU])
Streptozocin

Alkyl Sulfonates
Busulfan

Alkylating-Like Agents
Altretamine
Carboplatin
Cisplatin
Dacarbazine
Oxaliplatin

Antimetabolites
Folic Acid Antagonists
Methotrexate
Pemetrexed disodium

Pyrimidine Analogues
Azacitidine
Capecitabine
Cytarabine
Floxuridine
Fluorouracil injection (5-Fluorouracil [5-FU])
Gemcitabine hydrochloride

Purine Analogues
Cladribine
Clofarabine
Fludarabine
Mercaptopurine (6-MP)
Nelarabine
Pentostatin
Thioguanine (6-TG)

Ribonucleotide Reductase Inhibitors (Enzyme Inhibitors)
Hydroxyurea

Continued

BOX 32.2   Anticancer Drugs by Classification*—cont'd

Antitumorals
Anthracyclines
Daunorubicin hydrochloride
Daunorubicin liposomal
Doxorubicin
Epirubicin
Idarubicin
Mitoxantrone
Valrubicin

Other Antitumor Antibiotics
Bleomycin sulfate
Dactinomycin
Doxorubicin liposomal
Mitomycin

Plant Alkaloids
Antimicrotubules and Taxanes
Docetaxel
Paclitaxel

Camptothecin Analogues
Irinotecan
Topotecan

Epipodophyllotoxins
Etoposide
Teniposide

Immunomodulators
Alemtuzumab
Interleukin 2 (IL-2)
Rituximab
Thalidomide

Retinoids
Bexarotene

Vinca Alkaloids
Vinblastine sulfate
Vincristine sulfate
Vincristine, liposomal
Vinorelbine

Sex Hormones, Hormonal Agonists and Antagonists, Selective Estrogen Receptor Modulators, Luteinizing Hormone–Releasing Hormone Agonists, Aromatase Inhibitors, Enzymes, and Vaccines
Androgens
Fluoxymesterone

Hormonal Agonists and Antagonists
Abiraterone
Anastrozole
Bicalutamide
Enzalutamide
Exemestane
Flutamide
Fulvestrant
Goserelin acetate
Histrelin acetate implant
Letrozole
Leuprolide acetate
Medroxyprogesterone
Megestrol acetate
Mitotane
Nilutamide
Raloxifene
Tamoxifen citrate
Toremifene citrate

Enzymes
Asparaginase *Erwinia chrysanthemi*
Pegaspargase

Vaccines
Hepatitis B
Quadrivalent human papillomavirus subtypes 6, 11, 16, and 18
Human papillomavirus bivalent vaccine

High-Alert Medications
All chemotherapeutic agents are categorized as high-alert medications for all routes of drug delivery.

*See Chapter 33 for monoclonal antibodies and targeted therapies and Chapter 34 for biologic therapies.

Combination therapy increases the likelihood of affecting cancer cells in all phases of the cell cycle.

To maximize cell death, CCNS and CCS drugs are often combined to increase synergistic effects. Each individual drug used in combination therapy should have a proven tumoricidal activity, a different mode of action, and different dose-limiting toxicities. A combination of antineoplastic drugs has the advantage of decreasing drug resistance while increasing cancer cell destruction. Table 32.1 presents some of the combined anticancer drugs.

General Side Effects and Adverse Reactions
Anticancer drugs exert adverse effects on rapidly growing normal cells, such as skin and hair. These drugs can also affect cells in the gastrointestinal (GI) tract, mucous membranes, bone marrow, and reproductive system. Myelosuppression can occur when there is a significant decrease in the bone marrow activity that results in decreased white blood cells, platelets, and red blood cells. Following chemotherapy administration, the nadir—the time at which the blood count is at the lowest—typically occurs 7 to 10 days after treatment. Table 32.2 lists the general adverse effects anticancer drugs exert on the fast-growing cells of the body. Selected nursing measures and considerations are included. Because of the toxic effects of chemotherapy, care in handling of such drugs must be considered, and protective gear that includes gloves specific for handling chemotherapy drugs must be used.

Anticancer Therapy in Outpatient Settings
The administration of anticancer drugs in outpatient settings, such as in homes and oncology clinics, is both cost-effective and convenient. Although chemotherapy regimens have become

TABLE 32.1 Selected Combinations of Anticancer Drugs

Generic	Acronym*	Selected Uses
Cytarabine, daunorubicin, etoposide	ADE	Acute myelogenous leukemia
Fluorouracil, doxorubicin, cyclophosphamide	FAC	Breast cancer
Fluorouracil, epirubicin, cyclophosphamide	FEC	
Leucovorin, fluorouracil, irinotecan	FOLFIRI	Colorectal cancer
Leucovorin, fluorouracil, oxaliplatin	FOLFOX	
Capecitabine, irinotecan	XELIRI	Esophageal cancer, gastric cancer
Bortezomib (PS-341), doxorubicin, dexamethasone	PAD	Multiple myeloma
Carboplatin, paclitaxel	CARBOPLATIN-TAXOL	Non–small cell lung cancer
Cyclophosphamide, doxorubicin, vincristine, prednisone	CHOP	Non-Hodgkin lymphoma
Rituximab, cyclophosphamide, doxorubicin, vincristine, prednisone	R-CHOP	
Gemcitabine, cisplatin	(None)	Pancreatic cancer
Gemcitabine, fluorouracil, leucovorin	OFF	
Bleomycin, etoposide, cisplatin	BEP	Testicular cancer
Vinblastine, ifosfamide, cisplatin	VIP	

*Acronyms are based on the generic or trade name of the chemotherapy drugs used in a specific protocol (e.g., ABVD [Adriamycin, bleomycin, vinblastine, dacarbazine], FAC [fluorouracil, Adriamycin, cyclophosphamide]). Not all acronyms for combination chemotherapy treatments are listed.

TABLE 32.2 General Adverse Reactions to Anticancer Drugs

Adverse Reactions	Nursing Measures and Considerations
BONE MARROW SUPPRESSION, MYELOSUPPRESSION	
Low RBC count (anemia)	Assess for fatigue, shortness of breath, low blood pressure, increased heart rate, increased respiratory rate, and oliguria. Assess for cyanosis. Plan rest periods. Administer oxygen as prescribed. Elevate the head of the bed to facilitate breathing. Provide pain medication if pain is increasing oxygen consumption. Provide assistance with activities. Monitor for mental status changes. Anemia may be treated with ferrous sulfate or infusions of RBCs. EPO may be administered to stimulate RBC production. Monitor RBCs, hemoglobin, and hematocrit.
Low WBC count (leukopenia)	Susceptibility to infection increases as WBCs decrease. Patients should avoid people with infections and report fever, chills, URIs, or sore throat to their HCP. Hand hygiene before and after contact with the patient is important. Monitor for changes in body temperature; elevated temperature is considered a sign of infection. Avoid medications that may mask fever. Immediately report temperatures of 101°F (38.3°C) or above to the HCP. Appropriate cultures (e.g., blood, urine, sputum) are collected before antibiotics are started if applicable, and an antibiotic regimen is initiated. Assess for localized infections. Auscultate breath sounds. Colony-stimulating factors (e.g., filgrastim) may be administered to stimulate WBC production. Monitor WBCs, especially ANCs.
Low platelet count (thrombocytopenia)	Petechiae, bruising, bleeding of gums, and nosebleeds are signs of a low platelet count; report these signs to a HCP. Assess for bleeding, petechiae, and ecchymosis. Assess for occult bleeding in urine, feces, and emesis. Apply pressure to injection sites until bleeding has stopped. Platelet transfusions may be needed. Avoid medications that may promote bleeding (aspirin, heparin). Avoid invasive procedures (injections, indwelling urinary catheters, rectal temperature, and suppositories). Monitor platelet counts and bleeding time.
GASTROINTESTINAL DISTURBANCES	
Anorexia	Loss of appetite may be related to anemia, pain, fatigue, or altered taste caused by chemotherapy drugs. Provide small, frequent meals that are high in calories and protein. Plan rest periods. Address issues of pain control. Hard candy or ice chips may help relieve bitter taste.
Nausea and vomiting	Antineoplastic drugs often stimulate the CTZ, leading to nausea and vomiting, which can be caused by irritation of the GI tract; effects of radiation to chest, abdomen, or brain; anxiety; constipation; pain; electrolyte imbalances; or other medications. Grading scales are useful to assess severity. Provide antiemetics before, during, and after chemotherapy. Assess for GI upset, and medicate appropriately. Minimize noise, stimulation, and odors. Frequent mouth care is recommended. Monitor fluid balance and serum electrolytes.
Diarrhea	Diarrhea may be one of three types: *osmotic* (absorption defects), *secretory* (bacterial infection or neoplasm), or *exudative* (secondary to chemotherapy). Chemotherapeutic drugs most commonly associated with diarrhea are alkylating agents, antitumor antibiotics, and antimetabolites. Treatment (e.g., medications, diet changes) will depend on cause and severity.

Continued

TABLE 32.2   General Adverse Reactions to Anticancer Drugs—cont'd

Adverse Reactions	Nursing Measures and Considerations
GASTROINTESTINAL DISTURBANCES	
	Diarrhea may be caused by other medications, such as antibiotics; comorbid conditions (e.g., Crohn disease); or enteral (tube) feedings. Assess normal bowel habits, and monitor for electrolyte imbalances and dehydration. Administer appropriate antidiarrheal medications (antibiotics, anticholinergics, antispasmodics, psyllium, kaolin and pectin, or octreotide acetate). Teach patients to eat small, frequent meals; follow a low-residue diet; limit spicy, fatty foods; limit intake of salty foods, whole grains, fresh fruits and vegetables, and caffeinated and carbonated drinks; and avoid very hot or very cold foods (may stimulate peristalsis). Monitor intake and output.
Mucositis (stomatitis)	Many antineoplastic drugs cause changes in oral mucosa that generally occur 2 to 14 days after initiation of therapy. Assess for taste changes, tissue swelling, redness, pain, dry mouth, white patches, or a white coating on the oral mucosa. Mucositis ranges from mild to severe. Symptomatic treatment may include frequent mouth rinses, topical anesthetics, antibiotics, antifungal medication, saliva substitutes, and pain medication. Patients should avoid commercial mouthwashes that contain alcohol. A soft toothbrush is recommended. Offer ice chips or ice pops to help relieve pain. Assess intake and output. Evaluate caloric needs. A grading scale may be useful to assess severity.
OTHER	
Alopecia	Not all chemotherapeutic drugs cause hair loss. Hair thinning, patchy baldness, or complete alopecia may occur, depending on the drug. Hair on all areas of the body is affected. Hair loss may be gradual, progressing with each cycle of chemotherapy, or rapid. Hair regrowth usually occurs once chemotherapy is completed, although the texture may be changed. Before therapy, discuss potential hair loss and ways to address the discomforts (e.g., baldness and scalp hypothermia) due to hair loss (wigs, scarves, hats, or turbans). Assess for body image changes and concerns.
Fatigue	Fatigue may be caused by chemotherapy, sleep disturbances, emotional distress, depression, bone marrow suppression, infection, pain, or electrolyte imbalances.
	Assess fatigue using a visual analog grading scale (0 = no fatigue; 10 = worst fatigue). Address conditions that might be contributing to fatigue (lack of sleep, pain, depression). Plan ways to help patients conserve energy. Plan a well-balanced diet, and encourage participation in regular (but not strenuous) exercise and stress-reduction measures, such as relaxation and guided imagery.
Infertility	If infertility occurs, it may be permanent. Pretreatment counseling is advised.

ANC, Absolute neutrophil count; *CTZ,* chemoreceptor trigger zone; *EPO,* erythropoietin; *GI,* gastrointestinal; *HCP,* health care provider; *RBC,* red blood cell; *URI,* upper respiratory infection; *WBC,* white blood cell.
The list above is not all inclusive. Some more serious reactions are discussed in the prototype drug charts.

increasingly aggressive, most patients are not hospitalized unless they require close monitoring or become very ill. Patients receiving highly potent drugs will need to be closely monitored for severe adverse effects. When a chemotherapy drug is given, a health care provider qualified to administer anticancer drugs follows the policies provided by the oncologist and the health care agency. To reduce the nurse's exposure to hazardous chemotherapy drugs during administration, certain precautions should be followed to minimize occupational exposure:

- Use disposable powder-free gloves approved for handling chemotherapy, regardless of route of administration.
- Wear two pairs of gloves and change gloves every 30 minutes or when torn, punctured, or contaminated.
- Wear gowns with a front closure, long sleeves, and elastic or knit (closed) cuffs, and dispose of these after each use when administering IV chemotherapy.
- When there is a risk of aerosol exposure, follow the Occupational Safety and Health Administration (OSHA) respiratory protection standard. Surgical masks do *not* provide adequate respiratory protection.
- Use a face shield or a combination of a mask and face shield if there is a danger of splashing when administering chemotherapy or disposing of body fluids.

Cytotoxic drugs can be accidentally absorbed by inhalation, contact with skin or mucous membranes, or ingestion. For this reason, these guidelines should be followed:

1. Prepare chemotherapy in a separate work area. Use a plastic-backed absorbent pad to contain spills during preparation.
2. Wash hands before and after administration of chemotherapy.
3. Avoid hand-to-mouth or hand-to-eye contact while working with chemotherapy.
4. Refer to your agency's policy for priming IV tubing and disconnecting tubing after administration.
5. Wear gloves when disposing of body fluids (e.g., urine, feces, and emesis) of patients who have received chemotherapy in the previous 48 hours.
6. Refer to agency policy for disposal of used equipment.
7. Refer to agency policy for handling chemotherapy spills or exposure.

ALKYLATING DRUGS

One of the largest groups of anticancer drugs is the alkylating compounds. Alkylating drugs damage the cell's DNA by cross-linkage of DNA strands, abnormal base pairing, or DNA strand breaks, thus preventing the reproduction of cancer cells. Drugs in this group belong to the CCNS category and kill cells in all phases of the cell cycle. They are used to treat many different types of cancer, including leukemia, lymphoma, multiple myeloma, sarcoma, and solid tumors such as those of the breast, ovary, uterus, lung, bladder, and stomach. Even though alkylating agents are effective in all phases of the cell cycle, they are most effective in the G_0 phase. Alkylating drugs are divided into five different classes: (1) nitrogen mustards, (2) nitrosoureas, (3) alkyl sulfonates, (4) triazines, and (5) ethylenimines. Table 32.3

TABLE 32.3 Antineoplastics: Alkylating Drugs

Drug	Route and Dosage	Uses and Considerations
Nitrogen Mustards	Visually inspect parenteral products for particulate matter and discoloration prior to use. Observe and exercise precautions when handling, preparing, and administering cytotoxic drugs. The correct dose of chemotherapeutic drugs will vary from protocol to protocol. Consult appropriate references to verify doses.	
Bendamustine	CLL: A: IV: 100 mg/m^2 on days 1 and 2, repeated q28d for up to 6 cycles NHL: A: IV: 120 mg/m^2 on days 1 and 2, repeated q21d for up to 8 cycles	For CLL and NHL. Monitor for bone marrow depression. Assess for tumor lysis syndrome and skin reactions. Pregnancy category: D*; PB: 94%-96%; t½: 40 min
Chlorambucil	CLL: A: PO: 0.1-0.2 mg/kg/d (4-10 mg/d) for 3-6 wk Hodgkin disease: A/C: PO: 0.2 mg/kg/d NHL: A/C: PO: 0.1-0.2 mg/kg/d for 3-6 wk	For CLL, Hodgkin disease, and NHL. Monitor for bone marrow suppression or pancytopenia. Pregnancy category: D*; PB: 99%; t½: 1.5 h
Estramustine	A: PO: 14 mg/kg/d or 600 mg/m^2/d in 3-4 divided doses	For prostate cancer. Gynecomastia and impotence may occur. Pregnancy category: D*; PB: UK; t½: 20-24 h
Ifosfamide	A: IV: 1.2-2 g/m^2/d for 5 d in combination with mesna; repeat every 3 wk after recovery from hematologic toxicity. Mesna is usually given concomitantly to prevent hemorrhagic cystitis.	For testicular cancer. Monitor for hemorrhagic cystitis. Pregnancy category: D*; PB: negligible; t½: 7-15 h
Mechlorethamine hydrochloride	Hodgkin disease: A: IV: 0.2 mg/kg or 6 mg/m^2 as single dose CLL: A: IV: 6 mg/m^2 q4wk CML: A: IV: 0.4 mg/kg or 6 mg/m^2 monthly Other dosing regimen and routes are available.	For Hodgkin disease, leukemias, solid tumors, and effusions caused by cancer. This drug is contraindicated in patients with active infections. Pregnancy category: D*; PB: UK; t½: Minutes
Melphalan	Multiple myeloma: A: PO: 6 mg daily for 2-3 wk Maint: 2 mg/d; adjust 1-3 mg/d based on hematologic response A: IV: 16 mg/m^2 q2wk for 4 doses Maint: 16 mg/m^2 q4wk Ovarian cancer: A: PO: 200 mcg/kg/d for 5 d; repeat q4-5wk based on hematologic response	For multiple myeloma and ovarian cancer. *Do not confuse Alkeran with Leukeran or Myleran.* Pregnancy category: D*; PB: 20%-30%; t½: 1.25-1.5 h
Nitrosoureas Carmustine (BCNU)	Multiple myeloma and brain tumors: A: IV: 150-200 mg/m^2 single dose q6wk or 75-100 mg/m^2/d for 2 days q6wk C: IV: 200-250 mg/m^2 q4-6wk Hodgkin disease or NHL: A: IV: 100 mg/m^2/d q6wk	For Hodgkin disease, NHL, multiple myeloma, and brain tumors. Monitor for bone marrow suppression and pulmonary symptoms. Pregnancy category: D*; PB: UK; t½: 5-30 min
Lomustine (CCNU)	Hodgkin disease and malignant glioma: A/C: PO: 100-130 mg/m^2 q6wk	For Hodgkin disease and malignant gliomas. Monitor for bone marrow suppression and liver function. Pregnancy category: D*; PB: UK; t½: 16 h-2 d
Streptozocin	A/C: IV: 500 mg/m^2/d for 5 d q4-6wk; doses above 500 mg/m^2 are not recommended	*Do not confuse with streptomycin.* For pancreatic cancer. Pregnancy category: C*; PB: UK; t½: 30-45 min
Alkyl Sulfonates Busulfan	A: PO: 4-8 mg/d C: PO: 0.06-0.12 mg/kg/d	For myelocytic leukemia. Monitor for seizures and cerebral hemorrhage. Pregnancy category: D*; PB: 32%; t½: 2.5 h
Alkylating-Like Drugs Altretamine	A: PO: 260 mg/m^2/d in 4 divided doses after meals and at bedtime for 14 or 21 d in a 28-d cycle; drug holiday for ≥14 d then restart at 200 mg/m^2/d	For ovarian cancer. Pregnancy category: D*; PB: Weakly; t½: 4.7-10.2 h

Continued

TABLE 32.3   Antineoplastics: Alkylating Drugs—cont'd

Drug	Route and Dosage	Uses and Considerations
Carboplatin	New cancer: A: IV: 300 mg/m² in combination with cyclophosphamide q4wk for 6 cycles Recurrent cancer: A: IV: 360 mg/m² q4wk	For advanced ovarian cancer. Usually given as combination therapy. Pregnancy category: D*; PB: UK; t½: 1.5-2.5 h
Cisplatin	Bladder cancer: A: IV: 50-70 mg/m² q3-4wk Ovarian cancer: A: IV: 50-75 mg/m² q21d Testicular cancer: A/C: IV: 20 mg/m² for 5 d; repeat q3wk for 2 more cycles NSCLC: A: IV: 75 mg/m² q3wk	For bladder, ovarian, testicular, and NSCLC. Monitor for CNS function; reversible posterior leukoencephalopathy may occur. Pregnancy category: D*; PB: 90%; t½: 30-100 h, dose related
Dacarbazine	Melanoma: A: IV: 250 mg/m²/d for 5 d repeated q3wk Hodgkin disease: A/C: IV: 375 mg/m² days 1 and 15 q28d	For Hodgkin disease and malignant melanoma. Monitor hepatic function. Pregnancy category: C*; PB: Minimal; t½: 5 h
Oxaliplatin	A: IV: 85 mg/m² on day 1 q2wk for 12 cycles	For metastatic colorectal cancer. Used with 5-FU and leucovorin (FOLFOX4). Assess for pulmonary complications. Pregnancy category: D*; PB: >90%; t½: 391 h

*Pregnancy categories have been revised. See http://www.fda.gov/Drugs/DevelopmentApprovalProcess/DevelopmentResources/Labeling/ucm093 307.htm for more information.

Note: Chemotherapeutic doses and schedules will vary depending on protocol, body surface area (m²), age, functional status, and comorbid conditions. For a full discussion of body surface area in dosage calculation, see Chapter 11.

5-FU, 5-Fluorouracil; *A*, adult; *C*, child; *CLL*, chronic lymphocytic leukemia; *CML*, chronic myelogenous leukemia; *CNS*, central nervous system; *d*, day; *h*, hour; *IV*, intravenous; *maint*, maintenance; *min*, minute; *NHL*, non-Hodgkin lymphoma; *NSCLC*, non–small cell lung cancer; *PB*, protein binding; *PO*, by mouth; *q*, every; *t½*, half-life; *UK*, unknown; *wk*, week; *>*, greater than; *≥*, greater than or equal to.

lists some of the alkylating drugs, their uses, and considerations. Of the alkylating agents, nitrosoureas cross the blood-brain barrier, making them useful in the treatment of brain cancer. General adverse effects to anticancer drugs are discussed in Table 32.2. Additionally, alkylating agents given in high doses can cause long-term damage to the bone marrow, resulting in acute leukemia. The platinum (alkylating-like) drugs—cisplatin, carboplatin, and oxaliplatin—kill cells in a similar fashion but are less likely to cause leukemia later.

Cyclophosphamide

Cyclophosphamide, an alkylating agent, is an analogue of nitrogen mustard and has activity against many neoplastic diseases including Hodgkin and non-Hodgkin lymphoma (NHL), acute and chronic lymphocytic leukemia (CLL), multiple myeloma, breast and ovarian carcinoma, lung cancer, and retinoblastoma. The drug is also used for immunologic disorders such as lupus nephritis and has been shown to prevent progressive renal scarring, preserve renal function, induce renal remission, and decrease end-stage renal failure. This drug is a severe vesicant that causes tissue necrosis if it infiltrates into the tissues. Cyclophosphamide can be administered orally or intravenously. The patient should be well hydrated while taking cyclophosphamide to prevent hemorrhagic cystitis (bleeding due to severe bladder inflammation). Sodium 2-mercaptoethanesulfonate is a chemoprotectant drug often given with high-dose cyclophosphamide

to inactivate urotoxic metabolites to reduce the incidence of hemorrhagic cystitis.

⚡ PATIENT SAFETY

Patients should be well hydrated before and during therapy.

Do not confuse...
- **Myleran** with **Alkeran**
- **Cisplatin** with **carboplatin**
- **Paraplatin,** with **Platinol**
- **Cyclophosphamide** with **cyclosporine**

Pharmacokinetics Oral cyclophosphamide is well absorbed in the GI system. Cyclophosphamide is a prodrug that is activated and extensively metabolized by the liver. About 5% to 25% of the drug is eliminated by the kidney as unchanged drug, and its elimination half-life is 3 to 12 hours. Approximately 20% is bound to plasma protein, and this is not dose dependent. Some cyclophosphamide metabolites are greater than 60% protein bound. Less than 10%, most in the form of metabolites, are excreted in feces.

Pharmacodynamics Cyclophosphamide is an early antineoplastic drug used alone or with other drugs to treat a variety of cancers. Average time to peak plasma concentration (T_{max}) is 1 hour. Several drug interactions can occur with cyclophosphamide. Patients should report all medications they are taking, including over-the-counter (OTC) medicines and herbal supplements. Anthracycline (e.g., doxorubicin) has been reported to induce cardiotoxicity when taken with cyclophosphamide, and it exacerbates hemorrhagic cystitis. Other serious drug interactions can occur when taking cyclophosphamide concomitantly with aspirin, allopurinol, phenobarbital, warfarin, thiazide diuretics, and some psychiatric medications. Complementary and Alternative Therapies 32.1 lists herbal supplements that may also interact with cyclophosphamide.

Side Effects and Adverse Reactions

The side effects of cyclophosphamide reflect those seen in the general class of antineoplastic drugs. (For the general side effects, see Table 32.2). Hemorrhagic cystitis is a serious problem that can arise when high doses of cyclophosphamide are given. Patients who receive a high dose should be assessed for cardiomyopathy and syndrome of inappropriate antidiuretic hormone (SIADH) during treatment with this drug. In addition, cyclophosphamide may increase pigmentation of the skin or nail beds. Prototype Drug Chart 32.1 details the pharmacologic behavior of cyclophosphamide.

 NURSING PROCESS
Patient-Centered Collaborative Care
Alkylating Drugs: Cyclophosphamide

Assessment
- To avoid drug-drug interactions, obtain a detailed medication history that includes prescriptions, OTC medicines, antacids, dietary supplements, vitamins, and herbal supplements.
- Obtain a list of the patient's drug and food allergies.
- Obtain baseline information about the patient's physical status. Include height, weight, vital signs, cardiopulmonary assessment, intake and output, skin assessment, nutritional status, and information on any underlying disease.
- Assess baseline laboratory values (complete blood count [CBC], uric acid, chemistry panel) for future comparisons.
- Assess baseline results of pulmonary function tests, chest radiographs, electrocardiography (ECG), and renal and liver function studies.
- Assess the patient's current level of comprehension.

Nursing Diagnoses
- Infection, Risk for
- Bleeding, Risk for
- Body Image, Risk for Disturbed body image
- Knowledge, Deficient related to chemotherapeutic protocol

Planning
- The patient/family member/caretaker will verbalize understanding of the signs and symptoms of infection.
- The patient's white blood cell (WBC), red blood cell (RBC), and platelet counts will remain in the desired range.
- The patient will remain free from infection and hemorrhagic cystitis.

- The patient/family/caregiver will demonstrate understanding of protection from sun exposure.
- The patient/family/caregiver will demonstrate understanding of chemotherapeutic protocol (e.g., dose administration).

Nursing Interventions
- Monitor labs (CBC, blood urea nitrogen [BUN], creatinine, liver panel, and electrolytes) prior to drug administration and during treatment.
- Monitor the IV site frequently for irritation and phlebitis.
- Maintain strict medical asepsis during dressing changes and invasive procedures.
- Encourage small, frequent meals high in calories and protein.
- Monitor fluid intake and output and nutritional intake during therapy.
- Encourage patients to drink at least 2 L of fluid per day to promote excretion of cellular breakdown products and to reduce the risk of hemorrhagic cystitis.
- Assess the need for IV hydration.
- Maintain hydration before and during chemotherapy.
- Assess for signs and symptoms of hematuria, urinary frequency, or dysuria.
- Administer premedications as ordered 30 to 60 minutes before giving drugs.
- Provide drug information verbally and in print to the patient/family/caregiver.
- Encourage patients to use sunblock with a sun protection factor (SPF) of 50 or greater and to use other means to protect skin from sun exposure.

Patient Teaching
General
- Teach patients to take cyclophosphamide early in the day to prevent accumulation of drug in the bladder during the night.
- Remind patients to consult with a health care provider before administration of any vaccines.
- Advise patients to promptly report signs of infection (e.g., elevated temperature, fever, chills, sore throat, frequent urination or burning on urination, and redness/swelling/pain near a wound); bleeding (e.g., bleeding gums, petechiae, bruises, hematuria, blood in the stool); and anemia (e.g., increased fatigue, dyspnea, and orthostatic hypotension).
- Advise patients not to visit anyone who has a respiratory infection. A decreased WBC count puts patient at high risk for acquiring an infection.
- Emphasize protective precautions as necessary (e.g., hand washing and personal hygiene).
- Teach patients to empty their bladder every 2 to 3 hours.
- Teach methods of sun protection (e.g., sunblock with SPF 50 or greater, brimmed hats, and lightweight, long-sleeved shirts).

Side Effects
- Advise patients about good oral hygiene with a soft toothbrush for stomatitis; have patients use a soft toothbrush when the platelet count is less than 50,000/mm^3.
- Assess for use of alternative and complementary therapies that may interact with chemotherapy drugs.
- Advise patients to report any signs of bleeding.

Diet
- Advise patients to follow a diet low in purines—such as organ meats, beans, and peas—to alkalize urine.
- Advise patients to avoid citric acid.
- Offer patients food and fluids that may decrease nausea (e.g., cola, crackers, and ginger ale).
- Plan small, frequent meals.

Cultural Considerations
- Health care decisions are made by consensus in some cultures, and the family plays a key role in filtering the information given to a patient. Issues related to informed consent and full disclosure of medical information may cause distress in those who place the needs of the family above the needs of the individual. Interactions should be modified based on family structure, religious values and beliefs, time orientation, cultural health practices, and verbal and nonverbal communication.
- Cultural assessment tools can provide general guidelines for health care providers.
- Cytochrome P450 system variance may prohibit the conversion of cyclophosphamide into its active form more among African Americans than among Caucasians.
- Renal function among African Americans is poorer than among Caucasians.
- Despite lowering the dosage, Asians may develop febrile neutropenia.

Evaluation
- The patient is free from infection.
- The patient maintains the target weight.
- The patient maintains nutritional status.
- The patient does not develop hemorrhagic cystitis.
- The patient/family/caregiver education needs are met.

ANTIMETABOLITES

Molecularly, antimetabolites resemble natural substances, building blocks that not only synthesize but also recycle and break down organic compounds used by the body. However, antimetabolites interfere with various substances needed for normal cell function. Most antimetabolites are classified as CCS, and they exert their effects during the S phase (DNA synthesis and metabolism) of the cell cycle. Few antimetabolites (e.g., 5-fluorouracil [5-FU], floxuridine) have cytotoxic effects in multiple phases of the cell cycle. Antimetabolites are classified according to the substances with which they interfere. Substances can include folate, pyrimidine, purine analogues, and ribonucleotide reductase inhibitors. Table 32.4 lists the antimetabolite drugs, uses, and considerations.

🌿 COMPLEMENTARY AND ALTERNATIVE THERAPIES 32.1

Cyclophosphamide
- Use cautiously with garlic (antiplatelet activity), ginkgo (increased antiplatelet effect), echinacea (decreased effects of immunosuppressive drugs), ginseng (altered bleeding time), St. John's wort (may interfere with chemotherapy), and kava kava (increased risk for bleeding). Toxicity and actions of both cyclophosphamide and vitamin A are altered if given together. *Do not use with mistletoe because it may promote cancer growth.*
- Astragalus (Huang-qi; milk vetch root) stimulates the immune system and may help speed recovery from immunosuppressive chemotherapy. Astragalus has blood clot–fighting properties and may increase risk of bleeding when given with cyclophosphamide.

Fluorouracil
- Use cautiously with ginseng and St. John's wort (may interfere with chemotherapy). *Do not use with mistletoe because it may promote cancer growth.*
- Astragalus stimulates the immune system and may help speed recovery from immunosuppressive chemotherapy. Astragalus has blood clot–fighting properties and may increase risk of bleeding when given with 5-fluorouracil (5-FU).

Doxorubicin
- St. John's wort is a potent cytochrome P450 inducer and moderate P-glycoprotein inducer that may decrease the concentration of doxorubicin.
- Grapefruit is a potent cytochrome P3A4 inhibitor that may increase the concentration and effect of doxorubicin.
- Black cohosh and Dong-quai should be avoided in estrogen-dependent tumors.
- Many complementary therapies—such as acupuncture, art therapy, and music therapy—have been utilized to improve patients' sense of well-being.

Vincristine
- St. John's wort and echinacea are cytochrome P450 inducers, which causes decreased levels of vincristine. Many complementary therapies—such as acupuncture, art therapy, and music therapy—have been utilized to improve patients' sense of well-being.

Methotrexate, a folate antimetabolite, is used to treat malignant and nonmalignant conditions (e.g., rheumatoid arthritis, psoriasis). Methotrexate affects cells that have high metabolic rates, such as neoplasms, hair follicles, endothelium, cells of the GI tract, fetal cells, and bone marrow; it is used to treat leukemias and cancers of the GI tract, head and neck, breast, and ovaries. Because methotrexate causes apoptosis to fetal cells, it can be used for ectopic pregnancies. Methotrexate inhibits the biosynthesis of a purine nucleotide, 5-aminoimidazole-4-carboxamide ribonucleotide (AICAR) transformylase, which provides antiinflammatory properties that result in metabolites; AICARs are immunotoxic. Leucovorin can be given 12 to 24 hours after methotrexate administration (not simultaneously) to reduce AICAR concentrations, thereby diminishing the adverse effects of methotrexate. Leucovorin should not be referred to as *folinic acid* because it can be confused with *folic acid*, which can lead to severe methotrexate toxicity. Other interactions are seen with methotrexate. Nonsteroidal antiinflammatory drugs (NSAIDs) given just prior to, concomitantly with, or following intermediate or

PROTOTYPE DRUG CHART 32.1
Cyclophosphamide

Drug Class	Dosage
Alkylating drug: Nitrogen mustard Generic Name: Cyclophosphamide Pregnancy category: D*	Acute lymphocytic leukemia (ALL): A/C: IV: 300-1500 mg/m² A/C: PO: 1-5 mg/kg/d Breast cancer: A: IV: 500-1000 mg/m² q15d A: PO: 100-200 mg/m²/d Various protocols exist, including combination therapy. Dosage varies based on indicated use and response. Adjust dose if bone marrow suppression (myelosuppression) occurs.
Contraindications	**Drug-Lab-Food Interactions**
Absolute contraindications: Hypersensitivity, severe urinary outflow obstruction, bladder obstruction *Caution:* Myelosuppression, tumor lysis syndrome, liver or kidney disease, hemorrhagic cystitis, or heart failure. Many other precautions are necessary when administering cyclophosphamide.	Drug: Doxorubicin may potentiate cardiac toxicity, and busulfan may potentiate lung toxicity. Other antineoplastic and immunosuppressive drugs may have an additive effect on immunosuppressive activity. Drugs metabolized via cytochrome P450 can increase toxic effects of cyclophosphamide. Doxorubicin decreases digoxin level and increases drug action of barbiturates, chloramphenicol half-life, and effects of anticoagulant drugs. Duration of leukopenia may be prolonged if given with thiazide diuretics. Actions and toxicities of allopurinol, probenecid, colchicine, phenothiazines, potassium iodide, imipramine, warfarin, and succinylcholine are altered if given with cyclophosphamide. Toxicity is increased if given with corticosteroids, phenytoin, or sulfonamides. Many other possible drug-drug interactions are not listed here. Lab: Suppresses positive reaction to uric acid, purified protein derivative, mumps, candida. Cyclophosphamide may cause Papanicolaou test (Pap smear) to be falsely positive.
Pharmacokinetics	**Pharmacodynamics**
Absorption: PO: Well absorbed Distribution: PB: 20%, not dose dependent Metabolism: t½: 3-12 h Excretion: 5%-25% in urine unchanged; 4% in feces mostly as metabolites	PO/IV:Onset: 7 d PO/IV: Peak: 7-15 d PO/IV: Duration: 21 d
Therapeutic Effects/Uses	
Leukemias, breast and ovarian cancer, lymphomas, multiple myeloma, lung cancer, and retinoblastoma	
Mode of Action: Cell cycle–nonspecific alkylating drugs inhibit the protein synthesis by interfering with DNA replication by alkylation of DNA.	
Side Effects	**Adverse Reactions**
Nausea, vomiting, diarrhea, anorexia, leukopenia, febrile neutropenia, fever, weight loss, alopecia, amenorrhea, gonadal suppression, impaired wound healing, stomatitis, pain	Anaphylaxis, hematologic toxicity, pulmonary toxicity (pneumonitis, pulmonary fibrosis, pulmonary thrombosis), hemorrhagic cystitis, urotoxicity, nephrotoxicity, secondary neoplasm, cardiotoxicity, hepatotoxicity, tumor lysis syndrome

*Pregnancy categories have been revised. See http://www.fda.gov/Drugs/DevelopmentApprovalProcess/DevelopmentResources/Labeling/ucm093307.htm for more information.
Note: Chemotherapy drug doses are based on body weight and are prescribed either as milligrams per kilogram (mg/kg) or milligrams per meter squared (mg/m²). Doses will also vary based on drug protocol, type and stage of cancer, age, functional status, and comorbid conditions (e.g., heart disease).
A, Adult; *C,* child; *d,* day; *DNA,* deoxyribonucleic acid; *h,* hour; *IV,* intravenous; *q,* every; *PB,* protein binding; *PO,* by mouth; *t½,* half-life.

high doses of methotrexate have resulted in severe hematologic and GI toxicity. Furthermore, NSAIDs may mask fever, swelling, and other signs and symptoms of infection. Several corticosteroids can reduce the cytotoxicity of methotrexate. Protein-bound drugs such as salicylates (aspirin), sulfonylureas (glyburide), hydantoin (phenytoin) anticonvulsants, and sulfonamides can induce methotrexate toxicity. Penicillins, proton pump inhibitors, and probenecid, among other drugs, can cause methotrexate toxicity. Acidic food and drink can also cause elevated methotrexate concentrations.

Fluorouracil

Fluorouracil (5-FU), an antimetabolite agent similar to uracil with an addition of fluoride, is a component of chemotherapy for many cancers, including breast, colorectal, GI, and head and

neck. 5-FU is administered intravenously to treat solid tumors and is applied topically for superficial basal cell carcinoma and actinic keratosis. A microsponge delivery system for a cream-based 5-FU was approved in 2000 to provide a sustained release formulation administered once daily. It is not administered orally because of the inconsistent bioavailability.

⚡ PATIENT SAFETY

Obtain a complete medication list that includes over-the-counter (OTC), herbal preparations, and other alternative therapies.

Do not confuse...
- **Hydroxyurea** with **hydroxychloroquine**
- **Xeloda** with **Xenical**

TABLE 32.4   Antineoplastics: Antimetabolites

Drug	Route and Dosage	Uses and Considerations
FOLIC ACID ANTAGONISTS		
Visually inspect parenteral products for particulate matter and discoloration prior to use. Observe and exercise precautions when handling, preparing, and administering cytotoxic drugs. Chemotherapeutic drug dosages will vary from protocol to protocol. Consult appropriate references to verify doses.		
Methotrexate	ALL: A/C: PO/IM/IV: 3.3 mg/m^2/d for 4-6 wk followed by maintenance dosing NHL: A/C: IV: 200 mg/m^2 days 8 and 15 q21d in a combination regimen Head/Neck: A/C: IV: 40 mg/m^2 days 1 and 15 q21d A: PO: 25-50 mg/m^2 q7d C: PO: 7.5-30 mg/m^2 Osteogenic sarcoma: A/C: IV: 12 g/m^2 q2wk	For ALL, NHL, sarcomas, solid tumors, head and neck cancers, choriocarcinomas, lymphomas, and some autoimmune disorders. Older adults may be more sensitive to toxicity and adverse events. Pregnancy category: X*; PB: 50%-60%; t½: 10-12 h Leucovorin is used with high doses of methotrexate as rescue therapy to prevent fatal toxicity.
Pemetrexed	A: IV: 500 mg/m^2 day 1 of a 21-d cycle	For mesothelioma and non–small cell lung cancer. Folic acid and vitamin B12 IM injections are recommended to prevent hematologic and GI adverse reactions. Pregnancy category: D*; PB: 81%; t½: 3.5 h
PYRIMIDINE ANALOGUES		
Azacitidine	A: IV/Subcut: 75 mg/m^2/d for 7 d q4wk	For myelomonocytic syndrome (MDS). Absolutely contraindicated in those with mannitol hypersensitivity. Pregnancy category: D*; PB: UK; t½: 4 h
Capecitabine	Breast cancer: A: PO: 2500 mg/m^2/d in 2 divided doses for 2 wk repeated q3wk Colorectal cancer: A: PO: 1250 mg/m^2/d twice daily for 2 wk, repeated q3wk for a total of 8 cycles	For breast and colorectal cancer. Usually reserved for patients resistant to anthracyclines. Converted in tissue to 5-FU. Monitor for GI symptoms. Pregnancy category: D*; PB: <60%; t½: 0.75 h
Cytarabine	AML: A/C: IV: 100-200 mg/m^2/d continuous infusion for 7 d A/C: Subcut (maint): 100 mg/m^2/d for 5 d q28d ALL: A/C: IV: 1-3 g/m^2 every 12 h for 8-12 doses CML: A/C: IV: 200 mg/m^2/d continuous infusion for 9 d, but other doses have been used Carcinomatous meningitis: A/C: Intrathecal: 5-70 mg/m^2	For ALL, AML, CML, carcinomatous meningitis. Use preservative-free diluent. Pregnancy category: D*; PB: 15%; t½: 3-6 h in plasma; 2-11 h in CSF
Floxuridine	A: Intraarterial: 0.1-0.6 mg/kg/d continuous infusion	For colorectal cancer. Given as an intraarterial infusion into the hepatic artery; catabolized to 5-FU. Pregnancy category: D*; PB: UK; t½: UK, but CSF concentrations can be sustained for several hours
5-Fluorouracil (fluorouracil, 5-FU)	See Prototype Drug Chart 32.2.	
Gemcitabine hydrochloride	NSCLC and breast cancer: A: IV: 1250 mg/m^2 on days 1 and 8 of a 21-d cycle (usually given with another chemotherapeutic drug) Pancreatic cancer: A: IV: 1000 mg/m^2 weekly for up to 7 wk followed by 1 wk of rest Ovarian cancer: A: IV: 1000 mg/m^2 days 1 and 8 of a 21-d cycle	For breast, ovarian, pancreatic, and NSCLC. Pulmonary and cardiac toxicity may occur. Pregnancy category: D*; PB: 10%; t½: 32-94 min (sex and dose dependent)
PURINE ANALOGUES		
Cladribine	A: IV: 0.09-1 mg/kg/d continuous infusion for 7 d	For hairy cell leukemia. Chemical conversion to the active form takes place intracellularly. Pregnancy category: D*; PB: 20%; t½: 7 h

TABLE 32.4 Antineoplastics: Antimetabolites—cont'd

Drug	Route and Dosage	Uses and Considerations
PURINE ANALOGUES		
Clofarabine	C ≤21 years: IV: 52 mg/m² daily for 5 d repeated q2-6wk	For ALL. Safety and efficacy has not been established for those older than 21 years of age. Pregnancy category: D*; PB: 47%; t½: 5.2 h
Fludarabine	A: IV: 25 mg/m²/d for 5 d q28d A: PO: 40 mg/m²/d for 5 d q4wk	For CLL. Absolutely contraindicated in those with hemolytic anemia and renal disease. Pregnancy category: D*; PB: UK; t½: 7-12 h
Mercaptopurine (6-MP)	A: PO: 2.5-5 mg/kg/d followed by maintenance dosage	For ALL. Significant first-pass metabolism occurs following oral administration; significant metabolic variability. Pregnancy category: D*; PB: UK; t½: 1-2 h
Nelarabine	A: IV: 1500 mg/m² on days 1, 3, and 5 repeated q21d C: IV: 650 mg/m² for 5 consecutive days repeated q21d	For T-cell leukemia/lymphoma. Assess for neurologic symptoms. Pregnancy category: D*; PB: <25%; t½: 0.5-1 h
Pentostatin	A: IV: 4 mg/m² every other wk	*Do not confuse with pentosan.* For hairy cell leukemia. Monitor pulmonary, hepatic, and renal function; assess for seizures. Concomitant use with fludarabine is not recommended. Pregnancy category: D*; PB: 4%; t½: 2.6-15 h
Thioguanine (6-TG)	A/C: PO: 100 mg/m² q12h for 5-10 d	For AML. Not recommended for maintenance therapy or long-term continuous treatments due to liver toxicity. Pregnancy category: D*; PB: UK; t½: Variable
RIBONUCLEOTIDE REDUCTASE INHIBITORS (ENZYME INHIBITORS)		
Hydroxyurea	CML: A: PO: WBC-level based: For WBC >100,000/mm³, 50-75 mg/kg/d; maint: 10-30 mg/kg/d Head and Neck: A: PO: 80 mg/kg q3d	For CML and head and neck cancer.. Monitor for infection and bone marrow suppression. Pregnancy category: D*; PB: UK; t½: 3.5-4.5 h

*Pregnancy categories have been revised. See http://www.fda.gov/Drugs/DevelopmentApprovalProcess/DevelopmentResources/Labeling/ucm093 307.htm for more information.

Note: Chemotherapeutic doses and schedules will vary depending on protocol, body surface area (m²), age, functional status, and comorbid conditions. For a full discussion of body surface area in dosage calculation, see Chapter 11.

5-FU, 5-Fluorouracil; *A,* adult; *ALL,* acute lymphocytic leukemia; *AML,* acute myelogenous leukemia; *C,* child; *CLL,* chronic lymphocytic leukemia; *CSF,* cerebrospinal fluid; *CML,* chronic myelogenous leukemia; *d,* day; *GI,* gastrointestinal; *h,* hour; *IM,* intramuscular; *IV,* intravenous; *maint,* maintenance dose; *min,* minute; *NHL,* non-Hodgkin lymphoma; *NSCLC,* non–small cell lung cancer; *PB,* protein binding; *PO,* by mouth; *q,* every; *subcut,* subcutaneous; *t½,* half-life; *UK,* unknown; *WBC,* white blood cell; *wk,* weeks; *>,* greater than; *<,* less than ; *≤,* less than or equal to.

Pharmacokinetics 5-FU crosses the blood-brain barrier and is distributed widely throughout the body tissues. The concentration of 5-FU can be sustained for several hours in the cerebrospinal fluid (CSF). It is also effective for ascites and pleural effusions. The bioavailability and elimination half-life of IV 5-FU is nonlinear with high dosages, most likely due to saturation of metabolic processes. Approximately 15% is protein bound, and the rest (85%) is distributed throughout the body, including in the liver, GI mucosa, and peripheral WBCs. The major catabolizer is the liver; however, with continuous IV infusion, significant extrahepatic metabolism occurs. Following IV administration, the mean elimination half-life is 16 minutes, with a range of 8 to 20 minutes, and it is dose dependent. A small amount of unchanged 5-FU is eliminated by the biliary and renal systems. Following topical administration, approximately 6% is absorbed systemically. Also, 5-FU can be administered to patients with hepatic impairment with serum bilirubin less than 5 mg/dL without reducing the dose. No dose adjustments are needed for patients with renal impairment.

Pharmacodynamics 5-FU converts into multiple active metabolites, inhibiting normal cell growth by interfering with the cell's RNA and DNA. Cytotoxicity involving the DNA is noted during the S phase of the cell cycle during the first 24 hours after drug exposure. The cell's RNA is affected after 24 hours during the G1 phase. 5-FU is used alone or with other anticancer drugs and has a low therapeutic index. Dosing of 5-FU can vary from protocol to protocol. High IV boluses of 5-FU can result in severe hemorrhagic colitis or bone marrow suppression. Administering high doses as continuous therapy has reduced the incidences of hematologic toxicity. Complementary and Alternative Therapies 32.1 lists herbal supplements that may interact with fluorouracil.

Side Effects and Adverse Reactions

See Table 32-2 for general side effects. GI bleeding and bone marrow suppression can occur with high bolus doses of 5-FU, and patients who previously received myelosuppressive therapy and or radiation treatment have increased risk for bone marrow suppression. 5-FU can potentiate the effects of radiation therapy and should be discontinued at the first visible sign of WBCs less than 3500/mm³, a rapidly falling WBC count, or a platelet count below 100,000/mm³.

NURSING PROCESS
Patient-Centered Collaborative Care

Antimetabolites: Fluorouracil

Assessment
- To avoid drug-drug and drug-supplement interactions, conduct a detailed current medication history that includes prescriptions, OTC medicines, antacids, dietary supplements, vitamins, and herbal supplements.
- Obtain a list of drug and food allergies.
- Obtain baseline information about the patient's physical status. Include height, weight, vital signs, cardiopulmonary assessment, intake and output, skin assessment, daily activities status, nutritional status, and any underlying disease.
- Obtain baseline laboratory values (CBC, uric acid, and chemistry panel) to compare with future labs.
- Assess baseline results of pulmonary function tests, chest radiographs, ECGs, and renal and hepatic studies.
- Assess the ability for comprehension.

Nursing Diagnoses
- Infection, Risk for
- Bleeding, Risk for
- Imbalanced Nutrition, Risk for: Less Than Body Requirements
- Knowledge, Deficient related to chemotherapeutic protocol as evidenced by the inability to incorporate the health regimen into the current lifestyle

Planning
- The patient will be free of infection.
- Patient blood counts will remain in the desired range.
- The patient will remain free from signs and symptoms of bleeding.
- The patient's nutritional status will remain at the desired level.
- The patient/family/caregiver will demonstrate understanding of chemotherapeutic protocol (dose, administration, side effects, and adverse reactions).

Nursing Interventions
- Monitor the IV site frequently. Extravasation produces severe pain and can promote infection.
- Maintain strict medical asepsis during dressing changes and invasive procedures.
- Monitor blood counts and laboratory values.
- Administer an antiemetic 30 to 60 minutes before the drug to prevent nausea and emesis.
- Monitor fluid intake and output and nutritional intake.
- Offer the patient food and fluids that may decrease nausea (e.g., crackers, cola, and ginger ale).
- Assist with the planning of small, frequent meals.
- Record the number and consistency of stools; monitor perineal skin condition.

Patient Teaching
General
- Advise patients to promptly report signs of infection (fever, sore throat, chills, urinary frequency or burning on urination; redness, swelling, or pain near a wound); bleeding (bleeding gums, petechiae, bruises, hematuria, or blood in the stool); or signs of anemia (increased fatigue, dyspnea, or orthostatic hypotension).
- Teach patients to examine their mouth daily and report signs of stomatitis (soreness, ulcerations, or white patches in the mouth).
- Advise patient not to visit anyone who has a respiratory infection.
- Emphasize protective precautions such as hand washing and personal hygiene.
- Emphasize the importance of maintaining sound nutrition, and assist in the development of small, frequent meals high in calories and protein.

Side Effects
- Advise patients about good oral hygiene with a soft toothbrush for mucositis/stomatitis; have patients use a soft toothbrush when the platelet count is 50,000/mm³ or less. Instruct patients to rinse their mouth every 2 hours with normal saline and to avoid use of commercial mouthwashes that contain alcohol.
- Assess for use of alternative or complementary therapies that may interact with chemotherapy.

Diet
- Encourage small, frequent meals to decrease incidences of nausea and emesis.
- Encourage use of cool, bland foods when the patient is nauseated.
- Offer ice chips or ice pops to help relieve mouth pain.
- Encourage foods high in calories and protein.

Cultural Considerations
- Health care decisions are made by consensus in some cultures, and the family plays a key role in filtering information given to the patient. Issues related to informed consent and full disclosure of medical information may cause distress in cultural groups who place the needs of the family above the needs of the individual. Interactions should be modified based on family structure, religious values and beliefs, time orientation, cultural health practices, and verbal and nonverbal communication.
- Cultural assessment tools can provide general guidelines for health care providers.
- Hematologic toxicities that result in leukopenia and anemia are more common among African Americans than among Caucasians; however, other toxicities are decreased, including diarrhea, nausea, and vomiting.
- Asians may develop febrile neutropenia despite a lowered dosage.

Evaluation
- The patient is free from infection.
- Oral mucosa is free from erythema and swelling.
- Skin integrity remains intact.
- Patient/family/caregiver education needs are met.
- The patient's weight is maintained at the desired level.

PROTOTYPE DRUG CHART 32.2
Fluorouracil, 5-Fluorouracil (5-FU)

Drug Class	Dosage
Antimetabolite Pregnancy category*: D (systemic)/X (topical)	A: IV: 300-1000 mg/m^2/d for 4-5 d continuous infusion q4wk Topical: 1%-5% cream once or twice daily for 3-12 wk Various protocols exist, including topical; IV drugs are often used with other chemotherapeutic drugs.
Contraindications	**Drug-Lab-Food Interactions**
Bone marrow suppression, dihydropyrimidine dehydrogenase deficiency, infection, malnutrition, pregnancy *Caution:* GI bleeding, liver and renal impairment, biliary tract disease, coronary artery disease Many other precautions are present when administering fluorouracil.	Drug: Bone marrow depressants increase chances of toxicity. Avoid live virus vaccines, which may potentiate infection. Leucovorin may potentiate adverse effects of 5-FU. Drugs than can increase the systemic cytotoxicity of 5-FU include cimetidine, dipyridamole, interferon-alfa, and levamisole. Metronidazole may cause blood dyscrasias. Synergistic reaction can occur with cisplatin and 5-FU. Lab: May decrease albumin; may increase excretion of 5-HIAA in urine
Pharmacokinetics	**Pharmacodynamics**
Absorption: IV and topical: 5%-10% Distribution: PB: 15%; readily crosses the blood-brain barrier Metabolism (IV): t½: 8-20 min, dose dependent Excretion: 7%-20% via urine unchanged within 6 h; inactive metabolites via respiratory system as CO_2 and the urinary system as urea	IV onset: 1-9 d Topical onset: 2-3 d IV peak: 9-21 d Topical peak: 2-6 wk IV duration: 30 d Topical duration: 1-2 mo The above information provides two examples of pharmacodynamics. Clinical pharmacology is complex and is dependent on route of administration and patient condition.
Therapeutic Effects/Uses	
Basal cell carcinoma; breast, colorectal, pancreas, and gastric cancers; given in combination with levamisole after surgical resection in patients with Duke stage C colon cancer Mode of Action: Some cell cycle-specific effects during the S and G$_1$ phases; prevention of thymidine synthase production interferes with RNA synthesis and function and has some effects to DNA	
Side Effects	**Adverse Reactions**
Nausea, vomiting, anorexia, leukopenia, febrile neutropenia, fever, weight loss, alopecia, amenorrhea, gonadal suppression, impaired wound healing, stomatitis, pain, dry/cracked skin	Bone marrow suppression, bleeding, stomatitis, esophagopharyngitis, intractable vomiting, diarrhea, palmar-plantar erythrodysesthesia (hand and foot syndrome), cardiac toxicity, thrombocytopenia, myelosuppression, renal failure

*Pregnancy categories have been revised. See http://www.fda.gov/Drugs/DevelopmentApprovalProcess/DevelopmentResources/Labeling/ucm093307.htm for more information.

5-FU, Fluorouracil; *5-HIAA*, 5-hydroxyindoleacetic acid; *A*, adult; *CO₂*, carbon dioxide; *d*, day; *GI*, gastrointestinal; *h*, hour; *IV*, intravenous; *min*, minute; *mo*, months; *PB*, protein binding; *q*, every; *RNA*, ribonucleic acid; *t½*, half-life; *UK*, unknown; *wk*, week.

Prototype Drug Chart 32.2 details the pharmacologic behavior of 5-FU.

ANTITUMOR ANTIBIOTICS

Antitumor antibiotics are similar to natural antibiotics; however, they do *not* treat infections; instead, they interfere with DNA replication and RNA transcription of cancer cells. All antitumor antibiotics except for bleomycin have their major effects in all phases of the cell cycle (cell cycle nonspecific). Bleomycins affect cells during the G$_2$ phase. Types of antitumor antibiotics are anthracyclines (daunorubicin, doxorubicin, epirubicin, and idarubicin) and other antitumor antibiotics (actinomycin D, bleomycin, mitomycin C, and mitoxantrone). Antitumor antibiotics are used to treat leukemias and many solid tumors. Table 32.5 lists the antitumor antibiotics and their uses and considerations.

Adverse reactions to the antitumor antibiotics are similar to those of other antineoplastics and include alopecia, nausea, vomiting, stomatitis, and myelosuppression. Antitumor antibiotics are capable of causing vesication (blistering of tissue); exceptions to this are bleomycin and plicamycin. General adverse reactions to chemotherapeutic drugs are listed in Table 32.2.

Anthracyclines: Doxorubicin

Doxorubicin is an anthracycline antitumor antibiotic antineoplastic agent used to treat many solid and hematogenous tumors except for acute myelogenous leukemias (AMLs), due to the increased incidences of stomatitis and cardiotoxicity compared with other anthracyclines. Doxorubicin is a component of many combination chemotherapy treatments because of its broad antitumor activity and flexible dosing schedule. However, patients receiving IV doxorubicin must

TABLE 32.5 Antineoplastics: Antitumorals

Drug	Route and Dosage	Uses and Considerations
ANTHRACYCLINES		
Visually inspect parenteral products for particulate matter and discoloration prior to use. Observe and exercise precautions when handling, preparing, and administering cytotoxic drugs. Dosages of chemotherapeutic drugs vary from protocol to protocol. Consult appropriate references to verify dosages.		
Daunorubicin	AML: A ≤60 years: IV: 45 mg/m^2/d for 3 d for first course, then 2 d for subsequent courses A ≥60 years: IV: 30 mg/m^2/d for 3 d for first course, then 2 d for subsequent courses ALL: A: IV: 45 mg/m^2/d on days 1-3 Children dosages available.	Do not confuse with doxorubicin. For ALL and AML. Given with other antineoplastic drugs. Monitor for cardiotoxicity. Pregnancy category: D*; PB: 80%; t½: 45-55 h
Doxorubicin	See Prototype Drug Chart 32.3.	Do not confuse with daunorubicin.
Epirubicin	A: IV: 60-100 mg/m^2 q21d for 6 cycles	Adjuvant treatment for breast cancer. Assess for signs of infection. Pregnancy category: D*; PB: 77%; t½: 30 h
Idarubicin	AML: A: IV: 8-12 mg/m^2/d for 3 d APL: A: 12 mg/m^2/d for 3 d	For AML and APL. May cause red or orange urine discoloration. Pregnancy category: D*; PB: 97%; t½: 22 h
Mitoxantrone	AML: A: IV: 12 mg/m^2/d; duration of treatment is different for induction and consolidation therapy Prostate cancer: A: IV: 12-14 mg/m^2 q21d	Do not confuse with mitomycin. For AML and prostate cancer. Pregnancy category: D*; PB: 78%; t½: 23-215 h
Valrubicin	Intravesicular: A: 800 mg q1wk for 6 wk; *max:* 800 mg intravesically	For bladder cancer. Systemic exposure is dependent on the integrity of the bladder wall. Pregnancy category: C*; PB: UK; t½: UK
OTHER ANTITUMOR ANTIBIOTICS		
Bleomycin	Hodgkin disease and cervical, head and neck, and vulvar cancers: A/C: IV/IM/subcut: 5-20 units/m^2 1 or 2 times/wk; other dosing is available NHL and testicular cancer: A: IV/IM/subcut: 10-20 units/m^2 once a wk 1 or 2 times/wk	For head and neck cancer; Hodgkin disease; NHL; cervical, penile, testicular, and vulvar cancer; and malignant effusion. Monitor for pulmonary complications. Pregnancy category: D*; PB: 10%; t½: 2-4 h
Dactinomycin, actinomycin D	Choriocarcinoma: A: IV: 1250 mcg/m^2 q14d for 4 cycles Malignant melanoma: A: IA: 50 mcg/kg for legs; 35 mcg/kg for arms Rhabdomyosarcoma: A/C ≤21 y: 15 mcg/kg/d for 5 d Other dosing regimen available.	For testicular cancer, Ewing sarcoma, Wilms tumor, malignant melanoma, choriocarcinoma, and rhabdomyosarcoma. Nausea and vomiting may occur during first 24 h. Absolutely contraindicated with herpes infection or varicella. Pregnancy category: D*; PB: UK; t½: 36 h
Mitomycin	A: IV: 20 mg/m^2 q6-8wk	For gastric and pancreatic cancer. Monitor for pulmonary complications. Pregnancy category: D*; PB: UK; t½: 0.25-1.5 h

*Pregnancy categories have been revised. See http://www.fda.gov/Drugs/DevelopmentApprovalProcess/DevelopmentResources/Labeling/ucm093307.htm for more information.
Note: Chemotherapeutic doses and schedules vary depending on protocol, body surface area (m^2), age, functional status, and comorbid conditions. For a full discussion of body surface area in dosage calculation, see Chapter 11.
A, Adult; ALL, acute lymphocytic leukemia; *AML,* acute myelocytic leukemia; *APL,* acute promyelocytic leukemia; *C,* child; *d,* day; *h,* hour; *IA:* intra-arterial; *IM,* intramuscular; *IV,* intravenous; *max,* maximum dosage; *NHL,* non-Hodgkin lymphoma; *PB,* protein binding; *q,* every; *subcut,* subcutaneous; *t½,* half-life; *UK,* unknown; *wk,* week; ≥, greater than or equal to; ≤, less than or equal to.

be monitored for cardiotoxicity. Doxorubicin has a maximum dose of 550 mg/m^2 due to cardiotoxicity. Patients taking other cardiotoxic drugs, who are older, have preexisting cardiac problems, or have had radiation therapy to the chest are at increased risk for cardiotoxicity. Dexrazoxane, a chemoprotectant, is administered prior to anthracyclines to prevent cardiotoxicity. Cardiac function should be assessed prior to administering doxorubicin or other anthracyclines. Liposomal doxorubicin was developed to be carried by a liposomal carrier and decreases the incidence of severe toxicity; however, the dosages vary greatly from conventional doxorubicin, and the indications for use are different.

Pharmacokinetics Doxorubicin is administered intravenously and is distributed throughout the body tissues but does not cross the blood-brain barrier. It is extensively bound to DNA, 75% bound to plasma proteins, and not dose dependent up to 1.1 mcg/mL. Doxorubicin does not cross the placenta but appears to pass into breast milk. It is extensively metabolized by the liver into active (doxorubicinol) and inactive (hydroxylated conjugates or glucuronide) metabolites. Clearance of doxorubicinol from the blood decreases as the dose of conventional doxorubicin increases. The metabolites are excreted in the bile (50%), feces, and urine (<10%).

Pharmacodynamics Doxorubicin is part of standard regimens for breast, lung, gastric, and ovarian cancers; Hodgkin and non-Hodgkin lymphomas; sarcoma and myeloma; and acute lymphocytic leukemia (ALL). The terminal half-life for doxorubicin is 30 to 50 hours. The clearance of doxorubicin was found to be reduced in patients with elevated serum bilirubin levels; therefore dose reduction is recommended in patients with a bilirubin level greater than 1.2 mg/dL. Clearance was also reduced in patients whose weight was greater than 130% of ideal body weight. Administration of doxorubicin is not recommended to patients who received the maximum allowable dose of other anthracyclines. Cardiotoxicity is a major concern with doxorubicin. Mitochondrial damage to cardiac cells can be extensive and can cause cardiomyopathy, dysrhythmias, congestive heart failure (CHF), and cardiogenic shock. Mitochondrial damage occurs because superoxide radicals are not able to be converted back to oxygen; the heart is nearly devoid of glutathione peroxidase, an enzyme necessary for the conversion. Dexrazoxane is a parenteral chemoprotectant agent used to decrease anthracycline-associated cardiomyopathies; it is administered 30 minutes before the doxorubicin infusion. It is also used to treat anthracycline extravasation and is administered intravenously close to the affected area. Complementary and Alternative Therapies 32.1 lists herbal supplements that may also interact with doxorubicin.

⚡ PATIENT SAFETY

Monitor for cardiac toxicity and infection.

Do not confuse...
- **Doxorubicin** with **daunorubicin, doxorubicin liposomal,** or **idarubicin**

 NURSING PROCESS
Patient-Centered Collaborative Care

Antitumor Antibiotics: Doxorubicin

Assessment
- Conduct a detailed medication history that lists all concurrent medications and includes prescriptions, OTC medicines, antacids, dietary supplements, vitamins, and herbal supplements to avoid drug-drug and drug supplement interactions.
- Obtain baseline information about the patient's physical status. This should include height, weight, vital signs, cardiopulmonary assessment, intake and output, skin assessment, daily activities status (e.g., sleep-wake cycle, ability to perform activities of daily living [ADLs]), nutritional status, presence or absence of any underlying disease, and past or current use of medications and treatment.
- Assess laboratory values (CBC with differentials, uric acid, electrolytes, serum bilirubin, and hepatic and renal studies) and ECG for comparison with future labs.
- Obtain baseline data regarding the patient's psychosocial status that includes educational level, ability and desire to learn, support systems, past coping strategies, presence or absence of emotional difficulties, and self-care abilities.
- Assess patient and family knowledge related to the therapeutic regimen.

Nursing Diagnoses
- Infection, Risk for
- Decreased Cardiac Output, Risk for
- Impaired Skin Integrity, Risk for
- Knowledge, Deficient related to antineoplastic therapy as evidenced by inappropriate questions and behaviors

Planning
- The patient will remain free from infection.
- Patient laboratory values will remain in the desired range.
- The patient will be free from cardiac abnormalities.
- The patient's skin integrity will remain intact.
- The patient/family/caregiver will demonstrate understanding of the chemotherapy regimen, including side effects.
- The patient/family/caregiver will exhibit behavior appropriate for the chemotherapeutic protocol.

Nursing Interventions
- Maintain strict medical asepsis during dressing changes and invasive procedures.
- Assess cardiac status and check for any ECG abnormalities before and during treatment. Prepare to administer dexrazoxane.
- Monitor the IV site frequently, and stop the infusion immediately if signs of extravasation are apparent.
- Give drug through a large-bore, quickly running IV infusion. Monitor blood counts and laboratory values.
- Handle the drug with care during preparation, and avoid direct skin contact with the drug.

Patient Teaching
General
- Teach patients/family/caregivers when to call the health care provider.
- Explain to patients that the anticancer drug can decrease immune response and blood count.
- Emphasize protective precautions such as hand washing, personal hygiene, and avoiding people with respiratory infection.
Side Effects
- Teach patients about changes in urine color (pink or red) caused by this drug.
- Advise patients when to call a health care provider about cardiac abnormalities (chest pain, shortness of breath, or palpitations).

- Advise patients to promptly report signs of infection (fever, sore throat), bleeding (bleeding gums, petechiae, bruises, hematuria, or blood in stool), and anemia (increased fatigue, dyspnea, or orthostatic hypotension).
- Stress to patients the importance of notifying their health care provider immediately if burning or pain is experienced at the IV site.

Diet
- Encourage small, frequent, bland meals high in calories and protein.

🌐 Cultural Considerations

- Some cultural groups can lack understanding of Western approaches to health care. The need to respect patient autonomy and participation in the decision making is important, but at times health care decisions are made by consensus, and the family plays a key role. Interactions should be modified based on family structure, religious values and beliefs, time orientation, cultural health practices, and verbal and nonverbal communication.
- African Americans have a higher risk of cardiotoxicity than do Caucasians. Cardiotoxicity includes CHF, decreased cardiac function, and cardiac death.
- Asians may develop febrile neutropenia despite lowered dosages.

Evaluation
- The patient is free from infection.
- Cardiac function is maintained.
- The IV site remains free from extravasation.
- The patient and family educational needs are met.
- Side effects of therapy are controlled.

Side Effects and Adverse Reactions

Doxorubicin has adverse drug effects similar to those of other chemotherapeutic agents. Table 32.2 lists the common side effects and adverse reactions. One common side effect of doxorubicin includes a change of the urine color to pink or light red. Life-threatening effects include cardiotoxicity, CHF, severe myelosuppression, and ECG abnormalities. The amount of myelosuppression tends to be dose dependent, dose limiting, and reversible.

Prototype Drug Chart 32.3 presents the pharmacologic data for doxorubicin.

PLANT ALKALOIDS

Plant alkaloids are derived from plants and are cell cycle specific; they block cell division at the M phase of the cell cycle. The vinca alkaloids (vinblastine, vincristine, and vinorelbine) and the taxanes (docetaxel and paclitaxel) are considered antimicrotubule compounds that cause disruption and interference with vital cell functions when cells are dividing (mitosis), which leads to cell apoptosis. Microtubules also involve many nonmitotic functions and thereby affect malignant and nonmalignant cells.

The vinca alkaloids are derived from the periwinkle plant, and taxanes are derived from the yew tree. When the natural resources became scarce, a semisynthetic form of taxanes was developed. Epipodophyllotoxins (etoposide, teniposide) come from apple trees and interfere with topoisomerases, enzymes that separate strands of DNA during the S phase of the cell cycle. Another group of plant alkaloids, camptothecin analogues (irinotecan, topotecan) isolated from a Chinese tree are water soluble and have a broad range of antitumor properties. Retinoids (bexarotene), a natural derivative of vitamin A, is an important regulator for cell reproduction, proliferation, and differentiation. However, retinoids do not convert into the rhodopsin needed for night vision. Retinoids are given orally or topically. Table 32.6 lists the plant alkaloids and their uses and considerations.

Adverse reactions to plant alkaloids include leukopenia, hypersensitivity reactions, partial to complete alopecia, constipation, nausea, vomiting, diarrhea, and phlebitis. The plant alkaloids damage peripheral nerve fibers and may cause reversible or irreversible neurotoxicity. Signs and symptoms of neurotoxicity include a decrease in muscular strength numbness and tingling of fingers and toes (stocking-glove syndrome), constipation, and motor instability. Other adverse effects of these drugs include loss of deep tendon reflexes, muscle weakness, joint pain, and bone marrow suppression. Docetaxel may cause fluid retention. General adverse effects to chemotherapeutic drugs are listed in Table 32.2.

Vincristine

Vincristine was developed from the periwinkle plant and has an increased cellular retention compared with vinblastine. Neurotoxicity is a dose-limiting adverse effect of vincristine, whereas other vinca alkaloids have a dose-limiting myelosuppression. Vincristine is used for leukemias, breast carcinoma, NHL, multiple myeloma, soft-tissue and osteogenic sarcomas, and brain tumors.

Pharmacokinetics Vincristine is given parenterally. It is distributed widely throughout many tissues and binds to RBCs and platelets. Approximately 50% is metabolized by the liver and is excreted as metabolites or as the parent drug in the bile and feces. Approximately, three-fourths of the drug is eliminated through the biliary tree within 72 hours. The final elimination half-life is between 23 and 85 hours. Patients with significant biliary obstruction may need dose adjustment.

Pharmacodynamics Vincristine exerts cytotoxic effects by interfering with microtubules in the M phase in addition to having other effects, such as inhibition of RNA, DNA, and protein synthesis; inhibition of glycolysis; and disruption of cell membrane integrity. It has a high-volume distribution and rapid distribution half-life of less than 5 minutes due to extensive tissue binding. Vincristine does not cross the blood-brain barrier. Complementary and Alternative Therapies 32.1 lists herbal supplements that may also interact with vincristine.

Side Effects and Adverse Reactions

Vincristine is associated with neurotoxicity with an intracellular concentration above a certain critical threshold. Continuous infusion is associated with longer tissue exposure above the critical cytotoxic level. Neurotoxicity is a dose-limiting adverse effect, and neuropathy may occur with single weekly

PROTOTYPE DRUG CHART 32.3

Doxorubicin

Drug Class	Dosage
Antitumor antibiotic: Anthracycline Pregnancy category: D*	A: IV: 60-75 mg/m² once q21d as a single agent, 20-75 mg/m² q21-28d if used in combination with other drugs Various protocols exist, including combination therapy. Dose varies based on indicated use and response. Adjust dose with hepatic impairment.
Contraindications	**Drug-Lab-Food Interactions**
Anthracycline hypersensitivity, hepatic disease, myocardial infarction or severe myocardial insufficiency, neutropenia, those who received the maximum dose of doxorubicin or daunorubicin. *Caution:* Bone marrow suppression, extravasation, heart failure, impaired hepatic or renal function	Drug: Other cytotoxic drugs combined with doxorubicin may increase hematologic and GI toxicities. Cardiotoxicity may results with concomitant use with paclitaxel and verapamil. Hematologic toxicity can occur when used with cyclosporine and cyclophosphamide. Secondary malignancies have been noted with use of progesterone. Cytarabine has been known to cause necrotizing colitis. Lab: Abnormal hepatic function tests, may induce tumor-lysis syndrome and hyperuricemia, ECG changes; increases uric acid and may reduce neutrophil and RBC counts
Pharmacokinetics	**Pharmacodynamics**
Absorption: IV Distribution: PB: 70% Metabolism: t½: 20-48 h Excretion: 40% in bile and 5%-12% in urine	IV: Onset: 10 d Peak: 14 d Duration: 21-24 d
Therapeutic Effects/Uses	
Breast, gastric, lung, and ovarian cancers; hematogenous tumors; soft-tissue and bone sarcomas; leukemias; lymphomas Mode of Action: Inhibits DNA and RNA synthesis; has immunosuppressant activity; it is cell cycle specific for the S phase.	
Side Effects	**Adverse Reactions**
Complete alopecia, stomatitis, anorexia, nausea, vomiting, diarrhea, rash, reddish colored urine, hyperpigmentation of nail beds, dermal creases, fever, chills Dexrazoxane, a cytoprotectant drug, is used to treat extravasation and reduce the incidence and or severity of cardiotoxicity due to anthracycline toxicity.	Cardiotoxicity (cardiomyopathy, dysrhythmias, CHF, and cardiogenic shock); myelosuppression (hematologic toxicity [leukopenia, anemia, and thrombocytopenia])

*Pregnancy categories have been revised. See http://www.fda.gov/Drugs/DevelopmentApprovalProcess/DevelopmentResources/Labeling/ucm093307.htm for more information.
A, Adult *CHF*, congestive heart failure; *d*, day; *DNA*, deoxyribonucleic acid; *ECG*, electrocardiogram; *GI*, gastrointestinal; *h*, hour; *IV*, intravenous; *PB*, protein binding; *q*, every; *RBC*, red blood cell; *RNA*, ribonucleic acid; *t½*, half-life.

TABLE 32.6 Antineoplastics: Plant Alkaloids

Drug	Route and Dosage	Uses and Considerations
Antimicrotubules/Taxanes		
Visually inspect parenteral products for particulate matter and discoloration prior to use. Observe and exercise precautions when handling, preparing, and administering cytotoxic drugs. Chemotherapeutic drug dosages vary from protocol to protocol. Consult appropriate references to verify doses.		
Docetaxel	Breast cancer: A: IV: 60-100 mg/m² day 1, repeat q3wk All other cancers: A: IV: 75 mg/m² q3wk	For breast, gastric, prostate, and head and neck cancers and NSCLC. Monitor for pulmonary and cardiac complications. Pregnancy category: D*; PB: 94%; t½: 11 h
Paclitaxel	Breast cancer: A: IV: 175 mg/m² q3wk Ovarian, NSCLC, and Kaposi sarcoma: A: IV: 135 mg/m² q3wk	Do not confuse Taxol with Taxotere. For breast and ovarian cancers, NSCLC, and Kaposi sarcoma. Pregnancy category: D*; PB: 95%-98%; t½: 19 h
CAMPTOTHECIN ANALOGUES		
Irinotecan	A: IV: 125 mg/m² once a week for 4 wk Other dosing regimen is available	For colorectal cancer. Consider lower doses in older adults. Pregnancy category: D*; PB: 30%-68%; t½: 6-12 h
Topotecan	Ovarian cancer and SCLC: A: IV: 1.5 mg/m²/d for 5 d q21d Cervical cancer: A: IV: 0.75 mg/m² for 3 d q3wk	For cervical and ovarian cancers and SCLC. Do not give for severe renal impairment (creatinine >1.5 mg/dL). Pregnancy category: D*; PB: >35%; t½: 2-6 h (route dependent)

Continued

TABLE 32.6 Antineoplastics: Plant Alkaloids—cont'd

Drug	Route and Dosage	Uses and Considerations
EPIPODOPHYLLOTOXINS		
Etoposide	SCLC: A: IV: 35-50 mg/m²/d for 4-5d q21d for 4 cycles Testicular cancer: A: IV: 100 mg/m²/d for 5 d, repeat q3-4wk Other dosing regimen is available	For testicular cancer and SCLC. Contraindicated in known benzyl alcohol intolerance. Pregnancy category: D*; PB: 95%; t½: 5-10 h
Teniposide	C: IV: 165 mg/m² twice weekly for 8-9 doses	For ALL. Contraindicated with polyoxyethylated castor oil hypersensitivity. Pregnancy category: D*; PB: 99%; t½: 5 h
IMMUNOMODULATORS		
Thalidomide	ENL: A/C ≥12 y: PO: 100-300 mg/d at bedtime Multiple myeloma: A: PO: 200 mg/d at bedtime	For multiple myeloma and ENL. Do not administer to pregnant patients; severe birth defects occurred. Pregnancy category: X*; PB: 55%-66%; t½: 5.5-7.3 h
RETINOIDS		
Bexarotene	A: PO: 300 mg/m²/d (round to nearest 75 mg)	For cutaneous T-cell lymphoma. Do *not* administer to pregnant patients. Pregnancy category: X*; PB: >99%; t½: 7 h
VINCA ALKALOIDS		
Vinblastine	Breast cancer: A: IV: 4.5 mg/m²/d every 21 d NHL: A: IV: 4 mg/m² days 1 and 2, repeated q28d for 3 cycles Hodgkin disease: A: IV: 6 mg/m² days 1 and 15, repeated q28d C: IV: 2.5-6 mg/m²/d q1-2wk for 3-6 wk Other dosing regimen is available	For solid organ cancers, choriocarcinoma, cutaneous T-cell lymphoma, Hodgkin disease, and NHL. Usually given with combination therapy. Monitor for any pulmonary complications. Pregnancy category: D*; PB: 50%; t½: 23-85 h
Vincristine	See Prototype Drug Chart 32.4	
Vinorelbine	A: IV: 30 mg/m²/wk	For NSCLC. Dose must be adjusted with hepatic impairment. Pregnancy category: D*; PB: 79.6%-91.2%; t½: 27.7-43.6 h

*Pregnancy categories have been revised. See http://www.fda.gov/Drugs/DevelopmentApprovalProcess/DevelopmentResources/Labeling/ucm093307.htm for more information.

Note: Chemotherapeutic doses and schedules vary depending on protocol, body surface area (m²), age, functional status, and comorbid conditions. For a full discussion of body surface area in dosage calculation, see Chapter 11.

A, Adult; *ALL,* acute lymphocytic leukemia; *C,* child; *d,* day; *ENL,* erythema nodosum leprosum; *h,* hour; *IV,* intravenous; *NHL,* non-Hodgkin lymphoma; *NSCLC,* non–small cell lung cancer; *PB,* protein binding; *PO,* by mouth; *q,* every; *SCLC,* small cell lung cancer; *t½,* half-life; *UK,* unknown; *wk,* week: >, greater than; ≥, greater than or equal to.

vincristine doses but usually resolves within a week. If the total calculated dose is administered in divided doses, more severe neuritic pain occurs. Sensory loss, paresthesias, difficulty walking, hyporeflexia, and muscle wasting may occur and may become progressively worse as therapy continues. Neurologic symptoms usually resolve within 6 months; however, residual effects have been prolonged in some patients. Other adverse effects from vincristine include bronchospasm, hepatic venoocclusive disease, transient cortical blindness and optic atrophy with blindness, and bladder atony. Glutamic acid given with vincristine has been known to decrease the adverse effects. Nonneurologic symptoms are similar to those of other anticancer drugs.

Vincristine is a substrate for the cytochrome P450 system. Several drug interactions may occur with vincristine, so the

 NURSING PROCESS
Patient-Centered Collaborative Care

Plant Alkaloids: Vincristine

Assessment

- Conduct a detailed medication history that lists all concurrent medications and includes prescriptions, OTC medicines, antacids, dietary supplements, vitamins, and herbal supplements to avoid drug interactions.
- Obtain baseline information about the patient's physical status. This should include height, weight, vital signs, cardiopulmonary assessment, intake and output, skin assessment, daily activities status (i.e., ability to perform ADLs), sleep-wake cycle, nutritional status, presence or absence

of underlying symptoms of disease, and the use of current or past medications and treatments. Be especially aware of evidence of neurotoxicity such as peripheral neuropathy (numbness or tingling in fingers or toes), loss of deep tendon reflexes, foot drop, slapping gait, and difficulty walking.

- Assess baseline lab values (CBC, liver and renal function tests, serum sodium, and serum bilirubin) for comparison with future values.
- Assess temperature; fever may be an early sign of infection.
- Monitor for acute bronchospasm.
- Monitor bowel and urinary function. Autonomic neuropathy may lead to constipation, paralytic ileus, and bladder atony.
- Obtain baseline data regarding psychosocial status that includes the patient's educational level, ability and desire to learn, support systems, past coping strategies, presence or absence of emotional difficulties, and self-care abilities.

Nursing Diagnoses
- Injury, Risk for
- Breathing Pattern, Ineffective related to bronchospasm secondary to rapid infusion as evidenced by wheezes, dyspnea, and anxiety
- Infection, Risk for
- Constipation, Risk for
- Urinary Elimination, Risk for Altered
- Knowledge, Deficient related to antineoplastic therapy

Planning
- The patient will be free from neuropathic dysfunction.
- The patient will be free from respiratory complications (bronchospasm).
- The patient's laboratory values will remain in the desired range.
- The patient will maintain adequate bowel function.
- The patient will maintain adequate urinary function.
- The patient/family/caregiver will demonstrate understanding of the chemotherapy regimen, including side effects.

Nursing Interventions
- Assess for signs of respiratory distress during and after drug administration.
- Monitor for signs of peripheral neuropathy (numbness or tingling in hands or feet, sensory loss, loss of deep tendon reflexes, paresthesia, foot drop or wrist drop, ataxia).
- Assess the IV site carefully. Give drug through a large-bore, quickly running IV infusion.
- Monitor the IV site for extravasation, and if it occurs, stop the infusion immediately and follow the drug protocol for extravasation.
- Monitor blood counts and laboratory values.
- Maintain strict medical asepsis during dressing changes and invasive procedures.
- Administer stool softener or laxative as prescribed.
- Monitor fluid intake and output and nutritional intake.

Patient Teaching
General
- Teach patients the signs and symptoms of neurotoxicity: numbness or tingling in hands or feet, sensory loss, loss of deep tendon reflexes, paresthesia, foot or wrist drop, and ataxia.
- Emphasize the importance of notifying the health care provider of any breathing difficulties such as wheezing, shortness of breath, and anxiety.
- Advise patients to promptly report signs of infection (fever, sore throat), bleeding (bleeding gums, petechiae, bruises, hematuria, blood in the stool), and anemia (increased fatigue, dyspnea, orthostatic hypotension).
- Emphasize protective precautions such as hand washing and personal hygiene.
- Advise patient not to visit anyone who has a respiratory infection.

Side Effects
- Teach patients the signs of peripheral neuropathy.
- Teach patients the signs of respiratory compromise.
- Teach patients to report constipation, abdominal pain, and difficulty with urination.
- Teach patients the signs of drug extravasation into tissue, which can occur 3 to 4 weeks after administration of the drug.

Diet
- Encourage bulky high-fiber foods and moderate exercise to reduce the risk of constipation.
- Encourage adequate hydration to prevent electrolyte imbalances and renal toxicity.

Cultural Considerations
- In some cultural groups, health care decisions are made by consensus, and the family plays a key role in filtering information given to the patient. Issues related to informed consent and full disclosure of medical information may cause distress in cultural groups that place the needs of the family above the needs of the individual. Interactions should be modified based on family structure, religious values and beliefs, time orientation, cultural health practices, and verbal and nonverbal communication.
- Cultural assessment tools can provide general guidelines for health care providers.
- Older adults are at increased risk for hyponatremia and SIADH. Caution should be used when administering vincristine to older adults.
- Vincristine-associated toxicities are more pronounced among Caucasians than African Americans, which leads to more doses missed among Caucasians.
- Asians may develop febrile neutropenia despite a lowered dosage.

Evaluation
- The patient is free from infection.
- Bowel function is maintained.
- Electrolytes and renal function are maintained.
- Peripheral neuropathy did not occur.
- Extravasation and tissue necrosis did not occur.
- Patient/family/caregiver educational needs are met.

patient should report all medications being taken, including OTC medicines and herbal supplements. Other CYP3A4 inhibitors—including L-asparaginase, calcium channel blockers, amiodarone, statin drugs, proton pump inhibitors, and grapefruit juice—can decrease metabolism of vincristine, thereby increasing tissue exposure. CYP3A4 inducers such as phenytoin, barbiturates, and nafcillin decrease vincristine efficacy.

Prototype Drug Chart 32.4 details the pharmacologic behavior of vincristine.

⚡ PATIENT SAFETY

Serious drug interactions can occur. Obtain a complete medication list that includes over-the-counter preparations and herbal supplements.

Do not confuse...
- **Taxol** with **Taxotere** or **Paxil**
- **Vincristine** with **vinblastine**

IMMUNOMODULATORS

Chapter 25 provides information on other immunomodulators used as antiinflammatories. Thalidomide has antiangiogenic, immunomodulatory, and antitumor properties. The exact mechanism of action is unknown; however, thalidomide selectively reduces levels of tumor necrosis factor alpha (TNF-α) inhibits interleukin 12 (IL-12), increases IL-2, and increases interferon (IFN) gamma. Thalidomide is used to treat moderate to severe erythema nodosum leprosum (ENL; leprosy), and it is used with dexamethasone to treat patients with multiple myeloma. Thalidomide is well known for its teratogenicity, hence availability is limited. Other immunomodulators include monoclonal antibody therapy (rituximab, alemtuzumab, and nonspecific immunotherapies and adjuvants such as IL-2 and interferon-alfa) designed to strengthen the immune system to attack cancer cells. Table 32.2 provides information for general adverse effects from chemotherapeutic drugs.

📋 PROTOTYPE DRUG CHART 32.4

Vincristine

Drug Class	Dosage
Plant alkaloid/vinca alkaloid Pregnancy category: D*	A: IV: 1.4 mg/m² q7d for 4 wk C <10 kg: IV: 0.05 mg/m² q7d C ≥10 kg: IV: 0.05 mg/kg q7d Various protocols exist, including combination therapy. Dosage varies based on indicated use and response. Adjust dose if hepatic impairment.
Contraindications	**Drug-Lab-Food Interactions**
Demyelinating form of Charcot-Marie-Tooth syndrome, hypersensitivity to vincristine, pregnancy *Caution:* Liver impairment, history of viral infections, neurotoxicity, electrolyte imbalances, patients receiving radiation through ports (including liver), elderly *Hyaluronidase* may be given for extravasation.	Drug: Many drug-drug interactions exist. Vincristine can increase serum concentrations of methotrexate and bleomycin. Neurotoxicity can result if asparaginase or pegaspargase are coadministered with vincristine. Many drugs increase the concentration of vincristine; some include amiodarone, statin drugs, proton pump inhibitors, and testosterone. All these drugs inhibit the P-glycoprotein system. Lab: May increase serum uric acid, may cause leukopenia, may cause hyponatremia
Pharmacokinetics	**Pharmacodynamics**
Absorption: IV Distribution: PB: 44% Metabolism: Liver; t½: triphasic 19-155 h Excretion: 80% in feces; 10%-20% in urine	Onset: UK Peak: 4 d Duration: 7 d
Therapeutic Effects/Uses	
Hodgkin disease, non-Hodgkin lymphoma, neuroblastoma, rhabdomyosarcoma, Wilms tumor, acute lymphocytic leukemia	
Mode of Action: Affects cells in the M and S phase of the cell cycle-specific by inhibiting microtubule formation; inhibits cell division and RNA, DNA, and protein synthesis	
Side Effects	**Adverse Reactions**
Peripheral neuropathy, loss of deep tendon reflexes, phlebitis, constipation, cramps, nausea, vomiting, muscle weakness, reversible alopecia *Glutamic acid* may decrease adverse effects. *Leucovorin* may be given as a cytoprotectant from the toxic effects of vincristine.	Hepatic venoocclusive disease, neurotoxicity (dose dependent), sensory loss, hypotension, visual disturbances, ptosis, ileus, SIADH, hyponatremia, hyperuricemia, severe local reaction with extravasation, fever *Life threatening:* Intestinal necrosis, seizures, coma, acute bronchospasm, bone marrow suppression

*Pregnancy categories have been revised. See http://www.fda.gov/Drugs/DevelopmentApprovalProcess/DevelopmentResources/Labeling/ucm093307.htm for more information.

A, adult; *C,* child; *d,* day; *DNA,* deoxyribonucleic acid; *h,* hour; *IV,* intravenous; *PB,* protein binding; *q,* every; *RNA,* ribonucleic acid; *SIADH,* syndrome of inappropriate antidiuretic hormone; *t½,* half-life; *UK,* unknown; *wk,* weeks; <, less than; ≥, greater than or equal to.

TARGETED THERAPIES

Targeted cancer therapy is a relatively new approach to treating cancers. Chapter 33 provides in-depth information on this treatment modality.

LIPOSOMAL CHEMOTHERAPY

A more recent change in the delivery of chemotherapy involves the use of anticancer drugs packaged inside synthetic fat globules called liposomes. The fatty coating helps the chemotherapy drug remain in the system longer and increases the duration of therapeutic effects; it also decreases side effects such as hair loss, nausea, and cardiotoxicity. Encapsulated forms of liposomal doxorubicin, daunorubicin, vincristine, and cytarabine are examples of liposomal chemotherapy.

HORMONES AND HORMONAL AGONISTS AND ANTAGONISTS

Although hormones are not considered true chemotherapeutic agents, several classes of hormonal agents are used in the treatment of cancer. These hormones do not work in the same ways as standard chemotherapy drugs. Instead, the hormones mask the cancer cells and prevent them from using or producing hormones. These include corticosteroids, estrogens, antiestrogens, aromatase inhibitors, gonadotropin-releasing hormone, progestins, and antiandrogens.

Corticosteroids

Corticosteroids are natural hormones and hormonelike drugs used to treat many types of cancer and noncancerous illnesses. They are divided into glucocorticoids and mineralocorticoids. These steroids should not be confused with anabolic steroids. *Glucocorticoids* assist with protein metabolism; examples of such steroids are prednisone, methylprednisolone, hydrocortisone, and dexamethasone. Steroids suppress the inflammatory process associated with tumor growth. Additionally, they are also considered immunosuppressives, which depress the patient's immune system. Steroids are used to treat leukemias, multiple myeloma, inflammatory bowel disease (IBD), and transplant rejection among other diseases. Because steroids suppress both the immune and the inflammatory systems, it can mask infection. Other common adverse effects include delirium, elevated serum glucose, insomnia, irritability, and other psychological problems. Because of its deleterious effects, it is recommended to avoid the use of prednisone among older adults who are at high risk for delirium. Prednisone is the most common steroid prescribed and is four times as potent as a glucocorticoid. Prednisone has little mineralocorticoid activity. Other adverse effects include fluid retention, muscle weakness, irregular menstrual bleeding, atherosclerosis, and thrombosis among others. It is metabolized in the liver to the active metabolite prednisolone, and the drug is excreted in the urine.

Sex Hormones

The sex hormones (estrogen, androgen) and hormonelike agents are used to slow the growth of hormone-dependent tumors (e.g., prostate cancer and breast cancer). Exogenous estrogens maintain all the properties of endogenous estrogens, and estrogen therapy is a palliative treatment used to slow the progression of prostatic cancer by decreasing testosterone production. Estrogen has also been used for the improvement of bone metastasis. Examples of this group of drugs are conjugated estrogens. Synthetic progestin (e.g., hydroxyprogesterone caproate, megestrol, and medroxyprogesterone acetate) is used for renal and endometrial cancers. Both estrogen and progesterone are mainly metabolized by the liver, excreted through the biliary system, and eliminated by the kidneys. Adverse effects of estrogens and progestins include fluid retention, thrombosis, menstrual irregularities, and osteoporosis among others. Testosterone is the primary androgen synthesized by the cells in the testes, ovaries, and adrenal cortex. Exogenous androgen opposes the activity of estrogen and is most effective for palliative treatment of breast cancer among postmenopausal women.

Table 32.7 lists sex hormones, hormonal agonists and antagonists, selective estrogen receptor modulators, luteinizing hormone–releasing hormone agonists, aromatase inhibitors, miscellaneous enzymes, and vaccines and their uses and considerations.

Antiandrogens

Antiandrogens, such as bicalutamide and flutamide, and antiestrogens such as fulvestrant block the effects of testosterone and estrogen, respectively, thereby slowing or shrinking cancers.

Selective Estrogen Receptor Modulators

Selective estrogen receptor modulators (SERMs) such as tamoxifen and raloxifene have both estrogenic and antiestrogenic effects on various tissues. Tamoxifen is primarily used for breast cancer in both men and women. Raloxifene produces estrogenic effects in bone and lipids and has an antiestrogenic property in mammary tissues. It is used as a prophylactic against breast cancer in high-risk postmenopausal women with osteoporosis.

Luteinizing Hormone–Releasing Hormone Agonists

Luteinizing hormone–releasing hormone (LHRH), also known as *gonadotropin-releasing hormone* (GnRH) analogues or agonists (leuprolide, goserelin) suppress the secretion of follicle-stimulating hormone and luteinizing hormone from the pituitary gland. In men, the continued suppression of the male hormone decreases the size of the prostate gland and produces an improvement in symptoms. In women, continued suppression of LHRH decreases serum estradiol and reduces the size and function of the ovaries, uterus, and mammary glands.

Aromatase Inhibitors

Aromatases are enzymes that convert other hormones into estrogen, and aromatase inhibitors are drugs that stop the

TABLE 32.7   Antineoplastics: Sex Hormones, Hormonal Agonists and Antagonists, Selective Estrogen Receptor Modulators, Luteinizing Hormone–Releasing Hormone Agonists, Aromatase Inhibitors, Enzymes, and Vaccines

Drug	Route and Dosage	Uses and Considerations
Sex Hormones		
Visually inspect parenteral products for particulate matter and discoloration prior to use. Observe and exercise precautions when handling, preparing, and administering cytotoxic drugs. Chemotherapeutic drug dosages will vary from protocol to protocol. Consult appropriate references to verify doses.		
ANDROGENS		
Fluoxymesterone	Women: PO: 10-40 mg/d in divided doses	For breast cancer. Do *not* give to pregnant patients. Contraindicated with prostate cancer. Pregnancy category: X*; PB: UK; t½: 9.2 h
HORMONAL AGONISTS AND ANTAGONISTS		
Abiraterone	Men: PO: 1 g/d	For prostate cancer. Assess liver function. Pregnancy category: X*; PB: 99%; t½: 7-17 h
Anastrozole	A: PO: 1 mg/d	For advanced breast cancer. Monitor for cardiac toxicity and angioedema. Pregnancy category: D*; PB: 40%; t½: 50 h
Bicalutamide	Men: PO: 50 mg/d	For prostate cancer. Monitor for hepatotoxicity. Pregnancy category: X*; PB: 99%; t½: 6-10 d
Enzalutamide	A: PO: 160 mg/d	For prostate cancer. Given after docetaxel failure. Pregnancy category: X*; PB: 97%; t½: 2.8-10.2 d
Exemestane	Postmenopausal women: PO: 25 mg/d	For breast cancer. Adjuvant treatment for those who have estrogen receptor–positive early disease that and received tamoxifen. Pregnancy category: X*; PB: 90%; t½: 24 h
Flutamide	A: PO: 250 mg q8h; max daily dose: 750 mg	For prostate cancer. Assess for any suicidal thoughts or tendencies. Do not use with MAOIs. Pregnancy category: D*; PB: 95%; t½: UK
Fulvestrant	A: IM: 1 g on days 1, 15, and 29 and once monthly thereafter	For breast cancer. Avoid IV administration. Pregnancy category: D*; PB: 99%; t½: UK
Goserelin acetate	Subcut: 3.6 mg q28d Implants available for prostate cancer	For breast and prostate cancers. Slow absorption for first 8 days of therapy. Pregnancy category: X*; PB: <30%; t½: 4.2 h
Histrelin acetate implant	A men: Subcut implant: 50 mg q12mo	For prostate cancer. Contraindicated in children, females, and pregnancy. Proper surgical technique is critical to minimize adverse events. Pregnancy category: X*; PB: UK; t½: 3.92 h
Letrozole	Postmenopausal women: PO: 2.5 mg/d	For breast cancer. Dose adjustment is needed for severe hepatic impairment. Pregnancy category: X*; PB: UK; t½: 2 d
Leuprolide	Leuprolide acetate lyophilisate: A: Subcut: 1 mg/d Leuprolide acetate suspension: IM: Depot 7.5 mg q1mo	For prostate cancer. Cardiac, pulmonary, and hepatic toxicity can occur. Pregnancy category: X*; PB: 43%-49%; t½: 3 h
Medroxyprogesterone	A: IM: Depot 400-1000 mg/wk; attempt to decrease to 400 mg/mo	For endometrial and renal cell cancers. Monitor hepatic and renal function. Pregnancy category: X*; PB: >90%; t½: 30-50 d (dose dependent)
Megestrol acetate	Breast: A: PO: 40 mg qid Endometrial: A: PO: 40-320 mg/d divided doses	For breast and endometrial cancers. Risk for thromboembolism increases. Pregnancy category: X*; PB: >90%; t½: 15-105 h
Mitotane	A: PO: 2-6 g/d in 3-4 divided doses then 9-10 g/d	For adrenocortical cancer. Monitoring parameters include neurologic function and serum cortisol and potassium. Pregnancy category: C*; PB: UK; t½: 18-159 d
Nilutamide	A: PO: 300 mg/d for 30 d, then 150 mg/d maintenance dose	For prostate cancer. Absolutely contraindicated in hepatic and respiratory disease. Use with caution in Asians. Pregnancy category: C*; PB: UK: t½: 38-59 h
Raloxifene	Postmenopausal women: PO: 60 mg/d	For breast cancer prophylaxis. Increases risk of embolism and thromboembolism with estrogen products. Pregnancy category: X*; PB: UK; t½: 25.8-86.6 h
Tamoxifen citrate	A: PO: 20-40 mg bid	For breast cancer. May cause abnormal Papanicolaou and vaginal smears; regular gynecologic exams should be performed; uterine malignancy can occur. Pregnancy category: D*; PB: UK; t½: 5-7 d
Toremifene citrate	Women: PO: 60 mg/d	For breast cancer. Absolutely contraindicated in those with hypokalemia, hypomagnesemia, and prolonged QT intervals. Pregnancy category: D*; PB: >99%; t½: 5 d

TABLE 32.7 Antineoplastics: Sex Hormones, Hormonal Agonists and Antagonists, Selective Estrogen Receptor Modulators, Luteinizing Hormone–Releasing Hormone Agonists, Aromatase Inhibitors, Enzymes, and Vaccines—cont'd

Drug	Route and Dosage	Uses and Considerations
MISCELLANEOUS ENZYMES		
Asparaginase *Erwinia chrysanthemi*	To substitute pegaspargase: A/C: IV: 25,000 u/m^2 3/wk for 6 doses To substitute L-asparaginase *Escherichia coli*: A/C: IV: 25,000 u/m^2 for each scheduled dose of L-asparaginase	For ALL. Used as part of combination treatment. Assess for any pancreatic complications. Pregnancy category: C*; PB: UK; t½: 8-30 h
Pegaspargase	A/C: IV/IM: 2500 units/m^2 q14d	For ALL. Assess for any pancreatic complications or seizures. Pregnancy category: C*; PB: UK; t½: 3.24-5.07 d
VACCINES		
Hepatitis B virus (HBV)	A/C: IM: Given in a series of 3 doses at 0, 1, and 3 mo	As prophylaxis against HBV. Contraindicated with known yeast hypersensitivity. Pregnancy category: C*; PB: UK; t½: UK
Quadrivalent human papillomavirus (HPV; types 6, 11, 16, and 18) recombinant vaccine	A/C: IM: 0.5 mL given in a series of 3 doses (0, 2, and 6 mo)	As prophylaxis against HPV types 6, 11, 16, and 18 for prevention of cervical cancer. Contraindicated with known yeast hypersensitivity. Pregnancy category: B*; PB: UK; t1/2: UK
HPV bivalent vaccine	IM: 0.5 mL given in a series of 3 shots (0, 1, and 6 mo) in deltoid region of upper arm	As prophylaxis against HPV for prevention of cervical cancer and precancerous lesions associated with the most common cancer-causing HPV types. Pregnancy category: B*; PB: UK; t1/2: UK

*Pregnancy categories have been revised. See http://www.fda.gov/Drugs/DevelopmentApprovalProcess/DevelopmentResources/Labeling/ucm093 307.htm for more information.

Note: Chemotherapeutic doses and schedules vary depending on protocol, body surface area (m^2), age, functional status, and comorbid conditions. For a full discussion of body surface area in dosage calculation, see Chapter 11.

A, Adult; *ALL*, acute lymphocytic leukemia; *bid*, twice daily; *C*, child; *d*, day; *h*, hour; *IM*, intramuscular; *IV*, intravenous; *MAOI*, monoamine oxidase inhibitor; *max*, maximum; *mo*, month; *PB*, protein binding; *PO*, by mouth; *q*, every; *qid*, four times daily; *subcut*, subcutaneous; *t½*, half-life; *UK*, unknown; *wk*, week; *>*, greater than; *<*, less than.

enzyme from converting other hormones into estrogen. For example, in postmenopausal women, the ovaries no longer produce estrogen, but aromatase converts androgen to estrogen in this group of women. The aromatase inhibitors block the peripheral conversion of androgens to estrogens, thus suppressing the postmenopausal synthesis of estrogen and slowing tumor growth. Aromatase inhibitors are used in the treatment of hormonally sensitive breast cancer in postmenopausal women and premenopausal women who have had their ovaries removed. Anastrozole, letrozole, and exemestane are examples of aromatase inhibitors currently in use. Increasingly these agents are being used before tamoxifen in postmenopausal women with hormonally responsive metastatic breast cancer. Table 32.7 lists hormonal agents and their uses and considerations.

BIOLOGIC RESPONSE MODIFIERS

Biologic response modifiers (BRMs) enhance the body's immune system. Drugs that are BRMs are discussed further in Chapter 34.

MISCELLANEOUS CHEMOTHERAPY AGENTS

This category includes a number of antineoplastic agents in which the mechanism of action is unclear. Table 32.7 describes two, asparaginase and pegaspargase.

Vaccines

Vaccines used to prevent cancer can be considered specific immunotherapy. Recombinant vaccines include hepatitis B to prevent infection with the hepatitis B virus (HBV), which can cause liver cancer, and human papillomavirus (HPV) quadrivalent, HPV-9 valent, and HPV bivalent, given to males and females aged 9 to 26 years to prevent HPV infections that can cause cervical cancer in females and genital warts in males. Sipuleucel-T is composed of autologous blood mononuclear cells and antigen-presenting cells (APCs) fused in protein, and it is given to stimulate T-cell immunity against the prostate cancer antigen prostatic acid phosphatase. Sipuleucel-T is the first immunotherapy to treat prostate cancer.

CRITICAL THINKING CASE STUDY

A 63-year-old patient recently diagnosed with breast cancer is scheduled to receive combination chemotherapy consisting of IV fluorouracil (5-FU), epirubicin, and cyclophosphamide. The patient's treatment regimen consists of fluorouracil 500 mg/m^2, epirubicin 100 mg/m^2, and cyclophosphamide 500 mg/m^2 IV on day 1. This cycle is to be repeated every 21 days for 6 cycles.

1. Differentiate the mechanisms of action of fluorouracil, epirubicin, and cyclophosphamide.
2. Discuss the maximum lifetime dose and importance of lifetime dose for doxorubicin.
3. Describe the early signs of cardiotoxicity that could be seen after the administration of doxorubicin.

4. Determine a major side effect/adverse event for which the nurse should assess during therapy with 5-FU, epirubicin, and cyclophosphamide.

5. Describe nursing interventions for patients experiencing a major side effect/adverse event with 5-FU, epirubicin, and cyclophosphamide.

6. List five nursing actions to take as protective measures to avoid accidental exposure to chemotherapy drugs during administration.

NCLEX STUDY QUESTIONS

1. A patient is to receive a chemotherapy protocol that includes an alkylating agent, an antimetabolite, and an antitumor antibiotic. The patient asks the nurse why so much chemotherapy is needed. What is the nurse's best response?
   a. A protocol that uses a combination of chemotherapeutic agents works in the S phase to kill cells.
   b. Combination chemotherapy increases the extent of tumor cell killing.
   c. Combination chemotherapy uses drugs that work the same way.
   d. An outcome of the use of combination chemotherapy is that it has no dose-limiting toxicities.

2. A patient is scheduled to receive chemotherapy drugs that will cause myelosuppression. Which action by the nurse will be most important?
   a. Monitor for a change in temperature.
   b. Evaluate gastrointestinal function.
   c. Assess for evidence of cardiac compromise.
   d. Question the patient about changes in sense of taste.

3. The nurse is caring for a patient with colorectal cancer who is to receive fluorouracil. Which symptom will be most important for the nurse to report to the health care provider?
   a. Nausea
   b. Decreased appetite
   c. Bleeding gums
   d. Constipation

4. A patient in the outpatient oncology clinic complains of fatigue after receiving chemotherapy. Which initial nursing intervention will be most appropriate?
   a. Assess for other factors contributing to her fatigue, such as trouble sleeping.
   b. Encourage a high-protein, high-calorie diet, and design it with the patient.
   c. Refer the patient to a physical therapist to develop a strenuous exercise program.
   d. Encourage the patient to sleep as much as possible during the day to ease fatigue.

5. A patient in the outpatient oncology clinic has developed mucositis after receiving fluorouracil. Which statement made by the patient indicates the need for additional teaching about mucositis?
   a. I will frequently rinse out my mouth with normal saline.
   b. To relieve my mouth pain, I will use ice pops or ice chips.
   c. I will use mouthwash with alcohol to clean my mouth.
   d. Using a soft toothbrush will clean my teeth and freshen my breath.

6. A patient is scheduled to receive high-dose cyclophosphamide via an intravenous infusion as treatment for cancer. Which will be most important for the nurse to include when teaching the patient about cyclophosphamide?
   a. An indwelling urinary catheter will be placed.
   b. Drink at least 2 L of fluid per day.
   c. Empty the bladder every 4 to 6 hours.
   d. Limit fluid intake during chemotherapy.

7. A nurse is administering doxorubicin to a patient in the outpatient oncology clinic. Which information would be most important for the nurse to include in patient teaching?
   a. Blood counts will most likely remain normal.
   b. Complete alopecia rarely occurs with this drug.
   c. Report any shortness of breath, palpitations, or edema to the health care provider.
   d. Tissue necrosis usually occurs 2 to 3 days after administration.

8. A patient diagnosed with cancer is scheduled to receive vincristine. Which nursing assessment will have the highest priority when providing care for this patient?
   a. Degree of alopecia
   b. Increased digoxin levels
   c. Decreased phenytoin effects
   d. Peripheral neuropathy

9. A patient is experiencing mucositis (stomatitis) after receiving chemotherapy. Which symptomatic treatments will be appropriate? (Select all that apply.)
   a. Frequent mouth rinses
   b. Antiemetics
   c. Topical anesthetics
   d. Stress reduction
   e. Antibiotics

10. A nurse is teaching a patient who will receive chemotherapy that will cause thrombocytopenia. Which instructions will the nurse include in the patient's teaching plan? (Select all that apply.)
   a. Use an electric razor when shaving.
   b. Use a soft-bristled toothbrush.
   c. Use aspirin for pain or headache.
   d. Monitor oral temperature daily.
   e. Report any bleeding (gums, petechiae, bruises, hematuria, melena) to the health care provider.

Answers: 1, b; 2, a; 3, c; 4, a; 5, c; 6, b; 7, c; 8, c; 9, a, c, e; 10, a, b, e

Targeted Therapies to Treat Cancer

http://evolve.elsevier.com/McCuistion/pharmacology/

OBJECTIVES

- Identify the different forms of targeted therapy for cancers.
- Compare the mechanisms of action of targeted therapies for cancer with those of standard chemotherapy drugs.
- Explain the pharmacokinetics and pharmacodynamics for the different types of targeted therapy.

- Incorporate the nursing process related to the needs of patients receiving targeted therapies for cancer.
- Evaluate a focused teaching plan for patients, family, and caregivers for the different types of targeted therapies for cancer.

OUTLINE

KEY TERMS

Genes, inflammatory processes, infection, environment, and diet can influence cancer cells. Cancer cells grow out of control and can spread to distant parts of the body, invading normal tissues to the extent that tissues and vital organs can no longer function normally.

As discussed in Chapter 32, traditional chemotherapy is systemic, and its chemical makeup is cytotoxic such that it directly damages or kills normal cells and cancer cells. Chemotherapeutic drugs inhibit mitosis, which can damage the RNA and DNA and thus prevent cell division, eventually causing apoptosis, or programmed cell death. Even though traditional chemotherapy

treatments improve cancer control and increase long-term survival, adverse effects of traditional chemotherapy can be life-threatening. Furthermore, traditional chemotherapy's cancer cell–killing effect is limited by the dosages and scheduling regimens needed to reduce toxic side effects on normal cells. Drugs that molecularly target cells associated with cancer are currently the focus of many research.

In 1998, targeted therapy was first recognized as a potential cancer therapy against certain cell receptors. Targeted therapy for cancer treatment differs from traditional cancer chemotherapy in that targeted therapies are specific, deliberate, and

471

cytostatic, whereas most standard chemotherapies are not specific but rather are cytotoxic to normal and abnormal cells. Targeted therapy is the cornerstone of precision medicine because it directs the treatment according to the person's genes and proteins. The National Cancer Institute (NCI) defines *targeted therapy* as drugs or other substances that block the growth and spread of cancer by interfering with specific molecules involved in tumor growth, progression, and spread.

The ability to treat cancers with targeted therapy continues to expand. Currently, there are three approaches to targeted therapy. One approach is comparing individual proteins in cancer cells with those of normal cells. An example of a differentially expressed target is the human epidermal growth factor receptor 2 protein (*ERBB2*), which is expressed at high levels in breast and gastric cancers. Targeted therapy directed at *ERBB2* includes trastuzumab, which has been approved by the U.S. Food and Drug Administration (FDA) to treat certain breast and gastric cancers. A second approach is to identify mutant proteins that can cause cancer progression. An example of a mutant cell is the *BRAF* gene in its altered form, *BRAF V600E*, in melanomas. Vemurafenib targets this altered form of *BRAF* and has been approved to treat metastatic or inoperable melanomas. A third approach is looking for abnormal chromosomes present in cancer cells but not in normal cells. Chromosomal abnormalities can result in gene fusion, wherein parts of two different genes are incorporated as one gene. These fusion proteins can increase cancer development. Imatinib mesylate is one example of a therapy that targets the *BCR-ABL1* fusion protein responsible for the growth of some leukemic cells.

Targeted therapies do have limitations. One limitation is that cancers that do not have sufficient quantities of the specific molecular targets will not respond to targeted therapy. Another limitation involves cancer cells mutating and becoming drug resistant. Finally, yet another limitation of targeted therapy is the difficulty of developing drugs for some identified targets.

PATHOPHYSIOLOGY

Normal Cell-Growth Regulation

Genetic Control Over Cell Division

Some cancers are inherited, but others develop when genetic material becomes deranged or mutated. For malignancy to develop, cells must undergo more than one mutation; for this reason, malignancy may take years to develop. As depicted in Fig. 33.1, most if not all cells progress through the five phases of the cell cycle, which comprise a presynthesis phase (G_1), synthesis phase (S), postsynthesis phase (G_2), mitosis phase (M), and resting phase (G_0). Cells grow in size during the G_1 phase, DNA is copied during the S phase, the cell prepares to divide in the G_2 phase, and the cell divides in the M phase. A cell may remain in the G_0 phase for days to years, and under appropriate conditions, it will start participating in the cell cycle. Before entering a cell cycle, cells must pass through various **cellular checkpoints**, the function of which is to determine whether a cell has completed the necessary steps prior to progressing in the cell cycle. There are three major checkpoints in the cell cycle: one between the G_1 and S phases, one between G_2 and mitosis, and one during mitosis. A cell undergoes apoptosis if it is found to be defective at any one point during the cell cycle.

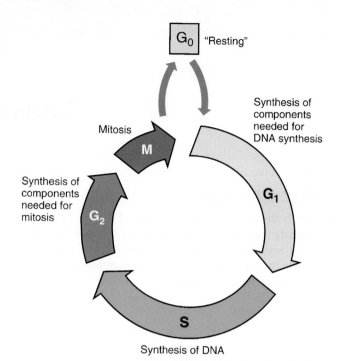

FIG. 33.1 The Cell Cycle. From Burcham, J., & Rosenthal, L. (2016). *Lehne's pharmacology for nursing care* (9th ed.). St. Louis: Elsevier.

Cellular communication and **signal transduction** are mechanisms in which cell-to-cell communication occurs locally or remotely by signal molecules sent to maintain homeostasis; to regulate growth and division; to develop and organize into tissues; and to coordinate cellular functions. Three primary means of cellular communications include direct contact with plasma membrane-bound receptors, remote contact with secreted signal molecules, and direct contact by way of gap junctions. Secreted signal molecules affect intercellular communication in a variety of ways, primarily by mechanisms that are contact dependent, paracrine, hormonal, and neurohormonal and also through neurotransmitters. Cells respond to external stimuli by activating a variety of signal **transduction pathways**, or signaling cascades. Fig. 33.2 illustrates a segment of a cell with one interconnecting signal transduction pathway that, when activated, leads to gene activation for those proteins that promote cell division. This pathway can be activated by (1) growth factors binding to cell receptors; (2) the interaction of certain drugs with the cell plasma membrane; (3) the presence of adhesion proteins; (4) changes in ion movement, especially sodium and calcium; (5) ligand binding; and (6) other cell-to-cell interactions. The signaling molecules in turn activate protein kinase pathways, increasing tyrosine kinase inside the cell.

A **tyrosine kinase (TK)** is an enzyme that activates other substances by adding a phosphate group (PO_4) to them, a process known as *phosphorylation*. Some families of TKs are unique to a cell type, whereas others may be present only in cancer cells that express a specific gene mutation. Regardless of how a pro–cell-division signal transduction pathway is activated, the result is an increase in TK levels that propagate the signal by activating many different transcription factors within the pathway.

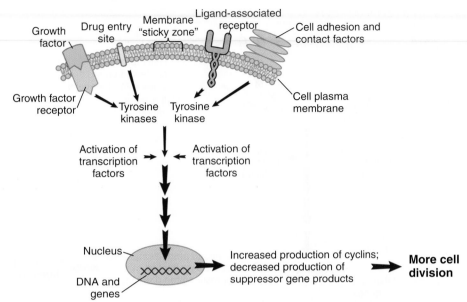

FIG. 33.2 Simplified example of a signal transduction pathway that promotes cell division.

Transcription factors are substances that enter the nucleus and signal the cell to begin mitosis. Many different types of substances serve as transcription factors. The overall response is a greater expression of oncogene products (cyclins) that promote cell division and reduced expression of **suppressor gene** products that inhibit cell division. When the cell responds to these mitotic signals, indicating cell division is needed and resources are adequate, the cell leaves the G_0 phase and enters the G_1 phase of the cell cycle. Once the cell enters the G_1 phase, the presence of specific cyclins determines whether it can progress to the next phase (Fig. 33.3).

Cyclins are a family of proteins that stimulate the cell to move through the cell cycle. Cyclins are the products of oncogenes, and most are activated when a phosphorous group is added to the cyclin chemical structure. (Removal of a phosphorous molecule from a cyclin [*dephosphorylation*] inhibits its activity.) Kinases that activate cyclins are called *cyclin-dependent kinases* (CDKs). CDKs combine with cyclins to form complexes that initiate cell mechanisms to complete cell division. The amount and type of cyclins and CDKs present in the cell during cell division vary by the phase of the cycle. These differences in types of cyclins and CDKs determine when or if a particular cell moves from one phase to the next. Of the cyclins identified, those in group D are the most studied and understood.

A common signal for entering and starting the cell cycle at G_1 is the combining of a cyclin-D with the appropriate CDK to form a cyclin-D/CDK complex (see Fig. 33.3). Movement of the cell from G_1 into other phases of the cell cycle is regulated by the continued presence of pro–cell-division transcription factors that promote DNA transcription and increased synthesis of specific pro–cell-division cyclins and CDKs.

In normal cells, the oncogenes that produce cyclins are carefully regulated by suppressor gene products so that cell division only occurs when it is needed and to the degree that it is needed. Proteins synthesized by suppressor genes determine how much oncogene expression is needed to allow cell division to occur without excessive cell division. Such control is exemplified by normal wound repair. For

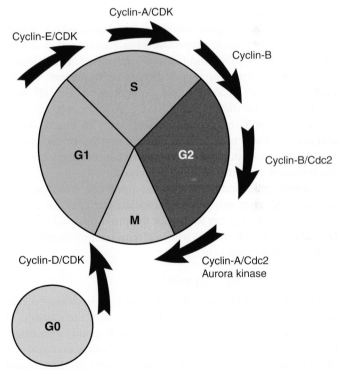

FIG. 33.3 Cyclin activity promoting progression through the cell cycle.

example, when a person falls and scrapes skin from the knee, the skin cells at the edge of the wound are signaled to divide and fill in the gap. When the wound area is closed, cell division normally stops; thereby, uncontrolled cell division does not occur.

When cell division is not needed, external signals—such as growth factor inhibitors and the surrounding of a cell plasma membrane with other cells—send signals that are inhibitory to the pro–cell-division signal transduction pathway (Fig. 33.4). The result of this inhibition leads to low levels of TKs and reduced levels of pro–cell-division transcription factors. In this

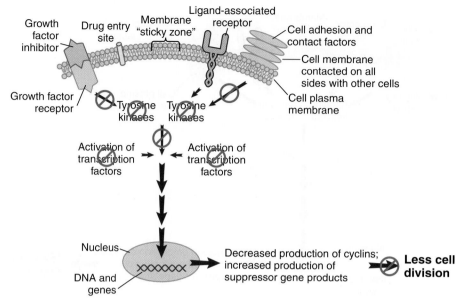

FIG. 33.4 External signals that inhibit the signal transduction pathway, resulting in greatly reduced cell division.

scenario, suppressor gene activity is increased, which results in production of more suppressor gene products that inhibit the synthesis of cyclins and CDKs by oncogenes. Even though many different types of suppressor genes are present, certain suppressor genes become active depending on the cell type. For example, the *BRCA1* suppressor gene appears to be most active in suppressing excessive cell division in breast, ovary, and genitourinary tract tissues. Without suppressor gene products, oncogenes would be overexpressed continually, leading to uncontrolled and unneeded cell division.

Internal cell conditions, such as poor cell nutrition and reduced energy stores, can inappropriately trigger the activation of suppressor genes to disrupt the pro–cell-division signal transduction pathway, even when external conditions indicate a need for cell division (Fig. 33.5).

Genetic Control Over Cell Death

As cells age, their function declines; function in damaged cells declines even earlier. In normal tissues that are capable of cell division, damaged cells and older cells respond to apoptosis (Fig. 33.6), or programmed cell death. Apoptosis is a natural way of removing aged cells from the body to ensure that tissues and organs contain healthy and optimally functional cells. Through genetic control, apoptosis prevents healthy, functional cells from self-destructing prematurely, and it eliminates older or damaged cells, thus preventing an overpopulation of cells that could reduce organ efficiency. Maintenance of optimally functional organs depends on a balance of cell division with apoptosis.

Telomeres are specialized, repetitive DNA sequences located at the ends of chromosomes. The signals for apoptosis may begin with the loss of these telomeres in aging cells. Telomeric DNA shortens with each cell division, eventually halting the dividing of cells (Fig. 33.7). When the cell has undergone its lifespan's worth of cell divisions, the telomeric DNA that capped the chromosomes disappears, allowing the ends to unravel and fragment. These processes then trigger genetic and other intracellular signals for

self-destruction through the action of autoenzymes of caspases. Activated caspases degrade the cell's internal structures, causing the plasma membrane to lyse the cell into small fragments that are then removed by the body's defense systems.

Growth Regulation and Cancer

Loss of Genetic Control of Cell Growth. Normal cells become cancer cells when external or internal conditions lead to gene damage. Cancer cells develop because of damaged suppressor genes, overproduction of cyclins and CDKs, or reactivation of telomeres that allow damaged cells prolonged life.

Excessive cell division from gene damage and mutations appears to be self-perpetuating, which leads to further gene mutations that:

- Allow one or more specific pro–cell-division signal transduction pathways to become more active.
- Allow greater expression of cancer cell membrane receptors that trigger pro–cell-division signal transduction pathways.
- Increase or amplify the production of specific TKs and transcription factors.

Loss of Apoptosis. The inability of cells to undergo apoptosis allows aged, damaged cells to undergo uncontrolled proliferation, resulting in tumor development, progression of tumors to cancer, and treatment resistance. A cell's resistance to apoptosis is multifactorial and involves expression of many antiapoptotic molecules. Mutations that occur in suppressor genes as a result of DNA damage inactivate the suppressor genes, preventing them from controlling oncogene activity. Some suppressor genes, such as the *TP53* gene, also regulate apoptosis. Inactivation of suppressor genes that regulate apoptosis makes cancer cells unresponsive to apoptotic signals. These cancer cells are now resistant to natural cell death, a feature known as *cellular immortality.* The lack of regulation for cell division and the loss of apoptosis result in cancer cells having no balance between cell division and apoptosis. This disequilibrium favors continuous cancer cell division.

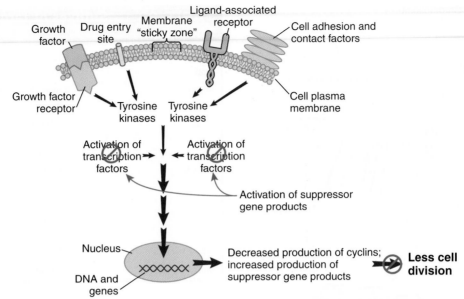

FIG. 33.5 Suppressor gene activity inhibiting the signal transduction pathway, resulting in greatly reduced cell division.

Autophagy and Resistance to Cancer. Intracellular homeostasis is maintained through autophagy, a process that involves lysosomal degradation and recycling of unnecessary or damaged cellular components. Autophagy can prevent cellular damage caused by chemotherapeutics by removing dysfunctional cellular parts and eliminating cellular stress. Autophagy has also been suggested as an important mechanism in the survival of tumor cells against apoptosis when exposed to certain anticancer drugs, leading to chemoresistance.

⚡ PATIENT SAFETY

Do not confuse...
- **Trastuzumab,** a chemotherapy drug, with **tositumomab,** a murine monoclonal antibody.
- **Bortezomib,** a chemotherapy drug for multiple myeloma and mantle cell lymphoma, with **bevacizumab,** a chemotherapy drug for colorectal, lung, ovary, and kidney cancers and glioblastoma.

TARGETED THERAPY DRUGS

Once a cell receives signals, the signal is relayed to other cells by a series of biochemical reactions. In cancer cells, the cells are stimulated to divide continuously without being prompted by external growth factors. **Signal transduction inhibitors (STIs)** block signals to cancerous cells by blocking signals passed from one molecule to another. They work at sites that are on the cell surface, at the intracellular level, or in the extracellular domain. Blocking various signals can affect cell division and can ultimately cause cell death. Targeted cancer therapies are STIs that block signal transduction among specific molecules, which blocks the growth and spread of cancerous cells. Drugs that target specific cells inhibit cancer cell division by blocking cancer membrane receptors and TK activities, interfering with signal transduction, stimulating immune system attacks on cancer cells, or inducing cells to undergo apoptosis. Targeted drugs

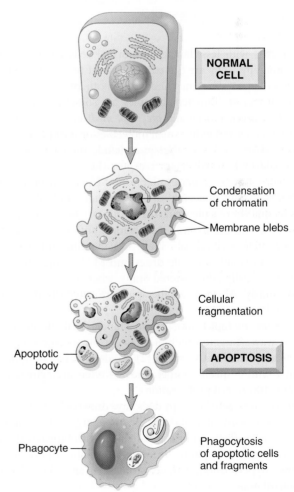

FIG. 33.6 Damaged cell undergoing normal apoptosis.

may be used as monotherapy (a single agent), in combination with traditional chemotherapy, and with radiotherapy.

Targeted therapies are more selective for specific molecular targets than cytotoxic anticancer drugs, thus they are able to kill

UNIT X Antineoplastics and Biologic Response Modifiers

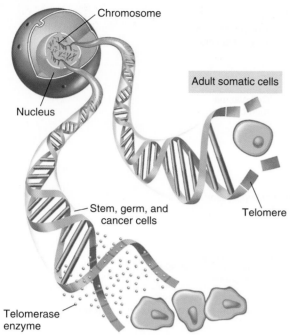

FIG. 33.7 Chromosome with telomeric DNA and chromosome end segment with telomeric DNA.

TABLE 33.1 Suffixes of Targeted Cancer Therapies

Suffix	Meaning
-mab	A monoclonal antibody
-momab	A monoclonal antibody composed of only murine (mouse) proteins
-imab	A monoclonal antibody composed of more human proteins (>60%) than murine proteins (~30%)
-zumab	A monoclonal antibody composed of mostly human proteins (95% or more) and only a few murine proteins (<5%)
-umab	A monoclonal antibody composed of only human proteins and no murine proteins
-nib	A tyrosine kinase inhibitor
-mib	A proteasome inhibitor

cancer cells with less damage to normal cells compared with chemotherapy. They are the cornerstone of precision medicine that uses a person's genes and proteins to prevent, diagnose, and treat cancer. Targeted therapies are sometimes known as *molecular targeted drugs* and *precision medicines*. Most targeted therapies consist of either small molecules or monoclonal antibodies (MAbs). Targeted therapies include angiogenesis inhibitors, epidermal growth factor receptor (EGFR)–TK inhibitors, BCR-ABL1 tyrosine kinase inhibitors, MAbs, and proteasome inhibitors. Small-molecule drugs are *not* antibodies. Most generic small-molecule drugs have *-nib* or *-mib* suffixes, such as imatinib and bortezomib. Monoclonal antibodies have *-mab* suffixes, such as rituximab. Table 33.1 identifies other suffixes common to small-molecule drugs and MAbs. Small-molecule drugs are usually administered orally, whereas MAbs are given intravenously. All targeted therapies are categorized as high-alert medications.

Targeted therapies differ from standard chemotherapy in several ways. Targeted therapies (1) act on specific molecular targets associated with cancer, (2) are deliberately designed to interact with a specific target, and (3) often are cytostatic by blocking tumor cell proliferation.

However, targeted therapy does have drawbacks. Cancer cells can become resistant, and drugs for some targets are difficult to develop. Side effects and risks associated with targeted therapy include diarrhea, hepatitis, thrombus formation, poor wound healing, hypertension, fatigue, stomatitis, and skin changes, among others.

The rapid identification of specific cancer cell targets in recent years has led to an increased development of targeted therapies. Management of patient issues related to targeted therapies is an evolving area of study. With many targeted therapies being new to the market, costs can be prohibitive.

Small-Molecule Compounds

Small-molecule compounds are one of the two main types of targeted therapy. Like most other types of drugs, they are chemicals that are small enough to have an intracellular effect, targeting the internal structures of cells. Small-molecule drugs are classified according to their actions; these include inhibiting enzymes, inducing apoptosis, and inhibiting formation of new vasculatures (angiogenesis). Table 33.2 lists the small-molecule inhibitors (SMIs) and their dosages, routes, uses, and considerations.

Angiogenesis Inhibitors/Vascular Endothelial Growth Factor Receptor Inhibitors

Angiogenesis inhibitors prevent new blood vessels from forming, which is required for tumors to grow. Some angiogenesis inhibitors interfere with the action of vascular endothelial growth factor (*VEGF*), a substance that stimulates new blood vessel formation. Others prevent the formation of platelet-derived growth factor (*PDGF*) that is intricate in the formation of new blood vessels and in the growth of preexisting blood vessels. Some angiogenesis inhibitors are also considered monoclonal antibodies (MAbs), such as bevacizumab. Prototype Drug Chart 33.1 lists specific drug information for bevacizumab.

Ziv-aflibercept. Ziv-aflibercept is a fully humanized recombinant fusion protein that inhibits angiogenesis. It is indicated in combination with 5-fluorouracil (5-FU), leucovorin, and irinotecan (FOLFIRI) for the treatment of metastatic colorectal cancer that is resistant to or has progressed after receiving an oxaliplatin-containing regimen.

Pharmacokinetics Ziv-aflibercept is administered by intravenous (IV) infusion. Its elimination half-life is approximately 6 days, which appears to be dose dependent. The steady state is also dose dependent, with the average steady state reached by the second dose in a 2-week regimen. The metabolic and elimination pathways are unknown. However, free ziv-aflibercept does not seem to be affected by mild to moderate hepatic or renal impairment.

Pharmacodynamics Ziv-aflibercept is an angiogenesis inhibitor that acts as a soluble receptor to bind vascular endothelial

TABLE 33.2   Small-Molecule Inhibitors

Drug Type and Name	Route and Dosage	Uses and Considerations
ANGIOGENESIS INHIBITORS/VASCULAR ENDOTHELIAL GROWTH FACTOR RECEPTOR INHIBITORS		
Bevacizumab (*VEGFR*/MAb; prototype)	See Prototype Drug Chart 33.1.	
Ziv-aflibercept (VEGFR)	A: IV: 4 mg/kg over 1 h, followed by FOLFIRI Steady state is reached by the second dose.	For metastatic colorectal cancer. Fully humanized angiogenesis inhibitor. Monitor ANC and UA. Discontinue for severe bleeding, GI perforation, fistula formation, wound dehiscence, hypertensive crisis/hypertensive encephalopathy, arterial thromboembolic events, and reversible posterior leukoencephalopathy syndrome. Pregnancy category: D*; PB: UK; t½: 6 d
EPIDERMAL GROWTH FACTOR RECEPTOR INHIBITORS		
Erlotinib (prototype)	See Prototype Drug Chart 33.2.	
Gefitinib	A: PO: 250 mg once daily Steady state is achieved in 10 d.	For NSCLC. Monitor LFTs, and increase the dose if used concomitantly with strong CYP3A4 inducers. Drug may be held for up to 14 d if patient develops poorly managed diarrhea, worsening ocular or pulmonary disorders, or worsening rash. Discontinue if GI perforation or interstitial lung disease is present. Pregnancy category: D*; PB: 90%; t½: 48 h
Osimertinib	A: PO: 80 mg/d	For NSCLC. Dose adjustment is required for treatment-related toxicities. Contraindicated in patients with interstitial lung disease/pneumonitis and symptomatic heart failure. Monitor ECG, ejection fraction, and serum electrolytes. Pregnancy category: UK*; PB: likely high based on physio-chemical properties; t½: 48 h
TYROSINE KINASE INHIBITORS/MULTIKINASE INHIBITORS		
Alectinib (TKI)	A: PO: 600 mg bid with food until disease progression or unacceptable toxicity occurs	For *ALK*-positive metastatic NSCLC in a patient who has progressed or is intolerant to crizotinib. Monitor LFTs, worsening respiratory symptoms, heart rate and blood pressure, and CPK levels. Pregnancy category: D*; PB: >99%; t½: 31-33 h
Dasatinib (MKI)	A: PO: Advanced CML, resistance or intolerance to prior therapy: 100-140 mg/d; can be increased to 180 mg/d if response is inadequate with the initial dose. Newly diagnosed CML: 100 mg/d; may be increased to 140 mg/d if response is inadequate.	For Ph+ CML and ALL. Adjust dose with concomitant use of a strong CYP3A4 inhibitor/inducer. Avoid grapefruit juice and concomitant use with H₂-receptor antagonists or proton pump inhibitors. Monitor CBC, serum electrolytes, and uric acid. Pregnancy category: D*; PB: 96%; t½: 3-5 h
Imatinib mesylate, STI-571 (TKI) prototype	See Prototype Drug Chart 33.3.	
Nilotinib (TKI)	A: PO: Resistance or intolerance to imatinib: 400 mg bid on an empty stomach Newly diagnosed Ph+ CML: 300 mg bid on an empty stomach	For Ph+ CML. No food should be given 1 hour after or 2 hours before dose is taken. Capsule may be opened and dispersed in 1 teaspoon of applesauce. Monitor ECG, CBC, electrolytes, LFTs, pancreatic functions, uric acid, and weight. *Absolute contraindications:* Hypokalemia, hypomagnesemia, long QT syndrome, and QT prolongation. Pregnancy category: D*; PB: 98%; t½: 17 h
Sorafenib (MKI)	A: PO: 400 mg bid; administer without food, at least 1 h before or 2 h after meal.	For hepatocellular, renal cell, and thyroid cancers. Adjust the dose if use is concomitant with a strong CYP3A4 inhibitor/inducer. Monitor CBC and LFTs. Pregnancy category: D*; PB: 99.5%: t½: 25-48 h

Continued

TABLE 33.2 Small-Molecule Inhibitors—cont'd

Drug Type and Name	Route and Dosage	Uses and Considerations
Sunitinib (MKI)	GIST and RCC: A: PO: 50 mg/d on a schedule of 4 wk on treatment followed by 2 wk off treatment PNET: A: PO: 37.5 mg/d; administer with or without food.	For GIST, PNET, and advanced RCC. Avoid concomitant use with a strong CYP3A4 inhibitor/inducer. Monitor UA and cardiac function. Pregnancy category: D*; PB: sunitinib 95%. metabolite 90%; t½: sunitinib 40-60 h, major metabolite 80-110 h
mTOR KINASE INHIBITORS (mTOR)/PROTEASOME INHIBITORS (PIs)		
Bortezomib (prototype)	See Prototype Drug Chart 33.4.	
Carfilzomib (PI)	A: IV: Progressive disease on or within 60 d after completing therapy: Cycle 1: 20 mg/m² on days 1 and 2; if tolerated, increase to 27 mg/m² on days 8, 9, 15, and 16. Treatment cycles are repeated q28d. Cycles 2-12: 27 mg/m² on days 1, 2, 8, 9, 15, and 16. Cycles 13 and beyond: 27 mg/m² on days 1, 2, 15, and 16 Relapsed multiple myeloma: Give carfilzomib as above with lenalidomide daily for 21 d of each cycle and dexamethasone on days 1, 8, 15, and 22 of each cycle. Treatment cycles are repeated q28d.	For relapsed multiple myeloma refractory to previous one to three lines of therapy, in combination with lenalidomide and dexamethasone. Premedicate with dexamethasone 30 min to 4 h prior to carfilzomib. Prehydrate and maintain hydration with oral and IV fluids. Monitor CBC, liver and renal function, and uric acid. Pregnancy category: D*; PB: 97%; t½: ≤1 h
Ixazomib (PI)	A: PO: 4 mg on days 1, 8, and 15 in combination with lenalidomide on days 1 through 21 and dexamethasone on days 1, 8, 15, and 22. Repeat treatment cycles q28d.	For relapsed multiple myeloma refractory to one previous therapy. Give with lenalidomide and dexamethasone, and adjust dose for hepatic or renal impairment. Adjust or hold dose for hematologic toxicity, moderate-grade rash, peripheral neuropathy, and other nonhematologic toxicity. Pregnancy category: D*; PB: 99%; t½: 9.5 d
Temsirolimus (mTOR)	A: IV: 25 mg given over 30-60 min once per wk	For advanced RCC. Premedicate with antihistamine intravenously approximately 30 min before the start of infusion. Two dilutions are required before IV infusion; use only the supplied diluent for initial dilution. Avoid strong CYP3A4 inducers/inhibitors. Dose reduction is required in patients with mild hepatic impairment. *Contraindication:* Moderate to severe hepatic impairment. Pregnancy category: D*; t½: 17 h

*Pregnancy categories have been revised. See http://www.fda.gov/Drugs/DevelopmentApprovalProcess/DevelopmentResources/Labeling/ucm093307.htm for more information.

A, adult; *ALL*, acute lymphoblastic leukemia; *ANC*, absolute neutrophil count; *bid*, twice daily; *CBC*, complete blood count; *CML*, chronic myelogenous leukemia; *CPK*, creatine phosphokinase; *CYP3A4*, cytochrome P3A4; *d*, day; *ECG*, electrocardiograph; *FOLFIRI*, folinic acid, fluorouracil, and irinotecan; *GI*, gastrointestinal; *GIST*, gastrointestinal stromal tumor; *h*, hour; *IV*, intravenous; *LFT*, liver function test; *MAb*, monoclonal antibody; *min*, minutes; *MKI*, multikinase inhibitor; *mTOR*, mechanistic target of rapamycin; *NSCLC*, non–small cell lung cancer; *PB*, protein bound; *Ph+*, Philadelphia-chromosome positive; *PI*, proteasome inhibitor; *PNET*, pancreatic neuroendocrine tumor; *PO*, oral; *q*, every; *RCC*, renal cell carcinoma; *t½*, half-life; *TKI*, tyrosine kinase inhibitor; *UA*, urinalysis; *UK*, unknown; *VEGFR*, vascular endothelial growth factor receptor; *wk*, week; *>*, greater than; *≤*, less than or equal to.

growth factors A and B and placental growth factors 1 and 2, which prevents other native receptors from binding. This action can result in decreased neovascularization and decreased vascular permeability.

Side effects and adverse reactions. Severe bleeding, including gastrointestinal (GI) bleeding, intractable bleeding, and pulmonary hemorrhage, has been noted. GI perforations, some fatal, have also been reported. Other adverse events include compromised wound healing and / or wound dehiscence, reversible posterior leukoencephalopathy syndrome (RPLS), hypertensive crisis, nephrotic syndrome, or thrombotic microangiopathy.

Common side effects include diarrhea, dizziness, asthenia, weight loss, and dehydration.

Drug interactions. No interactions have been reported.

Epidermal Growth Factor Receptor Inhibitors

The largest class of targeted therapy that attacks one particular molecular target is epidermal growth factor receptor (EGFR) inhibitor. These receptors are overexpressed, dysregulated, or mutated in many epithelial cancers. *EGFR* expression has been associated with poor prognosis, metastasis, chemotherapy resistance, hormonal therapy, and radiation therapy. The activation

PROTOTYPE DRUG CHART 33.1

Bevacizumab

Drug Class	**Dosage**
Monoclonal antibody/angiogenesis inhibitor (VEGF inhibitor)	A: IV:
Pregnancy category: D*	*Colorectal cancer:* 5 or 10 mg/kg q2wk in combination with 5-FU; or 5 or 7.5 mg/kg q2-3wk with fluoropyrimidine and irinotecan or fluoropyrimidine and oxaliplatin.
	NSCLC: 15 mg/kg q3wk with carboplatin and paclitaxel.
	Metastatic RCC: 10 mg/kg q2wk in combination with interferon-alfa.
	Progressive glioblastoma: 10 mg/kg q2wk on a 28-d cycle.
	Ovarian cancer: 10 mg/kg q2wk in combination with paclitaxel, topotecan, or pegylated liposomal doxorubicin.
	Cervical cancer: 15 mg/kg with cisplatin on day 2 in combination with paclitaxel q3wk
	Other treatment protocols exist (see full prescriber's information).
Contraindications	**Drug-Lab-Food Interactions**
No absolute contraindications. Warnings and precautions during treatment include serious bleeding (e.g., GI, intracranial), GI obstruction/perforation, wound dehiscence, and nephrotic syndrome.	Drug: When used as combination therapy with irinotecan, incidence of grade 3-4 diarrhea and neutropenia increased and serum concentration of irinotecan active metabolites increased. Concomitant use with sunitinib increased incidences of microangiopathic hemolytic anemia. Concomitant use with daunorubicin, doxorubicin, and epirubicin, among others, has an increased risk of cardiotoxicity.
Caution: Known murine protein hypersensitivity, hamster protein hypersensitivity, or sensitivity to any other component of the drug; preexisting hypertension, cardiovascular disease, renal disease, history of glaucoma (see full prescriber's information for a complete list).	Lab: None known
	Food: None known
Pharmacokinetics	**Pharmacodynamics**
Absorption: IV, bioavailability UK	Onset: UK
Distribution: PB: UK; steady state levels achieved at approx 100 d	Peak: UK
Metabolism: UK; t½: 11-50 d, dose dependent	Duration: UK
Excretion: Clearance of drug varies by weight, sex, and tumor burden.	

Therapeutic Effects/Uses

For cervical, colorectal, and ovarian cancers; metastatic RCC; NSCLC; and relapsed glioblastoma multiforme.

Mode of Action: Recombinant humanized monoclonal antibody binds to VEGF and prevents the binding of VEGF with its receptors, which are found on the surface of endothelial cells. The role of VEGF is critical in angiogenesis, the formation of new blood vessels. In human cancers, increased VEGF expression is associated with increased microvascular density, tumor growth, metastasis, and poor prognosis. The result of bevacizumab therapy is the reduction of microvascular growth and inhibition of metastatic disease progression.

Side Effects	**Adverse Reactions**
Hypertension, proteinuria, cephalgia, rhinitis, taste alteration, dry skin, rectal hemorrhage, lacrimation disorder, back pain, and exfoliative dermatitis	Perforation or fistula, thromboembolic events, hypertensive crisis/encephalopathy, nephrotic syndrome, infusion reactions, embryonic/fetal toxicity, ovarian failure, PRES, exogenous endophthalmitis, gallbladder perforation, and congestive heart failure have been associated with bevacizumab (see full prescriber's information for a complete list).

*Pregnancy categories have been revised. See http://www.fda.gov/Drugs/DevelopmentApprovalProcess/DevelopmentResources/Labeling/ucm093307.htm for more information.

5-FU, 5-Fluorouracil; *A,* adult; *d,* day; *GI,* gastrointestinal; *IV,* intravenous; *NSCLC,* non–small cell lung cancer; *PB,* protein bound; *PRES,* posterior reversible encephalopathy syndrome; *q,* every; *RCC,* renal cell cancer; *t½,* half-life; *UK,* unknown; *VEGF,* vascular endothelial growth factor; *wk,* week.

---

of *EGFR*s is important in cancer cell growth and proliferation. Most EGFR inhibitors also inhibit tyrosine kinase (TK) indirectly. However, two other classes of EGFR inhibitors target *EGFR* extracellularly (MAbs) and also target the receptor catalytic domain of *EGFR* (TK inhibitors). These two classes are further discussed under the headings *Monoclonal Antibodies* and *Tyrosine Kinase Inhibitors and Multikinase Inhibitors.* The EGFR inhibitors that inhibit TK indirectly include erlotinib, gefitinib, and osimertinib. As shown in Fig. 33.2, the growth factor receptors on the cell membrane can activate TKs, which then turn on signal transduction pathways that promote cell division. The EGFR inhibitors bind to different areas of the *EGFR*, blocking its activity so that it cannot activate TK. As a result, the downstream signal transduction

pathway for promotion of cell division is inhibited, and cell proliferation is severely limited. Table 33.2 lists the EGFR inhibitors and their dosages, routes, uses, and considerations. Prototype Drug Chart 33.2 lists the specific drug information for erlotinib.

Gefitinib. Gefitinib is a synthetic anilinoquinazoline that selectively inhibits the epidermal growth factor receptor tyrosine kinase (EGFR-TK). It is most commonly used in the management of locally or advanced metastatic non–small cell lung cancer (NSCLC).

Pharmacokinetics Gefitinib is taken orally and is absorbed slowly in the GI tract, with 60% reaching systemic circulation. Peak plasma level occurs 3 to 7 hours after dosing. No significant alteration in its bioavailability was noted when gefitinib was

PROTOTYPE DRUG CHART 33.2

Erlotinib

Drug Class	Dosage
Epidermal growth factor receptor inhibitor Pregnancy category: D*	*NSCLC*: 150 mg PO once daily *Pancreatic cancer*: 100 mg PO once daily as combination therapy. Take without food, 1 h before or 2 h after meal.
Contraindications	**Drug-Lab-Food Interactions**
No absolute contraindications. Precautions are warranted in patients who may become pregnant, are pregnant, or are breastfeeding; in those who have preexisting respiratory problems (pulmonary fibrosis may occur); or who are dehydrated or have liver impairment. Use cautiously in patients with history of peptic ulcer disease or diverticulitis (increases risk for GI perforation). Advise smokers to stop smoking while taking erlotinib; tobacco decreases the effectiveness of the drug.	Drug: Concomitant use with drugs that alter the pH of the upper GI tract is contraindicated (e.g., esomeprazole, lansoprazole, omeprazole, or pantoprazole). CYP3A4 inhibitors such as ketoconazole, atazanavir, clarithromycin, indinavir, itraconazole, nefazodone, nelfinavir, ritonavir, saquinavir, telithromycin, and voriconazole increase blood levels of erlotinib and may lead to increased adverse reactions or toxicities. Concomitant use with competitive inhibitors of CYP3A4, such as midazolam and statin drugs, can increase the competitor's concentration. CYP3A4 inducers such as rifampicin, dexamethasone, phenytoin, carbamazepine, phenobarbital, St. John's wort, H_2-receptor blockers, and proton pump inhibitors reduce the effectiveness of erlotinib. Lab: Erlotinib may increase INR and can lead to increased risk for bleeding. Food: Drug must be given on an empty stomach; administering with food increases the risk of side effects.
Pharmacokinetics	**Pharmacodynamics**
Absorption: Bioavailability is 60%. Distribution: 93% PB. Steady state levels are achieved in 7-8 d. Metabolism: Liver (CYP3A4 and CYP1A2 enzymes); t½: 36 h. Excretion: Mainly in feces, some renal elimination; 24% higher among smokers.	Give drug on an empty stomach, either 1 h before or 2 h after meals (administering with food increases risk for side effects). Administer at the same time each day between meals. Increase dose if used concomitantly with strong CYP3A4 inducers. Onset: Slowly absorbed with oral dosage with 60% bioavailability. Peak: 4 h; duration: UK
Therapeutic Effects/Uses	
Approved for treatment of NSCLC and pancreatic cancer. Mode of Action: Erlotinib selectively inhibits activation of *EGFR* tyrosine kinase, possibly blocking angiogenesis and cellular proliferation.	
Side Effects	**Adverse Reactions**
Diarrhea, skin changes (acne vulgaris, acneiform rash), alopecia, anorexia, anxiety, bone pain, cough, constipation, anorexia, diarrhea, fatigue, vomiting, pruritus.	Ocular changes (inflammation, corneal perforation), GI perforation, skin desquamation, renal failure, hepatic failure, interstitial pulmonary disease.

*Pregnancy categories have been revised. See http://www.fda.gov/Drugs/DevelopmentApprovalProcess/DevelopmentResources/Labeling/ucm093 307.htm for more information.

CYP, Cytochrome P; *d,* day; *GI,* gastrointestinal; *h,* hour; *H₂,* histamine 2; *INR,* international normalized ratio; *NSCLC,* non–small cell lung cancer; *PB,* protein bound; *PO,* by mouth; *t½,* half-life; *UK,* unknown.

taken with food. It is metabolized mainly by the hepatic system primarily through the CYP3A4 enzyme. Gefitinib is primarily excreted in the feces, mostly in the form of its metabolites. The elimination half-life is approximately 48 hours.

Pharmacodynamics Gefitinib reversibly binds to the adenosine triphosphate (ATP) binding site and completely inhibits autophosphorylation by EGFR-TK; EGFR-TK functions as a mediator of cell growth, differentiation, and death. This action results in blockage of downstream EGFR-TK–mediated signal transduction pathways, cell cycle arrest, and inhibition of angiogenesis.

Side effects and adverse reactions. Common side effects include skin reactions, diarrhea, anorexia, vomiting, and elevated transaminases. Gefitinib can cause conjunctivitis and abnormal eyelash growth, and rash occurs in about 47% of patients. Patients can also experience acne, pruritus, and nail disorders. Interstitial lung disease and GI perforation were also reported.

Drug interactions. Gefitinib is extensively metabolized by CYP3A4. Other drugs metabolized by the hepatic system can affect the concentrations of gefitinib and other drugs. Drugs that inhibit CYP3A4, increasing the gefitinib level, include thioridazine, amiodarone, bupropion, diphenhydramine, promethazine, and metoclopramide. Other CYP3A4 inhibitors, such as venlafaxine, may decrease the levels of gefitinib. Gefitinib can increase the concentration of other drugs that have a narrow therapeutic index, such as amitriptyline, warfarin, and eliglustat. Patients taking warfarin concomitantly with gefitinib had an elevated international normalized ratio (INR) and/or hemorrhage. CYP3A4 inducers—such as acetaminophen, butalbital, caffeine, and aspirin—can increase gefitinib metabolism, thereby decreasing concentrations of the drug. When given concomitantly with gefitinib, drugs that decrease gastric pH (e.g., omeprazole and lansoprazole) can lower plasma concentrations of gefitinib.

Osimertinib. Osimertinib is one of the newest FDA-approved EGFR-TK inhibitors for *T790M*-mutation positive NSCLC. Osimertinib was approved in November 2015.

Pharmacokinetics Osimertinib is taken orally, and absorption is dose dependent. High-fat, high-calorie meals increase the absorption rate by 14%. It is metabolized primarily by the hepatic system through the CYP3A isoenzyme and by oxidation and dealkylation. Osimertinib is primarily excreted in the feces and to a lesser extent in the urine. The elimination half-life is approximately 48 hours.

Pharmacodynamics Osimertinib is a CYP3A4 and CYP1A2 inducer that irreversibly binds to certain mutant forms of *EGFR* (*T790M*, *L858R*, and *exon 19* deletion). In vitro it exhibited inhibition of *ERBB2*, *ERBB3*, *ERBB4*, *ACK1*, and *BLK* receptors.

Side effects and adverse reactions. Common side effects include pancytopenia, rash, dry skin, anorexia, constipation, hyponatremia, nausea, pruritus, fatigue, cough, back pain, and stomatitis. Other side effects include eye disorders and cephalgia. Adverse reactions include venous thromboembolism, interstitial lung disease, pneumonitis, increased QTc, and cardiomyopathy.

Drug interactions. Osimertinib is a CYP3A inducer. Drugs metabolized by the liver can affect their concentrations and the osimertinib plasma level. Osimertinib can cause a prolonged QT interval. Other drugs that can prolong QT intervals, causing torsade de pointes, should be avoided or monitored closely when used concomitantly with osimertinib (e.g., thioridazine, beta agonists, chlorpromazine, ofloxacin, desipramine, moxifloxacin, metronidazole, promethazine, and trimethoprim or sulfamethoxazole-trimethoprim). CYP3A inhibitors such as aldesleukin, alfentanil, and ethanol can alter osimertinib concentration. Osimertinib can alter plasma concentration of other drugs, which can worsen adverse reactions and can alter the efficacy of drugs such as acetaminophen, amlodipine, amitriptyline, and alprazolam.

 NURSING PROCESS
Patient-Centered Collaborative Care

Angiogenesis Inhibitors, Vascular Endothelial Growth Factor Receptor Inhibitors, and Epidermal Growth Factor Receptor Inhibitors

Assessment
- To avoid drug interactions, obtain a detailed medication history that includes current prescriptions, over-the-counter (OTC) medicines, antacids, dietary supplements, vitamins, and herbal supplements.
- Obtain a list of all drug and food allergies.
- Obtain baseline information about the patient's physical status that includes height, weight, vital signs, cardiopulmonary assessment, intake and output, skin assessment, nutritional status, and any underlying diseases.
- Obtain baseline laboratory values (complete blood count [CBC], uric acid, chemistry panel) before and during treatment.
- Assess baseline results of pulmonary function tests, chest radiographs, electrocardiographs (ECGs), and renal and liver function studies.
- Assess patient's and caregiver's current level of comprehension related to the therapeutic regimen.

Nursing Diagnoses
- Skin Integrity, Risk for Impaired
- Infection, Risk for related to bone marrow suppression
- Knowledge, Deficient related to the targeted therapy regimen
- Injury, Risk for related to toxic effects of targeted therapy
- Sensory Perception, Risk for Disturbed Visual

Planning
- Skin will maintain its integrity.
- The patient will remain free from infection.
- The patient and family will verbalize understanding of targeted therapy as part of an anticancer treatment regimen.
- The patient and family will verbalize strategies to minimize risks related to targeted therapy–related side effects.
- The patient and family will demonstrate understanding of the importance of reporting targeted therapy–related side effects and adverse reactions.
- The patient's side effects will be managed to a tolerable level and are not life threatening.

Nursing Interventions
- Examine the patient's skin closely at each visit for the presence of erythema, rash, peeling, or blister formation; rate the severity of dermatologic reactions.
- Monitor for any evidence of infection, such as fever, chills, leukocytosis or leukopenia, and neutropenia.
- Assess for evidence of thromboembolic events.
- Monitor for any signs of perforation, such as abdominal pain/distension, absent bowel sounds, and changes in blood pressure and heart rate.
- Monitor lab values, such as renal function, hepatic function, CBC, chemistry, and urinalysis.
- Administer prescribed premedications according to established protocols for specific targeted therapies.
- Assess for any cardiac events, such as new chest pain and ECG changes.
- Assess for any pulmonary complications, such as dyspnea or cough.

Patient Teaching
- Advise patients to immediately report worsening of skin rash; severe or persistent diarrhea, nausea, anorexia, or vomiting; onset or worsening of unexplained shortness of breath or cough; or eye irritation.
- Advise patients to seek medical help immediately if chest pain, severe abdominal pain, or swelling associated with redness or pain in one leg occurs.
- Report symptoms of adverse effects or severe side effects promptly, especially fever, chills, persistent sore throat, swelling, weight gain, or increasing shortness of breath.
- Report symptoms of bleeding immediately, including black stools, coffee ground emesis, and easy bleeding or bruising.
- Advise patients to notify the health care provider if foaming of urine occurs (an indication of protein in the urine).

- To prevent excessive bleeding, teach patients to avoid taking nonsteroidal antiinflammatory drugs (NSAIDs) such as aspirin, celecoxib, ibuprofen, and naproxen.
- Teach patients ways to promote venous return and avoid deep venous thrombosis (DVT), such as avoiding dehydration, constrictive clothing, and smoking cigarettes.
- Remind women with childbearing potential to avoid pregnancy throughout treatment and for up to 12 months after treatment is completed.
- Advise breastfeeding women to stop breastfeeding during and for 60 days after therapy.
- Teach patients to avoid direct sunlight and tanning beds to prevent worsening of skin side effects.

Evaluation

- Patient, family, and caregiver education needs are met.
- The patient, family, and caregivers understand therapy-related side effects and adverse reactions.
- The patient, family, and caregivers understand strategies to minimize side effects and adverse reactions.
- Side effects are managed effectively.
- The patient is free from infection.
- The patient is free from injury, perforation, or internal fistula.

Tyrosine Kinase Inhibitors and Multikinase Inhibitors

Several types of targeted therapies inhibit tyrosine kinases. Specific drugs that cause this action as their main mechanism are referred to as tyrosine kinase inhibitors (TKIs). TKIs primarily exert their effects on an enzyme known as *BCR-ABL tyrosine kinase*. The *BCR-ABL* gene is an important pathogenesis for chronic myelogenous leukemia (CML). CML cells make abnormal active *BCR-ABL* tyrosine kinase enzyme. *BCR-ABL* tyrosine kinase enzymes are present in cancer cells that have a specific gene mutation known as the *Philadelphia chromosome*. When activated and expressed, *BCR-ABL* tyrosine kinase turns on a strong pro-cell-division signal transduction pathway that leads to the proliferation of cancer cells. TKIs prevent activation of tyrosine kinases, which then inhibits further activation of the signal transduction pathway and stops the proliferation of cancer cells. This action can control the disease but cannot eradicate it alone. As shown in Fig. 33.2 receptors on the cell membrane can activate TKs, which then turn on signal transduction pathways that promote cell division. Table 33.2 lists some of the TKI drugs and their uses and considerations. Of the TKIs, alectinib and nilotinib are further discussed under those headings in text. Prototype Drug Chart 33.3 lists specific drug information about the TKI imatinib.

The multikinase inhibitors (MKIs) are chemicals that directly inhibit the activity of multiple kinase enzymes in cancer cells. (Recall that kinases are enzymes that activate other proteins, including those that activate signal transduction pathways that promote cancer cell division.) Table 33.2 lists some of the MKIs and their dosages, routes, uses, and considerations. Of the MKIs, dasatinib, sorafenib, and sunitinib are discussed.

Alectinib. Alectinib is a TKI that targets anaplastic lymphoma kinase (*ALK*) and the RET proto-oncogene (*RET*). It is indicated for the treatment of patients with *ALK*-positive metastatic NSCLC who have progressed on or are intolerant to crizotinib.

Pharmacokinetics Alectinib is administered orally. Alectinib and its major metabolite, M4, are more than 99% bound to plasma proteins. Steady state is reached by day 7 of administration. Alectinib is metabolized by CYP3A4 to its major active metabolite, M4. The elimination half-lives for alectinib and M4 are 33 and 31 hours, respectively. Alectinib and its metabolite are excreted in the feces (84% and 6%, respectively). No significant effect was noted in patients with mild to moderate hepatic and renal impairment.

Pharmacodynamics Alectinib is a TKI that targets *ALK* and *RET*. Alectinib is a central nervous system (CNS)-active and highly selective ALK inhibitor that inhibits *ALK* phosphorylation and *ALK*-mediated activation of the downstream signaling proteins.

Side effects and adverse reactions. Common side effects include anemia, elevated transaminases, fatigue, constipation, bradycardia, edema, hypocalcemia, hypokalemia, and myalgia. Serious adverse events include hepatotoxicity, pneumonitis, bradycardia, and elevated creatine phosphokinase (CPK).

Drug interactions. No interactions with alectinib that require dose adjustment have been identified.

Nilotinib. Nilotinib is a TKI that has a high affinity for the ATP binding site of *BCR-ABL* kinase, inhibiting cell proliferation in cell lines and in primary Philadelphia-positive (Ph+) CML cells. It is indicated for the treatment of Ph+ CML that is resistant or intolerant to imatinib in the chronic or accelerated phase.

Pharmacokinetics Nilotinib is administered orally, and approximately 98% is protein bound in plasma. The elimination half-life is approximately 17 hours. Peak serum concentration occurs 3 hours after oral administration, and steady state is achieved on day 8. The bioavailability of the drug is significantly increased with food. Nilotinib is metabolized in the liver by CYP3A4; no active metabolites have been identified. The primary metabolic pathways are oxidation and hydroxylation. The majority of the drug was eliminated mainly in the feces within 7 days. Caution is advised in administering nilotinib to patients with hepatic impairment.

Pharmacodynamics Nilotinib is an oral TK that selectively inhibits *BCR-ABL* kinase. It is a competitor inhibitor at the ATP-binding site of *BCR-ABL* and prevents tyrosine phosphorylation of downstream intracellular signal transduction proteins. Blocking the TK prevents proliferation of cancer cells and induces cell death.

Side effects and adverse reactions. The most common adverse effects are pancytopenia, rash, pruritus, nausea, fatigue, cephalgia, and constipation. Severe adverse events include dysrhythmias due to prolonged QT interval, which can cause sudden cardiac death. Pulmonary toxicity has been reported in patients with CML.

Drug interactions. Concomitant administration of strong CYP3A4 inhibitors or inducers may significantly alter nilotinib concentrations. If CYP3A4 inhibitor drugs (e.g., ketoconazole, clarithromycin, ritonavir, fluoroquinolones, ibutilide, lithium) are unavoidable, dose reduction should be considered, and the QT interval should be monitored on a frequent basis. Electrolyte imbalances should be corrected before administering nilotinib.

Dasatinib. Dasatinib is an MKI approved for newly diagnosed Ph+ CML and acute lymphocytic leukemia (ALL); Ph+ CML in

PROTOTYPE DRUG CHART 33.3

Imatinib Mesylate, STI-571

Drug Class	Dosage
Signal transduction inhibitor/tyrosine kinase inhibitor Pregnancy category: D*	A: PO: For Ph+ leukemias; myelodysplastic syndrome, myeloproliferative disease; GI stromal tumors (GISTs), hypereosinophilic syndrome (HES) or chronic eosinophilic leukemia (CEL), aggressive systemic mastocytosis, metastatic dermatofibrosarcoma protuberans. Dose depends on disease; starting dose is 400 mg/d; may increase if no serious adverse reactions occur.. A ≤20 y/Adol/C >3 y: 260 mg/m²/d as a single dose or divided (morning and evening). Other protocols exist, including twice-daily dosing.

Contraindications	Drug-Lab-Food Interactions
Contraindicated among patients who may be or could become pregnant or who are breastfeeding. *Caution:* Patients with renal impairment, cardiac disease, hepatic impairment, bone marrow suppression, infection, and in children. Avoid concomitant strong CYP3A4 inducers. *See full prescriber's information for a complete list of contraindications.*	Drug: Any drug that *inhibits* CYP450 or CYP3A4 (e.g., nefazodone, itraconazole, fluvoxamine, fluconazole, erythromycin) can decrease the metabolism of imatinib and increases the concentration, leading to an increased incidence of adverse reactions. Any drug that *induces* CYP450 (e.g., St. John's wort, phenytoin, fosphenytoin, rifampin, barbiturates, dexamethasone, phenobarbital) can increase the metabolism of imatinib and decrease imatinib concentrations and clinical effects. Imatinib is a CYP450 inhibitor and serum concentrations of any drug that is metabolized by CYP450 (e.g., ergot alkaloids, carbamazepine, cyclosporine, quinidine, clonazepam, fentanyl, calcium channel blockers, sertraline, acetaminophen) can increase. Taking imatinib with thrombolytic agents, NSAIDs, platelet inhibitors, aspirin, and other anticoagulants/antiplatelets may increase risk of bleeding. Concomitant use of flibanserin and moderate CYP3A4 inhibitors, such as imatinib, is contraindicated due to severe hypotension and syncope. Lab: May affect serum levels of liver enzymes, CBC, electrolytes, renal function, and uric acid Food: Grapefruit juice increases imatinib plasma concentrations.

Pharmacokinetics	Pharmacodynamics
Absorption: Bioavailability is 98%. Distribution: 95% PB with extensive distribution. Metabolism: Mainly by CYP3A4; inhibits CYP2D6 and CYP3A4; t½: imatinib is 18 h, major metabolite is 40 h. Clearance is 8-14 L/h. Excretion: Mainly in the feces as metabolites.	Well absorbed following oral administration with Cmax achieved within 2-4 h. Imatinib should be taken with food and a large glass of water to decrease the risk of GI irritation. Drug may be dispersed in water or apple juice for patients who cannot swallow tablets. Suspension should be administered immediately after complete disintegration of the tablets. Onset: UK Peak: 2-4 h Duration: UK

Therapeutic Effects/Uses
Approved for ALL, CEL, CML, dermatofibrosarcoma protuberans, GIST, HES, myelodysplastic syndrome, and systemic mastocytosis. Mode of Action: Imatinib competitively inhibits the ATP binding site on *BCR-ABL* tyrosine kinase (TK) that results in inhibition of proliferation and induces apoptosis in *BCR-ABL*–positive cell lines and in fresh leukemic cells of Philadelphia-chromosome positive CML. Receptors for TKs include various growth factors (e.g., *EGF, PDGF, SGF, VEGF, NGF*). Imatinib also acts as a mediator for many nonreceptor TKs (e.g., G-protein–coupled receptors, B- and T-cell receptors, and interferon gamma receptors). Imatinib also interacts with lipids, proteins, and DNA. Imatinib inhibits proliferation in vitro and induces apoptosis in GIST cells, which express an activating *KIT* mutation. Imatinib inhibits CYP2C9, CYP2D6, and CYP3A4.

Side Effects	Adverse Reactions
Edema, fluid retention, GI irritation, nausea, vomiting, hematologic dyscrasias, hepatotoxicity, electrolyte abnormalities.	The most common adverse reactions include cerebral edema, cardiac tamponade, increased ICP and papilledema, pleural effusions, heart failure, renal failure, GI perforation and bleeding, avascular necrosis, cardiac events, and tumor lysis syndrome.

*Pregnancy categories have been revised. See http://www.fda.gov/Drugs/DevelopmentApprovalProcess/DevelopmentResources/Labeling/ucm093307.htm for more information.

A, Adult; *Adol*, adolescent; *ALL*, acute lymphoblastic leukemia; *ATP*, adenosine triphosphate; *C*, child; *CBC*, complete blood count; *CEL*, chronic eosinophilic leukemia; *Cmax*, maximum serum concentration; *CML*, chronic myelogenous leukemia; *CYP3A4*, cytochrome P3A4; *CYP450*, cytochrome P450; *d*, day; *EGF*, epidermal growth factor; *h*, hour; *GI*, gastrointestinal; *GIST*, gastrointestinal stromal tumor; *HES*, hypereosinophilic syndrome; *ICP*, intracranial pressure; *NGF*, nerve growth factor; *NSAID*, nonsteroidal antiinflammatory drug; *PDGF*, platelet-derived growth factor; *PB*, protein bound; *Ph+*, Philadelphia-chromosome positive; *PO*, oral; *SGF*, sarcoma growth factor; *t½*, half-life; *UK*, unknown; *VEGF*, vascular endothelial growth factor; *y*, year; *>*, greater than; *≤*, less than or equal to.

chronic, accelerated, or myeloid or lymphoid blast phases that is resistant or intolerant to prior therapy, including imatinib; and Ph+ ALL with resistance or intolerance to prior therapy.

Pharmacokinetics Dasatinib is an oral drug that is readily absorbed from the GI tract, and it can be taken with or without food. Dasatinib and its active metabolite are highly protein bound (96% and 93%, respectively). The drug is extensively metabolized in the liver by the CYP3A4 isoenzyme. Dasatinib is also a weak time-dependent inhibitor of CYP3A4. Unlike other tyrosine inhibitors, Dasatinib does not have the multidrug resistant protein, P-glycoprotein. Dasatinib is eliminated primarily through feces, with only minimal amounts recovered in the urine. Antacids slow the absorption.

Pharmacodynamics Dasatinib specifically targets *BCR-ABL* tyrosine kinase, *SRC* family kinases, and imatinib-resistant mutations mostly found in CML and ALL, possibly blocking angiogenesis and cell proliferation. Inhibiting the activity of these enzymes further inhibits activation of the signal transduction pathway, thereby stopping the proliferation of cancer cells. The drug has the greatest effects on Ph+-expressing cancer cells.

Side effects and adverse reactions. Dasatinib often causes electrolyte imbalances, especially hypokalemia, hypocalcemia, and hypophosphatemia. Other common side effects include diarrhea, cephalgia, fatigue, skin rash, nausea, vomiting, anorexia, arthralgia, pyrexia, and dyspnea, among others. Hemorrhage, vascular disorders, and severe dermatologic reactions have been associated with dasatinib. Another adverse reaction includes ECG abnormalities, especially prolonged QT intervals, and development of arrhythmias. Hematologic side effects of myelosuppression with anemia, thrombocytopenia, and neutropenia are relatively common and are usually reversible. Bleeding, including GI and intracranial bleeding, was reported that required treatment interruptions and transfusions.

Drug interactions. CYP3A4 enzyme inhibitors decrease dasatinib metabolism, resulting in an increased serum concentration and increased risk for toxicity. Other drugs that strongly increase the serum concentration of dasatinib include atazanavir, clarithromycin, indinavir, itraconazole, ketoconazole, nefazodone, nelfinavir, telithromycin, triazolobenzodiazepines, and voriconazole.

Drugs that enhance the activity of the CYP3A4 enzyme decrease dasatinib serum levels and reduce its effectiveness. Such drugs include aminoglutethimide, barbiturates, carbamazepine, dexamethasone, griseofulvin, nafcillin, phenytoin, primidone, and rifampin. Other drugs that appear to reduce the effectiveness of dasatinib include antacids, histamine 2 (H₂) receptor blockers, and proton pump inhibitors. Dasatinib may interfere with the metabolism of other drugs that use the CYP3A4 enzyme system, such as alfentanil, terfenadine, cisapride, cyclosporine, fentanyl, quinidine, tacrolimus, and ergot alkaloids.

Sorafenib. Sorafenib is an MKI that specifically targets serine/threonine and receptor TKs, which are activated because of gene mutations. Gene mutations are most commonly found in pancreatic cancer, colon cancer, and NSCLC. In addition, the drug may be used in hepatocellular carcinomas and renal cell carcinomas that overexpress the target.

Pharmacokinetics Sorafenib is an oral drug whose absorption and bioavailability are inhibited when taken with a high-fat meal. The drug is metabolized in the liver, mainly by the CYP3A4 enzyme system. It is 99.5% protein bound and reaches steady state within 7 days. The peak plasma level is about 3 hours; the mean half-life is 25 to 48 hours. Eight metabolites have been identified, with pyridine *N*-oxide being the major circulating active metabolite. The drug is eliminated in the feces unchanged and in the urine as glucuronidated metabolites (77% and 19%, respectively).

Pharmacodynamics Sorafenib inhibits multiple kinase receptors to inhibit cell proliferation and angiogenesis. Some of the targeted kinases include *RAF* kinase, *VEGF* receptors, platelet-derived growth factor receptor (*PDGFR*), and *RET*. When cytokines or growth factors activate these TK receptors, a protein-kinase–mediated cascade starts that leads to uncontrolled cellular proliferation. The inhibition of these signaling pathways decreased cancer cellular proliferation. In addition, sorafenib specifically inhibits two *VEGF* receptors, thereby inhibiting angiogenesis.

Side effects and adverse reactions. Sorafenib has many common adverse effects, such as hypertension, cephalgia, alopecia, pruritus, xerosis, exfoliative dermatitis, acne, flush, anorexia, nausea/vomiting, diarrhea, constipation, abdominal pain, dyspepsia, dysphagia, hand and foot syndrome, and mild neutropenia. More severe adverse events include QT prolongation, especially in patients with heart failure or electrolyte abnormalities and in those taking other drugs that prolong QT interval. Other severe adverse events were hemorrhage, especially in patients taking anticoagulants or antiplatelets; cardiac ischemia/infarction; GI perforation; and pulmonary toxicity.

Drug interactions. Sorafenib levels are not increased by the presence of other drugs, even those that inhibit the enzyme that metabolizes sorafenib. However, drugs that induce metabolizing enzyme activity can reduce the blood levels and the effectiveness of sorafenib. These include primidone, phenobarbital, rifampicin, phenytoin, carbamazepine, and dexamethasone. If drugs that prolong QT intervals—such as methadone, daunorubicin, epirubicin, and doxorubicin—are coadministered with sorafenib, close ECG monitoring is warranted. Sorafenib can increase the blood levels of repaglinide, amiodarone, ibuprofen, loperamide, irinotecan, propofol, and warfarin.

Sunitinib. Sunitinib is an MKI with antiangiogenic and antitumor activities. It selectively inhibits several receptor tyrosine kinase (RTKs). This inhibition results in regression of tumor growth, especially in advanced renal cell carcinoma (RCC); gastrointestinal stromal tumors (GISTs); and progressive, well-differentiated pancreatic neuroendocrine tumors in patients with unresectable or metastatic disease.

Pharmacokinetics Sunitinib is an oral MKI that is well absorbed with or without food. Sunitinib and its active metabolites are highly protein bound (95% and 90%, respectively). Sunitinib reaches peak plasma level in 6 to 12 hours. The drug and its metabolite are metabolized in the liver, mainly by the CYP3A4 enzyme system; elimination half-life is 40 to 60 hours, and the drug is eliminated primarily in the feces. No dose adjustment is warranted in patients with renal impairment or in patients with mild to moderate hepatic impairment.

Pharmacodynamics Sunitinib inhibits more than 80 receptor RTKs, including platelet-derived growth factor receptor (PDGFR), vascular endothelial growth factor receptor (*VEGFR*), stem cell factor receptor, and glial cell-line derived neurotrophic factor receptor. Additionally, it inhibits the phosphorylation of RTKs, and it has demonstrated inhibition of tumor growth, tumor regression, and tumor angiogenesis. Several adverse effects of sunitinib, including hair and skin discoloration, are associated with the inhibition of the multiple signaling pathways.

Side effects and adverse reactions. Side effects and adverse reactions are more widespread as a result of the number of different types of kinases sunitinib inhibits. Cardiovascular effects include hypertension, peripheral edema, left ventricular dysfunction, prolonged QT interval, and venous thromboembolism. GI effects include nausea, vomiting, diarrhea, stomatitis, and dyspepsia. Neuromuscular effects include fatigue, asthenia, headache, dizziness, peripheral neuropathy, mild arthralgia, limb pain, myalgia, and back pain. Liver impairment may occur with elevated liver enzymes and jaundice of the skin and sclera. Common integumentary changes include depigmentation of the skin, skin discoloration, rash, dry skin, and palmar-plantar erythrodysesthesia. Endocrine changes may include hypothyroidism and adrenal insufficiency, hematologic changes may include myelosuppression, and respiratory effects may include mild dyspnea and cough.

Drug interaction. Plasma concentration and the activity of sunitinib are increased by drugs that inhibit CYP3A4 enzyme levels, including atazanavir, clarithromycin, ketoconazole, itraconazole, nefazodone, nelfinavir, telithromycin, diltiazem, and verapamil. When these drugs are used during sunitinib therapy, side effects of sunitinib are more common and more severe. Drugs that increase sunitinib elimination and reduce its effectiveness include rifampin, phenytoin, phenobarbital, carbamazepine, dexamethasone, rifabutin, and rifapentin.

 NURSING PROCESS
Patient-Centered Collaborative Care
Tyrosine Kinase Inhibitors and Multikinase Inhibitors for Cancer Treatment

Assessment
- To avoid drug interactions, obtain a detailed current medication history that includes prescriptions, OTC medicines, antacids, dietary supplements, vitamins, and herbal supplements.
- Obtain a list of drug and food allergies.
- Obtain baseline information about the patient's physical status that includes height, weight, vital signs, cardiopulmonary assessment, intake and output, skin assessment, nutritional status, and any underlying diseases.
- Assess baseline laboratory values (CBC, uric acid, chemistry panel) to compare with future ones.
- Assess baseline results of pulmonary function tests, chest radiographs, ECGs, and renal and liver function studies.
- Assess the patient's and caregiver's current level of comprehension ability related to the therapeutic regimen.

Nursing Diagnoses
- Infection, Risk for
- Injury, Risk for
- Bleeding, Risk for
- Nutrition: Imbalanced, Risk for Less than Body Requirements
- Knowledge, Deficient related to the chemotherapeutic protocol

Planning
- The patient/family member/caretaker will verbalize understanding of the signs and symptoms of infection.

- The patient's white blood cell, red blood cell, and platelet counts will remain in the desired range.
- The patient will remain free from infection and from pulmonary, cardiac, and GI complications.
- The patient will verbalize ways to decrease GI disturbances to improve nutrition intake.
- The patient/family/caregiver will demonstrate understanding of the chemotherapeutic protocol (e.g., dose administration).

Nursing Interventions
- Monitor labs (CBC, blood urea nitrogen [BUN], creatinine, liver panel, and electrolytes) prior to administration and during treatment.
- Monitor for any signs of bleeding.
- Monitor for any dysrhythmias, decreased cardiac output, heart rate, and blood pressure.
- Monitor IV site frequently for irritation and phlebitis.
- Maintain strict medical asepsis during dressing changes and invasive procedures.
- Encourage small, frequent meals that are high in calories and protein.
- Monitor fluid intake and output, weight, and nutritional intake during therapy.
- Assess the need for IV hydration.
- Administer premedications as ordered 30 to 60 minutes before giving the drug.
- Provide drug information—such as therapeutic effects, side effects, and drug-drug/drug-food interactions—verbally and in print to the patient/family/caregiver.
- Monitor for any vision changes.

Patient Teaching
- Teach patients when to take medications as it relates to food intake.
- Teach patient to weigh daily and report a weight gain of more than 2 pounds in 1 day or 4 pounds in 1 week to the health care provider.
- Avoid alcohol and nonessential drugs that are metabolized by the liver or that have hepatotoxic effects (e.g., acetaminophen).
- Report symptoms of adverse effects or severe side effects promptly, especially fever, chills, persistent sore throat, swelling, weight gain, or increasing shortness of breath.
- Report symptoms of bleeding immediately, including black stools, coffee ground emesis, or easy bleeding or bruising.
- Report symptoms of stomach or abdominal pain, yellowing of eyes or skin, dark urine, or unusual fatigue.
- Remind women with childbearing potential to avoid pregnancy throughout treatment and for up to 12 months after treatment is complete.
- Advise breastfeeding patients to stop breastfeeding during and for 60 days after therapy.
- Teach patients to avoid grapefruit juice, which can increase blood levels of drug to a dangerous level, leading to worsening side effects or adverse events.

- Teach patients to avoid using St. John's wort while on treatment.

Evaluation
- Patient, family, and caregiver education needs are met.
- The patient, family, and caregivers understand therapy-related side effects and adverse reactions.
- The patient, family, and caregivers understand strategies to minimize side effects and adverse reactions.
- Side effects are managed effectively.
- The patient is free from infection.
- The patient's fluid balance and electrolytes are maintained at expected normal ranges.

mTOR Kinase Inhibitors and Proteasome Inhibitors

Mechanistic target of rapamycin (mTOR) is an atypical serine/threonine protein kinase that helps regulate cell growth, proliferation, and survival. Inhibitors of mTOR lead to G_1 arrest and apoptosis. They are not without adverse effects, which are common and include weakness, rash, mucositis, nausea, edema, anorexia, and fever. Effects on laboratory values include pancytopenia, hyperglycemia, hypercholesterolemia, hypertriglyceridemia, and hypophosphatemia. Severe adverse events include hepatic necrosis, pericardial effusion, cardiac tamponade, nephrotic syndrome, hemolytic uremic syndrome, and exfoliative dermatitis. Like other targeted drugs, adverse effects of mTOR and other CYP3A4 inhibitor drugs are increased when mTOR is administered concomitantly. CYP3A4 inducers can cause drug levels to decrease.

Proteasomes are multienzyme complexes that degrade proteins intracellularly. The degraded proteins can accumulate and can disrupt a cell's physiologic properties, such as regulating transcription, cell adhesion, apoptosis, and progression of mitosis. In cancer cells, proteasome inhibitors promote the accumulation of proteins that promote programmed cell death. It has limited action on normal, healthy cells. Table 33.2 lists the mTOR kinase inhibitors and the proteasome inhibitors. Prototype Drug Chart 33.4 lists specific drug information on bortezomib.

Temsirolimus. Temsirolimus is an inhibitor of mechanistic target of rapamycin (mTOR). When temsirolimus or sirolimus binds to the intracellular protein *FKBP-12*, a protein-drug complex forms that directly inhibits the activity of mTOR. Inhibition of mTOR greatly reduces the concentration of vascular endothelial growth factor (*VEGF*). In addition, by its inhibition of mTOR, a variety of downstream pro–cell-division signal transduction pathways are disrupted, especially in RCC cells. This drug is most commonly used to treat advanced RCC.

Pharmacokinetics Temsirolimus is administered by IV infusion. It is extensively metabolized in the liver by CYP3A4 into five active metabolites, including sirolimus. The half-life of temsirolimus is 17 hours, and the half-life of sirolimus is 54 hours. Temsirolimus and its metabolites are primarily excreted in the feces. Approximately 82% of total radioactivity was eliminated within 14 days. Serum concentration of the metabolite, sirolimus, peaked at 0.5 to 2 hours. Caution is advised in patients with

mild hepatic impairment. In patients with moderate to severe hepatic impairment, the drug is contraindicated.

Pharmacodynamics Temsirolimus and its metabolites bind to an intracellular protein to form a drug-protein complex that inhibits the activity of mTOR, and mTOR regulates messenger RNA (mRNA) translation through phosphorylation. Inhibition of mTOR activity resulted in G_1 growth arrest in treated RCC cells.

Side effects and adverse reactions. Hypersensitivity reactions to temsirolimus are common, and premedication with an IV antihistamine (e.g., diphenhydramine) is recommended. Adverse effects are common and include weakness, rash, mucositis, nausea, edema, anorexia, dyspnea, pain, elevated transaminases, pancytopenia, hyperlipidemia, diarrhea, hypophosphatemia, hypercholesterolemia, and hypertriglyceridemia. Hyperglycemia is also common in patients receiving temsirolimus; patients may require treatment with oral antidiabetic agents or with insulin. Respiratory adverse effects of interstitial pneumonitis or other interstitial lung disease are possible. Liver impairment and renal impairment have been reported. Cardiovascular effects of edema formation, chest pain, hypertension, venous thromboembolism, and thrombophlebitis are possible.

Drug interactions. Drugs that inhibit the CYP3A4 enzyme can lead to increased serum levels of temsirolimus, which increases the risk for severe side effects. These drugs include ketoconazole, clarithromycin, indinavir, itraconazole, nefazodone, telithromycin, voriconazole, diltiazem, fluconazole, verapamil, and cimetidine.

Drugs that induce CYP3A4 enzyme activity may lower temsirolimus blood serum levels and can reduce its effectiveness. These drugs include rifampin, carbamazepine, and phenytoin.

Patients taking antihypertensive drugs such as angiotensin-converting enzyme (ACE) inhibitors or angiotensin II–receptor antagonists during temsirolimus therapy are at increased risk for angioedema of the face and upper airways. The combination of temsirolimus and sunitinib may result in dose-limiting integumentary toxicities of erythematous maculopapular rash and gout/cellulitis that require hospitalization. The use of live vaccines such as intranasal influenza, measles, mumps, rubella, oral polio, bacille Calmette-Guérin (BCG), yellow fever, varicella, and typhoid vaccines should be avoided during treatment with temsirolimus.

Carfilzomib. Carfilzomib is a proteasome inhibitor that prevents the proliferation of cancerous cells and promotes apoptotic activity in solid and hematologic tumor cells. Carfilzomib is indicated in the treatment of multiple myeloma.

Pharmacokinetics Carfilzomib is administered intravenously, and in vitro, 97% of the drug is protein bound. Its metabolites have no known biologic activity. The elimination half-life was 1 hour or less. Carfilzomib is extensively metabolized in the plasma rather than in the liver. The drug clearance exceeded hepatic blood flow, suggesting a large extrahepatic clearance. About 25% of the drug's metabolite was excreted in the feces.

Pharmacodynamics Carfilzomib irreversibly binds to the N-terminal threonine-containing active sites of the 20S proteasome, unlike bortezomib. Carfilzomib may be more selective for the chymotrypsin protease, leading to more sustained and

PROTOTYPE DRUG CHART 33.4

Bortezomib

Drug Class	**Dosage**
Proteasome inhibitor	A: IV or Subcut:
Pregnancy category: D*	*Mantle cell lymphoma*: 1.3 mg/m^2 on days 1, 4, 8, and 11 followed by a 10-day rest period (days 12-21) for six 3-wk cycles in combination with rituximab, cyclophosphamide, doxorubicin, and prednisone.
	Multiple myeloma (FDA-designated orphan drug for multiple myeloma): Treatment is administered for nine 6-wk cycles. Cycles 1-4: Admin 1.3 mg/m^2/dose on days 1, 4, 8, and 11 followed by a 10-d rest period (days 12-21); then 1.3 mg/m^2/dose on days 22, 25, 29, and 32 followed by another 10-d rest period (days 33-42) in combination with melphalan and prednisone. Cycles 5-9: Admin 1.3 mg/m^2/dose on days 1, 8, 22, and 29 in combination with melphalan and prednisone.
	Other protocols exist. See full prescribing information.
	At least 72 h should elapse between consecutive doses of bortezomib. IV doses should be given as a bolus over 3-5 s.
	Subcut injections should be administered in the thigh or abdomen; rotate sites and *do not* admin to areas that are tender, bruised, erythematous, or indurated.
	Dose adjustment is needed for moderate to severe hepatic impairment; no adjustments are needed with renal impairment. Admin bortezomib after dialysis procedure; dialysis may reduce bortezomib blood levels.

Contraindications	**Drug-Lab-Food Interactions**
Absolute contraindications: Intrathecal administration, patients with mannitol, bortezomib, or boron hypersensitivity	Drug: Dialysis may reduce bortezomib drug level; bortezomib may increase serum levels of eliglustat, amobarbital, axitinib, and tamsulosin by inducing CYP2D6 metabolism.
Avoid during pregnancy; breastfeeding should be discontinued.	CYP3A4 inhibitor drugs (e.g., idelalisib, mefloquine, cimetidine, clarithromycin, cyclosporine, erythromycin, fluconazole, nifedipine) can increase the serum level of bortezomib if given concomitantly.
Caution: Cardiac, pulmonary, and liver disorders; bleeding dyscrasias; pancytopenia; dehydration; diabetes mellitus; herpes infection; bleeding; history of tumor lysis syndrome; and in neonates and children.	CYP2C19 inhibitor drugs can decrease the effects of clopidogrel and diazepam.
	Drugs metabolized by CYP3A4 (e.g., dexamethasone, diazepam, St. John's wort, phenobarbital) can decrease the level or effect of bortezomib. Bortezomib may increase the level or effect of omeprazole and pantoprazole through CYP2C19 metabolism.
	See full prescriber's information for a complete list of drug interactions.
	Lab: Bortezomib may alter other drug levels if given concomitantly (e.g., phenytoin and phenobarbital).
	Food: Green tea decreases bortezomib effects; grapefruit juice may increase the level of bortezomib.

Pharmacokinetics	**Pharmacodynamics**
Absorption: Bioavailability is unknown.	Onset: UK
Distribution: Range, 498 to 1884 L/m^2 distributed widely into peripheral tissues; >80% PB.	Peak: 509 ng/mL
Metabolism: CYP3A4, CYP2C19, and CYP1A2; t½: 40-193 h; dose dependent.	Duration: UK
Excretion: UK	

Therapeutic Effects/Uses

Mantle cell lymphoma (MCL) and multiple myeloma.

Mode of Action: Bortezomib is a signal transduction inhibitor and a reversible inhibitor of the 26S proteasome in mechanistic cells. Proteasome is a large multiprotein particle present in the cytosol and cell nucleus that regulates protein expression and degradation of damaged or obsolete proteins within the cell; it regulates the expression of proteins that mediate cell cycle progression, oncogenes, and apoptosis. Proteasome inhibition affects malignant cells more so than normal cells.

Side Effects	**Adverse Reactions**
See full prescriber's information for a complete list.	*See full prescriber's information for a complete list.*
Nausea, vomiting, diarrhea, constipation, anorexia, abdominal pain, dyspepsia, dysgeusia, hypotension, neuropathy, pancytopenia, rash, urticaria, vasculitis, pruritus, injection site reaction (e.g., pain, erythema, hematoma, skin irritation, and phlebitis), arthralgia, myalgia, back pain, bone pain, bone fractures, hyperglycemia, hypoglycemia, fatigue, fever, insomnia.	Severe sensory and peripheral neuropathy, cardiotoxicity, heart failure, QT prolongation, arrhythmias, pulmonary hypertension, acute respiratory distress syndrome, pneumonitis, interstitial pneumonia, GI perforation, GI toxicity, hepatotoxicity, toxic epidermal necrolysis, acute febrile neutrophilic dermatosis (Sweet syndrome).

*Pregnancy categories have been revised. See http://www.fda.gov/Drugs/DevelopmentApprovalProcess/DevelopmentResources/Labeling/ucm093 307.htm for more information.

A, Adult; *admin*, administer; *CYP*, cytochrome P; *d*, day; *FDA*, U.S. Food and Drug Administration; *GI*, gastrointestinal; *h*, hour; *IV*, intravenous; *PB*, protein bound; *s*, second; *Subcut*, subcutaneous; *t½*, half-life; *UK*, unknown; *wk*, week; *>*, greater than.

UNIT X Antineoplastics and Biologic Response Modifiers

selective proteasome activity. It has minimal cross-reactivity with other protease classes.

Side effects and adverse reactions. Adverse effects include fatigue, pancytopenia, dyspnea, diarrhea, pyrexia, cephalgia, cough, peripheral edema, nausea, vomiting, arthralgia, hypertension, asthenia, insomnia, and back pain. Cardiac toxicity (e.g., congestive heart failure, cardiac arrest, myocardial ischemia/infarction) has been reported. Pulmonary arterial hypertension and pulmonary edema were noted in some patients. Renal and hepatic toxicity was also noted, therefore close monitoring of renal and hepatic functions is warranted.

Drug interactions. Specific drug interactions have not been reported with this drug. Because carfilzomib is not metabolized by the liver, it is unlikely to be affected by concomitant administration of cytochrome P450 (CYP450) inhibitors and inducers.

Ixazomib. Ixazomib is a reversible proteasome inhibitor that binds and inhibits 20S proteasome. It is indicated for the treatment of multiple myeloma in patients who have received at least one prior therapy.

> **Pharmacokinetics** Ixazomib is administered orally and is highly bound to plasma proteins (99%) with distribution into erythrocytes. Terminal half-life is 9.5 days. The drug is metabolized by CYP450 isoenzymes and non-CYP proteins. Approximately 62% of the dose radioactivity was recovered in the urine and 22% in the feces. The concentration of the drug is decreased with food, therefore the drug should be given at least 1 hour before or at least 2 hours after food consumption.
>
> **Pharmacodynamics** Ixazomib is a reversible proteasome inhibitor that preferentially binds to the beta-5 subunit of the 20S proteasome, and it inhibits its chymotrypsin-like activity. It induces apoptosis of multiple myeloma cells and has a cytotoxic effect on myeloma cells in patients who relapsed after receiving prior therapies with other drugs.

Side effects and adverse reactions. Ixazomib causes multiple adverse effects that include pancytopenia, diarrhea, peripheral neuropathies, peripheral edema, back pain, upper respiratory tract infection, nausea, vomiting, dry eye, and grade 3 rash. Severe adverse effects include drug-induced hepatotoxicity, Stevens-Johnson syndrome, and grade 3 or 4 GI toxicity.

Drug interactions. Ixazomib is metabolized by CYP3A4; levels of ixazomib can be altered by drugs that induce or inhibit CYP3A4. Such drugs include carbamazepine, fosphenytoin, primidone, rifabutin, rifampin, and St. John's wort.

Monoclonal Antibodies

Monoclonal antibodies (MAbs) exert their effects mostly on specific cell-membrane surface proteins. All FDA-approved MAbs currently used in cancer treatment are given intravenously because the GI tract could alter the drug's structure and render it inactive. Ideal target antigens for cancer treatment should (1) be specific to tumor cells; (2) be located on the surface of the tumor cell and not shed into the bloodstream; (3) occur in high numbers; and (4) play a role in tumor cell survival.

MAb therapy is aimed specifically at tumor cells that express the target antigen. The side effects of MAbs are related to activation of the immune system, location of the target antigen, and

the type of MAb. Binding of a MAb to its specific target antigen on the cancer cell inactivates or destroys the cell by one or more of the following mechanisms:

- Causing neutralization of tumor cell growth by direct interference with normal biologic activities of the antigen, such as signal transduction of cell growth messages. This cytostatic process can slow growth of the tumor cells.
- Promoting antibody-dependent cell-mediated cytotoxicity (ADCC) that recruits effector cells such as phagocytes, T cells, and natural killer cells of the immune system to release cytokines that destroy the target cell.
- Initiating complement-dependent cytotoxicity (CDC) that activates the complement system, a cascade of naturally circulating blood proteins, thus enhancing immune system destruction of antibody-bound cells.
- Directly inducing apoptosis, or programmed cell death.

Fully human antibodies are engineered to contain only human antibody protein sequences. Murine MAbs are derived from mice. Mouse antibodies have a very short half-life in the human body, are not as effective as human antibodies in eliciting a response from the CDC and ADCC systems, and can cause development of human antimouse antibodies (HAMAs) that neutralize the mouse antibodies and render them ineffective against the tumor. Chimeric MAbs contain both human and mouse protein sequences (typically 70% human and 30% mouse). Humanized MAbs also contain human and gene mouse sequences; however, they are not considered chimeric because they contain more human sequences than do chimeric MAbs, usually 90% to 95% human and 5% to 10% mouse.

MAbs can also be transporters for other anticancer agents (e.g., chemotherapy agents, toxins, or radioisotopes). Although agents attached to conjugated antibodies specifically target tumor cells, nearby healthy cells can still be negatively affected, especially if radioisotopes are used. If the specific target antigen is found on normal cells, these antibodies also cause damage to these cells.

Table 33.3 lists some of the MAbs currently in use. Bevacizumab has angiogenesis-inhibiting properties. Prototype Drug Chart 33.1 lists specific information on bevacizumab. Prototype Drug Chart 33.5 lists specific drug information on rituximab.

Alemtuzumab

Alemtuzumab is an unconjugated, humanized MAb against the cell surface antigen CD52 that promotes antigen-dependent cell lysis of leukemic cells. CD52 is found on most B and T lymphocytes; on the majority of monocytes, macrophages, and natural killer (NK) cells; and on some granulocytes, stem cells, and mature spermatozoa. Although normal cells may express this antigen, malignant cells are much more sensitive to the destructive activity of this antibody. This drug is most commonly used for management of chronic lymphocytic leukemia (CLL) and multiple sclerosis (MS). However, alemtuzumab should be reserved for patients who have had an inadequate response to two or more drugs for the treatment of MS.

> **Pharmacokinetics** Alemtuzumab is administered as an IV infusion. Its average half-life is 12 days, and steady state levels are reached by about 6 weeks. Alemtuzumab is largely confined

TABLE 33.3 Monoclonal Antibodies

Drug Name and Type	Route and Dosage	Uses and Considerations
Alemtuzumab	Chronic lymphocytic leukemia: A: IV: Initially, 3 mg over 2 h once daily. When tolerated, escalate dose to 10 mg/d until infusion reactions are grade 2 or less, then start maintenance dose: 30 mg 3 × weekly on alternate days (e.g., Monday, Wednesday, Friday). Total therapy duration including dose escalation is 12 wk. MS with inadequate response to two or more previous treatments: A: IV: First treatment: 12 mg daily for 5 d Second treatment: 12 months later, 12 mg daily for 3 d (Not FDA approved for subcut use).	For CLL and MS. Premedicate 30 min before infusion with diphenhydramine and acetaminophen and an antiinfective prophylaxis to reduce risk of opportunistic infection. Monitor for infusion-related reaction. *Absolute contraindication:* HIV Pregnancy category: C*; PB: UK; t½: 12 d
Bevacizumab (*VEGFR*/MAb; prototype)	See Prototype Drug Chart 33.1.	
Cetuximab	A: IV: Initial infusion dose is 400 mg/m² over 2 h, then continue weekly infusions of 250 mg/m² over 60 min.	For colorectal and head and neck cancers. Monitor for infusion-related reactions and worsening symptoms of cardiac or respiratory problems. Pregnancy category: C*; PB: UK; t½: 41-213 h
Ibritumomab tiuxetan	A: IV: Given in two steps: Step 1: Day 1, admin rituximab 250 mg/m² with initial rate at 50 mg/h; increase as tolerated to a max of 400 mg/h. Step 2: Day 7, 8, or 9 repeat rituximab; within 4 h of second rituximab infusion, give ibritumomab 0.4 mCi/kg over 10 min; *max:* 32 mCi. Adjust dose for thrombocytopenia.	For untreated or relapsed/refractory follicular B-cell NHL. Premedicate with diphenhydramine and acetaminophen 30 min prior to each rituximab dose. Use actual body weight to calculate dose, not to exceed 32 mCi. *Do not* exceed 10% of the prescribed dose. *Do not* give Y-90 ibritumomab tiuxetan if platelets are <100,000 cells/mm³. Monitor CBC and platelet count. Pregnancy category: D*; PB: UK; t½: 30 h
Panitumumab	A: IV: 6 mg/kg admin over 60 min given once q2wk.	Fully human Ab against EGFR colorectal cancer. Not indicated for *RAS*-mutation–positive or *RAS*-mutation–unknown cancers. Monitor for acute or worsening dermatologic changes; monitor serum electrolytes. Pregnancy category: C*; PB: nonlinear, dose dependent; t½: 7.5 d
Trastuzumab	A: IV: Breast cancer: Week 1: 4 mg/kg over 90 min Week 2: If patient tolerates initial infusion, admin 2 mg/kg over 30 min once weekly. Other treatment protocols exist (see full prescriber's information). Gastric/GEJ adenocarcinoma given in combination with other chemotherapeutic drugs: Day 1: 8 mg/kg over 90 min. Day 22: 6 mg/kg over 30-90 min every 21 d.	*ERBB2*-positive metastatic breast cancer and not previously treated *ERBB2*-metastatic gastric or GEJ adenocarcinoma. *Do not* substitute trastuzumab for or with ado-trastuzumab emtansine. Monitor CBC and cardiac function; hold or adjust dose for LVEF ≥16% absolute decrease from baseline; may need to permanently discontinue. Monitor for infusion-related reactions such as fever, chills, and dyspnea. Pregnancy category: D*; PB: UK; t½: dose dependent, 6-16 d

*Pregnancy categories have been revised. See http://www.fda.gov/Drugs/DevelopmentApprovalProcess/DevelopmentResources/Labeling/ucm093307.htm for more information.

A, Adult; *Ab,* antibody; *admin,* administer; *CBC,* complete blood count; *CLL,* chronic lymphocytic leukemia; *d,* day; *EGFR,* epidermal growth factor receptor; *FDA,* U.S. Food and Drug Administration; *GEJ,* gastroesophageal junction; *h,* hour; *HIV,* human immunodeficiency virus; *IV,* intravenous; *LVEF,* left ventricular ejection fraction; *MAb,* monoclonal antibody; *max,* maximum dosage; *min,* minutes; *MS,* multiple sclerosis; *NHL,* non-Hodgkin lymphoma; *PB,* protein bound; *q,* every; *subcut,* subcutaneous, *t½,* half-life; *UK,* unknown; *VEGFR,* vascular endothelial growth factor receptor; *wk,* week; *Y-90,* yttrium-90; *<,* less than; *≥,* greater than or equal to.

to blood and interstitial spaces. MAbs bind to target cell surfaces and are destroyed along with the target cell; they are then cleared as debris from the blood and are eliminated in the feces.

Pharmacodynamics Alemtuzumab binds to leukemic cells that express the CD52 cell surface antigen and induces antibody-dependent lysis. Alemtuzumab seems to have preferential effects in the blood and bone marrow, as opposed to the spleen or lymph nodes, which indicates that alemtuzumab is most effective in hematologic disease. As an unconjugated MAb, this drug relies on inducing apoptotic signals and activation of mechanisms such as complement or T cells to attack and kill the target cells. Alemtuzumab is also associated with the release of tumor necrosis factor, interleukin 6, and interferon gamma.

PROTOTYPE DRUG CHART 33.5

Rituximab

Drug Class	Dosage

Monoclonal antibody
Pregnancy category: C*
	Relapsed/refractory low-grade or follicular, CD20-positive B-cell NHL:
	A: IV: 375 mg/m^2 once weekly for 4 doses; may be retreated for an additional 4 doses
	Combination chemotherapy treatment:
	A: IV: Day 1 of each cycle, 375 mg/m^2 for up to 8 infusions
	Maintenance therapy with Y-90 ibritumomab: Day 1, admin 250 mg/m^2; day 7, 8, or 9, admin second
	    rituximab dose within 4 h after Y-90 ibritumomab.
	CD20-positive CLL in combination with fludarabine and cyclophosphamide:
	Cycle 1: 375 mg/m^2 1 d before fludarabine and cyclophosphamide
	Cycles 2-6: 500 mg/m^2 plus fludarabine 25 mg/m^2/d on days 1-3 and cyclophosphamide 250 mg/m^2/d
	    on days 1-3, repeated every 28 d for 6 cycles
	RA, in combination with methotrexate: 1000 mg on days 1 and 15. Admin subsequent courses every
	    16-24 wk based on clinical evaluation. Admin methylprednisolone 30 min prior to each infusion for
	    RA. Premedicate 30 min before rituximab with diphenhydramine and acetaminophen.

Contraindications	**Drug-Lab-Food Interactions**

Patients who are or may become pregnant and those who
    are breastfeeding; those who have previously had
    hepatitis B; have active bacterial or viral infection; have
    moderate to severe renal, liver, and/or cardiac disease;
    and those with preexisting pulmonary fibrosis.
	Drug: Hypotension is potentiated when drug is coadministered with antihypertensive drugs. Bone
	    marrow suppression is potentiated when drug is coadministered with drugs that also cause bone
	    marrow suppression, increasing risk for infection and bleeding.
	Rituximab reduces effectiveness of vaccinations.
	Lab: None known
	Food: None known

Pharmacokinetics	**Pharmacodynamics**

Absorption: Bioavailability is 100% after IV infusion.
Distribution: Throughout extracellular fluid, bone marrow,
    and secondary lymphoid tissues (primarily the spleen); t½:
    first infusion, 76.3 h; fourth infusion, 205.8 h.
Metabolism: Degraded by circulating and liver-based
    phagocytic cells.
Excretion: As cellular debris in feces.
	Antibody binding specifically to the CD20 cell surface antigen on B lymphocytes.

Therapeutic Effects/Uses	
Relapsed or refractory, low-grade, or follicular CD20-positive B-cell NHL, CLL, RA, Wegener granulomatosis. Mode of Action: Binds to CD20-positive B lymphocytes and lymphoma cells, leading to complement-dependent cytotoxicity, antibody-dependent cellular cytotoxicity, and apoptosis.	
Side Effects	**Adverse Reactions**

Bone marrow suppression with pancytopenia, tumor lysis
    syndrome, hypotension, night sweats, joint and muscle
    aches, headaches, soreness at injection site.
	Infusion reactions, pulmonary fibrosis, cardiac dysrhythmias, heart failure, reactivation of dormant
	    viruses.

*Pregnancy categories have been revised. See http://www.fda.gov/Drugs/DevelopmentApprovalProcess/DevelopmentResources/Labeling/ucm093
307.htm for more information.
A, Adult; *admin*, administer; *CLL*, chronic lymphocytic leukemia; *d*, day; *h*, hour; *IV*, intravenous; *min*, minute; *NHL*, non-Hodgkin lymphoma; *RA*,
rheumatoid arthritis; *t½*, half-life; *wk*, week; *Y-90*, yttrium-90.

Side effects and adverse reactions. The most common side effect of alemtuzumab that is not related to infusion reactions or pancytopenia is fatigue. Another common side effect is flu-like symptoms. Subcutaneous injections, compared with IV infusion, have been shown to decrease the incidence of flu-like symptoms. Additional reactions include nausea, blood pressure changes, hyperglycemia, and hypoxia; these are common and often require premedication with antihistamines and acetaminophen. Alemtuzumab can cause severe lymphopenia and a rapid, sustained lymphocyte count decrease in addition to fatal autoimmune pancytopenia and prolonged myelo-suppression. Because of severe lymphopenia, patients are at increased risk for infections. Other adverse events include nonlethal arrhythmias, heart failure, cardiomyopathy, and decreased ejection fraction along with infusion reactions and

rash. Some patients have reduced reactions with subsequent infusions.

Drug interactions. Specific drug interactions have not been reported with this drug; however, concomitant administration of drugs with similar pharmacologic effects may cause additive side effects, including toxicity.

Cetuximab

Cetuximab is a recombinant, human/mouse chimeric MAb that binds specifically to the extracellular domain of the human *EGFR*. However, cetuximab differs in mechanism of action from small-molecule TK inhibitors (e.g., imatinib) that inhibit the TK activity of *EGFR* by interfering with ATP binding; cetuximab blocks the *EGFR* receptor. It is most commonly used for the management of colorectal and head and neck cancers.

Pharmacokinetics Cetuximab is administered as an IV infusion, and it exhibits nonlinear pharmacokinetics. The mean half-life ranged from 41 to 213 hours. Steady state half-life ranged from 75 to 188 hours. The pharmacokinetics do not seem to have any effect on patients with renal or hepatic impairments.

Pharmacodynamics Cetuximab still contains about 30% mouse protein. It binds specifically to *EGFR* on both normal and tumor cells and prevents formation of a ligand that usually attaches epidermal growth factor (*EGF*) to the receptor. This action prevents the receptor from binding to agonists that activate it. As a result, *EGFR*-TKs are not activated, and the signals are not conducted downstream. Other effects of this drug include inhibition of cell growth, induction of apoptosis, decreased proinflammatory cytokine and vascular growth factor production, and internalization of the *EGFR*. Cetuximab may make cancer cells more vulnerable to other cancer chemotherapy agents and radiation therapy. The drug is most effective in causing regression in tumors that have the wild-type *KRAS* oncogene and overexpress *EGFR*.

Side effects and adverse reactions. Cetuximab carries a black-box warning for infusion reactions, usually with the initial dosing, although severe reactions also have been reported during later infusions. Manifestations include rapid onset of airway obstruction, including bronchospasm, stridor, hoarseness, urticaria, and hypotension. Cetuximab is associated with dermatologic changes that typically involve the face, upper chest, and back. An acneiform rash occurred in 90% of patients, usually within the first 2 weeks of therapy. Most patients continued to have the rash for at least 28 days after therapy was discontinued.

Drug interactions. Minimal information is available on drug interactions, although cisplatin and radiation therapy increased the incidence of adverse events.

Ibritumomab Tiuxetan

Ibritumomab tiuxetan is a conjugated murine MAb. Yttrium-90 (Y-90), a pure beta-radionuclide ibritumomab, binds specifically to the human B lymphocytes that express the CD20 cell surface antigen. This drug is most commonly used for management of B-cell types of non-Hodgkin lymphoma (NHL).

Pharmacokinetics Ibritumomab tiuxetan is administered as an IV infusion. Its physical half-life is 64 hours, and its biologic half-life (determined by radioactivity detection) is 30 hours. The drug is excreted to a slight degree by the kidneys (7.2%) but is mostly eliminated in the feces. Y-90 decays by emission of beta particles with a half-life of 64.1 hours.

Pharmacodynamics Ibritumomab tiuxetan binds to the CD20 antigen on B lymphocytes and lymphoma cells. Following binding with the CD20 antigen, beta-wave radioactive emissions from the attached radionuclide, Y-90, induce cellular damage by the formation of free radicals in the target and neighboring cells. This cellular damage prevents cells from dividing.

Side effects and adverse reactions. Ibritumomab tiuxetan carries a black-box warning for infusion reactions, bone marrow suppression, and exfoliative dermatitis. Severe infusion reactions warrant discontinuing the drug. Less severe infusion reactions may be managed using premedication with antihistamines and acetaminophen. Some patients experienced reduced reactions with the second and subsequent infusions. Common adverse effects include pancytopenia, asthenia,

fever, chills, nausea, vomiting, cephalgia, abdominal pain, and infections.

Drug interactions. Ibritumomab tiuxetan increases the risk for bleeding or hemorrhage when used along with anticoagulant or antiplatelet drugs, including NSAIDs, aspirin, salicylate derivatives, thrombolytic therapy, and anticoagulants. Immunization with live viruses is not recommended for 12 months after therapy because of the patient's immunosuppressed state. No other formal studies have been conducted with other drugs to determine specific drug interactions.

Panitumumab

Panitumumab is a fully human MAb with a high affinity for the *EGFR* extracellularly. It is most commonly used in the management of advanced metastatic colorectal carcinomas that express or overexpress *EGFR*.

Pharmacokinetics Panitumumab is administered as an IV infusion. It is a small immunoglobulin that appears to be eliminated in the feces. The half-life ranged from 3.6 to 10.9 days, and the steady state was reached by the third infusion. Mild to moderate hepatic and renal impairment did not affect the drug's action.

Pharmacodynamics Panitumumab binds strongly to the *EGFR* when it is overexpressed on malignant cells. It binds specifically to the *EGFR* on both normal and tumor cells. As a result, *EGFR*-TKs are not activated, and the signals are not conducted downstream. Other effects of this drug include inhibition of cell growth, induction of apoptosis, and decreased proinflammatory cytokine and vascular growth factor production. Tumors must express *EGFR* for patients to be candidates for panitumumab.

Side effects and adverse reactions. Panitumumab carries a black-box warning for dermatologic toxicity. Manifestations usually occur within the first 2 weeks of therapy and include dry skin, skin fissures, erythema, acneiform rash, pruritus, exfoliation, and paronychia and other nail disorders. Electrolyte imbalances, specifically hypomagnesemia and hypocalcemia, may occur and require replacement. Severe diarrhea can occur when panitumumab is given along with irinotecan. Severe infusion reactions, including angioedema and anaphylaxis, have occurred with hypotension and bronchospasm. Although this reaction is rare, patients should be monitored closely throughout the infusion. Full resuscitative equipment should be available during infusion, including epinephrine, corticosteroids, IV antihistamines, bronchodilators, and oxygen.

Drug interactions. Panitumumab is not recommended for use in combination with other antineoplastic drug regimens because of the increased toxic reactions. No other information on drug interactions is available.

Tositumomab

Tositumomab is a murine MAb conjugated with the radioactive isotope Iodine I-131. Like rituximab and ibritumomab tiuxetan, the antibody portion of this drug binds specifically to the human B lymphocytes that express the CD20 cell surface antigen. This drug is most commonly used to manage B-cell NHL that does not respond to rituximab.

Pharmacokinetics Tositumomab is administered as four IV infusions in two distinct steps. It has a median blood clearance of 68.2 mg/hour (with a 485-mg dosage). The mean total-body effective half-life is 67 hours. The Iodine I-131 decays with beta and gamma emissions with a half-life of 8.04 days. The elimination of Iodine I-131 occurs by decay and is excreted in the urine. Whole body clearance was 67% of the injected dose, with elimination occurring mostly in the urine. Patients with high tumor burden, splenomegaly, or bone marrow involvement had faster clearance, shorter terminal half-life, and larger volume distribution.

Pharmacodynamics A tositumomab therapeutic regimen is administered as a two-step process. Each step consists of unlabeled tositumomab administered intravenously followed by Iodine I-131 tositumomab. The unlabeled tositumomab is given to decrease splenic targeting and to increase the terminal half-life of the Iodine I-131 tositumomab. The regimen induces cytotoxicity by combining the immunologic effects of antibody binding to nonmalignant B lymphocytes in the circulation, liver, and spleen. Actions of the antibody include the induction of complement-mediated cytolysis, antibody-dependent cellular cytotoxicity, and apoptosis. Radiation activity is cytotoxic not only to the cells bound by the radiolabeled antibody but also to adjacent normal cells, a process called the *cross-fire effect*. Together, these actions result in sustained depletion of circulating CD20-positive lymphocytes and lymphoma cells.

Side effects and adverse reactions. Tositumomab carries a black-box warning for fetal damage when used during pregnancy, for severe hypersensitivity reactions (anaphylaxis), severe bone marrow suppression, and radiation exposure. Specific tositumomab side effects and adverse effects include asthenia, headache, hypotension, nausea, vomiting, abdominal pain, diarrhea, hypothyroidism, cough, dyspnea, pleural effusion, and pneumonia. Toxicities associated with radioimmunotherapy can be acute, delayed, or long term. The most common acute toxicities are fever, rigors, fatigue, headache, and nausea, whereas hypotension and allergic reactions are less common. Delayed toxicities include shortness of breath, fever, signs of infection, inflammation, pain with urination, rash, sore joints, and bone marrow suppression. Long-term toxicities are myelodysplasia or acute leukemia, secondary malignancies, and hypothyroidism. Just as with other MAbs, this drug causes profound bone marrow suppression that may require dose interruptions or reductions, based on severity, and is more profound in patients who are also receiving standard cytotoxic chemotherapy. In addition, infusion reactions with fever, nausea, chills, blood pressure changes, hyperglycemia, and hypoxia are common and often require premedication with antihistamines and acetaminophen. Some patients have reduced reactions with subsequent infusions.

Drug interactions. Tositumomab increases the risk for bleeding or hemorrhage when used along with anticoagulant or antiplatelet therapy. When patients are immunosuppressed, immune response to vaccines and toxoids are decreased, and higher doses or more frequent boosters may be required. Other specific drug interactions have not been reported with this drug; however, concomitant administration of drugs with similar pharmacologic effects may cause additive side effects, including toxicity.

Trastuzumab

Trastuzumab is a monoclonal antibody that binds to the *ERBB2* protein on the surface of cancer cells. The *ERBB2* receptor is structurally related to *VEGFR*. The *ERBB2* receptor is overexpressed in some breast, ovarian, and colon cancers. Proliferation and angiogenesis of cancer cells are increased with the overexpression of *ERBB2* receptors. When the VEGF pathway is inhibited, tumor growth is suppressed. Trastuzumab is most commonly used in combination with chemotherapy agents to manage breast and gastric cancers that have demonstrated overexpression of the *ERBB2* receptor. Trastuzumab and ado-trastuzumab emtansine are not interchangeable.

> ⚡ **PATIENT SAFETY**
>
> **Do not confuse...**
> - **Trastuzumab** with **ado-trastuzumab emtansine**

Pharmacokinetics Trastuzumab is administered as a weekly IV infusion. Its half-life is 6 days. The steady state is reached within 9 weeks in patients with gastric cancer and 12 weeks in breast cancer patients. Elimination is unknown.

Pharmacodynamics Trastuzumab is a mostly humanized MAb that binds to the *ERBB2* protein on the surface of breast, ovarian, and colon cancer cells that overexpress this receptor. This drug specifically inhibits the proliferation of cancer cells that overexpress *ERBB2* receptors. In addition, binding of trastuzumab to the cancer cell receptor increases killing of these cells through attack by immune system cells, especially NK cells and monocytes.

Side effects and adverse reactions. Trastuzumab carries a black-box warning for cardiomyopathy manifesting as congestive heart failure when the drug is used as a monotherapy. This risk is increased when the drug is given in combination with other drugs that cause cardiotoxicity, such as the anthracyclines and cyclophosphamide. Another black-box warning includes infusion-related reactions (anaphylaxis) and pulmonary toxicity. Hypersensitivity reactions, including anaphylaxis, may occur but are not common. Trastuzumab is associated with headache, dizziness, hypotension, fever, chills, and nausea during the initial infusion. After the initial infusion, these symptoms typically do not recur. Other common side effects include headache, muscle aches, and loss of appetite.

Drug interactions. Trastuzumab can increase the incidence and severity of cardiac dysfunction in patients who receive trastuzumab in combination with anthracyclines and cyclophosphamide. Elevated INR can occur in patients taking warfarin concomitantly with trastuzumab. This drug may increase the myelosuppressive effects of other antineoplastic agents.

> ◎ **NURSING PROCESS**
> **Patient-Centered Collaborative Care**
>
> ### mTOR Inhibitors, Proteasome Inhibitors, and Monoclonal Antibodies
>
> **Assessment**
> - To avoid drug interactions, obtain a detailed current medication history that includes prescription drugs, OTC medicines, antacids, dietary supplements, vitamins, and herbal supplements.

- Obtain a list of the patient's drug and food allergies.
- Obtain baseline information about the patient's physical status. Include height, weight, vital signs, cardiopulmonary assessment, intake and output, skin assessment, nutritional status, and any underlying diseases.
- Assess baseline laboratory values (CBC, uric acid, chemistry panel) to compare with future ones.
- Assess baseline results of pulmonary function tests, chest radiographs, ECGs, and renal and liver function studies.
- Assess patient, family, and caregiver knowledge related to the therapeutic regimen.

Nursing Diagnoses
- Injury, Risk for
- Infection, Risk for
- Skin Integrity, Risk for Impaired
- Knowledge, Deficient related to the targeted therapy regimen
- Electrolyte Imbalance, Risk for

Planning
- The patient will remain free from infection.
- The patient and family will verbalize understanding of targeted therapy as part of an anticancer treatment regimen.
- The patient and family will verbalize strategies to minimize risks related to targeted therapy–related side effects.
- The patient and family will demonstrate understanding of the importance of reporting targeted therapy–related side effects and adverse reactions.
- The patient's side effects will be managed to a tolerable level and are not life threatening.

Nursing Interventions
- Assess for any cardiac events, such as new chest pain and ECG changes.
- Monitor appropriate labs according to established protocol for specific targeted therapy (e.g., CBC with differential, electrolytes, renal and hepatic function, glucose, phosphate).
- Assess for any bleeding, especially if the patient is taking anticoagulants, antiplatelets, or NSAIDs.
- Monitor liver function tests and renal function tests at baseline and at least once monthly during therapy.
- Examine the patient's skin closely at each visit for the presence of erythema, rash, peeling, or blister formation; rate the severity of dermatologic reactions, and determine whether infection is present in any nonintact skin.

- Administer prescribed premedications according to established protocols for specific targeted therapies (e.g., allopurinol, antiinfectives, antivirals, antihistamines).
- Have resuscitative equipment on standby as per protocol.
- Ensure appropriate supervising personnel are present according to protocols for specific targeted therapy.

Patient Teaching
- Report symptoms of bleeding immediately, including black stools, vomit that looks like coffee grounds, and easy bleeding or bruising.
- Report symptoms of adverse effects or severe side effects promptly, especially fever, chills, persistent sore throat, swelling, weight gain, or increasing shortness of breath.
- Report symptoms of liver impairment immediately, including stomach/abdominal pain, yellowing eyes or skin, dark urine, or unusual fatigue.
- Avoid alcohol and nonessential drugs that are cleared by the liver or that have hepatotoxic effects (e.g., acetaminophen).
- Remind women with childbearing potential to avoid pregnancy throughout treatment and for up to 12 months after treatment is completed.
- Advise breastfeeding patients to stop breastfeeding during and for 60 days after therapy.
- Teach diabetic patients to monitor their glucose more frequently, and advise them when to seek medical help.
- Advise the patient or a family member to immediately report convulsions, persistent headache, reduced eyesight, increased blood pressure, or blurred vision.
- Teach proper waste disposal to patients receiving monoclonal antibodies conjugated to radioisotopes (ibritumomab tiuxetan and tositumomab) to prevent unnecessary radiation exposure.

Evaluation
- Patient, family, and caregiver education needs are met.
- The patient, family, and caregiver understand therapy-related side effects and adverse reactions.
- The patient, family, and caregiver understand strategies to minimize side effects and adverse reactions.
- Side effects are managed effectively.
- The patient is free from infection.
- The patient's fluid balance and electrolytes are maintained at expected normal ranges.

CRITICAL THINKING CASE STUDY

MR is a 64-year-old man who was diagnosed with stage III B-cell non-Hodgkin lymphoma (NHL). He is scheduled to receive rituximab and a traditional chemotherapy regimen of cyclophosphamide, doxorubicin, vincristine, and prednisolone, a combination known as "CHOP." The dosage and schedule of rituximab for this patient is 375 mg/m^2 IV on day 1 before the first CHOP chemotherapy cycle, which will be administered on day 8. The next two doses will be administered 2 days before the third and fifth cycles, and the remaining two cycles of rituximab will be administered after the sixth cycle of CHOP on days 134 and 141. MR has a friend who is taking imatinib daily as an oral drug for chronic myelogenous leukemia. He asks why rituximab must be taken intravenously and, because he has an implanted port, if his spouse, who is a licensed practical nurse could administer it at home rather than him traveling to the clinic for his chemotherapy.

1. What is your best response about why rituximab must be administered intravenously?
2. How are rituximab and imatinib different?
3. Why can MR's spouse *not* administer rituximab at home?
4. What side effects are specific for rituximab?
5. What are the most common adverse effects of rituximab?
6. What should you teach this patient specifically in relation to rituximab therapy?

NCLEX STUDY QUESTIONS

1. A patient undergoing chemotherapy for breast cancer asks why she is not receiving trastuzumab like her sister. What is the nurse's best response?
   a. Your breast cancer cells are estrogen-receptor positive, and targeted therapy is not needed.
   b. You are much older than your sister and would not tolerate the treatment well.
   c. The drug is expensive, and your insurance does not cover it.
   d. Your cancer cells do not have the target for trastuzumab.

2. Which instruction is important for the nurse to include when teaching a patient about imatinib therapy?
   a. Do not drink grapefruit juice while taking this drug.
   b. Go immediately to the emergency department if you develop a headache while taking this drug.
   c. This drug will only work for about 2 months before your cancer develops resistance to it.
   d. Be sure to take this drug on an empty stomach, either 1 hour before or at least 3 hours after eating.

3. Which is the priority nursing diagnosis for patients receiving epidermal growth factor receptor inhibitors?
   a. Risk for thrombocytopenia related to bone marrow suppression and neutropenia
   b. Risk for impaired skin integrity related to skin side effects
   c. Risk for injury related to reduced platelet activity
   d. Disturbed body image related to alopecia

4. A nurse is monitoring several patients undergoing chemotherapy. Which of the following classes of targeted therapy would cause the nurse the most concern in regard to a possible infusion reaction?
   a. Tyrosine kinase inhibitors
   b. Multikinase inhibitors
   c. Monoclonal antibodies
   d. Proteasome inhibitors

5. A patient taking sunitinib reports that the skin on her hands and feet is red, painful, and has some blisters. What is the nurse's best action?
   a. The only action needed is to document the finding because this is a mild side effect.
   b. Advise the patient to wear gloves and mittens when going outdoors in cold weather.
   c. Advise the patient to avoid getting her hands wet and touching food.
   d. Notify the oncologist to determine if a dosage reduction is needed.

6. Which action is most important for the nurse to teach a patient taking tositumomab?
   a. Avoid drinking alcohol for 1 week after receiving this drug.
   b. Avoid smoking cigarettes for the entire treatment period.
   c. Use a separate bathroom and sit while urinating for 1 week after receiving this drug.
   d. Be sure to take this drug on an empty stomach, either 1 hour before or 2 hours after eating.

7. Which activity has a higher priority for the nurse to advise the patient to avoid while taking ixazomib?
   a. Drinking alcoholic beverages
   b. Taking aspirin or aspirin-containing drugs
   c. Socializing in crowds or with persons who are ill
   d. Taking the drug 1 hour before or 2 hours after food

8. A patient receiving a targeted therapy asks the nurse why St. John's wort must be avoided. What is the nurse's best response?
   a. This herbal drug increases blood levels of most targeted therapies and increases the risk for severe side effects or adverse reactions.
   b. This herbal drug decreases blood levels of most targeted therapies and reduces their effectiveness.
   c. Targeted therapies increase blood levels of St. John's wort, increasing the risk of an overdose of this herbal agent.
   d. Targeted therapies bind with St. John's wort in the intestinal tract, preventing absorption of both the drug and the herbal agent.

9. A patient taking imatinib voices concern about gaining 5 pounds in the past week. The nurse explains, knowing that:
   a. Weight gain is an expected side effect of this drug because it increases the appetite.
   b. Weight gain is an indication of slow metabolism and possible hypothyroidism.
   c. Weight gain is an indication of water retention and possible renal impairment.
   d. Weight gain is an indication of a drug interaction between imatinib and loop diuretics.

Answers: 1, d; 2, a; 3, b; 4, c; 5, d; 6, c; 7, d; 8, b; 9, c.

Biologic Response Modifiers

http://evolve.elsevier.com/McCuistion/pharmacology/

OBJECTIVES

- Compare the mechanisms of action of drugs classified as *biologic response modifiers* with those of standard chemotherapy drugs.
- Distinguish among the different types of biologic response modifiers with regard to indications, common side effects

and adverse effects, route of administration, and nursing responsibilities.
- Discuss three common side effects of interferons, colony-stimulating factors, and interleukin 2.
- Incorporate the nursing process related to the needs of patients receiving biologic response modifiers.

OUTLINE

KEY TERMS

The immune system recognizes and protects the body from foreign invaders, such as bacteria or viruses; it also destroys damaged, diseased, or abnormal cells, including cancer cells. When the body detects an invader, an immune response is triggered, and substances such as white blood cells (WBCs) and natural killer cells (NKCs) provide a certain level of protection. Biologic response modifiers (BRMs), also called *immunotherapies,* are a class of pharmacologic drugs used to enhance, direct, or restore the body's immune system. BRMs consist of substances naturally made in the body and those developed in the laboratory. They can kill cancer cells directly or indirectly. BRMs that target cancer cells directly are also called *targeted therapy,* and these are discussed in Chapter 33. Indirect therapies

stimulate the body's immune system and do not directly target cancer cells. Biologic therapies are used to treat the cancer or the side effects caused by other cancer treatments. Recombinant DNA, the genetic engineering process that combines two human DNA strands artificially, and hybridoma technology, the process that genetically makes monoclonal antibodies, are two advances that have led to commercial mass-production of BRMs (Fig. 34.1). Interferons (alfa, gamma, and beta), tumor necrosis factor (TNF), erythropoietin, vaccine therapy, colony-stimulating factors, interleukins, and monoclonal antibodies are some currently known BRMs. With the exception of monoclonal antibodies, BRMs are a complex set of proteins produced by the immune system (Fig. 34.2). Monoclonal antibodies are

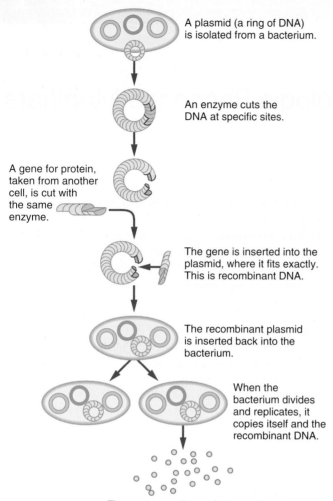

A plasmid (a ring of DNA) is isolated from a bacterium.

An enzyme cuts the DNA at specific sites.

A gene for protein, taken from another cell, is cut with the same enzyme.

The gene is inserted into the plasmid, where it fits exactly. This is recombinant DNA.

The recombinant plasmid is inserted back into the bacterium.

When the bacterium divides and replicates, it copies itself and the recombinant DNA.

The new gene directs the bacterium to make a new protein product, such as interferon.

FIG. 34.1 Recombinant DNA.

considered for targeted therapies and are further discussed in Chapter 33. Like chemotherapy, BRMs suppress the immune system; this immunocompromised state places patients at risk for complications such as infection. BRMs assist the immune system in several ways:

- They enhance the immune system's ability to kill abnormal cells (**immunomodulation**).
- They change cancer cells to make them behave more like healthy cells.
- They inhibit normal cells from changing into cancer cells.
- They enhance the body's ability to repair or replace damaged cells caused by other cancer treatments.
- They prevent cancer cells from **metastasizing** (spreading to other parts of the body).

New BRMs are always under development and investigation for clinical effectiveness. Several categories of these drugs have been approved by the U.S. Food and Drug Administration (FDA). Of the BRMs, interferons, colony-stimulating factors, and interleukin 2 are further discussed under those headings below.

INTERFERONS

Interferons (IFNs) are a family of proteins that occur naturally in the body, and they are also produced in the laboratory. Various subtypes of IFNs have different mechanisms of action with some overlapping actions. IFNs work directly on cancer cells to slow their growth or cause cancer cells to behave more like normal cells. Some IFNs also stimulate certain types of WBCs to fight cancer, which includes NKCs, T cells, and macrophages. The two main types of IFNs are type I and type II. *Type I interferons* include IFN-alfa (leukocyte IFN) and IFN beta (fibroblast and epithelial cell IFN). *Type II interferon* includes IFN gamma produced by CD4+, CD8+, NKCs, and lymphokine-activated killer (LAK) cells. Table 34.1 provides information on IFNs with their dosages, uses, and considerations.

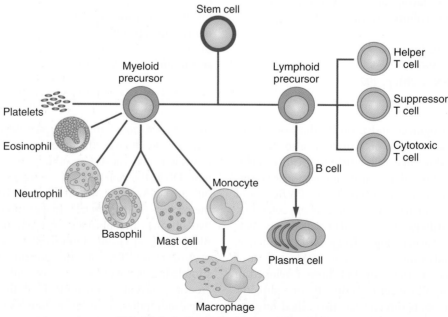

FIG. 34.2 Cells of the Immune System.

TABLE 34.1 Biologic Response Modifiers: Interferons

Generic Drug Name	Route and Dosage	Uses and Considerations
Interferon alfa-2b	Hairy cell leukemia: A: IM/Subcut: 2 million units/m² 3 times/wk for up to 6 mo Kaposi sarcoma: A: IM/Subcut: Initially: 30 million units/m² 3 times/wk until severe intolerance or maximal response after 16 wk Malignant melanoma as adjuvant treatment: A: IV: Induction: 20 million units/m² for 5 consecutive d/wk for 4 wk Subcut: Maint: 10 million units/m² 3 times/wk for 48 wk Follicular lymphoma (NHL): A: Subcut: 5 million units 3 times/wk for up to 18 mo	For hairy cell leukemia, adjuvant to surgical resection of malignant melanoma, follicular NHL, condyloma acuminata, AIDS-related Kaposi sarcoma, and chronic hepatitis B and non-A hepatitis. Monitor CBC, AST, ALT, ALP, LDH. Pregnancy category: C*; PB: UK; t½: 2-3 h
Interferon gamma	Body surface area: >0.5 m²: A/C: Subcut: 50 mcg/m² 3 times/wk Body surface area: <0.5 m²: A/C >1 y: Subcut: 1.5 mcg/kg/dose 3 times/wk	For chronic granulomatous disease. Pregnancy category: C*; PB: UK; t½: 0.5-6 h
Interferon beta-1b	Relapsing-remitting forms of MS: A: Subcut 250 mcg every other day. Incremental titration q2wk is recommended at 62.5 mcg every other day during wk 1 and 2, 125 mcg every other day during wk 3 and 4, and 187.5 mcg every other day during wk 5 and 6.	For MS. Pregnancy category: C*; PB: UK; t½: 8 min-4.3 h

*Pregnancy categories have been revised. See http://www.fda.gov/Drugs/DevelopmentApprovalProcess/DevelopmentResources/Labeling/ucm093307.htm for more information.

A, Adult; *AIDS*, acquired immunodeficiency syndrome; *ALP*, alkaline phosphatase; *ALT*, alanine aminotransferase; *AST*, aspartate aminotransferase; *C*, child; *CBC*, complete blood count; *d*, day; *h*, hour; *IM*, intramuscular; *IV*, intravenous; *LDH*, lactate dehydrogenase; *maint*, maintenance; *min*, minute; *mo*, month; *MS*, multiple sclerosis; *NHL*, non-Hodgkin lymphoma; *PB*, protein binding; *q*, every; *subcut*, subcutaneous; *t½*, half-life; *UK*, unknown; *wk*, week; *y*, year; *>*, greater than; *<*, less than.

Interferon Alpha

B-lymphocyte cells; non–B- and non–T-lymphocyte cells; and macrophages (mature monocytes) produce interferon alfa-2b (IFN-α-2b) endogenously in response to viral infection and other various exogenous inducers. Exogenous α-2b IFNs used as BRMs are considered second-generation IFNs. Interferon alfa-2a, a first-generation IFN, is currently not being marketed; however, both subtypes have similar actions. IFNs bind to cell receptors for biologic activities followed by activation of the tyrosine kinases (TKs). IFNs have been shown to have antiviral, antiproliferative, and immunomodulatory effects and they affect cellular differentiation, regulation of cell-surface major histocompatibility complex (MHC) antigen expression, and cytokine induction.

Interferon-α-2b is approved for hairy-cell leukemia, AIDS-related Kaposi sarcoma, malignant melanoma, and non-Hodgkin lymphoma (NHL); hepatitis B and C viruses; and human papillomavirus (HPV) infection. Additionally, it has been used in combination with antiviral or anticancer drugs in patients with Philadelphia-chromosome positive (Ph+) chronic myelogenous leukemia (CML), renal cell cancer (RCC), and T-cell leukemia/lymphoma.

Pharmacokinetics Interferon alpha-2b is administered parenterally via intravenous (IV), intramuscular (IM), or subcutaneous routes. Mean serum concentrations after IM and subcutaneous administration were similar. IFN is catabolized by the renal system. Maximum concentration occurs in 3 to 12 hours, and elimination half-life is 2 to 3 hours. Following the IV route, the half-life is reached in about 2 hours and is undetectable in the serum in about 4 hours. IFN- α-2b is not cleared by hemodialysis.

Pharmacodynamics IFN- α-2b has similar actions to native IFN-α. Endogenous IFNs are secreted by leukocytes in response to viral infection or various synthetic and biologic inducers. Once the IFN binds to cell surface receptors, tyrosine kinases are activated, which produce several IFN-stimulated enzymes that cause antiviral, antiproliferative, and immunomodulatory effects; cellular differentiation; regulation of cell-surface MHC antigen expression; and cytokine induction. Antiviral effects include inhibiting viral replication by inhibiting translation of viral proteins; inhibition of viral penetration and uncoating and/or viral assembly and release; and enhancement of the lytic (killing) effects of cytotoxic T lymphocytes. Viruses affected include hepatitis B, C, and D; herpes simplex virus types 1 and 2; human immunodeficiency virus (HIV); HPV; and rhinovirus, among others.

Antineoplastic effects may result from IFN's ability to induce a host response to the tumor (e.g., immunomodulatory effects), cause a cytostatic effect on tumor cells, and slow the rate of cell proliferation by enhancing or inhibiting the synthesis of specific proteins, modifying cell-surface antigen expression, and/or modulating the immune system. IFNs prolong all phases of the cell cycle and promote cells to enter the G_0 (resting) phase, which is thought to be important in treating hairy cell leukemia.

Side Effects and Adverse Reactions

Table 34.2 lists the common adverse effects for BRMs, including IFNs and any dosage adjustments or discontinuation of the drug for toxicity. The black-box warning includes the risk of fatal or life-threatening neuropsychiatric, autoimmune, ischemic, and infectious disorders. Patients must be closely monitored with periodic clinical and laboratory evaluations. Table 34.3 compares the black-box warnings for IFN, interleukin 2 (IL-2), and erythropoietin (EPO). While taking IFN-α, close monitoring of complete blood count (CBC), chest radiography (CXR), electrocardiography (ECG), liver function tests (LFTs), triglycerides, and thyroid function tests (TFTs) should be conducted.

Interactions

It is unknown whether IFN-α-2b is metabolized by the liver; therefore caution is advised when IFN-α-2b is taken with other drugs metabolized through the hepatic cytochrome P450 enzyme system. The effect of IFN on the CYP450 system might increase enzyme degradation or inhibit CYP450 system. IFN-α-2b with concomitant use of theophylline may result in a 100% increase in theophylline concentrations. Caution is also warranted when taking drugs (e.g., antiretroviral nonnucleoside reverse transcriptase inhibitors [NNRTIs] and antiretroviral protease inhibitors) that can cause liver toxicity because IFNs also can cause liver damage. Hearing loss has been associated with IV eflornithine in combination with IFN-α-2b. Other drugs that may interact with IFN include barbiturates, colchicine, chemotherapy, and hydroxyurea. No information is available on drug-food or drug-herbal interactions.

Interferon Beta

Interferon beta (IFN-β) is a type I interferon produced by fibroblasts, macrophages, and epithelial cells. It has both antiviral and immune regulatory activities, especially against herpesvirus, HPV, hepatitis B and C, and HIV. IFN-β-1a is indicated for the treatment of multiple sclerosis (MS); IFN-β-1a inhibits the proinflammatory cytokines responsible for triggering the autoimmune reaction that leads to MS. IFN-β-1a also reduces T-cell migration across the blood-brain barrier and increases the production of nerve growth factor, which promotes axonal recovery; this may result in remyelination.

TABLE 34.2 Adverse Effects and Dosage Modifications for Biologic Response Modifiers

Drug Class	Side Effects/Adverse Effects	Dose Adjustment or Discontinuation
Colony-stimulating factors: Erythropoietin (EPO)	Hypertension, flulike symptoms, rash, anaphylactoid reactions, antibody formation, arthralgia, myalgia, cephalgia, edema, red cell aplasia, thromboembolism, injection site reaction, urticaria, bronchospasm, cough, encephalopathy.	Stop treatment: Anaphylactoid reactions, red cell aplasia secondary to antibody formation. Adjust dosage: Hgb rise >1 g/dL in 2 wk, CKD
Colony-stimulating factors: Granulocyte colony–stimulating factor (G-CSF), granulocyte-macrophage colony–stimulating factor (GM-CSF)	Peripheral edema, flulike symptoms, chest pain, splenomegaly, anaphylactoid reactions, elevated hepatic enzymes, rash, cardiac arrhythmia, cephalgia, arthralgia, leukocytosis, asthenia, antibody formation, pulmonary disorders, capillary leak syndrome.	Stop treatment: Anaphylactoid reaction, capillary leak syndrome, ANC >10,000/mm³; ARDS, splenic involvement, sickle cell crisis, alveolar hemorrhage. Adjust dosage: Vasculitis, renal disorders
Erythropoietin-stimulating agents (ESAs; interferons)	Flulike symptoms (fever, chills, tachycardia, malaise, myalgia, cephalgia), chest pain, fatigue, depression, drowsiness, dizziness, irritability, paresthesia, insomnia, alopecia, skin rash, amenorrhea, nausea, diarrhea, vomiting, xerostomia, abdominal pain, pancytopenia, dyspnea, cough, pharyngitis, infection.	Stop treatment: Severe depression, hypersensitivity reactions, hematologic toxicity (ANC <500/mm³ or platelets <25,000/mm³); severe hepatic decompensation. Adjust dosages for other hematologic toxicity.
Interleukin (IL-2)	Hypotension, peripheral edema, tachycardia, SVT, flulike symptoms, rash, pruritus, electrolyte imbalances, diarrhea, vomiting, nausea, weight gain, anorexia, abdominal pain, pancytopenia, elevated liver function tests, weakness, renal impairment, respiratory disorders, antibody formation, infection.	See Table 34.5.

ANC, Absolute neutrophil count; *ARDS,* acute respiratory distress syndrome; *CKD,* chronic kidney disease; *Hgb,* hemoglobin; *SVT,* supraventricular tachycardia; *wk,* week; >, greater than; <, less than.

TABLE 34.3 U.S. Food and Drug Administration Black-Box Warnings for Interferon, Interleukin 2, and Erythropoietin

Interferon	Aldesleukin (IL-2)	Erythropoietin
Autoimmune disorders	Cardiac disease	Hgb concentration >11 g/dL
Infectious disorders	Coma	Myocardial infarction
Ischemic disorders	Capillary leak syndrome	Neoplastic disease
Neuropsychiatric disorders	Infection	Surgery
	Pulmonary disease	Thromboembolic disease
	Treatment requires a specialized setting and experienced clinician.	

Hgb, Hemoglobin; *IL,* interleukin; >, greater than.

Interferon Gamma

Interferon gamma (IFN-γ) is a type II interferon produced endogenously by activating T lymphocytes and NKCs, and it is genetically produced from *Escherichia coli*. IFN-γ regulates the immune system and interacts with other interleukins, and it has direct and indirect antiviral activities by affecting attachment, penetration, uncoating, transcription, assembly, and maturation of viruses. It is also the primary factor for macrophage activation to kill parasites and cancer cells. IFN-γ enhances antigen processing and presentation by increasing the expression of MHC; it also increases humoral immunity and the expression of tumor suppressor genes; and it enhances recruitment of leukocytes to the sites of inflammation. IFN-γ is used for the treatment of chronic granulomatous disease and osteopetrosis.

COLONY-STIMULATING FACTORS

Hematopoietic colony-stimulating factors (CSFs) are proteins that stimulate or regulate the growth, maturation, and differentiation of bone marrow stem cells. Like IFNs, CSFs are a subgroup of cytokines. Although CSFs are not directly tumoricidal, they are useful in cancer treatment. Chemotherapy depletes normal stem cells and the blood cells that they produce; CSFs promote the growth of these blood cells, which increases the opportunity to continue with chemotherapy. More specifically, CSFs have other functions:

- CSFs decrease the length of posttreatment neutropenia—the length of time neutrophils, a type of WBC, are decreased secondary to chemotherapy—thereby reducing the risk, incidence, and duration of infection.
- CSFs permit the delivery of higher doses of chemotherapy drugs. Myelosuppression, suppression of bone marrow activity, is often a dose-limiting toxicity of chemotherapy. Higher, possibly tumoricidal doses of these drugs cannot be administered because of potentially life-threatening side

effects. CSFs can minimize the myelosuppressive toxicity, thus allowing the delivery of the higher doses.

- CSFs reduce bone marrow recovery time after bone marrow transplantation.
- CSFs enhance macrophage or granulocyte tumor-, virus-, and fungus-destroying abilities.
- CSFs prevent severe thrombocytopenia after myelosuppressive chemotherapy.

CSFs have been used to treat patients with neutropenia secondary to disease or treatment and can be administered both intravenously and subcutaneously. The CSFs that are FDA approved for clinical use are erythropoietin-stimulating agents (ESAs), granulocyte colony–stimulating factors (G-CSFs), and granulocyte-macrophage colony–stimulating factors (GM-CSFs).

Erythropoietin-Stimulating Agents

Erythropoietin (EPO) is a glycoprotein produced by the kidney; it stimulates red blood cell (RBC) production in the bone marrow. Specifically, EPO stimulates the division and differentiation of committed RBC progenitors (parent cells destined to become circulating RBCs) in the bone marrow. RBCs contain hemoglobin, which is necessary to transport oxygen in the body.

Erythropoietin-stimulating agents (ESAs) include epoetin alfa and darbepoetin alfa. These recombinant ESAs are used when blood transfusions are not an option. ESAs are administered as an injection to stimulate RBC production in the bone marrow. They must be used cautiously and only as indicated because of the potential for serious complications (e.g., myocardial infarction, stroke, venous thromboembolism, thrombosis of vascular access, and tumor progression or recurrence) and even death. Table 34.2 lists the common adverse effects for BRMs, including ESAs, dosage adjustments, and whether discontinuation of the drug is warranted. Prototype Drug Chart 34.1 provides specific drug information for epoetin alfa.

📄 PROTOTYPE DRUG CHART 34.1

Epoetin Alfa (Erythropoietin)

Drug Class	Dosage

Biologic response modifier
Pregnancy category: C*
	Black Box Warning: ESAs increase the risk for death when given to target
	  Hgb >11 g/dL in cancer patients.
	A: Modify dose to keep target Hgb <11 g/dL.
	CKD: A/Adol ≥17 y: IV/Subcut: 50-100 units/kg 3 times/wk
	C/Adol <17 y: IV/Subcut: 50 units/kg 3 times/wk
	Dialysis patients: Initiate IV treatment when Hgb <10 g/dL.
	Anemia as a result of myelosuppression: A: Subcut: 150 units/kg 3 times/wk
	  or 40,000 units once/wk
	C ≥5 y: IV: 600 units/kg/wk

Contraindications	**Drug-Lab-Food Interactions**

Absolute contraindications:
Benzyl alcohol hypersensitivity
Black Box Warning:
Hgb concentration >11 g/dL; myocardial infarction; stroke; neoplastic disease;
  surgery; thromboembolic disease
Precautions:
Hypertension, anticoagulant therapy, cardiac disease, coagulopathy, dialysis, folate
  deficiency, heart failure, electrolyte imbalance, hyperparathyroidism, iron-deficiency
  hematologic disease, renal disease, seizure disorders, vitamin B12 deficiency
	Drug: Use with darbepoetin alfa has additive effects that increase adverse
	  reactions. Androgens have an additive effect to epoetin alfa. Probenecid
	  and amphotericin B may inhibit the response of epoetin.
	Lab: Inadequate iron stores interfere with the therapeutic response to epoetin
	  alfa. Monitor transferrin saturation and serum ferritin before and during
	  treatment. Administer iron therapy when serum ferritin is <100 mcg/L or
	  when transferrin saturation is <20%.
	Food: None known

Continued

PROTOTYPE DRUG CHART 34.1—cont'd

Epoetin Alfa (Erythropoietin)

Pharmacokinetics	Pharmacodynamics
Absorption: Subcut, IV	Onset: Several days
Distribution: PB: UK	Peak: 5-24 h (subcut); IV with more rapid peak
Metabolism: t½: Affected by renal function; 4-13 h in patients with CKD (IV); 20% less in those with normal renal function	Duration: UK
Excretion: Majority in feces, 10% in urine; dialysis does not remove EPO.	

Therapeutic Effects/Uses
Approved for use in the treatment of anemia to increase the Hgb concentration to the lowest level sufficient to avoid the need for RBC transfusions.
Mode of Action: Regulates the production of RBCs by stimulating the committed erythroid progenitor cells to divide and differentiate in the bone marrow to maintain optimal red cell mass for oxygen transport.

Side Effects	Adverse Reactions
Injection site reaction, myalgia, arthralgia, cephalgia, nausea, emesis, pruritus, cough, urticaria, dizziness, insomnia, anemia, fever, hypokalemia	Anaphylactoid reactions, angioedema, bronchospasm, MI, seizures, stroke, thromboembolism, red cell aplasia, hypertension, antibody formation, heart failure, encephalopathy

*Pregnancy categories have been revised. See http://www.fda.gov/Drugs/DevelopmentApprovalProcess/DevelopmentResources/Labeling/ucm093307.htm for more information.

A, Adult; *Adol*, adolescent; *C*, child; *CKD*, chronic kidney disease; *EPO*, erythropoietin; *ESA*, erythropoietin-stimulating agent; *h*, hour; *Hgb*, hemoglobin; *IV*, intravenous; *MI*, myocardial infarction; *PB*, protein binding; *RBC*, red blood cell; *subcut*, subcutaneous; *t½*, half-life; *UK*, unknown; *wk*, week; *y*, year; <, less than; >, greater than; ≥, greater than or equal to.

Pharmacokinetics EPO can be administered either subcutaneously or intravenously. The IV route for either drug results in a more rapid peak, whereas the subcutaneous route, with its delayed systemic absorption, gives a more sustained response. Serum half-life for darbepoetin alfa after IV administration is 22.1 hours in patients without chronic renal failure (CRF). With subcutaneous injections, peak plasma concentrations occur at 71 to 123 hours (in CRF, peak is 24 to 72 hours), and the half-life of darbepoetin alfa in patients with CRF ranges from 27 to 89 hours. The pharmacokinetics in children suggests darbepoetin is absorbed more rapidly after subcut injection when compared with adults.

Pharmacodynamics EPO stimulates erythropoiesis as endogenous EPO. Exogenous EPO stimulates the bone marrow in the production of RBCs to transport oxygen.

Side Effects and Adverse Reactions

Absolute contraindications for EPO include hypertension or hypersensitivity to albumin, hamster protein, or polysorbate 80. Black-box warnings include patients with a hemoglobin (Hgb) concentration greater than 11 g/dL, those who have had myocardial infarction (MI) or stroke, and patients with neoplastic or thromboembolic disease because of the increased risk of death. Other side effects and adverse reactions are similar to those of epoetin alfa. Table 34.3 compares the black-box warnings for IFNs, IL-2, and EPO.

Drug Interactions

⚡ Darbepoetin alfa and epoetin alfa should not be used concomitantly because of the danger of adverse reactions. Concurrent administration of androgens can increase the patient's response to EPO. In addition, the patient's iron stores should be repleted because inadequate iron interferes with EPO's therapeutic response.

Granulocyte Colony–Stimulating Factor

Endogenous granulocyte colony-stimulating factor (G-CSF) is produced by macrophages, endothelium, and other immune cells and stimulates the synthesis of neutrophils. Neutrophils are the most abundant WBCs that take part in the inflammatory response system, and their main function is to detect and destroy harmful bacteria. Recombinant DNA technology can produce CSFs for human granulocytes to be used for myelodysplastic syndrome (MDS) and for patients receiving myelosuppressive cancer chemotherapy, induction or consolidation chemotherapy for acute myeloid leukemia (AML), and bone marrow transplantation for cancer; for severe, chronic neutropenia; and to increase the hematopoietic stem cells in stem cell donors prior to leukapheresis. Two commercially available forms are filgrastim and pegfilgrastim. Unlike filgrastim, pegfilgrastim is administered once per chemotherapy cycle. Prototype Drug Chart 34.2 provides specific drug information for filgrastim.

Granulocyte-Macrophage Colony–Stimulating Factor

Granulocyte-macrophage colony–stimulating factor (GM-CSF), or *sargramostim*, belongs to a group of growth factors that support survival, proliferation, and differentiation (maturation) of hematopoietic progenitor cells. It induces partially committed progenitor (parent) cells to divide and differentiate in the granulocyte-macrophage pathway. GM-CSF, unlike G-CSF, is a multilineage factor that promotes proliferation of myelomonocytic, megakaryocytic, and erythroid progenitors. It is primarily produced by the bone marrow, B and T lymphocytes, and monocytes (immature macrophages). Commercially prepared GM-CSF came about through recombinant DNA technology and is FDA approved for use to reduce neutropenia and promote myeloid recovery in patients receiving myelosuppressive chemotherapy or bone marrow transplant (BMT), for mobilization of autologous peripheral blood progenitor cells, and in BMT failure or delayed engraftment. Prototype Drug Chart 34.3 provides specific drug information for sargramostim.

INTERLEUKIN 2

Interleukins are a group of signaling-molecule proteins produced by leukocytes, more specifically by T lymphocytes.

PROTOTYPE DRUG CHART 34.2

Filgrastim

Drug Class	Dosage
Granulocyte colony–stimulating factor Pregnancy category: C*	Chronic neutropenia, chemotherapy-induced neutropenia prophylaxis, following induction or consolidation therapy for AML; prophylaxis in nonmyeloid cancer A/C: IV/subcut: 5 mcg/kg/d HIV or drug therapy-induced neutropenia: C/A: Subcut: 5-10 mcg/kg/d 1 to 3 times weekly to maintain ANC of 2,000-10,000/mm^3. Refer to specific protocols.

Contraindications	Drug-Lab-Food Interactions
Absolute: Hypersensitivity to *Escherichia coli*–derived proteins or 24 h before or after cytotoxic chemotherapy Precaution: Pregnancy, lactation, latex hypersensitivity, leukemia, leukocytosis, obstetric delivery, pulmonary bleeding, radiation therapy, respiratory distress syndrome, sickle cell disease, vasculitis, thrombocytopenia	Drug: No clinically important drug interactions have been noted, but drugs that can increase the release of neutrophils (e.g., lithium) should be used with caution. Lab: Leukocytosis, thrombocytopenia, proteinuria, elevated LDH, and increased ALP Food: None known

Pharmacokinetics	Pharmacodynamics
Absolute bioavailability with subcut route is 60%-70%. Absorption: Subcut: Well absorbed Distribution: PB: UK Metabolism: t½: 1.8-3.5 h Excretion: Mainly by the kidneys; clearance is nonlinear and dependent on drug concentration and neutrophil count.	Onset: UK Peak: 2-8 h Duration: ANC decreases to baseline in approximately 4 d.

Therapeutic Effects/Uses

To decrease incidence of infection in patients with MDS; in those receiving myelosuppressive chemotherapeutic agents, including patients with AML undergoing induction or consolidation therapy; in aplastic anemia; and for mobilization of progenitor stem cells used in autologous transplant; also for treatment of patients with severe chronic neutropenia

Mode of Action: Increases production, maturation, and activation of neutrophils and enhances their migration and cytotoxicity

Side Effects	Adverse Reactions
Most common side effects include nausea, vomiting, arthralgia, alopecia, diarrhea, fever, fatigue, skin rash, anorexia, cephalgia, cough, chest pain, sore throat, constipation, dizziness, and dyspnea.	Splenomegaly, thrombocytopenia, MI, ARDS, splenic rupture, capillary leak syndrome, anaphylactoid reactions, glomerulonephritis, pulmonary bleeding/alveolar hemorrhage, and cutaneous vasculitis

*Pregnancy categories have been revised. See http://www.fda.gov/Drugs/DevelopmentApprovalProcess/DevelopmentResources/Labeling/ucm093307.htm for more information.

A, Adult; *ALP,* alkaline phosphatase; *AML,* acute myelogenous leukemia; *ANC,* absolute neutrophil count; *ARDS,* acute respiratory distress syndrome; *C,* child; *d,* day; *h,* hour; *IV,* intravenous; *LDH,* lactate dehydrogenase; *MDS,* myelodysplastic syndrome; *MI,* myocardial infarction; *PB,* protein binding; *subcut,* subcutaneous; *t½,* half-life; *UK,* unknown.

PROTOTYPE DRUG CHART 34.3

Sargramostim

Drug Class	Dosage
Granulocyte-macrophage colony–stimulating factor Pregnancy category: C*	Following reinfusion of BMT: A: 250 mcg/m^2/d subcut or IV over 24 h Following failed or delayed engraftment from BMT: A: 250 mcg/m^2/d subcut or IV over 2 h for 14 d; may repeat after having 7 d off therapy. If a third dose is warranted, give 500 mcg/m^2/d for 14 d after 7 d off therapy. Other dosing protocols are available.

Contraindications	Drug-Lab-Food Interactions
Absolute: Concomitant use with chemotherapy and/or radiation therapy or within 24 h of chemotherapy administration or within 12 h after last dose of radiation therapy; yeast hypersensitivity; excessive leukemic blasts ($\geq$ 10%) in the bone marrow or peripheral blood *Caution:* Pregnancy, lactation, cardiac arrhythmias, heart failure, leukemia, mannitol hypersensitivity, neonates, pulmonary disorders, leukocytosis	Drug: Drugs having synergistic effects may increase leukocytosis (e.g., lithium and corticosteroids); however, formal drug interaction data are currently not available. Sargramostim may increase the activity of zidovudine. Lab: Leukocytosis including neutrophilia, hyperbilirubinemia, elevated transaminases and serum creatinine Food: None known

Pharmacokinetics	Pharmacodynamics
Absorption: IV: Essentially complete Distribution: PB: UK Metabolism: t½: 1 h (IV); 2.7 h (subcut) Excretion: Mostly in urine as inactive protein fragments	Onset: 7-14 d Peak: 1-3 h (subcut) Duration: Baseline WBCs within 1 wk of stopping therapy

Therapeutic Effects/Uses

To accelerate growth and development of myeloid cell lines to shorten neutropenic state, to mobilize peripheral blood progenitor cells for collection, and for bone marrow graft failure or engraftment delay

Mode of Action: Stimulates the proliferation and differentiation of myeloid cell lines to enhance immune defense mechanism; enhances the function of mature granulocytes and monocytes; enhances bacteriocidal activity of neutrophils

Side Effects	Adverse Reactions
Generally well tolerated, but SEs may occur. Common SEs include arthralgia, myalgia, diarrhea, fatigue, chills, weakness, asthenia, cephalgia, malaise, unspecified chest pain, local irritation at injection site, peripheral edema, rash, and fever.	Pleural/pericardial effusion, capillary leak syndrome, anaphylactoid reactions, rigors, GI hemorrhage, dyspnea, hypotension

*Pregnancy categories have been revised. See http://www.fda.gov/Drugs/DevelopmentApprovalProcess/DevelopmentResources/Labeling/ucm093307.htm for more information.

A, Adult; *BMT,* bone marrow transplant; *C,* child; *d,* day; *GI,* gastrointestinal; *h,* hour; *IV,* intravenous; *PB,* protein binding; *SEs,* side effects; *subcut,* subcutaneous; *t½,* half-life; *UK,* unknown; *WBC,* white blood cell; *wk,* week; $\geq$, greater than or equal to.

TABLE 34.4 Interleukin 2*

Generic	Route and Dosage	Uses and Considerations
Aldesleukin	Two 5-d treatment periods are separated by a rest period. A: IV: 600,000 units/kg (0.037 mg/kg) over 15 min q8h; *max*: 14 doses. Following 9 d of rest, repeat the schedule for another 14 doses; *max*: 28 doses per course	For metastatic renal cancer and metastatic melanoma *Do not* give dexamethasone during treatment unless absolutely necessary; it may negate the effects of IL-2. Pregnancy category: C†

*Patients receiving IL-2 by any route, in any dose, and in any setting—inpatient or outpatient—should be monitored closely for signs of toxicity.
†Pregnancy categories have been revised. See http://www.fda.gov/Drugs/DevelopmentApprovalProcess/DevelopmentResources/Labeling/ucm093307.htm for more information.
A, Adult; *d,* day; *h,* hour; *IL,* interleukin; *IV,* intravenous; *max,* maximum; *min,* minute; *q,* every.

⚡ BOX 34.1 Absolute Contraindications for Aldesleukin

Angina
Cardiac arrhythmias
Cardiac disease
Cardiac tamponade
Coma
Gastrointestinal bleeding
Gastrointestinal perforation
Myocardial infarction
Organ transplant
Psychosis
Pulmonary disease
Renal failure
Respiratory insufficiency
Seizures
Ventricular tachycardia

Because interleukins are hormonelike glycoproteins manufactured by T lymphocytes, they are sometimes called lymphokines. Interleukins also increase the growth and activity of other T cells and B cells, which affect the immune response system. One of the most widely studied interleukins is interleukin 2 (IL-2). Table 34.4 provides information on IL-2 and includes dosages, uses, and considerations.

IL-2 is produced commercially through recombinant DNA technology as aldesleukin and is FDA approved for treatment of metastatic renal cell carcinoma and metastatic melanoma to induce proliferation and differentiation of B and T cells along with other cells involved in the immune system. Table 34.2 lists common adverse effects with IL-2 therapy.

Pharmacokinetics Aldesleukin is administered intravenously or subcutaneously and is rapidly distributed to the extravascular and extracellular spaces and to the liver, spleen, kidneys, and lungs. Following IV administration, the serum distribution and elimination half-life is 13 and 85 minutes, respectively. Following subcutaneous injection, the serum levels were slightly prolonged. Aldesleukin is cleared from the systemic circulation by the kidneys and is then metabolized into amino acids by the renal cells; the drug is also affected by the cytochrome P450 isoenzymes.

Pharmacodynamics Aldesleukin has essentially identical effects to those of endogenous IL-2. The interaction of the drug with the IL-2 receptors stimulates the cytokine cascade and involves various IFNs, interleukins, and tumor necrosis factors (TNFs). Along with these other cytokines, aldesleukin induces proliferation and differentiation of B and T lymphocytes, monocytes, macrophages, and natural killer cells, among others.

Side Effects and Adverse Reactions

The black-box warning includes patients with cardiac disease, coma, capillary leak syndrome, infection, and pulmonary disease and warns that the drug must be administered in a specialized care setting by an experienced clinician. Table 34.3 compares the black-box warnings for IFNs, IL-2, and EPO. Box 34.1 lists absolute contraindications for aldesleukin.

Conventional high-dose IV bolus aldesleukin is associated ❶ with significant adverse reactions that affect almost every organ system. Many of the adverse effects may be due to capillary leak syndrome, which results from extravasation of plasma proteins and fluid into the extravascular space and leads to vascular atony. Vascular tone is lost within 2 to 12 hours of starting aldesleukin and causes decreased arterial pressure and decreased organ perfusion, resulting in multiorgan dysfunction that leads to death. Once the drug is discontinued, the capillary leak syndrome resolves within a few hours. Other side effects and adverse reactions include hyperglycemia, diabetes, metabolic and respiratory acidosis, and electrolyte imbalance (e.g., hypomagnesemia and hypocalcemia). Because of the many potential adverse effects, patients must be selected with care, and those with significant cardiac, pulmonary, renal, hepatic, or central nervous system impairments must be excluded. Table 34.5 provides information on aldesleukin for dose interruption or discontinuation for drug toxicity.

Drug Interactions

Because of the number of serious adverse effects associated with aldesleukin therapy, almost any other drug represents a potential interaction. And because aldesleukin is associated with kidney and liver toxicity, other drugs known to cause such toxicity can exacerbate the impairment caused by aldesleukin (e.g., vancomycin, cyclosporine, nonsteroidal antiinflammatory drugs [NSAIDs], methotrexate, isoniazid [INH], and ethanol). Antihypertensives (e.g., beta blockers and calcium channel blockers) can worsen hypotension. The immune response from vaccines may be decreased if given to those who are immunocompromised and receiving aldesleukin.

⚡ PATIENT SAFETY

Do not confuse...
- **Interferon alfa-2a** with **interferon alfa-2b**
- **Interferon alfa** with **interferon-β** or **interferon gamma**
- **Interleukin 2** with **interferon 2**
- **Darbepoetin alfa** with **epoetin alfa**

TABLE 34.5 Aldesleukin* Dose Interruption or Discontinuation

Body System	Interruption†	Discontinue Permanently
Mental health	Any changes to mental status, including confusion or agitation	Coma or toxic psychosis lasting more than 48 h, poorly managed seizures
Skin, hair, and nails	New bullous dermatitis or worsening of preexisting skin condition; may treat with antihistamines; *do not* treat with topical steroids.	
❗ Cardiovascular	Atrial fibrillation, SVT, or bradycardia that is persistent, recurrent, or needs treatment SBP <90 mm Hg if it requires vasopressors ECG changes consistent with MI, ischemia, or myocarditis	Sustained ventricular tachycardia ≥5 beats Uncontrolled cardiac rhythm disturbances ECG changes that show MI or cardiac tamponade
Pulmonary	O_2 saturation <90%	Requiring intubation >72 h
Endocrine	Hypoglycemia	
Hematology	Sepsis	
GI/GU	Stool guaiac repeatedly >3-4+; serum creatinine >4.5 mg/dL or ≥4 mg/dL with severe volume overload, acidosis, or hyperkalemia; persistent oliguria, UO <10 mL/h for 16-24 h with increasing serum creatinine	Renal failure that requires dialysis >72 h; bowel ischemia or perforation or GI bleeding that requires surgery
Hepatobiliary	Hepatic failure, including encephalopathy, ascites, liver pain, hypoglycemia	

❗ *Aldesleukin must be withheld or interrupt a dose due to drug toxicity; *do not reduce dose.*
†May be resumed with dose adjustment once toxicity has resolved.
ECG, Electrocardiograph; *GI/GU,* gastrointestinal/genitourinary; *h,* hours; *MI,* myocardial infarction; O_2, oxygen; *SBP,* systolic blood pressure; *SVT,* supraventricular tachycardia; *UO,* urine output<, less than; >, greater than; ≥, greater than or equal to.

◎ NURSING PROCESS
Patient-Centered Collaborative Care

Biologic Response Modifiers

Assessment
- Conduct a detailed current medication history that includes prescriptions, over-the-counter (OTC) medicines, antacids, dietary supplements, vitamins, and herbal supplements.
- Obtain a list of the patient's drug and food allergies.
- Obtain baseline information about physical status that includes height, weight, vital signs, cardiopulmonary assessment, intake and output, skin assessment, nutritional status, and any underlying diseases.
- Obtain baseline laboratory values (CBC with differentials and platelet count, uric acid, chemistry panel, lipid panel, and thyroid panel) before and during treatment.
- ⚡ With erythropoietin-stimulating agents, assess serum ferritin and serum iron–transferrin saturation. Most patients will need supplemental iron.
- Assess baseline results of pulmonary function tests, chest radiographs, ECG, and kidney and liver function studies.
- Assess patient's and caregiver's level of comprehension and physical ability related to the therapeutic regimen.

Nursing Diagnoses
- Injury, Risk for
- Infection, Risk for
- Knowledge, Deficient related to immunotherapy regimen

Planning
- The patient and caregivers will verbalize signs and symptoms of significant reactions (e.g., wheezing; chest pain; swelling of face, neck, lips, throat, or tongue; emotional instability; altered speaking or thinking; and excessive weight gain or loss).
- The patient and caregivers will verbalize when to notify the health care provider or seek emergency treatment.
- The patient will remain free from infection.
- The patient and caregivers will verbalize understanding of immunotherapy as part of an anticancer treatment regimen.

Nursing Interventions
- Assess for any cardiac events, such as new chest pain and ECG changes.
- ⚡ Monitor appropriate labs according to established protocol for the specific immunotherapy (e.g., CBC with differential, electrolytes, renal and hepatic function, and glucose).
- Assess for bleeding, especially in patients taking anticoagulants, antiplatelets, or NSAIDs.
- Monitor renal and hepatic function at baseline and per treatment protocol.
- Examine the patient's skin closely at each visit for the presence of erythema, rash, peeling, or blister formation, and rate the severity of any dermatologic reactions.
- ⚡ During treatment, monitor patients for any indications of adverse effects such as fever, chills, hypoxia, wheezing, bradycardia or tachycardia, hypotension or hypertension, arrhythmia, or seizures.

- Premedicate patients with acetaminophen to reduce chills and fever and with diphenhydramine to reduce histamine effects.
- Have resuscitative equipment on standby as per protocol.
- Actively listen to patient and caregiver concerns, and explain in laymen's terms the immunotherapy being used as part of the patient's cancer treatment regimen.

Patient Teaching

- Report symptoms of bleeding immediately; these include black stools, vomit that looks like coffee grounds, easy bleeding/bruising, or hematuria.
- Report symptoms of adverse effects or severe side effects promptly, especially chest pain; swelling of the face, neck, tongue, or lips; weight gain or loss; increasing shortness of breath; fever or chills; convulsions; or difficulty speaking.

- Advise patients and caregivers to immediately report convulsions, persistent headache, reduced eyesight, increased blood pressure, or blurred vision.

Evaluation

- The patient is free of further injury related to immunotherapy.
- Side effects are managed effectively.
- The patient is free from infection.
- Patient, family, and caregiver education needs are met.
- The patient, family, and caregivers understand therapy-related side effects and adverse reactions.
- The patient, family, and caregivers understand strategies to minimize side effects and adverse reactions.

CRITICAL THINKING CASE STUDY

JW, a 75-year-old man, has metastatic non–small cell cancer of the lung. His past treatment regimen included external-beam chest irradiation and combination chemotherapy. Two weeks before hospitalization, JW received a course of carboplatin and paclitaxel as an outpatient. He was admitted to the hospital with neutropenia, thrombocytopenia, and anemia. Upon assessment, he was cachectic and weak but was able to perform activities of daily living with only minimal assistance. Admitting laboratory data were hemoglobin (Hgb) 6.9 g/dL, hematocrit (Hct) 20.6%, platelets $16 \times 10^3/\mu L$, a white blood cell (WBC) count of $6 \times 10^3/\mu L$ with absolute neutrophil

count (ANC) of $0.096 \times 10^3/\mu L$. JW was started on erythropoietin 40,000 units subcutaneously once a week and filgrastim, G-CSF 5 mcg/kg/day given subcutaneously. Parenteral antibiotic therapy was also initiated.

1. Why were filgrastim and erythropoietin (EPO) indicated?
2. What must be monitored closely in patients receiving EPO and why?
3. List three nursing diagnoses for this patient.
4. Identify three nursing actions for each of the nursing diagnoses identified in question 3 above.

NCLEX STUDY QUESTIONS

1. A patient is being seen regularly for treatment of chronic leukemia. The nurse understands that this patient has been treated with interferon-alfa. What is the primary action of this biologic response modifier?
   a. Enhancing immune function, producing white blood cells, producing antigen/antibody reaction
   b. Causing allergic reactions, producing red blood cells, producing interferon
   c. Immunomodulation, causing cytotoxic/cytostatic effects, differentiating stem cells
   d. Producing cytokines, producing interleukin, fighting infection

2. A patient diagnosed with malignant melanoma, a skin cancer, is treated with interferon alfa-2a. The nurse teaches this patient about which side effect that will make the patient uncomfortable?
   a. Increase in white blood cells
   b. Increase in red blood cells
   c. Flulike syndrome
   d. Gastrointestinal symptoms

3. A patient has anemia. The nurse reviews the list of medications and is aware that red blood cell production can be stimulated with which drug?
   a. Epoetin alfa
   b. Filgrastim
   c. Interleukin 2
   d. Sargramostim

4. The nurse is caring for a patient who has previously received a biologic response modifier as a subcutaneous injection. The patient will now be receiving a drug that is not often used in clinical practice because of its serious side effects and must be administered by intravenous infusion. Which drug meets this criterion?
   a. Epoetin alfa
   b. Interleukin 2
   c. Granulocyte colony–stimulating factor
   d. Granulocyte-macrophage colony–stimulating factor

5. A patient lives 120 miles from her oncologist's medical office and relies on her working son for transportation to and from the doctor's office. In developing a plan of care for the patient, the nurse understands that the order for pegfilgrastim was prescribed for what reason?
   a. Pegfilgrastim is eliminated via the kidneys.
   b. Pegfilgrastim is a pegylated filgrastim.
   c. Pegfilgrastim is not easily eliminated from the body.
   d. Pegfilgrastim requires injection once per chemotherapy cycle.

6. The nurse is caring for a patient who arrives at the outpatient office for a scheduled dose of an erythropoietin-stimulating agent to be administered. The patient arrives with the following laboratory values noted on the chart: hemoglobin, 12.8 mg/dL; platelet count, 148,000/mm^2; white blood cell count, 4800/mm^2. Which action is most appropriate for the nurse to implement?
   a. Discuss with the health care provider the potential need for a colony-stimulating factor such as granulocyte colony–stimulating factor based on the laboratory results.
   b. Contact the health care provider to discuss the laboratory results and a possible discontinuation of the ordered erythropoietin-stimulating agent.
   c. After comparing the patient's laboratory results with the previous results, discuss the laboratory values with the health care provider to determine whether a colony-stimulating factor such as interleukin 2 should be given.
   d. Discuss with the health care provider the potential need for more laboratory tests prior to administration of the erythropoietin-stimulating agent.

Answers: 1, a; 2, c; 3, a; 4, b; 5, d; 6, b.

Respiratory Drugs

The respiratory tract is divided into two major parts: the *upper respiratory tract,* which consists of the nares, nasal cavity, pharynx, and larynx, and the *lower respiratory tract,* which consists of the trachea, bronchi, bronchioles, alveoli, and alveolar-capillary membrane. Air enters through the upper respiratory tract and travels to the lower respiratory tract, where gas exchanges occur. Fig XI.1 illustrates these components.

Ventilation and *respiration* are distinct terms and should not be used interchangeably. Ventilation is the movement of air from the atmosphere through the upper and lower airways to the alveoli. *Respiration* is the process whereby gas exchange occurs at the alveolar-capillary membrane. Respiration has three phases:

1. *Ventilation* is the phase in which oxygen passes through the airways. With every inspiration, air is moved into the lungs, and with every expiration, air is transported out of the lungs.

2. *Perfusion* involves blood flow at the alveolar-capillary bed. Perfusion is influenced by alveolar

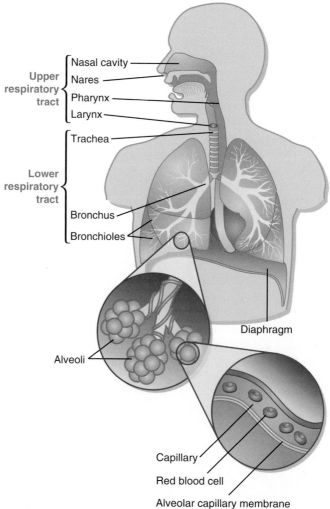

Upper respiratory tract
- Nasal cavity
- Nares
- Pharynx
- Larynx

Lower respiratory tract
- Trachea
- Bronchus
- Bronchioles

Diaphragm

Alveoli

Capillary

Red blood cell

Alveolar capillary membrane

FIG XI.1 Basic Structures of the Respiratory Tract.

pressure. For gas exchange to occur, the perfusion of each alveolus must be matched by adequate ventilation. Factors such as mucosal edema, secretions, and bronchospasm increase resistance to air flow and decrease ventilation and diffusion of gases.

3. *Diffusion,* the movement of molecules from higher to lower concentrations, takes place when oxygen passes into the capillary bed to be circulated and carbon dioxide leaves the capillary bed and diffuses into the alveoli for ventilatory excretion.

The chest cavity is a closed compartment bounded by 12 ribs, the diaphragm, thoracic vertebrae, sternum, neck muscles, and intercostal muscles between the ribs. The pleurae are membranes that encase the lungs. The lungs are divided into lobes; the right lung has three lobes, and the left lung has two lobes. The heart, which is not attached to the lungs, lies on the mid-left side in the chest cavity.

LUNG COMPLIANCE

Lung compliance is the lung volume based on the pressure in the alveoli. This volume determines the lung's ability to stretch. Factors that influence lung compliance include (1) connective tissue (collagen and elastin) and (2) surface tension in the alveoli, which is controlled by surfactant. Surfactant lowers the surface tension in the alveoli and prevents interstitial fluid from entering. Increased lung compliance is present with chronic obstructive pulmonary disease (COPD), and decreased lung compliance occurs with restrictive pulmonary disease. With low compliance, there is decreased lung volume resulting from increased connective tissue or increased surface tension. The lungs become "stiff," and it takes greater-than-normal pressure to expand lung tissue.

CONTROL OF RESPIRATION

Oxygen (O_2), carbon dioxide (CO_2), and hydrogen (H^+) ion concentration in the blood influence respiration. *Chemoreceptors* are sensors that are stimulated by changes in these gases and ions. The central chemoreceptors, located in the medulla near the respiratory center and cerebrospinal fluid, respond to an increase in CO_2 and a decrease in pH by increasing ventilation. However, if the CO_2 level remains elevated, the stimulus to increase ventilation is lost.

Peripheral chemoreceptors, located in the carotid and aortic bodies, respond to changes in oxygen (PO_2) levels. A low blood oxygen level (PO_2 <60 mm Hg) stimulates the peripheral chemoreceptors, which in turn stimulate the respiratory center in the medulla, and ventilation is increased. If oxygen therapy increases the oxygen level in the blood, the PO_2 may be too high to stimulate the peripheral chemoreceptors, and ventilation will be depressed.

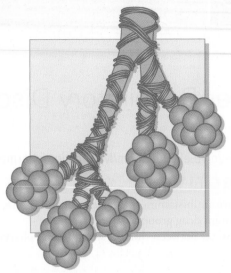

FIG XI.2 Bronchial smooth muscle fibers become more closely spaced as they near the alveoli.

BRONCHIAL SMOOTH MUSCLE

The tracheobronchial tube is composed of smooth muscle whose fibers spiral around the tracheobronchial tube, becoming more closely spaced as they near the terminal bronchioles (Fig. XI.2). Contraction of these muscles constricts the airway. The sympathetic and parasympathetic nervous systems affect the bronchial smooth muscle in opposite ways. The vagus nerve (parasympathetic nervous system) releases acetylcholine, which causes bronchoconstriction. The sympathetic nervous system releases epinephrine, which stimulates the beta$_2$ receptor in the bronchial smooth muscle, resulting in bronchodilation. These two nervous systems counterbalance each other to maintain homeostasis.

Cyclic adenosine monophosphate (cAMP) in the cytoplasm of bronchial cells increases bronchodilation by relaxing the bronchial smooth muscles. The pulmonary enzyme phosphodiesterase can inactivate cAMP. Drugs of the methylxanthine group (theophylline) inactivate phosphodiesterase, thus permitting cAMP to function.

This unit includes Chapter 35, Upper Respiratory Disorders, and Chapter 36, Lower Respiratory Disorders. Chapter 35 discusses drugs used to relieve cold symptoms, such as antihistamines, decongestants, antitussives, and expectorants. Drugs used to alleviate and control airway obstruction are presented in Chapter 36. These include the sympathomimetics (adrenergics), particularly the beta$_2$ adrenergics; methylxanthines such as theophylline; leukotriene receptor antagonists; glucocorticoids; cromolyn sodium; and mucolytics.

35

Upper Respiratory Disorders

OBJECTIVES

- Compare antihistamine, decongestant, antitussive, and expectorant drug groups.
- Differentiate between rhinitis, sinusitis, and pharyngitis.
- Describe the side effects of nasal decongestants and how they can be avoided.
- Apply the nursing process for drugs used to treat the common cold.

OUTLINE

KEY TERMS

Upper respiratory infections (URIs) include the common cold, acute rhinitis, sinusitis, and acute pharyngitis. The **common cold** is the most prevalent type of URI. Adults have an average of 2 to 4 colds per year, and children have an average of 4 to 12 colds per year. Incidence is seasonally variable: approximately 50% of the population experiences a winter cold and 25% experiences a summer cold. A cold is not considered a life-threatening illness, but it does cause physical and mental discomfort and lost time at work and school. The common cold is an expensive illness in the United States—more than $60 billion is spent each year on over-the-counter (OTC) cold and cough preparations in addition to missed time at work and school.

COMMON COLD, ACUTE RHINITIS, AND ALLERGIC RHINITIS

The common cold is caused by the rhinovirus and affects primarily the nasopharyngeal tract. **Acute rhinitis**, acute inflammation of the mucous membranes of the nose, usually accompanies the common cold. Acute rhinitis is not the same as **allergic rhinitis**, often called *hay fever,* which is caused by pollen or a foreign substance such as animal dander. Nasal secretions increase in both acute and allergic rhinitis.

A cold is most contagious 1 to 4 days before the onset of symptoms (the incubation period) and during the first 3 days of the cold. Transmission occurs more frequently from touching contaminated surfaces and then touching the nose or mouth than it does from contact with viral droplets released by sneezing.

The groups of drugs used to manage cold symptoms include antihistamines (H_1 blockers), decongestants (sympathomimetic amines), antitussives, and expectorants. These drugs can be used singly or in combination preparations.

Symptoms of the common cold include **rhinorrhea** (watery nasal discharge), nasal congestion, cough, and increased mucosal secretions. If a bacterial infection secondary to the cold occurs, infectious rhinitis may result, and nasal discharge becomes tenacious, mucoid, and yellow or yellow green. The nasal secretions are discolored by white blood cells and cellular debris that are by-products of the fight against the bacterial infection. Antibiotics used to treat bacterial respiratory infections are discussed in Chapter 26.

Antihistamines

Antihistamines, H_1 blockers or H_1 antagonists, compete with histamine for receptor sites and prevent a histamine response. The two types of histamine receptors, H_1 and H_2, cause different responses. When the H_1 receptor is stimulated, the extravascular smooth muscles—including those lining the nasal cavity—are constricted. With stimulation of the H_2 receptor, an increase in gastric secretions occurs, which is a cause of peptic ulcer (see Chapter 43). These two types of histamine receptors should not be confused. Antihistamines decrease nasopharyngeal secretions by blocking the H_1 receptor.

Although antihistamines are commonly used as cold remedies, these agents can also treat allergic rhinitis. However, the antihistamines are not useful in an emergency situation such as anaphylaxis. Most antihistamines are rapidly absorbed in 15 minutes, but they are not potent enough to combat anaphylaxis.

First-Generation Antihistamines

The antihistamine group can be divided into first and second generations. Most *first-generation antihistamines* cause drowsiness, dry mouth, and other anticholinergic symptoms, whereas *second-generation antihistamines* have fewer anticholinergic effects and a lower incidence of drowsiness. Many OTC cold remedies contain a first-generation antihistamine, which can cause drowsiness; therefore patients should be alerted not to drive or operate dangerous machinery when taking such medications. The anticholinergic properties of most antihistamines cause dryness of the mouth and decreased secretions, making them useful in treating rhinitis caused by the common cold. Antihistamines also decrease the nasal itching and tickling that cause sneezing.

The first-generation antihistamine diphenhydramine has been available for years and is frequently combined with other ingredients in cold remedy preparations. Its primary use is to treat rhinitis. Prototype Drug Chart 35.1 lists the pharmacologic behavior of diphenhydramine.

Pharmacokinetics Diphenhydramine can be administered orally, intramuscularly (IM), or intravenously (IV). It is well absorbed from the gastrointestinal (GI) tract, but systemic absorption from topical use is minimal. It is highly protein bound (98%) and has an average half-life of 2 to 8 hours. Diphenhydramine is metabolized by the liver and is excreted as metabolites in the urine.

Pharmacodynamics Diphenhydramine blocks the effects of histamine by competing for and occupying H_1 receptor sites. It has anticholinergic effects and should not be used by patients with narrow-angle glaucoma. Drowsiness is a major side effect of the drug; in fact, it is sometimes used in sleep-aid products. Diphenhydramine is also used as an antitussive to alleviate cough. Its onset of action can occur in as few as 15 minutes when taken orally and IM. Intravenous administration results in an immediate onset of action. The duration of action is 4 to 7 hours.

Diphenhydramine can cause central nervous system (CNS) depression if taken with alcohol, narcotics, hypnotics, or barbiturates.

⚡ PATIENT SAFETY

Do not confuse
• **Benadryl,** an antihistamine, with **benazepril,** an angiotensin-converting enzyme (ACE) inhibitor

📋 PROTOTYPE DRUG CHART 35.1
Diphenhydramine

Drug Class	Dosage
Antihistamine Pregnancy category: B*	A/C >12 y: PO: 25-50 mg q4-6h; *max:* 300 mg/d C 6-12 y: PO: 12.5-25 mg q4-6h; *max:* 150 mg/d A: IM/IV: 10-50 mg as single dose IV or IM q4-6h; *max:* 400 mg/d C: IM/IV: 5 mg/kg/d in 4 divided doses; *max:* 300 mg/d
Contraindications	**Drug-Lab-Food Interactions**
Acute asthmatic attack, severe liver disease, COPD, neonate *Caution:* Narrow-angle glaucoma, prostatic hypertrophy, pregnancy, breastfeeding, urinary retention	Drug: Increased CNS depression with alcohol, opioids, hypnotics, and barbiturates; avoid use with MAOIs
Pharmacokinetics	**Pharmacodynamics**
Absorption: PO: Well absorbed Distribution: PB: 98% Metabolism: t½: 2-8 h Excretion: In urine as metabolites	PO: Onset: 15-30 min Peak: 2-4 h Duration: 4-6 h IM: Onset: 15-30 min Peak: 1-4 h Duration: 4-7 h IV: Onset: Immediate Peak: 0.5-1 h Duration: 4-7 h
Therapeutic Effects/Uses	
To treat allergic rhinitis, the common cold, cough, sneezing, pruritus, and urticaria and to prevent motion sickness Mode of Action: Competes with histamine for binding at H_1-receptor sites and antagonizes histamine effects	
Side Effects	**Adverse Reactions**
Drowsiness, dizziness, headache, asthenia, agitation, insomnia, urinary retention, blurred vision, dry mouth and throat, hypotension, abdominal pain, restlessness, constipation, photosensitivity, palpitations	*Life threatening:* Agranulocytosis, hemolytic anemia, thrombocytopenia

*Pregnancy categories have been revised. See http://www.fda.gov/Drugs/DevelopmentApprovalProcess/DevelopmentResources/Labeling/ucm093307.htm for more information.
A, Adult; *C,* child; *CNS,* central nervous system; *COPD,* chronic obstructive pulmonary disease; *d,* day; *h,* hour; *IM,* intramuscular; *IV,* intravenous; *MAOI,* monoamine oxidase inhibitor; *max,* maximum; *min,* minute; *PB,* protein binding; *PO,* by mouth; *q4-6h,* every 4 to 6 hours; *t½,* half-life; *y,* years; *>,* greater than.

Side Effects of Most First-Generation Antihistamines.
The most common side effects of first-generation antihistamines are drowsiness, dizziness, fatigue, and disturbed coordination. Skin rashes and anticholinergic symptoms such as dry mouth, urine retention, blurred vision, and wheezing may also occur.

Second-Generation Antihistamines

The second-generation antihistamines are frequently called *nonsedating antihistamines* because they have little to no sedative effect. In addition, these antihistamines cause fewer anticholinergic symptoms. Although a moderate amount of alcohol and other CNS depressants may be taken with second-generation antihistamines, many clinicians advise against such use.

The second-generation antihistamines cetirizine, fexofenadine, and loratadine have half-lives between 7 and 30 hours.

Azelastine is a second-generation antihistamine that has a half-life of 22 hours and is administered by nasal spray. Table 35.1 lists the first- and second-generation antihistamines used to treat allergic rhinitis.

TABLE 35.1 Antihistamines for Treatment of Allergic Rhinitis

Drug	Route and Dosage	Uses and Considerations
First-Generation Antihistamines		
Alkylamine Derivatives		
Brompheniramine tannate	Chewable tablets: A/adol/C >12 y: PO: 12-24 mg/d; *max*: 48 mg/d C 6-11 y: PO: 12 mg/d; *max*: 24 mg/d	For allergic rhinitis and conjunctivitis, common cold, and pruritus. May cause drowsiness, dizziness, insomnia, nervousness, headache, blurred vision, dry mouth, GI distress, palpitations, and tachycardia. Pregnancy category: C*; PB: 39%-49%; t½: 11.8-34.7 h
Chlorpheniramine	Immediate release: A/adol/C >12 y: PO: 4 mg q4-6h; *max*: 24 mg/d C 6-11 y: PO: 2 mg q4-6h; *max*: 12 mg/d Extended release: A/adol/C >12 y: 12-18 mg bid; *max*: 36 mg/d	For allergic rhinitis and conjunctivitis, as well as the common cold. May cause drowsiness, dizziness, headache, nervousness, dry mouth, thick bronchial secretions, weakness, GI distress, diplopia, and urinary retention. Pregnancy category: C*; PB: 72%; t½: 10-24 h
Ethanolamine Derivatives		
Clemastine fumarate	A/adol/C >12 y: PO: 1.34-2.68 mg bid/tid; *max*: 8 mg/d	For common cold, allergic rhinitis, and urticaria. May cause drowsiness, dizziness, nervousness, headache, dry mouth, weakness, palpitations, tachycardia, blurred vision, urinary retention, and GI distress. Pregnancy category: B*; PB: UK; t½: 4-6 h
Diphenhydramine	See Prototype Drug Chart 35.1.	
Piperidine Derivatives		
Cyproheptadine	A/adol >15 y: PO: 4-20 mg/d in divided doses; *max*: 32 mg/d C 7-14 y: PO: 4 mg bid/tid; *max*: 16 mg/d C 2-6 y: PO: 2 mg bid/tid; *max*: 12 mg/d	For allergies (rhinitis, conjunctivitis, pruritus, and urticaria). May cause drowsiness, dry mouth, dizziness, headache, thick bronchial secretions, insomnia, blurred vision, nervousness, palpitations, tachycardia, urinary retention, and GI distress. Pregnancy category: B*; PB: UK; t½: 1-4 h
Piperazine Derivatives		
Levocetirizine	A/adol/C >12 y: PO: 2.5-5 mg/d in the evening; *max*: 5 mg/d C 6-11 y: PO: 2.5 mg/d in the evening; *max*: 2.5 mg/d	For allergic rhinitis and chronic urticaria. May cause drowsiness, dizziness, blurred vision, weakness, dysgeusia, diarrhea, and constipation. Pregnancy category: B*; PB: 91%-92%; t½: 8-9 h
Other Antihistamines		
Azelastine and fluticasone	A/adol/C >6 y: Nasal spray: 1 spray per nostril bid; *max*: 2 sprays/nostril/d	For allergic rhinitis. May cause drowsiness, headache, dysphonia, dysgeusia, and epistaxis. Pregnancy category: C*; PB: 88%-97%; t½: 8-25 h
Second-Generation Antihistamines		
Azelastine	Nasal spray: A/adol/C ≥12 y: 1-2 sprays in each nostril q12h; *max*: 4 sprays/nostril/d C <11 y: 1 spray in each nostril bid; *max*: 2 sprays/nostril/d	For allergic rhinitis and conjunctivitis, as well as pruritus. May cause drowsiness, headache, blurred vision, dysgeusia, dry mouth, weakness, and dysesthesia. Pregnancy category: C*; PB: 88%; t½: 22 h
Cetirizine	A/adol/C >6 y: PO: 5-10 mg/d; *max*: 10 mg/d Older adults: PO: 5 mg/d; *max*: 5 mg/d C 2-5 y: PO: 2.5-5 mg/d; *max*: 5 mg/d	For allergic rhinitis and urticaria. May cause drowsiness, dizziness, headache, insomnia, dry mouth, weakness, and GI distress. Pregnancy category: B*; PB: 93%; t½: 6.5 to 10 h
Fexofenadine	A/adol/C ≥12 y: PO: 60 mg bid or 180 mg qd; *max*: 180 mg/d	For allergic rhinitis and chronic urticaria. May cause headache, nausea, and vomiting. Pregnancy category: C*; PB: 60%-70%; t½: 14.4 h
Loratadine	A/adol/C >6 y: PO: 10 mg/d; *max*: 10 mg/d	For allergic rhinitis, pruritus, and urticaria. May cause drowsiness, dizziness, headache, weakness, dry mouth, nervousness, and tachycardia. Pregnancy category: UK*; PB: 97%; t½: 3-20 h

TABLE 35.1	Antihistamines for Treatment of Allergic Rhinitis—cont'd	
Drug	**Route and Dosage**	**Uses and Considerations**
Desloratadine	A/adol/C >12 y: PO: 5 mg/d; *max.* 5 mg/d C 6-11 y: PO: 2.5 mg/d; *max.* 2.5 mg/d C 1-5 y: PO: 1.25 mg/d; *max.* 1.25 mg/d	For allergic rhinitis, chronic urticaria, and pruritus. May cause drowsiness, dizziness, headache, irritability, weakness, insomnia, nausea, vomiting, and diarrhea. Pregnancy category: C*; PB: 82%-87%; t½: 20 to 30 h

*Pregnancy categories have been revised. See http://www.fda.gov/Drugs/DevelopmentApprovalProcess/DevelopmentResources/Labeling/ucm093 307.htm for more information.

A, Adult; *adol*, adolescent; *bid*, twice a day; *C*, child; *d*, day; *GI*, gastrointestinal; *h*, hour; *max*, maximum; *PB*, protein binding; *PO*, by mouth; *q*, every; *qd*, every day; *t½*, half-life; *tid*, three times a day; *UK*, unknown; *y*, years ; *>*, greater than; *≥*, greater than or equal to; *<*, less than.

 NURSING PROCESS
Patient-Centered Collaborative Care

Antihistamine: Diphenhydramine

Assessment
- Determine baseline vital signs.
- Obtain a drug history, and report if a drug-drug interaction is probable.
- Assess for signs and symptoms of urinary dysfunction, including retention, dysuria, and altered frequency.
- Note complete blood count (CBC) during drug therapy.
- Assess cardiac and respiratory status.
- Obtain a history of environmental exposures that includes drugs, recent foods eaten, and stress.

Nursing Diagnoses
- Airway Clearance, Ineffective related to nasal congestion
- Fluid Volume, Risk for Imbalanced
- Sleep Deprivation related to frequent coughing

Planning
- Patient will have decreased nasal congestion, mucosal secretions, and cough.
- Patient will sleep 6 to 8 hours per night.

Nursing Interventions
- Give the oral form of the drug with food to decrease gastric distress.
- Administer the intramuscular form in a large muscle. *Avoid subcutaneous injection.*

Patient Teaching
General
- ⚡ Warn patients to avoid driving a motor vehicle and performing other dangerous activities if drowsiness occurs or until stabilized on the drug.
- ⚡ Advise patients to avoid alcohol and other central nervous system depressants.
- Encourage patients to take drugs as prescribed. Notify a health care provider if confusion or hypotension occurs.
- Teach patients on prophylaxis for motion sickness to take the drug at least 30 minutes before the offending event and also before meals and at bedtime during the event.

- Inform breastfeeding mothers that small amounts of drug pass into breast milk. Because children are more susceptible to the side effects of antihistamines (e.g., unusual excitement or irritability), breastfeeding is not recommended while using these drugs.

Side Effects
- Advise family members or parents that children are more sensitive to the effects of antihistamines. Nightmares, nervousness, and irritability are more likely to occur in children.
- Inform older adults that they are more sensitive to the effects of antihistamines and are more likely to experience confusion, difficult or painful urination, dizziness, drowsiness, feeling faint, and dryness of the mouth, nose, or throat.
- Suggest using sugarless candy or gum, ice chips, or a saliva substitute for temporary relief of mouth dryness.

 Cultural Considerations
- Decrease language barriers by decoding jargon used in the health care environment for those with language difficulties and for those who are not in the health care field.

Evaluation
- Evaluate effectiveness of the drug in relieving allergic symptoms or as a sleep aid.

Nasal and Systemic Decongestants

Nasal congestion results from dilation of nasal blood vessels caused by infection, inflammation, or allergy. With this dilation, a transudation of fluid into the tissue spaces occurs that results in swelling of the nasal cavity. Nasal **decongestants** (sympathomimetic amines) stimulate the alpha-adrenergic receptors, producing vascular constriction (vasoconstriction) of the capillaries within the nasal mucosa. The result is shrinking of the nasal mucous membranes and a reduction in fluid secretion (runny nose).

Nasal decongestants are administered by nasal spray or drops or in tablet, capsule, or liquid form. Frequent use of decongestants, especially nasal spray or drops, can result in tolerance and **rebound nasal congestion**, rebound vasodilation instead of vasoconstriction. Rebound nasal congestion is caused by irritation of the nasal mucosa.

TABLE 35.2 Systemic and Nasal Decongestants (Sympathomimetic Amines)

Drug	Route and Dosage	Uses and Considerations
Oxymetazoline Hydrochloride	A/C >6 y: gtt or spray; 2-3 sprays in each nostril bid for <3 d	For nasal congestion. May cause dry nasal mucosa, nasal irritation, weakness, and nausea. Limit use to less than 3 days to avoid rebound congestion. Pregnancy category: C*; PB: UK; t½: UK
Phenylephrine Hydrochloride	A/C >12 y: Sol (0.25%) 2-3 sprays/gtts in each nostril q4h PRN <3 d A/C >12 y: PO: 10-20 mg q4-6h; *max.* 60 mg/d	For nasal congestion. May cause burning, stinging, sneezing, nausea, transient hypertension and headaches. Pregnancy category: C*; PB: UK; t½: 2.1-3.4 h
Pseudoephedrine	Regular release: A/adol: PO: 60 mg q4-6h; *max:* 240 mg/d C 6-11 y: 30 mg q4-6h; *max:* 120 mg/d C 2-5 y: 15 mg q4-6h; *max:* 60 mg/d Extended release: A/adol: PO: 120 mg q12h; *max:* 240 mg/d	For rhinitis, nasal congestion, and the common cold. May cause drowsiness, dizziness, headache, blurred vision, restlessness, insomnia, palpitations, dysrhythmia, hypertension, tachycardia, photosensitivity, and GI distress. Pregnancy category: C*; PB: UK; t½: 9-16 h
Tetrahydrozoline	A/C >6 y: Nasal: 2-4 sprays (0.1% sol) in each nostril q3-4h PRN C 2-6 y: Nasal: 2-3 sprays (0.05% sol) in each nostril q4-6h PRN	For nasal congestion. May cause transient stinging, sneezing, headache, blurred vision, tachycardia, and palpitations. Pregnancy category: C*; PB: UK; t½: UK

*Pregnancy categories have been revised. See http://www.fda.gov/Drugs/DevelopmentApprovalProcess/DevelopmentResources/Labeling/ucm093307.htm for more information.

A, Adult; *adol*, adolescent; *bid*, twice a day; *C*, child; *d*, day; *GI*, gastrointestinal; *gtts*, drops; *h*, hour; *max*, maximum; *PB*, protein binding; *PO*, by mouth; *PRN*, as necessary; *q4h*, every four hours; *sol*, solution; *t½*, half-life; *UK*, unknown; *y*, year; >, greater than; <, less than.

Systemic decongestants (alpha-adrenergic agonists) are available in tablet, capsule, and liquid form and are used primarily for allergic rhinitis, including hay fever and acute coryza (profuse nasal discharge). Examples of systemic decongestants are ephedrine, phenylephrine, oxymetazoline (Afrin), and pseudoephedrine. In the past, phenylpropanolamine (PPA) was used in many cold remedies; however, the U.S. Food and Drug Administration (FDA) ordered its removal from OTC cold remedies and weight-loss aids because reports suggest that the drug might cause stroke, hypertension, renal failure, and cardiac dysrhythmias. Ephedrine and pseudoephedrine are frequently combined with an antihistamine, analgesic, or antitussive in oral cold remedies. The advantage of systemic decongestants is that they relieve nasal congestion for a longer period than nasal decongestants; however, long-acting nasal decongestants are now available. Nasal decongestants usually act promptly and cause fewer side effects than systemic decongestants.

National regulatory measures control pseudoephedrine drug sales with individual limits of 3.6 g/day and 9 g within 30 days. Identifications are scanned with each purchase. The database is linked nationally and keeps a 2-year tally. Table 35.2 lists systemic and nasal decongestants and their dosages, uses, and considerations.

Side Effects and Adverse Reactions

The incidence of side effects is low with topical preparations such as nose drops. However, decongestants can make a patient jittery, nervous, or restless. These side effects decrease or disappear as the body adjusts to the drug.

Use of nasal decongestants for as little as 3 days could result in rebound nasal congestion. Instead of the nasal membranes constricting, vasodilation occurs, causing increased stuffy nose and nasal congestion. The nurse should emphasize the importance of limiting the use of nasal sprays and drops.

As with any alpha-adrenergic drug such as decongestants, blood pressure and blood glucose levels can increase. These drugs are contraindicated or used with extreme caution in patients with hypertension, cardiac disease, hyperthyroidism, and diabetes mellitus.

Drug Interactions

When using decongestants with other drugs, drug interactions can occur. Pseudoephedrine may decrease the effect of beta blockers. Taken together with monoamine oxidase inhibitors (MAOIs), decongestants may increase the possibility of hypertension or cardiac dysrhythmias. The patient should also avoid large amounts of caffeine (coffee, tea) because it can increase restlessness and palpitations caused by decongestants.

Intranasal Glucocorticoids

Intranasal glucocorticoids and steroids are effective for treating allergic rhinitis because they have an antiinflammatory action, thus decreasing the allergic rhinitis symptoms of rhinorrhea, sneezing, and congestion. The following are examples of intranasal steroids:

- Beclomethasone
- Budesonide
- Dexamethasone
- Flunisolide
- Fluticasone
- Mometasone
- Triamcinolone

TABLE 35.3 Intranasal Glucocorticoids

Drug	Route and Dosage	Uses and Considerations
Beclomethasone	Rhinitis: A/adol/C >12 y: 1-2 puffs/sprays bid C 6-12 y: 1 spray bid	For allergic rhinitis, nasal polyps, and asthma. May cause nasopharyngitis, candidiasis, dysphonia, hoarseness, epistaxis, and increased IOP. Pregnancy category: C*; PB: 87%; t½: 15 h
Budesonide	A/C >6 y: 1-2 sprays/d	For rhinitis and asthma. May cause dizziness, headache, weakness, dyspepsia, and epistaxis. Pregnancy category: B*; PB: 90%; t½: 2-3.6 h
Flunisolide	A/C >15 y: 2 sprays each nostril bid; max: 8 sprays/nostril/d C 6-14 y: 1-2 sprays bid; max: 8 sprays/nostril/d	For allergic rhinitis and asthma. May cause nasal burning/stinging, irritation, dryness, dysgeusia, dysphonia, hoarseness, and anosmia. Pregnancy category: C*; PB: UK; t½: 1.8-2 h
Fluticasone	A/adol/C >12 y: 2 sprays/d each nostril C 4-11 y: 1 spray/d	For allergic rhinitis. When symptoms decrease, reduce dose to 1 spray daily. May cause headache, epistaxis, dysphonia, candidiasis, fatigue, and GI distress. Pregnancy category: C*; PB: 91%; t½: 8-24 h
Mometasone furoate	A/adol/C >12 y: 2 sprays/d each nostril C 2-11 y: 1 spray/d	For allergic rhinitis, nasal congestion, and polyps. May cause headache, candidiasis, pharyngitis, and epistaxis. Pregnancy category: C*; PB: UK; t½: UK
Triamcinolone	A/adol/C >12 y: 2 sprays/d each nostril C 6-11 y: 1-2 sprays/d	For allergic rhinitis. Common side effects include headache and pharyngitis. Pregnancy category: C*; PB: UK; t½: 2-5 h

*Pregnancy categories have been revised. See http://www.fda.gov/Drugs/DevelopmentApprovalProcess/DevelopmentResources/Labeling/ucm093307.htm for more information.
A, Adult; adol, adolescent; bid, twice a day; C, child; d, day; GI, gastrointestinal; h, hour; IOP, intraocular pressure; max, maximum; PB, protein binding; t½, half-life; UK, unknown; y, year; >, greater than.

These drugs may be used alone or in combination with an H_1 antihistamine. The spray should be directed away from the nasal septum, and the patient should sniff gently. With continuous use, dryness of the nasal mucosa may occur.

Intranasal glucocorticoids undergo rapid deactivation after absorption. Most allergic rhinitis is seasonal; therefore the drugs are for short-term use unless otherwise indicated by the health care provider. Table 35.3 lists the intranasal glucocorticoids and their dosages, uses, and considerations.

Antitussives

Antitussives act on the cough-control center in the medulla to suppress the cough reflex. The cough is a naturally protective way to clear the airway of secretions or any collected material. A sore throat may cause coughing that increases throat irritation. If the cough is nonproductive and irritating, an antitussive may be taken. Hard candy may decrease the constant, irritating cough. Guaifenesin, a nonnarcotic antitussive, is widely used in OTC cold remedies. Prototype Drug Chart 35.2 lists the drug data related to dextromethorphan.

The three types of antitussives are nonopioid, opioid, or combination preparations. Antitussives are usually used in combination with other agents (Table 35.4).

Pharmacokinetics Dextromethorphan is available in numerous cold and cough remedy preparations in syrup or liquid form, chewable capsules, and lozenges. The drug is rapidly absorbed and exerts its effects 15 to 30 minutes after oral administration. Its protein-binding percentage is unknown, and the half-life is 1 hour. Dextromethorphan is metabolized by the liver and is excreted in the urine.

Pharmacodynamics Dextromethorphan, an expectorant, reduces the viscosity of tenacious secretions. This drug also acts as a nonopioid antitussive by changing a nonproductive cough to a less frequent, productive cough.

PROTOTYPE DRUG CHART 35.2
Dextromethorphan Hydrobromide

Drug Class	Dosage
Expectorant Pregnancy category: UK*	Immediate release: A/adol/C >12 y: PO: 10-20 mg q4h PRN; max: 120 mg/d C 6-11 y: 5-10 mg q4h PRN; max: 60 mg/d C 4-5 y: 2.5-7.5 mg q4-8h PRN; max: 30 mg/d Extended release: A/adol/C >12 y: PO: 60 mg q12h; max: 120 mg/d C 6-11 y: PO: 30 mg q12h; max: 60 mg/d

Contraindications	Drug-Lab-Food Interactions
Hypersensitivity Caution: Asthma, bronchitis, heart failure, tobacco smoking	No significant drug interactions occur with this drug.

Pharmacokinetics	Pharmacodynamics
Absorption: PO: Rapidly absorbed Distribution: PB: UK Metabolism: t½: 11 h Excretion: In urine	PO: Onset: 15-30 min Peak: 2-3 h Duration: 3-6 h

Therapeutic Effects/Uses
To ease expelling secretions from the lower respiratory tract and to produce a productive, less frequent cough
Mode of Action: Reduces viscosity and adhesiveness of tenacious secretions

Side Effects	Adverse Reactions
Dizziness, drowsiness, confusion, fatigue, ataxia, GI distress, nervousness	Nephrolithiasis, psychosis Life threatening: Respiratory depression, serotonin syndrome

*Pregnancy categories have been revised. See http://www.fda.gov/Drugs/DevelopmentApprovalProcess/DevelopmentResources/Labeling/ucm093307.htm for more information.
A, Adult; adol, adolescent; C, child; d, day; GI, gastrointestinal; h, hour; max, maximum; min, minute; PB, protein binding; PO, by mouth; PRN, as necessary; q4h, every 4 hours; t½, half-life; UK, unknown; y, year; >, greater than.

TABLE 35.4   Antitussives and Expectorants

Drug	Route and Dosage	Uses and Considerations
Opioid Antitussives		
Codeine CSS II	Cough: A/C >12 y: PO: 15-30 mg q6-8h; *max*: 120 mg/d	For cough and pain. May cause flushing, drowsiness, dizziness, euphoria, blurred vision, weakness, nausea, diarrhea, constipation, insomnia, headache, dependence, tolerance, withdrawal, and respiratory depression. Pregnancy category: C*; PB: 7%; t½: 3-4 h
Guaifenesin 200 mg and codeine 9 mg CSS V	A/C >12 y: PO: 2 capsules q4h PRN; *max*: 12 capsules/d C 6-12 y: PO: 1 capsule q4h PRN; *max*: 6 capsules/d	For cough and the common cold. May cause drowsiness, dizziness, headache, and GI distress. Pregnancy category: C*; PB: UK; t½: 1-4 h
Guaifenesin	Regular release: A/adol: PO: 200-400 q4h; *max*: 2400 mg/d C 6-11 y: PO: 100-200 mg q4h; *max*: 1200 mg/d C 2-5 y: PO: 50-100 mg q4h; *max*: 600 mg/d Extended release: A: PO: 600-1200 mg q12h; *max*: 2.4 g/d	For cough and the common cold. May cause drowsiness, dizziness, headache, nausea, vomiting, and diarrhea. Pregnancy category: C*; PB: UK; t½: 1 h
Homatropine 1.5 mg and hydrocodone 5 mg CSS III	A/adol: PO: Hydrocodone 5 mg and homatropine 1.5 mg q4-6h PRN; *max*: hydrocodone 30 mg and homatropine 9 mg/d C >6 y: PO: Hydrocodone 2.5 mg and homatropine 0.75 mg q4-6h PRN; *max*: hydrocodone 15 mg and homatropine 4.5 mg/d	For cough. May cause drowsiness, dizziness, euphoria, dry mouth, urinary retention, dysphoria, constipation, and dependence. Pregnancy category: C*; PB: UK; t½: 3.8 h
Nonopioid Antitussives		
Benzonatate	A/adol/C >10 y: PO: 100 mg tid PRN; *max*: 600 mg/d	For cough. May cause drowsiness, dizziness, headache, GI distress, and burning eyes. Pregnancy category: C*; PB: UK; t½: UK
Expectorants		
Dextromethorphan	See Prototype Drug Chart 35.2.	
Guaifenesin and dextromethorphan	A/adol: PO: Guaifenesin 200-400 mg and dextromethorphan 10-20 mg q4h PRN; *max*: guaifenesin 2400 mg and dextromethorphan 120 mg/d C 6-12 y: PO: Guaifenesin 200 mg and dextromethorphan 10 mg q4h PRN; *max*: guaifenesin 1200 mg and dextromethorphan 60 mg C 3-5 y: PO: Guaifenesin 100 mg and dextromethorphan 5 mg q4h PRN; *max*: guaifenesin 600 mg and dextromethorphan 30 mg	For common cold. May cause drowsiness, dizziness, headache, irritability, and nausea. Pregnancy category: C*; PB: UK; t½: 1-11 h

*Pregnancy categories have been revised. See http://www.fda.gov/Drugs/DevelopmentApprovalProcess/DevelopmentResources/Labeling/ucm093307.htm for more information.

A, Adult; *adol*, adolescent; *C*, child; *CSS*, Controlled Substances Schedule; *d*, day; *GI*, gastrointestinal; *h*, hour; *max*, maximum; *PB*, protein binding; *PO*, by mouth; *PRN*, as necessary; *q6h*, every 6 hours; *t½*, half-life; *tid*, three times a day; *UK*, unknown; *y*, year; *>*, greater than.

The onset of action for dextromethorphan is relatively fast, within 15 to 30 minutes, and its duration is 3 to 6 hours. Usually preparations that contain dextromethorphan can be used several times a day.

Expectorants

Expectorants loosen bronchial secretions so they can be eliminated by coughing. They can be used with or without other pharmacologic agents. Expectorants are found in many OTC cold remedies along with analgesics, antihistamines, decongestants, and antitussives. The most common expectorant in such preparations is guaifenesin. Hydration is the best natural expectorant. When taking an expectorant, patients should increase fluid intake to at least 8 glasses per day to help loosen mucus. Table 35.4 lists the dosages, uses, and considerations for antitussives and expectorants.

 NURSING PROCESS
Patient-Centered Collaborative Care

Common Cold

Assessment

- Determine whether the patient has a history of hypertension, especially if a decongestant is an ingredient in the cold remedy being taken.
- Note baseline vital signs. An elevated temperature of 99°F to 101°F (37.2°C to 38.3°C) may indicate a viral infection caused by a cold.
- Obtain a drug history, and report if a drug-drug interaction is probable. Dextromethorphan hydrochloride (HCl) given with MAOIs, narcotics, sedative-hypnotics, barbiturates, antidepressants, and alcohol may increase toxicity.
- Assess cardiac and respiratory status.

Nursing Diagnoses
- Airway Clearance, Ineffective related to nasal congestion
- Fluid Volume, Risk for Imbalanced
- Sleep Deprivation related to chronic coughing
- Fatigue related to sleep deprivation
- Infection, Risk for

Planning
- Patient's cough will be eliminated or diminished.
- Patient will be free from a secondary bacterial infection.

Nursing Interventions
- Monitor vital signs. Blood pressure can become elevated when a decongestant is taken, and dysrhythmias can also occur.
- Observe the color of bronchial secretions. Yellow or green mucus is indicative of a bronchial infection. Antibiotics may be needed.
- Warn patients that codeine preparations for cough suppression can lead to tolerance and physical dependence.

Patient Teaching
General
- Tell patients that hypotension and hyperpyrexia may occur when dextromethorphan is taken with MAOIs.
- Teach patients about proper use of nasal sprays and proper use of "puff" or squeeze products.
- Caution patients not to use more than one or two puffs four to six times a day for 5 to 7 days, because rebound congestion can occur with overuse.
- ⚡ Advise patients to read labels on OTC drugs and to check with a health care provider before taking cold remedies. This is especially important when taking other drugs or when a patient has a major health problem such as hypertension or hyperthyroidism. Also, acetaminophen may be in many products, promoting an overdose.
- Inform patients that antibiotics are *not* helpful in treating common cold viruses. However, they may be prescribed if a secondary infection occurs.
- Encourage older patients with heart disease, asthma, emphysema, diabetes mellitus, or hypertension to contact a health care provider concerning the selection of drug, including OTC drugs.
- Direct patients not to drive during initial use of a cold remedy containing an antihistamine because drowsiness is common.
- Tell patients to maintain adequate fluid intake. Fluids liquefy bronchial secretions to ease elimination with coughing.
- Teach patients not to take a cold remedy before or at bedtime. Insomnia may occur if it contains a decongestant.
- Encourage patients to get adequate rest.
- Inform patients that common cold and flu viruses are transmitted frequently by hand-to-hand contact or by touching a contaminated surface. Cold viruses can live on the skin for several hours and on hard surfaces for several days.

- Advise patients to avoid environmental pollutants, fumes, smoking, and dust to lessen irritating cough.
- Teach patients to perform three effective coughs before bedtime to promote uninterrupted sleep.
- Direct patients and parents to store drugs out of reach of children; request childproof caps.
- Advise patients to contact a health care provider if cough persists for more than 1 week or is accompanied by chest pain, fever, or headache.

Self-Administration
- Teach patients to self-administer medications such as nose drops and inhalants.
- Encourage patients to cough effectively, to take deep breaths before coughing, and to be in an upright position.

🌐 *Cultural Considerations*
- Allow patients to incorporate traditional, harmless remedies for treating the common cold into prescribed Western medical practices. Discuss practices that could cause harm.
- Identify conflicts in values and beliefs in treatment of the common cold.
- Present treatment methods to care for the common cold for patients from various cultural backgrounds, such as increasing fluid intake, getting adequate rest, and using disposable tissues to remove nasal and bronchial secretions.
- Advise patients to contact a health professional if cold persists and if body temperature is greater than 101°F (38.3°C).

Evaluation
- Evaluate effectiveness of drug therapy. Determine that the patient is free from nonproductive cough, has adequate fluid intake and rest, and is afebrile.

SINUSITIS

Sinusitis is an inflammation of the mucous membranes of one or more of the maxillary, frontal, ethmoid, or sphenoid sinuses. A systemic or nasal decongestant may be indicated. Acetaminophen, fluids, and rest may also be helpful. For acute or severe sinusitis, an antibiotic may be prescribed.

ACUTE PHARYNGITIS

Acute pharyngitis, inflammation of the throat or "sore throat," can be caused by a virus, beta-hemolytic streptococci ("strep throat"), or other bacteria. It can occur alone or with the common cold and rhinitis or acute sinusitis. Symptoms include elevated temperature and cough. A throat culture should be obtained to rule out beta-hemolytic streptococcal infection. If the culture is positive for beta-hemolytic streptococci, a 10-day course of antibiotics is often prescribed. Saline gargles, lozenges, and increased fluid intake are usually indicated. Acetaminophen may be taken to decrease elevated temperature. Antibiotics are *not* effective for viral pharyngitis.

CRITICAL THINKING CASE STUDY

GH, a 35-year-old patient, has allergic rhinitis. Her prescriptions include loratadine 5 mg/day and fluticasone two nasal inhalations per day. Previously she had taken OTC drugs and asked if she should continue to take the OTC drug with her prescriptions. She has never used a nasal inhaler before.

1. What additional information is needed from GH concerning her health problem?
2. What is your response to GH concerning the use of OTC drugs with her prescription drugs?

3. How would you instruct GH to use a nasal inhaler? Explain your answer.
4. What are the similarities and differences between loratadine and diphenhydramine? Could one of these antihistamines be more effective than the other? Explain your answer.
5. What could you suggest to decrease allergens such as dust mites in the home?

NCLEX STUDY QUESTIONS

1. A patient tells the nurse that he has started to take an over-the-counter antihistamine, diphenhydramine. In teaching about side effects, what is most important for the nurse to tell the patient?
   a. To avoid insomnia, do not to take this drug at bedtime.
   b. Avoid driving a motor vehicle until stabilized on the drug.
   c. Nightmares and nervousness are more likely in an adult.
   d. Medication may cause excessive secretions.
2. A patient complains of a sore throat and has been told it is due to beta-hemolytic streptococcal infection. The nurse anticipates that the patient has which acute condition?
   a. Rhinitis
   b. Sinusitis
   c. Pharyngitis
   d. Rhinorrhea
3. A patient is prescribed a decongestant nasal spray that contains oxymetazoline. What will the nurse teach the patient?
   a. Take this drug at bedtime because it may cause drowsiness.
   b. Directly spray the medication away from the nasal septum and gently sniff.
   c. This drug may be used in maintenance treatment for asthma.
   d. Limit use of the drug to 5 to 7 days to prevent rebound nasal congestion.
4. A patient has been prescribed guaifenesin. The nurse understands that the purpose of the drug is to accomplish what?
   a. Treat allergic rhinitis and prevent motion sickness
   b. Loosen bronchial secretions so coughing can eliminate them
   c. Compete with histamine for receptor sites, thus preventing a histamine response
   d. Stimulate alpha-adrenergic receptors, thus producing vascular constriction of capillaries in nasal mucosa

5. Beclomethasone has been prescribed for a patient with allergic rhinitis. What should the nurse teach the patient regarding this medication?
   a. This may be used for an acute attack.
   b. An oral form is available if the patient prefers to use it.
   c. Avoid large amounts of caffeine intake because an increased heart rate may occur.
   d. With continuous use, dryness of the nasal mucosa/lining may occur.
6. The nurse is teaching a patient about diphenhydramine. Which instructions should the nurse include in the patient's teaching plan? (Select all that apply.)
   a. Take medication on an empty stomach to facilitate absorption.
   b. Avoid alcohol and other central nervous system depressants.
   c. Notify a health care provider if confusion or hypotension occurs.
   d. Use sugarless candy, gum, or ice chips for temporary relief of dry mouth.
   e. Avoid handling dangerous equipment or performing dangerous activities until stabilized on the medication.

Answers: 1, b; 2, c; 3, d; 4, b; 5, d; 6, b, c, d, e.

36

Lower Respiratory Disorders

ⓔ http://evolve.elsevier.com/McCuistion/pharmacology/

OBJECTIVES

- Compare chronic obstructive pulmonary disease (COPD) and restrictive lung disease.
- Differentiate the drug groups used to treat COPD and asthma and the desired effects of each.
- Compare the side effects of beta$_2$-adrenergic agonists and methylxanthines.
- Describe the therapeutic serum or plasma theophylline level and the toxic level.

- Contrast the therapeutic effects of leukotriene antagonists, glucocorticoids, cromolyn, antihistamines, and mucolytics for COPD and asthma.
- Apply the nursing process for the patient taking drugs commonly used for COPD, including asthma, and for restrictive lung disease.

OUTLINE

KEY TERMS

Chronic obstructive pulmonary disease (COPD) and restrictive pulmonary disease are the two major categories of lower respiratory tract disorders. COPD is caused by airway obstruction with increased airway resistance of airflow to lung tissues. Four major pulmonary disorders cause COPD: (1) chronic bronchitis, (2) bronchiectasis, (3) emphysema, and (4) asthma. Chronic bronchitis, bronchiectasis, and emphysema frequently result in irreversible lung tissue damage. The lung tissue changes that result from an acute asthmatic attack are normally reversible; however, if the attacks are frequent and asthma becomes chronic, irreversible changes in the lung tissue may result. Patients with COPD usually have a decrease in forced expiratory volume in 1 second (FEV$_1$) as measured by pulmonary function tests.

Restrictive lung disease is a decrease in total lung capacity as a result of fluid accumulation or loss of elasticity of the lung. Pulmonary edema, pulmonary fibrosis, pneumonitis, lung tumors, thoracic deformities (scoliosis), and disorders that affect the thoracic muscular wall, such as myasthenia gravis, are among the types and causes of restrictive pulmonary disease.

Drugs discussed in this chapter are primarily used to treat COPD, particularly asthma. These drugs include **bronchodilators** (sympathomimetics [primarily beta$_2$-adrenergic agonists], methylxanthines [xanthines]), leukotriene antagonists, glucocorticoids, cromolyn, anticholinergics, and mucolytics. Some of these drugs may also be used to treat restrictive pulmonary diseases.

CHRONIC OBSTRUCTIVE PULMONARY DISEASE

Asthma is an inflammatory disorder of the airway walls associated with a varying amount of airway obstruction. This disorder is triggered by stimuli such as stress, allergens, and pollutants. When activated by stimuli, the bronchial airways become inflamed and edematous, leading to constriction of air passages. Inflammation aggravates airway hyperresponsiveness to stimuli, causing bronchial cells to produce more mucus, which obstructs air passages. This obstruction contributes to wheezing, coughing, dyspnea (breathlessness), and tightness in the chest, particularly at night or in the early morning.

Bronchial asthma, one of the COPD lung diseases, is characterized by bronchospasm (constricted bronchioles), wheezing, mucous secretions, and dyspnea. There is resistance to airflow caused by obstruction of the airway. In acute and chronic asthma, minimal to no changes are seen in the structure and function of lung tissues when the disease process is in remission. In chronic bronchitis, emphysema, and bronchiectasis, irreversible damage is done to the physical structure of lung tissue. Symptoms are similar to those of asthma in these three pulmonary disorders, except wheezing does not occur. Fig. 36.1 shows the overlapping symptoms of COPD conditions. Frequently, a steady deterioration occurs over a period of years.

Chronic bronchitis is a progressive lung disease caused by smoking or chronic lung infections. Bronchial inflammation and excessive mucous secretion result in airway obstruction. Productive coughing is a response to excess mucous production and chronic bronchial irritation. Inspiratory and expiratory rhonchi may be heard on auscultation. Hypercapnia (increased carbon dioxide retention) and hypoxemia (decreased blood oxygen) lead to respiratory acidosis.

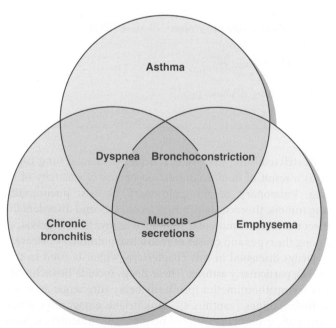

FIG. 36.1 Overlapping signs and symptoms of chronic obstructive pulmonary disease (COPD) conditions.

In bronchiectasis, dilation of the bronchi and bronchioles is abnormal secondary to frequent infection and inflammation. The bronchioles become obstructed by the breakdown of the epithelium of the bronchial mucosa, and tissue fibrosis may result.

Emphysema is a progressive lung disease caused by cigarette smoking, atmospheric contaminants, or lack of the alpha₁-antitrypsin protein that inhibits proteolytic enzymes that destroy alveoli (air sacs). Proteolytic enzymes are released in the lung by bacteria or phagocytic cells. The terminal bronchioles become plugged with mucus, causing a loss in the fiber and elastin network in the alveoli. Alveoli enlarge as many of the alveolar walls are destroyed. Air becomes trapped in the overexpanded alveoli, leading to inadequate gas exchange (oxygen and carbon dioxide).

Cigarette smoking is the most common risk factor for COPD, especially with chronic bronchitis and emphysema. There is no known cure for COPD at this time; however, it remains preventable in most cases. Because cigarette smoking is the most directly related cause, not smoking significantly prevents COPD from developing. Quitting smoking will slow the disease process.

Medications frequently prescribed for COPD include the following:

- Bronchodilators such as sympathomimetics (adrenergics), parasympatholytics (anticholinergic drugs, ipratropium bromide), and methylxanthines (caffeine, theophylline) are used to assist in opening narrowed airways.
- Glucocorticoids (steroids) are used to decrease inflammation.
- Leukotriene modifiers reduce inflammation in the lung tissue, and cromolyn acts as an antiinflammatory agent by suppressing the release of histamine and other mediators from the mast cells.
- Expectorants are used to assist in loosening mucus from the airways.
- Antibiotics may be prescribed to prevent serious complications from bacterial infections.

Bronchial Asthma

Bronchial asthma is a COPD characterized by periods of bronchospasm resulting in wheezing and difficulty breathing. Bronchospasm, or bronchoconstriction, results when the lung tissue is exposed to extrinsic or intrinsic factors that stimulate a bronchoconstrictive response. Factors that can trigger an asthmatic attack (bronchospasm) include humidity; air pressure changes; temperature changes; smoke; fumes (exhaust, perfume); stress; emotional upset; exercise; and allergies to animal dander, dust mites, food, and drugs (e.g., aspirin, ibuprofen, beta-adrenergic blockers). Reactive airway disease (RAD) is a cause of asthma that results from sensitivity stimulation from allergens, dust, temperature changes, and cigarette smoking.

Pathophysiology

Mast cells found in connective tissue throughout the body are directly involved in the asthmatic response, particularly to extrinsic factors. Allergens attach themselves to mast cells and basophils, resulting in an antigen-antibody reaction on the mast cells in the lung; thus the mast cells stimulate the release of chemical mediators such as histamines, cytokines, serotonin, eosinophil chemotactic factor of anaphylaxis (ECF-A), and leukotrienes. Eosinophil counts are usually elevated during an allergic reaction, which indicates that an inflammatory process is occurring. These chemical mediators stimulate bronchial constriction, mucous secretions, inflammation, and pulmonary congestion. Histamine and ECF-A are strong bronchoconstrictors. Bronchial smooth muscles are wrapped spirally around the bronchioles and contract as they are stimulated by these mediators. Exposure to an allergen results in bronchial hyperresponsiveness, epithelial shedding of the bronchial wall, mucous gland hyperplasia and hypersecretion, leakage of plasma that leads to swelling, and bronchoconstriction.

Fig. 36.2 shows factors that contribute to bronchoconstriction. Cyclic adenosine monophosphate (cyclic AMP, or cAMP), a cellular signaling molecule, is involved in many cellular activities and is responsible for maintaining bronchodilation. When histamine, ECF-A, and leukotrienes inhibit the action of cAMP, bronchoconstriction results. The sympathomimetic (adrenergic) bronchodilators and methylxanthines increase the amount of cAMP in bronchial tissue cells.

In an acute asthmatic attack, the short-acting sympathomimetics (beta$_2$-adrenergic agonists) are the first line of defense. They promote cAMP production and enhance bronchodilation. Long-acting sympathomimetics are used for maintenance. Sympathomimetics (adrenergics) are also discussed in Chapter 15.

SYMPATHOMIMETICS: ALPHA- AND BETA$_2$-ADRENERGIC AGONISTS

Sympathomimetics increase cAMP, causing dilation of the bronchioles. In an acute bronchospasm caused by anaphylaxis from an allergic reaction, the nonselective sympathomimetic epinephrine—an alpha$_1$, beta$_1$, and beta$_2$ agonist—is given subcutaneously to promote bronchodilation and elevate blood pressure. Epinephrine is administered in emergency situations to restore circulation and increase airway patency (see Chapter 55).

For bronchospasm associated with chronic asthma or COPD, selective beta$_2$-adrenergic agonists are given by aerosol or as a tablet. These drugs act primarily on the beta$_2$ receptors, therefore side effects are less severe than those of epinephrine, which acts on alpha$_1$, beta$_1$, and beta$_2$ receptors.

Albuterol

The newer beta-adrenergic drugs for asthma are more selective for beta$_2$ receptors. High doses or overuse of the beta$_2$-adrenergic agents for asthma may cause some degree of beta$_1$ response, such as nervousness, tremor, and increased pulse rate. The ideal beta$_2$ agonist is one that has a rapid onset of action, longer duration of action, and few side effects. Albuterol is a selective beta$_2$ drug that is effective for treatment and control of asthma by causing bronchodilation with a long duration of action. (See Prototype Drug Chart 15.2 for drug data related to albuterol.)

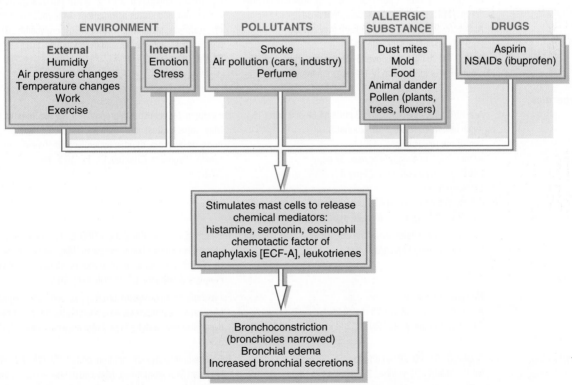

FIG. 36.2 Factors that contribute to bronchoconstriction. *NSAIDs,* nonsteroidal antiinflammatory drugs.

Metaproterenol

The beta-adrenergic agent metaproterenol has some beta$_1$ effect but is primarily used as a beta$_2$ agent. It can be administered orally or by inhalation with a metered-dose inhaler (MDI) or a nebulizer.

For long-term asthma treatment, beta$_2$-adrenergic agonists are frequently administered by inhalation. This route of administration usually delivers more of the drug directly to the constricted bronchial site. The effective inhalation drug dose is less than it would be by the oral route, and there are also fewer side effects using this route. The onset of action is 1 minute by oral inhalation, 5 to 30 minutes by nebulization, and 15 to 30 minutes when taken orally. The peak for inhalation and oral administration is 1 hour with a duration of 4 hours.

Use of an Aerosol Inhaler

If the beta$_2$ agonist is given by MDI or dry-powder inhaler (DPI), correct use of the inhaler and dosage intervals need to be explained to the patient. If the patient does not receive effective relief from the inhaler, either the technique is faulty or the canister is empty. A spacer device may be attached to the inhaler to improve drug delivery to the lung with less deposition in the mouth. If the patient does not use the inhaler properly to deliver the drug dose, the medication may be trapped in the upper airways. Because of drug inhalation, mouth dryness and throat irritation could result.

Excessive use of the aerosol drug can lead to tolerance and loss of drug effectiveness. Occasionally, severe paradoxic airway resistance (bronchoconstriction) develops with repeated, excessive use of sympathomimetic oral inhalation. Frequent dosing can cause tremors, nervousness, and increased heart rate. Table 36.1 lists the sympathomimetics used as bronchodilators.

Side Effects and Adverse Reactions

The side effects and adverse reactions of epinephrine include tremors, dizziness, hypertension, tachycardia, heart palpitations, cardiac dysrhythmias, and angina. The patient needs to be closely monitored when epinephrine is administered.

The side effects associated with beta$_2$-adrenergic drugs, such as albuterol, include tremors, headaches, nervousness, increased pulse rate, and palpitations (high doses). The beta$_2$ agonists may

TABLE 36.1	Adrenergic Bronchodilators and Anticholinergics	
Drug	**Route and Dosage**	**Uses and Considerations**
Alpha- and Beta-Adrenergics		
Ephedrine sulfate Alpha₁, beta₁, beta₂	Bronchospasm: A: PO: 25-50 mg q3-4h PRN; *max:* 150 mg/d A: Subcut/IM/IV: 12.5-25 mg; *max:* 150 mg/d	For asthma, acute bronchospasm, and hypotension. May cause restlessness, dizziness, headache, irritability, tremor, palpitations, tachycardia, dysrhythmias, and insomnia. Pregnancy category: C*; PB: UK; t½: 3-6 h
Epinephrine Alpha₁, beta₁, beta₂	A/adol/C >4 y: MDI: 1 puff (160-250 mcg), repeat once after 1 min PRN, wait 3-4 h for subsequent dose A: Subcut: 0.3-0.5 mg of 1:1000 sol; may repeat q5-10 min PRN × 3 for asthma A: IV: 0.1-0.25 mg slowly over 5-10 min, may repeat q5-15 min PRN or follow with IV 1-4 mcg/min infusion	For acute bronchospasm, asthma, anaphylaxis, angioedema, nasal congestion, and status asthmaticus. May cause restlessness, tremors, dizziness, sweating, weakness, hyperglycemia, GI distress, palpitations, tachycardia, and dysrhythmias. Pregnancy category: C*; PB: UK; t½: UK
Beta-Adrenergics		
Albuterol Beta₂	A/adol/C >4 y: Inhal MDI: 1 to 2 puffs q4-6h or 2 puffs 15 min before exercise; *max:* 12 inhal/d Immediate release: A/adol: PO: 2 to 4 mg q6-8h; *max:* 32 mg/d C 6-12 y: 2 mg q6-8h; *max:* 24 mg/d Extended release: A/adol: PO: 4 to 8 mg q12h; *max:* 32 mg/d C 6-12 y: PO: 4 mg q12h; *max:* 24 mg/d	For asthma, bronchospasm prophylaxis, and acute bronchospasm. May cause restlessness, tremors, headache, dizziness, palpitations, tachycardia, rhinitis, hyperglycemia, nausea, and bronchospasm. Pregnancy category: C*; PB: 10%; t½: 2.7-6 h
Formoterol Beta₂	A/adol/C >5 y: Inhalation: Inhale 20 mcg (one 2 mL unit) via nebulizer; max: 40 mcg/d	For asthma, chronic bronchitis, COPD, emphysema, and prophylaxis of exercise-induced bronchospasm. May cause dizziness, insomnia, tachycardia, chest pain, pharyngitis, sinusitis, and GI distress. Pregnancy category: C*; PB: UK; t1/2: 10 h
Levalbuterol Beta₂	Nebulizer inhalation: A/adol/C >12 y: 0.63 to 1.25 mg q6-8h C 6-11 y: 0.31 mg q6-8h PRN	For asthma, bronchospasm, prophylaxis, and acute bronchospasm. May cause restlessness, nasopharyngitis, nausea, headache, hyperglycemia, and tremors. Pregnancy category: C*; PB: UK; t½: 3.3-4 h
Metaproterenol sulfate Beta₁ (some) and beta₂	A/adol/C >9 y: PO: 20 mg tid/qid; *max:* 80 mg/d MDI: A/adol/C >12 y: Inhal: 2-3 inhal q3-4h; *max:* 12 inhal/d	For acute bronchospasm, asthma, and COPD. Allow 2 minutes between MDI inhalations. May cause headache, tremor, tachycardia, palpitations, and nausea. Pregnancy category: C*; PB: UK; t½: UK

TABLE 36.1   Adrenergic Bronchodilators and Anticholinergics—cont'd

Drug	Route and Dosage	Uses and Considerations
Salmeterol Beta₂	A/adol/C >4 y: Inhal: 1 puff (50 mcg) q12h Prevention of exercise-induced bronchospasm: A/adol/C >4 y: Inhal MDI: 1 puff at least 30 min before exercise	For asthma, COPD, and bronchospasm prophylaxis. May cause headache, pharyngitis, and musculoskeletal pain. Pregnancy category: C*; PB: 94%-98%; t½: 5 h
Terbutaline sulfate Beta₂	A/adol >15 y: PO: 2.5 to 5 mg tid; *max:* 15 mg/d Adol <15 y/C >12 y: PO: 2.5 mg tid; *max:* 7.5 mg/d A/adol >15 y: Subcut: 0.25 to 0.5 mg, may repeat in 15-30 min; *max:* 0.5 mg/4 h	For asthma, COPD, bronchospasm prophylaxis, and acute bronchospasm. May cause restlessness, tremors, dizziness, drowsiness, headache, palpitations, hyperglycemia, and hypokalemia. Pregnancy category: C*; PB: 25%; t½: 11-16 h
Arformoterol tartrate Beta₂	A: Inhal nebulizer: 15 mcg q12h; *max:* 30 mcg/d	For COPD. May cause restlessness, tremor, headache, sinusitis, chest pain, and diarrhea. Pregnancy category: C*; PB: 52%-65%; t½: 26 h
Indacaterol Beta₂	A: Oral inhal: 75 mcg/d; *max:* 1 inhal/d at the same time every day	For COPD. May cause cough, headache, hyperglycemia, and nasopharyngitis. Pregnancy category: C*; PB: 94%-96%; t½: 45.5-126 h
Olodaterol Beta₂	A: Inhal: 2 inhal/d (2.5 mcg each) at the same time every day	For COPD. May cause cough, nasopharyngitis, and URI. Pregnancy category: C*; PB: 60%; t½: 7.5 h
Anticholinergics Ipratropium bromide	COPD A: Inhal MDI: 2 puffs tid/qid, *max:* 12 inhal/d	For allergic rhinitis, common cold, COPD, and bronchospasm prophylaxis. Use with caution in patients with glaucoma. May cause headache, epistaxis, nasopharyngitis, and dyspnea. Pregnancy category: B*; PB: UK; t½: 1.5-2 h
Aclidinium	A: Oral MDI inhal: 1 inhal (400 mcg aclidinium) bid/tid; *max:* 2 inhal/d	For COPD bronchospasms. May cause headache and nasopharyngitis. Pregnancy category: C*; PB: UK; t½: 5-8 h
Tiotropium	See Prototype Drug Chart 36.1.	
Umeclidinium	A: Inhal: 1 inhal (62.5 mcg)/d at the same time every day	For COPD. May cause nasopharyngitis and URI. Pregnancy category: C*; PB: >90%; t½: 24 h
Monoclonal Antibody Omalizumab	A/adol/C >12 y: Subcut: 150-375 mg q2-4wk; dose and frequency based upon body weight and total IgE serum levels	For asthma. May cause rash, headache, pharyngitis, arthralgia, bone fractures, and infection. Pregnancy category: B*; PB: UK; t½: 24-26 d
Reslizumab	A: IV: 3 mg/kg infusion q4wk	For asthma.. May cause pharyngitis, musculoskeletal pain, antibody formation, and secondary malignancy. Pregnancy category: UK*; PB: UK; t½: 24 d
Combination Beta-Adrenergics and Anticholinergics Ipratropium and albuterol	A: Inhaled via nebulizer: 1 inhal (100 mcg albuterol, 20 mcg ipratropium) q6h; *max:* 6 inhal/d	For COPD. May cause headache, pharyngitis, tremor, infection, and palpitations. Pregnancy category: C*; PB: UK; t½: 2-4 h
Indacaterol and glycopyrrolate	A: Inhal: 1 capsule (27.5 mcg indacaterol and 31.2 mcg glycopyrrolate) bid in the morning and evening at the same time qd	For COPD. May cause cough, pharyngitis, and paradoxical bronchospasm. Pregnancy category: C*; PB: 38%-96%; t½: 33-126 h
Olodaterol and tiotropium	A: Inhal: 2 inhal/d at the same time qd (olodaterol 2.5 mcg and tiotropium 2.5 mcg each inhal)	For COPD. May cause cough, nasopharyngitis, headache, insomnia, chest and back pain, dyspepsia, abdominal pain, and paradoxic bronchospasm. Pregnancy category: C*; PB: UK; t½: UK
Umeclidinium and vilanterol	A: Inhal: 1 inhal/d (62.5 mcg umeclidinium/25 mcg vilanterol) at the same time qd	For COPD. May cause pharyngitis and diarrhea. Pregnancy category: C*; PB: 89%-94%; t½: 11-21.3 h

*Pregnancy categories have been revised. See http://www.fda.gov/Drugs/DevelopmentApprovalProcess/DevelopmentResources/Labeling/ucm093 307.htm for more information.

A, Adult; *adol,* adolescent; *bid,* two times a day; *C,* child; *COPD,* chronic obstructive pulmonary disease; *d,* day; *GI,* gastrointestinal; *h,* hour; *IgE,* immunoglobulin E; *IM,* intramuscular; *inhal,* inhalation; *IV,* intravenous; *max,* maximum; *MDI,* metered-dose inhaler; *min,* minute; *PB,* protein binding; *PO,* by mouth; *PRN,* as needed; *q,* every; *qd,* every day; *qid,* four times a day; *sol,* solution; *subcut,* subcutaneous; *t½,* half-life; *tid,* three times a day; *UK,* unknown; *URI,* upper respiratory infection; *wk,* week; *y,* year; *>,* greater than; *<,* less than.

increase blood glucose levels, so patients with diabetes should be taught to closely monitor their serum glucose levels. Side effects of beta₂ agonists may diminish after 1 week or longer. The bronchodilating effects may decrease with continued use.

It is believed that tolerance to these drugs can develop; if this occurs, the dose may need to be increased. Failure to respond to a previously effective dose may indicate worsening asthma that requires reevaluation before increasing the dose.

ANTICHOLINERGICS

Tiotropium is an anticholinergic drug used for maintenance treatment of bronchospasms associated with COPD. This drug is administered by inhalation only with the HandiHaler device (dry-powder capsule inhaler). Patients should discard any capsules that are opened and not used immediately. HandiHalers should be washed with warm water and dried. The most common adverse effects of tiotropium include dry mouth, constipation, vomiting, dyspepsia, abdominal pain, depression, insomnia, headache, joint pain, and peripheral edema. Chest pain has been reported following tiotropium administration. Prototype Drug Chart 36.1 lists the drug data related to tiotropium.

The anticholinergic drug ipratropium bromide is used to treat asthmatic conditions by dilating the bronchioles. Unlike other anticholinergics, ipratropium bromide has few systemic effects. It is administered by MDI.

The combination of ipratropium bromide with albuterol sulfate is used to treat COPD. The combination is more effective and has a longer duration of action than either agent used alone. These two agents combined increase the FEV₁, the index used to evaluate asthma and obstructive lung disease and the patient's response to bronchodilator therapy. Table 36.2 lists the inhalants for asthma control.

METHYLXANTHINE (XANTHINE) DERIVATIVES

The second major group of bronchodilators used to treat asthma is the methylxanthine (xanthine) derivatives, which include aminophylline, theophylline, and caffeine. Xanthines also stimulate the central nervous system (CNS) and respiration, dilate coronary and pulmonary vessels, and cause diuresis. Because of their effect on respiration and pulmonary vessels, xanthines are used in the treatment of asthma.

Theophylline

Theophylline relaxes the smooth muscles of the bronchi, bronchioles, and pulmonary blood vessels by inhibiting the enzyme phosphodiesterase, resulting in an increase in cAMP, which promotes bronchodilation.

Theophylline has a low therapeutic index and a narrow desired therapeutic range (5-15 mcg/mL). The serum or plasma theophylline concentration level should be monitored frequently to avoid severe adverse effects. Toxicity is likely to occur when the serum level is greater than 20 mcg/mL. Certain theophylline preparations can be given with sympathomimetic (adrenergic) agents, but the dose may need to be adjusted.

Theophylline was once used as the first-line drug for treating patients with chronic asthma and other COPDs. However, theophylline use has declined sharply because of a potential danger of serious adverse effects—including dysrhythmias, convulsions, and cardiorespiratory collapse—and efficacy has not been found to be greater than that of beta agonists or glucocorticoids. Because of its numerous adverse reactions, drug-drug interactions, and narrow therapeutic drug range, theophylline is prescribed mostly for maintenance therapy in patients with chronic stable asthma and other COPDs when other drugs have failed to show improvement. Theophylline drugs are *not* prescribed for patients with seizure disorders or cardiac, renal, or liver disease. Patients who receive theophylline preparations need to be closely monitored for serious side effects and drug interactions.

PROTOTYPE DRUG CHART 36.1

Tiotropium

Drug Class	Dosage
Anticholinergic Pregnancy category: C*	A: Oral inhalation: 2 inhal/d (2.5 mcg/actuation) at the same time qd
Contraindications	**Drug-Lab-Food Interactions**
Hypersensitivity *Caution:* Lactose hypersensitivity, narrow-angle glaucoma, bladder neck obstruction, renal impairment, cardiac dysrhythmias, breastfeeding, older adults	Drug: Increased anticholinergic effects with phenothiazines; decreased action of prokinetics (cisapride, metoclopramide, parasympathomimetics)
Pharmacokinetics	**Pharmacodynamics**
Absorption: Minimally absorbed PO Distribution: 72% PB Metabolism: t½: 5-6 d Excretion: In urine as metabolites	Inhalation: PO: Onset: 30 min Peak: 1-4 h Duration: 24 h
Therapeutic Effects/Uses	
For maintenance treatment of asthma and COPD Mode of Action: Blocks muscarinic cholinergic receptors and antagonizes acetylcholine action by inhibiting M3 receptor response to acetylcholine, thereby relaxing smooth muscle of bronchi; dilates bronchi	
Side Effects	**Adverse Reactions**
Insomnia, dizziness, depression, headache, sinusitis, nasopharyngitis, cough, dry mouth, nausea, vomiting, abdominal pain, constipation, urinary retention, hyperglycemia, myalgia, peripheral edema, blurred vision, oral ulceration, URI, UTI	Anaphylaxis, angioedema, dehydration, hyperglycemia, chest pain *Life threatening:* Cardiac dysrhythmias

*Pregnancy categories have been revised. See http://www.fda.gov/Drugs/DevelopmentApprovalProcess/DevelopmentResources/Labeling/ucm093307.htm for more information.

A, Adult; *COPD*, chronic obstructive pulmonary disease; *d*, day; *h*, hour; *inhal*, inhalations; *min*, minutes; *PB*, protein binding; *PO*, by mouth; *qd*, every day; *t½*, half-life; *URI*, upper respiratory infection; *UTI*, urinary tract infection.

Table 36.3 lists theophylline and its dosages, uses, and considerations.

Pharmacokinetics Theophylline is usually well absorbed after oral administration, but absorption may vary according to the specific dosage form. Theophylline is also well absorbed from oral liquids and uncoated plain tablets. Sustained-release dosage forms are slowly absorbed. Food and antacids may decrease the rate but not the extent of absorption; large volumes of fluid and high-protein meals may increase the rate of absorption. The dose size can also affect the rate of absorption: larger doses are absorbed more slowly. Theophylline can also be administered in intravenous (IV) fluids.

Theophylline drugs are metabolized by liver enzymes, and 90% of the drug is excreted by the kidneys. Tobacco smoking increases metabolism of theophylline drugs, thereby decreasing the half-life. The half-life is also shorter in children. With a short half-life, theophylline is readily excreted by the kidneys, so the dose may need to be increased to maintain a therapeutic serum/plasma range. In nonsmokers and older adults, the average half-life of theophylline is 6.5 to 10.5 hours, and the dose requirements may be decreased. However, in smokers and children,

the half-life is 4 to 5 hours, and the dose requirement may be increased. In premature infants, the half-life is 9.4 to 43 hours. In patients with heart failure (HF), cor pulmonale, COPD, or liver disease, the half-life is 24 hours. Kidney function may be decreased in older adults, so caution should be used regarding the theophylline dosage to avoid drug toxicity.

Pharmacodynamics Theophylline increases the level of cAMP, resulting in bronchodilation. The average onset of action is 30 minutes for oral preparations and 1 to 2 hours for sustained-release (SR) capsules. The peak action is 30 minutes for IV administration and 1 to 2 hours when taken orally.

Side Effects and Adverse Reactions

Side effects and adverse reactions to theophylline include anorexia, nausea and vomiting, gastric pain caused by increased gastric acid secretion, intestinal bleeding, nervousness, dizziness, headache, irritability, cardiac dysrhythmias, tachycardia, palpitations, marked hypotension, hyperreflexia, and seizures. Adverse CNS reactions—headaches, irritability, restlessness, nervousness, insomnia, dizziness, and seizures—are often more severe in children than in adults. To decrease the potential for side effects, patients should not take other xanthines while taking theophylline.

Theophylline toxicity is most likely to occur when serum concentrations exceed 20 mcg/mL. Theophylline can cause hyperglycemia, decreased clotting time, and, rarely, increased white blood cell count (leukocytosis). Because of the diuretic effect of xanthines, including theophylline, patients should avoid caffeinated products such as coffee, tea, cola, and chocolate, and they should increase fluid intake.

Rapid IV administration of aminophylline, a theophylline product, can cause dizziness, flushing, hypotension, severe bradycardia, and palpitations. To avoid severe adverse effects, IV theophylline preparations *must be administered slowly* via an infusion pump.

Drug Interactions

Beta blockers, cimetidine, propranolol, and erythromycin decrease the liver metabolism rate and increase the half-life and effects of theophylline; barbiturates and carbamazepine decrease its effects. In both situations, the theophylline dosage would need adjustment. Theophylline increases the risk of digitalis toxicity and decreases the effects of lithium. Phenytoin decreases theophylline levels. If theophylline and a beta-adrenergic

TABLE 36.2 Inhalants for Asthma Control

Categories	Inhalant Agents
Adrenergics	
Beta$_2$ and some beta$_1$	Metaproterenol sulfate
Beta$_2$	Albuterol
	Salmeterol
	Terbutaline sulfate
	Formoterol
	Indacaterol
	Olodaterol
	Arformoterol tartrate
Anticholinergics	Ipratropium bromide
	Aclidinium
	Tiotropium
	Umeclidinium
Antiinflammatory Drugs	
Cromolyn	Cromolyn
Glucocorticoids (corticosteroids)	Beclomethasone
	Budesonide
	Flunisolide
	Fluticasone

TABLE 36.3 Theophylline Preparations

Drug	Route and Dosage	Uses and Considerations
Aminophylline-theophylline ethylenediamine (Elixophyllin, Theo-24)	A: 16-60 y: IV: 0.4 mg/kg/h infusion Older adults >60 y: IV: 0.3 mg/kg/h infusion	For asthma exacerbations. Individual titration is based on serum theophylline levels. May cause restlessness, headache, insomnia, dizziness, nausea, vomiting, diarrhea, tremor, palpitations, and tachycardia. Therapeutic range: 5-15 mcg/L. Pregnancy category: C*; PB: 40%; t½: A: 6.5-10.5 h

*Pregnancy categories have been revised. See http://www.fda.gov/Drugs/DevelopmentApprovalProcess/DevelopmentResources/Labeling/ucm093307.htm for more information.
A, Adult; *h*, hour; *IV*, intravenous; *PB*, protein binding; *t½*, half-life; *y*, year; *>*, greater than.

agonist are given together, a synergistic effect can occur that can result in cardiac dysrhythmias.

LEUKOTRIENE RECEPTOR ANTAGONISTS AND SYNTHESIS INHIBITORS

Leukotriene (LT) is a chemical mediator that can cause inflammatory changes in the lung. The *cysteinyl leukotrienes* promote an increase in eosinophil migration, mucous production, and airway wall edema that results in bronchoconstriction. LT receptor antagonists and LT synthesis inhibitors, called *leukotriene modifiers,* are effective in reducing the inflammatory symptoms of asthma triggered by allergic and environmental stimuli. These drug groups are *not* recommended for treatment of acute asthmatic attacks, rather they are used for exercise-induced asthma. Three leukotriene modifiers—zafirlukast, zileuton, and montelukast—are available in the United States. These drugs are listed in Table 36.4.

Zafirlukast was the first drug in the class of leukotriene modifiers. It acts as an leukotriene receptor antagonist, reducing the inflammatory process and decreasing bronchoconstriction. It is administered orally, is absorbed rapidly, and has a moderate to moderately long half-life; it is given twice a day. Zileuton is a leukotriene synthesis inhibitor. It decreases the inflammatory process and decreases bronchoconstriction. Zileuton has a short half-life of 1 to 2.3 hours.

 NURSING PROCESS
Patient-Centered Collaborative Care
Bronchodilators

Assessment
- Obtain a medical and drug history; report probable drug-drug interactions.
- Note baseline vital signs and pulse oximetry for abnormalities and future comparisons.
- Assess for wheezing, decreased breath sounds, cough, and sputum production.
- Assess sensorium for confusion and restlessness caused by hypoxia and hypercapnia.
- Determine hydration; diuresis may result in dehydration in children and older adults.
- Assess serum theophylline levels. Toxicity occurs at a higher frequency with levels greater than 20 mcg/mL.

Nursing Diagnoses
- Breathing Pattern, Ineffective related to fatigue
- Airway Clearance, Ineffective related to retained secretions in the bronchi
- Gas Exchange, Impaired related to ineffective airway clearance
- Noncompliance with drug therapy related to inadequate financial resources
- Activity Intolerance related to fatigue and an imbalance between oxygen supply and demand

Planning
- The patient will be free from wheezing, and lung fields will be clear within 2 to 5 days.
- The patient will self-administer oral drugs and will use an inhaler as prescribed.

Nursing Interventions
- Monitor vital signs. Blood pressure and heart rate can increase greatly. Check for cardiac dysrhythmias.
- Provide adequate hydration. Fluids help loosen secretions.
- Monitor drug therapy.
- Observe for side effects.
- Administer medication after meals to decrease gastrointestinal (GI) distress.
- Administer medication at regular intervals around the clock to have a sustained therapeutic level.
- Do *not* crush enteric-coated (EC) or sustained-released (SR) tablets or capsules.
- ⚡ Check serum theophylline levels (normal level is 5-15 mcg/mL).

Patient Teaching
General
- Teach patients to monitor their pulse rate.
- Encourage patients to monitor the amount of medication remaining in the canister.
- Advise patients not to take over-the-counter (OTC) preparations without first checking with a health care provider. Some OTC products may have an additive effect.
- Encourage patients contemplating pregnancy to seek medical advice before taking a theophylline preparation.
- Advise patients to avoid smoking. Avoid marked sudden changes in smoking amounts, which could affect theophylline blood levels. Smoking increases drug elimination, which may require an increased drug dose.
- Discuss ways to alleviate anxiety, such as relaxation techniques and music.
- ⚡ Advise patients having asthmatic attacks to wear an identification bracelet or MedicAlert tag.
- Inform patients that certain complementary and alternative therapies may interact with theophylline (Complementary and Alternative Therapies 36.1).
- ⚡ Advise patients to notify a health care provider of aggressive or altered behavior and suicidal thoughts.
Self-Administration
- Teach patients to correctly use the inhaler or nebulizer. Caution against overuse because side effects and tolerance may result.
- Teach patients to monitor pulse rate and report to a health care provider any irregularities in comparison with baseline values.
Diet
- Advise patients that a high-protein, low-carbohydrate diet increases theophylline elimination. Conversely, a low-protein, high-carbohydrate diet prolongs half-life; dosage may need adjustment.

TABLE 36.4 Antiinflammatory Drugs for Chronic Obstructive Pulmonary Disease

Drug	Route and Dosage	Uses and Considerations
Leukotriene Modifiers (*Do Not* Administer for Acute Asthmatic Attack)		
Leukotriene Receptor Antagonists		
Zafirlukast	A/adol/C >12 y: PO: 20 mg bid 1 h before or 2 h after meals; *max:* 40 mg/d C 5-11 y: PO: 10 mg bid; *max:* 20 mg/d	For asthma. Reduces inflammation within bronchial tubes and airways. May cause headache, nausea, vomiting, and diarrhea. Pregnancy category: B*; PB: 99%; t½: 10 h
Montelukast	See Prototype Drug Chart 36.2.	
Leukotriene Synthesis Inhibitors		
Zileuton	Extended release: A/adol/C >12 y: PO: 1200 mg bid within 1 h after morning and evening meal; *max:* 2400 mg/d	For asthma. May cause headache, chills, asthenia, myalgia, and GI distress. Pregnancy category: C*; PB: 93%; t½: 1-2.3 h
Phosphodiesterase-4 Inhibitor		
Roflumilast	A: PO: 500 mcg/d	For COPD. May cause headache, nausea, diarrhea, weight loss, and suicidal ideation. This drug is contraindicated in moderate to severe liver impairment. Pregnancy category: C*; PB: 99%; t½: 17 h
Glucocorticoids (Corticosteroids)		
Intranasal Spray (See Chapter 35)		
Beclomethasone		
Qvar		
Budesonide		
Flunisolide		
Fluticasone		
Mometasone furoate		
Triamcinolone		
Aerosol Inhalation (See Chapter 46)		
Beclomethasone		
Flunisolide		
Budesonide		
Fluticasone		
Oral and Intravenous Administration (See Chapter 46)		
Cortisone acetate		
Dexamethasone		
Fludrocortisone acetate		
Hydrocortisone		
Methylprednisolone		
Prednisolone		
Prednisone		
Combination Drugs: Glucocorticoid and Beta₂ Agonist		
Fluticasone propionate and salmeterol	COPD: A:: Inhal DPI diskus (fluticasone 250 mcg and salmeterol 50 mcg): 1 inhal q12h; *max:* 2 inhal/d	For asthma and COPD. May cause headache, pharyngitis, nausea, vomiting, and musculoskeletal pain. Pregnancy category: C*; PB: 91%-98%; t½: 3-8 h
Fluticasone propionate and vilanterol	A: Inhal: 1 inhalation (fluticasone 100 mcg and vilanterol 25 mcg) at same time qd	For asthma and COPD. May cause headache, nasopharyngitis, candidiasis, fatigue, and insomnia. Pregnancy category: C*; PB: 93.7%-99.6%; t½: 21.3-24 h
Cromolyn (Do Not Use for Acute Asthmatic Attack)		
Cromolyn sodium	A/adol/C >5 y: MDI: 2 inhal (800 mcg/spray) q6h	For allergic rhinitis and conjunctivitis, asthma, and exercise-induced bronchospasm prophylaxis. May cause headache, bitter taste, cough, hoarseness, nausea, diarrhea, and myalgia. Pregnancy category: B*; PB: UK; t½: 80-90 min

*Pregnancy categories have been revised. See http://www.fda.gov/Drugs/DevelopmentApprovalProcess/DevelopmentResources/Labeling/ucm093307.htm for more information.

A, Adult; *adol,* adolescent; *bid,* twice a day; *C,* child; *COPD,* chronic obstructive pulmonary disorder; *d,* day; *DPI,* dry-powder inhaler; *GI,* gastrointestinal; *h,* hour; *inhal,* inhalation; *max,* maximum; *MDI,* metered-dose inhaler; *min,* minute; *PB,* protein binding; *PO,* by mouth; *q,* every; *qd,* every day; *t½,* half-life; *UK,* unknown; *y,* years; *>,* greater than.

Correct Use of a Metered-Dose Inhaler to Deliver Beta₂ Agonist

- Insert the medication canister into the plastic mouthpiece.
- Shake the inhaler well before use.
- Remove the cap from the mouthpiece.
- Hold the mouthpiece 1 to 2 inches from the mouth or place the inhaler mouthpiece in the mouth. A spacer may be used; discuss technique with a health care provider.
- Breathe out through the mouth, then take a *slow deep* breath in through the mouth; at the same time, push the top of the medication canister once.
- Hold the breath for a few seconds; exhale slowly through pursed lips.
- Wait 2 minutes if a second dose is required, and then repeat the procedure by first shaking the inhaler with the mouthpiece cap in place.
- Do a test spray into the air before administering the metered dose of a new inhaler or when the inhaler has not been used recently.

⊕ *Cultural Considerations*

- Respect cultural beliefs and practices concerning alternative ways to treat asthma or other COPDs, and incorporate alternative treatments into the patient care plan if they are harmless. If traditional practices and medicines are unsafe, explain in terms that can be understood by the patient.
- Advise patient to consult a health care provider of similar background and provide a written plan in the language the patient speaks and reads most easily if patient is from a different cultural background.

Evaluation

- Evaluate the effectiveness of the bronchodilator. The patient should be breathing without wheezing and should be unharmed from the side effects of the drug.
- Determine serum theophylline levels to ensure a therapeutic range.

📄 **PROTOTYPE DRUG CHART 36.2**

Montelukast

Drug Class	Dosage
Bronchodilator: Leukotriene receptor antagonist Pregnancy category: B*	A/adol >15 y: PO: 10 mg/d in the evening or at least 2 h before exercise Adol/C 6-14 y: PO: 5 mg/d in the evening or at least 2 h before exercise C 2-5 y: PO: 4 mg/d in evening
Contraindications	**Drug-Lab-Food Interactions**
Hypersensitivity, severe asthmatic attack, status asthmaticus, or acute bronchospasm *Caution:* Hepatic disease, depression, suicidal ideation, breastfeeding, pregnancy, corticosteroid withdrawal, alcoholism, older adults	Aspirin and NSAIDs block drug action; telithromycin, gemfibrozil, clopidogrel increase drug levels Lab: Abnormal liver function tests (ALT, AST)
Pharmacokinetics	**Pharmacodynamics**
Absorption: Well absorbed Distribution: 99% PB Metabolism: t½: 2.7-5.5 h Elimination: In feces and urine	PO: Onset: UK Peak: 3-4 h Duration: 24 h
Therapeutic Effects/Uses	
For treatment of allergic rhinitis and asthma, for exercise-induced bronchospasm prophylaxis Mode of Action: Binds with leukotriene receptors to inhibit smooth muscle contraction and bronchoconstriction	
Side Effects	**Adverse Reactions**
Headache, dizziness, drowsiness, restlessness, insomnia, confusion, depression, influenza, bruising, aggressive behavior	Angioedema, bleeding, seizures, edema, elevated liver enzymes *Life threatening:* Anaphylaxis, suicidal ideation, Stevens-Johnson syndrome

*Pregnancy categories have been revised. See http://www.fda.gov/Drugs/DevelopmentApprovalProcess/DevelopmentResources/Labeling/ucm093 307.htm for more information.

A, Adult; *adol,* adolescent; *ALT,* alanine aminotransferase; *AST,* aspartate aminotransferase; *C,* child; *d,* day; *h,* hour; *NSAID,* nonsteroidal antiinflammatory drug; *PB,* protein bound; *PO,* by mouth; *t½,* half-life; *UK,* unknown; *y,* year; *>,* greater than.

🌿 **COMPLEMENTARY AND ALTERNATIVE THERAPIES 36.1**

Lower Respiratory Disorders

- Ephedra may increase the effect of the theophylline group and may cause theophylline toxicity.
- St. John's wort may decrease montelukast concentration.

Montelukast has a short half-life of 2.7 to 5.5 hours and is considered safe for use in children 2 years of age and older (Prototype Drug Chart 36.2).

Leukotriene receptor antagonists and synthesis inhibitors should *not* be used during an acute asthmatic attack. They are only for prophylactic and maintenance drug therapy for chronic asthma.

⊚ NURSING PROCESS
Patient-Centered Collaborative Care
Leukotriene Receptor Antagonists

Assessment
- Obtain a medical, drug, and herbal history; report probable drug-drug or drug-herb interactions.
- Note baseline vital signs for identifying abnormalities and for future comparisons.
- Assess for wheezing, decreased breath sounds, cough, and sputum production.
- Assess sensorium for confusion and restlessness caused by hypoxia and hypercapnia.
- Assess for a history of phenylketonuria when montelukast is prescribed because children's chewable tablets contain phenylalanine.
- Determine hydration; diuresis may result in dehydration in children and older adults.

Nursing Diagnoses
- Airway Clearance, Ineffective related to retained secretions in bronchi
- Activity Intolerance related to imbalance between oxygen supply and demand
- Knowledge, Deficient of OTC drug interaction related to lack of exposure to information

Planning
- The patient will be free from wheezing, or wheezing will have significantly improved.
- The patient's lung fields will be clear within 2 to 5 days.
- The patient will take medications as prescribed.

Nursing Interventions
- Monitor respirations for rate, depth, rhythm, and type.
- Monitor lung sounds for rhonchi, wheezing, or rales.
- Observe lips and fingernails for cyanosis.
- Monitor drug therapy for effectiveness.
- Observe for side effects.
- Provide adequate hydration; fluids help loosen secretions.
- Monitor liver function tests; aspartate transaminase (AST) and alanine transaminase (ALT) may be elevated with zafirlukast and montelukast.
- Provide pulmonary therapy by chest clapping and postural drainage as appropriate.

Patient Teaching
General
- Advise patients that if an allergic reaction occurs (i.e., rash, urticaria), the drug should be discontinued and a health care provider should be notified.
- Monitor hepatic function tests periodically.
- Direct patients not to take St. John's wort without first checking with a health care provider because this product may decrease montelukast concentration.
- Warn patients that black or green tea and guarana taken with montelukast and zafirlukast may cause increased stimulation.

- Encourage patients to stop smoking.
- Discuss ways to alleviate anxiety (relaxation techniques, music).
- ⚡ Advise patients who have frequent or severe asthmatic attacks to wear an identification bracelet or a MedicAlert tag.
- Encourage patients contemplating pregnancy to seek medical advice before taking montelukast.
- Caution patients and their significant others not to open oral granule packets until they are ready to use them. After opening a packet, the dose must be administered within 15 minutes. If mixed with baby formula or an approved food (applesauce, carrots, rice, or ice cream), do *not* store for future use.
- Advise patients with known aspirin sensitivity to avoid a bronchoconstrictor response by avoiding aspirin and nonsteroidal antiinflammatory drugs (NSAIDs) while taking montelukast.

Self-Administration
- Teach patients not to use montelukast for reversal of an acute asthmatic attack because it is only recommended for prevention of acute attacks and for treatment of chronic asthma.
- Advise patients to continue to use the usual regimen of inhaled prophylaxis and short-acting rescue medication for exercise-induced bronchospasm.
- ⚡ Encourage patients to inform a health care provider if short-acting inhaled bronchodilators are needed more often than usual with montelukast.
- Tell patients to comply with the medication regimen even during symptom-free periods.
- Advise patients, especially children, that chewable tablets are to be chewed thoroughly because swallowing whole may alter absorption.

Diet
- Tell patients to take leukotriene receptor antagonists in the evening for maximum effectiveness.

 Cultural Considerations
- Use both hands to show respect when offering a prescription, instructions, or pamphlets to Asians and Pacific Islanders.

Evaluation
- Evaluate the effectiveness of the bronchodilators. The patient should be breathing without wheezing and without side effects of the drug.
- Evaluate tolerance to activity.

GLUCOCORTICOIDS (STEROIDS)

Glucocorticoids, members of the corticosteroid family, are used to treat respiratory disorders, particularly asthma. These drugs have an antiinflammatory action and are indicated if asthma is unresponsive to bronchodilator therapy or if the patient has an asthmatic attack while on maximum doses of theophylline or an adrenergic drug. It is thought that glucocorticoids have a synergistic effect when given with a beta$_2$ agonist.

Glucocorticoids can be given using the following methods:

- *MDI inhaler:* Beclomethasone
- *Tablet:* Dexamethasone, prednisone
- *Intravenous:* Dexamethasone

Inhaled glucocorticoids are not helpful in treating a severe asthmatic attack because it may take 1 to 4 weeks for an inhaled steroid to reach its full effect. When maintained on inhaled glucocorticoids, asthmatic patients demonstrate an improvement in symptoms and a decrease in asthmatic attacks. Inhaled glucocorticoids are more effective for controlling symptoms of asthma than are beta$_2$ agonists, particularly in the reduction of bronchial hyperresponsiveness. The use of an oral inhaler minimizes the risk for adrenal suppression associated with oral systemic glucocorticoid therapy. Inhaled glucocorticoids are preferred over oral preparations unless they fail to control the asthma.

The National Asthma Education and Prevention Program guidelines recommend systemic glucocorticoids—prednisone, prednisolone, dexamethasone, or methylprednisolone—for management of moderate to severe asthma exacerbations. Oral or IV administration of methylprednisolone 40 to 80 mg per day in 1 to 2 divided doses may be given for 3 to 10 days. With a single dose or short-term use, glucocorticoids may be discontinued abruptly after symptoms are controlled. Suppression of adrenal function does not usually occur within 1 to 2 weeks.

When severe asthma requires prolonged glucocorticoid therapy, weaning or tapering of the dose may be necessary to prevent an exacerbation of asthma symptoms and suppression of adrenal function. Previously, alternate-day therapy (ADT) with oral prednisone was used in some asthmatic patients. Currently, inhaled glucocorticoids are thought to be preferable in the treatment of most patients with asthma. Glucocorticoid preparations are discussed in detail in Chapter 46.

Glucocorticoids can irritate the gastric mucosa and should be taken with food to avoid ulceration. A combination inhalation drug containing the glucocorticoid fluticasone propionate and salmeterol is effective in controlling asthma symptoms by alleviating airway constriction and inflammation. This combination is used every day but requires only one inhalation in the morning and one at night. This drug does not replace fast-acting inhalers for sudden symptoms.

Side Effects and Adverse Reactions

Side effects associated with orally inhaled glucocorticoids are generally local (e.g., throat irritation, hoarseness, dry mouth, coughing) rather than systemic. Oral, laryngeal, and pharyngeal fungal infections have occurred but can be reversed with discontinuation and antifungal treatment. *Candida albicans* oropharyngeal infections may be prevented by using a spacer with the inhaler to reduce drug deposits in the oral cavity, rinsing the mouth and throat with water after each dose, and washing the apparatus (cap and plastic nose or mouthpiece) daily with warm water.

Oral and injectable glucocorticoids have many side effects when used long term, but short-term use usually causes no significant side effects. Most adverse reactions are seen within 2 weeks of glucocorticoid therapy and are usually reversible. Side effects that may occur include headache, euphoria, confusion, sweating, hyperglycemia, insomnia, nausea, vomiting, weakness, and menstrual irregularities. Adverse effects include depression, peptic ulcer, loss of bone density and development of osteoporosis, and psychosis.

When oral and IV steroids are used for prolonged periods, electrolyte imbalance, fluid retention (puffy eyelids, edema in the lower extremities, moon face, weight gain), hypertension, thinning of the skin, purpura, abnormal subcutaneous fat distribution, hyperglycemia, and impaired immune response are likely to occur.

CROMOLYN

Cromolyn sodium is used for prophylactic treatment of bronchial asthma, and it must be taken daily. It is not used for acute asthmatic attacks. Cromolyn does not have bronchodilator properties but instead acts by inhibiting release of histamine and other inflammatory mediators from mast cells to prevent an asthma attack. It's most common side effects include postnasal drip, irritation of the nose and throat, and a cough. These effects can be decreased by drinking water before and after using the drug.

Cromolyn is administered by oral inhalation via MDI or nebulizer and nasal inhalation via metered spray. It can be used with beta adrenergics and xanthine derivatives. Rebound bronchospasm is a serious side effect of cromolyn. The drug should not be discontinued abruptly because a rebound asthmatic attack can result.

Cromolyn has a low incidence of side effects but the drug is only moderately effective and many newer drugs have replaced cromolyn use. Table 36.4 lists antiinflammatory drugs for COPD, including LT receptor antagonists, LT synthesis inhibitors, phosphodiesterase-4 inhibitors, glucocorticoids, combination drugs (glucocorticoid and beta$_2$ agonist), and cromolyn.

DRUG THERAPY FOR ASTHMA ACCORDING TO SEVERITY

Chronic asthma may be controlled through a long-term medical treatment program and by a quick-relief program during an acute phase. The long-term program may vary according to the symptoms of the asthma and its severity, whereas the quick-relief therapy is the same for all classes of asthma.

DRUG THERAPY FOR ASTHMA ACCORDING TO AGE

Young Children

Cromolyn is used to treat the inflammatory effects of asthma in children. Oral glucocorticoids may be prescribed for the young child to control a moderate to severe asthmatic state. An inhalation dose of a glucocorticoid should be about 1 to 2 inhalations 4 times a day. If the condition is severe, selected young children may be ordered an oral beta$_2$-adrenergic agonist.

Older Adults

Drug selection and dosage need to be considered for the older adult with an asthmatic condition. Beta$_2$-adrenergic agonists and methylxanthines such as theophylline can cause tachycardia, nervousness, and tremors in older adults, especially those with cardiac conditions. Frequent use of glucocorticoids can increase the risk of the patient developing cataracts, osteoporosis, and diabetes mellitus. If a theophylline drug is ordered, dosages of glucocorticoids are normally decreased.

MUCOLYTICS

Mucolytics act as detergents to liquefy and loosen thick, mucous secretions so they can be expectorated. Acetylcysteine is administered by nebulization for bronchopulmonary disorders. With one important exception, *this drug should not be mixed with other drugs*. When patients with asthma or hyperactive airway disease produce increased secretions that obstruct bronchial airways, acetylcysteine may be administered as an adjunct to a bronchodilator, but these are *not* mixed together; the bronchodilator should be given 5 minutes *before* the mucolytic. Side effects include nausea and vomiting, stomatitis (oral ulcers), and "runny nose." Acetylcysteine may be diluted in soft drinks to minimize the risk of vomiting.

Dornase alfa is an enzyme that digests deoxyribonucleic acid (DNA) in thick sputum secretions of patients with cystic fibrosis (CF). This agent helps reduce respiratory infections and improves pulmonary function; such improvement usually occurs in 3 to 7 days with its use. Side effects include chest pain, sore throat, laryngitis, and hoarseness.

ANTIMICROBIALS

Antibiotics are used only if a bacterial infection results from retained mucous secretions. Trimethoprim-sulfamethoxazole is effective for the treatment of mild to moderate acute exacerbations of chronic bronchitis (AECBs) from infectious causes.

CRITICAL THINKING CASE STUDY

MA, a 55-year-old patient, was recently diagnosed with bronchial asthma. Her mother and three brothers also have asthma. In the past year, MA has had three asthmatic attacks that were treated with prednisone and an albuterol inhaler. At an office visit today, prednisone is prescribed for 4 weeks, and the order is written as follows: day 1, 1 tablet 4 times a day; day 2, 1 tablet 3 times a day; day 3, 1 tablet 2 times a day; day 4, 1 tablet in the morning; day 5, one-half tablet in the morning.

1. Explain the purpose for the use of prednisone during an asthmatic attack. Explain why the dosage is decreased (tapered) over a period of 5 days.
2. Can cromolyn sodium be substituted for prednisone during an asthmatic attack? Explain your answer.
3. MA is prescribed albuterol. What effect does albuterol have on controlling asthma?
4. For each drug dose, MA is to take two puffs of albuterol administered by the inhaler. What instructions should she be given concerning use of the inhaler?

To minimize the frequency of MA's asthmatic attacks, the health care provider prescribes aminophylline 1200 mg/day in divided doses. The albuterol inhalation is to be taken as needed. Nursing interventions include patient history of asthmatic attacks and physical assessment.

5. When taking the patient's history, what should the nurse include concerning asthmatic attacks? What physical assessment would suggest an asthmatic attack?
6. What type of drug is aminophylline? Why should the nurse ask MA if she smokes?
7. What are the side effects, adverse reactions, and drug interactions related to aminophylline?
8. What nonpharmacologic measures can the nurse suggest that may decrease the frequency of asthmatic attacks?
9. Which are appropriate rescue medications used for acute asthmatic attacks? Which drugs are used as preventive medications?

NCLEX STUDY QUESTIONS

1. Fluticasone propionate and salmeterol combination inhalation is ordered for a patient with chronic obstructive pulmonary disease. What does the nurse know about this medication? (Select all that apply.)
   a. It can be used to treat an acute attack.
   b. It is delivered as a dry-powder inhaler.
   c. It contains a beta$_1$ agonist and cromolyn.
   d. It is taken as one puff two times a day.
   e. It promotes bronchodilation.

2. A patient with chronic obstructive pulmonary disease has an acute bronchospasm. The nurse anticipates that the health care provider will prescribe which medication?
   a. Zafirlukast
   b. Epinephrine
   c. Dexamethasone
   d. Beclomethasone

3. A patient is prescribed aminophylline-theophylline. For what adverse effect should the nurse monitor the patient?
   a. Drowsiness
   b. Hypoglycemia
   c. Increased heart rate
   d. Decreased white blood cell count

4. A patient is receiving intravenous aminophylline. The nurse checks the patient's lab values and sees the serum theophylline level is 32 mcg/mL. What action should the nurse take?
   a. Assess the patient's breath sounds for improvement.
   b. Increase the dosage per sliding-scale directions.
   c. Notify the health care provider of the level.
   d. Have the laboratory collect another sample to verify the results.

5. A patient with chronic obstructive pulmonary disease is taking the leukotriene antagonist montelukast. The nurse is aware that this medication is given for which purpose?
   a. Maintenance treatment of asthma
   b. Treatment of acute asthmatic attack
   c. Reversing bronchospasm associated with chronic obstructive pulmonary disease
   d. Treatment of inflammation in chronic bronchitis

Answers: 1, b, d, e; 2, b; 3, c; 4, c; 5, a.

Cardiovascular Drugs

The cardiovascular system includes the heart, blood vessels (arteries and veins), and blood flow. Blood that is abundant in oxygen (O_2), nutrients, and hormones moves through vessels called *arteries,* which narrow to arterioles and then to capillaries. Capillaries transport nourished blood to body cells and absorb waste products, such as carbon dioxide (CO_2), urea, creatinine, and ammonia. The deoxygenated blood returns to the circulation by small venules and larger veins to be eliminated by the lungs and kidneys with other waste products (Fig. XII.1).

The heart's pumping action serves as the energy source that circulates blood to the cells of the body. Blockage of vessels can inhibit blood flow.

HEART

The heart is composed of four chambers including the right and left atria and the right and left ventricles (Fig. XII.2). The right atrium receives deoxygenated blood from the circulation, and the right ventricle pumps blood through the pulmonary artery to the lungs for gas exchange (carbon dioxide for oxygen). The left atrium receives oxygenated blood, and the left ventricle pumps the blood into the aorta for systemic circulation.

The heart muscle, called the *myocardium,* surrounds the ventricles and atria. The ventricles have thick walls, especially the left ventricle, to produce the muscular force needed to pump blood to the pulmonary and systemic circulations. The atria have thin walls, have less pumping action, and receive blood from the circulation and lungs.

The heart has a fibrous covering called the *pericardium,* which protects it from injury and infection. The *endocardium* is a three-layered membrane that lines the inner part of the heart chambers. Four valves—two atrioventricular (tricuspid and mitral) and two semilunar (pulmonic and aortic)—control blood flow between the atria and ventricles and between the ventricles and the pulmonary artery and the aorta. There are two main coronary arteries: the right coronary artery divides into branches that supply blood to the right atrium and both ventricles of the heart, and the left coronary artery divides near its origin to form the left circumflex artery and the anterior descending artery, which supply blood

to the left atrium and both ventricles of the heart. Blockage to one of these arteries can result in a myocardial infarction (MI), or heart attack.

CONDUCTION OF ELECTRICAL IMPULSES

The myocardium is capable of generating and conducting its own electrical impulses. The cardiac impulse normally originates in the *sinoatrial (SA) node* located in the posterior wall of the right atrium. The SA node is frequently called the *pacemaker,* because it regulates the heartbeat (firing of cardiac impulses), which is approximately 60 to 80 beats/min in the normal adult. The *atrioventricular (AV) node,* located in the posterior right side of the interatrial septum, has a continuous tract of fibers called the *bundle of His,* or the AV bundle. The AV node has an adult rate of 40 to 60 beats/min. If the SA node fails, the AV node takes over as the pacemaker, thus causing a slower heart rate; the AV node sends impulses to the ventricles. These two conducting systems, the SA and AV nodes, can act independently of each other. The ventricle can contract independently 30 to 40 times per minute.

Drugs that affect cardiac contraction include calcium, digitalis preparations, and quinidine and its related preparations. The autonomic nervous system (ANS) and drugs that stimulate or inhibit it influence heart contractions. The sympathetic nervous system and drugs that stimulate it *increase* heart rate; the parasympathetic nervous system and drugs that stimulate it *decrease* heart rate.

REGULATION OF HEART RATE AND BLOOD FLOW

The heart beats approximately 60 to 80 times per minute in an adult, pumping blood into the systemic circulation. As blood travels, resistance to blood flow develops, and arterial pressure increases. The average systemic arterial pressure, known as *blood pressure,* is 120/80 mm Hg. Arterial blood pressure is determined by peripheral resistance and *cardiac output,* which is the volume of blood expelled from the heart in 1 minute, calculated by multiplying the heart rate by the stroke volume. The average cardiac output is 4 to

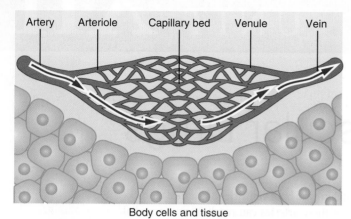

FIG. XII.1 Basic Structures of the Vascular System.

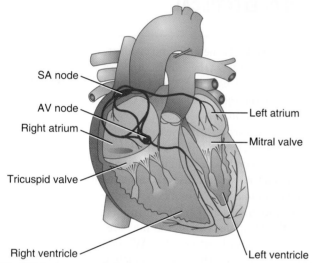

FIG. XII.2 Anatomy of the heart. *AV node,* Atrioventricular node; *SA node,* sinoatrial node.

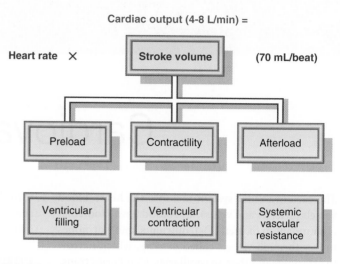

FIG. XII.3 Cardiac output and stroke volume.

8 L/min. *Stroke volume*, the amount of blood ejected from the left ventricle with each heartbeat, is approximately 70 mL/beat.

Three factors—preload, contractility, and afterload—determine the stroke volume (Fig. XII.3). *Preload* refers to the blood flow force that stretches the ventricle at the end of diastole. However, an increase in preload can increase stroke volume, and a decrease in preload can decrease stroke volume. *Contractility* is the force of ventricular contraction, and afterload is the resistance to ventricular ejection of blood, which is caused by opposing pressures in the aorta and systemic circulation. If afterload *increases,* stroke volume will *decrease,* and if afterload *decreases,* stroke volume will *increase.*

Specific drugs can increase or decrease preload and afterload, affecting both stroke volume and cardiac output. Most vasodilators decrease preload and afterload, thus decreasing arterial pressure and cardiac output.

CIRCULATION

There are two types of circulation, pulmonary and systemic. With *pulmonary circulation,* the heart pumps deoxygenated blood from the right ventricle through the pulmonary artery to the lungs. The pulmonary artery carries blood that has a high concentration of carbon dioxide. Oxygenated blood returns to the left atrium by the pulmonary vein.

With *systemic circulation,* also called *peripheral circulation,* the heart pumps blood from the left ventricle to the aorta and into the general circulation. Arteries and arterioles carry the blood to capillary beds. Nutrients in the capillary blood are transferred to cells in exchange for waste products. Blood returns to the heart through venules and veins.

BLOOD

Blood is composed of plasma, red blood cells (erythrocytes), white blood cells (leukocytes), and platelets. Plasma, made up of 90% water and 10% solutes, constitutes 55% of the total blood volume. The solutes in plasma include glucose, protein, lipids, amino acids, electrolytes, minerals, lactic and pyruvic acids, hormones, enzymes, oxygen, and carbon dioxide.

The major function of blood is to provide nutrients, including oxygen, to body cells. Most of the oxygen is carried on the hemoglobin of red blood cells (RBCs). White blood cells (WBCs) are the major defense mechanism of the body and act by engulfing microorganisms. They also produce antibodies. The platelets are large cells that cause blood to coagulate. RBCs have a life span of approximately 120 days, whereas the life span of a WBC is only 2 to 24 hours.

This unit is composed of five chapters that deal with drugs for cardiac disorders, diuretics and antihypertensive drugs, and drugs for circulatory disorders. Cardiac glycosides, antianginals, and antidysrhythmics are described in Chapter 37. Chapter 38 discusses the five categories of diuretics, and the four major categories of antihypertensive agents are presented in Chapter 39. The five groups of drugs covered in Chapters 40 and 41 are the anticoagulants, antiplatelets, thrombolytics, antihyperlipidemics, and peripheral vasodilators.

Cardiac Glycosides, Antianginals, and Antidysrhythmics

http://evolve.elsevier.com/McCuistion/pharmacology/

OBJECTIVES

- Differentiate the actions of cardiac glycosides, antianginal drugs, and antidysrhythmic drugs.
- Describe the signs and symptoms of digitalis toxicity.
- Compare the side effects and adverse reactions of nitrates, beta blockers, calcium channel blockers, quinidine, and procainamide.

- Apply the nursing process, including patient teaching, related to cardiac glycosides, antianginal drugs, and antidysrhythmic drugs.

OUTLINE

KEY TERMS

Three groups of drugs—cardiac glycosides, antianginals, and antidysrhythmics—are discussed in this chapter. Drugs in these groups regulate heart contraction, heart rate and rhythm, and blood flow to the myocardium (heart muscle).

CARDIAC GLYCOSIDES

Digitalis use began as early as CE 1200, making it one of the oldest drugs. It is still used in a purified form. Digitalis is obtained from the purple and white foxglove plant, and it can be poisonous. Digitalis preparations have come to be known for their effectiveness in treating heart failure (HF), also known as *cardiac failure* (CF), and previously referred to as congestive heart failure (CHF). When the heart muscle (*myocardium*) weakens and enlarges, it loses its ability to pump blood through the heart and into the systemic circulation. This is called heart failure, *pump failure*, or *chronic heart failure*. When compensatory mechanisms fail and the peripheral and lung tissues are congested, the condition is called *acute heart failure*. The causes of HF include chronic hypertension, myocardial infarction (MI), coronary artery disease (CAD), valvular heart disease, congenital heart disease, and arteriosclerosis.

Heart failure can be left-sided or right-sided. The patient has *left-sided HF* when the left ventricle does not contract sufficiently to pump the blood returned from the lungs and left atrium out through the aorta into the peripheral circulation; this causes excessive amounts of blood to back up into the lung tissue. Usually the patient has shortness of breath (SOB) and dyspnea. *Right-sided HF* occurs when the heart does not sufficiently pump the blood returned into the right atrium from the systemic circulation. As a result, the blood and its constituents are backed up into peripheral tissues, causing peripheral edema. Left-sided HF may lead to right-sided HF and vice versa. Myocardial hypertrophy resulting in *cardiomegaly,* increased heart size, can be a major problem associated with chronic HF.

In the cardiac physiology of HF, an increase in *preload* and *afterload* occurs. The increased preload results from an excess of blood volume in the ventricle at the end of diastole. This occurs because of a pathologic increase in the stretching and thickening of the ventricular walls, which allows a greater filling pressure associated with a weakened heart. Increased afterload is an additional pressure or force in the ventricular wall caused by excess resistance in the aorta. This resistance must be overcome to open the aortic valve so blood can be ejected into the circulation. The American College of Cardiology Foundation (ACCF) and the American Heart Association (AHA) have classified HF in stages according to its severity. Table 37.1 lists the stages of HF according to the ACCF/AHA. In the early stage of HF, there are no symptoms, and no structural heart damage occurs. Detailed information related to the staging process of HF can be found at http://www.heart.org/HEARTORG/Conditions/Heart Failure/Heart-Failure_UCM_002019_SubHomePage.jsp.

Naturally occurring cardiac glycosides are found in a number of plants, including *Digitalis*. Also called *Digitalis glycosides,* this group of drugs inhibits the sodium-potassium pump, which results in an increase in intracellular sodium. This increase leads to an influx of calcium, which causes the cardiac muscle fibers to contract more efficiently. Digitalis preparations have three effects on heart muscle: (1) a positive inotropic action *increases* myocardial contraction stroke volume, (2) a negative chronotropic action *decreases* heart rate, and (3) a negative dromotropic action *decreases* conduction of heart cells. The increase in myocardial contractility strengthens cardiac, peripheral, and kidney function by enhancing cardiac output, decreasing preload, improving blood flow to the periphery and kidneys, decreasing edema, and promoting fluid excretion. As a result, fluid retention in the lungs and extremities is decreased. Digoxin does not prolong life, rather it acts by increasing the force and velocity of myocardial systolic contraction.

Digoxin is a secondary drug for HF. First-line drugs used to treat acute HF include intravenous (IV) inotropic agents (dopamine and dobutamine) and phosphodiesterase inhibitors, such as milrinone. Other drugs prescribed for HF include oral diuretics, beta blockers, angiotensin-converting enzyme (ACE) inhibitors, angiotensin-receptor blockers (ARBs), calcium channel blockers, and vasodilators, all of which are more convenient to self-administer. Oral administration allows the patient to go home on these medications.

Cardiac glycosides are also used to correct atrial fibrillation, cardiac dysrhythmia with rapid uncoordinated contractions of atrial myocardium, and atrial flutter, cardiac dysrhythmia with rapid contractions of 200 to 300 beats/min. This is accomplished by the negative chronotropic effects (decreased heart rate) and negative dromotropic effects (decreased conduction through the atrioventricular [AV] node).

When digoxin cannot convert atrial fibrillation to normal heart rhythm, the goal is to slow the heart rate by decreasing electrical impulses through the AV node. For management of atrial fibrillation, a calcium channel blocker such as verapamil may be prescribed. To prevent thromboemboli resulting from atrial fibrillation, warfarin is prescribed concurrently with other drug therapy. Warfarin is discussed in Chapter 40.

Nonpharmacologic Measures to Treat Heart Failure

Nondrug therapy is an integral part of the regimen for controlling HF. The nondrug component of the regimen should be tailored to meet the needs of each patient, but the following

TABLE 37.1	The American College of Cardiology Foundation/American Heart Association Stages of Heart Failure
Stage	**Characteristics According to Stage**
A	High risk for heart failure without symptoms of structural heart disease
B	Some cardiac changes, such as decreased ejection fraction without symptoms of heart failure
C	Structural heart disease with symptoms of heart failure, such as fatigue, shortness of breath, edema, and decrease in physical activity
D	Severe structural heart disease and marked symptoms of heart failure at rest

are some general recommendations. The patient should limit salt intake to 2 g/day, approximately 1 teaspoon. Alcohol intake should be either decreased to 1 drink per day or completely avoided because excessive alcohol use can lead to cardiomyopathy. Fluid intake may be restricted. Smoking should be avoided because it deprives the heart of oxygen (O_2). Obesity may increase cardiovascular problems if it is associated with unhealthy behaviors, thus obese patients should modify their behaviors as needed. Saturated fat intake should be decreased. Mild exercise, such as walking or bicycling, is recommended.

Laboratory Tests

Atrial Natriuretic Hormone or Peptide. Reference values: 20 to 77 pg/mL; 20 to 77 ng/L (SI units). An elevated atriuretic hormone (ANH) or atrial natriuretic peptide (ANP) may confirm HF. ANH is secreted from the atria of the heart and acts as an antagonist to renin and aldosterone. Released during expansion of the atrium, it produces vasodilation and increases glomerular filtration rate (GFR). Results of ANH secretion include a large volume of urine that decreases blood volume and blood pressure.

Brain Natriuretic Peptide. Reference values: Desired value is less than 100 pg/mL; positive value is greater than 100 pg/mL. The brain natriuretic peptide (BNP) is primarily secreted from atrial cardiac cells and, when tested, aids in the diagnosis of HF. Diagnosing HF is difficult in persons with lung disease who are experiencing dyspnea and in those who are obese or older. An elevated BNP helps differentiate that dyspnea is due to HF rather than to lung dysfunction. Frequently the BNP is higher than 100 pg/mL in women who are 65 years of age or older. An 80-year-old woman may have a BNP of 160 pg/mL; however, the BNP is markedly higher (i.e., 400 pg/mL) in HF. BNP is considered a more sensitive test than ANP for diagnosing HF. Today, a bedside/emergency department machine can be used to measure BNP.

Digoxin

Prototype Drug Chart 37.1 gives the pharmacologic data for digoxin, a cardiac glycoside.

Pharmacokinetics The absorption rate of digoxin in oral tablet form is 70% to 80%. The rate is 75% to 85% in liquid form. The protein-binding power for digoxin is 20% to 30%. The half-life is 30 to 40 hours. Because of its long half-life, drug accumulation can occur. Side effects should be closely monitored to detect digitalis toxicity. Patients should be made aware of side effects that need to be reported to the health care provider. Serum digoxin levels are most commonly drawn when actual digitoxicity is suspected. This allows the health care provider to ascertain the extent of such toxicity and to confirm elimination of the

---

PROTOTYPE DRUG CHART 37.1

❶ Digoxin

Drug Class	Dosage
Cardiac glycoside Pregnancy category: C*	Heart failure: A/adol/C >10 y: PO: LD 10-15 mcg/kg in 3 divided doses; maint: 3.4-5.1 mcg/kg/d A/adol/C >10 y: IV/IM: LD 8-12 mcg/kg/d in 3 divided doses; maint: 2.4-3.6 mcg/kg/d

Contraindications	Drug-Lab-Food Interactions
Ventricular fibrillation *Caution:* AMI, AV block, hypertension, hypothyroidism, hyperthyroidism, renal and hepatic dysfunction, bradycardia, hypokalemia, electrolyte imbalance, older adults	Drug: Increased digoxin serum level with quinidine, flecainide, verapamil, indomethacin; decreased digoxin absorption with antacids, kaolin, pectin, psyllium, acarbose, colestipol; increased risk for digoxin toxicity with thiazide diuretics, loop diuretics, proton pump inhibitors Lab: Hypokalemia, hypomagnesemia, hypercalcemia can increase digitalis (digoxin) toxicity

Pharmacokinetics	Pharmacodynamics
Absorption: PO tablet: 70%-80%; PO liquid: 75%-85% Distribution: PB: 20%-30% Metabolism: t½: 30-40 h Excretion: 70% in urine; 30% by liver metabolism	PO: Onset: 30 min-2 h Peak: 2-6 h Duration: 3-4 d IV: Onset: 5-30 min Peak: 1-6 h Duration: UK

Therapeutic Effects/Uses
To treat heart failure, atrial fibrillation Mode of Action: Inhibits sodium-potassium ATPase, promoting increased force of cardiac contraction, cardiac output, and tissue perfusion; decreases ventricular rate

Side Effects	Adverse Reactions
Anorexia, nausea, vomiting, diarrhea, abdominal pain, headache, blurred or yellow vision, dizziness, weakness, confusion	Bradycardia *Life threatening:* Cardiac dysrhythmias, thrombocytopenia

*Pregnancy categories have been revised. See http://www.fda.gov/Drugs/DevelopmentApprovalProcess/DevelopmentResources/Labeling/ucm093307.htm for more information.

A, Adult; *adol,* adolescent; *AMI,* acute myocardial infarction; *ATPase,* adenosine triphosphatase; *AV,* atrioventricular; *C,* child; *d,* day; *h,* hour; *IM,* intramuscular; *IV,* intravenous; *LD,* loading dose; *maint,* maintenance; *min,* minute; *PB,* protein binding; *PO,* by mouth; *t½,* half-life; *UK,* unknown; *y,* year; *>,* greater than.

drug after it is stopped or decreased in dosage (see the Digitalis [Digoxin] Toxicity section later in this chapter).

Thirty percent of digoxin is metabolized by the liver, and 70% is excreted by the kidneys mostly unchanged. Kidney dysfunction can affect the excretion of digoxin. Thyroid dysfunction can alter the metabolism of cardiac glycosides. For patients with hypothyroidism, the dose of digoxin should be decreased; in hyperthyroidism, the dose may need to be increased.

Pharmacodynamics In patients with a failing heart, cardiac glycosides increase myocardial contraction, which increases cardiac output and improves circulation and tissue perfusion. Because these drugs decrease conduction through the AV node, the heart rate decreases. The onset and peak actions of oral and IV digoxin vary. The digoxin therapeutic serum level for dysrhythmias is 0.8 to 2.0 ng/mL. The target therapeutic serum level for heart failure is 0.5 to 1.0 ng/mL.

Digoxin can be administered orally or by the IV route. Table 37.2 lists the digitalis preparations and their dosages, uses, and considerations.

Digitalis (Digoxin) Toxicity

Overdose or accumulation of digoxin causes digitalis toxicity. Signs and symptoms include anorexia, diarrhea, nausea and vomiting, bradycardia (pulse rate below 60 beats/min), premature ventricular contractions, cardiac dysrhythmias, headaches, malaise, blurred vision, visual illusions (white, green, or yellow halos around objects), confusion, and delirium. Older adults are more prone to toxicity.

Cardiotoxicity is a serious adverse reaction to digoxin, and ventricular dysrhythmias result. Three cardiac-altered functions can contribute to digoxin-induced ventricular dysrhythmias: (1) suppression of AV conduction, (2) increased automaticity, and (3) a decreased refractory period in ventricular muscle. The antidysrhythmics phenytoin and lidocaine are effective in treating digoxin-induced ventricular dysrhythmias. Lidocaine should be limited to short-term treatment.

Antidote for Cardiac/Digitalis Glycosides

Digoxin-immune Fab may be given to treat severe digitalis toxicity. This agent binds with digoxin to form complex molecules that can be excreted in the urine, thus digoxin is unable to bind at the cellular site of action. Serum digoxin levels should be closely monitored, and signs and symptoms of digoxin toxicity should be reported promptly to the health care provider. Digitalis toxicity may result in first-degree, second-degree, or complete heart block.

Drug Interactions

Drug interaction with digitalis preparations can cause digitalis toxicity. Many of the potent diuretics, such as furosemide and hydrochlorothiazide, promote the loss of potassium from the body. The resultant hypokalemia, low serum potassium level, increases the effect of digoxin at its myocardial cell site of action, resulting in digitalis toxicity. Cortisone preparations taken systemically promote sodium retention and potassium excretion or loss and can also cause hypokalemia. Patients who take digoxin along with a potassium-wasting diuretic or a cortisone drug should consume foods rich in potassium or take potassium supplements to avoid hypokalemia and digitalis toxicity. Antacids can decrease digitalis absorption if taken at the same time. To prevent this problem, doses should be staggered.

! TABLE 37.2	Cardiac Glycosides and Inotropic Agents	
Drug	**Route and Dosage**	**Uses and Considerations**
Rapid-Acting Digitalis		
Digoxin	See Prototype Drug Chart 37.1.	
Phosphodiesterase Inhibitors (Positive Inotropic Bipyridines)		
Milrinone lactate	A: IV: Initially: 50 mcg/kg over 10 min; maint: 0.375-0.75 mcg/kg/min continuous infusion; *max.* 0.75 mcg/kg/min infusion	For heart failure. May cause headache, hypotension, tachycardia, and dysrhythmias. Pregnancy category: C*; PB: 70%; t½: 2.3 h
Atrial Natriuretic Peptide Hormones		
Nesiritide	A: IV bolus: 2 mcg/kg; maint: 0.01 mcg/kg/min infusion; *max:* 0.03 mcg/kg/min continuous infusion	For acute heart failure. May cause hypotension, headache, dizziness, ventricular tachycardia, and insomnia. Pregnancy category: C*; PB: UK; t½: 18 min
Antidote for Digitalis Toxicity		
Digoxin-immune Fab	A/adol/C: IV: 800 mg IV as a single dose or 400 mg then 400 mg more if needed	For digitalis overdose and toxicity, as well as cardiac glycoside–induced dysrhythmias. May cause anaphylaxis, orthostatic hypotension, atrial fibrillation, heart failure exacerbation, and hypokalemia. Pregnancy category: C*; PB: UK; t½: 15 h

*Pregnancy categories have been revised. See http://www.fda.gov/Drugs/DevelopmentApprovalProcess/DevelopmentResources/Labeling/ucm093307.htm for more information.

A, Adult; *adol*, adolescent; *C*, child; *h*, hours; *IV*, intravenous; *maint*, maintenance; *max*, maximum; *min*, minute; *PB*, protein binding; *t½*, half-life; *UK*, unknown.

NURSING PROCESS
Patient-Centered Collaborative Care

❶ *Cardiac Glycosides: Digoxin*

Assessment
- Obtain a drug and herbal history. Report if a drug-drug or drug-herb interaction is probable. If a patient is taking digoxin and a potassium-wasting diuretic or cortisone drug, hypokalemia can result, causing digitalis toxicity. A low serum potassium level enhances the action of digoxin. Patients taking a thiazide and/or cortisone with digoxin should take a potassium supplement.
- Obtain a baseline pulse rate for future comparisons. Apical pulse should be taken for a full minute and should be greater than 60 beats/min.
- Assess for signs and symptoms of digitalis toxicity. Common symptoms include anorexia, nausea, vomiting, bradycardia, cardiac dysrhythmias, and visual disturbances. Report symptoms immediately to the health care provider.

Nursing Diagnoses
- Cardiac Output, Decreased related to decreased cardiac pumping ability
- Tissue Perfusion, Ineffective Peripheral related to decreased cardiac pumping ability
- Anxiety related to threat to cardiac health status

Planning
- The patient will check the pulse rate daily before taking digoxin.
- The patient will report the pulse rate when it is less than 60 beats/min or when a marked decline in pulse rate occurs.
- The patient will eat foods high in potassium to maintain a desired serum potassium level (see Patient Teaching and Diet sections).

Nursing Interventions
- ⚡ Ascertain apical pulse rate before administering digoxin. Do *not* administer if pulse rate is below 60 beats/min.
- Determine signs of peripheral and pulmonary edema, which indicate HF is present.
- ⚡ Monitor serum digoxin level (normal therapeutic drug range is 0.8 to 2 ng/mL). A serum digoxin level greater than 2 ng/mL is indicative of digitalis toxicity.
- ⚡ Monitor serum potassium level (normal range is 3.5 to 5.0 mEq/L), and report if hypokalemia (<3.5 mEq/L) is present.

Patient Teaching
General
- Explain to patients the importance of adherence to drug therapy. A visiting nurse may ensure that medications are taken properly.
- Advise patients to avoid adverse drug interactions by not taking over-the-counter (OTC) drugs without first consulting a health care provider.
- Keep drugs out of reach of small children, and request childproof bottles.

- Teach patients and caregivers to check the pulse rate before administering drugs.
- Inform patients of possible herb-drug interactions (Complementary and Alternative Therapies 37.1).

Self-Administration
- Teach patients how to check the pulse rate before taking digoxin and to notify a health care provider if the pulse rate is irregular or less than 60 beats/min.

Side Effects
- ⚡ Instruct patients to report side effects: pulse rate less than 60 beats/min, nausea and vomiting, headache, diarrhea, and visual disturbances, including diplopia.

Diet
- Advise patients to eat foods high in potassium, such as fresh and dried fruits, fruit juices, and vegetables, including potatoes.

🌐 *Cultural Considerations*
- Analyze conflicts in values and beliefs, and use culturally consistent communication practices. It is essential that patients taking digoxin, diuretics, and potassium supplements for HF do not miss any doses of their medications. Patient should be fully aware of adverse effects and should readily report them to the health care provider.
- Validate the patient's understanding of purposes for taking these drugs. Be aware of potential cultural differences related to response to authority and involvement of family members. For example, Amish people often respect authority and may follow instructions without question, but family members must be involved in decision making.

Evaluation
- Evaluate the effectiveness of digoxin by noting the patient's response to a drug (decreased heart rate, decreased rales) and absence of side effects. Continue monitoring the pulse rate.

🌿 **COMPLEMENTARY AND ALTERNATIVE THERAPIES 37.1**

Cardiac Glycosides: Digoxin

- Ginseng may falsely elevate digoxin levels.
- St. John's wort decreases absorption of digoxin and thus decreases serum digoxin level.
- Psyllium may decrease digoxin absorption.
- Hawthorn may increase the effect of digoxin.
- Licorice can potentiate the effect of digoxin; it promotes potassium loss (hypokalemia), which increases the effect of digoxin, and it may cause digitalis toxicity.
- Aloe may increase the risk of digitalis toxicity. It increases potassium loss, which increases the effect of digoxin.
- Ma-huang, or ephedra, increases the risk of digitalis toxicity.
- Goldenseal may decrease the effects of cardiac glycosides and may increase the effects of antidysrhythmics.

❶ Phosphodiesterase Inhibitors

Phosphodiesterase inhibitors are another positive inotropic group of drugs given to treat acute HF. This drug group inhibits the enzyme phosphodiesterase (PDE), which promotes a positive inotropic response and vasodilation. A drug in this group is milrinone lactate. This drug increases stroke volume and cardiac output and promotes vasodilation. It is administered intravenously for no longer than 48 to 72 hours. Severe cardiac dysrhythmias might result from the use of PDE inhibitors, so the patient's electrocardiogram (ECG) and cardiac status should be closely monitored. Milrinone is a high-alert medication that may cause significant harm to a patient when given inappropriately.

OTHER AGENTS USED TO TREAT HEART FAILURE

Vasodilators, ACE inhibitors, angiotensin II–receptor antagonists (blockers), diuretics (thiazides, furosemide), spironolactone, and some beta blockers are other drug groups prescribed to treat HF.

Vasodilators can be used to treat HF. The vasodilators decrease venous blood return to the heart and result in a decrease in cardiac filling, ventricular stretching (preload), and oxygen demand on the heart. Arteriolar dilators act in three ways: they (1) reduce cardiac afterload, which increases cardiac output; (2) dilate the arterioles of the kidneys, which improves renal perfusion and increases fluid loss; and (3) improve circulation to the skeletal muscles.

ACE inhibitors are usually prescribed for HF. ACE inhibitors dilate venules and arterioles, which improves renal blood flow and decreases blood fluid volume. ACE inhibitors also moderately decrease the release of aldosterone, which in turn reduces sodium and fluid retention.

ACE inhibitors can increase potassium levels, so serum potassium levels should be monitored, especially if potassium-sparing diuretics such as spironolactone are being taken concurrently. Angiotensin II–receptor blockers (ARBs) such as valsartan and candesartan have been approved for HF in patients who cannot tolerate ACE inhibitors. Refer to Chapter 39 for a complete discussion of ACE inhibitors and ARBs.

Diuretics are the first-line drug treatment for reducing fluid volume. They are frequently prescribed with digoxin or other agents.

Spironolactone, a potassium-sparing diuretic, is used in treating moderate to severe HF. Aldosterone secretions are increased in HF. This promotes body loss of potassium and magnesium needed by the heart and increases sodium and water retention. Spironolactone blocks the production of aldosterone. This drug improves heart rate variability and decreases myocardial fibrosis by its cardioprotective effect of blocking aldosterone in the heart and blood vessels to promote cardiac remodeling. The recommended dose for HF is 12.5 to 25 mg/day. Occurrence of hyperkalemia (excess serum potassium) is rare unless the patient is receiving 50 mg/day and has renal insufficiency. However, the serum potassium level should be closely monitored.

In the past, all beta blockers were contraindicated for patients with HF because this drug class reduces cardiac contractility.

With dosage control, beta blockers (carvedilol, metoprolol, and bisoprolol) have been shown to improve cardiac performance. Doses should be low initially and gradually increased. It may take 1 to 3 months for a beneficial effect to develop. Refer to Chapters 15 and 39 for more information on beta blockers.

Nesiritide is an atrial natriuretic peptide hormone that inhibits antidiuretic hormone (ADH) by increasing urine sodium loss. Its effect in correcting HF is achieved by promoting vasodilation, natriuresis, and diuresis. It is useful for treating patients who have acute decompensated HF with dyspnea at rest or who have dyspnea with little physical exertion.

BiDil, a combination of hydralazine (for blood pressure) and isosorbide dinitrate (a dilator to relieve heart pain) has received U.S. Food and Drug Administration (FDA) approval for treating HF, especially in African Americans, who have more than twice the rate of HF as Caucasians; a research study has shown BiDil to be effective in treating HF in the African American population.

ANTIANGINAL DRUGS

Antianginal drugs are used to treat angina pectoris, a condition of acute cardiac pain caused by inadequate blood flow to the myocardium due to either plaque occlusions within or spasms of the coronary arteries. With decreased blood flow, there is a decrease in oxygen to the myocardium, which results in pain. Anginal pain is frequently described by the patient as tightness, pressure in the center of the chest, and pain radiating down the left arm. Referred pain felt in the neck and left arm commonly occurs with severe angina pectoris. Anginal attacks may lead to MI (heart attack). Anginal pain usually lasts for only a few minutes. Stress tests, echocardiogram, cardiac profile laboratory tests, and cardiac catheterization may be needed to determine the degree of blockage in the coronary arteries and then also to treat the condition.

Types of Angina Pectoris

The frequency of anginal pain depends on many factors, including the type of angina. There are three types of angina:

- *Classic (stable) angina* occurs with predictable stress or exertion.
- *Unstable (preinfarction) angina* occurs frequently with progressive severity unrelated to activity and is unpredictable regarding stress/exertion and intensity.
- *Variant (Prinzmetal, vasospastic) angina* occurs during rest.

The first two types are caused by a narrowing or partial occlusion of the coronary arteries; variant angina is caused by vessel spasm (vasospasm). It is common for a patient to have both classic and variant angina. Unstable angina often indicates an impending MI; it is an emergency that needs immediate medical intervention.

Nonpharmacologic Measures to Control Angina

A combination of pharmacologic and nonpharmacologic measures is usually necessary to control and prevent anginal attacks. Nonpharmacologic methods of decreasing anginal attacks are to avoid heavy meals, smoking, extreme weather changes, strenuous exercise, and emotional upset. Proper nutrition, moderate exercise (only after consulting with a health care provider), adequate rest, and relaxation techniques are used as preventive measures.

Types of Antianginal Drugs

Antianginal drugs increase blood flow either by increasing oxygen supply or by decreasing oxygen demand by the myocardium. Three types of antianginals are (1) nitrates, (2) beta blockers, and (3) calcium channel blockers. The major systemic effect of nitrates is a reduction of venous tone, which decreases the workload of the heart and promotes vasodilation. Beta blockers and calcium channel blockers decrease the workload of the heart and decrease oxygen demands.

Nitrates and calcium channel blockers are effective in treating variant (vasospastic) angina pectoris; beta blockers are not effective for this type of angina and may aggravate it. With stable angina, beta blockers can effectively be used to prevent angina attacks. Table 37.3 lists the effects of antianginal drug groups on angina.

With unstable angina, immediate medical care is necessary. Nitrates are usually given sublingually and intravenously as needed. If the cardiac pain continues, a beta blocker is given intravenously, and if the patient is unable to tolerate beta blockers, a calcium channel blocker may be substituted.

Nitrates

Nitrates were the first agents used to relieve angina. They affect coronary arteries and blood vessels in the venous circulation. Nitrates cause generalized vascular and coronary vasodilation, which increases blood flow through the coronary arteries to the myocardial cells. This group of drugs reduces myocardial ischemia but can cause hypotension.

⚡ PATIENT SAFETY

Do not confuse:
- **Nitrostat,** a nitroglycerin drug that promotes coronary vasodilation and thus increases blood flow to the coronary arteries, with **Nystatin,** an antifungal antibiotic that has fungistatic and fungicidal activity against yeasts and fungi

The sublingual (SL) nitroglycerin tablet, which is absorbed under the tongue, comes in various dosages, but the average prescribed dose is 0.4 mg following cardiac pain. If pain has not subsided then 911 should be called. The effects of SL nitroglycerin last for 30 to 60 minutes. The SL tablets decompose when exposed to heat and light, so they must be kept in their original, airtight glass containers. The tablets themselves are normally dispensed in these original glass containers, which have screw-cap tops that are *not* childproof to facilitate emergency use by older adults who may have reduced manual dexterity and are experiencing an anginal attack. After a dose of nitroglycerin, the patient may experience dizziness, faintness, or headache as a result of the peripheral vasodilation. If pain persists, the patient should immediately call for medical assistance.

Sublingual nitroglycerin is the most commonly used nitrate. It is not swallowed, because it undergoes first-pass metabolism by the liver, which decreases its effectiveness. Instead, it is readily absorbed into the circulation through the SL vessels. Nitroglycerin is also available in other forms: topical (ointment, transdermal patch), translingual, oral extended-release capsule and tablet, aerosol spray (inhalation), and IV. Prototype Drug Chart 37.2 summarizes the action of nitroglycerin (nitrates).

Among the various types of organic nitrates is *isosorbide dinitrate*, which can be administered in an SL tablet form and is also available as a chewable tablet, immediate-release tablet, and sustained-release tablet or capsule. *Isosorbide mononitrate* can be given orally in immediate- and sustained-release tablets.

Pharmacokinetics When taken sublingually, nitroglycerin is absorbed rapidly and directly into the internal jugular vein and the right atrium. Nitrates absorbed through the gastrointestinal (GI) tract are inactivated by first-pass metabolism in the liver. The nitroglycerin in the ointment and in the patch is absorbed slowly through the skin and is excreted primarily in the urine. The protein binding is 60%, and the half-life is 1 to 3 minutes.

Pharmacodynamics Nitroglycerin acts directly on the smooth muscle of blood vessels, causing relaxation and dilation. It decreases cardiac preload (amount of blood in the ventricle at the end of diastole) and afterload (peripheral vascular resistance) and reduces myocardial O_2 demand. With dilation of the veins, there is less blood return to the heart, and with dilation of the arteries, there is less vasoconstriction and resistance.

The onset of action of nitroglycerin depends on the method of administration. With SL use, the onset of action is rapid (1-3 minutes); it is slower with the transdermal method (40-60 minutes). The duration of action of the transdermal nitroglycerin patch is approximately 18 to 24 hours. Because nitroglycerin ointment is effective for only 4 to 8 hours, it must be reapplied three to four times a day. The use of nitroglycerin ointment has declined since the advent of the transdermal nitroglycerin patch, which is applied only once a day. It is important to note that the patch should be removed nightly to allow for an 8- to 12-hour nitrate-free interval. This is also true for most other forms of nitroglycerin. This is necessary to avoid tolerance associated with uninterrupted use or continued dosage increases of nitrate preparations. Table 37.4 lists the nitrates and their dosages, uses, and considerations.

TABLE 37.3   Effects of Antianginal Drug Groups on Angina

Drug Groups	Variant (Vasospastic) Anginas	Classic (Stable) Anginas
Nitrates	Relaxation of coronary arteries, which decreases vasospasms and increases oxygen supply	Dilation of veins, which decreases preload and decreases oxygen demand
Beta blockers	Not effective	Decrease heart rate and contractility, which decreases oxygen demand
Calcium channel blockers	Relaxation of coronary arteries, which decreases vasospasms and increases oxygen supply	Dilation of arterioles decreases afterload and decreases oxygen demand. Verapamil and diltiazem decrease heart rate and contractility.

PROTOTYPE DRUG CHART 37.2

Nitroglycerin

Drug Class	Dosage
Antianginal Pregnancy category: C*	Angina: A: PO/SL: 1 tab of 0.3, 0.4, or 0.6 mg; repeat q5min × 3 as needed; or 5-10 min prior to angina-provoking activities Extended release: A: PO: 2.5-6.5 mg, 3-4 times/d, *max.* 26 mg qid IV: Initially: 5 mcg/min infusion, titrate to 20 mcg/min until control achieved Ointment: 15-30 mg (2.5-5 cm or 1-2 inches) q6-8h while awake, remove at bedtime to provide 12 h nitrate-free interval Transdermal patch: 1 Patch qd, allow 12 h nitrate-free interval Translingual spray: 1-2 sprays on or under tongue q5min; *max.* 3 sprays in 15 min
Contraindications	**Drug-Lab-Food Interactions**
Increased intracranial pressure, anemia, cardiomyopathy, shock *Caution:* Renal or hepatic disease, AMI, hypotension, hypovolemia, head trauma, pregnancy, breastfeeding	Drug: Increased effect with alcohol, beta blockers, calcium channel blockers, antihypertensives, aspirin, benzodiazepines, vasodilators; decreased effects of heparin Herbs: Hawthorn increases nitroglycerin levels.
Pharmacokinetics	**Pharmacodynamics**
Absorption: SL: Greater than 75% absorbed; ointment and patch: slow absorption Distribution: PB: 60% Metabolism: t½: 1-3 min Excretion: Liver and urine	SL: Onset: 1-3 min Peak: 5 min Duration: 30-60 min ER cap: Onset: 20-45 min Duration: 8-12 h Ointment: Onset: 40-60 min Peak: 1 h Duration: 4-8 h Transdermal patch: Onset: 40-60 min Peak: 2 h Duration: 18-24 h IV: Onset: Immediate Duration: 3 min
Therapeutic Effects/Uses	
To control angina, AMI, hypertensive emergency, pulmonary edema, and heart failure Mode of Action: Decreases myocardial demand for oxygen; decreases preload by dilating veins, indirectly decreasing afterload	
Side Effects	**Adverse Reactions**
Nausea, vomiting, headache, blurred vision, dizziness, syncope, weakness, diaphoresis, flushing, pallor, rash, dry mouth, palpitations, paresthesia, peripheral edema, tolerance	Orthostatic hypotension, tachycardia, paradoxical bradycardia *Life threatening:* Circulatory collapse

*Pregnancy categories have been revised. See http://www.fda.gov/Drugs/DevelopmentApprovalProcess/DevelopmentResources/Labeling/ucm093307.htm for more information.
A, Adult; *AMI,* acute myocardial infarction; *cap,* capsule; *d,* day; *ER,* extended release; *h,* hour; *IV,* intravenous; *max,* maximum; *min,* minute; *PB,* protein binding; *PO,* by mouth; *q,* every; *qd,* every day; *qid,* four times daily; *SL,* sublingual; *t½,* half-life; *tab,* tablet.

Side Effects and Adverse Reactions

Headaches are one of the most common side effects of nitroglycerin, but they may become less frequent with continued use. Otherwise acetaminophen may provide some relief. Other side effects include hypotension, dizziness, weakness, and faintness. When nitroglycerin ointment or transdermal patches are discontinued, the dose should be tapered over several weeks to prevent the rebound effect of severe pain caused by myocardial ischemia, lack of blood supply to the heart muscle. In addition, *reflex tachycardia* may occur if the nitrate is given too rapidly. The heart rate increases greatly because of overcompensation of the cardiovascular system.

Drug Interactions

Beta blockers, calcium channel blockers, vasodilators, and alcohol can enhance the hypotensive effect of nitrates. IV nitroglycerin may antagonize the effects of heparin.

❶ Beta Blockers

Beta-adrenergic blockers block the beta₁- and beta₂-receptor sites. Beta blockers decrease the effects of the sympathetic nervous system by blocking the action of the catecholamines, epinephrine and norepinephrine, thereby decreasing the heart rate and blood pressure. Beta blockers are used as antianginal, antidysrhythmic, and antihypertensive drugs. Beta blockers are

! TABLE 37.4   Antianginals

Drug	Route and Dosages	Uses and Considerations
Nitrates		
Short Acting		
Nitroglycerin	See Prototype Drug Chart 37.2.	
Long Acting		
Isosorbide dinitrate	Immediate release: A: PO: Initially 5-20 mg bid/tid; maint: 10-40 mg bid/tid; *max*: 480 mg/d Sustained release: A: PO: Initially 40 mg/d; maint: 40-160 mg/d; *max*: 160 mg/d A: Sublingual: 2.5-5 mg 15 min prior to angina-causing activity	To prevent angina. May cause headaches, dizziness, hypotension, nausea, vomiting, and flushing. Pregnancy category: C*; PB: 28%; t½: 1 h
Isosorbide mononitrate	Immediate release: A: PO: 5-20 mg bid; *max*: 40 mg/d Extended release: A: PO: 30-60 mg am; *max*: 240 mg/d	To prevent angina. May cause headache, dizziness, hypotension, fatigue, flushing, GI distress, and tolerance. Pregnancy category: B, C*; PB: 4%; t½: 5 h
Beta-Adrenergic Blockers		
Atenolol (beta₁)	Angina: Regular release: A: PO: Initially 50 mg/d; maint: 25-100 mg/d; *max*: 200 mg/d	To treat angina, hypertension, and AMI. May cause hypotension, bradycardia, depression, fatigue, dizziness, and heart failure. Pregnancy category: D*; PB: 10%; t½: 6-7 h
Metoprolol tartrate (beta₁)	Regular release: A: PO: 50-100 mg in 2 divided doses; maint: 100-400 mg/d in 2 divided doses; *max*: 400 mg/d Extended release: A: PO: 100 mg/d; *max*: 400 mg/d	To treat angina, AMI, hypertension, and heart failure. May cause drowsiness, dizziness, fatigue, blurred vision, peripheral edema, erectile dysfunction, bradycardia, hypotension, and bronchospasm. Pregnancy category: C*; PB: 10%; t½: 3-4 h
Nadolol (beta₁ and beta₂)	Angina: A: PO: Initially 40 mg/d; maint: 40-80 mg/d; *max*: 240 mg/d	For angina and hypertension. May cause dizziness, bradycardia, hypotension, depression, bronchospasm, and fatigue. Pregnancy category: C*; PB: 30%; t½: 10-24 h
Propranolol Hydrochloride (beta₁ and beta₂)	Angina: Immediate release: A: PO: Initially 10-20 mg bid/qid; maint: 160-320 mg/d in 2-4 divided doses; *max*: 320 mg/d Extended release: A: PO: Initially 80 mg/d; maint: 160-320 mg/d; *max*: 320 mg/d	For angina, hypertension, AMI, dysrhythmias, and migraine prophylaxis. May cause dizziness, drowsiness, bradycardia, depression, agitation, insomnia, and bronchospasm. Pregnancy category: C*; PB: 90%; t½: 2-6 h
Calcium Channel Blockers		
Amlodipine	A: PO: Initially 5-10 mg/d; maint: 10 mg/d; *max*: 10 mg/d	For angina, CAD, and hypertension. May cause peripheral edema, dizziness, palpitations, flushing, and fatigue. Pregnancy category: C*; PB: 93%; t½: 30-50 h
Diltiazem Hydrochloride	Angina: Immediate release: A: PO: Initially 30 mg qid; maint: 180-360 mg/d in 3-4 divided doses; *max*: 360 mg/d Sustained release: A: PO: 120-180 mg/d; *max*: 480 mg/d	For angina, PSVT, atrial flutter or fibrillation, and hypertension. May cause headache, peripheral edema, dizziness, weakness, dyspnea, dyspepsia, bradycardia, and hypotension. Pregnancy category: C*; PB: 70%-80%; t½: 3.5-9 h
Felodipine	Hypertension: Extended release: A: PO: Initially 5 mg/d; maint: 2.5-10 mg/d; *max*: 10 mg/d Older adults: Initially 2.5 mg/d; *max*: 10 mg/d	To treat hypertension. May cause flushing, peripheral edema, palpitations, dizziness, weakness, and headache. Pregnancy category: C*; PB: >99%; t½: 11-16 h
Isradipine	Regular release: A: PO: Initially 2.5 mg bid; *max*: 10 mg/bid Extended release: A: PO: Initially 5 mg/d; *max*: 20 mg/d	To treat hypertension. May cause headache, palpitations, peripheral edema, fatigue, and dizziness. Pregnancy category: C*; PB: 95%; t½: 8 h
Nicardipine Hydrochloride	A: PO: Initially 20 mg tid; maint: 20-40 mg tid; *max*: 120 mg/d	For angina and hypertension. May cause peripheral edema, headache, dizziness, hypotension, flushing, weakness, nausea, and vomiting. Pregnancy category: C*; PB: 95%; t½: 11.5 h

Continued

! TABLE 37.4 Antianginals—cont'd

Drug	Route and Dosages	Uses and Considerations
Nifedipine	Angina: Immediate release: A: PO: Initially 10 mg tid; *max:* 180 mg/d Extended release: A: PO: 30-60 mg/d; *max:* 90 mg/d	For angina and hypertension. May cause dizziness, flushing, headache, peripheral edema, nausea, hypotension, palpitations, and weakness. Pregnancy category: C*; PB: 92%-98%; t½: 2-5 h
Nisoldipine	Extended release: A: PO: Initially 17 mg/d; maint: 17-34 mg/d; *max.* 34 mg/d Older adults: PO: Initially 8.5 mg/d; *max.* 34 mg/d	For hypertension. May cause headache, dizziness, flushing, and peripheral edema. Pregnancy category: C*; PB: 99%; t½: 7-12 h
Verapamil Hydrochloride	Angina: Immediate release: A: PO: Initially 80-120 mg q8h; *max:* 480 mg/d in 3-4 divided doses Extended release: A: PO: Initially 180 mg/d at bedtime; *max.* 540 mg/d	For angina, cardiac dysrhythmias, and hypertension. May cause peripheral edema, constipation, dizziness, headache, fatigue, and hypotension. Pregnancy category: C*; PB: 90%; t½: 5-12 h

*Pregnancy categories have been revised. See http://www.fda.gov/Drugs/DevelopmentApprovalProcess/DevelopmentResources/Labeling/ucm093 307.htm for more information.

A, Adult; *am*, in the morning; *AMI*, acute myocardial infarction; *bid*, twice a day; *CAD*, coronary artery disease; *d*, day; *GI*, gastrointestinal; *h*, hour; *maint*, maintenance; *max*, maximum; *min*, minute; *PB*, protein binding; *PO*, by mouth; *PSVT*, paroxysmal supraventricular tachycardia; *q8h*, every 8 hours; *qid*, four times a day; *SL*, sublingual; *SR*, sustained release; *tid*, three times a day; *t½*, half-life; *>*, greater than.

effective as antianginals because by decreasing the heart rate and myocardial contractility, they reduce the need for oxygen consumption and consequently reduce anginal pain. These drugs are most useful for classic (stable) angina.

Beta blockers should *not* be abruptly discontinued. The dose should be tapered over a specified number of days to avoid reflex tachycardia and recurrence of anginal pain. Patients who have decreased heart rate and blood pressure usually cannot take beta blockers. Patients who have second- or third-degree AV block should not take beta blockers.

Beta blockers, discussed in detail in Chapter 15 and 39, are subdivided into *nonselective* beta blockers that block beta₁ and beta₂ and *selective* (cardiac) beta blockers that only block beta₁. Examples of nonselective beta blockers are propranolol, nadolol, and pindolol. These drugs decrease the heart rate and can cause bronchoconstriction. The cardioselective beta blockers act more strongly on the beta₁ receptor, which decreases heart rate but avoids bronchoconstriction because of their lack of activity at the beta₂ receptor. Examples of selective beta blockers are atenolol and metoprolol. Selective beta blockers are the group of choice for controlling angina pectoris. Table 37.4 lists the beta blockers most frequently used for angina and their dosages, uses, and considerations.

Pharmacokinetics Beta blockers are well absorbed orally. Absorption of sustained-release capsules is slow. The half-life of propranolol is 2 to 6 hours. Of the selective beta blockers, atenolol has a half-life of 6 to 7 hours, and metoprolol has a half-life of 3 to 4 hours. Propranolol and metoprolol are metabolized and excreted by the liver. Half an *oral* dose of atenolol is absorbed from the GI tract, with the remainder excreted unchanged in feces.

Pharmacodynamics Because beta blockers decrease the force of myocardial contraction, oxygen demand by the myocardium is reduced. Therefore the patient can tolerate increased exercise with less oxygen requirement. Beta blockers are effective for classic (stable) angina.

The onset of action of the nonselective beta blocker propranolol is 30 minutes, its peak action is reached in 2 to 4 hours, and its duration is 12 to 24 hours. For the cardioselective beta blockers, the onset of action of atenolol is 60 minutes, its peak action occurs in 2 to 4 hours, and its duration of action is 24 hours. The onset of action of selective metoprolol is reached in 30 to 60 minutes, and the duration of action is approximately 3 to 6 hours.

Side Effects and Adverse Reactions. Both nonselective and selective beta blockers cause a decrease in heart rate and blood pressure. For the nonselective beta blockers, bronchospasm, behavioral or psychotic response, and impotence (with use of Inderal) are potential adverse reactions.

Vital signs need to be closely monitored in the early stages of beta-blocker therapy. When discontinuing use, the dosage should be tapered for 1 or 2 weeks to prevent a rebound effect such as reflex tachycardia or life-threatening cardiac dysrhythmias.

Calcium Channel Blockers

Calcium channel blockers (CCBs), or *calcium blockers,* were introduced in 1982 for the treatment of stable and variant angina pectoris, certain dysrhythmias, and hypertension. Calcium activates myocardial contraction, increasing the workload of the heart and the need for more oxygen. CCBs relax coronary artery spasm (variant angina) and relax peripheral arterioles (stable angina), decreasing cardiac oxygen demand. They also decrease cardiac contractility (negative inotropic effect that relaxes smooth muscle), afterload, and peripheral resistance, and they reduce the workload of the heart, which decreases the need for oxygen. CCBs achieve their effect in controlling variant (vasospastic) angina by relaxing coronary arteries and in controlling classic (stable) angina by decreasing oxygen demand. Fig. 37.1 shows the suggested steps for treating classic and variant angina pectoris. Table 37.4 presents the drug data for the CCBs used to treat angina and their dosages, uses, and considerations.

Pharmacokinetics Three calcium channel blockers—verapamil, nifedipine, and diltiazem—have been effectively used for the long-term treatment of angina. Eighty to ninety percent of

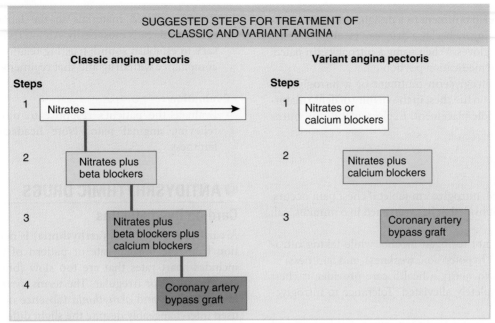

FIG. 37.1 Suggested steps for treating classic and variant angina pectoris.

CCBs are absorbed through the GI mucosa. However, first-pass metabolism by the liver decreases the availability of free circulating drug, and only 20% of verapamil, 45% to 65% of diltiazem, and 35% to 40% of nifedipine are bioavailable. All three drugs are highly protein bound (70% to 98%), and their half-lives are usually 2 to 12 hours.

Several other CCBs are available, such as nicardipine hydrochloride (HCl), amlodipine, felodipine, and nisoldipine. All are highly protein bound (greater than 93%). Nicardipine has the shortest half-life at 11.5 hours.

Pharmacodynamics Bradycardia is a common problem with the use of verapamil, the first calcium blocker. Nifedipine, the most potent of the calcium blockers, promotes vasodilation of the coronary and peripheral vessels, and hypotension can result. The onset of action is 10 minutes for verapamil and 30 minutes for nifedipine and diltiazem. Verapamil's duration of action is 6 to 8 hours when given orally and 10 to 20 minutes when given intravenously. The duration of action for nifedipine and diltiazem is 6 to 8 hours.

Side Effects and Adverse Reactions. The side effects of calcium blockers include headache, hypotension (more common with nifedipine and less common with diltiazem), dizziness, and flushing of the skin. Reflex tachycardia can occur as a result of hypotension. Peripheral edema may occur with several CCBs, including nicardipine, nifedipine, and verapamil. CCBs can cause changes in liver and kidney function, and serum liver enzymes should be checked periodically. CCBs are frequently given with other antianginal drugs such as nitrates to prevent angina.

In its immediate-release form (10- and 20-mg capsules), nifedipine has been associated with an increased incidence of sudden cardiac death, especially when prescribed in high doses for outpatients. This is not true of the sustained-release preparations. For this reason, immediate-release nifedipine is usually prescribed only as needed in the hospital setting for acute increases in blood pressure.

NURSING PROCESS
Patient-Centered Collaborative Care
Antianginals

Assessment
- Obtain baseline vital signs for future comparisons.
- Obtain health and drug histories. Nitroglycerin is contraindicated for marked hypotension or acute myocardial infarction (AMI).

Nursing Diagnoses
- Cardiac Output, Decreased related to poor myocardial perfusion
- Anxiety related to perceived threat of death
- Pain, Acute related to anginal pain due to inadequate coronary perfusion and lack of oxygen
- Activity Intolerance related to lack of oxygen due to poor blood perfusion to the heart and lungs

Planning
- The patient's angina pain will be controlled by nitroglycerin or other antianginals.

Nursing Interventions
- Monitor vital signs. Hypotension is associated with most antianginal drugs.
- Position the patient sitting or lying down when administering a nitrate for the first time. After administration, check vital signs while the patient is lying down and then sitting up. Have the patient rise slowly to a standing position.
- Offer sips of water before giving SL nitrates; dryness may inhibit drug absorption.
- Monitor effects of IV nitroglycerin. Report angina that persists.

- Apply nitroglycerin ointment to a designated mark on paper. Do *not* use fingers because drug can be absorbed; use tongue blade or gloves. When using a nitroglycerin patch, do not touch the medication portion.
- Do *not* apply nitroglycerin ointment or a nitroglycerin patch in any area on the chest in the vicinity of defibrillator-cardioverter paddle placement. Explosion and skin burns may result.

Patient Teaching
General
- ⚡ Administer SL nitroglycerin tablet if chest pain occurs. If pain has not subsided or has worsened in 5 minutes, call 911.
- Advise patients not to ingest alcohol while taking nitroglycerin to avoid hypotension, weakness, and faintness.
- Advise patients to notify a health care provider if chest pain is not completely alleviated. Tolerance to nitroglycerin can occur.
- ⚡ Inform patients not to discontinue beta blockers and calcium blockers without a health care provider's approval. Withdrawal symptoms (reflex tachycardia and pain) may be severe.

Self-Administration
- Demonstrate how SL nitroglycerin tablets are taken. The tablet is placed under the tongue for quick absorption. A stinging or biting sensation indicates that the tablet is fresh; however, with newer SL nitroglycerin tablets, the biting sensation may not be present.
- Teach patients to store medication bottles away from light in a dry place and to keep the drug in its original screw-cap, amber glass bottle. The amber color provides light protection, and the screw-cap closure protects from moisture in the air, which can easily reduce tablet potency.
- Teach patients about nitroglycerin patches, applied once a day, usually in the morning. Rotate skin sites. The patch is usually applied to the chest wall, but the thighs and arms may also be used. Avoid hairy areas.
- Advise patients to seek medical attention if nitroglycerin does not relieve pain.

Side Effects
- Suggest acetaminophen to patients for relief of headache, which commonly occurs when first taking nitroglycerin products and lasts about 30 minutes.
- ⚡ Place patients in a supine position with legs elevated if hypotension results from SL nitroglycerin.
- Instruct patients how to check their pulse rate.
- Advise patients taking beta blockers and calcium blockers to notify a health care provider if dizziness or faintness occurs because it may indicate hypotension.

🌐 *Cultural Considerations*
- Address cultural issues directly, especially in matters concerning dietary contributors to cardiac conditions. Family and community are important resources for promoting adherence to medication regimens and lifestyle changes.

- Provide printed materials in the language the patient speaks and reads most easily. An interpreter may be necessary to establish sound, trusting relationships and ensure compliance with drug and diet regimens.

Evaluation
- Evaluate the patient's response to nitrate products for relieving anginal pain. Note headache, dizziness, or faintness.

❶ ANTIDYSRHYTHMIC DRUGS

Cardiac Dysrhythmias

A cardiac dysrhythmia (arrhythmia) is defined as any deviation from the normal rate or pattern of the heartbeat. This includes heart rates that are too slow (bradycardia), too fast (tachycardia), or irregular. The terms *dysrhythmia* (disturbed heart rhythm) and *arrhythmia* (absence of heart rhythm) are used interchangeably despite the slight difference in meaning.

The ECG identifies the type of dysrhythmia. The *P wave* of the ECG reflects atrial activation, the *QRS complex* indicates ventricular depolarization, and the *T wave* reflects ventricular repolarization (return of cell membrane potential to resting after depolarization). The *PR interval* indicates AV conduction time, and the *QT interval* reflects ventricular action potential duration. Atrial dysrhythmias prevent proper filling of the ventricles and decrease cardiac output by 33%. Ventricular dysrhythmias are life threatening because ineffective filling of the ventricle and ineffective pumping results in decreased or absent cardiac output. With ventricular tachycardia, ventricular fibrillation is likely to occur, followed by death. Cardiopulmonary resuscitation (CPR) is necessary to treat these patients.

Cardiac dysrhythmias frequently follow an MI (heart attack) or can result from hypoxia (lack of oxygen to body tissues), hypercapnia (increased carbon dioxide in the blood), thyroid disease, coronary artery disease, cardiac surgery, excess catecholamines, or electrolyte imbalance.

Cardiac Action Potentials

Electrolyte transfer occurs through the cardiac muscle cell membrane. When sodium and calcium enter the cardiac cell, depolarization (myocardial contraction) occurs. Sodium enters rapidly to start the depolarization, and calcium enters later to maintain it. Calcium influx leads to an increased release of intracellular calcium from the sarcoplasmic reticulum, resulting in cardiac contraction. In the presence of myocardial ischemia, the contraction can be irregular.

Cardiac action potentials are transient depolarizations followed by repolarizations of myocardial cells. Fig. 37.2 illustrates the action potential of a ventricular cardiac cell (myocyte) during the course of a heartbeat. There are five phases: phase 0 is the rapid depolarization caused by an influx of sodium ions; phase 1 is initial repolarization, which coincides with termination of sodium ion influx; phase 2 is the plateau and is characterized by the influx of calcium ions, which prolong the action potential and promote atrial and

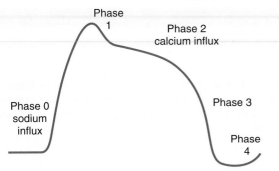

FIG. 37.2 Action potential of a ventricular myocyte during the course of a heartbeat.

ventricular muscle contraction; phase 3 is rapid repolarization caused by influx of potassium ions; and phase 4 is the resting membrane potential between heartbeats and is normally flat in ventricular muscle, but it begins to rise in the cells of the sinoatrial (SA) node as they slowly depolarize toward the threshold potential just before depolarization occurs, initiating the next heartbeat.

Types of Antidysrhythmic Drugs

The desired action of antidysrhythmic (antiarrhythmic) drugs is to restore the cardiac rhythm to normal. Box 37.1 describes the various mechanisms by which this is accomplished. Antidysrhythmics are high-alert drugs that may cause significant harm to the patient when given inappropriately.

The antidysrhythmics are grouped into four classes: (1) sodium (fast) channel blockers IA, IB, and IC; (2) beta blockers; (3) drugs that prolong repolarization; and (4) calcium (slow) channel blockers. Table 37.5 lists the classes, actions, and indications for cardiac antidysrhythmic drugs. Table 37.6 lists the commonly administered antidysrhythmics and their dosages, uses, and considerations.

Class I: Sodium Channel Blockers

A sodium channel blocker decreases sodium influx into cardiac cells. Responses to the drug are decreased conduction velocity in cardiac tissues; suppression of automaticity, which decreases the likelihood of ectopic foci; and increased recovery time (repolarization or refractory period). There are three subgroups of sodium channel blockers: those in *class IA* slow conduction and prolong repolarization (quinidine, procainamide, disopyramide); those in *class IB* slow conduction and shorten repolarization (lidocaine, mexiletine HCl); and *class IC* drugs prolong conduction with little to no effect on repolarization (flecainide).

Lidocaine, a class IB sodium channel blocker, was used in the 1940s as a local anesthetic and is still used for this purpose. It was later discovered to have antidysrhythmic properties as well. Lidocaine is still used by some cardiologists to treat acute ventricular dysrhythmias. It slows conduction velocity and decreases action potential amplitude. Onset of action (IV) is rapid. About one third of lidocaine reaches the general circulation, and a bolus of lidocaine is short-lived. Another class IB sodium channel blocker is mexiletine.

BOX 37.1 Pharmacodynamics of Antidysrhythmics

Mechanisms of Action
- Blocks adrenergic stimulation of the heart
- Depresses myocardial excitability and contractility
- Decreases conduction velocity in cardiac tissue
- Increases recovery time (repolarization) of the myocardium
- Suppresses automaticity (spontaneous depolarization to initiate beats)

TABLE 37.5 Classes, Actions, and Indications of Antidysrhythmic Drugs

Classes	Actions	Indications
Class I		
Sodium Channel Blockers		
IA	Slow conduction and prolong repolarization	Atrial and ventricular dysrhythmias, paroxysmal atrial tachycardia (PAT), supraventricular dysrhythmias
IB	Slow conduction and shorten repolarization	Acute ventricular dysrhythmias
IC	Prolong conduction with little to no effect on repolarization	Life-threatening ventricular dysrhythmias
Class II		
Beta blockers	Reduce calcium entry Decrease conduction velocity, automaticity, and recovery time (refractory period)	Atrial flutter and fibrillation, tachydysrhythmias, ventricular and supraventricular dysrhythmias
Class III		
Drugs that prolong repolarization	Prolong repolarization during ventricular dysrhythmias Prolong action potential duration	Life-threatening atrial and ventricular dysrhythmias resistant to other drugs
Class IV		
Calcium channel blockers	Block calcium influx Slow conduction velocity Decrease myocardial contractility (negative inotropic) Increase refraction in atrioventricular node	Supraventricular tachydysrhythmias; prevention of paroxysmal supraventricular tachycardia (PSVT)

Class II: Beta Blockers

The drugs in the second class, beta blockers, decrease conduction velocity, automaticity, and recovery time (refractory period). Examples are propranolol, acebutolol, esmolol, and sotalol. Beta blockers are more frequently prescribed for dysrhythmias than are sodium channel blockers. This drug class should be gradually reduced in dose upon discontinuation. Prototype Drug Chart 37.3 lists the drug data related to the beta blocker acebutolol hydrochloride, which can be prescribed to treat recurrent stable ventricular dysrhythmias.

! TABLE 37.6 Antidysrhythmics

Drug	Route and Dosage	Uses and Considerations
Class I		
Sodium Channel Blockers IA		
Disopyramide phosphate	A >18 y >50 kg: PO: 150-300 mg q6h; *max:* 800 mg/d A >18 y <50 kg: PO: 100 mg q6h; *max:* 800 mg/d Adol/C 5-12 y: PO: 6-15 mg/kg/d in divided doses q6h; *max:* 15 mg/kg/d Extended release: A >50 kg: PO: 300 mg q12h; *max:* 800 mg/d A <50 kg: PO: 200 mg q12h; *max:* 800 mg/d TDM: 2-5 mcg/mL	For ventricular tachycardia. May cause dizziness, headache, fatigue, blurred vision, dry mouth and eyes, urinary retention, nausea, flatulence, abdominal pain, and constipation. Pregnancy category: C*; PB: 90%; t½: 4-10 h
Procainamide Hydrochloride	Ventricular tachycardia: Loading dose: A: IV: 20-50 mg/min, then wait 10 min; maint: 1-4 mg/min infusion if needed C: IV: 15 mg/kg over 30-60 min TDM: 4-10 mcg/mL	For ventricular tachycardia and cardiopulmonary resuscitation. May cause GI distress and hypotension. Pregnancy category: C*; PB: 15%, t½: 2.5-5.2 h
Quinidine sulfate	Immediate release: A: PO: Initially 200-300 mg q6-8h Extended release: A: PO: 300-600 mg q8-12h TDM: 2-6 mcg/mL	For atrial, ventricular, and supraventricular dysrhythmias. May cause GI distress, headache, dizziness, fatigue, weakness, palpitations, and rash. Pregnancy category: C*; PB: 80%-90%; t½: 6-8 h
Sodium Channel Blockers IB		
Lidocaine	Dysrhythmias: A: IV: 50-100 mg bolus at 25-50 mg/min, may repeat in 5 min; *max:* 300 mg over 1 h, then IV 20-50 mcg/kg/min infusion	For ventricular dysrhythmias. May cause dizziness, restlessness, euphoria, drowsiness, blurred vision, metallic taste, and seizures. Pregnancy category: B, C*; PB: 60%-80%; t½: 1.5-2 h
Mexiletine Hydrochloride	A: PO: Initially 200 mg q8h; maint: 200-300 mg q8h; *max:* 1200 mg/d	For ventricular tachycardia. May cause weakness, GI distress, tremor, dizziness, headache, blurred vision, palpitations, chest pain, and ataxia. Pregnancy category: C*; PB: 50%-60%; t½: 10-12 h
Sodium Channel Blockers IC		
Flecainide	A: PO: Initially 50-100 mg q12h; maint: 150 mg q12h; *max:* 300 mg/d for atrial and supraventricular dysrhythmias, 400 mg/d for ventricular dysrhythmias	For atrial, ventricular, and supraventricular dysrhythmias. May cause dizziness, palpitations, headache, fatigue, visual impairment, tremor, dyspnea, dysrhythmia exacerbation, weakness, chest pain, HF, dysgeusia, and GI distress. Pregnancy category: C*; PB: 40%-50%; t½: 12-30 h
Propafenone Hydrochloride	Ventricular tachycardia: Immediate release: A: PO: 150 mg q8h; *max:* 900 mg/d Atrial fibrillation: Extended release: A: PO: 225 mg q12h; *max:* 850 mg/d	For atrial, ventricular, and supraventricular dysrhythmias. May cause dizziness, fatigue, headache, dysgeusia, GI distress, and blurred vision. Pregnancy category: C*; PB: 85%-97%; t½: 2-10 h
Class II		
Beta-Adrenergic Blockers		
Acebutolol Hydrochloride (beta₁ blocker)	See Prototype Drug Chart 37.3.	
Esmolol (beta₁ blocker)	SVT: A: IV: LD: 500 mcg/kg over 1 min; maint: 50 mcg/kg/min for 4 min; *max:* LD 500 mg/kg/min; maint 200 mcg/kg/min	To treat atrial flutter and fibrillation, SVT, and HTN. May cause bradycardia, hypotension, dizziness, sweating, infusion-site reaction, and nausea. Pregnancy category: C*; PB: 55%; t½: 9 min
Propranolol Hydrochloride (beta₁ and beta₂ blocker)	Atrial flutter/fibrillation: Immediate release: A: PO: Initially 10-30 mg tid/qid; *max:* 320 mg/d	For atrial and supraventricular dysrhythmias; AMI; angina; and HTN. May cause dizziness, drowsiness, agitation, insomnia, nightmares, bradycardia, depression, bronchospasm, and GI distress. Pregnancy category: C*; PB: 90%; t½: 2-6 h

! TABLE 37.6   Antidysrhythmics—cont'd

Drug	Route and Dosage	Uses and Considerations
Sotalol Hydrochloride (beta$_1$ and beta$_2$ blocker; also class III)	Atrial flutter/fibrillation: A: PO: 80 mg bid; maint: 120-160 qd/bid; *max:* 320 mg/d	For atrial flutter and fibrillation and ventricular tachycardia. May cause bradycardia, fatigue, dizziness, headache, chest pain, palpitations, weakness, edema, hypotension, HF, visual impairment, GI distress, and dyspnea. Pregnancy category: B*; PB: 0%; t½: 12 h
Class III ***Drugs That Prolong Repolarization***		
Adenosine	PSVT: A/adol/C >50 kg: IV: Initially 6 mg rapid bolus (1-2 s); repeat twice if needed with 12 mg, follow each dose with 20 mL saline flush C <50 kg: IV: 0.1 mg/kg rapid bolus, then give 0.2 mg/kg if needed, follow each dose with saline flush	For PSVT and Wolff-Parkinson-White syndrome. May cause headache, dizziness, flushing, dyspnea, GI distress, bradycardia, and chest pain. Pregnancy category: C*; PB: UK; t½: <10 s
Amiodarone Hydrochloride	A: PO: Initially 800-1600 mg/d for 1-3 wk, then 600-800 mg/d for 1 month; then reduce to lowest effective dose A: IV: 150 mg over 10 min, then 1 mg/min infusion for 6 h; maint: 0.5 mg/min	For life-threatening ventricular tachycardia and fibrillation. May cause dizziness, pulmonary toxicity, elevated hepatic enzymes, dysrhythmia exacerbation, hypotension, visual impairment, corneal deposits and degeneration, bradycardia, fatigue, confusion, peripheral neuropathy, blue-gray skin discoloration, tremors, involuntary movements, GI distress, and photosensitivity. Pregnancy category: D*; PB: >99%; t½: 26-107 d
Dofetilide	A: PO: Dose usually individualized based on ECG and renal function tests	For atrial flutter and fibrillation. May cause headache, dizziness, insomnia, chest pain, renal impairment, infection, dyspnea, and nausea. Monitor renal function. Pregnancy category: C*; PB: 60%-70%; t½: 10 h
Ibutilide	A >60 kg: IV: 1 mg over 10 min; may repeat with 1 mg in 10 min; *max:* 2 mg over 20 min A <60 kg: IV: 0.01 mg/kg given over 10 min; *max:* 2 mg in 20 min	For atrial flutter and fibrillation. May cause headache, palpitations, HF, dysrhythmia exacerbation, and ventricular tachycardia. Pregnancy category: C*; PB: 40%; t½: 2-12 h
Sotalol	Ventricular tachycardia: A: PO: 80 mg bid; maint: 120-320 mg/d; *max:* 640 mg/d	For atrial flutter and fibrillation and ventricular tachycardia. May cause visual impairment, bradycardia, fatigue, dizziness, headache, chest pain, palpitations, hypotension, HF, weakness, edema, GI distress, and dyspnea. Pregnancy category: B*; PB: 0%; t½: 12 h
Class IV ***Calcium Channel Blockers***		
Verapamil Hydrochloride	PSVT: A: IV: Initially 5-10 mg over 2 min, then in 30 min 10 mg if needed Atrial flutter/fibrillation: Regular-release tablets: A: PO: 240-320 mg/d in 3-4 divided doses	For angina, cardiac dysrhythmias, and HTN. May cause peripheral edema, constipation, dizziness, headache, fatigue, and hypotension. Pregnancy category: C*; PB: 90%; t½: 5-12 h
Diltiazem	PSVT: A: IV: 0.25 mg/kg IV bolus over 2 min, then after 15 min 0.35 mg/kg over 2 min if needed, then 10 mg/h inf if needed; *max:* 24 h inf	For angina, HTN, PSVT, and atrial flutter or fibrillation. May cause headache, peripheral edema, dizziness, weakness, dyspnea, bradycardia, and hypotension. Pregnancy category: C*; PB: 70%-80%; t½: 3.5-9 h
Others Digoxin	See Prototype Drug Chart 37.1.	
Dronedarone	A: PO: 400 mg bid with morning and evening meals; *max:* 800 mg/d	For atrial fibrillation. May cause rash, nausea, diarrhea, weakness, bradycardia, and prolonged QT interval. Avoid grapefruit and grapefruit juice. Pregnancy category: X*; PB: 98%; t½: 13-19 h

*Pregnancy categories have been revised. See http://www.fda.gov/Drugs/DevelopmentApprovalProcess/DevelopmentResources/Labeling/ucm093 307.htm for more information.

A, Adult; *adol,* adolescent; *AMI,* acute myocardial infarction; *bid,* two times a day; *C,* child; *d,* day; *ECG,* electrocardiogram; *GI,* gastrointestinal; *h,* hour; *HF,* heart failure; *HTN,* hypertension; *inf,* infusion; *IV,* intravenous; *LD,* loading dose; *maint,* maintenance; *max,* maximum; *min,* minute; *PB,* protein binding; *PO,* by mouth; *PSVT,* paroxysmal supraventricular tachycardia; *q,* every; *qd,* every day; *qid,* four times a day; *s,* second; *SVT,* supraventricular tachycardia; *t½,* half-life; *TDM,* therapeutic drug monitoring; *tid,* three times a day; *UK,* unknown; *wk,* week; *y,* year; *>,* greater than; *<,* less than.

PROTOTYPE DRUG CHART 37.3
❶ *Acebutolol Hydrochloride*

Drug Class	Dosage
Beta₁ blocker: Cardioselective beta-adrenergic antagonist Pregnancy category: B*	Premature ventricular contractions: A: PO: Initially 200 mg q12h; maint: 600-1200 mg/d in 2 divided doses; *max:* 1200 mg/d Older adults: PO: 200-400 mg/d; *max:* 800 mg/d
Contraindications	**Drug-Lab-Food Interactions**
AV heart block, bradycardia, heart failure, cardiogenic shock *Caution:* Surgery, renal and hepatic impairment, diabetes mellitus, hyperthyroidism, asthma, bronchitis, COPD, pulmonary edema, myasthenia gravis, PVD	Drug: Increased effects with diuretics, adenosine, amiodarone, class IC antidysrhythmics, cardiac glycosides, disopyramide; prolongs hypoglycemic effects of insulin and oral antidiabetics; antagonist effect with albuterol, metaproterenol, terbutaline Lab: May increase ALT, AST, ALP, ANA titer, BUN, lipoproteins, and potassium.
Pharmacokinetics	**Pharmacodynamics**
Absorption: Well absorbed Distribution: PB: 26% Metabolism: t½: 3-4 h Excretion: 80%-100% in bile, feces, and urine	Ventricular dysrhythmias: PO: Onset: 1-2 h Peak: 2-4 h Duration: 12-24 h
Therapeutic Effects/Uses	
To aid in treatment of premature ventricular contractions and hypertension Mode of Action: Blocks beta₁-adrenergic receptors in cardiac tissues	
Side Effects	**Adverse Reactions**
Dizziness, nausea, vomiting, anorexia, edema, headache, visual impairment, hypotension, diaphoresis, fatigue, insomnia, nightmares, anxiety, constipation, diarrhea, erectile dysfunction, depression	Palpitations, bradycardia, chest pain, hyperglycemia, hypoglycemia, lupus-like syndrome, elevated hepatic enzymes *Life threatening:* Agranulocytosis, dyspnea, thrombocytopenia, bronchospasm (high doses)

*Pregnancy categories have been revised. See http://www.fda.gov/Drugs/DevelopmentApprovalProcess/DevelopmentResources/Labeling/ucm093307.htm for more information.
A, Adult; *ALP,* alkaline phosphatase; *ALT,* alanine aminotransferase; *ANA,* antinuclear antibody; *AST,* aspartate aminotransferase; *AV,* atrioventricular; *BUN,* blood urea nitrogen; *COPD,* chronic obstructive pulmonary disease; *d,* day; *h,* hour; *maint,* maintenance; *max,* maximum; *PB,* protein binding; *PO,* by mouth; *PVD,* peripheral vascular disease; *q12h,* every 12 hours; *t½,* half-life.

Pharmacokinetics The cardioselective beta drug acebutolol is well absorbed in the GI tract. It is metabolized in the liver to active metabolites; 80% to 100% of the drug is eliminated in the bile via feces and in the urine. The half-life for the drug is 3 to 4 hours.

Pharmacodynamics Acebutolol is prescribed for ventricular dysrhythmias as well as for angina pectoris and hypertension. As an antidysrhythmic drug, the onset of action is 1 to 2 hours; peak time is 2 to 4 hours, and duration of action is 12 to 24 hours.

Class III: Drugs That Prolong Repolarization

Drugs in the third class prolong repolarization and are used in emergency treatment of ventricular dysrhythmias when other antidysrhythmics are ineffective. Amiodarone increases the refractory period (recovery time) and prolongs the action potential duration (cardiac cell activity).

Class IV: Calcium Channel Blockers

The fourth class consists of the calcium channel blockers verapamil and diltiazem. Verapamil is a slow (calcium) channel blocker that blocks calcium influx, thereby decreasing the excitability and (negative inotropic) contractility of the myocardium. It increases the refractory period of the AV node, which decreases ventricular response. Verapamil is contraindicated for patients with AV block or HF.

Side Effects and Adverse Reactions With Antidysrhythmic Drugs.
Quinidine, the first drug used to treat cardiac dysrhythmias, has many side effects that include nausea, vomiting, diarrhea, confusion, and hypotension. It can also cause heart block and neurologic and psychiatric symptoms. Procainamide causes less cardiac depression than quinidine.

High doses of lidocaine can cause cardiovascular depression, bradycardia, hypotension, seizures, blurred vision, and double vision. Less serious side effects may include dizziness, and confusion. The use of lidocaine is contraindicated in patients with advanced AV block, and it should be used with caution in patients with hepatic disorders or HF. Mexiletine has side effects similar to lidocaine, and both drugs are contraindicated for use in patients with cardiogenic shock or in those with second- or third-degree heart block.

The side effects of beta blockers are bradycardia and hypotension. Bretylium tosylate and amiodarone can cause nausea, vomiting, hypotension, and neurologic problems. The side effects of calcium blockers include nausea, vomiting, hypotension, and bradycardia.

It should be noted that *all* antidysrhythmic drugs are potentially prodysrhythmic. This is because of both the pharmacologic activity of the drug on the heart and the inherently unpredictable activity of a diseased heart, with or without the use of drugs. In some cases, life-threatening ventricular dysrhythmias can result from appropriate and skillful attempts at drug therapy to treat patients with heart disease. For these reasons, antidysrhythmic drug therapy is often initiated during continuous cardiac monitoring of the patient's heart rhythm in a hospital setting.

NURSING PROCESS
Patient-Centered Collaborative Care
❗ *Antidysrhythmics*

Assessment

- Obtain health and drug histories. The history may include shortness of breath, heart palpitations, coughing, chest pain (type, duration, and severity), previous angina or cardiac dysrhythmias, and drugs the patient currently takes.
- Obtain baseline vital signs and ECG for future comparisons.
- Monitor early cardiac enzyme results (aspartate aminotransferase [AST], lactate dehydrogenase [LDH], creatine phosphokinase) and cardiac-specific troponins for future comparisons.

Nursing Diagnoses

- Cardiac Output, Decreased related to cardiac dysrhythmia
- Anxiety related to irregular heartbeat
- Activity Intolerance, Risk for

Planning

- The patient will no longer experience abnormal sinus rhythm.
- The patient will comply with the antidysrhythmic drug regimen.

Nursing Interventions

- ⚡ Monitor vital signs because hypotension can occur.
- ⚡ Administer drug by IV push or bolus over a period of 2 to 3 minutes or as prescribed.
- Monitor ECG for abnormal patterns, and report findings such as premature ventricular contractions (PVCs), increased PR and QT intervals, and/or widening of the QRS complex. Increased QT interval is a risk factor for *torsades de pointes*.

Patient Teaching

General

- Teach patients to take prescribed drugs as ordered because drug compliance is essential.
- Provide specific instructions for each drug (e.g., photosensitivity for amiodarone).

Side Effects

- Tell patients to report side effects and adverse reactions to a health care provider, including dizziness, faintness, nausea, and vomiting.
- ⚡ Advise patients to avoid alcohol, caffeine, and tobacco. Alcohol can intensify a hypotensive reaction, caffeine increases catecholamine levels, and tobacco promotes vasoconstriction.

 Cultural Considerations

- Advise patients to focus on the relationship between certain dietary habits and cardiac disease. Discuss the importance of a drug regimen in terms that directly address cultural issues and accommodate patients' family values. An interpreter may be necessary to ensure understanding and compliance with drug and dietary regimens.

Evaluation

- Evaluate effectiveness of prescribed antidysrhythmics by comparing heart rates with baseline rates and assessing the patient's response to the drug.
- Report side effects and adverse reactions. Drug regimens may need to be adjusted, and drug-induced dysrhythmias may occur that can require discontinuation of a drug.

▮ CRITICAL THINKING CASE STUDY

ST, a 64-year-old patient, has heart failure that is being controlled with digoxin, furosemide, and a low-sodium diet. She is taking potassium chloride (KCl) 20 mEq per day orally. Three days ago, ST had flulike symptoms that included anorexia, nausea, lethargy, and diarrhea. Her fluid and food intake was diminished, and she refused to take the KCl, stating that the drug makes her sick. She has been taking the digoxin and furosemide daily.

The nurse's assessment during the home visit includes poor skin turgor, poor muscle tone, irregular pulse rate, and decreased bowel sounds. The nurse obtained a blood sample for serum electrolytes, and results indicated potassium (K) 2.9 mEq/L, sodium (Na) 137 mEq/L, and chloride (Cl) 96 mEq/L.

1. List reference values for serum potassium (K), serum sodium (Na), and serum chloride (Cl). Are ST's electrolyte levels within normal range? Explain your answer.

2. Match ST's physical findings with the corresponding electrolyte imbalance.

3. What are the reasons for the electrolyte imbalance?

4. ST said she was not taking KCl because the drug makes her sick. What information can you give her concerning the administration of potassium?

5. What is the effect of furosemide on digoxin when there is a potassium deficit? Explain your answer.

6. Why should the nurse assess ST for digitalis toxicity? List the signs and symptoms of digitalis toxicity.

7. ST should be monitored and educated about digoxin. What is the normal therapeutic range?

8. What important skill should the nurse teach ST about home monitoring while taking digoxin?

9. The nurse instructs ST to eat foods rich in potassium. Which foods are the richest sources of potassium?

NCLEX STUDY QUESTIONS

1. The patient is receiving digoxin for treatment of heart failure. Which finding would suggest to the nurse that the heart failure is improving?
   a. Pale and cool extremities
   b. Absence of peripheral edema
   c. Urine output of 60 mL every 4 hours
   d. Complaints of increasing dyspnea

2. The patient's serum digoxin level is 3.0 ng/mL. What does the nurse know about this serum digoxin level?
   a. It is in the high (elevated) range.
   b. It is in the low (decreased) range.
   c. It is within the normal range.
   d. It is in the low-average range.

3. The nurse is assessing a patient for possible evidence of digitalis toxicity. Which of these is included in the signs and symptoms for digitalis toxicity?
   a. Apical pulse rate of 100 beats/min
   b. Apical pulse of 72 beats/min with an irregular rate
   c. Apical pulse of 90 beats/min with an irregular rate
   d. Apical pulse of 48 beats/min with an irregular rate

4. A patient is taking a potassium-depleting diuretic and digoxin. The nurse expects that a low potassium level (hypokalemia) could have what effect on digoxin?
   a. Increases serum digoxin sensitivity level
   b. Decreases serum digoxin sensitivity level
   c. No effect on serum digoxin sensitivity level
   d. Causes a low-average serum digoxin sensitivity level

5. A patient takes an initial dose of a nitrate. Which symptom(s) will the nurse expect to occur?
   a. Nausea and vomiting
   b. Headaches
   c. Stomach cramps
   d. Irregular pulse rate

6. A patient is prescribed a beta blocker. Beta blockers are as effective as antianginals because they do what?
   a. Increase oxygen to the systemic circulation
   b. Maintain heart rate and blood pressure
   c. Decrease heart rate and decrease myocardial contractility
   d. Decrease heart rate and increase myocardial contractility

7. The health care provider is planning to discontinue a patient's beta blocker. Which instruction will the nurse give the patient regarding the beta blocker?
   a. The beta blocker should be abruptly stopped when another cardiac drug is prescribed.
   b. The beta blocker should not be abruptly stopped; the dose should be tapered down.
   c. The beta blocker dose should be maintained while taking another antianginal drug.
   d. Half the beta blocker dose should be taken for the next several weeks.

8. The beta blocker acebutolol is prescribed for dysrhythmias. What is the primary purpose of the drug?
   a. Increase beta$_1$ and beta$_2$ receptors in cardiac tissues
   b. Increase the flow of oxygen to cardiac tissues
   c. Block beta$_1$-adrenergic receptors in cardiac tissues
   d. Block beta$_2$-adrenergic receptors in cardiac tissues

9. A patient who has angina is prescribed nitroglycerin. Which are appropriate nursing interventions for nitroglycerin? (Select all that apply.)
   a. Have the patient sit or lie down when taking a nitroglycerin sublingual tablet.
   b. Teach the patient who has taken a tablet to call 911 in 5 minutes if chest pain persists.
   c. Apply the nitroglycerin patch to a hairy area to protect skin from burning.
   d. Call the health care provider after taking five tablets if chest pain persists.
   e. Warn the patient against ingesting alcohol while taking nitroglycerin.

Answers: 1, b; 2, a; 3, d; 4, a; 5, b; 6, c; 7, b; 8, c; 9, a, b, e.

38

Diuretics

http://evolve.elsevier.com/McCuistion/pharmacology/

OBJECTIVES

- Compare the action and uses of thiazide, loop, and potassium-sparing diuretics.
- Differentiate side effects and adverse reactions related to thiazide, loop, and potassium-sparing diuretics.

- Explain the nursing interventions—including patient teaching—related to thiazide, loop, and potassium-sparing diuretics.
- Apply the nursing process for the patient taking thiazide, loop, and potassium-sparing diuretics.

OUTLINE

KEY TERMS

Diuretics are used for two main purposes: to decrease hypertension (lower blood pressure) and to decrease edema, typically peripheral and pulmonary, in heart failure (HF) and renal or liver disorders. Hypertension is a blood pressure greater than 140/90 mm Hg. Diuretics discussed in this chapter are used either alone or in combination to decrease blood pressure and edema.

Diuretics produce increased urine flow, or diuresis, by inhibiting sodium and water reabsorption from the kidney tubules. Most sodium and water reabsorption occurs throughout the renal tubular segments (proximal, loop of Henle [descending loop and ascending loop], and collecting tubule). Diuretics can affect one or more segments of the renal tubules. Fig. 38.1 illustrates the renal tubule along with the normal process of water and electrolyte reabsorption and diuretic effects on the tubules.

Every 1.5 hours, the total volume of the body's extracellular fluid (ECF) goes through the kidneys (glomeruli) for cleansing; this is the first process for urine formation. Small particles such as electrolytes, drugs, glucose, and waste products from protein metabolism are filtered in the glomeruli. Larger products such as protein and blood cells are not filtered with normal renal function, and they remain in the circulation. Sodium and water are the largest filtrate substances.

Normally, 99% of the filtered sodium that passes through the glomeruli is reabsorbed; 50% to 55% of sodium reabsorption occurs in the proximal tubules, 35% to 40% occurs in the loop of Henle, 5% to 10% occurs in the distal tubules, and less than 3% occurs in the collecting tubules. Diuretics that act on the tubules closest to the glomeruli have the greatest effect in causing natriuresis, sodium loss in the urine. A classic example is the osmotic diuretic mannitol. The diuretic effect depends on the drug reaching the kidneys and its concentration in the renal tubules.

Diuretics have an antihypertensive effect because they promote sodium and water loss by blocking sodium and chloride reabsorption. This causes a decrease in fluid volume, which

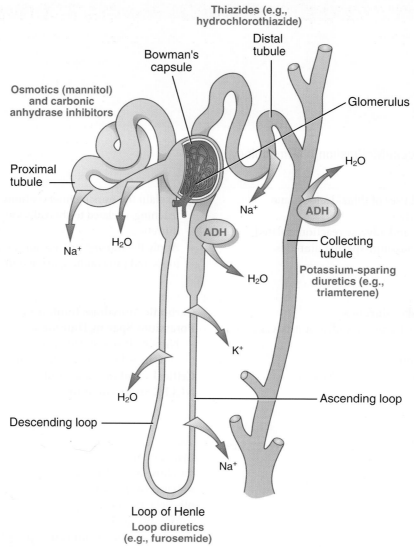

FIG. 38.1 Diuretics act on different segments of the renal tubule. Osmotic, mercurial, and carbonic anhydrase inhibitor diuretics affect the proximal tubule; loop diuretics affect the loop of Henle; thiazides affect the distal tubule; and potassium-sparing diuretics act primarily on the collecting tubules. ADH, Antidiuretic hormone; H_2O, water; K^+, potassium; Na^+, sodium.

lowers blood pressure. With fluid loss, edema—fluid retention in body tissues—should decrease, but if sodium is retained, water is also retained, and blood pressure increases.

Many diuretics cause the loss of other electrolytes, including potassium, magnesium, chloride, and bicarbonate. The diuretics that promote potassium excretion are classified as potassium-wasting diuretics, and those that promote potassium retention are called potassium-sparing diuretics.

The following five categories of diuretics are effective in removing water and sodium:
- Thiazide and thiazide-like diuretics
- Loop or high-ceiling diuretics
- Osmotic diuretics
- Carbonic anhydrase inhibitors
- Potassium-sparing diuretics

Thiazide, loop, and potassium-sparing diuretics are most frequently prescribed for hypertension and for edema associated with HF. Except for those in the potassium-sparing group, all diuretics are potassium wasting.

Combination diuretics that contain both potassium-wasting and potassium-sparing drugs have been marketed primarily for the treatment of hypertension. Combinations have an additive effect in reducing blood pressure and are discussed in more detail in the Potassium-Sparing Diuretics section later in this chapter. Chapter 39 takes a closer look at the combinations of antihypertensive agents with hydrochlorothiazide.

THIAZIDES AND THIAZIDE-LIKE DIURETICS

The first thiazide, chlorothiazide, was marketed in 1957 and was followed a year later by hydrochlorothiazide. There are numerous thiazide and thiazide-like preparations. Thiazides act on the distal convoluted renal tubule, beyond the loop of Henle, to promote sodium, chloride, and water excretion. Thiazides are used

TABLE 38.1   Diuretics

Drug	Route and Dosage	Uses and Considerations
Thiazides		
Short Acting		
Chlorothiazide	Hypertension: A/adol: PO: 500-1000 mg/d in 1-2 divided doses; *max*: 2 g/d Infants/C <12y: PO: 10-20 mg/kg/d in 1-2 divided doses; *max*: 20 mg/kg/d A: IV: 500-1000 mg qd/bid in 1-2 divided doses given slowly or as an infusion; *max*: 2 g/d	For hypertension, edema, HF, ascites, and nephrotic syndrome. May cause headache, dizziness, blurred vision, orthostatic hypotension, constipation, hypokalemia, hyperglycemia, GI distress, renal dysfunction, and Stevens-Johnson syndrome. Pregnancy category: C*; PB: UK; t½: 45-120 min
Hydrochlorothiazide	See Prototype Drug Chart 38.1.	
Intermediate Acting		
Bendroflumethiazide with nadolol	A: PO: Initially 1 tablet (40 mg nadolol and 5 mg bendroflumethiazide); *max*: 80 mg nadolol/5 mg bendroflumethiazide	For hypertension and edema. May cause dizziness, fatigue, hypokalemia, hyponatremia, hyperglycemia, hyperuricemia, blurred vision, bradycardia, and Stevens-Johnson syndrome. Pregnancy category: C*; PB: nadolol: 30%; bendroflumethiazide: 95%; t½: nadolol: 10-24 h; bendroflumethiazide: 3 h
Long Acting		
Methyclothiazide	Hypertension/edema: A: PO: 2.5-5 mg/d; *max*: 5 mg/d for hypertension; 10 mg/d for edema Adol/C: PO: 0.05-0.2 mg/kg/d; *max*: 0.2 mg/kg/d	For hypertension and edema. May cause orthostatic hypotension, headache, dizziness, weakness, hypokalemia, GI distress, photosensitivity, and Stevens-Johnson syndrome. Pregnancy category: B*; PB: UK; t½: UK
Thiazide-Like Diuretics		
Chlorthalidone	Hypertension: A: PO: Initially 25 mg/d; maint: 25-50 mg/d; *max*: 50 mg/d C: PO: 2 mg/kg 3 times weekly Edema: A: PO: Initially 50-100 mg/d; maint: 150-200 mg/d; *max*: 200 mg/d C: PO: 2 mg/kg 3 times weekly	For hypertension and edema. May cause dizziness, orthostatic hypotension, hyperglycemia, GI distress, hyperuricemia, photosensitivity, electrolyte imbalances, and Stevens-Johnson syndrome. Pregnancy category: B*; PB: 75%; t½: 40-60 h
Indapamide	A: PO: 1.25-2.5 mg/d; *max*: 5 mg/d	For hypertension and edema. May cause dizziness, headache, anxiety, weakness, GI distress, photosensitivity, hypokalemia, muscle cramps, and Stevens-Johnson syndrome. Pregnancy category: B*; PB: 71%-79%; t½: 14-18 h
Metolazone	Hypertension: A: PO: 2.5-5.0 mg/d; *max*: 5 mg/d C: PO: 0.2-0.4 mg/kg/d in divided doses; *max*: 0.4 mg/kg/d Edema: A: PO: 5-10 mg/d; *max*: 20 mg/d	For hypertension and edema. May cause headache, blurred vision, orthostatic hypotension, GI distress, hypokalemia, hyperglycemia, hyperuricemia, and Stevens-Johnson syndrome. Pregnancy category: B*; PB: 33%; t½: 14 h

*Pregnancy categories have been revised. See http://www.fda.gov/Drugs/DevelopmentApprovalProcess/DevelopmentResources/Labeling/ucm093 307.htm for more information.

A, Adult; *adol*, adolescent; *bid*, twice a day; *C*, child; *d*, day; *GI*, gastrointestinal; *h*, hour; *HF*, heart failure; *IV*, intravenous; *maint*, maintenance; *max*, maximum; *min*, minute; *PB*, protein binding; *PO*, by mouth; *qd*, every day; *t½*, half-life; *UK*, unknown; *y*, year; <, less than.

to treat hypertension and peripheral edema. They are not effective for immediate diuresis and should not be used to promote fluid loss in patients with severe renal dysfunction. Table 38.1 lists thiazide and thiazide-like diuretics and their dosages, uses, and considerations. Drug dosages for hypertension and edema are similar.

Thiazide diuretics are used primarily for patients with normal renal function. If the patient has a renal disorder and creatinine clearance is less than 30 mL/min, the effectiveness of the thiazide diuretic is greatly decreased. Thiazides cause a loss of sodium, potassium, and magnesium, but they promote calcium reabsorption. Hypercalcemia (calcium excess) may result, and the condition can be hazardous to the patient who is digitalized

or has cancer that causes hypercalcemia. Thiazides affect glucose tolerance, so hyperglycemia can also occur. Thiazides should be used cautiously in patients with diabetes mellitus. Laboratory test results, such as electrolytes and glucose, need to be monitored.

Hydrochlorothiazide has been combined with selected angiotensin-converting enzyme (ACE) inhibitors, beta blockers, alpha blockers, angiotensin II blockers, and centrally acting sympatholytics to control hypertension. Prototype Drug Chart 38.1 outlines the pharmacologic data for hydrochlorothiazide.

Pharmacokinetics Thiazides are well absorbed from the gastrontestinal (GI) tract. Hydrochlorothiazide has moderate protein-binding power. The half-life of the thiazide drugs is

PROTOTYPE DRUG CHART 38.1

Hydrochlorothiazide

Drug Class	Dosage
Thiazide diuretic Pregnancy category: B*	Hypertension: A: PO: 12.5-50 mg/d; *max:* 50 mg/d Edema: A: PO: 25-100 mg/d in single or divided doses; *max:* 100 mg/d C/infants >6 mo: PO: 2 mg/kg/d in divided doses; *max:* 2 mg/kg/d C/infants <6 mo: PO: 2-3 mg/kg/d in divided doses; *max.* 3 mg/kg/d
Contraindications Renal failure, hypersensitivity *Caution:* Hepatic and renal dysfunction, diabetes mellitus, gout, systemic lupus erythematosus, electrolyte imbalance, hypotension	**Drug-Lab-Food Interactions** Drug: Increased digitalis toxicity with digitalis if hypokalemia is present; increased renal toxicity with aspirin; increased potassium loss with steroids; decreased effect of antidiabetics; decreased thiazide absorption and effects with NSAIDs, cholestyramine, and colestipol Lab: Increased serum calcium, glucose, uric acid; decreased serum potassium, sodium, magnesium
Pharmacokinetics Absorption: Readily absorbed from GI tract Distribution: PB: 40%-65% Metabolism: t½: 5.6-14.8 h Excretion: In urine	**Pharmacodynamics** PO: Onset: 2 h Peak: 4 h Duration: 6-12 h
Therapeutic Effects/Uses To increase urine output and to treat hypertension, edema, HF, nephrotic syndrome, and ascites Mode of Action: Action is on the renal distal tubules, promoting sodium, potassium, and water excretion and decreasing preload and cardiac output; also decreases edema; acts on arterioles and causes vasodilation, thus decreasing blood pressure	
Side Effects Dizziness, headache, weakness, nausea, vomiting, diarrhea, abdominal pain, hyperglycemia, constipation, rash, photosensitivity, blurred vision, paresthesias, hyperuricemia, muscle cramps	**Adverse Reactions** Orthostatic hypotension, hyponatremia, gout *Life threatening:* Severe hypokalemia, aplastic anemia, hemolytic anemia, thrombocytopenia, agranulocytosis, renal failure, Stevens-Johnson syndrome

*Pregnancy categories have been revised. See http://www.fda.gov/Drugs/DevelopmentApprovalProcess/DevelopmentResources/Labeling/ucm093307.htm for more information.
A, Adult; *C,* child; *d,* day; *GI,* gastrointestinal; *h,* hour; *HF,* heart failure; *max,* maximum; *mo,* month; *NSAID,* nonsteroidal antiinflammatory drug; *PB,* protein binding; *PO,* by mouth; *t½,* half-life; >, greater than; <, less than.

longer than that of the loop diuretics. For this reason, thiazides should be administered in the morning to avoid nocturia (nighttime urination) and sleep interruption.

Pharmacodynamics Thiazides act directly on arterioles to cause vasodilation, which can lower blood pressure. Other action includes the promotion of sodium chloride and water excretion, resulting in a decrease in vascular fluid volume and a concomitant decrease in cardiac output and blood pressure. The onset of action of hydrochlorothiazide occurs within 2 hours. Peak concentration times are long (4 hours). Thiazides are divided into three groups according to their duration of action: (1) short acting (duration <12 hours), (2) intermediate acting (duration 12–24 hours), and (3) long acting (duration >24 hours).

Side Effects and Adverse Reactions. Side effects and adverse reactions of thiazides include electrolyte imbalances (hypokalemia, hypercalcemia, hypomagnesemia, and bicarbonate loss), hyperglycemia (elevated blood glucose), hyperuricemia (elevated serum uric acid level), and hyperlipidemia (elevated blood lipid level). Signs and symptoms of hypokalemia should be assessed, and serum potassium levels must be closely monitored. Potassium supplements are frequently needed. Serum calcium and uric acid levels should be checked because thiazides block calcium and uric acid excretion. Thiazides affect the metabolism of carbohydrates, and hyperglycemia can result, especially in patients with high to high-normal blood glucose levels. Thiazides can increase serum cholesterol, low-density lipoprotein, and triglyceride levels. A drug may be ordered to lower blood lipids. Other side effects include dizziness, headache, nausea, vomiting, constipation, urticaria, or hives (rare) and blood dyscrasias (rare). Table 38.2 summarizes the serum chemistry abnormalities that can occur with thiazide use.

Contraindications. Thiazides are contraindicated for use in renal failure. Symptoms of severe kidney impairment or shutdown include oliguria, a marked decrease in urine output; elevated blood urea nitrogen (BUN); and elevated serum creatinine.

Drug Interactions. Of the numerous thiazide drug interactions, the most serious occurs with digoxin. Thiazides can cause hypokalemia, which enhances the action of digoxin, and digitalis toxicity can occur. Potassium supplements are frequently prescribed, and serum potassium levels are monitored. Thiazides also induce hypercalcemia, which enhances the action of digoxin, resulting in possible digitalis toxicity. Signs and symptoms of digitalis toxicity—bradycardia, nausea, vomiting, and visual changes—should be reported. Thiazides enhance the action of lithium, and lithium toxicity can occur. Thiazides potentiate the action of other antihypertensive drugs, which may be used to advantage in combination drug therapy for hypertension.

TABLE 38.2 Serum Chemistry Abnormalities Associated With Thiazides

Serum Chemistry Parameter	Abnormal Results
Electrolytes, Normal Levels	
Potassium, 3.5-5.0 mEq/L	Hypokalemia (low serum potassium); potassium is excreted from the distal renal tubule.
Magnesium, 1.5-2.5 mEq/L	Hypomagnesemia (low serum magnesium); potassium and sodium loss prompt magnesium loss.
Calcium, 8.6-10.2 mg/dL	Hypercalcemia (elevated serum calcium); thiazides may block calcium excretion.
Chloride, 96-106 mEq/L	Hypochloremia (low serum chloride); sodium and potassium losses produce chloride loss.
Bicarbonate, 24-28 mEq/L	Minimal bicarbonate loss occurs from the proximal tubule.
Uric acid, 2.8-8.0 mg/dL	Hyperuricemia (elevated uric acid); thiazides can block uric acid excretion.
Blood glucose, 70-99 mg/dL	Hyperglycemia (increased blood glucose); thiazides increase fasting blood glucose levels and those of the prediabetic state.
Blood Lipids Cholesterol: <200 mg/dL LDL: <100 mg/dL Triglyceride: <150 mg/dL	Elevated cholesterol, LDL, and triglycerides

LDL, Low-density lipoprotein.

NURSING PROCESS
Patient-Centered Collaborative Care

Diuretics: Thiazides

Assessment
- Assess vital signs, weight, urine output, and serum chemistry values (electrolytes, glucose, uric acid) for baseline levels.
- Check peripheral extremities for the presence of edema. Note pitting edema.
- Obtain a history of drugs and herbal supplements taken daily. Review for drugs and herbs that may cause a drug interaction (digoxin, corticosteroids, antidiabetics, ginkgo, licorice).

Nursing Diagnoses
- Fluid Volume, Risk for Deficient
- Elimination, Impaired Urinary related to kidney dysfunction
- Fluid Volume, Excess related to body fluid retention

Planning
- The patient's blood pressure will be decreased or will return to a normal value.
- The patient's edema will be decreased.
- The patient's serum chemistry levels will remain within normal ranges.

Nursing Interventions
- ⚡ Monitor vital signs and serum electrolytes, especially potassium, glucose, uric acid, and cholesterol levels. Report changes. If a patient is taking digoxin and hypokalemia occurs, digitalis toxicity frequently results.
- Observe for signs and symptoms of hypokalemia such as muscle weakness, leg cramps, and cardiac dysrhythmias.
- Monitor the patient's weight daily. A weight gain of 2.2 lb is equivalent to 1 L of body fluids.
- Note urine output to determine fluid loss or retention.

Patient Teaching
General
- Emphasize the need for adherence to the therapy plan. The patient may not feel better for some time or may not feel worse if treatment is missed or discontinued.
- Suggest that the patient take the drug early in the morning to avoid sleep disturbance resulting from nocturia.
- Instruct patients to keep drugs out of reach of small children. Request a childproof bottle.
- Inform patients that certain herbal products may interact with thiazide diuretics. (Complementary and Alternative Therapies 38.1).

Self-Administration
- Instruct patients or family members on how to take blood pressure and record daily results.

Side Effects
- ⚡ Instruct patients to slowly change positions from lying to standing because dizziness may occur as a result of orthostatic (postural) hypotension.
- Advise patients who may be prediabetic to have blood glucose checked periodically because large doses of hydrochlorothiazide increase blood glucose levels.
- Suggest that patients use sunblock when in direct sunlight to prevent photosensitivity.

Diet
- Teach patients to eat foods rich in potassium (fruits, fruit juices, and vegetables). Potassium supplements may be ordered.
- Instruct patients to take drugs with food to avoid GI upset (anorexia, nausea, vomiting, diarrhea).

 Cultural Considerations
- Respect cultural practices and values. If a patient from a different background tells the health care provider that she or he does not eat fruits and vegetables, the nurse may have two options: to encourage the patient to eat fruits and vegetables or to contact the health care provider so that an adequate potassium supplement can be prescribed to overcome potassium loss. An interpreter may be necessary.
- Emphasize the importance of patients taking potassium supplements with potassium-wasting diuretics. In addition, advise patients of the consequences and dangers of *not* taking potassium supplements or lacking appropriate nutrition while taking potassium-wasting diuretics. Monitor serum potassium levels.

Evaluation
- Evaluate the effectiveness of drug therapy. The patient's blood pressure and edema will be reduced, and blood chemistry will remain within normal range.
- Determine an absence of side effects and adverse reactions to therapy.

 COMPLEMENTARY AND ALTERNATIVE THERAPIES 38.1

Diuretics

- When taken with a potassium-wasting diuretic such as a thiazide, aloe can decrease the serum potassium level, thereby causing hypokalemia.
- Gingko may increase blood pressure when taken with a thiazide diuretic.
- Licorice can increase potassium loss, leading to hypokalemia.
- Hawthorn may potentiate hypotension.

LOOP (HIGH-CEILING) DIURETICS

The loop, or high-ceiling, diuretics act on the thick ascending loop of Henle to inhibit chloride transport of sodium into the circulation and inhibit passive reabsorption of sodium. Sodium and water are lost, together with potassium, calcium, and magnesium. Loop diuretics can affect blood glucose and can increase uric acid levels. Drugs in this group are extremely potent and cause marked depletion of water and electrolytes. This high diuretic potential is the reason they are often called *high-ceiling diuretics* or *potassium-wasting diuretics*. The effects of loop diuretics are dose related; that is, increasing the dose increases the effect and response of the drug. More potent than thiazides for promoting diuresis, inhibiting reabsorption of sodium two to three times more effectively, loop diuretics are less effective as antihypertensive agents.

Loop diuretics should not be prescribed if a thiazide could alleviate body fluid excess. If furosemide alone is not effective in removing body fluid, a thiazide may be added. Furosemide is usually administered as an oral dose in the morning or intravenously when the patient's condition warrants immediate removal of body fluid, for example, in cases of acute heart failure or pulmonary edema.

Loop diuretics can increase renal blood flow up to 40%. Furosemide is a frequently prescribed diuretic for patients whose creatinine clearance is less than 30 mL/min and for those with end-stage renal disease. This group of diuretics causes excretion of calcium, unlike thiazides, which inhibit calcium loss.

The first loop diuretic marketed was ethacrynic acid, followed by furosemide and then bumetanide, which is more potent than furosemide on a milligram-for-milligram basis. Furosemide and bumetanide are derivatives of sulfonamides. Ethacrynic acid, a phenoxyacetic acid derivative, is a seldom-chosen loop diuretic. It is usually reserved for patients who are allergic to sulfa drugs. Prototype Drug Chart 38.2 lists the drug data for the loop diuretic furosemide.

Pharmacokinetics Loop diuretics are rapidly absorbed by the GI tract. These drugs are highly protein bound with half-lives that vary from 1 to 5 hours. Loop diuretics compete for protein-binding sites with other highly protein-bound drugs.

Pharmacodynamics Loop diuretics have a great saluretic (sodium chloride–losing) or natriuretic (sodium-losing) effect and can cause rapid diuresis, decreasing vascular fluid volume and causing a decrease in cardiac output and blood pressure. Because furosemide is more potent than thiazide diuretics, it causes a vasodilatory effect; thus renal blood flow increases before diuresis. Furosemide is used when other conservative measures, such as sodium restriction and use of less potent diuretics, fail. The oral dose of furosemide is usually twice that of an intravenous (IV) dose.

The onset of action of loop diuretics occurs within 30 to 60 minutes. The onset of action for IV furosemide is 5 minutes. The duration of action is shorter than that of the thiazides.

Side Effects and Adverse Reactions. The most common side effects of loop diuretics are fluid and electrolyte imbalances such as hypokalemia, hyponatremia, hypocalcemia, hypomagnesemia, and hypochloremia. Hypochloremic metabolic alkalosis may result, which can worsen hypokalemia, and orthostatic hypotension can occur. Thrombocytopenia, skin disturbances, and transient deafness are rarely seen. Table 38.3 lists the physiologic and laboratory changes associated with loop diuretics.

Drug Interactions. The major drug interaction is with digitalis preparations. If the patient takes digoxin with a loop diuretic, digitalis toxicity can result. Hypokalemia enhances the action of digoxin and increases the risk for digitalis toxicity. The patient needs potassium replacement with food or supplements. Serum potassium levels should be closely monitored, especially when the patient is taking high dosages of loop diuretics. Table 38.4 lists the data for the four loop diuretics.

 NURSING PROCESS
Patient-Centered Collaborative Care

Diuretics: Loop

Assessment
- Obtain a history of drugs taken daily. Note if the patient is taking a drug that may interact with a loop diuretic, such as alcohol, aminoglycosides, anticoagulants, corticosteroids, lithium, amphotericin B, or digitalis. Recognize that furosemide is highly protein bound and can displace other protein-bound drugs such as warfarin.
- Assess vital signs, serum electrolytes, weight, and urine output for baseline levels.
- Compare the patient's drug dose with the recommended dose, and report any discrepancy.
- Note whether the patient is hypersensitive to sulfonamides.

Nursing Diagnoses
- Fluid Volume, Risk for Deficient
- Electrolyte Imbalance, Risk for

Planning
- The patient's edema and/or hypertension will be decreased.
- The patient's serum chemistry levels will remain within normal ranges.

PROTOTYPE DRUG CHART 38.2

Furosemide

Drug Class	Dosage
Loop diuretic Pregnancy category: C*	Peripheral edema: A: PO: 20-80 mg single dose/d; may repeat in 6-8 h; maint: 40-120 mg/d; *max:* 600 mg/d C: PO: 1-2 mg/kg q6-12 h; *max:* 6 mg/kg/dose A: IM/IV: 20-40 mg; repeat 20 mg in 2 h; *max:* 6 g/d IV C/infants: IM/IV: 1-2 mg/kg q6-12h; *max:* 6 mg/kg/dose
Contraindications	**Drug-Lab-Food Interactions**
Presence of severe electrolyte imbalances, hypovolemia, anuria, hepatic coma, hypersensitivity to sulfonamides *Caution:* HF, diabetes mellitus, hypotension, systemic lupus erythematosus, gout, patients with hearing impairment, nephrotoxocity	Drug: Increased orthostatic hypotension with alcohol; increased ototoxicity with aminoglycosides; increased bleeding with anticoagulants; increased potassium loss with steroids, amphotericin B, amiodarone; increased digitalis toxicity and cardiac dysrhythmias with digoxin and hypokalemia; increased lithium toxicity; increased amphotericin B ototoxicity and nephrotoxicity Food: Licorice may increase potassium loss. Lab: Increased BUN, blood/urine glucose, serum uric acid, ammonia; decreased potassium, sodium, calcium, magnesium, chloride serum levels Complementary and Alternative Therapies: Hawthorn may potentiate hypotension, and ginseng may decrease the action of loop diuretics.
Pharmacokinetics	**Pharmacodynamics**
Absorption: PO: Absorbed erratically from oral dose Distribution: PB: 95% Metabolism: t½: 0.5-1 h Excretion: In urine, some in feces; crosses the placenta	PO: Onset: 30-60 min Peak: 1-2 h Duration: 6-8 h IV: Onset: 5 min Peak: 20-30 min Duration: 2 h

Therapeutic Effects/Uses

To treat HF, renal dysfunction, hypertension, nephrotic syndrome, and acute pulmonary and peripheral edema

Mode of Action: Inhibition of sodium and water reabsorption from loop of Henle and distal renal tubules; potassium, magnesium, and calcium also may be excreted.

Side Effects	Adverse Reactions
Nausea, diarrhea, electrolyte imbalances, dizziness, abdominal cramping, constipation, rash, headache, weakness, blurred vision, muscle cramps, photosensitivity, paresthesias, hyperuricemia	Hypokalemia, hyponatremia, hypomagnesemia, orthostatic hypotension, hyperglycemia, gout, hearing loss, hypercholesterolemia *Life-threatening:* Renal failure, aplastic anemia, thrombocytopenia, agranulocytosis, Stevens-Johnson syndrome

*Pregnancy categories have been revised. See http://www.fda.gov/Drugs/DevelopmentApprovalProcess/DevelopmentResources/Labeling/ucm093307.htm for more information.

A, Adult; *BUN,* blood urea nitrogen; *C,* child; *d,* day; *GI,* gastrointestinal; *h,* hour; *HF,* heart failure; *IM,* intramuscular; *IV,* intravenous; *maint,* maintenance dose; *max,* maximum; *min,* minute; *PB,* protein binding; *PO,* by mouth; *q6-12h,* every 6 to 12 hours; *t½,* half-life.

Nursing Interventions

- Monitor urinary output to determine body fluid gain or loss. Urinary output should be at least 30 mL/h or 600 mL/24 h.
- Notify a health care provider if urine output does not increase; a severe renal disorder may be present.
- Weigh the patient to determine fluid loss or gain. A loss of 2.2 lb is equivalent to a fluid loss of 1 L.
- Monitor vital signs, and be alert for marked decreases in blood pressure.
- Administer IV furosemide slowly; hearing loss may occur if it is rapidly injected.
- ⚡ Observe for signs and symptoms of hypokalemia (<3.5 mEq/L), such as muscle weakness, abdominal distension, leg cramps, and/or cardiac dysrhythmias.
- Monitor serum potassium levels, especially when a patient is taking digoxin. Hypokalemia enhances the action of digitalis, causing digitalis toxicity.

Patient Teaching

General

- Advise patients to take furosemide in the morning and *not* in the evening to prevent sleep disturbance and nocturia.

Side Effects

- Teach patients to rise slowly from lying or sitting to standing to prevent dizziness resulting from fluid loss.

Diet

- Suggest taking furosemide with food to avoid nausea.

 Cultural Considerations

- Respect cultural practices and values. If a patient from a different background tells a health care provider that she or he does not eat fruits and vegetables, the nurse may have two options: encourage the patient to eat fruits and vegetables or contact the health care provider so that an adequate potassium supplement can be prescribed to overcome potassium loss. An interpreter may be necessary.

- Emphasize the importance of patients taking the potassium supplement with a potassium-wasting diuretic. In addition, advise patients of the consequences and dangers of not taking potassium supplements or lacking appropriate nutrition while taking potassium-wasting diuretics.

Evaluation
- Evaluate effectiveness of the drug action, such as decreased fluid retention or fluid overload, decreased respiratory distress, and increased cardiac output.
- Check for side effects and increased urine output.

TABLE 38.3   Physiologic and Laboratory Changes Associated With Loop Diuretics

Physiologic/Laboratory Changes	Possible Effects of Loop (High-Ceiling) Diuretics
Physiologic Changes	
Hypotension	Postural (orthostatic) hypotension can result because of ECFV deficit.
Ototoxicity	Hearing impairment, although rare, may occur. It is more common with use of ethacrynic acid. Diuretics in other categories are not considered ototoxic. *Caution:* Avoid taking a loop diuretic with a drug that can be ototoxic, such as an aminoglycoside.
Skin disturbances	Pruritus, urticaria, exfoliative dermatitis, and purpura may occur in some persons allergic to the drug or when taking a loop diuretic in high doses over a long period.
Photosensitivity	When exposed to sun or a sunlamp for a prolonged time, severe sunburn could result. Patient should use sunblock and avoid long sun exposures.
Hypovolemia	Excess extracellular fluid is lost through increased urine excretion.
Laboratory Changes	
Hypokalemia, hypomagnesemia, hyponatremia, hypocalcemia, hypochloremia	Potassium, magnesium, sodium, calcium, and chloride are lost from the body from increased urine excretion. Chloride, an anion, is attached to the cations potassium and sodium; thus chloride is lost along with potassium and sodium.
Hyperglycemia	Increased glycogenolysis may contribute to elevated blood glucose level. Patients with diabetes should closely monitor blood glucose levels when taking a loop diuretic.
Hyperuricemia	Elevated uric acid levels are common in patients susceptible to gout.
Elevated BUN and creatinine	These elevations may result from ECFV loss. Hemoconcentration can cause elevated BUN and creatinine levels, which are reversible when fluid volume returns to normal levels.
Thrombocytopenia, leukopenia	Decreases in platelet and white blood cell counts are rare, but they should be closely monitored.
Elevated lipids	Loop diuretics can decrease HDL and increase LDL. Patients with elevated cholesterol levels should have their HDL and LDL levels checked. Regardless of the lipid effects, loop diuretics are useful for patients with serious fluid retention caused by a cardiac condition such as HF.

BUN, Blood urea nitrogen; *ECFV*, extracellular fluid volume; *HDL*, high-density lipoprotein; *HF*, heart failure; *LDL*, low-density lipoprotein.

TABLE 38.4   Diuretics: Loop, Osmotics, and Carbonic Anhydrase Inhibitors

Drug	Route and Dosage	Uses and Considerations
Loop		
Bumetanide	A: PO: 0.5-2.0 mg/d; *max:* 10 mg/d A: IM/IV: Initially 0.5-1 mg/dose slowly over 2 min, may give a 2nd and 3rd dose at 2-3 h intervals if needed; *max:* 10 mg/d	For edema and HF. May cause orthostatic hypotension, hypokalemia, hyponatremia, hyperglycemia, hyperuricemia, renal impairment, and Stevens-Johnson syndrome. Pregnancy category: C*; PB: 96%; t½: 1-1.5 h
Ethacrynic acid	A: PO: Initially 50-100 mg/d; maint: 50-200 mg in divided doses; *max:* 400 mg/d C: PO: Initially 1 mg/kg/d; *max:* 3 mg/kg/d A: IV: 0.5-1 mg/kg/dose, may repeat after 2-4 h; *max:* 100 mg/dose C: IV: 1 mg/kg/dose; *max:* 1 mg/kg/dose or 3 mg/kg/d	For pulmonary and peripheral edema, ascites, and HF. May cause headache, blurred vision, injection site reaction, orthostatic hypotension, fatigue, anxiety, GI distress, electrolyte imbalance, hyperglycemia, hyperuricemia, and ototoxicity. Moderate to high doses may cause ototoxicity. Pregnancy category: B*; PB: 95%; t½: 2-4 h
Furosemide	See Prototype Drug Chart 38.2.	
Torsemide	Hypertension: A: PO: Initially: 5 mg/d; maint: 5-10 mg/d; *max:* 10 mg/d HF/edema: A: PO/IV: 10-20 mg/d; *max:* 200 mg/d	For hypertension, HF, and ascites. May cause headache, weakness, orthostatic hypotension, GI distress, hypokalemia, hyperglycemia, hypercholesterolemia, hyperuricemia, and Stevens-Johnson syndrome. Pregnancy category: B*; PB: 99%; t½: 3.5 h

TABLE 38.4 Diuretics: Loop, Osmotics, and Carbonic Anhydrase Inhibitors—cont'd

Drug	Route and Dosage	Uses and Considerations
Osmotics		
Mannitol	ICP/IOP: A: IV: Initially 1-2 g/kg followed by 0.25-1 g/kg q4h; infused over 30-60 min	For cerebral and peripheral edema, oliguria, urologic irrigation, and increased ICP. May cause headache, blurred vision, dry mouth, electrolyte imbalance, pulmonary edema, blood pressure fluctuations, injection site reaction, polyuria, and renal failure. Pregnancy category: C*; PB: UK; t½: 4.7 h
Carbonic Anhydrase Inhibitors		
Acetazolamide	Edema: A: PO/IV: 250-375 mg in morning for 2 d; allow 1-2 d drug free, then give qod; *max:* 1000 mg/d	For edema, absence seizures, and glaucoma. May cause headache, drowsiness, dizziness, hyperglycemia, hyperuricemia, electrolyte imbalance, crystalluria, paresthesias, photosensitivity, metabolic acidosis, and Stevens-Johnson syndrome. Pregnancy category: C*; PB: 90%; t½: 10-15 h
Methazolamide	A: PO: 50-100 mg bid/tid; *max:* 300 mg/d	For glaucoma. May cause drowsiness, fatigue, paresthesias, tinnitus, hearing loss, GI distress, metallic taste, photosensitivity, hypokalemia, weakness, and Stevens-Johnson syndrome. Pregnancy category: C*; PB: 55%; t½: 14 h

*Pregnancy categories have been revised. See http://www.fda.gov/Drugs/DevelopmentApprovalProcess/DevelopmentResources/Labeling/ucm093307.htm for more information.
A, Adult; *bid,* twice a day; *C,* child; *d,* day; *GI,* gastrointestinal; *h,* hour; *HF,* heart failure; *ICP,* intracranial pressure; *IM,* intramuscular; *IOP,* intraocular pressure; *IV,* intravenous; *maint,* maintenance dose; *max,* maximum; *min,* minute; *PB,* protein binding; *PO,* by mouth; *q4h,* every 4 hours; *qod,* every other day; *t½,* half-life; *tid,* three times a day; *UK,* unknown.

OSMOTIC DIURETICS

Osmotic diuretics increase the osmolality (concentration) and sodium reabsorption in the proximal tubule and loop of Henle. Sodium, chloride, potassium (to a lesser degree), and water are excreted. This group of drugs is used to prevent kidney failure, decrease intracranial pressure (ICP, such as in cerebral edema), and decrease intraocular pressure (IOP, such as in glaucoma). Mannitol is a potent osmotic, potassium-wasting diuretic frequently used in emergency situations such as ICP and IOP. In addition, mannitol can be used with cisplatin and carboplatin in cancer chemotherapy to induce a frank diuresis and decrease side effects of treatment.

Mannitol is the most frequently prescribed osmotic diuretic, followed by urea. Diuresis occurs within 1 to 3 hours after IV administration. Table 38.4 describes mannitol.

Side Effects and Adverse Reactions. The side effects and adverse reactions of mannitol include fluid and electrolyte imbalance, pulmonary edema from rapid shift of fluids, nausea and vomiting, tachycardia from rapid fluid loss, and acidosis. Crystallization of mannitol in the vial may occur when the drug is exposed to a low temperature; the vial should be warmed to dissolve the crystals. The mannitol solution should not be used for IV infusion if crystals are present and have not been dissolved.

Contraindications. Mannitol must be given with extreme caution to patients who have heart disease and HF. It should be immediately discontinued if the patient develops HF or renal failure.

CARBONIC ANHYDRASE INHIBITORS

The carbonic anhydrase inhibitors acetazolamide and methazolamide block the action of the enzyme *carbonic anhydrase,* which is needed to maintain the body's acid-base balance (hydrogen and bicarbonate ion balance). Inhibition of this enzyme causes increased sodium, potassium, and bicarbonate excretion. With prolonged use, metabolic acidosis can occur.

This group of drugs is used primarily to decrease IOP in patients with open-angle (chronic) glaucoma. These drugs are not used in narrow-angle or acute glaucoma. Other uses include diuresis, management of epilepsy, and treatment of high-altitude or acute mountain sickness. Table 38.4 presents the drug data for carbonic anhydrase inhibitor diuretics. Such drugs may also be used for patients in metabolic alkalosis who need a diuretic. Carbonic anhydrase inhibitors may be alternated with a loop diuretic.

Side Effects and Adverse Reactions. Acetazolamide can cause fluid and electrolyte imbalance, metabolic acidosis, nausea, vomiting, anorexia, confusion, orthostatic hypotension, and crystalluria. Hemolytic anemia and renal calculi can also occur. These drugs are contraindicated during the first trimester of pregnancy.

POTASSIUM-SPARING DIURETICS

Potassium-sparing diuretics, which are weaker than thiazides and loop diuretics, are used as mild diuretics or in combination with another diuretic such as hydrochlorothiazide or an antihypertensive drug. Continuous use of potassium-wasting diuretics requires a daily oral potassium supplement because the kidneys excrete potassium, sodium, and body water. However, potassium supplements are *not* used when the patient takes a potassium-sparing diuretic; in fact, serum potassium excess, called hyperkalemia, results when a potassium supplement is taken with a potassium-sparing diuretic. The serum potassium should be periodically monitored when the patient continuously takes a potassium-sparing diuretic. If the serum potassium level is greater than 5.0 mEq/L, the patient should discontinue the potassium-sparing diuretic and restrict foods high in potassium.

Potassium-sparing diuretics act primarily in the collecting duct renal tubules and late distal tubule to promote sodium and water excretion and potassium retention. The drugs interfere with the sodium-potassium pump controlled by the mineralocorticoid hormone aldosterone (sodium retained and potassium excreted).

Spironolactone, an aldosterone antagonist discovered in 1958, was the first potassium-sparing diuretic. Aldosterone is a mineralocorticoid hormone that promotes sodium retention and potassium excretion. Spironolactone blocks the action of aldosterone and inhibits the sodium-potassium pump (i.e., potassium is retained and sodium is excreted). Spironolactone has been prescribed by cardiologists for patients with cardiac disorders because of its potassium-retaining effect. As a result of the action of spironolactone, the heart rate is more regular, and the possibility of myocardial fibrosis is decreased. The effects of spironolactone may take 48 hours.

Amiloride, triamterene, and eplerenone are additional, commonly prescribed potassium-sparing diuretics. Amiloride and eplerenone are effective as antihypertensive agents. Triamterene is useful in the treatment of edema caused by HF or cirrhosis of the liver. Low doses of spironolactone and eplerenone are effective for chronic HF. Spironolactone, amiloride, triamterene, and eplerenone should not be taken with ACE inhibitors and angiotensin II receptor blockers (ARBs) because they can also increase serum potassium levels. Prototype Drug Chart 38.3 provides the pharmacologic data for spironolactone.

When potassium-sparing diuretics are used alone, they are less effective than when used in combination to reduce body fluid and sodium. These drugs are usually combined with a potassium-wasting diuretic, primarily hydrochlorothiazide or a loop diuretic. The combination of potassium-sparing and potassium-wasting diuretics intensifies the diuretic effect and prevents potassium loss. The common combination diuretics contain spironolactone and hydrochlorothiazide, amiloride and hydrochlorothiazide, and triamterene and hydrochlorothiazide. Table 38.5 lists the potassium-sparing diuretics and the combination potassium-wasting and potassium-sparing diuretics.

Side Effects and Adverse Reactions. The main side effect of potassium-sparing diuretics is hyperkalemia. Caution must be used when giving potassium-sparing diuretics to patients with poor renal function because the kidneys excrete 80% to 90% of potassium. Urine output should be at least 600 mL/day. Patients should *not* use potassium supplements while taking potassium-sparing diuretics, unless the serum potassium level is low. If a potassium-sparing diuretic is given with antihypertensive ACE inhibitors, hyperkalemia could become severe or life threatening because both drugs retain potassium. Monitoring serum potassium levels is essential to safe drug therapy. Headache, dizziness, weakness, GI disturbances (anorexia, nausea, vomiting, diarrhea) hyperuricemia, muscle cramps, numbness, and tingling of the hands and feet can occur.

PROTOTYPE DRUG CHART 38.3

Spironolactone

Drug Class	Dosage
Potassium-sparing diuretic Pregnancy category: C*	Edema: A: PO: 25-200 mg/d in divided doses; *max:* 400 mg/d Hypertension: A: PO: 50-100 mg/d; *max:* 400 mg/d
Contraindications Renal failure, hyperkalemia *Caution:* Renal or hepatic dysfunction, diabetes mellitus, HF	**Drug-Lab-Food Interactions** Drug: Increased serum potassium level with potassium supplements; increased effects of antihypertensives and lithium *Life threatening:* Hyperkalemia if given with an ACE inhibitor Lab: Increased serum potassium level; may increase BUN, AST, alkaline phosphatase levels; decreased serum sodium, chloride
Pharmacokinetics Absorption: PO: Rapidly absorbed from GI tract Distribution: PB: 90% Metabolism: t½: 1.3-2 h Excretion: In urine, mostly as metabolites and bile	**Pharmacodynamics** PO: Onset: UK Peak: UK Duration: 2-3 d or longer
Therapeutic Effects/Uses For peripheral and pulmonary edema, circulatory overload, hypertension, HF, ascites, hypokalemia Mode of Action: Acts on distal renal tubules to promote sodium and water excretion and potassium retention	
Side Effects Nausea, vomiting, diarrhea, dizziness, headache, weakness, muscle cramps	**Adverse Reactions** *Life threatening:* Severe hyperkalemia, thrombocytopenia, agranulocytosis, hepatotoxicity, Stevens-Johnson syndrome

*Pregnancy categories have been revised. See http://www.fda.gov/Drugs/DevelopmentApprovalProcess/DevelopmentResources/Labeling/ucm093307.htm for more information.
A, Adult; *ACE,* angiotensin-converting enzyme; *AST,* aspartate aminotransferase; *BUN,* blood urea nitrogen; *d,* day; *GI,* gastrointestinal; *h,* hour; *HF,* heart failure; *max,* maximum; *PB,* protein binding; *PO,* by mouth; *t½,* half-life; *UK,* unknown.

TABLE 38.5   Diuretics: Potassium-Sparing

Drug	Route and Dosage	Uses and Considerations
Single Agents		
Amiloride Hydrochloride	A: PO: 5-10 mg/d; *max:* 20 mg/d	For hypokalemia, hypertension, HF, and edema. May cause headache, dizziness, GI distress, weakness, severe hyperkalemia, hypochloremia, hyponatremia, and metabolic acidosis. Monitor serum potassium. Pregnancy category: B*; PB: 40%; t½: 6-9 h
Eplerenone	A: PO: 25-50 mg/d; *max:* 100 mg/d for hypertension; 50 mg/d for HF	For hypertension, HF, and acute MI. May cause hyperkalemia, hyponatremia, hypertriglyceridemia, and hypercholesterolemia. Pregnancy category: B*; PB: 50%; t½: 4-6 h
Spironolactone	See Prototype Drug Chart 38.3.	
Triamterene	A: PO: Initially 50-100 mg bid; *max:* 300 mg/d	For edema, ascites, and hypokalemia. May cause headache, dizziness, weakness, GI distress, electrolyte imbalance, hyperuricemia, photosensitivity, and dysrhythmias. Pregnancy category: C*; PB: 67%; t½: 1-2 h
Combinations		
Amiloride Hydrochloride and Hydrochlorothiazide	A: PO: 1-2 tab/d (amiloride 5 mg/HCTZ 50 mg); *max:* 10 mg amiloride, 100 mg HCTZ	For hypertension, HF, and edema. May cause headache, dizziness, GI distress, weakness, muscle cramps, electrolyte imbalance, and hyperuricemia. Pregnancy category: B*; PB: 40% amiloride, 40%-68% HCTZ; t½: 6-9 h amiloride, 5.6-14.8 h HCTZ
Spironolactone and Hydrochlorothiazide	A: PO: Initially 1 tab (25 mg spironolactone/25 mg HCTZ); maint: 100 mg/d of each; *max:* 200 mg/d of each	For edema and HTN. May cause electrolyte imbalance, hyperuricemia, muscle cramps, hyperglycemia, and hypercholesterolemia. Pregnancy category: C*; PB: 90% spironolactone, 40%-68% HCTZ; t½: 1.3-2 h spironolactone, 5.6-14.8 h HCTZ
Triamterene and Hydrochlorothiazide	A: PO: Initially 1 cap pc (37.5 mg triamterene, 25 mg hydrochlorothiazide; maint: 1-2 cap pc; *max:* 75 mg triamterene, 50 mg HCTZ	For edema and HTN. May cause blurred vision, orthostatic hypotension, gout, hyperglycemia, electrolyte imbalance, hyperuricemia, and hypercholesterolemia. Pregnancy category: C*; PB: 67% triamterene, 40%-68% HCTZ; t½: 1-2 h triamterene, 5.6-14.8 h hydrochloride

*Pregnancy categories have been revised. See http://www.fda.gov/Drugs/DevelopmentApprovalProcess/DevelopmentResources/Labeling/ucm093 307.htm for more information.

A, Adult; *bid*, twice a day; *cap*, capsule; *d*, day; *GI*, gastrointestinal; *h*, hour; *HCTZ*, hydrochlorothiazide; *HF*, heart failure; *HTN*, hypertension; *maint*, maintenance dose; *max*, maximum; *MI*, myocardial infarction; *PB*, protein binding; *pc*, after meals; *PO*, by mouth; *t½*, half-life; *tab*, tablet.

◉ NURSING PROCESS
Patient-Centered Collaborative Care

Diuretics: Potassium Sparing

Assessment
- Obtain a history of drugs taken daily. Note whether the patient is taking a potassium supplement or using a salt substitute.
- Assess vital signs, serum electrolytes, weight, and urinary output for baseline levels.
- Compare the patient's drug dose with the recommended dose, and report any discrepancy.

Nursing Diagnoses
- Fluid Volume, Risk for Deficient
- Electrolyte Imbalance, Risk for

Planning
- The patient's fluid retention and blood pressure will be decreased.
- The patient's serum electrolytes will remain within normal ranges.

Nursing Interventions
- Note the half-life of spironolactone. With a long half-life, the drug is usually administered once a day, sometimes twice a day.
- Monitor urinary output; it should increase. Report if urine output is less than 30 mL/h or less than 600 mL/day.

- Record vital signs and report any abnormal changes.
- ⚡ Observe for signs and symptoms of hyperkalemia (serum potassium >5.0 mEq/L). Nausea, diarrhea, abdominal cramps, numbness and tingling of the hands and feet, leg cramps, tachycardia and later bradycardia, peaked narrow T wave on electrocardiogram, or oliguria may signal hyperkalemia.
- Administer spironolactone in the morning and not in the evening to avoid nocturia.

Patient Teaching
General
- Teach patients to take spironolactone with or after meals to avoid nausea.
- Encourage patients not to discontinue the drug without consulting a health care provider.

Side Effects
- Caution patients to avoid exposure to direct sunlight because spironolactone can cause photosensitivity.
- Advise patients to report possible side effects such as rash, dizziness, weakness, and GI upset.

Diet
- Advise patients with high serum potassium levels to avoid foods rich in potassium when taking potassium-sparing diuretics.

🌐 *Cultural Considerations*
- Use both hands to show respect when offering a prescription, instructions, or pamphlets to Asians and Pacific Islanders.

Evaluation
- Evaluate the effectiveness of potassium-sparing diuretics (e.g., triamterene). Fluid retention (edema) should be decreased or absent.

- Determine whether urine output has increased and whether serum potassium level is within the normal range.

CRITICAL THINKING CASE STUDY

JQ, a 58-year-old patient, has been recently diagnosed with hypertension. His resting blood pressure is 158/92. He is prescribed hydrochlorothiazide 50 mg/day and is told to eat foods rich in potassium.

1. How does hydrochlorothiazide differ from furosemide? What are their similarities and differences?
2. Why is it necessary for JQ to eat foods rich in potassium when taking hydrochlorothiazide? Explain your answer.
3. What nursing interventions should be considered while JQ takes hydrochlorothiazide?

After 1 month on hydrochlorothiazide therapy, JQ becomes weak and complains of nausea and vomiting. His muscles are

"soft," and his serum potassium level is 3.3 mEq/L. JQ's diuretic is changed to triamterene and hydrochlorothiazide. Again, he is advised to eat foods rich in potassium.

4. Explain the rationale for changing JQ's diuretic.
5. Should JQ receive a potassium supplement? Explain your answer.
6. What nursing interventions should the nurse follow for JQ?
7. What care plan should the nurse develop for JQ in relation to patient teaching?
8. What medical follow-up care is needed for JQ?

NCLEX STUDY QUESTIONS

1. A patient is taking hydrochlorothiazide 50 mg/day and digoxin 0.25 mg/day. The nurse plans to monitor the patient for which potential electrolyte imbalance?
   a. Hypocalcemia
   b. Hypokalemia
   c. Hyperkalemia
   d. Hypermagnesemia
2. The nurse knows that which statement is correct regarding nursing care of a patient receiving hydrochlorothiazide? (Select all that apply.)
   a. Monitor patients for signs of hypoglycemia.
   b. Administer ordered potassium supplements.
   c. Monitor serum potassium and uric acid levels.
   d. Assess blood pressure before administration.
   e. Notify the health care provider if a patient has had oliguria for 24 hours.
   f. Assess for decreased cholesterol and triglyceride levels.
3. A patient has heart failure, and a high dose of furosemide is ordered. What suggests a favorable response to furosemide?
   a. A decrease in level of consciousness occurs, and the patient sleeps more.
   b. Respiratory rate decreases from 28/min to 20/min, and the depth increases.
   c. Increased congestion is heard in breath sounds, and the patient complains of shortness of breath.
   d. Urine output is 50 mL/4 h, and intake is 200 mL.
4. What does the nurse know to be correct concerning the use of mannitol in patients?
   a. It decreases intracranial pressure.
   b. It increases intraocular pressure.
   c. It causes sodium and potassium retention.
   d. It causes diuresis in several days.

5. What should the nurse do when a patient is taking furosemide?
   a. Instruct the patient to change positions quickly when getting out of bed.
   b. Assess blood pressure before administration.
   c. Administer the drug at bedtime for maximum effectiveness.
   d. Teach the patient to avoid fruits to prevent hyperkalemia.
6. For the patient taking a diuretic, a combination such as triamterene and hydrochlorothiazide may be prescribed. The nurse realizes that this combination is ordered for which purpose?
   a. To decrease serum potassium level
   b. To increase serum potassium level
   c. To decrease glucose level
   d. To increase glucose level
7. The patient has been receiving spironolactone 50 mg/day for heart failure. The nurse should closely monitor the patient for which condition?
   a. Hypokalemia
   b. Hyperkalemia
   c. Hypoglycemia
   d. Hypermagnesemia

Answers: 1, b; 2, b, c, d, e; 3, b; 4, a; 5, b; 6, b; 7, b.

39

Antihypertensives

http://evolve.elsevier.com/McCuistion/pharmacology/

OBJECTIVES

- Differentiate the pharmacologic action of the various categories of antihypertensive drugs.
- Compare the side effects and adverse reactions to sympatholytics, direct-acting vasodilators, and angiotensin antagonists.
- Apply the nursing process related to antihypertensives including nursing interventions and teaching.
- Describe the blood pressure guidelines for determining hypertension.

OUTLINE

KEY TERMS

HYPERTENSION

Hypertension is an increase in blood pressure such that the systolic pressure is greater than 140 mm Hg and the diastolic pressure is greater than 90 mm Hg. Essential hypertension is the most common type, affecting 90% of persons with high blood pressure. The exact origin of essential hypertension is unknown; however, contributing factors may include hyperlipidemia, African American race, diabetes, aging, stress, excessive alcohol ingestion, smoking, obesity, and a family history of hypertension. Ten percent of hypertension cases are related to renal and endocrine disorders and are classified as secondary hypertension. Hypertension is the most common condition leading to myocardial infarction (MI), stroke, renal failure, and death.

Selected Regulators of Blood Pressure

The kidneys and blood vessels strive to regulate and maintain a "normal" blood pressure. The kidneys regulate blood pressure by control of fluid volume and via the renin-angiotensin-aldosterone system (RAAS; Fig. 39.1). Kidneys control sodium and water elimination and retention, which affects cardiac output and systemic arterial blood pressure. Renin from the renal cells stimulates production of angiotensin II, a potent vasoconstrictor that causes the release of aldosterone, an adrenal hormone that promotes sodium retention and thereby water retention. Retention of sodium and water causes fluid volume to increase, elevating blood pressure.

The baroreceptors in the aorta and carotid sinus and the vasomotor center in the medulla also assist in the regulation

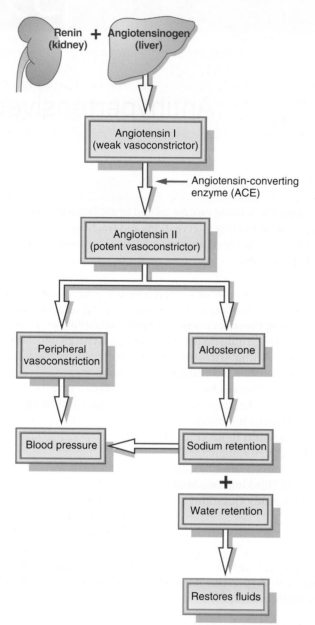

FIG. 39.1 The renin-angiotensin-aldosterone system (RAAS). Renin, an enzyme located in the juxtaglomerular cells of the kidney, is released when blood pressure decreases. This diagram shows how the RAAS restores fluid balance and stabilizes blood pressure.

of blood pressure. Catecholamines such as norepinephrine, released from the sympathetic nerve terminals, and epinephrine, released from the adrenal medulla, increase blood pressure through vasoconstrictive activity.

Other hormones that contribute to blood pressure regulation are antidiuretic hormone (ADH), atrial natriuretic peptide (ANP) hormone, and brain natriuretic peptide (BNP) hormone. ADH is produced by the hypothalamus and is stored and released by the posterior pituitary gland (neurohypophysis). This hormone stimulates the kidneys to conserve and retain water when there is a fluid volume deficit. When there is fluid overload, ADH secretion is inhibited, and the kidneys then excrete more water.

Physiologic Risk Factors

Certain physiologic risk factors contribute to hypertension. A diet high in saturated fat and simple carbohydrates can increase blood pressure. Carbohydrate intake can affect sympathetic nervous activity. Alcohol increases renin secretions, causing the production of angiotensin II. Obesity affects the sympathetic and cardiovascular systems by increasing cardiac output, stroke volume, and left ventricular filling. Two thirds of hypertensive persons are obese. Normally weight loss can decrease hypertension, as can mild to moderate sodium restriction.

Cultural Responses to Antihypertensive Agents

African Americans are more likely to develop hypertension at an earlier age than Caucasians. African Americans also have a higher mortality rate from hypertension than the Caucasian population. The use of beta-adrenergic blockers (beta blockers) and angiotensin-converting enzyme (ACE) inhibitors is less effective for the control of hypertension in African Americans unless the drug is combined or given with a diuretic. This group is susceptible to low-renin hypertension, therefore they do not respond well to beta blockers and ACE inhibitors. The antihypertensive drugs that are effective for African Americans are alpha$_1$ blockers and calcium channel blockers (calcium blockers). African American patients do respond to diuretics as the initial monotherapy for controlling hypertension. Caucasian patients usually have high-renin hypertension and respond well to all antihypertensive agents.

Asian Americans are twice as sensitive as Caucasians to beta blockers and other antihypertensives. A reduction in antihypertensive dosing is frequently needed. Native Americans have a reduced or lower response to beta blockers compared with Caucasians. Monitoring blood pressure and drug dosing should be an ongoing assessment for patients in these cultural groups.

Hypertension in Older Adults

Approximately 70 million American adults have hypertension, which is 29% of the adult population, about one in three people. Only approximately 52% of hypertensive individuals have this condition under control. Of individuals over 60 years of age, 65% have developed hypertension. Typically, in the age range of 18 to 49, males have more prevalence of hypertension than females. By age 70, the prevalence of hypertension in Caucasian males is 50%, whereas the female prevalence is 55%. Both systolic and diastolic hypertension are associated with increased cardiovascular morbidity and mortality. With antihypertensive therapy, the greatest decrease in cardiovascular disorders is 34% for stroke and 19% for coronary heart disease.

One of the troublesome side effects of the use of antihypertensive agents in older adults, especially frail or institutionalized persons, is orthostatic (postural) hypotension. This episode of sudden low blood pressure presents as dizziness due to blood pooling in the lower extremities when an individual changes to an upright position. In older adults, the sympathetic nervous system does not respond as quickly to correct the situation, especially when potentiated by antihypertensive drug administration. If orthostatic hypotension occurs, the antihypertensive drug dose may need to be decreased or another antihypertensive drug may need to be used. Older adults with hypertension should be instructed to modify their lifestyle and activities. This includes restricting dietary sodium to 2400 mg daily, avoiding tobacco, modifying diet, exercising, and decreasing stress.

NONPHARMACOLOGIC CONTROL OF HYPERTENSION

A sufficient decrease in blood pressure can be accomplished by nonpharmacologic methods. There are many nonpharmacologic ways to decrease blood pressure, but if the systolic pressure is greater than 140 mm Hg, antihypertensive drugs are generally ordered. Nondrug methods to decrease blood pressure include stress-reduction techniques, exercise, salt restriction, decreased alcohol ingestion, and smoking cessation.

When hypertension cannot be controlled by nonpharmacologic means, antihypertensive drugs are prescribed. However, nonpharmacologic methods should be combined with antihypertensive drugs to control hypertension.

GUIDELINES FOR HYPERTENSION

Blood pressure guidelines for determining hypertension have been revised and are contained in the Eighth Report of the Joint National Committee on Prevention, Detection, Evaluation, and Treatment of High Blood Pressure, or JNC 8, from 2014. The purpose of these guidelines is to decrease the risk of cardiovascular disease (CVD) in the American population. The guideline for normal blood pressure is less than 120/80 mm Hg. *Prehypertension* is defined as systolic blood pressure (SBP) of 120 to 139 and diastolic blood pressure (DBP) of 80 to 89. *Stage 1 hypertension* falls between 140/90 and 159/99, and *stage 2 hypertension* is 160/100 or greater.

Two out of three patients with hypertension have uncontrolled blood pressure or are not optimally treated. SBP is more important than DBP as a CVD risk. According to the JNC 8, a blood pressure of 140/90 is the goal for the population younger than 60 years, with a target of 150/90 for those above 60.

PHARMACOLOGIC CONTROL OF HYPERTENSION

An individualized approach to the treatment of hypertension is used by many health care providers. All drugs are considered *initial agents* when first prescribed for hypertension. Reduction of other cardiovascular risk factors and the use of fewer drugs (i.e., substituting instead of adding drugs) at the lowest effective doses are emphasized. Often more than one antihypertensive is used to control blood pressure, which also may lead to fewer adverse effects.

Antihypertensive drugs, used either singly or in combination with other drugs, are classified into six categories: (1) diuretics, (2) sympatholytics (sympathetic depressants), (3) direct-acting arteriolar vasodilators, (4) ACE inhibitors, (5) angiotensin II–receptor blockers (ARBs), and (6) calcium channel blockers.

Diuretics

Diuretics promote sodium depletion, which decreases extracellular fluid volume (ECFV). Diuretics are effective as first-line drugs for treating mild hypertension. Hydrochlorothiazide is the most frequently prescribed diuretic for controlling mild hypertension by decreasing excess fluid volume. It can be used alone for recently diagnosed or mild hypertension, or it can be used with other antihypertensive drugs. Many antihypertensive drugs can cause fluid retention; therefore diuretics are often administered together with antihypertensive agents. The various types of diuretics are discussed in Chapter 38.

Thiazide diuretics are not recommended for patients with renal insufficiency (creatinine clearance <30 mL/min). The loop (high-ceiling) diuretics such as furosemide are usually recommended because they do not depress renal blood flow. Loop diuretics are not used if hypertension is the result of RAAS involvement because they tend to elevate serum renin level immediately. Instead of a single thiazide drug, a combination of potassium-wasting and potassium-sparing diuretics may be useful; less potassium excretion would occur. In addition, thiazides can be combined with other antihypertensive drugs to increase their effectiveness. Box 39.1 lists the combinations of thiazides with other drugs. Many drug products on the market include combinations of thiazide diuretics and potassium-sparing diuretics, beta blockers, ACE inhibitors, or ARBs. ACE inhibitors tend to increase serum potassium (K) levels, so when they are combined with a thiazide diuretic, serum potassium loss is minimized.

Sympatholytics (Sympathetic Depressants)

The sympatholytics comprise five groups of drugs: (1) beta-adrenergic blockers, (2) centrally acting alpha$_2$ agonists, (3) alpha-adrenergic blockers, (4) adrenergic neuron blockers (peripherally acting sympatholytics), and (5) alpha$_1$- and beta$_1$-adrenergic blockers. Beta-adrenergic blockers block the beta receptors, and alpha-adrenergic blockers block the alpha receptors.

❶ Beta-Adrenergic Blockers

Beta-adrenergic blockers, frequently called *beta blockers*, are used as antihypertensive drugs or in combination with a diuretic. Beta blockers are also used as antianginals and antidysrhythmics and are discussed in this context in Chapter 37.

Beta (β+ and β−)-adrenergic blockers reduce cardiac output by diminishing the sympathetic nervous system response to decrease basal sympathetic tone. With continued use of beta blockers, vascular resistance is diminished, and blood pressure is lowered. Beta blockers reduce heart rate, contractility, and renin release. The hypotensive response is greater in patients with higher renin levels.

African American hypertensive patients do not respond well to beta blockers alone for the control of hypertension. Instead, hypertension in the African American population can be controlled by combining beta blockers with diuretics.

There are many types of beta blockers. Nonselective beta blockers, such as propranolol and carvedilol, inhibit beta$_1$ (heart) and beta$_2$ (bronchial) receptors. Heart rate slows,

BOX 39.1   Combination of Thiazides With Antihypertensive Drugs and Other Combinations

Thiazide With Potassium-Sparing Diuretics
- Hydrochlorothiazide with spironolactone
- Hydrochlorothiazide with amiloride
- Hydrochlorothiazide with triamterene

Thiazide With Beta Blockers
- Hydrochlorothiazide with bisoprolol fumarate
- Hydrochlorothiazide with metoprolol
- Bendroflumethiazide with nadolol

Tenoretic
- Chlorthalidone (thiazide-like diuretic) with atenolol

Thiazide With Angiotensin-Converting Enzyme Inhibitors
- Hydrochlorothiazide with benazepril
- Hydrochlorothiazide with captopril
- Hydrochlorothiazide with enalapril maleate
- Hydrochlorothiazide with fosinopril
- Hydrochlorothiazide with lisinopril
- Hydrochlorothiazide with moexipril
- Hydrochlorothiazide with quinapril

Thiazide With Angiotensin II Antagonists
- Hydrochlorothiazide with candesartan
- Hydrochlorothiazide with eprosartan
- Hydrochlorothiazide with irbesartan
- Hydrochlorothiazide with losartan
- Hydrochlorothiazide with olmesartan
- Hydrochlorothiazide with telmisartan
- Hydrochlorothiazide with valsartan

Thiazide With Centrally Acting Alpha$_2$ Agonist
- Chlorthalidone with clonidine
- Hydrochlorothiazide with methyldopa

Combination of Angiotensin-Converting Enzyme Inhibitors With Calcium Channel Blocker
- See Table 39.3.

Combination of Calcium Channel Blocker With Statin Drug
- Amlodipine with atorvastatin

blood pressure decreases secondary to the decrease in heart rate, and bronchoconstriction occurs because of unopposed parasympathetic tone. Cardioselective beta blockers are preferred because they act mainly on the beta$_1$—rather than the beta$_2$—receptors and bronchoconstriction is less likely to occur. Acebutolol, atenolol, betaxolol, bisoprolol, and metoprolol are cardioselective beta blockers that block beta$_1$ receptors.

Cardioselectivity does not confer absolute protection from bronchoconstriction. In tests measuring forced expiratory volume in 1 second (FEV$_1$) as a measure of $\beta-$ reactivity, only atenolol demonstrated true protection. Other cardioselective beta blockers were only partially effective. Studies also show that at the upper end of the dosage range, cardioselectivity is less effective. In patients with preexisting bronchospasm or other pulmonary disease, beta blockers—even those considered to be cardioselective—should be used with caution. Some experts regard this as a relative contraindication. The real value of beta selectivity is in maintaining renal blood flow and minimizing the hypoglycemic effects of beta blockade.

The combination of beta blockers with hydrochlorothiazides is packaged together in tablet form (see Box 39.1). Usually the hydrochlorothiazide dose is 12.5 to 25 mg.

Beta blockers tend to be more effective in lowering blood pressure in patients who have an elevated serum renin level. The cardioselective prototype drug metoprolol is presented in Prototype Drug Chart 39.1.

Beta blockers should not be used by patients with second- or third-degree atrioventricular (AV) block or sinus bradycardia. A noncardioselective beta blocker such as propranolol should not be given to a patient with chronic obstructive pulmonary disease (COPD).

Pharmacokinetics Metoprolol is well absorbed from the gastrointestinal (GI) tract. Its half-life is short, and its protein-binding power is low.

Pharmacodynamics Cardioselective beta-adrenergic blockers block beta$_1$ receptors, thereby decreasing heart rate and blood pressure. The nonselective beta blockers block beta$_1$ and beta$_2$ receptors, which can result in bronchial constriction. Beta blockers cross the placental barrier and are excreted in breast milk.

The onset of action of oral beta blockers is usually 60 minutes or less, and the duration of action is usually 24 hours with some exceptions. The peak for extended release is usually 1 to 7 hours, and the duration is typically 24 hours. When beta blockers are administered intravenously, the onset of action is immediate, peak time is 20 minutes, and duration of action is approximately 4 to 10 hours.

Side Effects and Adverse Reactions. Side effects and adverse reactions include decreased pulse rate; markedly decreased blood pressure; and with noncardioselective beta$_1$ and beta$_2$ blockers, bronchospasm. Beta blockers should not be abruptly discontinued because rebound hypertension, angina, dysrhythmias, and MI can result. Beta blockers can cause dizziness, insomnia, depression, fatigue, nightmares, and sexual dysfunction. Table 39.1 lists the beta blockers used to treat hypertension and their dosages, uses, and considerations.

Noncardioselective beta blockers inhibit the liver's ability to convert glycogen to glucose in response to hypoglycemia. Because of this side effect, beta blockers should be used with caution in patients with diabetes mellitus. In addition, bradycardia is a very common adverse effect of beta blockers.

! PROTOTYPE DRUG CHART 39.1

Metoprolol

Drug Class Antihypertensive: beta₁ blocker Pregnancy category: C *	**Dosage** Hypertension: Regular release: A: PO: Initially 100 mg/d in divided doses; maint: 100-450 mg in divided doses; max: 450 mg/d in divided doses Extended release: A: PO: 25-100 mg/d; max: 400 mg/d C 6-16 y: PO: 0.2-2 mg/kg/d; max: 2 mg/kg/d
Contraindications Hypersensitivity, heart block, cardiogenic shock, hypotension, acute HF, bradycardia Caution: Hepatic or thyroid dysfunction, asthma, peripheral vascular disease, diabetes mellitus, COPD, cerebrovascular disease, depression	**Drug-Lab-Food Interactions** Drug: Increases bradycardia and heart block with digitalis, clonidine, SSRIs, MAOIs, cimetidine; increased hypotensive effect with other antihypertensives, alcohol, anesthetics; NSAIDs decrease effect of beta blockers. Lab: Increased hepatic enzymes
Pharmacokinetics Absorption: PO: 95% Distribution: PB: 10% Metabolism: t½: 3-4 h Excretion: In urine	**Pharmacodynamics** Immediate release: PO: Onset: 30-60 min Peak: 1-2 h Duration: 6.4 h Extended release: PO: Onset UK Peak: 7 h Duration: 24 h
Therapeutic Effects/Uses To control hypertension, acute myocardial infarction, angina, and HF Mode of Action: Promotes blood pressure reduction via a beta₁-blocking effect	
Side Effects Fatigue, weakness, dizziness, dysgeusia, dry mouth, nausea, vomiting, diarrhea, drowsiness, headache, blurred vision, insomnia, short-term memory loss, peripheral edema, tinnitus, erectile dysfunction, depression	**Adverse Reactions** Bradycardia, hypotension, stroke, thrombocytopenia, diabetes mellitus Life threatening: AV heart block, bronchospasm, agranulocytosis, HF

*Pregnancy categories have been revised. See http://www.fda.gov/Drugs/DevelopmentApprovalProcess/DevelopmentResources/Labeling/ucm093307.htm for more information.
A, Adult; AV, atrioventricular; C, child; COPD, chronic obstructive pulmonary disease; d, day; h, hour; HF, heart failure; maint, maintenance; MAOI, monoamine oxidase inhibitor; max, maximum; min, minute; NSAID, nonsteroidal antiinflammatory drug; PB, protein binding; PO, by mouth; SSRI, selective serotonin reuptake inhibitor; t½, half-life; UK, unknown; y, year.

! TABLE 39.1   Antihypertensives: Beta Blockers and Central Alpha₂ Agonists

Drug	Route and Dosage	Uses and Considerations
Beta-Adrenergic Blockers		
Acebutolol hydrochloride Cardioselective beta₁	Hypertension: A: PO: Initially 400 mg/d in 1-2 divided doses; maint: 400-800 mg/d; max: 1200 mg/d Older A: Initially 200 mg/d; max: 800 mg/d	For hypertension and PVCs. May cause dizziness, headache, fatigue, hypotension, bradycardia, nausea, and constipation/diarrhea. Closely monitor vital signs. Pregnancy category: B, D*; PB: 26%; t½: 3-4 h
Atenolol Cardioselective beta₁	Hypertension: A: PO: Initially 25-50 mg/d; max: 100 mg/d C: PO: Initially 0.8-1 mg/kg/d; maint: 0.8-1.5 mg/kg/d; max: 2 mg/kg/d	For hypertension, angina, and prophylaxis and treatment of AMI. May cause hypotension, heart failure, bradycardia, fatigue, dizziness, depression, and supraventricular tachycardia. Pregnancy category: D*; PB: 10%; t½: 6-7 h
Betaxolol hydrochloride Cardioselective beta₁	Hypertension: A: PO: Initially 10 mg/d; maint: 10-20 mg/d; max: 20 mg/d Older A: PO: Initially 5 mg/d; max: 20 mg/d	For hypertension, glaucoma, and ocular hypertension. May cause headache, dizziness, bradycardia, fatigue, nausea, and chest pain. Discontinue over a 2-week period. Pregnancy category: C*; PB: 50%; t½: 15 h
Bisoprolol fumarate Beta₁ blocker	A: PO: Initially 2.5-5 mg/d; max: 20 mg/d	For hypertension. May cause drowsiness, headache, fatigue, sweating, bradycardia, hypotension, peripheral edema, elevated hepatic enzymes, and bronchospasm. Pregnancy category: C*; PB: 30%; t½: 9-12 h
Carvedilol Alpha blocker, nonselective beta₁ and beta₂	Hypertension: A: PO: Initially 6.25 mg bid; max: 50 mg/d Extended release: A: PO: Initially 20 mg/d in the morning; max: 80 mg/d	For treating hypertension, AMI, and heart failure. May cause dizziness, drowsiness, weakness, orthostatic hypotension, weight gain, diarrhea, edema, bradycardia, and hyperglycemia. Pregnancy category: C, D*; PB: 98%; t½: 7-11 h

Continued

Drug	Route and Dosage	Uses and Considerations
Metoprolol Cardioselective beta₁	See Prototype Drug Chart 39.1.	
Nadolol Nonselective beta₁ and beta₂	A: PO: Initially 40 mg/d; maint: 40-80 mg/d; *max:* 320 mg/d for HTN	For hypertension and angina. May cause dizziness, drowsiness, fatigue, bradycardia, hypotension, palpitations, cold extremities, and dysrhythmias. Pregnancy category: C*; PB: 30%; t½: 10-24 h
Pindolol Nonselective beta₁ and beta₂	A: PO: Initially 5 mg bid; maint: 10-30 mg/d in 2-3 divided doses; *max:* 60 mg/d in divided doses	For hypertension. May cause dizziness, fatigue, visual impairment, nervousness, insomnia, arthralgia, myalgia, edema, bradycardia, hypotension, cold extremities, and elevated hepatic enzymes. Pregnancy category: B*; PB: 40%-60%; t½: 3-4 h
Propranolol Nonselective beta₁ and beta₂	Hypertension: Immediate release: A: PO: Initially 40 mg bid; maint: 160-480 mg/d in 2-3 divided doses; *max:* 640 mg/d Extended release: A: PO: 80 mg/d; maint: 120-160 mg/d; *max:* 640 mg/d	For hypertension, AMI, angina, and dysrhythmias and for migraine prophylaxis. May cause dizziness, sleep disorders, visual impairment, bradycardia, cool extremities, hyperkalemia, seizures, and agitation. Bronchospasm may occur due to the beta₂-blocker effect. Pregnancy category: C*; PB: 90%; t½: 2-6 h
Central Alpha₂ Agonists		
Clonidine hydrochloride	A: PO: Initially 0.1 mg bid; maint: 0.2-0.6 mg/d; *max:* 2.4 mg/d A: Transdermal patch: Initially 1 patch (0.1 mg/24 h) q7d	For hypertension. May cause drowsiness, dizziness, confusion, dry mouth, fatigue, headache, nightmares, irritability, orthostatic hypotension, and erythema. Pregnancy category: C*; PB: 20%-40%; t½: 12-16 h PO, 20 h transdermal
Guanfacine hydrochloride	A: PO: Initially 1 mg/d at bedtime; maint: 2-3 mg/d; *max:* 4 mg/d	For hypertension. May cause drowsiness, dry mouth, headache, dizziness, fatigue, abdominal pain, constipation, diarrhea, orthostatic hypotension, bradycardia, and depression. Pregnancy category: B*; PB: 70%; t½: 10-30 h
Methyldopa	A: PO: Initially 250 mg bid-tid; maint: 500-2000 mg/d in 2-4 divided doses; *max:* 3 g/d Hypertensive urgency/emergency: IV: 250-500 mg q6h over 30-60 min; *max:* 4 g/d	For hypertension, hypertensive urgency, and emergency. May cause orthostatic hypotension, drowsiness, weakness, bradycardia, psychosis, depression, and agranulocytosis. Take with food if GI upset occurs. Pregnancy category: B*; PB: 10%-15%; t½: 2 h

*Pregnancy categories have been revised. See http://www.fda.gov/Drugs/DevelopmentApprovalProcess/DevelopmentResources/Labeling/ucm093 307.htm for more information.

A, Adult; *AMI*, acute myocardial infarction; *bid*, twice a day; *C*, child; *d*, day; *GI*, gastrointestinal; *h*, hour; *HTN*, hypertension; *IV*, intravenous; *maint*, maintenance; *max*, maximum; *min*, minutes; *PB*, protein binding; *PO*, by mouth; *PVCs*, premature ventricular contractions; *q*, every; *t½*, half-life; *tid*, three times a day.

◎ NURSING PROCESS
Patient-Centered Collaborative Care
❶ *Antihypertensives: Beta Blockers*

Assessment
- Obtain a medication and herbal history from the patient. Report if a drug-drug or drug-herbal interaction is probable.
- Obtain vital signs. Report abnormal blood pressure and bradycardia, and compare vital signs with baseline findings.
- Check laboratory values related to renal and liver function periodically. Elevated blood urea nitrogen (BUN) and serum creatinine may be caused by beta blockers or a cardiac disorder. Elevated cardiac enzymes, such as aspartate transaminase (AST) and lactate dehydrogenase (LDH), may be caused by beta blockers or cardiac disorder.

Nursing Diagnoses
- Cardiac Output, Decreased related to variations in blood pressure readings
- Noncompliance with drug regimen related to cost of multiple drugs ordered
- Sexual Dysfunction related to a side effect of beta blockers
- Knowledge, Deficient related to inexperience with beta blockers

Planning
- The patient's blood pressure will be decreased or will return to a normal value.
- The patient states he or she will take medication as prescribed.
- The patient will verbalize the importance of following the beta-blocker regimen.

Nursing Interventions
- Monitor vital signs, especially blood pressure and pulse.
- Monitor laboratory results, especially BUN, serum creatinine, AST, and LDH.

Patient Teaching
General
- ⚡ Encourage patients to comply with the drug regimen. Advise that abrupt discontinuation of antihypertensive drugs may cause rebound hypertension.
- Inform patients that herbs can interfere with beta blockers (Complementary and Alternative Therapies 39.1).
- ⚡ Advise patients to avoid over-the-counter (OTC) drugs without first checking with a health care provider. Many OTC drugs carry warnings against use in presence of hypertension or concurrent use with antihypertensives.

- Suggest that patients wear a MedicAlert bracelet or carry a card indicating their health problem and prescribed drugs.
- Teach patients in trauma situations to inform a health care provider of drugs taken daily, such as a beta blocker. Beta blockers block compensatory effects of the body to the shock state. Glucagon may be needed to reverse the effects so the patient can be resuscitated.

Self-Administration
- Teach patients or family members how to take a radial pulse and blood pressure and to report abnormal findings to a health care provider.

Side Effects
- Advise patients that antihypertensives may cause dizziness (orthostatic hypotension). Warn patients to rise slowly from lying or sitting to a standing position.
- Advise patients to report dizziness, slow pulse rate, changes in blood pressure, heart palpitation, confusion, or GI upset to a health care provider.
- Alert patients with diabetes mellitus to possible hypoglycemic symptoms.
- Inform patients that antihypertensives may cause sexual dysfunction (e.g., impotence).

Diet
- Teach patients and family members nonpharmacologic methods to decrease blood pressure, such as a low-salt diet, relaxation techniques, exercise, smoking cessation, and decreased alcohol ingestion (limit to 1 drink for females and 2 drinks for males daily).
- Advise patients to report constipation. Foods high in fiber, a stool softener, and increased water intake (except in patients with heart failure) are usually indicated.

Cultural Considerations
- Explain to African American patients that monotherapy with beta blockers is generally less effective in controlling their hypertension. However, taking a diuretic together with a beta blocker can increase effectiveness of therapy.

Evaluation
- Evaluate the effectiveness of the drug therapy (decreased blood pressure, absence of side effects).
- Determine that the patient is adhering to the drug regimen.

COMPLEMENTARY AND ALTERNATIVE THERAPIES 39.1

Antihypertensives

- Ma-huang (ephedra) decreases or counteracts the effect of antihypertensive drugs. When taken with beta blockers, hypertension may continue or increase.
- Ephedra increases hypertension when taken with beta blockers.
- Black cohosh increases the hypotensive effect of antihypertensive drugs.
- Hawthorn may increase the effects of beta blockers and angiotensin-converting enzyme (ACE) inhibitors.
- Licorice antagonizes the effects of antihypertensive drugs.
- Goldenseal may increase the effects of antihypertensive drugs.
- Parsley may potentiate hypotension when taken with an antihypertensive drug.

Centrally Acting Alpha₂ Agonists

Centrally acting alpha$_2$ agonists decrease the sympathetic response from the brainstem to the peripheral vessels. They stimulate the alpha$_2$ receptors, which in turn decreases sympathetic activity; increases vagus activity; decreases cardiac output; and decreases serum epinephrine, norepinephrine, and renin release. All of these actions result in reduced peripheral vascular resistance and increased vasodilation. This group of drugs has minimal effects on cardiac output and blood flow to the kidneys. Beta blockers are not given with centrally acting sympatholytics because accentuation of bradycardia during therapy can occur, as can rebound hypertension upon discontinuing therapy.

Drugs in this group include methyldopa, clonidine, and guanfacine. Methyldopa was one of the first drugs widely used to control hypertension. In high doses, methyldopa and clonidine can cause sodium and water retention. Frequently methyldopa and clonidine are administered with diuretics. Clonidine is available in a transdermal preparation that provides a 7-day duration of action. Transdermal patches are replaced every 7 days and may be left on while bathing; skin irritations may occur. Guanfacine has effects similar to clonidine. Guanfacine has a long half-life and usually is taken once a day. Table 39.1 lists centrally acting alpha$_2$ agonists along with beta blockers.

Side Effects and Adverse Reactions. Side effects and adverse reactions of alpha$_2$ agonists include drowsiness, dry mouth, dizziness, and slow heart rate (bradycardia). Methyldopa should not be used in patients with impaired liver function, and serum liver enzymes should be monitored periodically in all patients. This group of drugs must not be abruptly discontinued because a rebound hypertensive crisis can result. If the drug needs to be stopped immediately, another antihypertensive drug is usually prescribed to avoid rebound hypertensive symptoms such as restlessness, tachycardia, tremors, headache, and increased blood pressure. Rebound hypertension is less likely to occur with guanfacine. The nurse should emphasize the need to take the medication as prescribed. This group of drugs can cause sodium and water retention, resulting in peripheral edema. A diuretic may be ordered with methyldopa or clonidine to decrease water and sodium retention (edema). Patients who are pregnant or contemplating pregnancy should avoid clonidine. Methyldopa is frequently used to treat chronic or pregnancy-induced hypertension; however, it crosses the placental barrier, and small amounts may enter the breast milk of a lactating patient.

Alpha-Adrenergic Blockers

This group of drugs blocks the alpha-adrenergic receptors (alpha blockers), resulting in vasodilation and decreased blood pressure. They help maintain the renal blood flow rate. Alpha blockers are useful in treating hypertension in patients with lipid abnormalities. They decrease the very-low-density lipoprotein (VLDL) and the low-density lipoprotein (LDL) responsible for the buildup of fatty plaques in the arteries (atherosclerosis). In addition, they increase high-density lipoprotein (HDL) levels. Alpha blockers are safe for patients with diabetes because they do not affect glucose metabolism. They also do not affect respiratory function.

The selective alpha$_1$-adrenergic blockers—prazosin, terazosin, and doxazosin—are used mainly to reduce blood pressure and can be used to treat benign prostatic hypertrophy (BPH). Prazosin is a commonly prescribed drug. Terazosin and doxazosin have longer half-lives than prazosin, and they are normally given once at bedtime. When prazosin is taken with alcohol or other antihypertensives, the hypotensive state can be intensified. These drugs, like the centrally acting alpha$_2$ agonists, cause sodium and water retention with edema, therefore diuretics are frequently given concomitantly to decrease fluid accumulation in the extremities.

Pharmacokinetics Prazosin is absorbed through the GI tract, but a large portion of prazosin is lost during hepatic first-pass metabolism. The half-life is short, so the drug should be administered twice a day. Prazosin is highly protein bound, and when it is given with other highly protein-bound drugs, the patient should be assessed for adverse reactions.

Pharmacodynamics Selective alpha-adrenergic blockers dilate the arterioles and venules, decreasing peripheral resistance and lowering blood pressure. With prazosin, the heart rate is only slightly increased, whereas with nonselective alpha blockers such as phenoxybenzamine, the blood pressure is greatly reduced, and reflex tachycardia can occur. Nonselective alpha blockers are more effective for acute hypertension; selective alpha blockers are more useful for long-term essential hypertension.

The onset of action of prazosin occurs between 30 minutes and 2 hours. The duration of action of prazosin is less than 24 hours. Table 39.2 presents drug data for selective and nonselective alpha blockers.

Side Effects and Adverse Reactions. Side effects of prazosin, doxazosin, and terazosin include orthostatic hypotension (dizziness, faintness, lightheadedness, and increased heart rate, which may occur with first dose), nausea, headache, drowsiness, nasal congestion caused by vasodilation, edema, and weight gain.

Side effects of phentolamine include hypotension, reflex tachycardia caused by the severe decrease in blood pressure, nasal congestion caused by vasodilation, and GI disturbances.

Drug Interactions. Drug interactions occur when alpha-adrenergic blockers are taken with antiinflammatory drugs and nitrates, such as nitroglycerin taken for angina. Peripheral edema is intensified when prazosin and an antiinflammatory drug are taken daily. Nitroglycerin taken for angina lowers blood pressure. If prazosin is taken with nitroglycerin, syncope (faintness) caused by a decrease in blood pressure can occur. The selective alpha-adrenergic blocker prazosin is shown in Prototype Drug Chart 39.2.

! TABLE 39.2	**Antihypertensives: Sympatholytics—Alpha-Adrenergic and Peripherally Acting Blockers and Direct-Acting Vasodilators**	
Drug	**Route and Dosage**	**Uses and Considerations**
Selective Alpha-Adrenergic Blockers		
Doxazosin mesylate	Hypertension: A: PO: Initially: 1 mg/d at bedtime; *max:* 16 mg/d	For hypertension and BPH. May cause orthostatic hypotension, headache, dizziness, drowsiness, fatigue, weakness, and GI upset. Pregnancy category: C*; PB: 98%; t½: 22 h
Prazosin hydrochloride	See Prototype Drug Chart 39.2.	
Terazosin hydrochloride	Hypertension: A: PO: Initially: 1 mg at bedtime; maint: 1-5 mg/d; *max:* 20 mg/d in divided doses q12h	For hypertension, and BPH. May cause dizziness, drowsiness, nasal congestion, headache, weakness, orthostatic hypotension, bradycardia, peripheral edema, and depression. Pregnancy category: C*; PB: 90%-94%; t½: 9-12 h
Nonselective Alpha-Adrenergic Blockers		
Phenoxybenzamine hydrochloride	A: PO: Initially: 10 mg bid; maint: 20-40 mg bid/tid	For hypertension associated with pheochromocytoma. May cause orthostatic hypotension, tachycardia, dizziness, weakness, gastritis, and nasal congestion. Pregnancy category: C*; PB: UK; t½: 24 h
Adrenergic Neuron Blockers (Peripherally Acting Sympatholytics)		
Reserpine	A: PO: Initially: 0.05-0.1 mg/d for 1-2 wk; maint: 0.1-0.25 mg/d; *max:* 0.5 mg/d for adults, 0.25 mg/d for older adults	For hypertension. May cause anxiety, dizziness, drowsiness, nightmares, GI distress, hypotension, bradycardia, and pseudoparkinsonism. Pregnancy category: C*; PB: 98%; t½: 50-100 h
Alpha$_1$- and Beta$_1$-Adrenergic Blockers		
Labetalol hydrochloride	Hypertension: A: PO: Initially: 100 mg bid; maint: 200-400 mg/d; *max:* 2.4 g/d Hypertensive emergency: A: IV: 20 mg over 2 min; may give 40-80 mg q10min PRN; *max:* 300 mg/d	For hypertension, hypertensive emergency, preeclampsia, and eclampsia. May cause orthostatic hypotension, dizziness, headache, weakness, erectile/ejaculation dysfunction, depression, and nausea. Pregnancy category: C*; PB: UK; t½: 2.5-8 h

TABLE 39.2 Antihypertensives: Sympatholytics—Alpha-Adrenergic and Peripherally Acting Blockers and Direct-Acting Vasodilators—cont'd

Drug	Route and Dosage	Uses and Considerations
Direct-Acting Vasodilators		
Hydralazine hydrochloride	A: PO: Initially: 10 mg qid; maint: 50 mg qid; *max.* 300 mg/d Hypertensive urgency/emergency: A: IV: 10-20 mg bolus, may repeat q4-6h	For hypertension, hypertensive urgency and emergency, preeclampsia, and eclampsia. May cause angina, headaches, tachycardia, hypotension, palpitations, and GI distress. Closely monitor vital signs. Pregnancy category: C*; PB: 87%; t½: 3-7 h
Minoxidil	Hypertension: A/adol: PO: Initially: 5 mg/d; maint: 10-40 mg/d; *max:* 100 mg/d Older A: PO: Initially: 2.5 mg/d; *max:* 100 mg/d C <12 y: PO: Initially: 0.2 mg/kg/d; maint: 0.25-1 mg/kg/d; *max:* 50 mg/d	For hypertension and alopecia. May cause headache, hypotension, tachycardia, angina, peripheral edema, and excess hair growth. Pregnancy category: C*; PB: 0%; t½: 4 h
Nitroprusside	Hypertensive emergency: A: IV: Initially: 0.25-0.3 mcg/kg/min in D₅W; maint: 0.25-10 mcg/kg/min; *max:* 10 mcg/kg/min for 10 min	For hypertensive urgency and emergency and for HF. Drug is good for 24 h but decomposes in light, so container must be wrapped in opaque material, such as aluminum foil. Discard drug if red, green, or blue. Measure cyanide and thiocyanate levels. May cause confusion, hypotension, bradycardia, tachycardia, dizziness, headache, palpitations, ataxia, seizures, cyanide or thiocyanate toxicity, and methemoglobinemia. Pregnancy category: C*; PB: UK; t½: 2 min

*Pregnancy categories have been revised. See http://www.fda.gov/Drugs/DevelopmentApprovalProcess/DevelopmentResources/Labeling/ucm093307.htm for more information.
A, Adult; *adol*, adolescent; *bid*, twice a day; *BPH*, benign prostatic hyperplasia; *C*, child; *d*, day; *D₅W*, dextrose 5% in water; *GI*, gastrointestinal; *h*, hour; *HF*, heart failure; *IV*, intravenous; *maint*, maintenance; *max*, maximum; *min*, minute; *PB*, protein binding; *PO*, by mouth; *PRN*, as needed; *q*, every; *qid*, four times a day; *t½*, half-life; *tid*, three times a day; *UK*, unknown; *wk*, week; *y*, year; *<*, less than.

PROTOTYPE DRUG CHART 39.2

Prazosin Hydrochloride

Drug Class Antihypertensive: Alpha-adrenergic blocker Pregnancy category: C*	**Dosage** A: PO: Initially 1 mg bid/tid; maint: 6-15 mg/d; *max:* 20 mg/d in divided doses Older A: PO: Initially 1 mg qd/bid; *max.* 20 mg/d
Contraindications Hypersensitivity *Caution:* Angina, orthostatic hypotension, syncope, ocular surgery, priapism, pregnancy, breastfeeding	**Drug-Lab-Food Interactions** Drug: Increased hypotensive effect with other antihypertensives, nitrates, diuretics, alcohol; decreased effects with NSAIDs Lab: Increased hepatic enzymes
Pharmacokinetics Absorption: GI: 60% (5% to circulation) Distribution: PB: 97% Metabolism: t½: 2-4 h Excretion: In bile and feces, 10% in urine	**Pharmacodynamics** PO: Onset: 0.5-2 h Peak: 2-4 h Duration: <24 h
Therapeutic Effects/Uses To control hypertension Mode of Action: Dilates peripheral blood vessels by blocking alpha-adrenergic receptors	
Side Effects Dizziness, drowsiness, nervousness, blurred vision, tinnitus, fatigue, weakness, headache, depression, dry mouth, nausea, vomiting, diarrhea, abdominal pain, constipation, peripheral edema, erectile dysfunction, urinary incontinence	**Adverse Reactions** Orthostatic hypotension, palpitations, tachycardia, pancreatitis, elevated liver enzymes

*Pregnancy categories have been revised. See http://www.fda.gov/Drugs/DevelopmentApprovalProcess/DevelopmentResources/Labeling/ucm093307.htm for more information.
A, Adult; *bid*, twice a day; *d*, day; *h*, hour; *GI*, gastrointestinal; *maint*, maintenance; *max*, maximum; *NSAID*, nonsteroidal antiinflammatory drug; *PB*, protein binding; *PO*, by mouth; *qd*, every day; *t½*, half-life; *tid*, three times a day; *<*, less than.

Adrenergic Neuron Blockers (Peripherally Acting Sympatholytics)

Adrenergic neuron blockers are potent antihypertensive drugs that block norepinephrine release from the sympathetic nerve endings, causing a decrease in norepinephrine release that results in a lowering of blood pressure. A decrease occurs in both cardiac output and peripheral vascular resistance. Reserpine, the most potent drug, is used to control severe hypertension. Orthostatic hypotension is a common side effect, so the patient should be advised to rise slowly from a reclining or sitting position. The adrenergic neuron blockers are considered the last choices for treatment of chronic hypertension because these drugs can cause orthostatic hypotension. Use of reserpine may cause vivid dreams, nightmares, and suicidal ideation. The drugs in this group can cause sodium and water retention, and they can be taken alone or with a diuretic to decrease peripheral edema.

❶ Alpha₁- and Beta₁-Adrenergic Blockers

This group of drugs blocks both the $alpha_1$ and $beta_1$ receptors. Labetalol is an example of an alpha/beta blocker. Blocking the $alpha_1$ receptor causes vasodilation, which decreases resistance to blood flow. The effect on the alpha receptor is stronger than the effect on the beta receptor; therefore blood pressure is lowered, and pulse rate is moderately decreased. By blocking the cardiac $beta_1$ receptor, both heart rate and AV contractility are decreased. Large doses of alpha/beta blockers could block $beta_2$-adrenergic receptors, thus increasing airway resistance. Patients who have severe asthma should *not* take large doses of labetalol. Table 39.2 lists two alpha/beta blockers.

◎ NURSING PROCESS
Patient-Centered Collaborative Care

Antihypertensives: Alpha-Adrenergic Blockers

Assessment
- Obtain a medication history from the patient that includes current drugs. Report if drug-drug or drug-herbal interaction is probable. Prazosin is highly protein bound and can displace other highly protein-bound drugs.
- Obtain baseline vital signs and weight for future comparisons.
- Check urinary output. Report if it is decreased (less than 600 mL/day) because drug is contraindicated if renal disease is present.

Nursing Diagnoses
- Activity Intolerance, Risk for
- Knowledge, Deficient related to drug regimen
- Sexuality Pattern, Ineffective related to beta-blocker or other drug therapy

Planning
- The patient's blood pressure will decrease.
- The patient will follow the proper drug regimen.

Nursing Interventions
- Monitor vital signs. The desired therapeutic effect of prazosin may not fully occur for 4 weeks. A sudden marked decrease in blood pressure and tachycardia should be reported.
- Check daily for fluid retention in extremities and weight gain. Prazosin may cause sodium and water retention.

Patient Teaching
General
- ⚡ Advise patients to comply with the drug regimen. Explain that abrupt discontinuation of antihypertensive drugs may cause rebound hypertension.
- Inform patients that orthostatic hypotension may occur. Explain that before rising, patients should sit and dangle their feet. Drugs may be taken at bedtime to avoid orthostatic hypotension.
- Teach patients to self-monitor daily weights. Prazosin may lead to edema.
Self-Administration
- Teach patients or family members how to take and record blood pressure. A blood pressure chart should be established, and blood pressure changes should be reported.
Side Effects
- Caution patients that dizziness, lightheadedness, and drowsiness may occur, especially when a drug is first initiated. If these symptoms occur, a health care provider should be notified.
- Inform male patients that impotence may occur if high doses of drug are prescribed. This problem should be reported to the health care provider.
- Tell patients to report if edema is present in the morning. Water retention is a problem with alpha blockers.
- ⚡ Inform patients not to take OTC cold, cough, or allergy medications without first contacting the health care provider.
Diet
- Encourage patients to decrease salt intake unless otherwise indicated by the health care provider.

🌐 *Cultural Considerations*
- Explain to African American patients with hypertension that they can take alpha-adrenergic blockers and calcium channel blockers but should avoid taking beta blockers because these agents are not generally effective in controlling their hypertension. However, taking a diuretic together with a beta blocker increases effectiveness for these patients.
- Caution Asian patients that they are twice as sensitive to the effects of propranolol regarding blood pressure and heart rate, so the dose should be decreased or another antihypertensive drug may be given.

Evaluation
- Evaluate the effectiveness of the drug in controlling blood pressure; side effects should be absent.
- Evaluate the patient's adherence to the medication schedule.
- Evaluate the patient's knowledge of the medication.

Common side effects of these drugs include orthostatic hypotension, GI disturbances, nervousness, dry mouth, and fatigue. Large doses of labetalol may cause AV heart block.

Direct-Acting Arteriolar Vasodilators

Vasodilators are potent antihypertensive drugs. Direct-acting vasodilators act by relaxing the smooth muscles of the blood vessels, mainly the arteries, causing vasodilation. Vasodilators promote an increase in blood flow to the brain and kidneys. With vasodilation, the blood pressure decreases and sodium and water are retained, resulting in peripheral edema. Diuretics can be given with a direct-acting vasodilator to decrease the edema.

Two direct-acting vasodilators, hydralazine and minoxidil, are used for moderate to severe (dose-related) hypertension. These two drugs cause little orthostatic hypotension because of minimum dilation of the arterioles. However, reflex tachycardia and release of renin can occur secondary to vasodilation and decreased blood pressure. Beta blockers are frequently prescribed with arteriolar vasodilators to decrease the heart rate; this counteracts the effect of reflex tachycardia.

❶ Nitroprusside is prescribed for acute hypertensive emergency. This is a very potent vasodilator that rapidly decreases blood pressure. Nitroprusside acts on both arterial and venous vessels. Table 39.2 lists direct-acting vasodilators.

Side Effects and Adverse Reactions. The effects of hydralazine are numerous and include reflex tachycardia, palpitations, edema, nasal congestion, headache, dizziness, GI bleeding, lupus-like symptoms, and neurologic symptoms (tingling, numbness). Minoxidil has similar side effects, as well as tachycardia, edema, and excess hair growth. In addition, it can precipitate an anginal attack.

Nitroprusside can cause reflex tachycardia, palpitations, restlessness, agitation, nausea, and confusion. Nitroprusside is discussed in greater detail in Chapter 55.

Angiotensin-Converting Enzyme Inhibitors

When ACE is inhibited, it in turn inhibits the formation of angiotensin II (vasoconstrictor) and blocks the release of aldosterone. Aldosterone promotes sodium retention and potassium excretion. When aldosterone is blocked, sodium is excreted along with water, and potassium is retained. ACE inhibitors cause little change in cardiac output or heart rate, and they lower peripheral resistance. (Fig. 39.1 illustrates the RAAS.) These drugs can be used in patients who have elevated serum renin levels.

The ACE inhibitors are used primarily to treat hypertension; some of these agents are also effective in treating heart failure. The ACE inhibitors are benazepril, captopril, enalapril maleate, fosinopril, lisinopril, moexipril, perindopril, quinapril, ramipril, and trandolapril, which are all presented in Table 39.3. These drugs can be used for first-line antihypertensive therapy, but thiazide diuretics are recommended by JNC 8.

African Americans and older adults do not respond to ACE inhibitors with the desired reduction in blood pressure, but when

TABLE 39.3   Antihypertensives: Angiotensin-Converting Enzyme Inhibitors and Angiotensin II–Receptor Blockers

Drug	Route and Dosage	Uses and Considerations
Angiotensin Antagonists (ACE Inhibitors)		
Benazepril hydrochloride	A: PO: Initially 10 mg/d; maint: 20-40 mg/d in 1-2 divided doses; *max:* 80 mg/d Adol/C >6 y: PO: 0.2 mg/kg/d; maint: 0.1-0.6 mg/kg/d; *max.* 40 mg/d	To treat hypertension. May cause headache, dizziness, hypotension, palpitations, peripheral edema, erectile dysfunction, constipation, and Stevens-Johnson syndrome. Pregnancy category: D*; PB: 95%; t½: 10-11 h
Captopril	Hypertension: A: PO: Initially 12.5-25 mg bid/tid; maint: 25-150 mg bid/tid; *max:* 450 mg/d	For hypertension. post MI, diabetic nephropathy, and HF. May cause dysgeusia, flushing, pruritis, rash, and Stevens-Johnson syndrome. Pregnancy category: C, D*; PB: 25%; t½: 2 h
Enalapril maleate	A/adol: PO: Initially 2.5-5 mg/d; maint: 10-40 mg/d in 1-2 divided doses; *max:* 40 mg/d C/infants >1 month: PO: Initially 0.08 mg/kg/d; *max.* 0.58 mg/kg/d	For hypertension and HF. May cause hypotension, dizziness, headache, renal dysfunction, neutropenia, agranulocytosis, thrombocytopenia, dysrhythmias, and Stevens-Johnson syndrome. Pregnancy category: D*; PB: 50%; t½: 11 h
Fosinopril	Hypertension: A/adol>16 y: PO: Initially 10 mg/d; maint: 20-40 mg/d in 1-2 divided doses; *max:* 80 mg/d C 6-16 y >50 kg: PO: 5-10 mg/d; *max.* 40 mg/d	For hypertension and HF. May cause dizziness, cough, weakness, angina, and hypotension. Pregnancy category: D*; PB: 99.4%; t½: 11.5 h
Lisinopril	Hypertension: A: PO: Initially 10 mg/d; maint: 20-40 mg/d; *max:* 80 mg/d C >6 y: PO: Initially 0.07 mg/kg/d; *max.* 40 mg/d	For hypertension, AMI, and HF. May cause hypotension, headache, dizziness, syncope, and hyperkalemia. Pregnancy category: D*; PB: UK; t½: 12 h
Moexipril	A: PO: Initially 7.5 mg/d; maint: 7.5-30 mg/d; *max:* 30 mg/d in divided doses	For hypertension. May increase serum lithium levels, causing toxicity. May cause dizziness and hypotension. Pregnancy category: C, D*; PB: 50%-90%; t½: 1.3 h
Perindopril erbumine	Hypertension: A: PO: Initially 4 mg/d; maint: 4-8 mg/d in 1-2 divided doses; *max:* 16 mg/d Older adults: Initially 4 mg/d; *max:* 8 mg/d	For hypertension and to prevent MI. May cause cough, headache, dizziness, weakness, back pain, hypotension, and hyperkalemia. Pregnancy category: D*; PB: 10%-60%; t½: 0.8-10 h

Continued

TABLE 39.3 Antihypertensives: Angiotensin-Converting Enzyme Inhibitors and Angiotensin II–Receptor Blockers—cont'd

Drug	Route and Dosage	Uses and Considerations
Quinapril hydrochloride	Hypertension: A: PO: Initially 10-20 mg/d; maint: 20-80 mg/d in 1-2 divided doses; *max:* 80 mg/d Older adults: PO: Initially 5-10 mg/d; *max:* 80 mg/d	For hypertension and HF. May cause dizziness, headache, myalgia, and cough. Pregnancy category: C, D*; PB: 97%; t½: 1-3 h
Ramipril	Hypertension: A: PO: Initially 2.5 mg/d; *max:* 20 mg/d	For hypertension, AMI, HF, and prevention of stroke. May cause dizziness, headache, hypotension, hyperkalemia, and cough. Pregnancy category: C*; PB: 73%; t½: 3-17 h
Trandolapril	Hypertension: A: PO: Initially 1 mg/d for Caucasians, 2 mg/d for African Americans: maint: 2-4 mg/d; *max:* 8 mg/d	For hypertension, AMI, and HF. May cause dizziness, syncope, cough, dyspepsia, bradycardia, hypotension, hyperkalemia, hypocalcemia, and hyperuricemia. Pregnancy category: C, D*; PB: 80%; t½: 6-10 h

Combinations of ACE Inhibitors With Calcium Blockers

Drug	Route and Dosage	Uses and Considerations
Benazepril with amlodipine	A: PO: Initially amlodipine 2.5-10 mg/d and benazepril 10-40 mg/d; *max:* amlodipine 10 mg/d and benazepril 40 mg/d	For hypertension. May cause headache, hypotension, peripheral edema, and cough. Pregnancy category: D*; PB: 93%-95%; t½: 10-50 h
Trandolapril and verapamil	A: PO: Trandolapril 2-8 mg/d and verapamil 180-240 mg/d; *max:* 8 mg/d trandolapril and 240 mg/d verapamil	For hypertension. May cause dizziness, cough, hypotension, ileus, hyperkalemia, and headache. Pregnancy category: D*; PB: 80%-90%; t½: 2-10 h
Perindopril arginine and amlodipine besylate	A: PO: Initially perindopril 3.5 mg/d and amlodipine 2.5 mg/d; *max:* perindopril 14 mg/d and amlodipine 10 mg/d	For hypertension. May cause dizziness, headache, cough, peripheral edema, weakness, syncope, bradycardia, hypotension, dysrhythmias, and hyperkalemia. Pregnancy category: D*; PB: 10%-93%; t½: 1-50 h

Angiotensin II–Receptor Blockers (ARBs)

Drug	Route and Dosage	Uses and Considerations
Candesartan	Hypertension: A: PO: Initially 16 mg/d; maint: 8-32 mg/d in 1-2 divided doses; *max:* 32 mg/d C >6 y >50 kg: PO: Initially 8-16 mg/d in 1-2 divided doses; maint: 4-32 mg/d; *max:* 32 mg/d C >6 y <50 kg: PO: Initially 4-8 mg/d in 1-2 divided doses; maint: 2-16 mg/d; *max:* 16 mg/d	For hypertension and HF. May cause dizziness, hypotension, hyperkalemia, hyperglycemia, elevated hepatic enzymes, and URI. Pregnancy category: C, D*; PB: 99%; t½: 9-12 h
Eprosartan	A: PO: Initially 600 mg/d; maint: 400-800 mg/d in 1-2 divided doses; *max:* 900 mg/d	For hypertension. May cause cough, URI, and hypotension. Pregnancy category: C, D*; PB: 98%; t½: 5-9 h
Irbesartan	Hypertension: A: PO: Initially 150 mg/d; maint: 150-300 mg/d; *max:* 300 mg/d	For hypertension, diabetic nephropathy, and proteinuria. May cause cough, fatigue, orthostatic hypotension, pyrosis, and GI distress. Pregnancy category: C, D*; PB: 90%; t½: 11-15 h
Losartan potassium	Hypertension: A/adol: PO: Initially 50 mg/d; maint: 25-100 mg/d in 1-2 divided doses; *max:* 100 mg/d C >6 y: PO: 0.7 mg/kg/d; *max:* 1.4 mg/kg/d	For hypertension, diabetic nephropathy, proteinuria, and to prevent stroke. May cause fatigue, dizziness, weakness, cough, hypotension, chest pain, anemia, and infection. Pregnancy category: C, D*; PB: 98%; t½: 2 h
Olmesartan medoxomil	A/C >6 y >35 kg: PO: Initially 20 mg/d; maint: 20-40 mg/d; *max:* 40 mg/d C >6 y <35 kg: PO: Initially 10 mg/d; *max:* 20 mg/d	For hypertension. May cause dizziness, headache, peripheral edema, hypotension, hyperglycemia, and diarrhea. Pregnancy category: C, D*; PB: 99%; t½: 13 h
Telmisartan	Hypertension: A: PO: Initially 40 mg/d; maint: 20-80 mg/d; *max:* 80 mg/d	For hypertension and to prevent MI and CVA. May cause URI, orthostatic hypotension, and rhabdomyolysis. Pregnancy category: C, D*; PB: 99.5%; t½: 24 h
Valsartan	See Prototype Drug Chart 39.3.	
Azilsartan	A: PO: Initially 40 mg/d; maint: 40-80 mg/d; *max:* 80 mg/d	For hypertension. May cause orthostatic hypotension, dizziness, fatigue, and diarrhea. Pregnancy category: D*; PB: 99%; t½: 11 h

Aldosterone Receptor Antagonists

Drug	Route and Dosage	Uses and Considerations
Eplerenone	Hypertension: A: PO: 50 mg/d; may increase to 50 mg bid; *max:* 100 mg/d	For hypertension, HF, and AMI. May cause dizziness, bradycardia, hyponatremia, hypertriglyceridemia, and abnormal vaginal bleeding. Pregnancy category: B*; PB: 50%; t½: 4-6 h

TABLE 39.3   Antihypertensives: Angiotensin-Converting Enzyme Inhibitors and Angiotensin II–Receptor Blockers—cont'd

Drug	Route and Dosage	Uses and Considerations
Direct Renin Inhibitors		
Aliskiren	A: PO: Initially 150 mg/d; maint: 150-300 mg/d; *max*: 300 mg/d	For hypertension. May cause hypotension, hyperkalemia, peripheral edema, diarrhea, renal failure, and Stevens-Johnson syndrome. Pregnancy category: D*; PB: UK; t½: 24 h

*Pregnancy categories have been revised. See http://www.fda.gov/Drugs/DevelopmentApprovalProcess/DevelopmentResources/Labeling/ucm093 307.htm for more information.

A, Adult; *ACE*, angiotensin-converting enzyme; *adol*, adolescent; *AMI*, acute myocardial infarction; *bid*, two times a day; *C*, child; *CVA*, cerebrovascular accident; *d*, day; *h*, hour; *HF*, heart failure; *maint*, maintenance; *max*, maximum; *MI*, myocardial infarction; *PB*, protein binding; *PO*, by mouth; *t½*, half-life; *tid*, three times a day; *UK*, unknown; *URI*, Upper respiratory infection; *y*, year; *>*, greater than.

taken with a diuretic, blood pressure will usually be lowered. ACE inhibitors should not be given during pregnancy because they reduce placental blood flow. For patients with renal insufficiency, reduction of the drug dose (except for fosinopril) is necessary.

With the exception of moexipril, which should be taken on an empty stomach for maximum effectiveness, ACE inhibitors can be administered with food.

Side Effects and Adverse Reactions. The primary side effect of ACE inhibitors is a constant, irritated cough. Other side effects include nausea, vomiting, diarrhea, headache, dizziness, fatigue, insomnia, serum potassium excess (hyperkalemia), and tachycardia. The persistent, nonproductive "ACE cough" may be relieved upon discontinuance of the drug. Often an ARB may be substituted without cough as a side effect. The major adverse effects are first-dose hypotension and hyperkalemia. Hypotension results because of the vasodilating effect. First-dose hypotension is more common in patients also taking diuretics. Angioedema—swelling of the face, tongue, lips, mucous membranes, and larynx and extremity edema—may occur due to hypersensitivity and has a higher incidence in African Americans. This may occur within hours or 1 week after the first dose. Angioedema may be reversed with drug discontinuance. When laryngeal edema occurs, the patient may require rescue epinephrine.

Contraindications. ACE inhibitors should not be given during pregnancy because harm to the fetus due to reduction in placental blood flow could occur. This group of drugs should not be taken with potassium-sparing diuretics such as spironolactone or with salt substitutes that contain potassium because of the risk of hyperkalemia (serum potassium excess).

◎ NURSING PROCESS
Patient-Centered Collaborative Care

Antihypertensives: Angiotensin-Converting Enzyme Inhibitors

Assessment
- Obtain a drug and herbal history from the patient of current drugs taken. Report if a drug-drug or drug-herb interaction is probable.
- Obtain baseline vital signs for future comparisons.
- Check laboratory values for serum protein, albumin, blood urea nitrogen (BUN), creatinine, potassium, and white blood cell count to compare with future serum levels.

Nursing Diagnoses
- Knowledge, Deficient related to drug regimen
- Anxiety related to hypertensive state
- Falls, Risk for

Planning
- Patient's blood pressure will be within the desired range.
- Patient will be free from moderate to severe side effects.

Nursing Interventions
- Monitor blood pressure. A sudden drop in blood pressure should be reported.
- Monitor laboratory tests related to renal function (BUN, creatinine, protein) and blood glucose levels. *Caution:* Watch for hypoglycemic reactions in patients with diabetes mellitus. Urine protein may be checked in the morning using a dipstick.
- Report to a health care provider any bruising, petechiae, or bleeding. These may indicate a severe adverse reaction to an angiotensin antagonist such as captopril.

Patient Teaching
General
- Warn patients not to abruptly discontinue use of captopril without notifying a health care provider. Rebound hypertension could result.
- Inform patients not to take OTC drugs such as cold medications without first contacting a health care provider.
- Advise patients not to use salt substitutes that contain potassium.
- Warn pregnant patients and those contemplating becoming pregnant not to take ACE inhibitors or ARBs; they can cause harm to the fetus.
- Teach patients to rise slowly to avoid orthostatic hypotension.
Self-Administration
- Teach patients or family members how to take and record blood pressure. A blood pressure chart should be established, and blood pressure changes should be reported.
Side Effects
- Explain to patients that dizziness and/or lightheadedness may occur during the first week of captopril therapy. If dizziness persists, a health care provider should be notified.

- Monitor the patient for the following side effects: angi-oedema, cough dysgeusia, weakness, hyperkalemia, ortho-static hypotension, and renal impairment.
- Advise patients to report any occurrence of bleeding.

Diet

- Teach patients to take captopril 20 minutes to 1 hour be-fore a meal. Food decreases 35% of captopril absorption.
- Warn patients that the taste of food may be diminished during the first month of drug therapy.
- Advise patients to avoid foods high in potassium because hyperkalemia is an adverse effect of ACE inhibitors.

Cultural Considerations

- Explain to African American patients that they may not respond well to ACE inhibitors unless the drug is taken with a diuretic.

Evaluation

- Evaluate the effectiveness of the drug therapy (absence of severe side effects, blood pressure returns to desired range).
- Evaluate the patient's renal function.

Angiotensin II–Receptor Blockers

Angiotensin II–receptor blockers (ARBs) are similar to ACE inhibitors in that they prevent the release of aldosterone, a sodium-retaining hormone. They act on the renin-angiotensin-aldosterone system (RAAS). The difference between ARBs and ACE inhibitors is that ARBs block angiotensin II from the angiotensin I (AT_1) receptors found in many tissues, whereas ACE inhibitors inhibit the angiotensin-converting enzyme in the formation of angiotensin II. ARBs cause vasodilation and decrease peripheral resistance. They do not cause the constant, irritated cough ACE inhibitors can. Like ACE inhibitors, ARBs should not be taken during pregnancy.

Losartan, valsartan, irbesartan, candesartan, eprosartan, olmesartan, azilsartan, and telmisartan are examples of ARBs. These agents block the vasoconstrictor effects of angiotensin II at the receptor site. The combination of losartan potassium and hydrochlorothiazide tablets, valsartan and hydrochlorothiazide tablets, and others should not cause serum potassium excess or loss. ARBs may be used as a first-line treatment for hypertension.

Prototype Drug Chart 39.3 gives the pharmacologic data related to valsartan.

⚡ PATIENT SAFETY

Do not confuse:

- **Diovan** (valsartan), an angiotensin II–receptor blocker, and **Dioval** (estradiol), an estrogen hormone. If both drugs are in the home, caution must be taken to select the correct drug, especially by the male patient taking Diovan and the female patient taking Dioval.

Pharmacokinetics Valsartan is prescribed primarily to manage hypertension. The combination drug Diovan HCT contains valsartan plus a low dose of hydrochlorothiazide. It is rapidly absorbed in the GI tract and undergoes first-pass metabolism in the liver to form active metabolites. It is highly protein bound and should not be given during pregnancy, especially during the second and third trimesters. The half-life is approximately 6 hours, and the drug is excreted in urine and feces.

Pharmacodynamics Valsartan is a potent vasodilator. It blocks the binding of angiotensin II to the AT_1 receptors found in many tissues. Its peak time is approximately 6 hours, and it has a long duration of action (24 hours).

📄 PROTOTYPE DRUG CHART 39.3

Valsartan

Drug Class	Dosage
Antihypertensive: Angiotensin II–receptor blocker Pregnancy category: D*	Hypertension: A: PO: Initially 80-160 mg/d; maint: 80-320 mg/d; *max:* 320 mg/d C 6-16 y: PO: Initially 1.3 mg/kg/d; *max:* 2.7 mg/kg/d
Contraindications	**Drug-Lab-Food Interactions**
Hypersensitivity *Caution:* Renal and hepatic impairments, hypotension, heart failure, hypovolemia, hyperkalemia, pregnancy, breastfeeding	Drug: Antihypertensives, diuretics, MAOIs, and alcohol may increase hypotensive effects; ACE inhibitors and aspirin may increase hyperkalemia and renal dysfunction; digoxin and NSAIDs may increase renal dysfunction; lithium may increase lithium toxicity. Lab: May increase AST, ALT, ALP, bilirubin, BUN, creatinine, Hct, Hgb
Pharmacokinetics	**Pharmacodynamics**
Absorption: Rapidly absorbed, 10%-35% in blood circulation Distribution: PB: 95% Metabolism: t½: 6 h Excretion: 13% in urine and 83% in bile/feces	PO: Onset: 2 h Peak: 6 h Duration: 24 h
Therapeutic Effects/Uses	
To treat hypertension and heart failure Mode of Action: Potent vasodilator that inhibits binding of angiotensin II	

PROTOTYPE DRUG CHART 39.3—cont'd

Valsartan

Side Effects	Adverse Reactions
Dizziness, drowsiness, cough (rare), palpitations, blurred vision, headache, diarrhea, abdominal and back pain, arthralgia, fatigue, erectile dysfunction	Orthostatic hypotension, hyperkalemia, rhabdomyolysis, elevated hepatic enzymes *Life threatening:* Renal dysfunction, neutropenia

*Pregnancy categories have been revised. See http://www.fda.gov/Drugs/DevelopmentApprovalProcess/DevelopmentResources/Labeling/ucm093307.htm for more information.
A, Adult; *ACE,* angiotensin-converting enzyme; *ALP,* alkaline phosphatase; *ALT,* alanine aminotransferase; *AST,* aspartate aminotransferase; *BUN,* blood urea nitrogen; *C,* child; *d,* day; *h,* hour; *Hct,* hematocrit; *Hgb,* hemoglobin; *maint,* maintenance dose; *MAOI,* monoamine oxidase inhibitor; *max,* maximum; *NSAID,* nonsteroidal antiinflammatory drug; *PB,* protein binding; *PO,* by mouth; *t½,* half-life; *y,* years.

Like ACE inhibitors, ARBs are less effective for treating hypertension in African American patients. In addition, like ACE inhibitors, ARBs may cause angioedema. These agents can be taken with or without food and are suitable for patients with mild hepatic insufficiency.

Direct Renin Inhibitors

The first U.S. Food and Drug Administration (FDA)-approved direct renin inhibitor for treating hypertension is aliskiren, which binds with renin and causes a reduction of angiotensin I, angiotensin II, and aldosterone levels (see Fig. 39.1). It is effective for mild and moderate hypertension. Aliskiren can be used alone or with another antihypertensive agent. It has an additive effect in reducing blood pressure when combined with a thiazide diuretic or an ARB. This drug, when used as monotherapy, has not proven to be as effective in reducing blood pressure in the African American population.

Calcium Channel Blockers

Slow calcium channels are found in the myocardium (heart muscle) and vascular smooth muscle (VSM) cells. Free calcium increases muscle contractility, peripheral resistance, and blood pressure. Calcium channel blockers, also called *calcium antagonists* and *calcium blockers,* block the calcium channel in the VSM, promoting vasodilation. The large central arteries are not as sensitive to calcium blockers as coronary and cerebral arteries and the peripheral vessels. Calcium blockers are highly protein bound but have a short half-life. Slow-release preparations decrease the frequency of administration. Table 39.4 lists the calcium blockers in three groups: diphenylalkylamine

TABLE 39.4 Antihypertensives: Calcium Channel Blockers

Drug	Route and Dosage	Uses and Considerations
Phenylalkylamines Verapamil	Hypertension: Regular release: A: PO: Initially 80 mg tid; *max.* 480 mg/d Older A: PO: Initially 40 mg tid; *max.* 480 mg/d Extended release: A: PO: Initially 180 mg/d in morning; maint: 180-240 mg/d; *max:* 480 mg/d Older A: PO: Initially 120 mg/d in morning; *max.* 480 mg/d	For hypertension, angina, and dysrhythmia. May cause dizziness, headache, hypotension, fatigue, edema, and constipation. Pregnancy category: C*; PB: 90%; t½: 2-10 h
Benzothiazepines Diltiazem hydrochloride	Hypertension: Extended release: A: PO: Initially 120-240 mg/d; maint: 240-360 mg/d; *max:* 540 mg/d	For hypertension, angina, and dysrhythmia. May cause headache, peripheral edema, dizziness, dyspepsia, bradycardia, and hypotension. Pregnancy category: C*; PB: 70%-80%; t½: 3.5-9 h
Dihydropyridines Amlodipine	Hypertension: A: PO: Initially 5 mg/d; maint: 5-10 mg/d; *max.* 10 mg/d Older A: PO: Initially 2.5 mg/d; maint: 2.5-10 mg/d; *max.* 10 mg/d Adol/C >6 y: PO: 2.5-5 mg/d; *max:* 5 mg/d	For hypertension, CAD, and angina. May cause peripheral edema, palpitations, flushing, and fatigue. Pregnancy category: C*; PB: 93%; t½: 30-50 h
Felodipine	A: PO: Initially 5 mg/d; maint: 2.5-10 mg/d; *max.* 10 mg/d Older A: PO: Initially 2.5 mg/d; *max.* 10 mg/d	For hypertension. May cause peripheral edema, palpitations, dizziness, infection, weakness, and headache. Pregnancy category: C*; PB: 99%; t½: 11-16 h

Continued

TABLE 39.4 Antihypertensives: Calcium Channel Blockers—cont'd

Drug	Route and Dosage	Uses and Considerations
Isradipine	Regular release: A: PO: Initially 2.5 mg bid; maint: 5-10 mg bid; *max:* 10 mg/d Extended release: A: PO: 5 mg/d; *max:* 20 mg/d	For hypertension. May cause headache, dizziness, palpitations, fatigue, and peripheral edema. Pregnancy category: C*; PB: 95%; t½: 8 h
Nicardipine hydrochloride	Hypertension: Regular release: A: PO: Initially 20 mg tid; maint: 20-40 mg tid; *max:* 120 mg/d Sustained release: A: PO: Initially 30 mg bid; maint: 30-60 mg bid; *max:* 120 mg/d A: IV: Initially 5 mg/h infusion; *max:* 15 mg/h	For hypertension and angina. May cause headache, dizziness, hypotension, palpitations, tachycardia, flushing, weakness, peripheral edema, nausea, and vomiting. Pregnancy category: C*; PB: 95%; t½: 2-4 h
Nifedipine	Hypertension: Extended release: A: PO: 30-60 mg/d; *max:* 90 mg/d	For hypertension and angina. Common side effects include dizziness, headache, weakness, flushing, peripheral edema, palpitations, nausea, pyrosis, and Stevens-Johnson syndrome. Pregnancy category: C*; PB: 92%-98%; t½: 2-5 h
Nisoldipine	Extended release: A: PO: Initially 17 mg/d; maint: 17-34 mg/d; *max:* 34 mg/d Older A: PO: Initially 8.5 mg/d; *max:* 34 mg/d	For hypertension. May cause pharyngitis, headache, dizziness, flushing, and peripheral edema. Pregnancy category: C*; PB: 99%; t½: 7-12 h

*Pregnancy categories have been revised. See http://www.fda.gov/Drugs/DevelopmentApprovalProcess/DevelopmentResources/Labeling/ucm093307.htm for more information.
A, Adult; *bid,* twice a day; *C,* child; *CAD, coronary artery disease; d,* day; *h,* hour; *IV,* intravenous; *maint,* maintenance; *max,* maximum; *PB,* protein binding; *PO,* by mouth; *t½,* half-life; *tid,* three times a day; *y,* year; *>,* greater than.

(verapamil), benzothiazepine (diltiazem), and dihydropyridines (amlodipine and others).

Verapamil is used to treat chronic hypertension, angina pectoris, and cardiac dysrhythmias. Verapamil and diltiazem act on the arterioles and the heart. The dihydropyridines are the largest group of calcium channel blockers; most of these are used to control hypertension.

Nifedipine decreases blood pressure in older adults and in those with low serum renin values. Nifedipine and verapamil are potent calcium blockers. In its immediate-release form (10- and 20-mg capsules), nifedipine has been associated with an increased incidence of profound hypotension, MI, and death, especially in older adults; therefore only extended-release preparations of nifedipine are recommended for chronic hypertension. For this reason, immediate-release nifedipine is usually prescribed for acute rises in blood pressure only on an as-needed basis in the hospital setting. Like the vasodilators, calcium channel blockers can cause reflex tachycardia, although it is more prevalent with nifedipine.

Pharmacokinetics Like other calcium blockers, amlodipine is highly protein bound. It is gradually absorbed via the GI tract. Because the half-life of amlodipine is longer than that of other calcium blockers, it is taken once a day.

Pharmacodynamics Amlodipine may be used alone or with other antihypertensive drugs. Peripheral edema may occur because of its vasodilator effect, so persons with edema may need to take another type of antihypertensive drug. This drug has a long duration of action, so it is prescribed only once a day. Amlodipine may be combined with the ACE inhibitor benazepril (Lotrel).

Normally, beta blockers are not prescribed with calcium blockers, because both drugs decrease myocardium contractility. Calcium blockers lower blood pressure better in African Americans than do drugs in other categories.

Side Effects and Adverse Reactions. The side effects and adverse reactions of calcium channel blockers include flushing, headache, dizziness, ankle edema, bradycardia, and AV block.

CRITICAL THINKING CASE STUDY

GG, a 72-year-old African American patient, has heart failure and diabetes. Her vital signs are blood pressure 176/94, pulse 92, and respirations 30. Her medications include hydrochlorothiazide 50 mg/day and atenolol 50 mg/day.

1. Why was hydrochlorothiazide prescribed for GG? Explain the effects of hydrochlorothiazide on blood pressure.
2. Abnormal electrolytes and other laboratory test results may occur when taking hydrochlorothiazide. Would

the following serum electrolyte and laboratory values be expected to *increase* or *decrease*?
a. Sodium
b. Potassium
c. Calcium
d. Magnesium
e. Glucose
f. Uric acid

3. Why should GG's blood glucose level be monitored while she is taking hydrochlorothiazide?
4. What cultural response does a health care provider need to keep in mind when prescribing antihypertensive agents? Explain your answer.
5. Atenolol is what type of antihypertensive? Would atenolol be effective in lowering GG's blood pressure if given as the only antihypertensive drug? Explain your answer.
6. How effective is the combination of hydrochlorothiazide and atenolol for controlling GG's blood pressure? Explain your answer.
7. When using a combination drug therapy to correct hypertension, would the dosage for each drug be the same? Explain your answer.
8. When abruptly discontinuing beta blockers for hypertension without the patient taking another antihypertensive, what might occur? Explain how adverse effects can be avoided.
GG's blood glucose is 229. Her drugs for controlling hypertension are changed to prazosin 10 mg three times daily. Her cholesterol and LDL are elevated, and her serum potassium level is 3.2 mEq/L.
9. Why were GG's hydrochlorothiazide and atenolol discontinued? Explain your answer.
10. What type of antihypertensive is prazosin? Explain the physiologic action of prazosin for lowering the blood pressure.
11. Does prazosin have an effect on the blood glucose level? What effect could prazosin have on GG's abnormal lipid levels? Explain your answer.
GG's ankles have become edematous. Hydrochlorothiazide is again prescribed.
12. Why was hydrochlorothiazide again added to the drug regimen?
13. Is the daily prazosin dose within the safe therapeutic prescribed range for GG? Explain your answer. (You may refer to Prototype Drug Chart 39.2.)
14. List the groups of antihypertensive drugs that can cause sodium and water retention.

NCLEX STUDY QUESTIONS

1. A patient's blood pressure is 130/84. The health care provider plans to suggest nonpharmacologic methods to lower blood pressure. Which should the nurse include in teaching? (Select all that apply.)
   a. Stress-reduction techniques
   b. An exercise program
   c. Salt restriction
   d. Smoking cessation
   e. A diet with increased protein
2. A patient has developed mild hypertension. The nurse acknowledges that the first-line drug for treating this patient's blood pressure might be which drug?
   a. Diuretic
   b. Alpha blocker
   c. Angiotensin-converting enzyme inhibitor
   d. Alpha/beta blocker
3. An African American patient has developed hypertension. The nurse is aware that which group(s) of antihypertensive drugs are *less effective* in African American patients?
   a. Diuretics
   b. Calcium channel blockers and vasodilators
   c. Beta blockers and angiotensin-converting enzyme inhibitors
   d. Alpha blockers
4. The nurse knows that which diuretic is most frequently combined with an antihypertensive drug?
   a. Chlorthalidone
   b. Hydrochlorothiazide
   c. Bendroflumethiazide
   d. A potassium-sparing diuretic
5. The nurse is administering a beta blocker to a patient. Which is the most important assessment to perform before administration?
   a. Urine output
   b. Apical pulse
   c. Potassium level
   d. Serum level of medication
6. Captopril has been ordered for a patient. The nurse should teach the patient that the most commonly occurring side effect of an angiotensin-converting enzyme drug is which of the following?
   a. Nausea and vomiting
   b. Dizziness and headaches
   c. Upset stomach
   d. Constant, irritating cough
7. A patient is prescribed losartan. The nurse teaches the patient that an angiotensin II-receptor blocker acts by doing what?
   a. Inhibiting angiotensin-converting enzyme
   b. Blocking angiotensin II from angiotensin I receptors
   c. Preventing the release of angiotensin I
   d. Promoting the release of aldosterone
8. During an admission assessment, a patient states that she takes amlodipine. The nurse should inquire about which signs and symptoms to determine whether the patient has any common side effects of a calcium channel blocker? (Select all that apply.)
   a. Insomnia
   b. Dizziness
   c. Headache
   d. Angioedema
   e. Ankle edema
   f. Hacking cough

Answers: 1, a, b, c, d; 2, a; 3, c; 4, b; 5, b; 6, d; 7, b; 8, b, c, e.

40

Anticoagulants, Antiplatelets, and Thrombolytics

e http://evolve.elsevier.com/McCuistion/pharmacology/

OBJECTIVES

- Compare the actions of anticoagulants, antiplatelets, and thrombolytics.
- Differentiate the side effects and adverse reactions of anticoagulants, antiplatelets, and thrombolytics.

- Apply the nursing process, including patient teaching, for anticoagulants and thrombolytics.

OUTLINE

KEY TERMS

Various drugs are used to maintain or restore circulation. The three major groups of these drugs are (1) anticoagulants, (2) antiplatelets (antithrombotics), and (3) thrombolytics. The *anticoagulants* prevent the formation of clots that inhibit circulation. The *antiplatelets* prevent platelet aggregation, clumping together of platelets to form a clot. The *thrombolytics*, appropriately called *clot busters*, attack and dissolve blood clots that have already formed. Each of these three drug groups are discussed separately.

PATHOPHYSIOLOGY: THROMBUS FORMATION

Thrombosis is the formation of a clot in an arterial or venous vessel. The formation of an arterial thrombus could be caused by blood stasis (decreased circulation), platelet aggregation on the blood vessel wall, or blood coagulation. Arterial clots are usually made up of both white and red clots with the white clots, *platelets,* initiating the process, followed by fibrin formation and the trapping of red blood cells in the fibrin mesh. Blood clots found in the veins are from platelet aggregation with fibrin that attaches to red blood cells. Both types of thrombus can be dislodged from the vessel and become an *embolus,* a blood clot moving through the bloodstream.

Platelets do not usually stick together unless there is a break in the endothelial lining of a blood vessel. When platelets adhere to the broken surface of an endothelial lining, they synthesize thromboxane A_2, which is a product of prostaglandins and a potent stimulus for platelet aggregation, clumping of platelet cells. The platelet receptor protein that binds fibrinogen, *glycoprotein IIb/IIIa* (GP IIb/IIIa), also promotes platelet aggregation. Thromboxane A_2 and adenosine diphosphate (ADP) increase the activation of this receptor.

The thrombus inhibits blood flow, and the fibrin, platelets, and red blood cells (erythrocytes) surround the clot, building its size and structure. As the clot occludes the blood vessel, tissue ischemia occurs.

The venous thrombus usually develops because of slow blood flow, and the venous clot can form rapidly. Small pieces of the venous clot can detach and travel to the pulmonary artery and then to the lung. Inadequate oxygenation and gas exchange in the lungs is the end result.

Oral and parenteral anticoagulants, such as warfarin and heparin, act primarily to prevent venous thrombosis, whereas antiplatelet drugs act to prevent arterial thrombosis. However, both groups of drugs suppress thrombosis in general.

❶ ANTICOAGULANTS

Anticoagulants are used to inhibit clot formation. Unlike thrombolytics, they do *not* dissolve clots that have already formed but rather act prophylactically to prevent new clots from forming. Anticoagulants are used in patients with venous and arterial disorders that put them at high risk for clot formation. Venous problems include deep venous thrombosis (DVT) and pulmonary embolism (PE), and arterial problems include coronary thrombosis, or myocardial infarction (MI); presence of artificial heart valves; and cerebrovascular accidents (CVAs), or stroke.

Heparin

Anticoagulants are administered orally or parenterally, both subcutaneously and by the intravenous (IV) route. Heparin, introduced in 1938, is a natural substance in the liver that prevents clot formation. It was first used in blood transfusions to prevent clotting. Heparin is indicated for a rapid anticoagulant effect when a thrombosis occurs because of a DVT, PE, or an evolving stroke. Heparin is also used in open-heart surgery to prevent blood from clotting and in the critically ill patient with disseminated intravascular coagulation (DIC), which occurs when fibrin clots form within the vascular system. These clots consume proteins and platelets, depleting clotting factors and causing excess bleeding. However, the primary use of heparin is to prevent venous thrombosis, which can lead to PE or stroke.

Heparin combines with antithrombin III, which accelerates the anticoagulant cascade of reactions that prevents thrombosis formation. By inhibiting the action of thrombin, conversion of fibrinogen to fibrin does not occur, and the formation of a fibrin clot is prevented (Fig. 40.1).

Heparin is poorly absorbed through the gastrointestinal (GI) mucosa, and much is destroyed by heparinase, a liver enzyme. Because heparin is poorly absorbed orally, it is given subcutaneously for prophylaxis or by IV to treat acute thrombosis. It can be administered as an IV bolus or in IV fluid for continuous infusion. Heparin prolongs clotting time. Partial thromboplastin time (PTT) and activated partial thromboplastin time (aPTT) are laboratory tests used to detect deficiencies of certain clotting factors, and these tests are used to monitor heparin therapy. Heparin can decrease the platelet count, causing thrombocytopenia. If hemorrhage occurs during heparin therapy, the anticoagulant antagonist protamine sulfate is given by IV. Protamine sulfate can be an anticoagulant, but in the presence of heparin, it is an antagonist that reverses the action of

heparin. Before discontinuing heparin, oral therapy with warfarin therapy is begun.

Low–Molecular-Weight Heparins

These derivatives of standard heparin were introduced to prevent venous thromboembolism. Studies have shown that by extracting only the low–molecular-weight fractions of standard heparin through depolymerization, the equivalent of anticoagulation can be achieved with a lower risk of bleeding. Low–molecular-weight heparins (LMWHs) produce more stable responses at recommended doses. As a result, frequent laboratory monitoring of aPTT is not required, because LMWH does not have the standard effect of heparin. Heparin prevents coagulation by combining with antithrombin III to inactivate factor Xa and thrombin. LMWH inactivates the Xa factor, but it is less able to inactivate thrombin.

The examples of LMWHs include enoxaparin, dalteparin, and tinzaparin.

The anticoagulant fondaparinux is a synthetically engineered antithrombotic designed to be effective as a once-daily subcutaneous injection. Categorized as a *selective factor Xa inhibitor*, fondaparinux is closely related in structure to heparin and LMWHs and is used for the same purposes.

These agents are most commonly prescribed to prevent DVT and acute PE after orthopedic or abdominal surgery. Hip and knee replacement anticoagulant therapy often includes

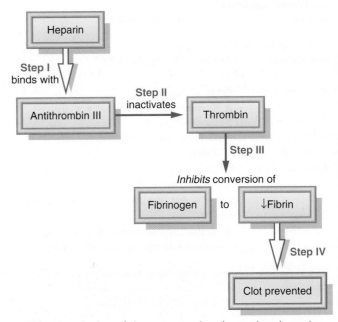

FIG. 40.1 Action of the parenteral anticoagulant heparin.

enoxaparin, and abdominal surgery includes dalteparin. The drugs can be administered at home because aPTT monitoring is not necessary, whereas heparin must be given in the hospital. LMWHs are administered subcutaneously once or twice a day, depending on the drug or drug regimen, and they are available in prefilled syringes with attached needles. The patient or family member is taught how to administer the subcutaneous injection, which is usually given in the abdomen. The average treatment period lasts 7 to 10 days. The LMWH is usually started in the hospital within 24 hours after surgery (Table 40.1).

The half-life of LMWHs is two to four times longer than that of heparin. Patients should be instructed not to take antiplatelet drugs such as aspirin while taking LMWHs or heparin. Bleeding because of LMWH use is less likely to occur than when heparin

is given. LMWH overdose is rare; if bleeding occurs, protamine sulfate is the anticoagulant antagonist used. The dosage is 1 mg of protamine sulfate for every 100 units of unfractionated heparin or LMWH given to be neutralized.

Contraindications

The LMWHs are contraindicated for patients with strokes, peptic ulcers, and blood anomalies. These drugs should not be given to patients having eye, brain, or spinal surgery.

❶ Direct Thrombin Inhibitors: Parenteral Anticoagulants II

Parenteral anticoagulants directly inhibit thrombin from converting fibrinogen to fibrin. These drugs differ from heparin-like

---

⚠ TABLE 40.1   Anticoagulants and Anticoagulant Antagonists

Drug	Route and Dosage	Uses and Considerations
Anticoagulants		
Heparins		
Heparin sodium	See Prototype Drug Chart 40.1.	
Low–Molecular-Weight Heparins (LMWHs)		
Dalteparin	Prophylaxis before surgery: A: Subcut: 2500-5000 units/d for 5-10 d starting 1-2 h before surgery DVT treatment: A: Subcut: 200 units/kg/d for 1 month, then 150 units/kg/d for months 2-6	For DVT and PE prophylaxis and treatment, prophylaxis of thrombosis, and unstable angina. May cause bleeding, pain at the injection site, elevated liver enzymes, and thrombocytopenia. Pregnancy category: B*; PB: <10%; t½: 3-5 h
Enoxaparin sodium	DVT prophylaxis: A: Subcut: 30 mg q12h for at least 10 days	For prophylaxis of AMI, thrombosis, and unstable angina and for prophylaxis and treatment of PE and DVT. May cause bleeding, hematoma, fever, anemia, peripheral edema, and elevated liver enzymes. Pregnancy category: B*; PB: UK; t½: 3-6 h
Tinzaparin	DVT: A: Subcut: 175 units/kg/d	For DVT, PE, cerebral thromboembolism, and prophylaxis of thrombosis. May cause bleeding, hematoma, and elevated hepatic enzymes. Pregnancy Category B; PB: 90%; t½: 3-4 h
Oral Anticoagulants		
Warfarin	See Prototype Drug Chart 40.1.	
Selective Factor Xa Inhibitors		
Fondaparinux	A: Subcut: 2.5-10 mg/d for 5-9 d	For prophylaxis and treatment of DVT and PE. May cause bleeding, anemia, and insomnia. Pregnancy category: B*; PB: 94%; t½: 18 h
Rivaroxaban	Stroke prophylaxis: A: PO: 20 mg/d with evening meal; *max:* 30 mg/d DVT and PE prophylaxis: A: PO: 15 mg bid for 21 d, then 20 mg/d for 6 months	For prophylaxis of DVT, PE, and stroke and for atrial fibrillation. May cause bleeding and back pain. Pregnancy category: C*; PB: 92%-95%; t½: 5-9 h
Apixaban	DVT, PE: A: PO: 10 mg bid for 7 d then 5 mg bid for 6 months; *max:* 10 mg/d	To prevent and treat DVT and PE and for prevention of stroke and atrial fibrillation. May cause bleeding, hematoma, and anemia.. Pregnancy category: B*; PB: 87%; t½: 12 h
Edoxaban	DVT, PE: A: PO: 30-60 mg/d after 5-10 d of initial therapy with parenteral anticoagulant; *max:* 60 mg/d	For treatment of DVT, PE, and nonvalvular atrial fibrillation and stroke prophylaxis. May cause bleeding, elevated hepatic enzymes, and anemia. Pregnancy category: C*; PB: 55%; t½: 10-14 h
Direct-Acting Thrombin Inhibitors: Anticoagulants II (Intravenous)		
Argatroban	A: IV: 2 mcg/kg/min infusion; adjust dose to maintain aPTT 1.5-3 times baseline	For PCI, HIT, prophylaxis and treatment of DVT and PE; prophylaxis of coronary artery thrombosis. May cause bleeding, hypotension, chest pain, bradycardia, tachycardia, headache, GI distress, back pain, dyspnea, and cardiac arrest. Pregnancy category: B*; PB: 54%; t½: 39-51 min

Drug	Route and Dosage	Uses and Considerations
! TABLE 40.1	**Anticoagulants and Anticoagulant Antagonists—cont'd**	
Bivalirudin	PCI: A: IV bolus: 0.75 mg/kg; then IV infusion of 1.75 mg/kg/h during and within 4 h postprocedure; *max.* 1.75 mg/kg/h infusion	For thrombosis prophylaxis in PCI, unstable angina, and HIT. May cause bleeding, headache, hypotension, GI distress, insomnia, anxiety, back and pelvic pain, and bradycardia. Pregnancy category: B*; PB: 0%; t½: 25 min
Desirudin	A: Subcut: 15 mg q12h for 9-12 d, give first dose 5-15 min before surgery	For DVT prophylaxis. May cause bleeding, hematoma, injection site reaction, and anemia. Pregnancy category: C*; PB: UK; t½: 2-3 h
Dabigatran	A: PO: 150 mg bid; *max:* 300 mg/d	For prevention of stroke and for prophylaxis and treatment of atrial fibrillation, DVT, and PE. May cause bleeding and GI distress. Pregnancy category: C*; PB: 35%; t½: 12-17 h
Anticoagulant Antagonists		
Protamine sulfate	A: IV: Initially: 1 mg/100 units heparin to be neutralized; *max:* 100 mg in 2-h period	To neutralize heparin in hemorrhage; antidote to heparin overdose and toxicity. May cause hypotension, flushing, and bradycardia. Pregnancy category: C*; PB: UK; t½: 7.4 min
Phytonadione	Bleeding: A: IV: 1-10 mg slow infusion, hold warfarin therapy	For vitamin K deficiency, bleeding prophylaxis and treatment, and hypoprothrombinemia; antidote for warfarin overdose and toxicity. May cause hypersensitivity, dizziness, flushing, dysgeusia, sweating, tachycardia, and hypotension. Pregnancy category: C*; PB: UK; t½: UK

*Pregnancy categories have been revised. See http://www.fda.gov/Drugs/DevelopmentApprovalProcess/DevelopmentResources/Labeling/ucm093 307.htm for more information.

A, Adult; *AMI,* acute myocardial infarction; *aPTT,* activated partial thromboplastin time; *bid,* twice a day; *d,* day; *DVT,* deep vein thrombosis; *GI,* gastrointestinal; *h,* hour; *HIT,* heparin-induced thrombocytopenia; *IV,* intravenous; *max,* maximum; *min,* minute; *PB,* protein binding; *PCI,* percutaneous coronary intervention; *PE,* pulmonary embolism; *PO,* by mouth; *q12h,* every 12 hours; *subcut,* subcutaneous; *t½,* half-life; *UK,* unknown; *<,* less than.

anticoagulants. Argatroban and bivalirudin are given intravenously; bivalirudin binds with and inhibits free-flowing thrombin. Desirudin is administered subcutaneously, and dabigatran is an oral anticoagulant that does *not* require routine coagulation monitoring (see Table 40.1). These drugs are more expensive than the other anticoagulants.

Oral Anticoagulants

Oral anticoagulants inhibit hepatic synthesis of vitamin K, thus affecting the clotting factors II, VII, IX, and X. Warfarin is an oral anticoagulant that is synthesized from dicumarol. Warfarin is used mainly to prevent thromboembolic conditions such as thrombophlebitis, PE, and embolism formation caused by atrial fibrillation, which can lead to stroke. Oral anticoagulants prolong clotting time and are monitored by the prothrombin time (PT), a laboratory test that measures the time it takes blood to clot in the presence of certain clotting factors, which warfarin affects. This laboratory test is usually performed immediately before administering the next drug dose until the therapeutic level has been reached. Today, the international normalized ratio (INR) is the laboratory test most frequently used to report PT results. It was introduced to account for variability in reported PTs from different laboratories. Reagents used in the PT test are compared with an international reference standard and reported as the INR; normal INR is 1.3 to 2. Patients on warfarin therapy are maintained at an INR of 2 to 3. The desired INR for patients who have a mechanical heart valve or recurrent systemic embolism is 2.5 to 3.5, but the desired level could be as high as 4.5.

Monitoring INR at regular intervals is required for the duration of drug therapy. Warfarin has a long half-life and very long duration. Drug accumulation can occur and can lead to external or internal bleeding, so the nurse must observe for petechiae, ecchymosis, tarry stools, and hematemesis and must teach the patient to do the same at home.

The antidote for warfarin overdose is vitamin K, but it takes 24 to 48 hours to be effective. Usually a low dose of oral vitamin K may be recommended for patients with an INR of 5.5. If excessive vitamin K is given, it may take warfarin 1 to 2 weeks before it can be effective again. For acute bleeding, fresh frozen plasma is indicated.

Parenteral and oral anticoagulants (heparin and warfarin) are presented in Prototype Drug Chart 40.1.

Pharmacokinetics Heparin is poorly absorbed through the GI mucosa, and much is destroyed by heparinase, a liver enzyme. Heparin is given parenterally, either subcutaneously for prophylactic anticoagulant therapy or by IV (bolus or continuous infusion) for an immediate response. Warfarin, an oral anticoagulant, is well absorbed through the GI mucosa; food will delay but not inhibit absorption.

The half-life of heparin is dose related; high doses prolong the half-life. The half-life of warfarin is 20 to 80 hours, in contrast to 1 to 5 hours for heparin. Because warfarin has a long half-life and is highly protein bound, the drug can have cumulative effects. Bleeding can occur, especially if another highly protein-bound drug is administered together with warfarin. Kidney and liver disease prolong the half-life of both heparin and warfarin. Warfarin is metabolized to inactive metabolites that are excreted in urine and bile.

Pharmacodynamics Heparin, administered for acute thromboembolic disorders, prevents thrombus formation and embolism. It has been effectively used to treat DIC, which causes multiple thrombi in small blood vessels. Warfarin is effective for long-term anticoagulant therapy. The PT level should be 1.5 to 2 times the reference value to be therapeutic, or INR should be 2.0 to 3.0. INR has effectively replaced the use of PT, because PT can vary from laboratory to laboratory and reagent to reagent. Higher INR levels (up to 3.5) are usually required for patients with prosthetic heart valves, cardiac valvular disease, and recurrent emboli. Heparin does not cross the placental barrier, unlike warfarin; warfarin use is not recommended during pregnancy.

! PROTOTYPE DRUG CHART 40.1
Heparin and Warfarin Sodium

Drug Class	Dosage
Anticoagulant Pregnancy category: C* (heparin) Pregnancy category: X* (warfarin)	Heparin: A: Subcut: 8000-10,000 units q4-6h based on aPTT q12h A: IV: 80 units/kg bolus; maint: 18 units/kg/h infusion based on aPTT C >1 y: IV: 75 units/kg bolus; maint: 20 units/kg/h infusion based on aPTT Warfarin: A: PO: 0.5-7 mg/d based on INR; target INR 2-3.5
Contraindications Heparin: Bleeding disorder, hypersensitivity *Caution:* Peptic ulcer, hepatic or renal disease, hemophilia, DIC, diverticulitis, head trauma, HIT, thrombocytopenia Warfarin: Hematologic disorders, eclampsia, alcoholism, bleeding, head trauma, psychosis *Caution:* Diabetes mellitus, leukemia, anemia, hepatic and renal impairment, peptic ulcer, atrial fibrillation	**Drug-Lab-Food Interactions** Drug: Heparin: Increased effect with aspirin, NSAIDs, thrombolytics, probenecid, antibiotics, SSRIs; decreased effect with nitroglycerin, protamine sulfate Warfarin: Increased effect with amiodarone, aspirin, NSAIDs, sulfonamides, thyroid drugs, allopurinol, histamine$_2$ blockers, oral hypoglycemics, metronidazole, miconazole, methyldopa, diuretics, oral antibiotics, vitamin E; decreased effect with barbiturates, laxatives, phenytoin, estrogens, vitamins C and K, oral contraceptives, rifampin Lab: May increase AST, ALT Food: Decrease diet rich in vitamin K
Pharmacokinetics Absorption: Heparin: Subcut or IV; warfarin: PO: Well absorbed Distribution: PB: Heparin: >80%; warfarin: 97% Metabolism: t½: Heparin: IV 1-5 h; warfarin: 20-80 h Excretion: Heparin: Slowly in urine and reticuloendothelial system; warfarin: in urine and bile	**Pharmacodynamics** Heparin: Subcut: Onset: 20-30 min Peak: UK Duration: UK IV: Onset: Immediate Peak: 5-10 min Duration: 2-6 h Warfarin: PO: Onset: 24-72 h Peak: 36-72 h, 5-7 d full effect Duration: 2-5 d
Therapeutic Effects/Uses Heparin/warfarin: To prevent thrombosis associated with PE, MI, unstable angina, prosthetic heart valves, DVT, and PCI; Heparin: To treat DIC; Warfarin: To treat atrial fibrillation Mode of Action: Heparin inhibits thrombin, which prevents conversion of fibrinogen to fibrin; warfarin depresses hepatic synthesis of vitamin K clotting factors (II [prothrombin], VII, IX, and X).	
Side Effects Heparin: Itching, chills, injection-site reaction, priapism Warfarin: Headache, GI distress, alopecia, fever, weakness, priapism	**Adverse Reactions** Heparin: Hypersensitivity, bleeding, anemia, elevated hepatic enzymes, osteoporosis, stroke, *Life threatening:* Hemorrhage, HIT Warfarin: Purple-toe syndrome, bone fracture, hypotension, chest pain, elevated hepatic enzymes *Life threatening:* Hemorrhage

*Pregnancy categories have been revised. See http://www.fda.gov/Drugs/DevelopmentApprovalProcess/DevelopmentResources/Labeling/ucm093307.htm for more information.
A, Adult; *ALT,* alanine transaminase; *aPTT,* activated partial thromboplastin time; *AST,* aspartate transaminase; *C,* child; *d,* day; *DIC,* disseminated intravascular coagulation; *DVT,* deep venous thrombosis; *GI,* gastrointestinal; *h,* hour; *HIT,* heparin-induced thrombocytopenia; *INR,* international normalized ratio; *IV,* intravenous; *maint,* maintenance; *MI,* myocardial infarction; *min,* minute; *NSAIDs,* nonsteroidal antiinflammatory drugs; *PB,* protein binding; *PCI,* percutaneous coronary intervention; *PE,* pulmonary embolism; *PO,* by mouth; *q,* every; *SSRI,* selective serotonin reuptake inhibitor; *subcut,* subcutaneous; *t½,* half-life; *UK,* unknown; *y,* years; *>,* greater than.

IV heparin has a rapid onset; its peak time of action is reached in minutes, and its duration of action is short. After an IV heparin dose, the patient's clotting time will return to normal in 2 to 6 hours. Subcutaneous heparin is more slowly absorbed through the blood vessels in fatty tissue. Warfarin has a long onset of action, peak concentration, and duration of action, so drug accumulation may occur.

Table 40.2 gives the summary comparison between heparin and warfarin, including methods of administration, drug action, uses, contraindications, laboratory tests, side effects, adverse reactions, and antidotes.

Side Effects and Adverse Reactions. Bleeding (hemorrhage) is the major adverse effect of warfarin. Patients should be monitored closely for signs of bleeding such as petechiae, ecchymosis, and hematemesis. Laboratory testing of PT or INR should be scheduled at recommended intervals.

Drug Interactions. Because warfarin is highly protein bound, it is affected by drug interactions. Aspirin, nonsteroidal antiinflammatory drugs (NSAIDs), other types of antiinflammatory drugs, sulfonamides, phenytoin, cimetidine, allopurinol, and oral hypoglycemic drugs for diabetes can displace warfarin

TABLE 40.2 Comparison of Parenteral and Oral Anticoagulants

Factors to Consider	Heparin	Warfarin (Coumadin)
Methods of administration	Subcutaneously Intravenously	Primarily orally
Drug actions	Binds with antithrombin III, which inactivates thrombin and clotting factors, inhibiting fibrin formation	Inhibits hepatic synthesis of vitamin K, which decreases prothrombin and the clotting factors VII, IX, and X
Uses	Treatment of venous thrombosis, PE, thromboembolic complications (e.g., heart surgery, DIC)	Treatment of DVT, PE, TIA; prophylactic for cardiac valves
Contraindications/ cautions	Hemophilia, peptic ulcer, severe (stage 3 or 4) hypertension, severe liver or renal disease, dissecting aneurysm	Hemophilia, peptic bleeding ulcer, blood dyscrasias, severe liver or kidney disease, AMI, alcoholism
Laboratory tests	PTT: 60-70 s Anticoagulant therapeutic level: 1.5 to 2 × control in seconds	PT: 11-15 s Anticoagulant therapeutic level: 1.25 to 2.5 × control in seconds
	aPTT: 20-35 s Anticoagulant: aPTT: 30-85 s	INR: 1.3-2 Anticoagulant: INR 2-3 Prosthetic heart valves: INR up to 3.5
Side effects/ adverse effects	Bleeding, hemorrhage, hematoma, severe hypotension	Bleeding, hemorrhage, GI bleeding, ecchymoses, hematuria
Antidote	Protamine sulfate	Phytonadione (vitamin K)

AMI, acute myocardial infarction; *aPTT*, activated partial thromboplastin time; *DIC*, disseminated intravascular coagulation; *DVT*, deep venous thrombosis; *GI*, gastrointestinal; *INR*, international normalized ratio; *PE*, pulmonary embolism; *PT*, prothrombin time; *PTT*, partial thromboplastin time; *s*, second; *TIA*, transient ischemic attack.

from the protein-bound site and can cause more free-circulating anticoagulant. Numerous other drugs also increase the action of warfarin, and bleeding is likely to occur. Acetaminophen should be used instead of aspirin by patients taking warfarin. For frank bleeding resulting from excess free drug, parenteral vitamin K is given as a coagulant to decrease bleeding and promote clotting. However, caution must be used with this approach because the prothrombin can remain depressed for prolonged periods.

Table 40.1 lists the pharmacologic data for the anticoagulants.

❶ *Factor Xa Inhibitors: Oral Anticoagulants.* Four oral anticoagulants—fondaparinux, rivaroxaban, apixaban, and edoxaban—form a category called *factor Xa inhibitors.* These drugs do not require routine coagulation monitoring and are given once or twice daily (see Table 40.1).

Anticoagulant Antagonists

Bleeding occurs in about 10% of patients taking oral anticoagulants. Phytonadione, an antagonist of warfarin, is vitamin K_1 and is used for warfarin overdose or uncontrollable bleeding.

NURSING PROCESS
Patient-Centered Collaborative Care

Anticoagulants: Warfarin and Heparin

Assessment
- Obtain a history of abnormal clotting or health problems that affect clotting, such as severe alcoholism or severe liver or renal disease. Warfarin is contraindicated for patients with blood dyscrasias, peptic ulcer, CVA, hemophilia, or severe hypertension. Use with caution in patients with acute traumatic injury.
- Gather a drug history that includes a complementary and alternative therapy history of current drugs and products that the patient takes. Report if drug-drug or drug-herb interaction or other interaction with complementary and alternative therapy is probable. Warfarin is highly protein bound and can displace other highly protein-bound drugs, or warfarin could be displaced, which may result in bleeding.
- Develop a flowchart that lists PT or INR and warfarin dosages. A baseline PT or INR should be obtained before warfarin is administered.

Nursing Diagnoses
- Injury, Risk for
- Knowledge, Deficient related to lack of previous exposure to side effects of anticoagulants and their action

Planning
- The patient's PT will be 1.25 to 2.5 times the control level, or INR will be 2 to 3.
- The patient will not have excessive bleeding.
- The patient's aPTT level will be within a therapeutic range.

Nursing Interventions
- Monitor vital signs. An increased pulse rate followed by a decreased systolic pressure can indicate a fluid volume deficit resulting from external or internal bleeding.
- ⚡ Monitor PT or INR for warfarin and aPTT for heparin before administering anticoagulant. PT should be 1.25 to 2.5 times the control level, or INR should be 2 to 3, except for patients with prosthetic heart valves, in whom INR may be up to 3.5. Monitor platelet count because anticoagulants can decrease it.
- Examine the patient's mouth, nose (epistaxis), urine (hematuria), and skin (petechiae, purpura) for bleeding. Watch older adults closely for bleeding; their skin is thin, and capillary beds are fragile.
- Check stools periodically for occult blood.
- Keep anticoagulant antagonists available, protamine sulfate for heparin and vitamin K for warfarin, when the drug dose is increased or indications of frank bleeding are evident. Fresh frozen plasma may be needed for transfusion.

Patient Teaching
General
- Teach patients to inform their dentist when taking an anticoagulant. Contacting a health care provider may be necessary.

- Advise patients to use a soft toothbrush to prevent gums from bleeding.
- Warn patients to shave with an electric razor. Bleeding from shaving cuts may be difficult to control.
- Advise patients to have laboratory tests such as PT or INR performed as ordered by a health care provider. The warfarin dose is regulated according to INR derived from PT.
- Suggest that patients carry a medical identification card or wear a MedicAlert bracelet that lists the patient's name, telephone number, and the drug taken.
- Encourage patients *not* to smoke. Smoking increases drug metabolism, so warfarin dose may need to be increased. If a patient insists on smoking, notify the health care provider.
- Tell patients to check with a health care provider before taking over-the-counter (OTC) drugs. Aspirin should *not* be taken with warfarin because it intensifies warfarin's action, and bleeding is apt to occur. Suggest that patients use acetaminophen.
- Inform patients that many herbal products interact with anticoagulants and may increase bleeding (Complementary and Alternative Therapies 40.1). Closely monitor INR or PT.
- ⚡ Teach patients to control external hemorrhage from accidents or injuries by applying firm, direct pressure for at least 5 to 10 minutes with a clean, dry, absorbent material.

Side Effects
- Warn patients to report frank or occult bleeding such as petechiae, ecchymosis, purpura, tarry stools, bleeding gums, epistaxis, or expectoration of blood.

Diet
- Advise patients to avoid large amounts of green, leafy vegetables; broccoli; legumes; soybean oil (rich in vitamin K); coffee, tea, cola (caffeine); excessive alcohol; and certain herbs and nutritional supplements (coenzyme Q10) or to be very consistent with their intake. Coenzyme Q10, fish oils, substances high in vitamin K, St. John's wort, ginseng, and vitamin C may decrease the effectiveness of warfarin. Garlic, ginger, kava kava, green tea, chamomile tea, ginkgo biloba, and acute alcohol intoxication also decrease warfarin effectiveness.

🌐 Cultural Considerations
- Provide instructions in the language the patient speaks and reads most easily. Certain cultural groups may lack understanding of Western approaches to health problems, drug therapy, adverse effects, and follow-up care concerning thrombophlebitis or other conditions that cause thrombus formation.
- Identify conflicts in cultural values and beliefs of patient regarding methods for treating a vascular problem. Respect traditional practices, and incorporate them into the care plan if harmless. If a method may be harmful, initiate explanations along with the nursing plan.

Evaluation
- Evaluate the effectiveness of drug therapy. The patient's PT or INR values are within the desired range, and the patient is free from significant side effects.

🌿 COMPLEMENTARY AND ALTERNATIVE THERAPIES 40.1
Anticoagulants: Warfarin and Heparin
- Dong quai, feverfew, garlic, ginger, green tea, chamomile tea, ginkgo, and bilberry may increase bleeding when taken with anticoagulants such as warfarin. Warfarin has an additive effect and increases the international normalized ratio (INR) and prothrombin time (PT).
- Excessive doses of anise may interfere with anticoagulants.
- Ginseng may decrease the effects of warfarin, thereby decreasing INR.
- Alfalfa may decrease anticoagulant activity.
- Goldenseal may decrease the effects of heparin and oral anticoagulants.
- Hawthorn increases the action of anticoagulants.
- Valerian may decrease the effects of warfarin.

Usually 5 to 10 mg of vitamin K_1 is given by slow intravenous infusion at once, and if it fails to control bleeding, fresh whole blood or fresh frozen plasma or platelets are generally given.

ANTIPLATELET DRUGS

Antiplatelets are used to prevent thrombosis in the arteries by suppressing platelet aggregation. Heparin and warfarin prevent thrombosis in the veins.

Antiplatelet drug therapy is mainly for prophylactic use in (1) prevention of MI or stroke for patients with a family history of these, (2) prevention of repeat MI or stroke, and (3) prevention of stroke for patients having transient ischemic attacks (TIAs).

Long-term, low-dose aspirin therapy has been found to be both an effective and inexpensive treatment for suppressing platelet aggregation. Aspirin inhibits cyclooxygenase (COX), an enzyme needed by platelets to synthesize thromboxane A_2 (TxA_2). For patients with a family history of stroke or MI, the recommended aspirin dose is 50 to 325 mg/day for stroke prophylaxis and 75 to 162 mg/day for MI prophylaxis. Because aspirin has prolonged antiplatelet activity, it should be discontinued at least 7 days before surgery.

Other antiplatelet drugs include anagrelide, clopidogrel, dipyridamole, prasugrel, ticagrelor, vorapaxar, cangrelor, abciximab, eptifibatide, and tirofiban. Clopidogrel and dipyridamole have effects similar to those of aspirin, but they are known as *adenosine diphosphate (ADP) antagonists,* and they affect platelet aggregation. Cilostazol inhibits platelet aggregation and is a vasodilator that may be used for intermittent claudication. Ticagrelor 90 mg twice a day is taken in conjunction with aspirin 75 to 100 mg in a maintenance regimen. Doses greater than 100 mg of aspirin should be avoided. Table 40.3 lists the antiplatelet drugs and their dosages, uses, and considerations.

Clopidogrel is an antiplatelet drug frequently used after MI or stroke to prevent a second event. It may be prescribed singly or with aspirin. It has been stated that clopidogrel and aspirin are more effective in inhibiting platelet aggregation if used together than if used as separate antiplatelet therapies. Prototype Drug Chart 40.2 lists the pharmacologic data for clopidogrel.

TABLE 40.3   Antiplatelets

Drug	Route and Dosage	Uses and Considerations
Anagrelide Hydrochloride	A: PO: Initially 0.5 mg qid or 1 mg bid for 1 wk; maint: 1.5-3 mg/d; *max:* 10 mg/d, 2.5 mg/dose Adol/C >7 y: PO: 0.5 mg/d; maint: 0.5 mg qd-qid; *max.* 10 mg/d, 2.5 mg/dose	For treatment of thrombocytosis, chronic myelogenous leukemia, and polycythemia vera. May cause headache, dizziness, palpitations, peripheral edema, tachycardia, pain, GI distress, weakness, and dyspnea. Pregnancy category: C*; PB: UK; t½: 3-4 d
Aspirin (ASA)	Thromboembolus prophylaxis: A: PO: 75-100 mg/d Stroke prophylaxis: A: PO: 50-325 mg/d MI prophylaxis: A: PO: 75-162 mg/d TDM: Salicylate toxicity is >300 mcg/mL	For prevention and treatment of stroke, prophylaxis of MI, and thromboembolism. May cause bleeding, GI distress, and Reye syndrome. Pregnancy category: UK*; PB: 90%-95%; t½: 15-20 min
Cilostazol	A: PO: 50-100 mg bid; *max.* 200 mg/d	For intermittent claudication and PVD. Smoking may decrease serum levels. May cause headache, diarrhea, GI distress, nasopharyngitis, dizziness, infection, palpitations, and peripheral edema. Pregnancy category: C*; PB: 95%-98%, t½: 11-13 h
Clopidogrel	See Prototype Drug Chart 40.2.	
Dipyridamole	Thromboembolism prophylaxis: A: PO: 75-100 mg qid in combination with warfarin *or* 75 mg tid/qid in combination with ASA; *max:* 400 mg/d	For prevention of thromboembolism associated with prosthetic heart valves. May cause dizziness, headache, GI distress, and chest pain. Pregnancy category: B*; PB: 91%-99%; t½: 12 h
Prasugrel	A: PO: Loading dose: 60 mg; maint: 10 mg/d in combination with ASA	For PCI, prevention of thrombotic cardiovascular events, and treatment of AMI and unstable angina. May cause headache, dizziness, bleeding, nausea, back pain, and hypercholesterolemia. Pregnancy category: B*; PB: 98%; t½: 2-15 h
Ticagrelor	A: PO: Loading dose: 180 mg; maint: 90 mg bid with ASA 75-100 mg/d; *max:* 180 mg/d tricagrelor and 100 mg/d ASA	For PCI, prevention and treatment of unstable angina, and AMI. May cause headache, dizziness, bradycardia, bleeding, and dyspnea. Pregnancy category: C*; PB: 99%: t½: 7 h
Vorapaxar	A: PO: 2.08 mg/d in combination with ASA and/or clopidogrel; *max.* 2.08 mg/d	A new protease-activated receptor-1 antagonist for prevention of thrombosis, MI, PAD, and stroke. May cause bleeding and anemia. Pregnancy category: B*; PB: 99%; t½: 5-13 d
Cangrelor	A: IV: Initially 30 mcg/kg bolus prior to PCI, follow immediately with infusion of 4 mcg/kg/min for at least 2 h or duration of PCI, whichever is longer	A new, nonthienopyridine antiplatelet for prevention of thrombosis in PCI and MI. May cause bleeding. Pregnancy category: C*; PB: 97%-98%; t½: 3-6 min
Combination of Antiplatelet Drugs		
Dipyridamole and aspirin	Stroke prevention: Extended release: A: PO: 1 cap (ASA 25 mg and dipyridamole 200 mg) bid in morning and evening; *max.* ASA 50 mg and dipyridamole 400 mg/d	For stroke prevention, ischemic stroke, and TIA. May cause headache, GI distress, fatigue, bleeding, arthralgia, and back pain. Pregnancy category: D*; PB: 91%-99%; t½: Dipyridamole 12 h, ASA 15-20 min
Antiplatelets: Glycoprotein (GP) IIb/IIIa Receptor Antagonists		
Abciximab	A: IV bolus: 0.25 mcg/kg given 10-60 min before PCI; follow with continuous infusion of 0.125 mcg/kg/min for 12 h; *max:* 10 mcg/min infusion; 0.25 mg/kg bolus	To prevent thrombosis in PCI, unstable angina, and AMI. May cause headache, hypotension, hypersensitivity, bleeding, back and chest pain, and GI distress. Pregnancy category: C*; PB: UK; t½: 10 min
Eptifibatide	PCI: A: IV bolus: 180 mcg/kg, then 2 mcg/kg/min infusion until hospital discharge or 18-24 h; *max:* 15 mg/h infusion or 180 mcg/kg bolus	For prevention of thrombosis in PCI, unstable angina, and AMI. May cause hypotension and bleeding. Pregnancy category: B*; PB: 25%; t½: 1.5-2 h
Tirofiban	A: IV: 25 mcg/kg bolus over 5 min followed by 0.15 mcg/kg/min infusion for 18-24 h	For unstable angina and AMI. May cause bleeding, pelvic pain, and bradycardia. Pregnancy category: B*; PB: 65%; t½: 1.7-2 h

*Pregnancy categories have been revised. See http://www.fda.gov/Drugs/DevelopmentApprovalProcess/DevelopmentResources/Labeling/ucm093 307.htm for more information.

A, Adult; *adol,* adolescent; *AMI,* acute myocardial infarction; *ASA,* acetylsalicylic acid (aspirin); *bid,* twice daily; *C,* child; *cap,* capsule; *d,* day; *ER,* extended release; *GI,* gastrointestinal; *h,* hour; *IV,* intravenous; *maint,* maintenance; *max,* maximum; *MI,* myocardial infarction; *min,* minute; *PAD,* peripheral artery disease; *PB,* protein binding; *PCI,* percutaneous coronary intervention; *PO,* by mouth; *PVD,* peripheral vascular disease; *qd,* every day; *qid,* four times a day; *t½,* half-life; *TDM,* therapeutic drug monitoring; *TIA,* transient ischemic attack; *tid,* three times a day; *UK,* unknown; *wk,* week; *y,* years; *>,* greater than.

PROTOTYPE DRUG CHART 40.2
Clopidogrel Bisulfate

Drug Class	Dosage
Antiplatelet Pregnancy category: B*	A: PO: LD: 300 mg and then 75 mg/d in combination with aspirin 75-325 mg/d up to 12 months
Contraindications	**Drug-Lab-Food Interactions**

Intracranial hemorrhage, GI bleeding
Caution: Hepatic and renal disease, surgery, peptic ulcer,
   MI, stroke, thrombotic thrombocytopenia purpura,
   bleeding from trauma
	Drug: May increase bleeding when taken with NSAIDs, anticoagulants, omeprazole, antineoplastics, azole
	   antifungals, SSRIs, and barbiturates; interferes with metabolism of phenytoin, warfarin, fluvastatin, ta-
	   moxifen, tolbutamide, NSAIDs, torsemide, calcium channel blockers, morphine, and amiodarone; increases
	   effects of valsartan, rosuvastatin, glipizide, glyburide; effects are decreased with grapefruit juice.
	Lab: Prolongs bleeding time
	Herb: May increase bleeding when taken with ginger, garlic, ginkgo, feverfew, green tea

Pharmacokinetics	**Pharmacodynamics**

Absorption: Rapid
Distribution: PB: 94%-98%
Metabolism: t½: 6 h
Excretion: 50% in urine and 50% in feces
	PO: Onset: 2 h for dose of 300-600 mg/d,
	   2 d for dose of 50-100 mg/d
	Peak: 6 h for dose of 300-600 mg/d,
	   5-7 d for dose of 50-100 mg/d
	Duration: UK

Therapeutic Effects/Uses	
To prevent thrombosis associated with unstable angina, AMI, stroke, TIA Mode of Action: Inhibits platelet aggregation and prevents ADP from binding with the ADP platelet receptor	
Side Effects	**Adverse Reactions**
Abdominal pain, flulike symptoms, dizziness, confusion, epistaxis, headaches, GI distress, bleeding, rash, pruritus	Hypotension, hypertension, bronchospasm, elevated hepatic enzymes, peptic ulcer *Life threatening:* Agranulocytosis, aplastic anemia, thrombocytopenia, pancytopenia, Stevens-Johnson syndrome

*Pregnancy categories have been revised. See http://www.fda.gov/Drugs/DevelopmentApprovalProcess/DevelopmentResources/Labeling/ucm093307.htm for more information.
A, Adult; *ADP*, adenosine diphosphate; *AMI*, acute myocardial infarction; *d*, day; *GI*, gastrointestinal; *h*, hour; *LD*, loading dose; *MI*, myocardial infarction; *PB*, protein binding; *PO*, by mouth; *NSAID*, nonsteroidal antiinflammatory drug; *SSRI*, serotonin reuptake inhibitor; *t½*, half-life; *TIA*, transient ischemic attack; *UK*, unknown.

Pharmacokinetics Clopidogrel is rapidly absorbed and has a high protein-binding power. Studies have not established a relationship between the concentration of the main metabolite and platelet aggregation. The half-life is 6 hours; it is usually prescribed once a day. Excretion of the drug metabolite occurs equally in the urine and in feces.

Pharmacodynamics Clopidogrel prevents platelet aggregation by blocking the binding of ADP to the platelet ADP receptor. ADP-mediated activation of the glycoprotein (GP) IIb/IIIa complex inhibits platelet aggregation. Clopidogrel prolongs bleeding time, therefore it should be discontinued for 7 days preceding surgery. The onset of action of clopidogrel is dependent upon dosage. The peak time is 1 hour. The drug should not be taken if the patient has a bleeding peptic ulcer, any active bleeding, or intracranial hemorrhage.

Abciximab, eptifibatide, and tirofiban are used primarily for acute coronary syndromes (unstable angina or non–Q-wave MI) and for preventing reocclusion of coronary arteries following percutaneous transluminal coronary angioplasty (PTCA). These drugs are usually given before and after PTCA. The drug of choice for angioplasty is abciximab. Abciximab, eptifibatide, and tirofiban block the binding of fibrinogen to the GP IIb/IIIa receptor on the platelet surface. They are called *platelet glycoprotein IIb/IIIa receptor antagonists.* Following IV infusion, the antiplatelet effects at low levels for abciximab persist for up to 10 days; for eptifibatide and tirofiban, the antiplatelet effects last for 4 hours.

Complementary and alternative therapy products can interact with antiplatelet drugs (Complementary and Alternative Therapies 40.2).

COMPLEMENTARY AND ALTERNATIVE THERAPIES 40.2
Antiplatelets

Dong quai, feverfew, garlic, and ginkgo biloba interfere with platelet aggregation. When these herbs are taken with an antiplatelet drug such as aspirin, increased bleeding may occur.

❶ THROMBOLYTICS

Thromboembolism, occlusion of an artery or vein caused by a thrombus or embolus, results in ischemia (deficient blood flow) that causes necrosis (death) of the tissue distal to the obstructed area. It takes approximately 1 to 2 weeks for the blood clot to disintegrate by natural fibrinolytic mechanisms. If a new thrombus or embolus can be dissolved more quickly, tissue necrosis is minimized, and blood flow to the area is reestablished faster. This is the basis for thrombolytic therapy.

Thrombolytics have been used since the early 1980s to promote the fibrinolytic mechanism (converting plasminogen to plasmin, which destroys the fibrin in the blood clot). The thrombus, or blood clot, disintegrates when a thrombolytic drug is administered as soon as possible after symptoms of an acute myocardial infarction (AMI), acute heart attack. Ideally, the thrombolytic should be administered within 3 to 4 hours or within 30 minutes after arriving at the hospital for treatment. However, benefits may

! PROTOTYPE DRUG CHART 40.3

Alteplase

Drug Class	Dosage
Thrombolytic agent Pregnancy category: C*	PE treatment: A: IV: 100 mg infusion over 2 h Ischemic CVA treatment: A: IV: 0.9 mg/kg (give 10% of dose as bolus over 1 min then 90% as an infusion over 1 h)
Contraindications	**Drug-Lab-Food Interactions**
Internal bleeding, bleeding disorders, aneurysm, recent CVA, surgery or trauma, bacterial endocarditis, severe liver dysfunction, severe uncontrolled hypertension, brain tumor, head trauma *Caution:* Cardiac dysrhythmias, hepatic or renal disease, CABG, peptic ulcer disease, diabetic retinopathy, older adults, pregnancy	Drug: Increased bleeding when taken with anticoagulants, NSAIDs, cefotetan, plicamycin, SNRIs, SSRIs, and cephalosporins; decreased effect when taken with aminocaproic acid, aprotinin Lab: Decrease in plasminogen, fibrinogen, hematocrit, and hemoglobin Complementary and Alternative Therapies: Increased bleeding with ginkgo biloba, garlic, feverfew, ginger, green tea, omega-3 fatty acids
Pharmacokinetics	**Pharmacodynamics**
Absorption: Direct IV Distribution: PB: UK Metabolism: t½: 5 min Excretion: Urine	A: IV: Onset: Immediate Peak: 5-10 min Duration: 1 h
Therapeutic Effects/Uses	
To promote fibrinolysis associated with thrombosis, AMI, PE, ischemic stroke, occluded IV catheter Mode of Action: Alteplase promotes conversion of plasminogen to plasmin, an enzyme that digests the fibrin matrix of clots. Alteplase also initiates fibrinolysis.	
Side Effects	**Adverse Reactions**
Bleeding, epistaxis, hypotension, infection, GI distress, rash	Anaphylactoid reactions, laryngeal edema, angioedema; cholesterol microembolization hypertension, MI, cerebral edema, rhabdomyolysis, bleeding, bradycardia, tachycardia, heart failure, seizures *Life threatening:* Stroke; dysrhythmias; pulmonary edema

*Pregnancy categories have been revised. See http://www.fda.gov/Drugs/DevelopmentApprovalProcess/DevelopmentResources/Labeling/ucm093307.htm for more information.
A, Adult; *AMI*, acute myocardial infarction; *CABG*, coronary artery bypass graft; *CVA*, cerebrovascular accident; *GI*, gastrointestinal; *h*, hours; *IV*, intravenous; *MI*, myocardial infarction; *min*, minute; *NSAIDs*, nonsteroidal antiinflammatory drugs; *PB*, protein binding; *PE*, pulmonary embolism; *SNRI*, selective norepinephrine reuptake inhibitor; *SSRI*, selective serotonin reuptake inhibitor; *t½*, half-life; *UK*, unknown.

be seen when administered within 12 hours after initial symptoms. Necrosis resulting from the blocked artery is prevented or minimized, and hospitalization time may be decreased. The need for cardiac bypass or coronary angioplasty can be evaluated soon after thrombolytic treatment. A thrombolytic drug should be administered within 3 hours of a thrombolic stroke. These drugs are also used for PE, DVT, noncoronary arterial occlusion from an acute thromboembolism, and thrombolic stroke.

Commonly used thrombolytics include alteplase, also known as *tissue plasminogen activator* (tPA), and tenecteplase (TNK tPA). Alteplase is clot specific and binds to the fibrin surface of a clot, promoting the conversion of plasminogen to plasmin. Plasmin, an enzyme, digests the fibrin in the clot. Plasmin also degrades fibrinogen, prothrombin, and other clotting factors. These drugs all induce fibrinolysis (fibrin breakdown). Prototype Drug Chart 40.3 lists the pharmacologic data for alteplase.

Anticoagulants and antiplatelet drugs increase the risk of hemorrhage, therefore they should be avoided until the thrombolytic effect has passed. The health care provider needs to determine whether the patient has taken any of these drugs before seeking treatment.

Pharmacokinetics The commercial preparation of alteplase is identical to natural human tissue plasminogen activator (tPA),

the enzyme that converts plasminogen to plasmin. Alteplase is initially administered with 10% of dose as an IV bolus over 1 minute and 90% of dose is then infused over 60 minutes. A total dose of 90 mg is the recommended maximum; a larger dose could result in risk for intracranial bleeding. Allergic reactions to alteplase occur less frequently than with other thrombolytics.

Pharmacodynamics Alteplase is similar to natural human tissue plasminogen activator. It promotes thrombolysis by converting plasminogen to plasmin, which degrades fibrin, fibrinogen, and factors V, VIII, and XII. Peak action of alteplase occurs in 5 to 10 minutes. The duration of action is 1 hour.

Side Effects and Adverse Reactions. Allergic reactions can complicate thrombolytic therapy. Anaphylaxis (vascular collapse) occurs more frequently with streptokinase than with the other thrombolytics. If the drugs are administered through an intracoronary catheter after MI, reperfusion dysrhythmia or hemorrhagic infarction at the myocardial necrotic area can result. The major complication of thrombolytic drugs is hemorrhage. The antithrombolytic drug aminocaproic acid is used to stop bleeding by inhibiting plasminogen activation, which inhibits thrombolysis.

Table 40.4 lists the thrombolytic drugs and their dosages, uses, and considerations.

! TABLE 40.4 Thrombolytics

Drug	Route and Dosage	Uses and Considerations
Thrombolytics		
Tenecteplase	A: IV: *Max:* 30-50 mg bolus over 5 s; administer within 30 min of arrival to hospital; *max:* 50 mg/dose	To promote fibrinolysis associated with coronary artery thrombosis and AMI. May cause bleeding, hematoma. Pregnancy category: C*; PB: UK; t½: 20 to 24 min
Alteplase	See Prototype Drug Chart 40.3.	
Plasminogen Inactivators		
Aminocaproic acid	A: PO/IV: LD: 4-5 g over first h; follow with 1 g/h for 8 h or until bleeding is controlled; *max:* 30 g/d	To control excessive bleeding and hyperfibrinolysis. May cause orthostatic hypotension, dysrhythmias, headache, vision impairment, dizziness, GI distress, and thrombocytopenia. Pregnancy category: C*; PB: 0%; t½: 2 h

*Pregnancy categories have been revised. See http://www.fda.gov/Drugs/DevelopmentApprovalProcess/DevelopmentResources/Labeling/ucm093307.htm for more information.

A, Adult; *AMI*, acute myocardial infarction; *d*, day; *GI*, gastrointestinal; *h*, hour; *IV*, intravenous; *LD*, loading dose; *max*, maximum; *min*, minutes; *PB*, protein binding; *PO*, by mouth; *s*, seconds; *t½*, half-life; *UK*, unknown.

◎ NURSING PROCESS
Patient-Centered Collaborative Care
Thrombolytics

Assessment
- Assess baseline vital signs for comparison with future values.
- Check baseline complete blood count (CBC), PT, or INR values before administration of thrombolytics.
- Obtain a medical and drug history. Contraindications for use of thrombolytics include recent CVA, active bleeding, severe hypertension, and anticoagulant therapy. Report if a patient takes aspirin or NSAIDs. Thrombolytics are contraindicated for patients with a recent history of traumatic injury, especially head injury.

Nursing Diagnoses
- Cardiac Output, Decreased related to excessive bleeding
- Anxiety related to fear of the unknown secondary to coronary artery disease
- Tissue Integrity, Impaired related to a thrombus or embolus secondary to heart attack or stroke
- Injury, Risk for

Planning
- The patient's blood clot will be dissolved.
- The patient's vital signs will be monitored for stability during and after thrombolytic therapy.
- The patient will not have excessive bleeding from thrombolytic therapy.

Nursing Interventions
- Monitor vital signs. Increased pulse rate followed by decreased blood pressure usually indicates blood loss and impending shock. Record vital signs, and report changes.
- Observe for signs and symptoms of active bleeding from the mouth or rectum. Hemorrhage is a serious complication of thrombolytic treatment. Aminocaproic acid can be given as an intervention to stop bleeding.
- ⚡ Examine the patient for active bleeding for 24 hours after thrombolytic therapy has been discontinued: this should be done every 15 minutes for the first hour, and then every 30 minutes until the eighth hour, and then hourly.
- ⚡ Observe for signs of allergic reaction to thrombolytics, such as itching, hives, flushing, fever, dyspnea, bronchospasm, hypotension, and/or cardiovascular collapse.
- Avoid administering aspirin or NSAIDs for pain or discomfort when the patient is receiving a thrombolytic. Acetaminophen can be substituted.
- Monitor the electrocardiogram (ECG) for presence of reperfusion dysrhythmias as the blood clot is dissolving; antidysrhythmic therapy may be indicated.
- Avoid venipuncture/arterial sticks.

Patient Teaching
General
- Explain thrombolytic treatment to patients and family. Be supportive.
Side Effects
- Advise patients to report any side effects such as lightheadedness, dizziness, palpitations, nausea, pruritus, or urticaria.

⊕ Cultural Considerations
- If a patient from a different cultural background does not comply with a drug regimen, consult a health care provider of similar background, and provide a written plan in the language the patient speaks and reads most easily.

Evaluation
- Determine the effectiveness of drug therapy: the clot should have dissolved, and vital signs should be stable with no signs or symptoms of active bleeding, and the patient is pain free.

CRITICAL THINKING CASE STUDY

TM, a 57-year-old man, has thrombophlebitis in the right lower leg. IV heparin, 5000 units by bolus, was given. Following the IV bolus, heparin 5000 units given subcutaneously every 6 hours was prescribed. Other therapeutic means to decrease pain and alleviate swelling and redness were also prescribed, and an aPTT test was ordered.

1. Was TM's heparin order within the safe daily dosage range?
2. What are the various methods for administering heparin?
3. Why was an aPTT test ordered? How would you determine whether TM is within the desired range? Explain your answer.

    After 5 days of heparin therapy, TM was prescribed oral warfarin 5 mg daily. An INR test was ordered.

4. What is the pharmacologic action of warfarin? Is the warfarin dose within the safe daily dosage range? Explain your answer.
5. What are the half-life and protein binding for warfarin? If a patient takes a drug that is highly protein bound, would there be a drug interaction? Explain your answer.
6. Why was an INR ordered for TM? What is the desired range?
7. What serious adverse reactions could result with prolonged use or large doses of warfarin?
8. What patient teaching interventions should the nurse include? List three interventions.
9. Months later, TM has hematemesis. What nursing action should be taken?

NCLEX STUDY QUESTIONS

1. A patient is placed on heparin, and the nurse acknowledges that heparin is effective for preventing clot formation in patients who have which disorder(s)? (Select all that apply.)
    a. Coronary thrombosis
    b. Acute myocardial infarction
    c. Deep vein thrombosis
    d. Hemorrhagic stroke
    e. Disseminated intravascular coagulation

2. A patient who received heparin begins to bleed. The nurse anticipates that the health care provider will order which antidote?
    a. Protamine sulfate
    b. Phytonadione
    c. Aminocaproic acid
    d. Potassium chloride

3. A patient is prescribed enoxaparin. The nurse knows that low–molecular-weight heparin has what kind of half-life?
    a. A longer half-life than heparin
    b. A shorter half-life than heparin
    c. The same half-life as heparin
    d. A four-times shorter half-life than heparin

4. The nurse is teaching a patient about clopidogrel. Which information will the nurse include in the patient's teaching plan?
    a. Constipation may occur.
    b. Hypotension may occur.
    c. Bleeding may increase when taken with aspirin.
    d. Normal dose is 25-mg tablet per day.

5. A patient had an orthopedic surgery and is prescribed enoxaparin. What would the nurse teach the patient and/or family members about this low–molecular-weight heparin before discharge?
    a. How to administer the medication intramuscularly
    b. Prothrombin time and international normalized ratio monitoring will be done weekly.
    c. Avoidance of green leafy vegetables is recommended.
    d. Watch for bleeding or excessive bruising.

6. A patient is being changed from an injectable anticoagulant to an oral anticoagulant. Which anticoagulant does the nurse realize is administered orally?
    a. Enoxaparin
    b. Warfarin
    c. Bivalirudin
    d. Dalteparin

7. A patient is taking warfarin 5 mg/day for atrial fibrillation. The patient's international normalized ratio is 3.8. The nurse would consider the international normalized ratio to be what?
    a. Within normal range
    b. Elevated range
    c. Low range
    d. Low-average range

8. Cilostazol is being prescribed for a patient with coronary artery disease. The nurse understands that which of the following is the major purpose for antiplatelet drug therapy?
    a. Dissolve the blood clot
    b. Decrease tissue necrosis
    c. Inhibit hepatic synthesis of vitamin K
    d. Suppress platelet aggregation

9. A patient is to undergo a coronary angioplasty. The nurse acknowledges that which drug is used primarily for preventing reocclusion of coronary arteries following coronary angioplasty?
    a. Clopidogrel
    b. Abciximab
    c. Warfarin
    d. Cilostazol

10. A patient is admitted to the emergency department with an acute myocardial infarction. Which drug does the nurse expect the health care provider to order for prevention of tissue necrosis following blood clot blockage in a coronary artery?
    a. Heparin sodium
    b. Clopidogrel
    c. Alteplase
    d. Aminocaproic acid

Answers: 1, a, b, c, d, e; 2, a; 3, a; 4, c; 5, d; 6, b; 7, b; 8, d; 9, b; 10, c.

41

Antihyperlipidemics and Drugs to Improve Peripheral Blood Flow

ⓔ http://evolve.elsevier.com/McCuistion/pharmacology/

OBJECTIVES

- Describe the action of the two main drug groups: antihyperlipidemics and drugs that improve peripheral blood flow.
- Compare the side effects and adverse reactions of antihyperlipidemics.
- Differentiate the side effects and adverse reactions of peripheral vasodilators and blood viscosity reducer agents.
- Apply the nursing process, including patient teaching, for antihyperlipidemics and blood viscosity reducer agents.

OUTLINE

KEY TERMS

Various drugs are used to maintain or decrease blood lipid concentrations and promote dilation of vessels. Drugs that lower blood lipids are called *antihyperlipidemics, antilipidemics, antilipemics,* and *hypolipidemics.* In this chapter, drugs used to lower lipoproteins are called antihyperlipidemics. Drugs that improve blood flow are called peripheral vasodilators as they dilate vessels that have been narrowed by vasospasm and blood viscosity reducer agents, which decrease viscosity of blood and increase erythrocyte flexibility.

LIPOPROTEINS

Lipids—cholesterol, triglycerides, and phospholipids—are bound in the inner shell of protein, a carrier that transports lipids in the bloodstream. When there is an excess of one or more lipids in the blood, the condition is known as hyperlipidemia or *hyperlipoproteinemia.* The four major categories of lipoprotein are high-density lipoprotein (HDL), low-density lipoprotein (LDL), very-low-density lipoprotein (VLDL), and chylomicrons. HDL, also known as "friendly" or "good" lipoprotein, is the smallest and densest lipoprotein, meaning that it contains more protein and less fat than the others. The function of HDL is to remove cholesterol from the bloodstream and deliver it to the liver for excretion in bile. LDL, the "bad" lipoprotein, contains 50% to 60% of cholesterol in the bloodstream. With an elevated LDL, the risk is greater for developing atherosclerotic plaques and heart disease. VLDL carries mostly triglycerides and less cholesterol. The chylomicrons are large particles that transport fatty acids and cholesterol to the liver. They are composed mostly of triglycerides.

Serum cholesterol and triglyceride measurements are frequently part of a regular physical examination or readmission evaluation and are used as baseline test results. If the levels are high, a 12- to 14-hour fasting lipid profile may be ordered. When cholesterol, triglycerides, and LDL are elevated, the patient is at increased risk for coronary artery disease (CAD). Table 41.1 lists the various serum lipids and their reference values (normal serum levels) according to risk classification.

TABLE 41.1 Serum Lipid Values

Lipids	Desirable (mg/dL)	LEVEL OF RISK FOR CAD		
		Low Risk (mg/dL)	Moderate Risk (mg/dL)	High Risk (mg/dL)
Cholesterol	150-200	200	200-240	>240
Triglycerides	40-150	Values vary with age.	Values vary with age.	>190
Lipoproteins				
LDL	<100	100-130	130-159	>160
HDL	>60	50-60	35-50	<35

CAD, Coronary artery disease; *HDL,* high-density lipoproteins; *LDL,* low-density lipoproteins; >, greater than; <, less than.

APOLIPOPROTEINS

Apolipoproteins are within the lipoprotein shell and contain apolipoprotein (apo) A-1, B, and E. The major component of apoA-1 is HDL. The major component of apoB is LDL, which exists in two forms, apoB-100 and apoB-48. ApoB-100 has VLDL as well as LDL and is a better indicator of risk for CAD than LDL alone.

NONPHARMACOLOGIC METHODS OF CHOLESTEROL REDUCTION

Before drugs to lower LDL and raise HDL are prescribed, non-drug therapy should be initiated to decrease cholesterol. Saturated fats and cholesterol in the diet should be reduced. Total fat intake should be 30% or less of caloric intake, and cholesterol intake should be 300 mg/day or less. The patient should be advised to read labels on containers and buy appropriate foods. Patients should choose lean meats, especially chicken and fish.

In many cases, diet alone will not lower blood lipid levels. Because 75% to 85% of serum cholesterol is endogenously (internally) derived, dietary modification alone will typically lower total cholesterol levels by only 10% to 30%. This and the fact that adherence to dietary restrictions is often short-lived explains why many patients do not respond to diet modification alone.

Exercise is an important aspect of the nonpharmacologic method to reduce cholesterol and increase HDL. For the older adult, exercise can be walking and bicycling. Smoking is another risk factor that should be eliminated. Smoking increases LDL cholesterol and decreases HDL.

If nonpharmacologic methods are ineffective for reducing LDL and VLDL cholesterol, and hyperlipidemia remains, anti-hyperlipidemic drugs are prescribed to lower blood lipid levels. It must be emphasized to the patient that dietary changes need to be made, and an exercise program followed, even after drug therapy is initiated. The type of antihyperlipidemics ordered depends on the lipoprotein phenotype (Table 41.2).

ANTIHYPERLIPIDEMICS

Drugs that lower lipid levels include bile-acid sequestrants, fibrates (fibric acid), nicotinic acid, cholesterol absorption inhibitors, and hepatic 3-hydroxy-3-methylglutaryl-coenzyme A (HMG-CoA) reductase inhibitors, better known as *statins*. The statin drugs have fewer adverse effects and are well tolerated.

One of the first antihyperlipidemics, cholestyramine is a bile-acid sequestrant that reduces LDL cholesterol (LDL-C) levels by binding with bile acids in the intestine. It is effective against hyperlipidemia type II. This group may be used as an adjunct to the statins. The drug comes in a gritty powder that is mixed thoroughly in water or juice. Colestipol is another resin antihyperlipidemic similar to cholestyramine. Both are effective in lowering cholesterol. Colesevelam, another bile acid sequestrant similar to cholestyramine and colestipol, is an agent that has fewer side effects (less constipation, flatulence, and cramping). Colesevelam also has less effect on the absorption of fat-soluble vitamins than the older agents and is usually the first-choice bile-acid sequestrant drug.

Gemfibrozil is a fibric acid derivative that is more effective for reducing triglyceride and VLDL levels than for reducing LDL. It is used primarily to reduce hyperlipidemia type IV, but it can also be used for type II hyperlipidemia. This drug is highly protein bound and should not be taken with anticoagulants because they compete for protein sites. The anticoagulant dose should be reduced during antihyperlipidemic therapy, and the international normalized ratio (INR) should be closely monitored. Fenofibrate has similar actions and some of the same side effects as gemfibrozil. If taken with warfarin, bleeding might occur. Both fenofibrate and gemfibrozil are highly protein bound.

Niacin (vitamin B3) reduces VLDL and LDL. Niacin is actually very effective at lowering cholesterol levels, and its effect on the lipid profile is highly desirable. Because it has numerous side effects and large doses are required, as few as 20% of patients can initially tolerate niacin. However, with proper counseling, careful drug titration, and concomitant use of aspirin, this number can be increased to as much as 60% to 70%.

Ezetimibe is a cholesterol absorption inhibitor that acts on the cells in the small intestine to inhibit cholesterol absorption. It decreases cholesterol from dietary absorption, reducing serum cholesterol, LDL, triglycerides, and apoB levels. Ezetimibe causes only a small increase in HDL. It must be combined with a statin (e.g., simvastatin) for optimum effect.

Statins

The statin drugs inhibit the enzyme HMG-CoA reductase in cholesterol biosynthesis, thus statins are called *HMG-CoA reductase inhibitors*. By inhibiting cholesterol synthesis in the liver, this group of antihyperlipidemics decreases the concentration of cholesterol, decreases LDL, and slightly increases HDL cholesterol. Reduction of LDL cholesterol may be seen as early

TABLE 41.2 Hyperlipidemia: Lipoprotein Phenotype

Type*	Major Lipids
I	Increased chylomicrons and increased triglycerides; uncommon
IIA	Increased low-density lipoprotein (LDL) and increased cholesterol; common
IIB	Increased very low-density lipoprotein (VLDL), increased LDL, increased cholesterol and triglycerides; very common
III	Moderately increased cholesterol and triglycerides; uncommon
IV	Increased VLDL and markedly increased triglycerides; very common
V	Increased chylomicrons, VLDL, and triglycerides; uncommon

*Types II and IV are commonly associated with coronary artery disease.

as 2 weeks after initiating therapy. The statin group has been useful in decreasing CAD and reducing mortality rates.

Numerous statins have been approved since statins were first introduced. The present group of statins includes atorvastatin calcium, fluvastatin, lovastatin, pravastatin sodium, simvastatin, and rosuvastatin. Lovastatin was the first statin used to decrease cholesterol. It is effective for lowering LDL (hyperlipidemia type II) within several weeks. Gastrointestinal (GI) disturbances, headaches, muscle cramps, and fatigue are early complaints. With all statins, serum liver enzymes should be monitored, and an annual eye examination is needed because cataract formation may result. The patient should report immediately any muscle aches or weakness, which can lead to rhabdomyolysis, a muscle disintegration that can become fatal.

The statins have actions in decreasing serum cholesterol, LDL, VLDL, and triglycerides, and they slightly elevate HDL. Atorvastatin, lovastatin, rosuvastatin, and simvastatin are more effective at lowering LDL than the other statins. Rosuvastatin and atorvastatin are at the top of the list of most prescribed drugs in the United States.

The statin drugs can be combined with other drugs to decrease blood pressure and blood clotting and to enhance the antihyperlipidemic effect. Examples are atorvastatin and amlodipine, simvastatin and ezetimibe, and atorvastatin and ezetimibe. Table 41.3 lists these combination drugs and their dosages, uses, and considerations.

If antihyperlipidemic therapy is withdrawn, cholesterol and LDL levels return to pretreatment levels. The patient taking an antihyperlipidemic drug should understand that antihyperlipidemic therapy is a lifetime commitment for maintaining a decrease in serum lipid levels. Abruptly stopping the statin drug could cause a threefold rebound effect that may cause death from acute myocardial infarction (AMI).

Laboratory Tests

Reference values for homocysteine, an amino acid, are 4 to 17 mmol/L (fasting). Homocysteine is a by-product of protein and is found in eggs, chicken, beef, and cheddar cheese. A high level of homocysteine has been linked to cardiovascular disease, stroke, and Alzheimer disease. It may also promote

blood clotting, and it has been stated that an increase in serum homocysteine can damage the inner lining of blood vessels and promote a thickening and loss of flexibility in the vessel. Three vitamins that can lower serum homocysteine levels are vitamin B6 (pyridoxine), vitamin B12 (cyanocobalamin), and folic acid.

High-sensitivity C-reactive protein (hsCRP) reference values are less than 0.175 mg/L; low risk is less than 1 mg/L, moderate risk is 1 to 3 mg/L, and high risk is less than 3 mg/L. The standard C-reactive protein (CRP) is produced in the liver in response to tissue injury and inflammation. The hsCRP is a highly sensitive test for detecting the inflammatory protein that can be associated with cardiovascular and peripheral vascular disease. This test is frequently ordered along with cholesterol screening. Approximately one third of persons who have had a heart attack have normal cholesterol levels and normal blood pressure. A positive hsCRP test can indicate that the patient is at high risk for CAD, making it a valuable test for predicting CAD. This test can detect an inflammatory process caused by the buildup of atherosclerotic plaque in the arterial system, particularly the coronary arteries.

Prototype Drug Chart 41.1 lists the pharmacologic data for a frequently prescribed antihyperlipidemic, rosuvastatin.

Pharmacokinetics Rosuvastatin decreases LDL by 46% at a dose of 10 mg. It is highly protein bound, so it usually is prescribed as a once-daily dose. Rosuvastatin has a half-life of 20 hours.

Pharmacodynamics The positive effect of lowering lipids with rosuvastatin is seen in about 2 weeks. The peak time after a dose of rosuvastatin is 3 to 5 hours; however, it takes 2 to 4 weeks to achieve therapeutic effect. When the patient is taking high doses of rosuvastatin or any other statin, myopathy and rhabdomyolysis—disintegration of striated muscle fibers—may occur. If the patient complains of muscle pain or tenderness, it should be reported immediately.

Side Effects and Adverse Reactions. Side effects and adverse reactions of cholestyramine include constipation and peptic ulcer. Constipation can be decreased or alleviated by increasing intake of fluids and foods high in fiber. Early signs of peptic ulcer are nausea and abdominal discomfort, followed later by abdominal pain and distension. To avoid GI discomfort, the drug must be taken with and followed by sufficient fluids.

The many side effects of niacin—which include GI disturbances, flushing of the skin, abnormal liver function (elevated serum liver enzymes), hyperglycemia, and hyperuricemia—decrease its usefulness. However, as mentioned, aspirin and careful drug titration can reduce side effects to a manageable level in most patients.

The statin drugs can cause a dose-related increase in liver enzyme levels. Serum liver enzyme levels (alkaline phosphatase [ALP], alanine aminotransferase [ALT], gamma-glutamyl transferase [GGT]) should be monitored. Baseline liver enzyme studies should be obtained before initiating statin therapy. A slight transient increase in serum liver enzyme levels may be within normal range for the patient, but it should be rechecked in 1 week or so. Patients with acute hepatic disorders should not take a statin drug.

The serious skeletal muscle adverse effect, rhabdomyolysis, has been reported with use of the statin drug class, although it is rare. Patients should be advised to promptly report to the health

TABLE 41.3 Antihyperlipidemics

Generic	Route and Dosage	Uses and Considerations
BILE-ACID SEQUESTRANTS		
Cholestyramine	A: PO: Initially 4 g 1-2 times daily before meals; mix powder in 60-180 mL of fluid; maint: 4-16 g daily in 2 divided doses; *max:* 24 g daily Adol: PO: Initially, 2-4 g bid; maint: 8 g/d in 2 divided doses ac; *max:* 8 g daily C >6 y: PO: 80 mg/kg/d tid; *max:* 8 g daily	For hypercholesterolemia and hyperlipoproteinemia. May cause GI upset, constipation, steatorrhea, osteoporosis, vitamin A, D, or K deficiency, and bleeding. Pregnancy category: C*; PB: UK; t½: UK
Colesevelam	A: PO: Initially 3 tabs (625 mg/tab) bid or 6 tabs daily with liquid and meals; maint: 4-6 tabs daily; *max:* 7 tabs daily	For hypercholesterolemia and hyperlipoproteinemia. May cause headache, dyspepsia, constipation, weakness, and hypertriglyceridemia. Pregnancy category: B*; PB: UK; t½: UK
Colestipol hydrochloride	A: PO: Initially 5 g/d or bid, may increase at 1- to 2-month intervals; maint: 5-20 g daily in divided doses; *max:* 30 g daily	For hypercholesterolemia and hyperlipoproteinemia. May cause headache, constipation, GI distress, vitamin K deficiency, and GI bleeding. Pregnancy category: C*; PB: UK; t½: UK
FIBRATES (FIBRIC ACID)		
Fenofibrate	A: PO: 50-150 mg daily with meals; *max:* 150 mg daily	For hypercholesterolemia and hypertriglyceridemia. May cause dizziness, headache, weakness, abdominal pain, pulmonary embolus, and photosensitivity. Pregnancy category: C*; PB: 99%; t½: 20 h
Gemfibrozil	A: PO: 600 mg bid 30 min before morning and evening meals; *max:* 1200 mg daily	For hyperlipoproteinemia and hypertriglyceridemia. May cause dizziness, headache, dyspepsia, abdominal pain, cholelithiasis, and diarrhea. Pregnancy category: C*; PB: 95%; t½: 1.5 h
NIACIN		
Niacin	A: PO: Initially 250 mg daily following evening meal; may increase q4-7d; maint: 1.5-3 g daily after meals in 3 divided doses; *max:* 6 g daily	For atherosclerosis, hyperlipoproteinemia, and hypertriglyceridemia. May cause warmth, flushing, hypotension, dizziness, headache, cough, pruritus, GI distress, hyperglycemia, and elevated hepatic enzymes. Pregnancy category: C*; PB: <20%; t½: 20-48 min
CHOLESTEROL ABSORPTION INHIBITORS		
Ezetimibe	A/adol/C >10 y: PO: 10 mg daily; *max:* 10 mg daily	For hypercholesterolemia and hyperlipoproteinemia. May cause diarrhea, arthralgia, abdominal and back pain, URI, and rhabdomyolysis. Pregnancy category: C*; PB: 90%; t½: 22 h
STATINS (HMG-CoA REDUCTASE INHIBITORS)		
Atorvastatin calcium	A: PO: Initially 10-20 mg daily; maint: 10-80 mg daily; *max:* 80 mg daily Adol/C >10 y: PO: 10 mg daily; *max:* 20 mg daily	For hypercholesterolemia, hyperlipoproteinemia, and hypertriglyceridemia. May cause insomnia, dyspepsia, nausea, diarrhea, abdominal pain, arthralgia, myalgia, nasopharyngitis, diabetes mellitus, increased hepatic enzymes, renal dysfunction, and rhabdomyolysis. Pregnancy category: X*; PB: 98%; t½: 14 h
Fluvastatin sodium	Regular release: A: PO: Initially 20-40 mg daily at bedtime; maint: 20-80 mg daily; *max:* 40 mg bid Adol/C >10 y: PO: Initially 20 mg daily; maint: 20-40 mg daily; *max:* 80 mg daily Extended release: A/C >10 y: PO: 20-80 mg daily; *max:* 80 mg daily	For hypercholesterolemia, hyperlipoproteinemia, and hypertriglyceridemia. May cause headache, abdominal pain, dyspepsia, diarrhea, constipation, myalgia, elevated hepatic enzymes, and rhabdomyolysis. Pregnancy category: X*; PB: 98%; t½: Immediate release 2.5-2.7 h, extended release 9 h
Lovastatin	Immediate release: A: PO: 10-20 mg daily with evening meal; maint: 10-80 mg daily; *max:* 80 mg daily Adol/C >10 y: PO: Initially 10-20 mg daily with evening meal; maint: 10-40 mg daily; *max:* 40 mg daily Extended release: A: PO: 20-60 mg daily at bedtime; *max:* 60 mg daily	For atherosclerosis, hypercholesterolemia, and hyperlipoproteinemia. May cause headache, sinusitis, infection, flatulence, arthralgia, back pain, weakness, erectile dysfunction, elevated hepatic enzymes, and rhabdomyolysis. Pregnancy category: X*; PB: 95%; t½: 1.1-1.7 h
Pravastatin sodium	A: PO: Initially 40 mg daily; maint: 10-80 mg daily; *max:* 80 mg daily Adol 14-18 y: PO: 40 mg daily C 8-13 y: PO: 20 mg daily	For atherosclerosis, hypercholesterolemia, hyperlipoproteinemia, and hypertriglyceridemia. May cause headache, GI distress, fatigue, muscular-skeletal pain, elevated hepatic enzymes, and rhabdomyolysis. Pregnancy category: X*; PB: 50%; t½: 2-3 h

Continued

TABLE 41.3   Antihyperlipidemics—cont'd

Generic	Route and Dosage	Uses and Considerations
STATINS (HMG-CoA REDUCTASE INHIBITORS)		
Rosuvastatin	See Prototype Drug Chart 41.1.	
Simvastatin	A: PO: Initially 10-20 mg daily in evening; maint: 5-40 mg daily in evening; *max:* 40 mg daily Adol/C >10 y: PO: Initially 10 mg daily in evening; maint: 10-40 mg daily; *max:* 40 mg daily	For hypercholesterolemia, hyperlipoproteinemia, and hypertriglyceridemia. May cause headache, dizziness, sinusitis, insomnia, edema, GI distress, constipation, myalgia, elevated hepatic enzymes, rhabdomyolysis, URI, and atrial fibrillation. Pregnancy category: X*; PB: 95%; t½: 1.9 h
Pitavastatin	A: PO: Initially 2 mg daily; maint: 1-4 mg daily; *max:* 4 mg daily	For hypercholesterolemia, hyperlipoproteinemia, and hypertriglyceridemia. May cause myalgia, back pain, constipation, diarrhea, and elevated hepatic enzymes. Pregnancy category: X*; PB: 99%; t½: 12 h
MISCELLANEOUS ANTILIPEMICS		
Icosapent ethyl	A: PO: 2 g q12h; *max:* 4 g daily with food	For hypertriglyceridemia. May cause arthralgia, prolonged bleeding time, ecchymosis, and epistaxis. Pregnancy category: C*; PB: 99%; t½: 89 h
Lomitapide	A: PO: Initially 5 mg daily 2 h after evening meal, may increase to 10 mg in 2 wk; maint: 10-60 mg daily; *max:* 60 mg daily	For hypercholesterolemia. May cause dizziness, fatigue, chest pain, GI distress, steatosis, weight loss, flatulence, elevated liver enzymes, nasopharyngitis, and influenza. Pregnancy category: X*; PB: 99.8%; t½: 39.7 h
Mipomersen	A: Subcut: 200 mg/wk; *max:* 200 mg/wk	For hypercholesterolemia. May cause headache, fatigue, nausea, injection site reaction, antibody formation, erythema, elevated hepatic enzymes, and influenza, Pregnancy category: B*; PB: 90%; t½: 1-2 mo
Alirocumab	A: Subcut: Initially 75 mg q2wk; *max:* 150 mg q2wk	For hypercholesterolemia. May cause myalgia, diarrhea, antibody formation, infection, injection site reaction, nasopharyngitis, and influenza. Pregnancy category: NA*; PB: UK; t½: 17-20 d
Evolocumab	A: Subcut: 140 mg q2wk or 420 mg q1mo; *max:* 420 mg/mo	For atherosclerosis and hypercholesterolemia. May cause dizziness, headache, infection, influenza, arthralgia, myalgia, diarrhea, and injection site reaction. Pregnancy category: NA*; PB: UK; t½: 11-17 d
COMBINATION ANTIHYPERLIPIDEMIC DRUGS		
Amlodipine and atorvastatin	A: PO: Initially 5-10 mg amlodipine and 10-20 mg atorvastatin daily; maint: 10 mg amlodipine and 10-80 mg atorvastatin daily; *max:* 10 mg amlodipine and 80 mg atorvastatin daily	For hypercholesterolemia, hyperlipoproteinemia, and hypertriglyceridemia. May cause headache, fatigue, nasopharyngitis, nausea, diarrhea, arthralgia, and peripheral edema. Pregnancy category: X*; PB: amlodipine 93%, atorvastin 98%; t½: amlodipine 30-50 h, atorvastin 14 h
Ezetimibe and simvastatin	A: PO: Initially 10 mg ezetimibe and 10-20 mg simvastatin daily; maint: 10 mg ezetimibe and 40 mg simvastatin daily; *max:* 10 mg ezetimibe and 40 mg simvastatin daily	For hypercholesterolemia and hyperlipoproteinemia. May cause headache, diarrhea, myalgia, URI, influenza, elevated hepatic enzymes, and rhabdomyolysis. Pregnancy category: X*; PB: ezetimibe 90%, simvastatin 95%; t½: ezetimibe 22 h, simvastatin 1.9 h
Ezetimibe and atorvastatin	A: PO: Initially 10 mg ezetimibe and 10-20 mg atorvastatin daily; maint: 10 mg ezetimibe and 10-80 mg atorvastatin daily; *max:* 10 mg ezetimibe and 80 mg atorvastatin daily	For hypercholesterolemia and hyperlipoproteinemia. May cause pharyngitis, dyspepsia, arthralgia, and elevated hepatic enzymes. Pregnancy category: X*; PB: ezetimibe 90%, atorvastatin 98%; t½: ezetimibe 22 h, atorvastatin 14 h

*Pregnancy categories have been revised. See http://www.fda.gov/Drugs/DevelopmentApprovalProcess/DevelopmentResources/Labeling/ucm093307.htm for more information.

A, Adult; *ac,* before meals; *adol,* adolescent; *bid,* twice a day; *C,* child; *d,* day; *GI,* gastrointestinal; *h,* hour; *HMG-CoA,* 3-hydroxy-3-methylglutaryl-coenzyme A; *maint,* maintenance; *max,* maximum; *min,* minute; *mo,* months; *NA,* not applicable; *PB,* protein binding; *PO,* by mouth; *q,* every; *subcut,* subcutaneously; *t½,* half-life; *tab,* tablet; *tid,* three times a day; *UK,* unknown; *URI,* upper respiratory infection; *wk,* weeks; *y,* year; *<,* less than; *>,* greater than.

PROTOTYPE DRUG CHART 41.1

Rosuvastatin

Drug Class	Dosage
Antihyperlipidemic: HMG-CoA reductase inhibitor Pregnancy category: X*	A: PO: Initially 5-10 mg daily; maint: 5-40 mg/d; *max:* 40 mg daily
Contraindications	**Drug-Lab-Food Interactions**
Hepatic disease, pregnancy, breastfeeding *Caution:* Alcoholism, diabetes mellitus, seizures, renal impairment, Asian population, older adults	Drug: Decreased effect with antacids, phenytoin, and propranolol; may increase digoxin level, oral contraceptive efficacy; increased drug effects with macrolide antibiotics and antifungals
Pharmacokinetics	**Pharmacodynamics**
Absorption: Rapid Distribution: PB: 88% Metabolism: t½: 20 h Excretion: Primarily in feces	PO: Onset: UK Peak: 3-5 h Duration: UK
Therapeutic Effects/Uses	
To decrease cholesterol levels and serum lipids, especially LDL and triglycerides, for treatment of atherosclerosis, hypercholesterolemia, hyperlipoproteinemia, and hypertriglyceridemia. Mode of action: Inhibits HMG-CoA reductase, the enzyme necessary for hepatic production of cholesterol	
Side Effects	**Adverse Reactions**
Headache, flushing, dizziness, weakness, myalgia, arthralgia, abdominal pain, constipation, peripheral neuropathy, photosensitivity	Rhabdomyolysis (rare), myopathy, hyperglycemia, elevated hepatic enzymes, renal failure, hepatotoxicity, leukopenia, thrombocytopenia

*Pregnancy categories have been revised. See http://www.fda.gov/Drugs/DevelopmentApprovalProcess/DevelopmentResources/Labeling/ucm093307.htm for more information.
A, Adult; *d*, day; *h*, hour; *HMG-CoA*, 3-hydroxy-3-methyl glutaryl-coenzyme A; *LDL*, low-density lipoprotein; *maint*, maintenance; *max*, maximum dosage; *PB*, protein binding; *PO*, by mouth; *t½*, half-life; *UK*, unknown.

care provider any unexplained muscle tenderness or weakness, especially if accompanied by fever or malaise. Table 41.3 lists the pharmacologic data for antihyperlipidemics.

 NURSING PROCESS
Patient-Centered Collaborative Care

Antihyperlipidemics (Statins)

Assessment
- Assess vital signs and baseline serum chemistry values (cholesterol, triglycerides, aspartate aminotransferase [AST], ALT, and creatine phosphokinase [CPK]).
- Obtain a medical history. Statin drugs are contraindicated for patients with liver disorders and have been designated pregnancy category X.

Nursing Diagnoses
- Tissue Integrity, Impaired related to atherosclerosis because of hyperlipidemia
- Anxiety related to elevated cholesterol levels because of possible CAD
- Knowledge, Deficient related to inexperience with statin medications

Planning
- The patient's cholesterol level will be less than 200 mg/dL in 6 to 8 weeks.
- The patient will be able to choose foods low in fat, cholesterol, and complex sugars.

Nursing Interventions
- Monitor the patient's blood lipid levels—cholesterol, triglycerides, LDL, and HDL—every 6 to 8 weeks for the first 6 months after statin therapy, then every 3 to 6 months. For a lipid-level profile, the patient should fast for 12 to 14 hours. The desired values are less than 200 mg/dL for cholesterol; less than 150 mg/dL for triglyceride, although this can vary; less than 100 mg/dL for LDL; and more than 60 mg/dL for HDL. Cholesterol levels higher than 240 mg/dL, LDL levels higher than 160 mg/dL, and HDL levels below 35 mg/dL can lead to severe cardiovascular events or cerebrovascular accident (CVA).
- Monitor laboratory tests for liver function (ALT, ALP, and GGT). Antihyperlipidemic drugs can cause liver disorders.
- Observe for signs and symptoms of GI upset. Taking the drug with sufficient water or with meals may alleviate some of the discomfort.

Patient Teaching
General
- Emphasize the need to comply with the drug regimen to lower blood lipids.
- Inform patients that it may take several weeks before blood lipid levels decline.
- Explain that laboratory tests for blood lipids—cholesterol, triglycerides, LDL, and HDL—are usually ordered every 3 to 6 months.
- Advise patients to have serum liver enzymes monitored as indicated by their health care provider. Lovastatin, pravastatin, and simvastatin are contraindicated in acute hepatic disease and pregnancy.

- Instruct patients to have an annual eye examination and to report changes in visual acuity.
- Advise patients taking gemfibrozil that the drug may increase their risk for bleeding if they are also taking an oral anticoagulant, so bleeding should be reported. Drug dosage can be changed, or another antihyperlipidemic may be ordered.
- Instruct patients to take nicotinic acid with meals to decrease GI discomfort.

Self-Administration
- Teach patients to mix cholestyramine/colestipol powder well in water or juice.

Side Effects of Cholestyramine, Colestipol, and Niacin
- Advise patients that constipation may occur with cholestyramine and colestipol. Increasing fluid intake and food bulk should help alleviate the problem.
- Explain to patients that flushing is common with niacin and should decrease with continued use of the drug. Usually the drug is started at a low dose.
- Advise patients that large doses of niacin can cause vasodilation and produce dizziness and faintness (syncope).

Side Effects of Ezetimibe
- Explain to patients that ezetimibe may cause headaches and GI upset. If it continues, notify the health care provider.

Side Effects of Statins
- Explain to patients that serum liver enzyme levels are periodically monitored.
- ⚡ Encourage patients to promptly report any unexplained muscle tenderness or weakness that may be caused by rhabdomyolysis.
- ⚡ Caution patients not to abruptly stop taking their statin drug because a serious rebound effect might occur that could lead to AMI and possible death. Before stopping a statin, the patient should talk to his or her health care provider.

Diet
- Explain to patients that GI discomfort is a common problem with most antihyperlipidemics. Suggest increasing fluid intake when taking the medication.
- Encourage patients to consume foods that are low in animal fats, cholesterol, and complex sugars. Lovastatin and other antihyperlipidemics are adjuncts to, not substitutes for, a low-fat diet.

🌐 Cultural Considerations
- Respect the patient's beliefs about how to control his or her cholesterol level.
- Avoid criticizing traditional practices. Explanations and modifications to the plan of care may be necessary if the method the patient uses is ineffective or unsafe.

Evaluation
- Evaluate effectiveness of the antihyperlipidemic drug. The patient's cholesterol level should be within the desired range.
- Determine that the patient is maintaining a low-fat, low-cholesterol diet.

DRUGS TO IMPROVE PERIPHERAL BLOOD FLOW

A common problem in older adults is peripheral arterial disease (PAD), also called *peripheral vascular disease* (PVD). It is characterized by numbness and coolness of the extremities, claudication (pain and weakness of a limb when walking but no symptoms at rest), and possible leg ulcers. The primary cause is arteriosclerosis and hyperlipidemia, resulting in atherosclerosis, after which the arteries become occluded.

Peripheral vasodilators increase blood flow to the extremities. They are used in peripheral vascular disorders of venous and arterial vessels. They are more effective for disorders that result from vasospasm (Raynaud disease) than from vessel occlusion or arteriosclerosis (arteriosclerosis obliterans, thromboangiitis obliterans [Buerger disease]). In Raynaud disease, cold exposure or emotional upset can trigger vasospasm of the toes and fingers; these patients have benefited from vasodilators. Patients with diabetes mellitus are more likely to have PAD by two to four times the usual rate and are at risk of intermittent claudication.

Individuals with PAD who are treated with HMG-CoA reductase inhibitors (statins) for dyslipidemia may see an improvement in intermittent claudication symptoms as well as a decrease in serum lipids. Also, patients with PAD who are hypertensive see improvement for both conditions when taking the antihypertensive drug ramipril, an angiotensin-converting enzyme (ACE) inhibitor. The alpha blocker prazosin and the calcium channel blocker nifedipine have been used as peripheral vasodilators. The antiplatelet drugs clopidogrel and aspirin have been used to decrease PAD symptoms. Another antiplatelet drug, cilostazol, has been approved by the U.S. Food and Drug Administration (FDA) for treating intermittent claudication. It decreases arterial thrombi. Ginkgo biloba, taken with an antiplatelet drug, has been used to treat intermittent claudication because of its vasodilating and antioxidant effects, although this product has not been approved by the FDA. Most of the drugs used for treating PAD do not cure the health problem, but they can aid in relieving PAD symptoms.

Cilostazol

Cilostazol is an antiplatelet that has a dual purpose of inhibiting platelet aggregation as well as causing vasodilation to treat intermittent claudication. Prototype Drug Chart 41.2 lists the pharmacologic data for cilostazol.

Pharmacokinetics Cilostazol is a direct-acting vasodilator that is absorbed from the GI tract. It has a half-life of 11 to 13 hours and is usually taken two times a day.

Pharmacodynamics Cilostazol causes arterial vasodilation, especially within the femoral vasculature. Common adverse effects include headache, diarrhea, and abnormal stools. This drug has an onset of action within 2 to 12 weeks.

Side Effects and Adverse Reactions. Lightheadedness, dizziness, tachycardia, palpitations, and GI distress may occur. The effectiveness of peripheral vasodilators in increasing blood flow by vasodilation is questionable in the presence of arteriosclerosis. These drugs may decrease some of the symptoms of

PROTOTYPE DRUG CHART 41.2

Cilostazol

Drug Class	Dosage
Direct-acting vasodilator Pregnancy category: C*	A: PO: 50-100 mg q12h 30 min before or 2 h after meals; *max:* 200 mg daily Administer with full glass of water. Do not administer with grapefruit juice.
Contraindications	**Drug-Lab-Food Interactions**
Class III-IV congestive heart failure, hypersensitivity, bleeding disorders, thrombocytopenia *Caution:* Hepatic and renal disease, tobacco smokers, pregnancy, older adults	Drug: Increased effects with aspirin, cimetidine, clarithromycin, erythromycin, enoxaparin, ticlopidine, warfarin Food: Grapefruit and green tea will increase levels; ginger and *Ginkgo biloba* may prolong bleeding time; St. John's wort will decrease effect.
Pharmacokinetics	**Pharmacodynamics**
Absorption: PO: Readily absorbed Distribution: PB: 95%-98% Metabolism: t½: 11-13 h Excretion: In urine (74%), feces (20%)	PO: Onset: 2-12 wk Peak: UK Duration: UK
Therapeutic Effects/Uses	
To treat peripheral vascular disease and intermittent claudication Mode of Action: Acts directly to inhibit platelet aggregation and cause vasodilation, especially in femoral vasculature	
Side Effects	**Adverse Reactions**
Dizziness, headache, nasopharyngitis, nausea, vomiting, flatulence, diarrhea, melena, back and abdominal pain, peripheral edema, increased susceptibility to infection, cough	Tachycardia, palpitations, thrombocytopenia, leucopenia, aplastic anemia, agranulocytosis, elevated hepatic enzymes, dysrhythmias

*Pregnancy categories have been revised. See http://www.fda.gov/Drugs/DevelopmentApprovalProcess/DevelopmentResources/Labeling/ucm093307.htm for more information.
A, Adult; *h,* hour; *max,* maximum dosage; *min,* minutes; *PB,* protein binding; *PO,* by mouth; *q,* every; *t½,* half-life; *UK,* unknown; *wk,* weeks.

TABLE 41.4   Peripheral Vasodilators

Generic	Route and Dosage	Uses and Considerations
DIRECT-ACTING VASODILATORS		
Ergoloid mesylates	A: PO/SL: 1 mg tid; *max:* 3 mg daily	For Alzheimer disease and vascular dementia. May cause dizziness, headache, flushing, nasal congestion, orthostatic hypotension, GI distress, and blurred vision. Pregnancy category: X*; PB: UK; t½: 2.6-5.1 h
Cilostazol	See Prototype Drug Chart 41.2.	
BLOOD VISCOSITY REDUCER AGENT		
Pentoxifylline	Extended release: A: PO: 400 mg tid with meals; *max:* 1200 mg daily	For claudication. May cause nausea, vomiting, areflexia, tachycardia, and GI bleeding. Pregnancy category: C*; PB: UK; t½: 0.4-0.8 h

*Pregnancy categories have been revised. See http://www.fda.gov/Drugs/DevelopmentApprovalProcess/DevelopmentResources/Labeling/ucm093307.htm for more information.
A, Adult; *GI,* gastrointestinal; *h,* hour; *max,* maximum; *PB,* protein binding; *PO,* by mouth; *SL,* sublingual; *t½,* half-life; *tid,* three times a day; *UK,* unknown.

cerebrovascular insufficiency. Table 41.4 lists the peripheral vasodilators and their dosages, uses, and considerations.

Pentoxifylline

Pentoxifylline, classified as a *hemorrheologic agent* or *blood viscosity reducer agent,* improves microcirculation and tissue perfusion by decreasing blood viscosity and improving the flexibility of erythrocytes, thus increasing tissue oxygenation. It inhibits aggregation of platelets and red blood cells, and because it decreases blood viscosity, it helps to increase flow through peripheral vessels. A derivative of the xanthine group,

pentoxifylline has been approved by the FDA for patients with intermittent claudication, and it has been prescribed for those with Buerger disease resulting from arterial occlusions. However, in one research study, pentoxifylline was not determined to be more effective than a placebo.

Reactions to an overdose of pentoxifylline include tachycardia, areflexia, and GI bleeding. The drug should be taken with food, and the patient should avoid smoking because nicotine increases vasoconstriction. Patients taking an antihypertensive drug along with pentoxifylline may need to have the antihypertensive dosage decreased to avoid side effects.

NURSING PROCESS
Patient-Centered Collaborative Care

Peripheral Vasodilators: Cilostazol

Assessment
- Obtain baseline vital signs for future comparison.
- Assess for signs of inadequate blood flow to the extremities: pallor, coldness of extremities, and pain.

Nursing Diagnoses
- Tissue Integrity, Impaired related to insufficient blood supply
- Pain, Acute related to inadequate blood flow to extremity

Planning
- Blood flow to the patient's extremities will improve, and pain will be controlled.

Nursing Interventions
- Monitor vital signs, especially blood pressure and heart rate. Tachycardia and orthostatic hypotension can be problematic with peripheral vasodilators.

Patient Teaching
General
- Inform patients that a desired therapeutic response may take 1.5 to 3 months.
- Advise patients not to smoke because smoking increases vasospasm.

- Instruct patients to use aspirin or aspirin-like compounds only with the health care provider's approval. Salicylates help prevent platelet aggregation.

Side Effects
- Encourage patients to change position slowly but frequently to avoid orthostatic hypotension. Orthostatic hypotension is common when taking high doses of a vasodilator.
- Instruct patients to report side effects of cilostazol, such as flushing, headaches, and dizziness.

Diet
- Suggest that patients with GI disturbances take cilostazol with meals.
- Advise patients not to ingest alcohol with a vasodilator because it may cause a hypotensive reaction.

 Cultural Considerations
- Do not assume that lack of eye contact means that a patient is not listening or does not care. It might indicate respect. The more traditional and older individuals in some cultures may not maintain eye contact.

Evaluation
- Evaluate effectiveness of cilostazol therapy; blood flow is increased in extremities, and pain has subsided.
- The patient should experience no side effects from the prescribed drug.

CRITICAL THINKING CASE STUDY

JH had a myocardial infarction (MI) 3 years ago. He was prescribed gemfibrozil 600 mg twice daily before meals, but his cholesterol remained between 220 and 240 mg/dL, and his LDL was 140 mg/dL. His anticholesterol drug was changed to simvastatin 20 mg/day in the evening.

1. How does simvastatin differ from gemfibrozil?
2. Why do you think JH's cholesterol drug, gemfibrozil, was changed to simvastatin?
3. While JH is taking simvastatin, which group of serum levels should be monitored?

4. How long after taking simvastatin should JH's cholesterol and lipoproteins be checked?
5. What is the maximum dose for simvastatin?
6. JH complains of muscle pain and muscle weakness. What might this indicate?
7. Could JH receive both gemfibrozil and simvastatin? Explain your answer.
8. JH is on vacation and does not have enough simvastatin tablets. What should he do?

NCLEX STUDY QUESTIONS

1. A patient has a serum cholesterol level of 265 mg/dL, a triglyceride level of 235 mg/dL, and a low-density lipoprotein of 180 mg/dL. What do these serum levels indicate?
   a. Hypolipidemia
   b. Normolipidemia
   c. Hyperlipidemia
   d. Alipidemia
2. The nurse knows that a patient's total cholesterol level should be within which range?
   a. 150 to 200 mg/dL
   b. 200 to 225 mg/dL
   c. 225 to 250 mg/dL
   d. Greater than 250 mg/dL

3. A patient has a low-density lipoprotein of 175 mg/dL and a high-density lipoprotein of 30 mg/dL. What teaching should the nurse implement for this patient?
   a. Discuss medications ordered, dietary changes, and exercise.
   b. No changes in lifestyle are needed; continue with the current plan.
   c. Discuss how to have fat intake be 40% of caloric intake.
   d. Begin keeping a food diary, and schedule lab work to be repeated in 6 months.

4. Which laboratory test value does the nurse realize can contribute to the development of cardiovascular disease and stroke?
   a. Decreased antidiuretic hormone
   b. Increased homocysteine level
   c. Decreased triglycerides
   d. Increased high-density lipoprotein level

5. A patient is taking lovastatin. Which serum level is most important for the nurse to monitor?
   a. Blood urea nitrogen
   b. Complete blood count
   c. Cardiac enzymes
   d. Hepatic enzymes

6. For what severe skeletal muscle adverse reaction should the nurse observe in a patient taking rosuvastatin?
   a. Myasthenia gravis
   b. Rhabdomyolysis
   c. Dyskinesia
   d. Agranulocytosis

7. A patient is taking ezetimibe and asks the nurse how it works. The nurse should explain that ezetimibe does what?
   a. Inhibits absorption of dietary cholesterol in the intestines
   b. Binds with bile acids in the intestines to reduce low-density lipoprotein levels
   c. Inhibits 3-hydroxy-3-methylglutaryl-coenzyme A reductase, which is necessary for cholesterol production in the liver
   d. Forms insoluble complexes and reduces circulating cholesterol in the blood

8. A patient is diagnosed with peripheral arterial disease. He is prescribed pentoxifylline. What does the nurse realize are the effects of pentoxifylline? (Select all that apply.)
   a. May lead to hypertension and bradycardia
   b. Improves microcirculation and tissue perfusion
   c. Decreases blood viscosity and improves flexibility of erythrocytes
   d. Alleviates intermittent claudication
   e. Commonly causes an adverse effect of rhabdomyolysis
   f. Allows vasodilation of arteries in skeletal muscles

Answers: 1, c; 2, a; 3, a; 4, b; 5, d; 6, b; 7, a; 8, b, c, d.

Gastrointestinal Drugs

The gastrointestinal (GI) system, or GI tract, comprises the alimentary canal and the digestive tract and begins at the oral cavity and ends at the anus. Major structures of the GI system are (1) the oral cavity (mouth, tongue, and pharynx), (2) the esophagus, (3) the stomach, (4) the small intestine (duodenum, jejunum, and ileum), (5) the large intestine (cecum, colon, and rectum), and (6) the anus. The accessory organs and glands that contribute to the digestive process are (1) the salivary glands, (2) the pancreas, (3) the gallbladder, and (4) the liver (Fig. XIII.1). The main functions of the GI system are digestion of food particles and absorption of the digestive contents—nutrients, electrolytes, minerals, and fluids—into the circulatory system for cellular use. Digestion and absorption take place in the small intestine and to a lesser extent in the stomach. Undigested material passes through the lower intestinal tract with the aid of peristalsis to the rectum and anus, where it is excreted as feces, or stool.

ORAL CAVITY

The oral cavity, or mouth, starts the digestive process by (1) breaking up food into smaller particles; (2) adding saliva, which contains the enzyme amylase for digesting starch (the beginning of the digestive process); and (3) swallowing, a voluntary movement of food that becomes involuntary (peristalsis) in the esophagus, stomach, and intestines. Swallowing occurs in the pharynx (throat), which connects the mouth and esophagus.

ESOPHAGUS

The esophagus, a tube that extends from the pharynx to the stomach, is composed of striated muscle in its upper portion and smooth muscle in its lower portion. The inner lining of the esophagus is a mucous membrane that secretes mucus. The peristaltic process of contraction begins in the esophagus and ends in the lower large intestine. There are two sphincters, the *superior esophageal (hyperpharyngeal) sphincter* and the *lower esophageal sphincter.* The lower esophageal sphincter prevents gastric reflux into the esophagus, a condition called *reflux esophagitis.*

STOMACH

The stomach is a hollow organ that lies between the esophagus and the intestine. The body of the stomach has lesser and greater curvatures. It can hold 1000 to 2000 mL of gastric contents and empties in 2 to 6 hours (average is 3 to 4 hours), depending on gastric content and motility. Two sphincters—the *cardiac sphincter,* which lies at the upper opening of the stomach, and the *pyloric sphincter,* located at the lower portion of the stomach or the head of the duodenum—regulate the entrance of food into the stomach.

The interior lining of the stomach has mucosal folds that contain glands that secrete gastric juices. The four types of cells in the stomach mucosa that secrete these juices are (1) *chief cells,* which secrete the proenzyme pepsinogen (pepsin); (2) *parietal cells,* which secrete hydrochloric acid (HCl); (3) *gastrin-producing cells,* which secrete gastrin, a hormone that regulates enzyme release during digestion; and (4) *mucus-producing cells* that release mucus to protect the stomach lining, which extends into the duodenum.

SMALL INTESTINE

The small intestine begins at the pyloric sphincter of the stomach and extends to the ileocecal valve at the cecum. Most drug absorption occurs in the duodenum, but lipid-soluble drugs and alcohol are absorbed from the stomach. The lower digestive process begins in the stomach, but most of the digestive contents are absorbed from the small intestine. The duodenum releases the hormone secretin, which suppresses gastric acid secretion and causes the intestinal juices to have a higher pH than the gastric juices. The intestinal cells also release the hormone cholecystokinin, which in turn stimulates the release of pancreatic enzymes and the contraction of the gallbladder to release bile into the duodenum. Hormones, bile, and pancreatic enzymes (trypsin, chymotrypsin, lipase, and amylase) complete the digestion of carbohydrates, protein, and fat in preparation for absorption.

LARGE INTESTINE

The large intestine accepts undigested material from the small intestine, absorbs water, secretes mucus,

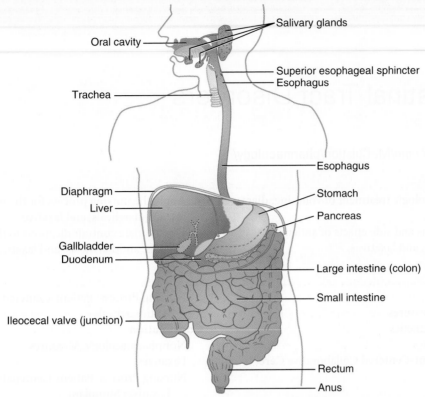

FIG. XIII.1 The Gastrointestinal System and Alimentary Canal.

and with peristaltic contractions moves the remaining intestinal contents to the rectum for elimination. Defecation completes the process.

DRUGS FOR GASTROINTESTINAL DISORDERS

Vomiting, diarrhea, and constipation are GI problems that frequently require drug intervention. Chapter 42, Gastrointestinal Tract Disorders, describes the antiemetics used to control vomiting. This chapter also discusses emetics used to eliminate ingested toxins and drugs, antidiarrheal drugs, and laxatives. The nursing process is considered in relation to each of these drug groups.

Chapter 43, Antiulcer Drugs, discusses drugs used to prevent and treat peptic ulcers, both gastric and duodenal. These drugs include tranquilizers, anticholinergics, antacids, histamine$_2$ blockers, proton pump inhibitors, a pepsin inhibitor, and a prostaglandin analogue antiulcer drug.

42

Gastrointestinal Tract Disorders

OBJECTIVES

- Compare the pharmacologic treatment of vomiting, diarrhea, and constipation.
- Differentiate the actions and side effects of antiemetics, emetics, antidiarrheals, and laxatives.
- Apply the nursing process for the patient taking antiemetics, antidiarrheals, and laxatives.
- Differentiate contraindications to the use of antiemetics, emetics, antidiarrheals, and laxatives.

OUTLINE

Vomiting
   Nonpharmacologic Measures
   Nonprescription Antiemetics
   Prescription Antiemetics
   Nursing Process: Patient-Centered Collaborative Care—
      Antiemetics
Emetics
Diarrhea
   Nonpharmacologic Measures
   Travelers' Diarrhea
   Antidiarrheals

Nursing Process: Patient-Centered Collaborative Care—
     Antidiarrheals
Constipation
   Nonpharmacologic Measures
   Laxatives
   Nursing Process: Patient-Centered Collaborative Care—
      Laxative: Stimulant
   Nursing Process: Patient-Centered Collaborative Care—
      Laxative: Bulk Forming
Critical Thinking Case Study
NCLEX Study Questions

KEY TERMS

adsorbents, p. 612
antidiarrheals, p. 611
antiemetics, p. 605
cannabinoids, p. 609
cathartics, p. 613
chemoreceptor trigger zone (CTZ), p. 604
constipation, p. 613
diarrhea, p. 610

emetics, p. 610
emollients, p. 616
laxatives, p. 613
opiates, p. 611
osmotics, p. 614
purgatives, p. 613
selective chloride channel activators, p. 616
vomiting center, p. 604

Drug groups used to correct or control vomiting, diarrhea, and constipation are antiemetics, emetics, antidiarrheals, and laxatives. Each of these drug groups is discussed separately. Drugs used to treat peptic ulcers are discussed in Chapter 43.

VOMITING

Vomiting (emesis), the expulsion of gastric contents, has a multitude of causes, including motion sickness, viral and bacterial infection, food intolerance, surgery, pregnancy, pain, shock, effects of selected drugs (e.g., antineoplastics, antibiotics), radiation, and disturbances of the middle ear that affect equilibrium. Nausea, a queasy sensation, may or may not precede the expulsion. The cause of the vomiting must be identified. Antiemetics can mask the underlying cause of vomiting and should not be used until the cause has been determined, unless the vomiting is so severe as to cause dehydration and electrolyte imbalance.

Two major cerebral centers—the **chemoreceptor trigger zone (CTZ)**, which lies near the medulla, and the **vomiting center** in the medulla—cause vomiting when stimulated (Fig. 42.1). The CTZ receives most of the impulses from drugs, toxins, and the vestibular center in the ear and transmits them to the vomiting center. The neurotransmitter dopamine stimulates the CTZ, which in turn stimulates the vomiting center. Levodopa, a drug with dopamine-like properties, can cause vomiting by stimulating the CTZ. Some sensory impulses—such as odor, smell, taste, and gastric mucosal irritation—are transmitted directly to the vomiting center. The neurotransmitter acetylcholine is also a vomiting stimulant. When the vomiting center is stimulated, the motor neuron responds by causing contraction of the diaphragm, the anterior abdominal muscles, and the stomach. The glottis closes, the abdominal wall moves upward, and vomiting occurs.

Nonpharmacologic measures should be used first when nausea and vomiting occur. If the nonpharmacologic measures

604

are not effective, antiemetics are combined with nonpharmacologic measures. The two major groups of antiemetics are *nonprescription* (antihistamines, bismuth subsalicylate, and phosphorated carbohydrate solution) and *prescription* (antihistamines, dopamine antagonists, benzodiazepines, serotonin antagonists, glucocorticoids, cannabinoids, and miscellaneous antiemetics).

Nonpharmacologic Measures

The nonpharmacologic methods of decreasing nausea and vomiting include administration of weak tea, flat soda, gelatin, Gatorade, and Pedialyte (for use in children). Crackers and dry toast may be helpful. When dehydration becomes severe, intravenous (IV) fluids are needed to restore body fluid balance.

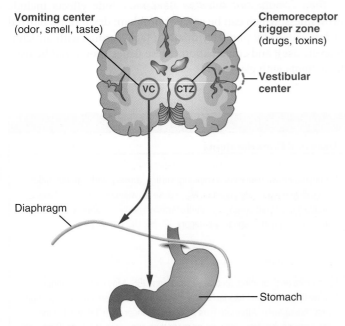

FIG. 42.1 The chemoreceptor trigger zone and vomiting center.

Nonprescription Antiemetics

Nonprescription antiemetics (antivomiting agents) can be purchased as over-the-counter (OTC) drugs. These drugs are frequently used to prevent motion sickness but have minimal effect on controlling severe vomiting resulting from anticancer agents (antineoplastics), radiation, and toxins. To prevent motion sickness, the antiemetic should be taken 30 minutes before travel. These drugs are not effective in relieving motion sickness if taken after vomiting has occurred.

Selected antihistamine antiemetics—such as dimenhydrinate, cyclizine hydrochloride, meclizine hydrochloride, and diphenhydramine hydrochloride—can be purchased without a prescription to prevent nausea, vomiting, and dizziness (vertigo) caused by motion. These drugs inhibit vestibular stimulation in the middle ear. Diphenhydramine is also used to prevent or alleviate allergic reactions to drugs, insects, and food by acting as an antagonist to histamine$_1$ (H$_1$) receptors.

The side effects of antihistamine antiemetics are similar to those of anticholinergics and include drowsiness, dryness of the mouth, and constipation. Table 42.1 lists the nonprescription antiemetics used for vomiting caused by motion sickness. Diphenhydramine characteristics are explained in Prototype Drug Chart 35.1.

Several nonprescription drugs, such as bismuth subsalicylate, act directly on the gastric mucosa to suppress vomiting. They are marketed in liquid and chewable tablet forms and can be taken for gastric discomfort or diarrhea. Phosphorated carbohydrate solution, a hyperosmolar carbohydrate, decreases nausea and vomiting by changing the gastric pH; it may also decrease smooth-muscle contraction of the stomach. Its effectiveness as an antiemetic has not been verified. Patients with diabetes mellitus should avoid this drug because of its high sugar content.

Antiemetics that were once frequently used for the treatment of nausea and vomiting during pregnancy are no longer recommended because they may cause harm to the fetus.

TABLE 42.1	Nonprescription Antiemetics: Antihistamine	
Drug	**Route and Dosage**	**Uses and Considerations**
Motion Sickness		
Cyclizine hydrochloride	A/adol/C >12 y: PO: 50 mg tablet q4-6h, 30 min prior to travel; *max:* 200 mg/d C 6-11 y: PO: 25 mg q6-8h; *max:* 75 mg/d	For prevention and treatment of motion sickness associated with dizziness, nausea, and vomiting. Avoid concurrent alcohol use. May cause drowsiness, blurred vision, fatigue, dry mouth, nasal dryness, headache, and urinary retention. Pregnancy category: B*; PB: UK; t½: 13 h
Dimenhydrinate	A/adol/C >12 y: PO: Initially 50 mg 30-60 min prior to travel; maint: 50-100 mg q4-6h PRN; *max:* 400 mg/d C 6-11 y: PO: 25-50 mg q6-8h PRN; *max:* 150 mg/d C 2-5 y: 12.5-25 mg q6-8h PRN; *max:* 75 mg/d	To prevent and treat motion sickness, dizziness, nausea, and vomiting. May cause drowsiness, dizziness, headache, restlessness, dry mouth and eyes, blurred vision, urinary retention, tachycardia, and hypotension. Pregnancy category: B*; PB: 78%; t½: 3.5 h
Meclizine hydrochloride	Motion sickness: A/adol/C >12 y: PO: 25-50 mg 1 h before travel; may repeat q24h PRN; *max:* 100 mg/d	Prevention and treatment of nausea, vomiting, vertigo, and motion sickness. May cause drowsiness, headache, fatigue, blurred vision, and dry mouth. Pregnancy category: B*; PB: UK; t½: 5-6 h

*Pregnancy categories have been revised. See http://www.fda.gov/Drugs/DevelopmentApprovalProcess/DevelopmentResources/Labeling/ucm093307.htm for more information.

A, Adult; *adol*, adolescent; *C*, child; *d*, day; *h*, hour; *maint*, maintenance dose; *max*, maximum; *min*, minute; *PB*, protein binding; *PO*, by mouth; *PRN*, as needed; *q*, every; *t½*, half-life; *UK*, unknown; *y*, year; *>*, greater than.

Instead, nonpharmacologic methods are used when possible to alleviate nausea and vomiting during pregnancy. Ginger and Red Raspberry leaf tea have been used effectively but are not regulated by the U.S. Food and Drug Administration (FDA). When antiemetics are necessary, a delayed release combination of pyridoxine and doxylamine is usually preferred. If vomiting becomes severe and threatens the well-being of the mother and fetus, an antiemetic such as promethazine or metoclopramide can be administered. Other antiemetics may be prescribed cautiously.

Prescription Antiemetics

Common prescription antiemetics are classified into the following groups: (1) antihistamines, (2) anticholinergics, (3) dopamine antagonists, (4) benzodiazepines, (5) serotonin antagonists, (6) glucocorticoids, (7) cannabinoids (for patients with certain diagnoses, such as cancer), and (8) miscellaneous. Many of these drugs act as antagonists to dopamine, histamine, serotonin, and acetylcholine, which are associated with vomiting. Antihistamines and anticholinergics act primarily on the vomiting center; they also act by decreasing stimulation of the CTZ and vestibular pathways. The cannabinoids act on the cerebral cortex. Phenothiazines, the miscellaneous antiemetics (e.g., metoclopramide), and trimethobenzamide act on the CTZ. Drug combination therapy is commonly used to manage chemotherapy-induced nausea and vomiting. Lorazepam, glucocorticoids, and serotonin (5-HT$_3$)-receptor antagonists are quite effective in combination therapy. Lorazepam, haloperidol, and glucocorticoids are not approved by the FDA as antiemetics but are extremely effective when combined for this unlabeled use.

Antihistamines and Anticholinergics

Only a few prescription antihistamines and anticholinergics are used in the treatment of nausea and vomiting. Table 42.2 lists these drugs and their dosages, uses, and considerations.

Side Effects and Adverse Reactions. Side effects include drowsiness, which can be a major problem; dry mouth; blurred vision caused by pupillary dilation; tachycardia (with anticholinergic use); and constipation. These drugs should *not* be used by patients with glaucoma.

TABLE 42.2	Prescription Antiemetics	
Drug	**Route and Dosage**	**Uses and Considerations**
Prescription Antihistamines		
Hydroxyzine	Postoperative nausea/vomiting: A: IM: 25-100 mg single dose; *max:* 400 mg/d C: IM: 1.1 mg/kg single dose; *max:* 2 mg/kg	For postoperative nausea and vomiting, vertigo, anxiety, and sedation induction. Give deep in large muscle. May cause drowsiness, dizziness, fatigue, headache, blurred vision, dry mouth, tardive dyskinesia, urinary retention, and constipation. Pregnancy category: X*; PB: UK; t½: 14-25 h
Promethazine	See Prototype Drug Chart 42.1.	
Anticholinergics		
Scopolamine	Motion sickness: A: PO: 250-800 mcg 1 h before antiemetic needed A: Transdermal patch: 1.5 mg patch (1 mg dose over 3 d); apply patch to a hairless area behind the ear at least 4 h before travel and q3d as needed.	For nausea and vomiting, motion sickness, and IBS. May cause dizziness, drowsiness, fatigue, headache, dry mouth, blurred vision, urinary retention, and constipation. Alternate ears if using for longer than 3 d, wash hands after applying patch, and wear no more than one patch at a time. Pregnancy category: C*; PB: UK; t½: 8 h
Dopamine Antagonists		
Phenothiazines		
Prochlorperazine maleate	Nausea and vomiting: A: PO/IM/IV: 5-10 mg tid/qid PRN (give deep in the muscle); *max:* 40 mg/d SR: 10-15 mg q12h PR: 25 mg bid; *max:* 50 mg/d	For nausea, vomiting, schizophrenia, and anxiety. May cause drowsiness, dizziness, insomnia, headache, blurred vision, extrapyramidal symptoms, dry mouth, and urinary retention. Not approved for patients with dementia-related psychosis. Pregnancy category: C*; PB: 91%-99%; t½: 6-10 h
Promethazine	See Prototype Drug Chart 42.1.	
Butyrophenones		
Droperidol	A: IM/IV: Initially 0.625-2.5 mg; *max:* 2.5 mg/initial dose C 2-12 y: IM/IV: 0.1 mg/kg; *max:* 0.1 mg/kg initial dose	For prevention and treatment of postoperative nausea and vomiting. May cause hypotension, tachycardia, dizziness, drowsiness, restlessness, dysrhythmias, and extrapyramidal symptoms. *Black Box Warning:* Not approved for patients with dysrhythmias. Pregnancy category: C*; PB: 85%-90%: t½: 2.3 h
Benzodiazepines		
Lorazepam	Chemo-induced nausea/vomiting: A: IV: 0.025 mg/kg 45 min prior to chemo C: IV: 0.04-0.05 mg/kg q6h 30 min prior to chemo	For prevention of chemo-induced nausea and vomiting and for anxiety, insomnia, procedural sedation, amnesia induction, and status epilepticus. May cause dizziness, drowsiness, amnesia, injection site reaction, suicidal ideation, and dependence. Pregnancy category: D*; PB: 91%; t½: 12 h

TABLE 42.2 Prescription Antiemetics—cont'd

Drug	Route and Dosage	Uses and Considerations
Serotonin (5-HT₃) Receptor Antagonists		
Granisetron	Chemo-induced nausea/vomiting: A: PO: 1 mg bid (1 h before and 12 h later); *max.* 2 mg/d A/adol/C >2 y: IV: 10 mcg/kg 30 min before chemo, may repeat during first 24 h for breakthrough nausea/vomiting; *max.* 40 mcg/kg A: Transdermal patch: Apply 1 patch (3.1 mg/24 h) at least 24-48 h prior to chemo; remove patch no sooner than 24 h after chemo completion.	For prevention and treatment of radiation- and chemo-induced nausea and vomiting. May cause dizziness, headache, weakness, constipation, and leukopenia. Pregnancy category: B*; PB: 65%; t½: 6.23 h PO, 5-7.7 h IV
Ondansetron hydochloride	A: PO: 8-24 mg 30 min before chemo; may repeat in 8 h, then q12h for 1-2 d after chemo; *max.* 24 mg/d Adol/C >12 y: PO: 8 mg 30 min before chemo; may repeat in 8 h, then q8-12h for 1-5 d after chemo A/adol/C/infants >6 mo: IV: 0.15 mg/kg (150 mcg/kg) infused over 15 min 30 min before chemo, then q4h × 2	For postoperative and chemo- and radiation-induced nausea and vomiting. May cause dizziness, drowsiness, agitation, headache, fatigue, diarrhea, and constipation. Pregnancy category: B*; PB: 70%-76%; t½: 3.1-5.8 h
Palonosetron	Postoperative nausea/vomiting: A: IV: 0.075 mg over 10 s before induction as a single dose; *max.* 0.25 mg/single dose	To prevent postoperative and chemo-induced nausea and vomiting. May cause headache, constipation, and prolonged QT. Pregnancy category: B*; PB: 62%; t½: 40 h
Cannabinoids		
Dronabinol CSS III	Chemo-induced nausea: A/C: PO: 5 mg/m² 1-3 h before chemo, then q2-4h after; *max.* 15 mg/m²/dose or 6 doses/d	For anorexia and chemo-induced nausea and vomiting. May cause drowsiness, dizziness, impaired cognition, euphoria, dysphoria, emotional lability, paranoia, and GI distress. Pregnancy category: C*; PB: 97%; t½: 25-30 h
Miscellaneous		
Metoclopramide hydrochloride	Postoperative: A: IM/IV: 10-20 mg at end of surgery, may repeat q4-6h	For prevention and treatment of postoperative and chemo-induced nausea and vomiting, diabetic gastroparesis, and GERD. Avoid alcohol and CNS depressants. May cause drowsiness, fatigue, restlessness, headache, seizures, suicidal ideation, and extrapyramidal symptoms. Pregnancy category: B*; PB: 30%; t½: 2.5-6 h
Trimetho-benzamide hydrochloride	A: PO: 100-300 mg tid/qid PRN; *max.* 1200 mg/d A: IM: 200 mg tid/qid PRN; *max.* 800 mg/d	For nausea and vomiting. Avoid with CNS depressants and if sensitive to benzocaine or similar local anesthetics. May cause drowsiness, dizziness, headache, hypotension, blurred vision, seizures, extrapyramidal symptoms, and diarrhea. Pregnancy category: C*; PB: UK; t½: 7-9 h
Aprepitant	Postoperative nausea/vomiting: A: PO: 40 mg within 3 h before anesthesia induction	For prevention of postoperative and chemo-induced nausea and vomiting. May cause dizziness, fatigue, headache, weakness, hypotension, neutropenia, hiccups, dyspepsia, diarrhea, and constipation. Pregnancy category: B*; PB: 95%; t½: 9-13 h
Netupitant and palonosetron	A: PO: 1 capsule (netupitant 300 mg/palonosetron 0.5 mg) 1 h prior to chemo	For prevention of chemo-induced nausea and vomiting. May cause headache, weakness, dyspepsia, and constipation. Pregnancy category: C*; PB: 62%-99.5%; t½: 40-109 h
Rolapitant	A: PO: 180 mg day 1, 1-2 h and 30 min prior to chemo	For prevention of chemo-induced nausea and vomiting. May cause dizziness, anorexia, neutropenia, hiccups, GI distress, stomatitis, and UTI. Pregnancy category: UK; PB: 99.8%; t½: 169-183 h

*Pregnancy categories have been revised. See http://www.fda.gov/Drugs/DevelopmentApprovalProcess/DevelopmentResources/Labeling/ucm093 307.htm for more information.

A, Adult; *adol*, adolescent; *bid*, twice a day; *C*, child; *chemo*, chemotherapy; *CNS*, central nervous system; *CSS*, Controlled Substances Schedule; *d*, day; *GERD*, gastroesophageal reflux disease; *GI*, gastrointestinal; *h*, hour; *IBS*, irritable bowel syndrome; *IM*, intramuscular; *IV*, intravenous; *max*, maximum; *min*, minute; *mo*, month; *PB*, protein binding; *PO*, by mouth; *PR*, per rectum; *PRN*, as needed; *q*, every; *qid*, four times a day; *s*, second; *SR*, sustained release; *t½*, half-life; *tid*, three times a day; *UK*, unknown; *UTI*, urinary tract infection; *y*, year; *>*, greater than.

Dopamine Antagonists

These agents suppress emesis by blocking dopamine (D2) receptors in the CTZ. The categories of dopamine antagonists include phenothiazines, butyrophenones, and benzodiazepines. Common side effects of dopamine antagonists are extrapyramidal symptoms, or extrapyramidal syndrome (EPS), caused by blocking dopamine receptors, and hypotension. See Chapter 22 for a more detailed description of EPS and phenothiazines.

Phenothiazine Antiemetics

Selected piperazine phenothiazines are used to treat nausea and vomiting resulting from surgery, anesthetics, chemotherapy, and radiation sickness. They act by inhibiting the CTZ. When used in patients with cancer, these drugs are commonly given the night before treatment, the day of treatment, and for 24 hours after treatment. Not all phenothiazines are effective antiemetic agents. When prescribed for vomiting, the

PROTOTYPE DRUG CHART 42.1

❶ *Promethazine Hydrochloride*

Drug Class	Dosage
Antiemetic: Phenothiazine Pregnancy category: C*	Nausea/vomiting: A/adol/C 6-12 y: PO/PR/IM/IV: 12.5-25 mg q4-6h PRN; *max.* 100 mg/d C >2 y: PO/PR/IM/IV: 0.25-1 mg/kg q4-6h PRN; *max.* 25 mg/dose
Contraindications Hypersensitivity *Caution:* Narrow-angle glaucoma, intestinal obstruction, blood dyscrasias, bone marrow depression, cardiovascular disease, liver dysfunction, COPD, hypertension, older adults and debilitated patients	**Drug-Lab-Food Interactions** Drug: Increases CNS depression and anticholinergic effects when taken with alcohol and other CNS depressants; lowers seizure threshold with phenytoin and tramadol Lab: False pregnancy test
Pharmacokinetics Absorption: PO: Easily absorbed from GI tract Distribution: PB: 80%-93% Metabolism: t½: 10-14 h Excretion: In urine and feces	**Pharmacodynamics** PO: Onset: 15-60 min Peak: UK; duration: 4-6 h IM: Onset: 20 min Peak: UK; duration: 4-6 h IV: Onset: 3-5 min Peak: UK; duration: 4-6 h PR: Onset: 15-60 min Peak: UK; duration: 4-6 h
Therapeutic Effects/Uses	
To treat and prevent motion sickness, nausea, vomiting, and sedation induction Mode of Action: Blocks H_1 receptor sites and inhibits CTZ	
Side Effects Drowsiness, dizziness, confusion, anorexia, dry mouth, constipation, blurred vision, excitability, photosensitivity, hypertension, hypotension, urinary retention, fatigue, injection site reaction, incoordination, slate gray skin hyperpigmentation, erectile/ejaculation dysfunction	**Adverse Reactions** Extrapyramidal syndrome, seizures *Life threatening:* Agranulocytosis, leukopenia, thrombocytopenia, NMS, respiratory depression

*Pregnancy categories have been revised. See http://www.fda.gov/Drugs/DevelopmentApprovalProcess/DevelopmentResources/Labeling/ucm093307.htm for more information.
A, Adult; *adol*, adolescent; *C*, child; *CNS*, central nervous system; *COPD*, chronic obstructive pulmonary disorder; *CTZ*, chemoreceptor trigger zone; *d*, day; *GI*, gastrointestinal; *h*, hour; *H1*, histamine 1; *IM*, intramuscular; *IV*, intravenous; *max*, maximum; *min*, minute; *NMS*, neuroleptic malignant syndrome; *PB*, protein binding; *PO*, by mouth; *PR*, per rectum; *PRN*, as needed; *q4-6h*, every 4 to 6 hours; *t½*, half-life; *UK*, unknown; *y*, year; *>*, greater than.

drug dosage is usually smaller than is used for psychiatric disorders.

Chlorpromazine and prochlorperazine edisylate were the first phenothiazines used for both psychosis and vomiting. Promethazine, a phenothiazine introduced as an antihistamine in the 1940s, has a sedative effect and can also be used for motion sickness and management of nausea and vomiting.

❶ When promethazine is administered intravenously, it is a high-alert medication that may cause significant harm to the patient if given incorrectly. Prototype Drug Chart 42.1 lists the pharmacologic data for promethazine.

Pharmacokinetics Promethazine is readily absorbed in the gastrointestinal (GI) tract. It has 80% to 93% protein-binding capacity. Promethazine is metabolized by the liver and is excreted in urine and feces.

Pharmacodynamics Promethazine blocks H_1-receptor sites on effector cells and impedes histamine-mediated responses. The onset of action of oral promethazine is 15 to 60 minutes, and onset with intramuscular (IM) administration is 20 minutes. The duration of action is from 4 to 6 hours. The onset of action of IV promethazine is 3 to 5 minutes; the duration of action is the same as for the oral preparation.

Drug and Laboratory Interactions. Central nervous system (CNS) depression increases when promethazine is taken with

alcohol, narcotics, sedative-hypnotics, and general anesthetics. Anticholinergic effects increase when promethazine is combined with antihistamines, anticholinergics such as atropine, and other phenothiazines. Promethazine may interfere with urinary pregnancy tests, producing false results.

Side Effects and Adverse Reactions. Phenothiazines have antihistamine and anticholinergic properties. The side effects of phenothiazine antiemetics are moderate sedation, hypotension, extrapyramidal symptoms, CNS effects (restlessness, weakness, dystonic reactions, agitation), and mild anticholinergic symptoms (dry mouth, urinary retention, and constipation). Because the dose is lower for vomiting than for psychosis, the side effects are not so severe. Promethazine is relatively free of extrapyramidal symptoms at antiemetic doses. Table 42.2 lists the pharmacologic data for phenothiazines and other prescription antiemetics.

Butyrophenones

Haloperidol and droperidol, like phenothiazines, block the D2 receptors in the CTZ. They are used to treat postoperative nausea and the vomiting and emesis associated with toxins, cancer chemotherapy, and radiation therapy. Antiemetic doses of haloperidol are smaller than those required for antipsychotic effects. Like phenothiazines, haloperidol and droperidol are likely to cause extrapyramidal symptoms if used for an extended time. Hypotension may result, therefore blood pressure should be monitored.

Benzodiazepines

Select benzodiazepines indirectly control nausea and vomiting that may occur with cancer chemotherapy. Lorazepam is the drug of choice. Previously, diazepam was the preferred benzodiazepine, but lorazepam effectively provides emesis control, sedation, anxiety reduction, and amnesia when used in combination with a glucocorticoid and serotonin (5-HT$_3$)-receptor antagonist.

Serotonin-Receptor Antagonists

Serotonin antagonists suppress nausea and vomiting by blocking the serotonin (5-HT$_3$) receptors in the CTZ and blocking the afferent vagal nerve terminals in the upper GI tract.

Serotonin antagonists—ondansetron, granisetron, dolasetron, and palonosetron—are the most effective of all antiemetics in suppressing nausea and vomiting caused by cancer chemotherapy–induced emesis or emetogenic anticancer drugs. Ondansetron (the first serotonin antagonist), granisetron, and dolasetron do *not* block the dopamine receptors, therefore they do not cause extrapyramidal symptoms as do the phenothiazine antiemetics. These drugs can be administered orally and intravenously. They are also effective in preventing nausea and vomiting before and after surgery. Common side effects include headache, diarrhea, dizziness, and fatigue.

Glucocorticoids (Corticosteroids)

Dexamethasone and methylprednisolone are two agents that are effective in suppressing emesis associated with cancer chemotherapy. Because these glucocorticoids are administered intravenously and for only a short while, side effects normally associated with glucocorticoids are minimized. Glucocorticoids are discussed in Chapter 46.

Cannabinoids

Cannabinoids, the active ingredients in *Cannabis,* were approved for clinical use in 1985 to alleviate nausea and vomiting resulting from cancer treatment. These agents may be prescribed for patients receiving chemotherapy who do not respond to or are unable to take other antiemetics. They are contraindicated for patients with psychiatric disorders. Cannabinoids can be used as an appetite stimulant for patients with acquired immunodeficiency syndrome (AIDS). The cannabinoid dronabinol is described in Table 42.2.

Side Effects and Adverse Reactions. Side effects that can occur as a result of cannabinoid use include mood changes, euphoria, drowsiness, dizziness, headaches, depersonalization, nightmares, confusion, incoordination, memory lapse, dry mouth, orthostatic hypotension or hypertension, and tachycardia. Less common symptoms are depression, anxiety, and manic psychosis.

Miscellaneous Antiemetics

Trimethobenzamide is in the class of miscellaneous antiemetics because it does not act strictly as an antihistamine, anticholinergic, or phenothiazine. The drug suppresses impulses to the CTZ.

Side Effects and Adverse Reactions. The side effects and adverse reactions of the miscellaneous antiemetics are drowsiness and anticholinergic symptoms such as dry mouth, increased heart rate, urine retention, constipation, and blurred vision. Trimethobenzamide can cause hypotension, diarrhea, and extrapyramidal symptoms that include abnormal involuntary movements, postural disturbances, and alterations in muscle tone.

Metoclopramide

Metoclopramide suppresses emesis by blocking the dopamine receptors in the CTZ. It is used in the treatment of postoperative emesis, cancer chemotherapy, and radiation therapy. High doses can cause sedation and diarrhea. With this agent, the occurrence of extrapyramidal symptoms is more prevalent in children than in adults. Metoclopramide should not be given if the patient has GI obstruction, hemorrhage, or perforation.

Table 42.2 lists pharmacologic data for the miscellaneous antiemetics along with other prescription antiemetics.

⚡ PATIENT SAFETY

Do not confuse:
- **Antivert,** an antiemetic, with **Axert,** an antimigraine drug
- **Lorazepam,** which controls nausea and vomiting, with **alprazolam,** an anxiolytic
- **Hydroxyzine,** an antiemetic, with **hydralazine,** an antihypertensive drug

◎ NURSING PROCESS
Patient-Centered Collaborative Care
Antiemetics

Assessment
- Determine a history of the onset, frequency, and amount of vomiting and contents of the vomitus. If appropriate, elicit from the patient possible causative factors such as food (e.g., seafood, mayonnaise, pregnancy, exposure to virus).
- Obtain a history of present health problems. Patients with glaucoma should avoid many of the antiemetics.
- Record vital signs for abnormalities and for future comparisons.
- Assess urinalysis before and during therapy.
- Assess the patient for dehydration due to excess fluid loss from vomiting.

Nursing Diagnoses
- Nutrition, Imbalanced: Less than Body Requirements related to inability to ingest food
- Fluid Volume, Risk for Deficient

Planning

- The patient will adhere to nonpharmacologic methods or the drug regimen to alleviate vomiting.
- The patient's underlying cause of vomiting will be corrected.
- The patient will retain small amounts of food and fluid.

Nursing Interventions

- Check vital signs. If vomiting is severe, dehydration may occur, and shocklike symptoms may be present.
- Monitor bowel sounds for hypoactivity or hyperactivity.
- Provide mouth care after vomiting. Encourage patients to maintain oral hygiene.

Patient Teaching
General

- Instruct patients to store drugs in airtight, light-resistant containers if required.
- Tell patients to avoid OTC preparations.
- Warn patients not to consume alcohol while taking antiemetics. Alcohol can intensify the sedative effect.
- ⚡ Advise pregnant patients to avoid antiemetics during the first trimester because of possible teratogenic effects on the fetus. Encourage these patients to seek medical advice about OTC and prescription antiemetics.

Side Effects

- Tell the patient to report sore throat, fever, and mouth sores; notify the health care provider, and have blood drawn for a complete blood count (CBC).
- ⚡ Alert patients to avoid driving a motor vehicle or engaging in dangerous activities because drowsiness is common with antiemetics. If drowsiness becomes a problem, a decrease in dosage may be indicated.
- Caution patients with hepatic disorders to seek medical advice before taking phenothiazines. Instruct patients to report dizziness.
- Suggest to patients nonpharmacologic methods of alleviating nausea and vomiting such as flat soda, weak tea, crackers, and dry toast.

🌐 *Cultural Considerations*

- Respect patients' cultural beliefs and alternative methods for treating nausea and vomiting. Discuss with patients the safety of their methods, other nondrug methods, and the purpose of the antiemetic if prescribed.
- Procure an interpreter when needed to assist non–English-speaking patients to understand the drug schedule for prescribed antiemetics and their side effects.

Evaluation

- Evaluate the effectiveness of nonpharmacologic methods and antiemetics by noting the absence of vomiting. Identify any side effects that may result from drugs.

EMETICS

Emetics are drugs used to induce vomiting. When an individual has consumed certain toxic substances, induced vomiting (emesis) may be indicated to expel the substance before absorption occurs. Vomiting can be induced in a number of ways without using drugs, such as putting a finger in the back of the throat.

Vomiting should not be induced if caustic substances such as ammonia, chlorine bleach, lye, toilet cleaners, or battery acid have been ingested. Regurgitating these substances can cause additional injury to the esophagus. To prevent aspiration, vomiting should also be avoided if petroleum distillates are ingested; these include gasoline, kerosene, paint thinners, and lighter fluid. Activated charcoal is given when emesis is contraindicated (Table 42.3).

DIARRHEA

Diarrhea, frequent liquid stool, is a symptom of an intestinal disorder. Causes include (1) foods (spicy, spoiled), (2) fecal impaction, (3) bacteria (*Escherichia coli, Salmonella*) or viruses (parvovirus, rotavirus), (4) toxins, (5) drug reactions, (6) laxative abuse, (7) malabsorption syndrome caused by lack of digestive enzymes, (8) stress and anxiety, (9) bowel tumor, and (10) inflammatory bowel disease such as ulcerative colitis or Crohn disease. Diarrhea can be mild to severe. Antidiarrheals should not be used for more than 2 days and should not be used if fever is present.

Because intestinal fluids are rich in water, sodium, potassium, and bicarbonate, diarrhea can cause minor or severe dehydration and electrolyte imbalances. The loss of bicarbonate places the patient at risk for developing metabolic acidosis. Patients with diarrhea should avoid milk products and foods rich in fat. Diarrhea can develop very quickly and can be life threatening to young patients and older adults, who may not be able to compensate for the fluid and electrolyte losses.

Nonpharmacologic Measures

The cause of diarrhea should be identified. Nonpharmacologic treatment for diarrhea is recommended until the underlying cause can be determined. This includes use of clear liquids and oral solutions such as Gatorade (for adults) and Pedialyte or Rehydralyte (for children) and IV electrolyte solutions. Antidiarrheal drugs are frequently used in combination with nonpharmacologic treatment.

Travelers' Diarrhea

Travelers' diarrhea, also called *acute diarrhea*, is usually caused by *E. coli.* It ordinarily lasts less than 2 days; however, if it becomes severe, fluoroquinolone antibiotics are usually prescribed. Loperamide may be used to slow peristalsis and decrease the frequency of defecation, but it can also slow the exit of the organism from the GI tract. Travelers' diarrhea can be reduced by drinking bottled water, washing fruit, and eating cooked vegetables. Meats should be cooked until well done.

TABLE 42.3 Adsorbents

Drug	Route and Dosage	Uses and Considerations
Adsorbents		
Charcoal, activated	A: PO: 50-100 g in 6-8 oz of water q4-6h PRN C: PO: 1-2 g/kg/dose in 6-8 oz of water q4-6h PRN C <1 y: PO: 1 g/kg repeat q4-6h PRN	Promotes absorption of poison/toxic/overdose substances. Administer within 30 min of ingesting substance. May cause tongue discoloration, black stool, abdominal pain, diarrhea, and constipation. Pregnancy category: C*; PB: NA; t½: NA

*Pregnancy categories have been revised. See http://www.fda.gov/Drugs/DevelopmentApprovalProcess/DevelopmentResources/Labeling/ucm093307.htm for more information.
A, Adult; *C*, child; *min*, minute; *NA*, not applicable; *PB*, protein binding; *PO*, by mouth; *PRN*, as necessary; *q4-6h*, every 4 to 6 hours; *t½*, half-life; *UK*, unknown; *y*, year; *<*, less than.

PROTOTYPE DRUG CHART 42.2
Diphenoxylate With Atropine

Drug Class Antidiarrheal Pregnancy category: C* CSS V	**Dosage** A/adol: PO: 2.5-5 mg tid/qid PRN; *max:* 20 mg/d
Contraindications Severe diarrhea due to pseudomembranous colitis, obstructive jaundice, children <2 y *Caution:* Severe hepatic disease, electrolyte imbalance; dehydration, ulcerative colitis	**Drug-Lab-Food Interactions** Drug: Increased CNS depression with alcohol, antihistamines, opioids, sedative-hypnotics; MAOIs may enhance hypertensive crisis Lab: Increased serum liver enzymes, amylase
Pharmacokinetics Absorption: PO: Well absorbed Distribution: PB: UK Metabolism: t½: 3-14 h Excretion: In feces and urine	**Pharmacodynamics** PO: Onset: 45-60 min Peak: 2 h Duration: 3-4 h
Therapeutic Effects/Uses To treat diarrhea by slowing intestinal motility Mode of Action: Inhibits gastric motility by exerting effect on smooth muscle cells of GI tract	
Side Effects Drowsiness, dizziness, confusion, euphoria, headache, restlessness, nausea, vomiting, constipation, dry mouth, weakness, flushing, rash, urine retention	**Adverse Reactions** Angioedema, pancreatitis, tachycardia *Life threatening:* Paralytic ileus, toxic megacolon, anaphylaxis

*Pregnancy categories have been revised. See http://www.fda.gov/Drugs/DevelopmentApprovalProcess/DevelopmentResources/Labeling/ucm093307.htm for more information.
A, Adult; *adol*, adolescent; *CNS*, central nervous system; *CSS*, Controlled Substances Schedule; *d*, day; *GI*, gastrointestinal; *h*, hour; *MAOI*, monoamine oxidase inhibitor; *max*, maximum; *min*, minute; *PB*, protein binding; *PO*, by mouth; *PRN*, as necessary; *qid*, four times a day; *t½*, half-life; *tid*, three times a day; *UK*, unknown; *y*, year; *<*, less than.

Antidiarrheals

There are various antidiarrheals for treating diarrhea and decreasing hypermotility (increased peristalsis). Usually, an underlying cause of the diarrhea needs to be corrected as well. The antidiarrheals are classified as (1) opiates and opiate-related agents, (2) somatostatin analogues, (3) adsorbents, and (4) miscellaneous antidiarrheals.

Opiates and Opiate-Related Agents

Opiates decrease intestinal motility thereby decreasing peristalsis. Constipation is a common side effect of opium preparations. Codeine is an example. Opiates are frequently combined with other antidiarrheal agents. Opium antidiarrheals can cause CNS depression when taken with alcohol, sedatives, or tranquilizers. The duration of action of opiates is approximately 2 hours.

Diphenoxylate with atropine is an opiate that has less potential for causing drug dependence than other opiates such as codeine. Difenoxin is an active metabolite of diphenoxylate, but it is more potent than diphenoxylate. Both drugs are combined with atropine to decrease abdominal cramping, intestinal motility, and hypersecretion. Diphenoxylate with atropine is frequently prescribed for travelers' diarrhea, and difenoxin with atropine is prescribed to treat nonspecific and chronic diarrhea. With prolonged use of these drugs, physical dependence may occur. Diphenoxylate antidiarrheal products are approximately 50% atropine, which will discourage drug abuse. Prototype Drug Chart 42.2 lists the pharmacologic data for diphenoxylate with atropine.

Loperamide is structurally related to diphenoxylate but causes less CNS depression than diphenoxylate and difenoxin. It can be purchased as an OTC drug, and it protects against

TABLE 42.4   Antidiarrheals: Opiates and Opiate-Related, Adsorbents, and Miscellaneous Agents

Drug	Route and Dosage	Uses and Considerations
Opiates and Opiate-Related		
Deodorized opium tincture CSS II	A: PO: 6 mg qid mixed with water	For diarrhea. Avoid taking with alcohol and CNS depressants. May cause drowsiness, dizziness, confusion, weakness, hypotension, constipation, and tolerance. Pregnancy category: C*; PB: UK; t½: 1.5-4 h
Difenoxin and atropine CSS IV	A/adol/C >12 y: PO: Initially 2 mg, then 1 mg after each loose stool; *max:* 8 mg/d	For diarrhea. Avoid use in patients with narrow-angle glaucoma. May cause dizziness, drowsiness, dry mouth, flushing, headache, and fatigue. Pregnancy category: C*; PB: UK; t½: UK
Diphenoxylate and atropine CSS V	A: PO: Initially 5 mg tid-qid until control achieved, then reduce to 2.5 mg bid-tid if needed; *max:* 20 mg/d	For diarrhea. Avoid use in patients with narrow-angle glaucoma. May cause dizziness, drowsiness, dry mouth, headache, nausea, and vomiting. Pregnancy category: C*; PB: UK; t½: 3-14 h
Loperamide hydrochloride	A: PO: Initially 4 mg, then 2 mg after each loose stool; *max:* 16 mg/d	For diarrhea. May cause drowsiness, dizziness, dry mouth, fatigue, headache, and GI distress. Pregnancy category: C*; PB: 97%; t½: 10.8 h
Adsorbents		
Bismuth subsalicylate	A: PO: 2 tab (524 mg) q30-60min PRN; *max:* 8 doses/d	For diarrhea, dyspepsia, and pyrosis. May cause dizziness, drowsiness, headache, weakness, anxiety, confusion, tinnitus, tongue discoloration, hearing loss, and stool discoloration. Pregnancy category: C*; PB: UK; t½: UK
Miscellaneous		
Crofelemer	A: PO: 125 mg bid; *max:* 250 mg/d	For diarrhea in patients with HIV/AIDS. May cause flatulence, nausea, abdominal pain, arthralgia, hyperbilirubinemia, and pharyngitis. Pregnancy category: C*; PB: UK; t½: UK
Eluxadoline	A: PO: 75-100 mg bid; *max:* 200 mg/d	For treatment of IBS with diarrhea. May cause nausea, vomiting, abdominal pain, constipation, and pharyngitis. Pregnancy category: UK*; PB: 81%; t½: 3.7-6 h
Rifaximin	Travelers' diarrhea: A/adol/C >12 y: PO: 200 mg tid for 3 d; *max:* 600 mg/d	For treatment of IBS, travelers' diarrhea, and hepatic encephalopathy. May cause dizziness, headache, depression, fatigue, nausea, abdominal pain, ascites, myalgia, peripheral edema, and anemia. Pregnancy category: UK*; PB: 67.5%; t½: 3.2-6.1 h

*Pregnancy categories have been revised. See http://www.fda.gov/Drugs/DevelopmentApprovalProcess/DevelopmentResources/Labeling/ucm093307.htm for more information.
A, Adult; *adol*, adolescent; *AIDS*, acquired immunodeficiency syndrome; *bid*, twice a day; *C*, child; *CNS*, central nervous system; *CSS*, Controlled Substances Schedule; *d*, day; *GI*, gastrointestinal; *h*, hour; *HIV*, human immunodeficiency virus; *IBS*, irritable bowel syndrome; *max*, maximum; *min*, minute; *PB*, protein binding; *PO*, by mouth; *PRN*, as needed; *q*, every *qid*, four times a day; *t½*, half-life; *tab*, tablet; *tid*, three times a day; *UK*, unknown; *y*, year; *>*, greater than.

diarrhea, reduces fecal volume, and decreases intestinal fluid and electrolyte losses.

Patients with severe hepatic impairment should not take products that contain diphenoxylate, difenoxin, or loperamide. Children and older adults who take diphenoxylate are more susceptible to respiratory depression than are other age groups.

Pharmacokinetics Diphenoxylate with atropine is well absorbed from the GI tract. The diphenoxylate is metabolized by the liver mainly as metabolites. There are two half-lives: 3 hours for diphenoxylate and 3 to 14 hours for the diphenoxylate metabolites. The drug is excreted in the feces and urine.

Pharmacodynamics Diphenoxylate with atropine is an opium agonist with anticholinergic properties (atropine) that decreases GI motility (peristalsis). It has a moderate onset of action of 45 to 60 minutes, and the duration of action is 3 to 4 hours. Many side effects are caused by the anticholinergic atropine. Patients with severe glaucoma should take another antidiarrheal that does not have an anticholinergic effect. If this drug is taken with alcohol, narcotics, or sedative-hypnotics, CNS depression can occur.

Adsorbents

Adsorbents act by coating the wall of the GI tract and adsorbing bacteria or toxins that cause diarrhea. Adsorbent antidiarrheals include kaolin and pectin. These agents are combined as a mild or moderate antidiarrheal that can be purchased without a prescription and used in combination with other antidiarrheals. Bismuth subsalicylate is considered an adsorbent because it adsorbs bacterial toxins. Bismuth subsalicylate is an OTC drug commonly used to treat travelers' diarrhea, and it can also be used as an antacid for gastric discomfort. Colestipol and cholestyramine are prescription drugs that have been used to treat diarrhea due to excess bile acids in the colon. They are effective, although they have not been approved by the FDA for this purpose. Table 42.4 lists the pharmacologic data for antidiarrheal adsorbents.

Miscellaneous Antidiarrheals

Various miscellaneous antidiarrheals are prescribed to control diarrhea. This group includes rifaximin. Table 42.4 includes these other antidiarrheals.

NURSING PROCESS
Patient-Centered Collaborative Care
Antidiarrheals

Assessment
- Obtain a history of any viral or bacterial infection, drugs taken, and foods ingested that could be contributing factors to diarrhea. Many antidiarrheals are contraindicated if the patient has liver disease, narcotic dependence, ulcerative colitis, or glaucoma.
- Check vital signs to provide a baseline for future comparisons and to determine body fluid and electrolyte losses.
- Determine frequency and consistency of bowel movements.
- Assess bowel sounds. Hyperactive sounds can indicate increased intestinal motility.
- Report if a patient has a narcotic drug history. If opiate or opiate-related antidiarrheals are given, drug misuse or abuse may occur.

Nursing Diagnoses
- Diarrhea related to laxative abuse
- Nutrition, Imbalanced: Less than Body Requirements related to misconceptions regarding OTC drugs
- Fluid Volume, Risk for Imbalanced

Planning
- The patient will have bowel movements that are formed.
- The patient's body fluids will be restored.

Nursing Interventions
- Record vital signs. Report tachycardia or systolic blood pressure decreases of 10 to 15 mm Hg. Monitor respirations. Opiates and opiate-related drugs can cause CNS depression.
- Monitor frequency of bowel movements and bowel sounds. Notify a health care provider if intestinal hypoactivity occurs when taking a drug.
- ⚡ Check for signs and symptoms of dehydration resulting from persistent diarrhea. Fluid replacement may be necessary. With prolonged diarrhea, check serum electrolytes.
- Administer antidiarrheals cautiously to pregnant patients and those with glaucoma, liver disorders, or ulcerative colitis.
- ⚡ Recognize that a drug may need to be withheld if diarrhea continues for more than 48 hours or acute abdominal pain develops.

Patient Teaching
- Instruct patients not to take sedatives, tranquilizers, or other narcotics with antidiarrheal drugs. CNS depression may occur.
- Tell patients to avoid OTC preparations; they may contain alcohol and can promote liver damage, and concurrent use with loratadine and loperamide may lead to significant interaction.

- Counsel patients to take drugs only as prescribed. Advise that drugs may be habit-forming and that they should not exceed the recommended dose.
- Encourage patients to drink clear liquids.
- Advise patients not to ingest fried foods or milk products until diarrhea has stopped.
- Teach patients that constipation can result from overuse of antidiarrheal drugs.

 Cultural Considerations
- Do not assume that lack of eye contact means that a patient is not listening or does not care. It might indicate respect. The more traditional and older individuals in some cultures may not maintain eye contact.

Evaluation
- Evaluate the effectiveness of the drug; diarrhea has stopped.
- Monitor long-term use of opiates and opiate-related drugs for possible abuse and physical dependence.
- Continue to monitor vital signs and report abnormal changes.

CONSTIPATION

Constipation, the accumulation of hard fecal material in the large intestine, is a relatively common complaint and a major problem for older adults. Insufficient water intake and poor dietary habits are contributing factors. Other causes include (1) fecal impaction, (2) bowel obstruction, (3) chronic laxative use, (4) neurologic disorders (paraplegia), (5) ignoring the urge to defecate, (6) lack of exercise, and (7) select drugs such as anticholinergics, narcotics, and certain antacids.

Nonpharmacologic Measures

Nonpharmacologic management includes diet (high fiber), water, exercise, and routine bowel habits. A "normal" number of bowel movements ranges between one and three per day to three per week. What is normal varies from person to person; the nurse should determine what normal bowel habits are for each patient. At times a laxative may be needed, but the patient should also use nonpharmacologic measures to prevent constipation.

Laxatives

Laxatives and cathartics are used to eliminate fecal matter. Laxatives promote a soft stool, cathartics result in a soft to watery stool with some cramping, and frequently dosage determines whether a drug acts as a laxative or cathartic. Because these terms are often used interchangeably, *laxative* will cover both classes in this chapter. Purgatives are harsh cathartics that cause a watery stool with abdominal cramping. There are four types of laxatives: (1) osmotics (saline), (2) stimulants (contact or irritants), (3) bulk-forming, and (4) emollients (stool softeners).

Laxatives should be avoided if there is any question that the patient may have intestinal obstruction; if abdominal pain is severe; or if symptoms of appendicitis, ulcerative colitis, or diverticulitis are present. Most laxatives stimulate peristalsis. Laxative abuse from chronic use is a common problem, especially in older adults. Laxative dependence can become a problem, so patient teaching is an important nursing responsibility.

Osmotic (Saline) Laxatives

Osmotics, hyperosmolar laxatives, include salts or saline products, lactulose, and glycerin. Saline products consist of sodium or magnesium, and a small amount is systemically absorbed. Serum electrolytes should be monitored to avoid electrolyte imbalance. Hyperosmolar salts pull water into the colon and increase water in the feces to increase bulk, which stimulates peristalsis. Saline cathartics cause a semiformed to watery stool according to low or high doses. Good renal function is needed to excrete any excess salts. Saline cathartics are contraindicated for patients with heart failure.

Osmotic laxatives contain electrolyte salts, including (1) sodium salts (sodium phosphate or Phospho-Soda, sodium biphosphate) and (2) magnesium salts (magnesium hydroxide [Milk of Magnesia], magnesium citrate). High doses of salt laxatives are used for bowel preparation for diagnostic and surgical procedures. Another laxative used for bowel preparation is polyethylene glycol (PEG) with electrolytes. With PEG, however, a large volume of solution—approximately 3 to 4 L over 3 hours—must be ingested. Patients may be advised to keep PEG refrigerated to make it more palatable. The positive aspect is that the solution is an isotonic, nonabsorbable osmotic substance that contains sodium salts and potassium chloride, thus it can be used by patients with renal impairment or cardiac disorders.

Lactulose, another saline laxative that is not absorbed, draws water into the intestines to form a soft stool. It decreases the serum ammonia level and is useful in liver diseases, such as cirrhosis. Glycerin acts like lactulose, increasing water in the feces in the large intestine. The bulk that results from the increased water in the feces stimulates peristalsis and defecation.

Side Effects and Adverse Reactions. Adequate renal function is needed to excrete excess magnesium. Patients who have renal insufficiency should avoid magnesium salts. Hypermagnesemia can result from continuous use of magnesium salts, causing symptoms such as drowsiness, weakness, paralysis, complete heart block, hypotension, flush, and respiratory depression.

The side effects of excess lactulose use include flatulence, diarrhea, abdominal cramps, nausea, and vomiting. Patients who have diabetes mellitus should avoid lactulose because it contains glucose and fructose.

Stimulant (Contact) Laxatives

Stimulant (contact or irritant) laxatives increase peristalsis by irritating sensory nerve endings in the intestinal mucosa. Types include those that contain bisacodyl, senna, and castor oil (purgative). Bisacodyl is the most frequently used and abused laxative and can be purchased OTC. Bisacodyl and several others of these drugs are used to empty the bowel before diagnostic tests (barium enema). Prototype Drug Chart 42.3 lists the pharmacologic data for the stimulant laxative bisacodyl.

PROTOTYPE DRUG CHART 42.3
Bisacodyl

Drug Class	Dosage
Laxative: Stimulant Pregnancy category: C*	A/adol/C >12 y: PO: 5-15 mg/d single dose; *max:* 15 mg/d C 6-11 y: PO: 5 mg; *max:* 5 mg/d A/adol/C >12 y: supp PR: 10 mg/d C 6-11 y: 5 mg (½ supp)
Contraindications Hypersensitivity, fecal impaction, intestinal/biliary obstruction, GI bleeding, appendicitis, abdominal pain, nausea, vomiting *Caution:* Diarrhea, diverticulitis, electrolyte imbalance, ulcerative colitis	**Drug-Lab-Food Interactions** Drug: Decreased effect with antacids, histamine₂ blockers, proton pump inhibitors Food: Milk
Pharmacokinetics Absorption: Minimal (5%-15%) Distribution: PB: UK Metabolism: t½: UK Excretion: In bile and urine	**Pharmacodynamics** PO: Onset: 6-8 h Peak: N/A Duration: N/A PR: Onset: 15-60 min Peak: N/A Duration: N/A
Therapeutic Effects/Uses Bowel preparation, prevention and short-term treatment for constipation Mode of Action: Increases peristalsis by direct effect on smooth muscle of intestine	
Side Effects Dizziness, anorexia, nausea, vomiting, abdominal cramps, diarrhea, rectal burning	**Adverse Reactions** Dependence, fluid and electrolyte imbalance

*Pregnancy categories have been revised. See http://www.fda.gov/Drugs/DevelopmentApprovalProcess/DevelopmentResources/Labeling/ucm093307.htm for more information.
A, Adult; *adol,* adolescent; *C,* child; *d,* day; *GI,* gastrointestinal; *h,* hour; *max,* maximum; *min,* minute; *N/A,* not applicable; *PB,* protein binding; *PO,* by mouth; *PR,* per rectum; *supp,* suppository; *t½,* half-life; *UK,* unknown; *y,* year; *>,* greater than.

Castor oil is a harsh laxative (purgative) that acts on the small bowel and produces a watery stool. The action is quick, within 2 to 6 hours, so the laxative should not be taken at bedtime. Castor oil is not FDA approved to correct constipation, rather it is used mainly for bowel preparation.

Pharmacokinetics The contact laxative bisacodyl is minimally absorbed from the GI tract. It is excreted in feces, but because of the small amount of bisacodyl absorption, a portion is excreted in urine.

Pharmacodynamics Bisacodyl promotes defecation by irritating the colon, causing defecation; psyllium compounds increase fecal bulk and peristalsis. The onset of action of oral bisacodyl occurs within 6 to 8 hours, and with the suppository (rectal administration), it occurs within 15 to 60 minutes.

Side Effects and Adverse Reactions. Side effects include nausea, abdominal cramps, weakness, and reddish-brown urine caused by excretion of phenolphthalein, senna, or cascara.

With excessive and chronic use of bisacodyl, fluid and electrolyte imbalances—especially of potassium and calcium—are likely to occur. Systemic effects occur infrequently because absorption of bisacodyl is minimal. Mild cramping and diarrhea are side effects of bisacodyl.

Castor oil should not be used in early pregnancy because it stimulates uterine contractions, and spontaneous abortion may result. Prolonged use of senna can damage nerves, which may result in loss of intestinal muscular tone. Table 42.5 lists the osmotic and stimulant laxatives with their dosages, uses, and considerations.

TABLE 42.5 Laxatives: Osmotics (Saline), Stimulants, and Selective Chloride Channel Activators

Drug	Route and Dosage	Uses and Considerations
Osmotics: Saline		
Glycerin	A/adol/C >6 y: PR: 1 supp, retain 15 min C <6 y: PR: 1 infant supp, retain 15 min	For constipation. Use with caution in patients with cardiac, renal, or liver disease and older adults or dehydrated patients. May cause cramps, perianal irritation, and weakness. Pregnancy category: C*; PB: UK; t½: UK
Lactulose	Constipation: A: PO: 15-30 mL/d, may increase to 60 mL/d PRN	For constipation and hepatic encephalopathy. May cause belching, flatulence, nausea, vomiting, diarrhea, abdominal pain, metabolic acidosis, hypokalemia, and hypernatremia. Pregnancy category: B*; PB: UK; t½: UK
Magnesium citrate	Constipation: A/adol/C >12 y: PO: 150-300 mL in single or divided dose C 6-12 y: PO: 100-150 mL in single or divided dose C 2-5 y: PO: 60-120 mL in single or divided dose	For constipation and bowel preparation. May cause drowsiness, nausea, vomiting, diarrhea, dehydration, and electrolyte imbalance. Pregnancy category: B*; PB: UK; t½: UK
Magnesium hydroxide	A/adol/C >12 y: PO: 15-60 mL/d C 6-11 y: PO: 15-30 mL/d C 2-5 y: PO: 5-15 mL/d	For constipation, dyspepsia, and pyrosis. Take with a glass of water in morning or evening. May cause chalky taste, nausea, vomiting, diarrhea, dehydration, and hypermagnesemia. Pregnancy category: B*; PB: UK; t½: UK
Magnesium oxide (Mag-Ox)	A: PO: 2-4 g at bedtime with 8 oz water	For constipation, dyspepsia, and bowel preparation. Contraindicated in patients with renal failure. May cause flushing, sweating, hypotension, hypermagnesemia, and diarrhea. Pregnancy category: A*; PB: UK; t½: UK
Stimulants		
Bisacodyl	See Prototype Drug Chart 42.3.	
Castor oil	A/adol/C >12 y: PO: 15-60 mL/d PRN C 2-11 y: PO: 5-15 mL/d PRN	For bowel preparation and constipation. May cause hypotension, dizziness, nausea, diarrhea, steatorrhea, pruritus ani, abdominal cramps, and electrolyte imbalance. Pregnancy category: X*; PB: UK; t½: UK
Senna	Constipation: A/adol/C >12 y: PO: 1-2 tab or 10-15 mL syrup with full glass of water at bedtime; *max:* 4 tab bid or 15 mL bid C 6-11 y: PO: 1 tab or 5-7.5 mL at bedtime; *max:* 2 tabs bid or 7.5 mL bid C 2-5 y: PO: ½ tab or 2.5-3.75 mL at bedtime; *max:* 1 tab bid or 3.75 mL bid	For constipation and bowel preparation. May cause weakness, nausea, vomiting, diarrhea, and abdominal cramps. Prolonged use may cause fluid and electrolyte imbalances. Pregnancy category: C*; PB: UK; t½: UK
Selective Chloride Channel Activator		
Lubiprostone	A: PO: 24 mcg bid with food and water; *max:* 48 mcg/d	For treatment of constipation, IBS, and opioid-induced constipation. May cause headache, nausea, diarrhea, abdominal distension and pain, and flatulence. Pregnancy category: C*; PB: 94%; t½: 0.9-1.4 h

Continued

TABLE 42.5 Laxatives: Osmotics (Saline), Stimulants, and Selective Chloride Channel Activators—cont'd

Drug	Route and Dosage	Uses and Considerations
Miscellaneous		
Linaclotide	Constipation: A: PO: 145 mcg/d on empty stomach at least 30 min prior to first meal; *max.* 290 mcg/d	For constipation and IBS. May cause headache, flatulence, abdominal distension and pain, diarrhea, dehydration, and URI. Pregnancy category: C*; PB: UK; t½: UK
Naloxegol	A: PO: 12.5-25 mg/d am on empty stomach 1 h prior to first meal; *max.* 25 mg/d	For opiate agonist–induced constipation. May cause headache, flatulence, nausea, vomiting, diarrhea, and abdominal pain. Pregnancy category: C*; PB: 4.2%; t½: 6-11 h

*Pregnancy categories have been revised. See http://www.fda.gov/Drugs/DevelopmentApprovalProcess/DevelopmentResources/Labeling/ucm093 307.htm for more information.

A, Adult; *adol*, adolescent; *am*, in the morning; *bid*, twice a day; *C*, child; *d*, day; *h*, hour; *IBS*, irritable bowel syndrome; *max*, maximum; *min*, minute; *PB*, protein binding; *PO*, by mouth; *PR*, per rectum; *PRN*, as needed; *supp*, suppository; *t½*, half-life; *tab*, tablet; *UK*, unknown; *URI*, upper respiratory infection; *y*, year; *>*, greater than; *<*, less than.

Bulk-Forming Laxatives

Bulk-forming laxatives are natural fibrous substances that promote large, soft stools by absorbing water into the intestine, increasing fecal bulk and peristalsis. These agents are nonabsorbable. Defecation usually occurs within 8 to 24 hours; however, it may take up to 3 days after drug therapy is started for the stool to be soft and well formed. Powdered bulk-forming laxatives, which sometimes come in flavored and sugar-free forms, should be mixed in a glass of water or juice, stirred, drunk immediately, and followed by a half to a full glass of water. Insufficient fluid intake can cause the drug to solidify in the GI tract, which can result in intestinal obstruction. This group of laxatives does not cause laxative dependence and may be used by patients with diverticulosis, irritable bowel syndrome (IBS), and ileostomy and colostomy.

Polycarbophil, polyethylene glycol, methylcellulose, and psyllium are examples of bulk-forming laxatives. Patients with hypercalcemia should avoid calcium polycarbophil because of the significant amount of calcium in the drug. Prototype Drug Chart 42.4 lists the pharmacologic data for the bulk-forming laxative psyllium.

> **Pharmacokinetics** The bulk-forming laxative psyllium is a nondigestible and nonabsorbent substance that becomes a viscous solution when mixed with water. Because it is not absorbed, there is no protein binding or half-life for the drug. Psyllium is excreted in the feces.

> **Pharmacodynamics** The onset of action for psyllium is 12 to 72 hours. Peak action is 1 to 3 days. The duration of action is unknown.

Side Effects and Adverse Reactions. Bulk-forming laxatives are not systemically absorbed, therefore there is no systemic effect. If bulk-forming laxatives are excessively used, nausea, vomiting, flatus, or diarrhea may occur. Abdominal cramps may occur if the drug is used in dry form.

Chloride Channel Activators

Selective chloride channel activators are a new category of laxatives used to treat idiopathic constipation in adults. The first drug in this category is lubiprostone, manufactured by Sucampo Pharmaceuticals. Lubiprostone activates chloride channels in the lining of the small intestine, leading to an increase in intestinal fluid secretion and motility. By enhancing the passage of stool, lubiprostone relieves constipation and accompanying symptoms of abdominal discomfort, pain, and bloating. Lubiprostone is contraindicated for patients with a history of mechanical GI obstruction, Crohn disease, diverticulitis, and severe diarrhea. Adverse effects of lubiprostone include nausea that seems to be dose dependent, diarrhea, headache, abdominal distension, and flatulence.

Emollients (Stool Softeners)

Emollients are lubricants and stool softeners (surface-acting or wetting drugs) used to prevent constipation. These drugs decrease straining during defecation. Lubricants such as mineral oil increase water retention in the stool. Mineral oil absorbs the essential fat-soluble vitamins A, D, E, and K. Some of the minerals can be absorbed into the lymphatic system.

Stool softeners work by lowering surface tension and promoting water accumulation in the intestine and stool. They are frequently prescribed for patients after myocardial infarction or surgery. They are also given before administration of other laxatives in treating fecal impaction. Docusate calcium, docusate sodium, and docusate sodium with senna are examples of stool softeners.

Side Effects and Adverse Reactions. Side effects of mineral oil include nausea, vomiting, diarrhea, and abdominal cramping. This laxative is not indicated for children, older adults, or patients with debilitating diseases because they might aspirate the mineral oil, resulting in lipid pneumonia. The docusate group of drugs may cause mild cramping.

Contraindications. Contraindications to the use of laxatives include pregnancy and inflammatory disorders of the GI tract such as appendicitis, ulcerative colitis, undiagnosed severe pain that could be caused by inflammation within the intestine (diverticulitis, appendicitis), along with spastic colon or bowel obstruction. Laxatives are contraindicated when any of these conditions is suspected. Table 42.6 lists the laxatives and their dosages, uses, and considerations.

PROTOTYPE DRUG CHART 42.4

Psyllium

Drug Class	Dosage
Laxative: Bulk forming	A/adol: PO: 1 rounded tsp in 8 oz water followed by 8 oz water 1-3 times/d
Pregnancy category: B*	C >6 y: PO: ½ rounded tsp in 8 oz water, followed by at least 4 oz water 1-3 times/d

Contraindications	Drug-Lab-Food Interactions
Hypersensitivity, fecal impaction, intestinal obstruction, abdominal pain, GI bleeding, dysphagia, appendicitis	Drug: Decreased absorption of oral anticoagulants, aspirin, and digoxin
Caution: Older adults	

Pharmacokinetics	Pharmacodynamics
Absorption: Not absorbed	PO: Onset: 12-72 h
Distribution: PB: N/A	Peak: UK
Metabolism: t½: N/A	Duration: UK
Excretion: In feces	

Therapeutic Effects/Uses	
To control constipation	
Mode of Action: Acts as a bulk-forming laxative by drawing water into the intestine	

Side Effects	Adverse Reactions
Anorexia, nausea, vomiting, abdominal cramps, flatulence, diarrhea	Esophageal or intestinal obstruction if not taken with adequate water
	Life threatening: Bronchospasm, anaphylaxis

*Pregnancy categories have been revised. See http://www.fda.gov/Drugs/DevelopmentApprovalProcess/DevelopmentResources/Labeling/ucm093307.htm for more information.
A, Adult; *adol,* adolescent; *C,* child; *d,* day; *GI,* gastrointestinal; *h,* hour; *N/A,* not applicable; *PB,* protein binding; *PO,* by mouth; *t½,* half-life; *tsp,* teaspoon; *UK,* unknown; *y,* year; *>,* greater than.

TABLE 42.6 Laxatives: Bulk Forming, Emollients, and Evacuants

Drug	Route and Dosage	Uses and Considerations
Bulk Forming		
Polycarbophil	A/adol: PO: 1 g 1-4 times/d; *max:* 6 g/d C 6-12 y: PO: 500 mg/d 1-4 times/d; *max:* 2 g/d C 3-5 y: PO: 500 mg 1-2 times/d; *max:* 1 g/d	For constipation and IBS, administer with a full glass of water. May cause nausea, vomiting, flatulence, abdominal cramps, and distension. Pregnancy category: C*; PB: NA; t½: NA
Polyethylene glycol	A/adol >17 y: PO: 17 g (1 Tbsp) in 4-8 oz water qd; *max:* 34 g/d	For constipation and bowel preparation. May cause nausea, flatulence, diarrhea, abdominal cramps, and distension. Pregnancy category: C*; PB: NA; t½: NA
Methylcellulose	A/adol/C >12 y: PO: 2 g powder (1 heaping Tbsp) 1-3 times/d in 8-10 oz of water or 2 caplets 6 times/d; *max:* 3 doses/d or 12 caplets/d C 6-12 y: 1 g powder (½ Tbsp) qd with 8 oz of water or 1 caplet 6 times/d; *max:* 3 doses/d or 6 caplets/d	For constipation. Take immediately after mixing in water. May cause nausea, vomiting, diarrhea, abdominal cramps, and GI obstruction. Pregnancy category: C*; PB: NA; t½: NA
Psyllium hydrophilic mucilloid	See Prototype Drug Chart 42.4.	
Emollient: Stool Softeners		
Docusate calcium; docusate sodium	Docusate calcium: A/adol/C >12 y: PO: 240 mg/d Docusate sodium: A/adol/C >12 y: PO: 50-200 mg/d C 2-11 y: 25-100 mg/d	For constipation. May cause throat irritation, diarrhea, and abdominal cramps. Pregnancy category: C*; PB: NA; t½: NA
Docusate sodium with senna	A/adol/C >12 y: PO: 2-4 tabs/d C 6-11 y: PO: 1-2 tabs/d C 2-5 y: PO: 1 tab/d	For constipation. May cause weakness, dependence, electrolyte imbalance, abdominal cramps, and diarrhea. Pregnancy category: C*; PB: NA; t½: NA
Emollient: Lubricant		
Mineral oil	A/adol/C >12 y: PO: 30-90 mL/d C 6-11 y: PO: 10-30 mL/d	For constipation and fecal impaction. May be useful for those with cardiac disorders and following anorectal surgery. Avoid prolonged use because vitamins A, D, E, and K may be lost; may cause dizziness, weakness, nausea, diarrhea, abdominal cramps, fecal urgency/incontinence, skin irritation, and anal leakage. Pregnancy category: UK*; PB: NA; t½: NA

Continued

TABLE 42.6 Laxatives: Bulk Forming, Emollients, and Evacuants—cont'd

Drug	Route and Dosage	Uses and Considerations
Evacuant/Bowel Preparation		
Polyethylene glycol–electrolyte solution	A: PO: 240 mL q10-15min for total of 4 L	For constipation and bowel preparation. May cause disordered sleep, dizziness, weakness, thirst, nausea, vomiting, abdominal cramps and distension, fecal urgency, dehydration, and electrolyte imbalance. Pregnancy category: C*; PB: NA; t½: NA

*Pregnancy categories have been revised. See http://www.fda.gov/Drugs/DevelopmentApprovalProcess/DevelopmentResources/Labeling/ucm093307.htm for more information.

A, Adult; *adol*, adolescent; *C*, child; *d*, day; *GI*, gastrointestinal; *IBS*, irritable bowel syndrome; *max*, maximum; *NA*, not applicable; *PB*, protein binding; *PO*, by mouth; *q10-15 min*, every 10 to 15 minutes; *qd*, every day; *t½*, half-life; *tab*, tablet; *Tbsp*, tablespoon; *UK*, unknown; *y*, year; *>*, greater than.

NURSING PROCESS
Patient-Centered Collaborative Care
Laxative: Stimulant

Assessment
- Obtain a history of constipation and possible causes (insufficient water or fluid intake, diet deficient in bulk or fiber, inactivity), frequency and consistency of stools, and general health status.
- Record baseline vital signs for identification of abnormalities and for future comparisons.
- Evaluate renal function.
- Assess electrolyte balance of patients who frequently use laxatives.

Nursing Diagnoses
- Constipation related to ignoring urge to defecate
- Fluid Volume, Risk for Deficient
- Knowledge, Deficient related to overuse of laxatives
- Health Maintenance, Ineffective related to lack of ability to make thoughtful judgments

Planning
- The patient will have a normal bowel elimination pattern.
- The patient will exercise, eat foods high in fiber, and have adequate fluid intake to avoid constipation.

Nursing Interventions
- Monitor fluid intake and output.
- Note signs and symptoms of fluid and electrolyte imbalances that may result from watery stools. Habitual use of laxatives can cause fluid volume deficit, electrolyte losses, and loss of the urge to defecate.

Patient Teaching
General
- Encourage patients to increase water intake (if not contraindicated), which will decrease hard, dry stools.
- ⚡ Advise patients to avoid overuse of laxatives, which can lead to fluid and electrolyte imbalances and drug dependence. Suggest exercise to help increase peristalsis.
- Teach patients not to chew tablets but to swallow them whole.

- Direct patients to store suppositories at less than 86°F (30°C).
- Counsel patients to take drugs only with water to increase absorption.
- Educate patients not to take the drug within 1 hour of any other drug.
- Warn patients that the drug is not for long-term use; bowel tone may be lost.
- Encourage patients to time administration of the drug so as not to interfere with activities or sleep.

Side Effects
- Advise patients to discontinue use if rectal bleeding, nausea, vomiting, or cramping occurs.

Diet
- Inform patients to consume foods high in fiber such as bran, whole grains, and fruits.

Cultural Considerations
- Provide explanation and written information as needed related to the use and abuse of stimulant laxatives. Respect values and beliefs of patients from various cultural groups, and incorporate their traditional practices into the treatment plan when possible.

Evaluation
- Determine the effectiveness of nonpharmacologic methods for alleviating constipation.
- Evaluate the patient's use of laxatives in managing constipation. Identify laxative abuse.

NURSING PROCESS
Patient-Centered Collaborative Care
Laxative: Bulk Forming

Assessment
- Obtain a history of constipation and possible causes (insufficient water or fluid intake, diet deficient in bulk or fiber, inactivity), frequency and consistency of stools, and general health status.
- Record baseline vital signs for identification of abnormalities and for future comparisons.
- Assess renal function, urine output, blood urea nitrogen (BUN), and serum creatinine.

Nursing Diagnoses
- Constipation related to inadequate fiber in diet
- Fluid Volume, Risk for Deficient

Planning
- The patient will have a normal bowel elimination pattern.
- The patient will exercise, eat foods high in fiber, and have adequate fluid intake to avoid constipation.

Nursing Interventions
- ⚡ Check fluid intake and output. Note signs and symptoms of fluid and electrolyte imbalances that may result from watery stools. Habitual use of laxatives can cause fluid volume deficit and electrolyte losses.
- Monitor bowel sounds.
- Identify the cause of constipation.
- Avoid inhalation of psyllium dust.

Patient Teaching
General
- Teach patients to mix the agent with water immediately before use to avoid GI obstruction.
- Advise patients *not* to swallow the agent in dry form.
- Counsel patients to avoid overuse of laxatives, which can lead to fluid and electrolyte imbalances and laxative dependence. Suggest exercise to help increase peristalsis.
- ⚡ Advise patients to avoid inhaling psyllium dust; it may cause watery eyes, runny nose, and wheezing.

Side Effects
- Encourage patients to discontinue use if nausea, vomiting, cramping, or rectal bleeding occurs.

Diet
- ⚡ Instruct patients to mix the drug in 8 to 10 oz of water and to stir and drink it immediately. At least one glass of extra water should follow. Insufficient water can cause the drug to solidify, which can lead to dry, hard stools; fecal impaction; and esophageal obstruction.
- Encourage patients to increase foods rich in fiber such as bran, grains, vegetables, and fruits.
- Advise patients to increase water intake to at least 8 oz of fluids per day, which will decrease hard, dry stools.

🌐 Cultural Considerations
- Respect patients' cultural beliefs and alternative methods for treating constipation. Suggest nonpharmacologic methods that might be of benefit.
- Provide additional explanation about use and abuse of laxatives, and provide written materials in a language that the patient speaks and reads most easily.

Evaluation
- Determine the effectiveness of nonpharmacologic methods for alleviating constipation.
- Evaluate patients' use of laxatives in managing constipation.
- Identify laxative abuse.

CRITICAL THINKING CASE STUDY

CS, a 34-year-old woman, has been vomiting for 48 hours. In the last 12 hours, CS has had vomiting and diarrhea. Prochlorperazine 10 mg was administered intramuscularly.

1. What nonpharmacologic measures should the nurse suggest when vomiting occurs?
2. Why was CS given prochlorperazine intramuscularly and not orally or rectally? Prochlorperazine should be given deep into the muscle. Why?
3. What electrolyte imbalances may occur as a result of vomiting and diarrhea? Explain how they can be replaced.
4. What are the side effects of prochlorperazine? Could these occur to CS? Explain your answer.
5. Could a serotonin antagonist be given to CS instead of prochlorperazine? Explain your answer.

CS was prescribed diphenoxylate with atropine 2.5 mg initially, then 1 mg after each loose stool.

6. Is the diphenoxylate with atropine dosage for CS within the normal prescribed range? Explain your answer.
7. What clinical conditions are contraindicated for the use of diphenoxylate with atropine?
8. What are some combination drugs that may be prescribed to control diarrhea? Give their advantages and disadvantages.
9. Explain the similarities of two OTC antidiarrheals. Explain how frequently they should be administered.
10. Do you think CS should receive an adsorbent? Explain your answer.

NCLEX STUDY QUESTIONS

1. A patient complains of constipation and requires a laxative. In providing teaching for this patient, the nurse reviews the common causes of constipation, including which cause?
   a. Motion sickness
   b. Poor dietary habits
   c. Food intolerance
   d. Bacteria (*Escherichia coli*)

2. A patient with nausea is taking ondansetron. She asks the nurse how this drug works. The nurse is aware that this medication has which action?
   a. Enhances histamine$_1$ receptor sites
   b. Blocks serotonin receptors in the chemoreceptor trigger zone
   c. Blocks dopamine receptors in the chemoreceptor trigger zone
   d. Stimulates anticholinergic receptor sites

3. A patient who has constipation is prescribed a bisacodyl suppository. Which explanation will the nurse use to explain the action of bisacodyl?
   a. Acts on smooth intestinal muscle to gently increase peristalsis
   b. Absorbs water into the intestines to increase bulk and peristalsis
   c. Lowers surface tension and increases water accumulation in the intestines
   d. Pulls salts into the colon and increases water in the feces to increase bulk
4. A patient is using scopolamine to prevent motion sickness. About which common side effect should the nurse teach the patient?
   a. Diarrhea
   b. Vomiting
   c. Insomnia
   d. Dry mouth

5. When metoclopramide is given for nausea, the nurse plans to caution the patient to avoid which substance?
   a. Milk
   b. Coffee
   c. Alcohol
   d. Carbonated beverages
6. The nurse is administering difenoxin with atropine to a patient. Which should be included in the patient teaching regarding this medication? (Select all that apply.)
   a. Caution the patient to avoid laxative abuse.
   b. Record the frequency of bowel movements.
   c. Caution the patient against taking sedatives concurrently.
   d. Encourage the patient to increase fluids.
   e. Instruct the patient to avoid this drug if he or she has narrow-angle glaucoma.
   f. Teach the patient that the drug acts by drawing water into the intestine.

Answers: 1, b; 2, b; 3, a; 4, d; 5, c; 6, a, b, c, d, e.

Antiulcer Drugs

OBJECTIVES

- Explain the predisposing factors for peptic ulcers.
- Differentiate between peptic ulcer, gastric ulcer, duodenal ulcer, and gastroesophageal reflux disease (GERD).
- Compare the actions of the seven groups of antiulcer drugs used in the treatment of peptic ulcer: tranquilizers, anticholinergics, antacids, histamine$_2$ blockers, proton pump inhibitors, pepsin inhibitors, and prostaglandin analogues.

- Plan patient teaching for anticholinergic, antacid, and histamine$_2$ blocker drug groups.
- Differentiate among the side effects of anticholinergics and systemic and nonsystemic antacids.
- Apply the nursing process, including teaching, to antiulcer drugs.

OUTLINE

KEY TERMS

Peptic ulcer is a broad term for an ulcer that occurs in the esophagus, stomach, or duodenum within the upper gastrointestinal (GI) tract. Ulcers are more specifically named according to the site of involvement: esophageal, gastric, or duodenal. Duodenal ulcers occur 10 times more frequently than gastric and esophageal ulcers. The release of hydrochloric acid (HCl) from the parietal cells of the stomach is influenced by histamine, gastrin, and acetylcholine. Peptic ulcers occur when there is a hypersecretion of hydrochloric acid and pepsin, which erode the GI mucosal lining.

The gastric secretions in the stomach strive to maintain a pH of 2 to 5. Pepsin, a digestive enzyme, is activated at a pH of 2, and the acid-pepsin complex of gastric secretions can cause mucosal damage. If the pH of gastric secretions increases to 5, the activity of pepsin declines. The gastric mucosal barrier (GMB) is a thick, viscous, mucous material that provides a barrier between the mucosal lining and acidic gastric secretions. The GMB maintains the integrity of the gastric mucosal lining and is a defense against corrosive substances. The two sphincter muscles—the *cardiac,* located at the upper portion of the stomach, and the *pyloric,* located at the lower portion of the stomach—act as barriers to prevent reflux of acid into the esophagus and duodenum. Fig. 43.1 shows common sites of peptic ulcers.

An esophageal ulcer results from reflux of acidic gastric secretions into the esophagus as a result of a defective or incompetent cardiac sphincter. A gastric ulcer frequently occurs because of a breakdown of the GMB. A duodenal ulcer is

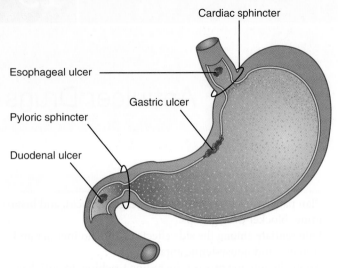

FIG. 43.1 Common sites of peptic ulcers.

TABLE 43.1	**Predisposing Factors for Peptic Ulcer Disease**
Predisposing Factors	**Effects**
Mechanical disturbances	Hypersecretion of acid and pepsin; inadequate GMB mucous secretion; impaired GMB resistance; hypermotility of the stomach; incompetent (defective) cardiac or pyloric sphincter
Genetic influences	Increased number of parietal cells in the stomach; susceptibility of mucosal lining to acid penetration; susceptibility to excess acetylcholine and histamine; excess hydrochloric acid caused by external stimuli
Environmental influences	Foods and liquids containing caffeine; fatty, fried, and highly spiced foods; alcohol; nicotine, especially from cigarette smoking; stressful situations; pregnancy; massive trauma; major surgery
Helicobacter pylori	A gram-negative bacterium, *H. pylori*, infects gastric mucosa and can cause gastritis, gastric ulcer, and duodenal ulcer. If not eradicated, peptic ulcer may return as frequently as every year. *H. pylori* can lead to atrophic gastritis in some patients. Serology and special breath tests can detect the presence of *H. pylori*.
Drugs	NSAIDs, including aspirin and aspirin compounds, ibuprofen, and indomethacin; corticosteroids; potassium salts; antineoplastic drugs

GMB, Gastric mucosal barrier; *NSAIDs,* nonsteroidal antiinflammatory drugs.

caused by hypersecretion of acid from the stomach passing into the duodenum because of (1) insufficient buffers to neutralize gastric acid in the stomach, (2) a defective or incompetent pyloric sphincter, or (3) hypermotility of the stomach. **Gastroesophageal reflux disease (GERD)** is inflammation or erosion of the esophageal mucosa caused by a reflux of gastric acid content from the stomach into the esophagus.

PREDISPOSING FACTORS IN PEPTIC ULCER DISEASE

The nurse needs to assist the patient in identifying possible causes of the ulcer and to teach ways to alleviate it. Predisposing factors include mechanical disturbances, genetic influences, bacterial organisms, environmental factors, and certain drugs. Healing of an ulcer takes 4 to 8 weeks. Complications can occur as the result of scar tissue. Table 43.1 lists the predisposing factors for peptic ulcers and their effects.

The classic symptom of peptic ulcers is gnawing, aching pain. With a gastric ulcer, pain occurs 30 minutes to 1.5 hours after eating, and with a duodenal ulcer, pain occurs 2 to 3 hours after eating. Small, frequent meals of nonirritating foods decrease the pain. With treatment, pain usually subsides in 10 days; however, the healing process may take 1 to 2 months.

A **stress ulcer** usually follows a critical situation such as extensive trauma, such as burns, or major surgery (e.g., cardiac surgery). Prophylactic use of antiulcer drugs decreases the incidence of stress ulcers.

Helicobacter pylori

Helicobacter pylori, a gram-negative bacillus, is linked with the development of peptic ulcer and is known to cause gastritis, gastric ulcer, and duodenal ulcer. When a peptic ulcer recurs after antiulcer therapy, and the ulcer is not caused by nonsteroidal antiinflammatory drugs (NSAIDs) such as aspirin or ibuprofen, the patient should be tested for the presence of *H. pylori,* which may have infected the gastric mucosa. In the past, endoscopy and a biopsy of the gastric antrum were needed to check for

H. pylori. Currently, a noninvasive breath test—the Meretek UBT (urea breath test)—can detect *H. pylori.* This test consists of drinking a liquid containing 13C urea and breathing into a container. If *H. pylori* is present, the bacterial urease hydrolyzes the urea, releasing 13CO$_2$, which is detected by a spectrometer. This test is 90% to 95% effective for detecting *H. pylori* and also notes progress in treatment. In addition, a blood test may be performed to check for antibodies to *H. pylori,* and a stool test may be done to check for antigens to determine whether the immune system has been triggered to fight *H. pylori.*

There are various protocols for treating *H. pylori* infection, but antibacterial agents are the treatment of choice. The use of only one antibacterial agent is not effective for eradicating *H. pylori* because the bacterium can readily become resistant to that drug. Treatment to eradicate this bacterial infection includes using a dual-, triple-, or quadruple-drug therapy program in a variety of drug combinations—such as with amoxicillin, tetracycline, clarithromycin, omeprazole, lansoprazole, metronidazole, bismuth subsalicylate, or ranitidine bismuth citrate—on a 7- to 14-day treatment plan. The combination of drugs differs for each patient according to the patient's drug tolerance. A common treatment protocol is the triple therapy of metronidazole (or amoxicillin), omeprazole (or lansoprazole), and clarithromycin (MOC). The drug regimen eradicates more than 90% of peptic ulcers caused by *H. pylori* (Complementary and Alternative Therapies 43.1).

One of the proton pump inhibitors (PPIs), such as omeprazole or lansoprazole, is frequently used as a component of combination drug therapy because each suppresses acid secretion by inhibiting the enzyme hydrogen or potassium adenosine triphosphatase

COMPLEMENTARY AND ALTERNATIVE THERAPIES 43.1

Tetracycline

St. John's wort may increase the risk for photosensitivity when taken with tetracycline.

TABLE 43.2 Pharmacologic Agents Used to Treat *Helicobacter pylori* Infection

Drug	Route and Dosage	Uses and Considerations
Antiinfective Agents		
Metronidazole hydrochloride	A: PO: 250 mg qid	To treat numerous organisms, including *H. pylori;* used in combination with other drugs to treat *H. pylori*
Amoxicillin	A: PO: 1000 mg bid	Used in triple- or quadruple-drug therapy for *H. pylori*
Clarithromycin	A: PO: 500 mg bid	Used in dual- and triple-drug therapy for *H. pylori*
Tetracycline	A: PO: 500 mg qid	Used in triple- and quadruple-drug therapy for *H. pylori*
Proton Pump Inhibitors (PPIs)		
Omeprazole	A: PO: 20 mg bid or 40 mg/d	Used in dual-, triple-, and quadruple-drug therapy for *H. pylori*
Lansoprazole	A: PO: 30 mg bid	Used in dual- and triple-drug therapy for *H. pylori*
Esomeprazole	A: PO: 40 mg/d	Used in therapy for *H. pylori*
Pantoprazole	A: PO: 40 mg/d	Used in therapy for *H. pylori*
Rabeprazole	A: PO: 20 mg bid	Used in therapy for *H. pylori*

A, Adult; *bid,* twice a day; *d,* day; *PO,* by mouth; *qid,* four times a day.

(ATPase), which makes gastric acid. These agents block the final steps of acid production. If triple therapy fails to eradicate *H. pylori,* quadruple therapy using two antibiotics, a PPI, and a bismuth or histamine$_2$ (H$_2$) blocker is recommended. After completion of the treatment regimen, 6 weeks of standard acid suppression—such as H$_2$ blocker therapy—is recommended. Table 43.2 lists agents used to treat *H. pylori* with their dosages, uses, and considerations.

Gastroesophageal Reflux Disease

Gastroesophageal reflux disease (GERD), also called *reflux esophagitis,* is an inflammation of the esophageal mucosa caused by reflux of gastric acid content into the esophagus. Its main cause is an incompetent lower esophageal sphincter. Smoking tends to accelerate the disease process.

Medical treatment for GERD is similar to the treatment for peptic ulcers. This includes use of the common antiulcer drugs to neutralize gastric contents and reduce gastric acid secretion. Drugs used in treatment include H$_2$ blockers such as ranitidine and PPIs such as omeprazole, lansoprazole, rabeprazole, pantoprazole, or esomeprazole. A PPI relieves symptoms faster and maintains healing better than an H$_2$ blocker. Once the strictures are relieved by dilation, they are less likely to recur if the patient was taking PPIs rather than an H$_2$ blocker.

Effective management of GERD keeps the esophageal mucosa healed and the patient free from symptoms, but GERD is a chronic disorder that requires continuous care.

NONPHARMACOLOGIC MEASURES FOR MANAGING PEPTIC ULCER AND GASTROESOPHAGEAL REFLUX DISEASE

Nonpharmacologic measures, along with drug therapy, are an important part of treatment for a GI disorder. Once the GI problem is resolved, the patient should continue to follow nonpharmacologic measures to avoid recurrence of the condition.

Avoiding tobacco and alcohol can decrease gastric secretions. With GERD, nicotine relaxes the lower esophageal sphincter, permitting gastric acid reflux. Obesity enhances GERD, so weight loss is helpful in decreasing symptoms. The patient should avoid hot, spicy, and greasy foods, which could aggravate the gastric problem. Certain drugs like NSAIDs, which include aspirin, should be taken with food or in a decreased dosage. Glucocorticoids can cause gastric ulceration and should be taken with food.

To relieve symptoms of GERD, the patient should raise the head of the bed, not eat before bedtime, and wear loose-fitting clothing.

> ⚡ **PATIENT SAFETY**
>
> **Do not confuse:**
> - **Ranitidine,** an H$_2$ blocker, with **rimantadine,** an antiviral, or **amantadine,** an antiviral and antiparkinsonism agent
> - **Zantac,** an H$_2$ blocker, with **Xanax,** an anxiolytic

ANTIULCER DRUGS

The seven groups of antiulcer agents are (1) tranquilizers, which decrease vagal activity; (2) anticholinergics, which decrease acetylcholine by blocking the cholinergic receptors; (3) antacids, which neutralize gastric acid; (4) H$_2$ blockers, which block the H$_2$ receptor; (5) PPIs, which inhibit gastric acid secretion, regardless of acetylcholine or histamine release; (6) the pepsin inhibitor sucralfate; and (7) the prostaglandin E$_1$ analogue misoprostol, which inhibits gastric acid secretion and protects the mucosa. Currently, tranquilizers and anticholinergics are used infrequently due to potential adverse effects and much more effective drugs on the market. Fig. 43.2 shows the action of the antiulcer drug groups, each of which is discussed separately.

Tranquilizers

Tranquilizers have minimal effect in preventing and treating ulcers; however, they reduce vagal stimulation and decrease anxiety. A combination of the anxiolytic chlordiazepoxide and the anticholinergic clidinium bromide may be used in the treatment of ulcers. Adverse effects may include edema, ataxia, confusion, extrapyramidal syndrome (EPS), and agranulocytosis.

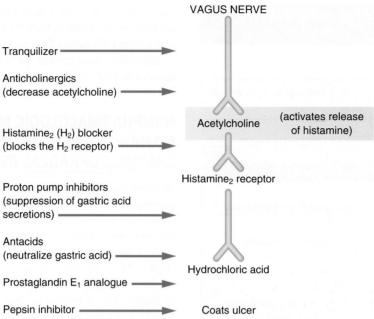

FIG. 43.2 Actions of the antiulcer drug groups.

TABLE 43.3	Antiulcer Drugs: Anticholinergics	
Drug	**Route and Dosage**	**Uses and Considerations**
Clidinium bromide and chlordiazepoxide hydrochloride	Ulcer: A: PO: 1-2 cap (clidinium 2.5 mg, chlordiazepoxide 5 mg) tid/qid ac and at bedtime; *max.* clidinium 20 mg/d, chlordiazepoxide 40 mg/d Older A: PO: 1 cap bid; *max.* clidinium 20 mg/d, chlordiazepoxide 40 mg/d	For treatment of gastric ulcer, IBS, and enterocolitis. May cause drowsiness, confusion, dry mouth, blurred vision, nausea, constipation, edema, and ataxia. Pregnancy category: D*; PB: 96%; t½: 2.4-20 h
Glycopyrrolate	Ulcer: A/adol/C >12 y: PO: 1-2 mg bid/tid; *max:* 6 mg/d A/adol >16 y: IM/IV: 100-200 mcg q4h as needed; *max:* 6 mg/d	For gastric and duodenal ulcers, bradycardia, and aspiration prophylaxis. May cause dry mouth, blurred vision, headache, flushing, anhidrosis, palpitations, seizures, erectile dysfunction, urinary retention, and constipation. Pregnancy category: B*; PB: UK; t½: 0.5-3 h
Propantheline	A: PO: 15 mg tid 30 min ac and 30 mg at bedtime Older A: PO: 7.5 mg bid/tid ac	For duodenal ulcers. May cause headache, dizziness, blurred vision, confusion, palpitations, hypotension, anhidrosis, urinary retention, dysphagia, and constipation. Pregnancy category: C*; PB: UK; t½: 1.6 h

*Pregnancy categories have been revised. See http://www.fda.gov/Drugs/DevelopmentApprovalProcess/DevelopmentResources/Labeling/ucm093 307.htm for more information.

A, Adult; *ac,* before meals; *adol,* adolescent; *bid,* twice a day; *C,* child; *cap,* capsule; *d,* day; *h,* hour; *IBS,* irritable bowel syndrome; *IM,* intramuscular; *IV,* intravenous; *max,* maximum; *min,* minutes; *PB,* protein binding; *PO,* by mouth; *q4h,* every 4 hours; *qid,* four times a day; *t½,* half-life; *tid,* three times a day; *UK,* unknown; *y,* years; *>,* greater than.

Anticholinergics

Anticholinergics (antimuscarinics, parasympatholytics) and antacids were the drugs of choice for peptic ulcers for many years. However, anticholinergic use declined with the introduction of H₂ blockers in 1975. These drugs relieve pain by decreasing GI motility and secretion. They act by inhibiting acetylcholine and blocking histamine and hydrochloric acid. Anticholinergics delay gastric emptying time, so they are used more frequently for duodenal ulcers than for gastric ulcers. The anticholinergic propantheline bromide inhibits gastric secretions in the treatment of peptic ulcers.

Anticholinergics should be taken before meals to decrease the acid secretion that occurs with eating. Antacids can slow the absorption of anticholinergics and therefore should be taken 2 hours after anticholinergic administration.

Table 43.3 lists selected anticholinergic drugs used to treat peptic ulcer. Anticholinergics should be used as adjunctive therapy and not as the only antiulcer drug. Anticholinergics are discussed in more detail in Chapter 16.

Side Effects and Adverse Reactions

Anticholinergics have many side effects, including dry mouth, decreased secretions, headache, blurred vision, drowsiness, dizziness, lethargy, palpitations, bradycardia, tachycardia, urinary retention, and constipation. Because anticholinergics decrease GI motility, gastric emptying time is delayed, which can stimulate gastric secretions and aggravate the ulceration.

Antacids

Antacids promote ulcer healing by neutralizing hydrochloric acid and reducing pepsin activity; they do not coat the ulcer. There are two types of antacids: those that have a *systemic* effect and those that have a *nonsystemic* effect.

Sodium bicarbonate, a systemically absorbed antacid, was one of the first antiulcer drugs. Because it has many side effects (sodium excess, causing hypernatremia and water retention; metabolic alkalosis caused by excess bicarbonate; and acid rebound [excess acid secretion]), sodium bicarbonate is seldom used to treat peptic ulcers.

Calcium carbonate is most effective in neutralizing acid; however, one third to one half of the drug can be systemically absorbed and can cause acid rebound. Hypercalcemia and Burnett syndrome, formerly called *milk-alkali syndrome*, can result from excessive use of calcium carbonate. Burnett syndrome is intensified if milk products are ingested with calcium carbonate. It is identified by the presence of alkalosis, hypercalcemia, and in severe cases, by crystalluria and renal failure.

The nonsystemic antacids are composed of alkaline salts such as aluminum (aluminum hydroxide) and magnesium (magnesium hydroxide, magnesium trisilicate). A small degree of systemic absorption occurs with these drugs, mainly of aluminum. Magnesium hydroxide has greater neutralizing power than aluminum hydroxide. Magnesium compounds can cause diarrhea, and aluminum and calcium compounds can cause constipation with long-term use. A combination of magnesium and aluminum salts neutralizes gastric acid without causing severe diarrhea or constipation. Simethicone, an antigas agent, is found in many antacids. Prototype Drug Chart 43.1 lists the pharmacologic data for aluminum hydroxide antacids.

Pharmacokinetics Aluminum hydroxide was one of the first antacids used to neutralize hydrochloric acid. Aluminum products are frequently used to lower high serum phosphate (hyperphosphatemia). Because aluminum hydroxide alone can cause constipation, and magnesium products alone can cause diarrhea, combination drugs such as aluminum hydroxide and magnesium hydroxide have become popular because they decrease these side effects.

Only a small amount of aluminum hydroxide is absorbed from the GI tract. It is primarily bound to phosphate and excreted in the feces. The small portion that is absorbed is excreted in the urine.

Pharmacodynamics Aluminum hydroxide neutralizes gastric acid, including hydrochloric acid, and increases the pH of gastric secretions; an elevated pH inactivates pepsin. The onset of action is fairly rapid, but the duration of action varies, depending on whether the antacid is taken with or without food. If the antacid is taken after a meal, the duration of action may be up to 3 hours because food delays gastric emptying time. Frequent dosing may be necessary if the antacid is given during a fasting state or early in the course of treatment.

PROTOTYPE DRUG CHART 43.1
Aluminum Hydroxide

Drug Class	Dosage
Antiulcer: Antacid Pregnancy category: C*	Hyperacidity: A: PO: 640 mg (10 mL) 5-6 times/day between meals and at bedtime

Contraindications	Drug-Lab-Food Interactions
Hypersensitivity to aluminum products, hypophosphatemia *Caution:* Diarrhea, hepatic and renal disease, older adults, children, pregnancy	Drug: Decreased effects with tetracycline, phenothiazine, isoniazid, phenytoin, digitalis, quinidine, amphetamines, fluoroquinolones, and captopril; may increase effects of benzodiazepines, glipizide, and glyburide Lab: Increased urine pH

Pharmacokinetics	Pharmacodynamics
Absorption: PO: Small amount absorbed Distribution: PB: UK Metabolism: t½: UK Excretion: In feces; small amount in urine	PO: Onset: 15-30 min Peak: 0.5 h Duration: 1-3 h

Therapeutic Effects/Uses
To treat hyperacidity, gastric and duodenal ulcer, and reflux esophagitis; to reduce hyperphosphatemia
Mode of Action: Neutralizes gastric acidity

Side Effects	Adverse Reactions
Anorexia, constipation, weakness, impaired cognition	Hypophosphatemia, hypercalcemia, hemorrhoids, osteoporosis, nephrolithiasis; long-term use can result in GI obstruction.

*Pregnancy categories have been revised. See http://www.fda.gov/Drugs/DevelopmentApprovalProcess/DevelopmentResources/Labeling/ucm093307.htm for more information.

A, Adult; *GI*, gastrointestinal; *h*, hour; *min*, minute; *PB*, protein binding; *PO*, by mouth; *t½*, half-life; *UK*, unknown.

The ideal dosing interval for antacids is 1 and 3 hours after meals (maximum acid secretion occurs after eating) and at bedtime. Antacids taken on an empty stomach are effective for 30 to 60 minutes before passing into the duodenum. Chewable tablets should be followed by water. Liquid antacids should also be taken with water (2 to 4 oz) to ensure that the drug reaches the stomach; however, no more than 4 ounces of water should be taken because water quickens gastric emptying time.

Antacids that contain magnesium salts are contraindicated in patients with impaired renal function because of the risk for hypermagnesemia. Magnesium is primarily excreted by the kidneys; however, hypermagnesemia is usually not a problem unless a patient with renal insufficiency is ingesting magnesium. Prolonged use of aluminum hydroxides can cause hypophosphatemia (low serum phosphate), osteoporosis, nephrolithiasis, and osteomalacia. If hyperphosphatemia occurs because of poor renal function, aluminum hydroxide can be given to decrease the phosphate level. In patients with renal insufficiency, aluminum salt ingestion can cause encephalopathy from accumulation of aluminum in the brain. Table 43.4 lists the antacids and their dosages, uses, and considerations.

TABLE 43.4   Antiulcer Drugs: Antacids

Drug	Route and Dosage	Uses and Considerations
Aluminum hydroxide	See Prototype Drug Chart 43.1.	
Calcium carbonate	Dyspepsia: A: PO: Chew 1-4 tabs (400-800 mg), may repeat q1-2h PRN; *max.* 3200 mg/d	To treat pyrosis, dyspepsia, hypocalcemia, and hyperphosphatemia and for osteoporosis prophylaxis. May cause hypercalcemia, hypophosphatemia, eructation, constipation, flatulence, and acid rebound. Pregnancy category: C*; PB: 40%; t½: UK
Calcium carbonate and magnesium hydroxide	Regular strength: A: PO: Chew 2-4 tabs PRN; *max.* 12 tabs/d Ultra strength: 2-3 tabs PRN; *max.* 7 tabs/d	To treat pyrosis and dyspepsia. May cause hypercalcemia, hypermagnesemia, hypophosphatemia, eructation, flatulence, constipation, and acid rebound. Pregnancy category: C*; PB: 40%; t½: UK
Magnesium hydroxide and aluminum hydroxide	A: PO: 10-20 mL qid; *max.* 80 mL/d	To treat gastric and duodenal ulcers, dyspepsia, pyrosis, and GERD. May cause nausea, vomiting, constipation, hypercalcemia, hypermagnesemia, and hypophosphatemia. Pregnancy category: B*; PB: UK; t½: UK
Magnesium hydroxide 200 mg and aluminum hydroxide 200 mg with simethicone 25 mg	A/C >12 y: PO: 10-20 mL or 2-4 tsp between meals and at bedtime Extra strength: A/C >12 y: PO: 1-2 tabs between meals and at bedtime	To treat dyspepsia, pyrosis, and flatulence. May cause hypercalcemia, hypermagnesemia, hypophosphatemia, nausea, vomiting, diarrhea, constipation, dehydration, and GI obstruction. Pregnancy category: C*; PB: UK; t½: UK
Magnesium trisilicate with aluminum hydroxide	A/adol/C >12 y: PO: 2-4 tab (magnesium hydroxide 14.2 mg and aluminum hydroxide 80 mg) qid; *max:* 16 tab/d	To treat dyspepsia, pyrosis, and GERD. May cause hypercalcemia, hypermagnesemia, hypophosphatemia, nausea, vomiting, constipation, and GI obstruction. Pregnancy category: UK*; PB: UK; t½: UK
Sodium bicarbonate	Dyspepsia: A: PO: 300 mg-2 g 1-4 times/d	To treat dyspepsia, pyrosis, hyperkalemia, and metabolic acidosis. May cause flatulence, peripheral edema, hypernatremia, metabolic alkalosis, tremor, and seizure. Pregnancy category: C*; PB: UK; t½: UK

*Pregnancy categories have been revised. See http://www.fda.gov/Drugs/DevelopmentApprovalProcess/DevelopmentResources/Labeling/ucm093 307.htm for more information.

A, Adult; *adol*, adolescent; *C*, child; *d*, day; *GERD*, gastroesophageal reflux disease; *GI*, gastrointestinal; *max*, maximum; *PB*, protein binding; *PO*, by mouth; *PRN*, as needed, *q1-2h*, every 1 to 2 hours; *qid*, four times a day; *t½*, half-life; *tab*, tablet; *UK*, unknown; *y*, years; *>*, greater than.

⊙ NURSING PROCESS
Patient-Centered Collaborative Care
Antiulcer: Antacids

Assessment
- Evaluate patient pain, including the type, duration, severity, and frequency.
- Check renal function.
- Assess for fluid and electrolyte imbalances, especially serum phosphate and calcium levels.
- Obtain a drug history, and report probable drug-drug interactions.

Nursing Diagnoses
- Pain, Acute related to repeated spicy food and alcohol ingestion
- Health Maintenance, Ineffective related to misuse of antacids
- Knowledge, Deficient related to misinterpretation of information

Planning
- The patient's abdominal pain will decrease after 1 to 2 weeks of antiulcer drug management.

Nursing Interventions
- Avoid administering antacids with other oral drugs because antacids can delay their absorption. Do not give an antacid with tetracycline, digoxin, or quinidine because it binds with and inactivates most of the drug. Antacids are given 1 to 2 hours after other medications.
- Shake suspensions well before administering, and follow them with water.
- Monitor electrolytes and urinary pH, calcium, and phosphate levels.

Patient Teaching
General
- ⚡ Teach patients to report pain, coughing, or vomiting of blood.
- Encourage patients to drink 2 oz of water after taking an antacid to ensure that the drug reaches the stomach.
- Direct patients to take antacids 1 to 3 hours after meals and at bedtime. Instruct patients not to take antacids at mealtime; they slow gastric emptying time, causing increased GI activity and gastric secretions.
- Advise patients to notify a health care provider if constipation or diarrhea occurs; the antacid may have to be changed. Self-treatment should be avoided.
- ⚡ Warn that taking an unlimited amount of the antacid is contraindicated.
- Warn patients to avoid taking antacids with milk or foods high in vitamin D.
- Advise patients to avoid taking antacids within 1 to 2 hours of other oral medications because they may interfere with absorption.

- Guide patients on a sodium-restricted diet to check antacid labels for sodium content.
- Alert patients to consult with a health care provider before taking self-prescribed antacids for longer than 2 weeks.
- Inform patients on the use of relaxation techniques.

Self-Administration
- Teach patients how to take antacids correctly. Chewable tablets must be thoroughly chewed and followed with water. With liquid antacids, patients should follow the antacid with 2 to 4 oz of water. Increased amounts of water with antacids increases gastric emptying time.

Side Effects
- Direct patients to avoid foods and beverages that can cause gastric irritation (high-fat or spicy meals; caffeine-containing coffee and soda; alcohol).
- Explain to patients that stools may become speckled or white.

Cultural Considerations
- Respect patients' cultural beliefs and alternative methods for treating GI discomfort.
- Discuss with patients the safety of those methods and the use of drugs prescribed to heal and lessen the symptoms.
- Recognize that patients of various cultural backgrounds may need guidance in understanding the disease process of their GI disturbance. Use of a written plan of care with modifications should be considered.

Evaluation
- Determine the effectiveness of the antiulcer treatment and the presence of side effects. The patient should be free of pain, and healing should progress.

Histamine$_2$ Blockers

The **histamine$_2$ (H$_2$) receptor antagonists**, or H$_2$ blockers, are popular drugs used in the treatment of gastric and duodenal ulcers. Histamine$_2$ blockers prevent acid reflux in the esophagus (reflux esophagitis). These drugs block the H$_2$ receptors of the parietal cells in the stomach thus reducing gastric acid secretion and concentration. Antihistamines used to treat allergic conditions act against histamine$_1$ (H$_1$); they are not the same as H$_2$ blockers.

The first H$_2$ blocker was cimetidine, introduced in 1975. Cimetidine, which has a short half-life and a short duration of action, blocks about 70% of acid secretion for 4 hours. Good kidney function is necessary because approximately 50% to 80% of the drug is excreted unchanged in the urine. In patients with renal insufficiency, the dose and frequency may need to be reduced. Antacids can be given 1 hour before or after cimetidine as part of an antiulcer drug regimen; however, if they are given at the same time, the effectiveness of the H$_2$ blocker is decreased.

Three H$_2$ blockers—ranitidine, famotidine, and nizatidine—are more potent than cimetidine. In addition to blocking gastric acid secretions, they promote healing of the ulcer by eliminating its cause. Their duration of action is longer, decreasing the frequency of dosing, and they have fewer side effects and fewer

PROTOTYPE DRUG CHART 43.2
Ranitidine

Drug Class	Dosage
Antiulcer: Histamine$_2$ blocker Pregnancy category: B*	Dyspepsia/pyrosis: A: PO: 75-150 mg q12h; *max*: 300 mg/d

Contraindications	Drug-Lab-Food Interactions
Hypersensitivity, severe *Caution:* Pregnancy, breastfeeding, renal or liver disease, older adults, children	Drug: Decreased absorption with antacids; decreased effects of ketoconazole, cephalosporins, sulfonylureas; toxicity with metoprolol Lab: Increased serum alkaline phosphatase

Pharmacokinetics	Pharmacodynamics
Absorption: PO: Well absorbed, 50% Distribution: PB: 15% Metabolism: t½: 2-3 h Excretion: In urine and feces	PO: Onset: 15 min Peak: 2-3 h Duration: 8-12 h IM/IV: Onset: 10-15 min Peak: 15 min Duration: 8-12 h

Therapeutic Effects/Uses
To prevent and treat gastric and duodenal ulcers, pyrosis, dyspepsia, esophagitis, GERD, and Zollinger-Ellison syndrome
Mode of Action: Inhibits gastric acid secretion by inhibiting histamine at histamine$_2$ receptors in parietal cells

Side Effects	Adverse Reactions
Headache, dizziness, drowsiness, confusion, nausea, vomiting, diarrhea or constipation, abdominal pain, depression, rash, blurred vision, malaise, erectile dysfunction, weakness	*Life threatening:* Elevated hepatic enzymes, cardiac dysrhythmias, bradycardia, blood dyscrasias

*Pregnancy categories have been revised. See http://www.fda.gov/Drugs/DevelopmentApprovalProcess/DevelopmentResources/Labeling/ucm093307.htm for more information. *A*, Adult; *d*, day; *GERD*, gastroesophageal reflux disease; *h*, hour; *IM*, intramuscular; *IV*, intravenous; *max*, maximum; *min*, minute; *PB*, protein binding; *PO*, by mouth; *q12h*, every 12 hours; *t½*, half-life.

drug interactions than cimetidine. Prototype Drug Chart 43.2 lists the pharmacologic data for ranitidine, the most frequently prescribed H$_2$ blocker.

Pharmacokinetics Ranitidine is 5 to 12 times more potent than cimetidine but is less potent than famotidine. It is rapidly absorbed and reaches its peak concentration after a single dose in 2 to 3 hours. Ranitidine has a low protein-binding power and a short half-life. With liver disease, the half-life of ranitidine is prolonged. About 50% of the absorbed drug is excreted unchanged in the urine.

Ulcer healing occurs in 4 weeks for 70% of patients and in 8 weeks for 90% of patients taking ranitidine. Large doses of ranitidine are effective for controlling Zollinger-Ellison syndrome, whereas cimetidine is not effective in controlling the symptoms of this disorder.

Pharmacodynamics Ranitidine inhibits histamine at the H$_2$ receptor site. The drug is effective in treating gastric and duodenal ulcers and can be used prophylactically. It is also useful in relieving symptoms of reflux esophagitis, preventing stress

TABLE 43.5　Antiulcer Drugs: Histamine₂ Blockers

Drug	Route and Dosage	Uses and Considerations
Cimetidine	Dyspepsia, pyrosis: A/adol/C >12 y: PO: 200 mg bid 30 min ac; *max.* 400 mg/d GERD, ulcers: A/ adol >16 y: PO: 800 mg bid C <15 y: PO: 20-40 mg/kg/d divided doses Peptic ulcer: A/adol >16 y: PO: 800 mg/d at bedtime A/adol >16 y: IV/IM: 300 mg q6h C <15 y: PO/IV/IM: 20-40 mg/kg/d divided q6h	To treat gastric and duodenal ulcers, *Helicobacter pylori* infection, pyrosis, and dyspepsia. May cause headache, dizziness, drowsiness, agitation, gynecomastia, and diarrhea. Pregnancy category: B*; PB: 20%; t½: 2 h
Famotidine	Ulcers: A: PO: 20-40 mg bid up to 12 weeks; *max.* 40 mg/d A: IV: 20 mg q12h; *max.* 40 mg/d	To treat gastric and duodenal ulcers, dyspepsia, *H. pylori* infection, pyrosis, GERD, and esophagitis. May cause dizziness, headache, confusion, agitation, diarrhea, constipation, erectile dysfunction, and palpitations. Pregnancy category: B*; PB: 15%-20%; t½: 2.5-3.5 h
Nizatidine	A: PO: 150 mg q12h or 300 mg at bedtime for 8 weeks; *max.* 300 mg/d	To treat gastric and duodenal ulcers, dyspepsia, *H. pylori* infection, pyrosis, GERD, and esophagitis. May cause dizziness, cough, irritability, headache, fever, rhinitis, and diarrhea. Do not give within 1 h of antacids. Pregnancy category: B*; PB: 35%; t½: 1-2 h
Ranitidine	See Prototype Drug Chart 43.2.	

*Pregnancy categories have been revised. See http://www.fda.gov/Drugs/DevelopmentApprovalProcess/DevelopmentResources/Labeling/ucm093 307.htm for more information.

A, Adult; *ac*, before meals; *adol*, adolescent; *bid*, twice daily; *C*, child; *d*, day; *GERD*, gastroesophageal reflux disease; *h*, hour; *IM*, intramuscular; *IV*, intravenous; *max*, maximum; *min*, minute; *PB*, protein binding; *PO*, by mouth; *q*, every; *t½*, half-life; *y*, years; >, greater than; <, less than.

ulcers that can occur following major surgery, and preventing aspiration pneumonitis that can result from aspiration of gastric acid secretions.

Ranitidine has a longer onset of action and duration of action (up to 12 hours) than cimetidine. Because the duration of action of cimetidine is only 4 to 5 hours, it is frequently given three to four times a day.

Famotidine is 50% to 80% more potent than cimetidine and is five to eight times more potent than ranitidine. It is indicated for short-term use (4 to 8 weeks) for duodenal ulcer and for Zollinger-Ellison syndrome.

Nizatidine is an H₂ blocker that can relieve nocturnal gastric acid secretion for 12 hours. This drug is similar to famotidine and ranitidine, and none of these agents suppresses the metabolism of other drugs. To prevent recurrence of duodenal ulcers, administer nizatidine 150 mg twice a day at bedtime or famotidine 20 mg twice a day at bedtime. Both nizatidine and famotidine have similar protein-binding times and half-lives.

Table 43.5 lists the H₂ blockers and their dosages, uses, and considerations.

Side Effects and Adverse Reactions. Side effects and adverse reactions of H₂ blockers include headache, dizziness, constipation, pruritus, skin rash, gynecomastia, decreased libido, and impotence. Ranitidine and famotidine have fewer side effects than cimetidine.

Drug and Laboratory Interactions. Cimetidine interacts with many drugs. By inhibiting hepatic drug metabolism, it enhances the effects of oral anticoagulants, theophylline, caffeine, phenytoin, diazepam, propranolol, phenobarbital, and calcium channel blockers. Cimetidine can cause an increase in blood urea nitrogen (BUN), serum creatinine, and serum alkaline phosphatase. Neither cimetidine nor ranitidine should be taken with antacids because their H₂ blocking action could be decreased. Ranitidine can increase the effect of oral anticoagulants.

 NURSING PROCESS
Patient-Centered Collaborative Care

Antiulcer: Histamine₂ Blocker

Assessment
- Determine the patient's pain, including the type, duration, severity, frequency, and location.
- Evaluate GI complaints.
- Check mental status.
- Assess fluid and electrolyte imbalances, including intake and output.
- Monitor gastric pH (>5 is desired), BUN, and creatinine.
- Determine a drug history, and report probable drug-drug interactions.

Nursing Diagnoses
- Pain, Acute related to excess gastric secretion

Planning
- The patient's abdominal pain will decrease after 1 to 2 weeks of drug therapy.

Nursing Interventions
- Administer drug just before meals or at bedtime to decrease food-induced acid secretion.
- ⚡ Be alert that older adults have less gastric acid and need reduced doses of the drug. Metabolic acidosis must be prevented.
- Administer IV drug in 20 to 100 mL of solution.

Patient Teaching
General
- ⚡ Teach patients to report pain, coughing, or vomiting of blood.

- Advise patients to avoid smoking because it can hamper the effectiveness of the drug.
- Remind patients that the drug must be taken exactly as prescribed to be effective.
- Direct patients to separate ranitidine and antacid dosage by at least 1 hour.
- ⚡ Warn patients not to drive a motor vehicle or engage in dangerous activities until stabilized on the drug.
- Tell patients that drug-induced impotence and gynecomastia are reversible.
- Educate patients in the use of relaxation techniques to decrease anxiety.

Diet
- Teach patients to eat foods rich in vitamin B12 to avoid deficiency as a result of drug therapy.
- Alert patients to avoid foods and liquids that cause gastric irritation, such as caffeine-containing beverages, alcohol, and spices.

🌐 Cultural Considerations
- Respect patients' cultural beliefs and alternative methods for treating GI discomfort. Discuss the safety of these methods and the use of drugs prescribed to heal and lessen symptoms.
- Recognize that patients of various cultural backgrounds may need guidance in understanding the disease process of their GI disturbance. Use of a written plan of care with modifications should be considered.

Evaluation
- Determine the effectiveness of drug therapy and the presence of any side effects or adverse reactions. The patient should be free of pain, and healing should progress.

Proton Pump Inhibitors (Gastric Acid Secretion Inhibitors, Gastric Acid Pump Inhibitors)

PPIs suppress gastric acid secretion by inhibiting the hydrogen/potassium ATPase enzyme system located in the gastric parietal cells. They tend to inhibit gastric acid secretion up to 90% more than the H_2 blockers (histamine antagonists). These agents block the final step of acid production.

Omeprazole was the first PPI marketed, followed by lansoprazole, rabeprazole, pantoprazole, esomeprazole, and dexlansoprazole, a delayed-release oral capsule. These agents are effective in suppressing gastric acid secretions and are used to treat peptic ulcers and GERD. With lansoprazole, ulcer relief usually occurs in 1 week. Rabeprazole is more effective in treating duodenal ulcers than gastric ulcers, but it is most effective for treating GERD and hypersecretory disease (Zollinger-Ellison syndrome). Pantoprazole is prescribed to treat short-term erosive GERD. Intravenous (IV) pantoprazole is also reported as effective in treating Zollinger-Ellison syndrome. Esomeprazole has the highest success rate for healing erosive GERD, more so than omeprazole. Omeprazole promotes irreversible hydrogen or potassium ATPase inhibition until new enzyme is synthesized, which could take days, whereas rabeprazole causes

PROTOTYPE DRUG CHART 43.3
Esomeprazole

Drug Class	Dosage
Antiulcer: Proton pump inhibitor Pregnancy category: B and C*	GERD: A/C >12 y: PO: 20-40 mg/d 1 h before first meal of d for 4 weeks C 1-11 y: PO: 5-10 mg/d 1 h before first meal of d for 4 weeks
Contraindications Hypersensitivity *Caution:* Hepatic disease, pregnancy, breastfeeding, diarrhea, bone fractures, osteoporosis, older adults	**Drug-Lab-Food Interactions** Drug: May decrease theophylline levels; may interfere with absorption of ampicillin, ketoconazole, digoxin, diazepam, phenytoin, carbamazepine; statins increase PPI absorption and bioavailability. Food: Food decreases peak levels.
Pharmacokinetics Absorption: Rapidly absorbed in GI tract Distribution: PB: 97% Metabolism: t½: 1.5 h Excretion: Primarily in urine, also in bile and feces	**Pharmacodynamics** PO: Onset: 2 h Peak: 1.5-3 h Duration: 24 h
Therapeutic Effects/Uses	
To treat duodenal ulcers, GERD, esophagitis, dyspepsia, pyrosis, *Helicobacter pylori* infection, and Zollinger-Ellison syndrome and to prevent NSAID-induced ulcers Mode of Action: Suppresses gastric acid secretion by inhibiting hydrogen/potassium ATPase enzyme in gastric parietal cells	
Side Effects	**Adverse Reactions**
Headache, dizziness, drowsiness, blurred vision, fatigue, thirst, dry mouth, appetite stimulation, anorexia, nausea, eructation, flatulence, diarrhea, constipation, rash, erectile dysfunction	Elevated AST, ALT, GI bleeding, anemia, leukopenia, thrombocytopenia, depression

*Pregnancy categories have been revised. See http://www.fda.gov/Drugs/DevelopmentApprovalProcess/DevelopmentResources/Labeling/ucm093307.htm for more information.
A, Adult; *ALT*, alanine aminotransferase; *AST*, aspartate aminotransferase; *ATP*, adenosine triphosphate; *C*, child; *d*, day; *GERD*, gastroesophageal reflux disease; *GI*, gastrointestinal; *h*, hour; *NSAID*, nonsteroidal antiinflammatory drug; *PB*, protein binding; *PO*, by mouth; *PPI*, proton pump inhibitor; *t½*, half-life; *y*, years; *>*, greater than.

reversible ATPase inhibition. Dexlansoprazole is prescribed to treat erosive esophagitis and symptomatic nonerosive GERD. All PPIs in large doses can be combined with antibiotics to treat *H. pylori*. Prototype Drug Chart 43.3 lists the pharmacologic data for esomeprazole.

⚡ PATIENT SAFETY

Do not confuse:
- **Protonix**, a PPI, with **Lotronex**, a serotonin 5-HT₃ receptor antagonist used for irritable bowel syndrome
- **AcipHex**, a PPI, with **Aricept**, an Alzheimer drug
- **Nexium**, a PPI, with **Nexavar**, a biologic response modifier
- **Rabeprazole**, a PPI, with **aripiprazole**, an atypical antipsychotic
- **Misoprostol**, an antiulcer agent, with **mifepristone**, a postcoital contraceptive agent

TABLE 43.6 Antiulcer Drugs: Proton Pump Inhibitors, Pepsin Inhibitors, and Prostaglandin Analogues

Drug	Route and Dosage	Uses and Considerations
Proton Pump Inhibitors (Gastric Acid Secretion Inhibitors)		
Esomeprazole magnesium	See Prototype Drug Chart 43.3.	
Lansoprazole	GERD: Delayed release: A/adol/C >12 y: PO: 15-30 mg/d 30-60 min ac; *max.* 30 mg/d	To treat duodenal and gastric ulcers, GERD, dyspepsia, *Helicobacter pylori* infection, esophagitis, pyrosis, and Zollinger-Ellison syndrome, and for NSAID-induced ulcer prophylaxis. May cause headache, abdominal pain, diarrhea, and constipation. Pregnancy category: B*; PB: 97%; t½: 1.5 h
Omeprazole	Ulcer: Delayed release: A/adol >17 y: PO: 20 mg/d; *max.* 40 mg/d	To treat gastric and duodenal ulcer, GERD, esophagitis, dyspepsia, pyrosis, Zollinger-Ellison syndrome, and *H. pylori* infection. May cause headache, vomiting, diarrhea, and abdominal pain. Pregnancy category: C*; PB: 95%; t½: 30-60 min
Pantoprazole	GERD: A: PO/IV: 40 mg/d for 8 wk	For esophagitis, gastric and duodenal ulcers, Zollinger-Ellison syndrome, and GERD. May cause headache, dizziness, edema, constipation, and diarrhea. Pregnancy category: B*; PB: 99%; t½: 3.5-10 h
Rabeprazole	Duodenal ulcer/GERD: Delayed release: A/adol/C >12 y: PO: 20 mg/d up to 4-8 wk; *max.* 40 mg/d for A, 20 mg/d for adol/C C 1-11 y: PO: 5-10 mg/d; *max.* 10 mg/d	For duodenal ulcer, GERD, Zollinger-Ellison syndrome, esophagitis, and *H. pylori* infection. May cause headache, nausea, and diarrhea. Pregnancy category: C*; PB: 96.3%; t½: 1-2 h
Dexlansoprazole	GERD: Delayed release: A: PO: 30-60 mg/d for up to 4-8 wk; *max.* 60 mg/d	For esophagitis, pyrosis, and GERD. May cause abdominal pain and diarrhea. May be given without regard to food. Pregnancy category: B*; PB: 96%-98%; t½: 1-2 h
Pepsin Inhibitor		
Sucralfate	See Prototype Drug Chart 43.4.	
Prostaglandin Analogue		
Misoprostol	A: PO: 100-200 mcg qid with meals and at bedtime; *max.* 800 mcg/d	For prevention of NSAID-induced ulcer; may be taken during NSAID therapy, including with aspirin. May cause diarrhea, abdominal pain, chills, shivering, and hyperthermia. Pregnancy category: X*; PB: 85%; t½: UK
Combinations of Proton Pump Inhibitors With Antacids		
Omeprazole and sodium bicarbonate	Ulcer: A: PO: Omeprazole 20-40 mg/sodium bicarbonate 1100 mg 1 h ac; *max.* omeprazole 40 mg/d and sodium bicarbonate 1100 mg/d	To treat gastric and duodenal ulcers, GERD, esophagitis, and pyrosis and to prevent stress gastritis. May cause headache, pyrexia, diarrhea, constipation, hypernatremia, hypokalemia, hyperglycemia, and hypotension. Pregnancy category: C*; PB: 95%; t½: 1 h
Esomeprazole and naproxen	A: PO: 1 tablet (esomeprazole 20 mg and naproxen 375 mg or esomeprazole 20 mg and naproxen 500 mg) bid; *max.* esomeprazole 40 mg/d and naproxen 1000 mg/d	To prevent NSAID-associated gastric ulcers. May cause headache, dizziness, nausea, dry mouth, flatulence, diarrhea, and tinnitus. Pregnancy category: C/D*; PB: 97%-99%; t½: esomeprazole 1.2-1.5 h, naproxen 15 h

*Pregnancy categories have been revised. See http://www.fda.gov/Drugs/DevelopmentApprovalProcess/DevelopmentResources/Labeling/ucm093307.htm for more information.

A, Adult; *ac*, before meals; *adol*, adolescent; *bid*, two times a day; *C*, child; *d*, day; *GERD*, gastroesophageal reflux disease; *h*, hour; *IV*, intravenous; *max*, maximum; *min*, minute; *NSAID*, nonsteroidal antiinflammatory drug; *PB*, protein binding; *PO*, by mouth; *qid*, four times a day; *t½*, half-life; *UK*, unknown; *wk*, week; *y*, year; *>*, greater than.

Two combination medications involving PPIs are omeprazole with sodium bicarbonate and esomeprazole with naproxen. These combinations are used to treat GERD, erosive esophagitis, and gastric or duodenal ulcers.

Pharmacokinetics and Pharmacodynamics The duration of action for esomeprazole is 24 hours. These drugs have a short half-life and are highly protein bound (97%). PPIs should usually be taken before meals. Caution should be used in patients with hepatic impairment, and liver enzymes should

be monitored. Possible side effects include headache, dizziness, diarrhea, abdominal pain, and rash. Prolonged use of PPIs may increase the risk for cancer, although this has only been proven in mice, not humans.

Table 43.6 lists the PPIs and their dosages, uses, and considerations.

Drug Interactions. PPIs can enhance the action of digoxin, oral anticoagulants, certain benzodiazepines, and phenytoin because they interfere with liver metabolism of these drugs.

PROTOTYPE DRUG CHART 43.4
Sucralfate

Drug Class	Dosage
Antiulcer: Pepsin inhibitor Pregnancy category: B*	Ulcer: A: PO: 1 g qid 1 h before meals and at bedtime for 4-8 weeks

Contraindications	Drug-Lab-Food Interactions
Hypersensitivity *Caution:* Renal impairment, diabetes mellitus, dysphagia, pregnancy, breastfeeding, older adults	Drug: Decreased effects with tetracycline, phenytoin, digoxin; altered absorption with fluoroquinolones, antacids, ketoconazole, furosemide, lansoprazole, thyroid hormones

Pharmacokinetics	Pharmacodynamics
Absorption: PO: Minimal absorption (<5%) Distribution: PB: UK Metabolism: t½: 6-20 h Excretion: In urine	PO: Onset: 1-2 h Peak: UK Duration: 6 h

Therapeutic Effects/Uses
To prevent gastric mucosal injury from drug-induced ulcers (aspirin, NSAIDs); to treat duodenal ulcers
Mode of Action: In combination with gastric acid, forms a protective covering on the ulcer surface

Side Effects	Adverse Reactions
Dizziness, drowsiness, headache, nausea, flatulence, constipation, dry mouth, rash, pruritus	Hyperglycemia, hypophosphatemia

*Pregnancy categories have been revised. See http://www.fda.gov/Drugs/DevelopmentApprovalProcess/DevelopmentResources/Labeling/ucm093307.htm for more information.

A, Adult; *h,* hour; *NSAID,* nonsteroidal antiinflammatory drug; *PB,* protein binding; *PO,* by mouth; *qid,* four times a day; *t½,* half-life; *UK,* unknown; <, less than.

Pepsin Inhibitors (Mucosal Protective Drugs)

Sucralfate, a complex of sulfated sucrose and aluminum hydroxide, is classified as a pepsin inhibitor, or *mucosal protective drug.* It is nonabsorbable and combines with protein to form a viscous substance that covers the ulcer and protects it from acid and pepsin. This drug does not neutralize acid or decrease acid secretions.

The dosage of sucralfate is 1 g, usually four times a day before meals and at bedtime. If antacids are added to decrease pain, they should be given either 30 minutes before or 30 minutes after the administration of sucralfate. Because sucralfate is not systemically absorbed, side effects are few; however, it can cause constipation. If the drug is stored at room temperature in an airtight container, it will remain stable for up to 2 years. Prototype Drug Chart 43.4 lists the pharmacologic data for sucralfate.

Pharmacokinetics Less than 5% of sucralfate is absorbed by the GI tract. It has a half-life of 6 to 20 hours, and 90% of the drug is excreted in feces.

Pharmacodynamics Sucralfate promotes healing by adhering to the ulcer surface. Onset of action occurs within 30 minutes, and duration of action is short. Sucralfate decreases the absorption of tetracycline, phenytoin, fat-soluble vitamins, and the antibacterial agents ciprofloxacin and norfloxacin. Antacids decrease the effects of sucralfate.

NURSING PROCESS
Patient-Centered Collaborative Care
Antiulcer: Pepsin Inhibitors

Assessment
- Evaluate the patient's pain, including the type, duration, severity, and frequency. Ulcer pain usually occurs after meals and during the night.
- Determine the patient's renal function. Report urine output of less than 600 mL/day or less than 30 mL/hour.
- Assess for fluid and electrolyte imbalances.
- Measure gastric pH (>5 is desired).

Nursing Diagnosis
- Pain, Acute related to excess gastric secretion

Planning
- The patient will have relief of abdominal pain after 1 to 2 weeks of antiulcer drug management.

Nursing Interventions
- Administer drug on an empty stomach.
- Administer antacid 30 minutes before or 30 minutes after sucralfate. Allow 1 to 2 hours to elapse between sucralfate and other prescribed drugs; sucralfate binds with certain drugs (e.g., tetracycline, phenytoin), reducing their effect.

Patient Teaching
General
- Advise patients to take the prescribed drug exactly as ordered. Therapy usually requires 4 to 8 weeks for optimal ulcer healing. Advise patients to continue to take the drug even if they are feeling better.
- Increase fluids, dietary bulk, and exercise to relieve constipation.
- Educate patients in use of relaxation techniques.
- Monitor for severe, persistent constipation.
- Emphasize the need for follow-up medical care.
- Emphasize cessation of smoking as indicated.
Side Effects
- ⚡ Direct patients to report pain, coughing, or vomiting of blood.
Diet
- Teach patients to avoid liquids and foods that can cause gastric irritation, such as caffeine-containing beverages, alcohol, certain fats, and spices.

Cultural Considerations

- Greet the patient by name with the appropriate title (e.g., Mr., Ms., Dr.). Wait until the patient gives permission to use his or her first name.
- Orthodox Jewish men do not touch women other than their wives, so their failure to take a hand offered in greeting should not be interpreted as impoliteness.

Evaluation

- Determine the effectiveness of the antiulcer treatment and the presence of any side effects. The patient should be free of pain, and healing should progress.

Prostaglandin Analogue Antiulcer Drug

Misoprostol, a synthetic prostaglandin analogue, is a drug used to prevent and treat peptic ulcer. It appears to suppress gastric acid secretion and to increase cytoprotective mucus in the GI tract. It causes a moderate decrease in pepsin secretion. Misoprostol is considered as effective as cimetidine. Patients who complain of gastric distress from NSAIDs such as aspirin or indomethacin prescribed for long-term therapy can benefit from misoprostol. When a patient takes high doses of NSAIDs, misoprostol is frequently recommended for the duration of the NSAID therapy. Misoprostol is contraindicated during pregnancy and for women of childbearing age.

Table 43.6 lists the pharmacologic data for the PPIs, pepsin inhibitors, and a prostaglandin analogue.

CRITICAL THINKING CASE STUDY

JH, a 48-year-old patient, complains of a gnawing, aching pain in the abdominal area that usually occurs several hours after eating. He says that over-the-counter antacids help somewhat but that the pain has recently intensified. Diagnostic tests indicate that he has a duodenal ulcer.

1. Differentiate between peptic ulcer, gastric ulcer, and duodenal ulcer. Explain your answer.
2. What are the predisposing factors related to peptic ulcers? What additional information do you need from JH?
3. What nonpharmacologic measures can you suggest to alleviate symptoms related to peptic ulcer?

The health care provider prescribed aluminum hydroxide and magnesium hydroxide 20 mL to be taken 2 hours after meals and ranitidine 150 mg twice a day. The dose of magnesium hydroxide and aluminum hydroxide with simethicone is to be taken either 1 hour before or 1 hour after the ranitidine.

4. JH asks the nurse the purposes for magnesium hydroxide and aluminum hydroxide with ranitidine. What is the nurse's best response?

5. Why does the health care provider suggest that the patient take ranitidine with meals? Why should magnesium hydroxide, aluminum hydroxide, and ranitidine not be taken at the same time?
6. In what ways are ranitidine and cimetidine the same, and how do they differ? Explain your answer.
7. As part of patient teaching, the nurse discusses side effects of ranitidine with JH. What is the most effective way to present this information? Develop a plan.

JH states that he drinks beer at lunch and has two gin and tonics in the afternoon. He states that the drinks help him relax.

8. What nursing intervention should be taken in regard to JH's alcohol intake and smoking?
9. What foods should he avoid?

A week later JH states that he discontinued the prescribed medications because he "felt better." However, the pain recurred, and he asked whether he should resume taking the medications.

10. What is the nurse's best response? What should be included in the patient teaching?

NCLEX STUDY QUESTIONS

1. A patient is diagnosed with peptic ulcer disease. The nurse realizes that which of these is a predisposing factor for this condition?
   a. *Helicobacter pylori*
   b. Hyposecretion of pepsin
   c. Decreased hydrochloric acid
   d. *Escherichia coli*
2. A student nurse is preparing to administer sucralfate to a patient. Which statement by the student nurse demonstrates understanding of sucralfate's mode of action?
   a. Sucralfate neutralizes gastric acidity.
   b. Gastric acid secretion is decreased by inhibiting histamine at histamine$_2$ receptors in parietal cells.
   c. Gastric acid secretion is suppressed by inhibiting the hydrogen/potassium adenosine triphosphatase enzyme.
   d. Sucralfate combines with protein to form a viscous substance that forms a protective covering over the ulcer.

3. A patient is taking ranitidine. What information should the nurse teach the patient about this drug? (Select all that apply.)
   a. Drug-induced erectile dysfunction is irreversible.
   b. The drug must be administered 30 minutes before meals.
   c. The drug must be administered separately from an antacid by at least 1 hour.
   d. The drug must always be administered with magnesium hydroxide.
   e. Smoking should be avoided while taking this drug.
   f. Foods high in vitamin B12 should be increased in the diet.
4. When a patient complains of pain accompanying a peptic ulcer, why should the nurse give an antacid?
   a. Antacids decrease gastrointestinal motility.
   b. Antacids decrease gastric acid secretion.
   c. Antacids strengthen the lower esophageal sphincter's action.
   d. Antacids neutralize hydrochloric acid and reduce pepsin activity.

5. A patient is taking famotidine to inhibit gastric secretions. Which side effects of famotidine will the nurse teach the patient? (Select all that apply.)
   a. Dizziness
   b. Headaches
   c. Hypokalemia
   d. Hyperkalemia
   e. Blurred vision
   f. Erectile dysfunction

6. The patient is taking esomeprazole magnesium for erosive gastroesophageal reflux disease. Which should the nurse include in patient teaching?
   a. Take the medication daily with breakfast.
   b. Healing should occur in 1 week.
   c. This medication decreases stomach acid secretion.
   d. A blood test to check kidney function should be done.

Answers: 1, a; 2, d; 3, c; 4, f; 5, a, b, d; 6, c.

Eye, Ear, and Skin Drugs

Unit XIV discusses in detail the agents used to treat disorders of the eye, ear, and skin. Chapter 44, Eye and Ear Disorders, presents medications used to treat eye disorders, particularly glaucoma and ocular infections. Drugs used to treat ear disorders are also covered. Drugs used to treat eye and ear disorders are also discussed in other chapters; antibiotics are covered in Chapter 26. Chapter 45, Dermatologic Disorders, presents the drugs used to treat skin conditions such as acne, psoriasis, and burns.

OVERVIEW OF THE EYE

Protected within the orbits of the skull, the eyeballs are controlled by the third, fourth, and sixth cranial nerves and are connected to six extraocular muscles. The eye has three layers: (1) the cornea and sclera; (2) the choroid, iris, and ciliary body; and (3) the retina. Fig. XIV.1 illustrates the basic structures of the eye.

The cornea, the anterior covering of the eye, is transparent and allows light to enter the eye. It has no blood vessels and receives nutrition from the aqueous humor. An abraded cornea is susceptible to infection. Loss of corneal transparency is usually caused by increased intraocular pressure (IOP).

The sclera is the opaque, white fibrous envelope of the eye. Within the sclera are the posterior and anterior chambers. The posterior chamber has a blind spot around the optic nerve that is insensitive to light. The lens is held in place by ligaments and separates these two chambers. The normally transparent lens focuses light on the retina by changing its shape through a process called *accommodation*.

The anterior chamber, filled with aqueous humor secreted by the ciliary body, lies in front of the lens. The fluid flows into the anterior chamber through a space between the lens and iris. The excess fluid drains into the canal of Schlemm. An increase in IOP, resulting in glaucoma, occurs with increased production or decreased drainage of aqueous humor.

The choroid, iris, and ciliary body—the thickened part of the vascular covering of the eye that provides attachment to ligaments and support to the lens—constitute the second layer. The choroid absorbs light,

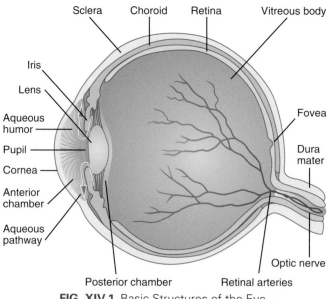

FIG. XIV.1 Basic Structures of the Eye.

and the iris surrounds the pupil and gives the eye its color. By dilating and constricting, the iris controls the quantity of light that reaches the lens.

The retina, the third layer, consists of nerves, rods, and cones that serve as visual sensory receptors. The retina is connected to the brain via the optic nerve.

The eyebrows, eyelashes, eyelids, tears, and corneal and conjunctival reflexes all serve to protect the eye. Bilateral blinking occurs every few seconds during waking hours to keep the eye moist and free of foreign material.

OVERVIEW OF THE EAR

The ear is divided into the external, middle, and inner ear. Fig. XIV.2 illustrates the basic structures of the ear.

The *external ear* consists of the pinna and the external auditory canal. The external auditory canal transmits sound to the tympanic membrane (eardrum), a transparent partition between the external and middle ear. The eardrum in turn transmits sound to the bones of the middle ear; it also serves a protective function.

The *middle ear,* an air-filled cavity, contains three auditory ossicles—the malleus, incus, and stapes—that transmit sound waves to the inner ear. The tip of the malleus is attached to the eardrum; its head is attached to the incus, which is attached to the stapes. The eustachian tube provides a direct connection to the nasopharynx and equalizes air pressure on both sides of the eardrum to prevent it from rupturing. Swallowing, yawning, and chewing gum help the eustachian tube relieve pressure changes during airplane flights.

The *inner ear* is a series of labyrinths (canals) that consist of a bony section and a membranous section. The vestibule, cochlea, and semicircular canals make up the bony labyrinth. The vestibular area is responsible for maintaining equilibrium and balance. The cochlea is the principal hearing organ.

Professional evaluation of ear problems is essential, because hearing loss can result from untreated disorders. External ear disorders can be treated with over-the-counter products, whereas prescription drugs are required to treat middle ear disorders.

OVERVIEW OF THE SKIN

Skin, the largest organ of the body, consists of two major layers: the *epidermis* is the outer layer of skin, and the *dermis* is the layer of skin beneath the epidermis. The functions of the skin include (1) protecting the body from the environment, (2) aiding in body temperature control, and (3) preventing body fluid loss.

The epidermis has four layers: (1) the basal layer, or *stratum germinativum,* the deepest layer lying over the dermis; (2) the spinous layer, or *stratum spinosum*; (3) the granular layer, or *stratum granulosum*; and (4) the cornified layer, or *stratum corneum,* the outer layer of the epidermis. As the epidermal cells migrate to the surface, they die, and their cytoplasm converts to keratin (hard and rough texture), forming keratinocytes. Eventually the keratinocytes slough off as new layers of epidermal cells migrate upward.

The dermis has two layers: the *papillary layer* lies next to the epidermis, and the *reticular layer* is the deeper layer of the dermis. The dermal layers consist of fibroblasts, collagen fibers, and elastic fibers. The collagen and elastic fibers give the skin its strength and elasticity. Within the dermal layer are sweat glands, hair follicles, sebaceous glands, blood vessels, and sensory nerve terminals. Fig. XIV.3 shows the layers of the skin.

The subcutaneous tissue, primarily fatty tissue, lies under the dermis. Besides fatty cells, subcutaneous tissue contains blood and lymphatic vessels, nerve fibers, and elastic fibers. It supports and protects the dermis.

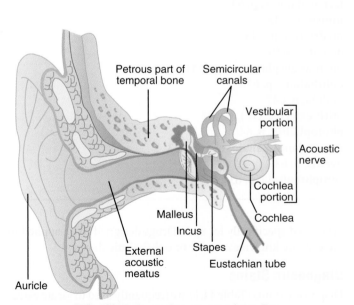

FIG. XIV.2 Basic Structures of the Ear.

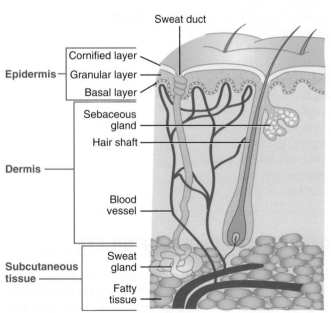

FIG. XIV.3 Basic Structures of the Skin.

44

Eye and Ear Disorders

ⓔ http://evolve.elsevier.com/McCuistion/pharmacology/

OBJECTIVES

- Describe the drug groups commonly used for disorders of the eye and ear.
- Discuss the mechanisms of action, routes, side effects and adverse reactions, and contraindications for selected drugs in each group.

- Discuss the nursing process related to drugs used in treating and managing disorders of the eye and ear.
- Identify patient teaching needed for eye and ear drugs.

OUTLINE

KEY TERMS

DRUGS FOR DISORDERS OF THE EYE

Problems associated with the eyes may occur as the result of injuries, infections, or specific noninfectious eye disorders such as glaucoma and macular degeneration. Most drugs used to treat these conditions are topical medications in formulations developed specifically for eyes. Drugs designed to be applied to the eyes are known as ocular or ophthalmic drugs.

Diagnostic Stains

Diagnostic stains (Table 44.1) are frequently used to locate extraocular lesions or foreign objects, evaluate dry eyes, or evaluate

TABLE 44.1 Diagnostic Stains for Eye Disorders

Diagnostic Aid	Purpose
Fluorescein sodium, ophthalmic	Stains the anterior segment of the eye to visualize the anterior ocular surface for defects and for contact lens fitting.
	When viewed through the cobalt blue filter of the ophthalmoscope or under a Wood lamp, corneal scratches and lesions fluoresce a bright yellow green.
Rose bengal, ophthalmic	Stains the anterior segment of the eye to visualize defects or dry eye.
	Defective and normal cells are stained a pink-violet color.
	Staining of normal cells and stinging and mild tissue toxicity limit use.
Lissamine green	Stains the anterior segment of the eye to visualize defects and dry eyes.
	Defective cells are stained green.

extraocular changes. Stains may be combined with local anesthetics to allow examination that is more thorough by alleviating pain associated with the examination. Patients should be informed that these drugs will cause discoloring of the external eye and will dissipate over several hours; they may also stain nasal secretions if the lacrimal ducts (tear ducts) are patent, and they discolor soft contact lenses. Contact lenses should be removed before administration, and the eye should be rinsed with sterile normal saline solution after the procedure. Contact lenses can be replaced after 1 hour.

Topical Anesthetics

Topical anesthetics are used in selected aspects of a comprehensive eye examination and in a variety of ophthalmic procedures. Ophthalmic anesthetics act by locally blocking the pain signals at the eye's nerve endings. The two most common topical ophthalmic anesthetics are proparacaine hydrochloride (HCl) and tetracaine HCl. Both medications, available in solutions, are administered as drops. Ophthalmic anesthetics should be administered by a trained clinician.

Corneal anesthesia usually starts occurring within 15 seconds and lasts about 15 minutes. The blink reflex is temporarily lost, therefore the corneal epithelium may become dry. Protecting the eye from irritating chemicals, foreign bodies, and corneal scratches is important. The patient must be instructed that the affected eye will be insensitive to touch and to not rub, touch, or wipe the affected eye. Contact lenses may be reinserted after the anesthetic has completely worn off, usually after 20 minutes.

Antiinfectives

Antiinfectives (Table 44.2) are frequently used for eye infections. Conjunctivitis, an inflammation of the membrane (conjunctiva) covering the eye and inner eyelids, is the most common eye condition. Conjunctivitis is also called "pink eye" and can occur because of bacteria, viruses, and allergens. Bacterial conjunctivitis usually requires antiinfective therapy to either kill

or inhibit the spread of bacteria. Some ocular viral infections (e.g., cytomegalovirus [CMV] and herpes simplex virus [HSV]) may require antiviral therapy. Examples of other ocular conditions caused by pathogens treated with ophthalmic antiinfective drugs include the following:
- **Blepharitis**, infection of the margins of the eyelid
- **Chalazion**, infection of the meibomian glands of the eyelids that may produce cysts, causing blockage of the ducts
- Bacterial and fungal **endophthalmitis**, infection and inflammation of structures of the inner eye
- **Hordeolum**, a local infection of eyelash follicles and glands on lid margins, also known as a *stye*
- Infectious **keratitis**, corneal infection and inflammation
- Infectious **uveitis**, infection of the vascular layer of the eye (ciliary body, choroid, and iris)

Before administering ophthalmic antiinfectives, the nurse should screen the patient for previous allergic reactions. Noninfectious conjunctivitis and local skin and eye irritation are possible side effects of ophthalmic antiinfective drugs.

Antiinflammatories

Inflammatory conditions of the eye not related to infectious pathogens often require treatment with antiinflammatory drugs (Table 44.3). If the inflammation is secondary to a bacterial or fungal infection, an antibiotic or antifungal agent is included in the medication regimen. Some ocular antiinflammatories are combined with antibacterials. Many antiinflammatories are not appropriate in patients with ocular viral infections.

Inflammation associated with keratoconjunctivitis sicca, causing lymphocytes to damage the lacrimal gland, results in fibrosis and loss of tear production; this can lead to **xerophthalmia** (dry eyes). Immunomodulators, such as cyclosporine ophthalmic emulsion, is an immunosuppressant that relieves xerophthalmia by a mechanism that is different from over-the-counter (OTC) lubricants. Ophthalmic cyclosporine acts as a partial immunomodulatory that causes apoptosis of lymphocytes and allows tear production to resume.

Ophthalmic nonsteroidal antiinflammatory drugs (NSAIDs) such as diclofenac sodium and ketorolac tromethamine inhibit miosis by preventing the formation of ocular prostaglandins. Most of these drugs are used for management or prevention of ocular inflammation before and following eye surgery. Unlike corticosteroids, NSAIDs do not affect **intraocular pressure (IOP)** (IOP is further discussed in Glaucoma and Ocular Hypertension Drugs). However, ocular NSAIDs can increase bleeding tendencies and delay corneal healing. Topical NSAIDs are not expected to increase cardiovascular risk, hepatic reactions, or other systemic adverse effects; however, ocular NSAIDs can cause bleeding of ocular tissues.

Ophthalmic corticosteroids such as dexamethasone and prednisolone acetate are another type of antiinflammatory. Corticosteroids are used to treat a number of eye conditions, such as allergic conjunctivitis, herpes zoster keratitis (not herpes *simplex* keratitis), corneal abrasion, postoperative ocular inflammation, and optic neuritis. ⚡ Ocular corticosteroids can mask infections and delay healing and are contraindicated in persons with untreated ocular infections.

TABLE 44.2   Ophthalmic Antiinfectives

Generic	Route and Dosage†	Uses and Considerations
ANTIBACTERIALS		
Ciprofloxacin HCl, 0.3% ophthalmic solution and ointment	Bacterial conjunctivitis: Sol: A/C >1 y: 1-2 gtt q2h while awake for 2 d, then q4h while awake for 5 d Bacterial conjunctivitis: Oint: A/C >2 y: ½-inch ribbon tid for 2 d, then ½-inch ribbon bid for 5 d Corneal ulcer: Sol: A/C >1 y: Day 1: 2 gtt q15min for 6 h, then 2 gtt q30min Day 2: 2 gtt q1h Days 3-14: 2 gtt q4h	For bacterial conjunctivitis and corneal ulceration. Pregnancy category: C*
Gentamicin sulfate, 0.3% ophthalmic solution and ointment	Sol 0.3%: A/C: 1-2 gtt q4h; may increase to 2 gtt q1h for severe infections Oint 0.3%: A/C: ½-inch ribbon 2-3 times daily	For blepharitis, blepharoconjunctivitis, bacterial conjunctivitis, corneal ulcer, dacryocystitis, keratitis, keratoconjunctivitis, acute meibomianitis, and bacterial and fungal corneal lesion/abrasion. May cause ototoxicity (of the eighth cranial nerve) that could be permanent. Pregnancy category: C*
Levofloxacin, 0.5% ophthalmic solution	A: 1-2 gtt q2h; *max:* 8 doses/d for 1-2 d, then q4h; *max:* 4 doses/d for 5 d	For bacterial conjunctivitis and corneal ulcers. (Systemic therapy is required for treatment of hordeolum, dacryocystitis, and meibomianitis.) Pregnancy category: C*
Neomycin, polymyxin B sulfate, bacitracin; ophthalmic	Oint: A: ½-inch ribbon q3-4h for 7-10 d Max dose: 8 applications/d for 10 d	For bacterial conjunctivitis, blepharitis, blepharoconjunctivitis, keratitis, and keratoconjunctivitis. A triple antibiotic is effective against many gram-positive and -negative microorganisms. Pregnancy category: C*
Ofloxacin, 0.3% ophthalmic solution	Bacterial conjunctivitis: A/C: 1 gtt q2-4h while awake for 2 d, then 1-2 gtt qid for 5 d Bacterial corneal ulcer: A/C: 1-2 gtt q30min while awake and q4-6h after retiring; days 3-6: 1-2 gtt q1h while awake; days 7-9: 1-2 gtt qid	For bacterial conjunctivitis, bacterial corneal ulcer. Pregnancy category: C*
Sulfacetamide, 10% ophthalmic solution and ointment	Sol: A/C >2 mo: 1-2 gtt q1-3h while awake, less frequently at night Oint: A/C >2 mo: Small ribbon 4 times during the day and at bedtime	For chlamydial conjunctivitis, corneal ulcer, and other superficial ophthalmic infections; not effective against fungal, viral, or all types of bacterial infection. Continued use may result in nonsusceptible microorganism overgrowth. Ointment may be applied at night with the ophthalmic solution. Ophthalmic sulfonamides are incompatible with preparations that contain silver salts (e.g., silver nitrate). Ointment may delay corneal wound healing. Purulent exudates that contain PABA can inactivate the drug's antibacterial activity. Pregnancy category: C*
Tobramycin, 0.3% ophthalmic solution and ointment	Sol: A/C ≥2 mo: 1-2 gtt q4h; for severe infection, apply 2 gtt hourly until improvement is seen, then decrease frequency. Oint: A/C: ≥2 mo: 1 cm q8-12h. For severe infections, apply q3-4h	For superficial external ocular infections. Tobramycin may delay healing of corneal abrasion or lesions. Pregnancy category: B* (ophthalmic products only)
ANTIFUNGALS		
Natamycin, 5% ophthalmic suspension	A: 1 gtt q1-2h for 3-4 d, then 1 gtt q3-4h for 14-21 d; *max:* 24 gtt/d	For external ocular fungal infections. Drops possess no antibacterial or antiviral activity, and prolonged treatment may result in bacterial or viral infection. Patients allergic to cheese may have sensitivity to natamycin. Pregnancy category: C*
ANTIVIRALS		
Trifluridine, 1% ophthalmic solution	A/C ≥6 y: 1 gtt q2h while awake; *max:* 9 gtt/d until corneal ulcer is reepithelialized, then 1 gtt q4h for 7 d; *max:* 21-d treatment	For herpetic ophthalmic infections and keratoconjunctivitis caused by HSV-1 and HSV-2. Treatment longer than 21 d can result in ocular toxicity. Pregnancy category: C*

*Pregnancy categories have been revised. See http://www.fda.gov/Drugs/DevelopmentApprovalProcess/DevelopmentResources/Labeling/ucm09 3307.htm for more information.

†To minimize systemic absorption, gently apply pressure on inner canthus.

A, Adult; *bid,* twice a day; *C,* child; *d,* day; *HSV,* herpes simplex virus; *gtt,* drops; *h,* hour; *HCl,* hydrochloride; *max,* maximum; *min,* minute; *mo,* months; *Oint,* ointment; *PABA,* para-aminobenzoic acid; *q,* every; *qid,* four times a day; *sol,* solution; *tid,* three times a day; *y,* year ; *>,* greater than; *≥,* greater than or equal to.

TABLE 44.3 Ophthalmic Antiinflammatories

Generic	Route and Dosage	Uses and Considerations
IMMUNOSUPPRESSANTS		
Cyclosporine, 0.05% ophthalmic emulsion	A/C ≥16 y: 1 gtt q12h	For xerophthalmia due to ocular inflammation associated with keratoconjunctivitis sicca. Artificial tears may be used concomitantly with cyclosporine ocular drops, allowing 15 min between the products. _Absolute contraindication:_ Patients with active ocular infection. Emulsion must be thoroughly mixed by inverting the bottle a few times to obtain a uniform, white, opaque emulsion prior to using. Pregnancy category: C*
NONSTEROIDAL ANTIINFLAMMATORY DRUGS (NSAIDS)		
Diclofenac sodium, 0.1% ophthalmic solution	24 h after cataract surgery: A: 1 gtt qid for 2 wk Corneal refractive surgery: A: 1-2 gtt within 1 h of surgery, then 1-2 gtt q15min after surgery, then qid 4-6 h after surgery for up to 3 d	For postoperative inflammation after cataract surgery and ocular pain/photophobia following corneal refractive surgery. Use a separate bottle for each eye. May increase ocular bleeding and delay healing. Pregnancy category: C*
Flurbiprofen sodium, 0.03% ophthalmic solution	A: 1 gtt q30min starting 2 h before surgery for a total dose of 4 gtt	For prevention of intraoperative miosis. If eye involvement is bilateral, one bottle per eye should be used to avoid cross-contamination. May increase ocular bleeding and delay healing. Concomitant use with ocular corticosteroid can cause corneal erosion. Pregnancy category: C*
Ketorolac tromethamine, ophthalmic solution	Allergic conjunctivitis: Sol 0.5%: A/C ≥3 y: 1 gtt qid After cataract surgery (first 24 h): Sol 0.5%: A/C ≥2 y: 1 gtt qid for 2 wk Following cataract surgery: Sol 0.45%: A: 1 gtt bid 1 d before surgery; continue on day of surgery and for 2 wk Corneal refractive surgery: Sol 0.4%: A/C ≥3 y: 1 gtt qid for 4 d	For relief of ocular itching due to allergic conjunctivitis, postoperative inflammation after cataract surgery, and postoperative corneal refractive surgery. Use separate bottle for each eye to prevent cross-contamination. Ocular NSAIDs may result in keratitis; use for longer than 14 d postoperatively may cause corneal adverse events. May increase ocular bleeding and delay healing. Pregnancy category: C*
CORTICOSTEROIDS		
Dexamethasone, 0.1% ophthalmic solution	A/C: 1-2 gtt q1h while awake and q2h at night; taper to q4h	For corticosteroid-responsive ocular disorders (e.g., allergic conjunctivitis, herpes zoster ocular infection, optic neuritis, corneal injury). Can cause increased IOP, which is reversible. Can also cause optic neuritis and visual defects. Pregnancy category: C*
Loteprednol etabonate, 0.2% and 0.5% ophthalmic suspension; 0.5% ophthalmic gel and ointment	Allergic conjunctivitis: Susp 0.2%: A: 1 gtt qid Steroid-responsive disorders: Susp 0.5%: A: 1-2 gtt qid; may increase to 1 gtt qh if needed 24 h after ocular surgery: Susp/gel 0.5%: 1-2 gtt qid for 2 wk _or_ Oint 0.5%: ½-inch qid for 2 wk 24 h after ocular surgery for postoperative pain: Oint 0.5%: ½-inch qid for 2 wk _or_ Gel 0.5%: 1-2 gtt qid for 2 wk	For allergic conjunctivitis, steroid-responsive ophthalmic disorders including iritis, keratitis, ocular pain, and postoperative ocular inflammation _Do not_ discontinue prematurely; ophthalmologic exam should be done after 14 d of therapy. Pregnancy category: C*
Prednisolone sodium phosphate 1% ophthalmic solution	Dosage must be individualized and is variable depending on nature and severity. A: 1-2 gtt qh while awake, q2h during the night; maint: 1 gtt q4-6h; taper as indicated	For corticosteroid-responsive ocular disorders (e.g., allergic conjunctivitis, herpes zoster ocular infection, optic neuritis, corneal injury, postoperative ocular inflammation). Can mask other infections. May delay healing. _Contraindication:_ Most cornea and conjunctiva viral infection, unless appropriate antiviral therapy is coadministered, and ocular fungal infection. Pregnancy category: C*

Continued

TABLE 44.3 Ophthalmic Antiinflammatories—cont'd

Generic	Route and Dosage	Uses and Considerations
OPHTHALMIC ANTIBACTERIAL AND CORTICOSTEROID COMBINATIONS		
Refer to individual drug information for general considerations.		
Neomycin sulfate/polymyxin B sulfate/dexamethasone, ophthalmic suspension and ointment	Severe disease: Susp: A/C ≥2 y: 1-2 gtt q1h Mild disease: Susp: A/C ≥2 y: 1-2 gtt q4-6h, taper gradually; *max.* 48 gtt/d Oint: A: ½-inch ribbon tid/qid; *max:* ½-inch oint qid	For external ocular inflammation and abrasion Pregnancy category: C*
Gentamicin sulfate/prednisolone acetate, ophthalmic suspension and ointment	Susp: A: 1 gtt bid-qid; *max:* 24 gtt/d Oint: A: ½-inch qd-tid; *max:* ½-inch tid	For external ocular inflammation and abrasion Pregnancy category: C*
Tobramycin/dexamethasone, ophthalmic suspension and ointment	Susp: A: 1-2 gtt q4-6h Oint: A/C ≥2 y: ½-inch ribbon q6-8h	External ocular inflammation and abrasion Pregnancy category: C*
OPHTHALMIC ALLERGY TREATMENT DRUGS		
Azelastine HCl, 0.05% ophthalmic solution	A/C ≥3 y: 1 gtt bid	For ocular pruritus due to allergic conjunctivitis. Drug can cause cephalgia, fatigue, dysgeusia, conjunctivitis, abnormal vision, and xerophthalmia. Pregnancy category: C*
Cromolyn sodium, 4% ophthalmic solution	A/C >4 y: 1-2 gtt 4-6 times/d at regular intervals	For allergic conjunctivitis. Transient ocular irritation may occur during therapy. Pregnancy category: B*
Emedastine difumarate, ophthalmic solution	A/C ≥3 y: 1 gtt up to 4 times/d; *max:* 4 gtt/d	For ocular pruritus due to allergic conjunctivitis. Cephalgia may occur along with asthenia, blurred vision, dysgeusia, and ocular irritation. *Do not* confuse emedastine with epinastine. Pregnancy category: B*
Epinastine, 0.05% ophthalmic solution	A/C ≥3 y: 1 gtt bid	For ocular pruritus due to allergic conjunctivitis. Does not cross the blood-brain barrier. May cause ocular irritation and worsen pruritus. Continue treatment through period of allergen exposure, even when symptoms are absent. *Do not* confuse epinastine with emedastine. Pregnancy category: C*
Ketotifen fumarate	A/C ≥3 y: 1 gtt q8-12h	For ocular pruritus due to allergic conjunctivitis. Cephalgia and rhinitis may occur. Pregnancy category: C*
Olopatadine HCl, 0.2% ophthalmic solution	A/C ≥3 y: 1 gtt bid at an interval of 6-8 h	For allergic conjunctivitis. Cephalgia or dysgeusia may occur during therapy. Use until offending allergen is terminated. Pregnancy category: C*

*Pregnancy categories have been revised. See http://www.fda.gov/Drugs/DevelopmentApprovalProcess/DevelopmentResources/Labeling/ucm093 307.htm for more information.

A, Adult; *bid*, twice daily; *C*, child; *d*, day; *gtt*, drops; *h*, hour; *HCl*, hydrochloride; *IOP*, intraocular pressure; *maint*, maintenance; *max*, maximum; *min*, minute; *Oint*, ointment; *q*, every; *qid*, four times daily; *Sol*, solution; *Susp*, suspension; *tid*, thrice daily; *wk*, week; *y*, year ; >, greater than; ≥, greater than or equal to.

Corticosteroids can worsen glaucoma by reducing the outflow of aqueous humor and increasing IOP; the effects are usually reversible upon discontinuation of the drug. Prolonged use can cause open-angle glaucoma, ocular nerve damage, or visual defects. Refer to Chapter 24 for more information on corticosteroids.

When allergies are the cause of eye inflammation, ophthalmic allergy drugs are commonly prescribed to treat the underlying cause. These allergy drugs contain antihistamines and mast cell stabilizers. Antihistamines block histamine from activating histamine receptors in the tissues. Degranulation of mast cells releases histamine and other inflammatory mediators; mast cell stabilizers prevent mast cells from degranulating. Ocular sensations that include burning, stinging, and blurred vision are common adverse effects reported. Other adverse effects include cephalgia, dysgeusia, and rhinitis.

Decongestants

Eye inflammation typically presents with redness due to vascular congestion of the conjunctiva. Ophthalmic decongestants such as phenylephrine, naphazoline, and tetrahydrozoline stimulate alpha-adrenergic receptors in the arterioles of the conjunctiva, vasoconstricting (narrowing) the blood vessels and thereby decreasing congestion. Many ocular decongestants are available without prescription. If these are absorbed in significant amounts, their sympathetic nervous system effects may pose problems for patients with increased IOP and hypertension. ⚡ Ocular decongestants are contraindicated in patients with angle-closure glaucoma because these drugs may contribute to acute angle-closure, a medical emergency.

Lubricants

Eye lubricants moisten eyes to alleviate discomfort such as the burning and irritation associated with xerophthalmia. They are also used to moisten contact lenses and artificial eyes. During anesthesia and in acute or chronic central nervous system (CNS) disorders that result in unconsciousness or decreased blinking, lubricants keep eyes moist and maintain the integrity of the epithelial surface of the eye.

Many brands and forms of ocular lubricants (artificial tears) are available OTC without a prescription. Although these agents are typically safe, the nurse must be alert to potential allergic reactions to preservatives found in lubricants.

Glaucoma and Ocular Hypertension Drugs

In the anterior chamber of the eye, aqueous humor, a clear fluid, flows continuously in and out of the chamber. As aqueous humor is formed, excess fluid drains through the trabecular meshwork structure of the eye and out the canal of Schlemm, with a much smaller fraction of the fluid exiting through the uveoscleral structure at the root of the iris (Fig. 44.1A). Overproduction of the fluid or improper drainage causes IOP to increase, and this buildup of pressure can damage the optic nerve and result in glaucoma. Without treatment, permanent vision loss can occur.

There are two types of glaucoma, open-angle and angle-closure. In open-angle glaucoma, the trabecular network is open but becomes clogged (see Fig. 44.1B). Over time, as blockage of the trabecular network worsens, the IOP gradually increases, which damages the optic nerve.

In angle-closure glaucoma, also known as closed-angle or narrow-angle glaucoma, the iris is situated close to the drainage angle blocking the trabecular network (see Fig. 44.1C). Because the excess aqueous humor cannot drain, it builds up within the eye and increases IOP. When the drainage angle is completely blocked, eye pressure increases quickly, and the vision becomes suddenly blurred; this is a medical emergency and must be treated immediately. Management of angle-closure glaucoma is often surgical; however, pharmacologic management is sometimes indicated. ⚡ Anticholinergic drugs (see Chapter 16) can cause mydriasis and can worsen angle-closure glaucoma.

Glaucoma is further classified as either primary or secondary. Primary glaucoma occurs because of a pathologic change within the eye that happens without a known cause. Primary open-angle glaucoma (POAG), the most common type of glaucoma, is a chronic condition that develops slowly over time as the trabecular meshwork becomes clogged for unknown reasons. Secondary glaucoma occurs in response to a known cause such as injury, disease, or medication. Although a number of drugs can increase the risk of secondary glaucoma, those that cause pupillary dilation are particularly problematic because they give the iris more flexibility to move toward the drainage angle, blocking the trabecular meshwork. People who are at risk for glaucoma should avoid decongestants. Certain herbal preparations (e.g., goldenseal, ephedra, and bitter orange)

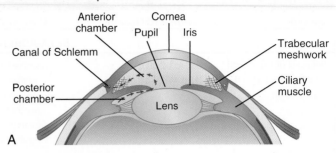
Normal flow of aqueous humor

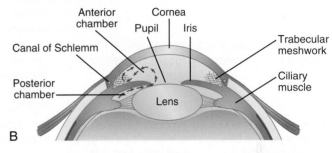
Open-angle glaucoma

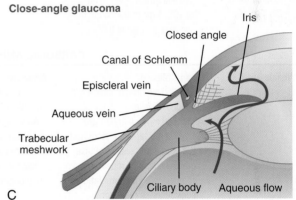
Close-angle glaucoma

FIG. 44.1 A, Normal flow of aqueous humor. B, Open-angle glaucoma. C, Closed-angle glaucoma.

can also create problems when given to patients who have glaucoma.

> ⚡ **PATIENT SAFETY**
>
> Herbs that should be avoided in patients with glaucoma include bitter orange, blood root, celandine, coffee, corkwood, ephedra, goldenseal, and jimsonweed. Because all herbs have inherent risks, it is important to receive approval from the patient's health care provider before recommending herbal preparations.

Drugs for glaucoma (Table 44.4) belong to one of six drug categories: (1) prostaglandin analogues, (2) beta-adrenergic blockers, (3) alpha-adrenergic agonists, (4) cholinergic agents, (5) carbonic anhydrase inhibitors, or (6) systemic hyperosmotic drugs. Prostaglandin analogues and beta-adrenergic blockers are typically first-line therapy, followed by alpha-adrenergic agonists. Each category acts in different ways to decrease IOP. Even though damage due to glaucoma cannot be reversed, treatments may prevent further damage.

TABLE 44.4 Glaucoma Drugs

Generic	Route and Dosage	Uses and Considerations
BETA-ADRENERGIC BLOCKERS		
Betaxolol HCl, 0.5% ophthalmic solution or 0.25% suspension	Sol: A: 1-2 gtt q12h Susp: A/C: 1 gtt q12h	Selective beta blocker for chronic open-angle glaucoma and ocular hypertension (increased IOP). The ophthalmic drug has not been shown to have significant effects on heart rate, blood pressure, or pulmonary function; however, such preparations can be absorbed systemically with the same adverse reactions and drug interactions. May have additive effects in patients receiving oral beta blockers. *Absolute contraindications:* AV block, bradycardia, cardiogenic shock, HF Pregnancy category: C*
Carteolol HCl, 1% ophthalmic solution	A: 1 gtt q12h	Nonselective beta blocker for chronic open-angle glaucoma or ocular hypertension. Conjunctival hyperemia and eye irritation may occur. *Absolute contraindications:* AV block, bradycardia, cardiogenic shock, HF Pregnancy category: C*
Levobunolol HCl, 0.25% or 0.5% ophthalmic solution	A: 1-2 gtt of 0.25% bid or 1-2 gtt of 0.5% once daily	Nonselective beta blocker for increased IOP for open-angle glaucoma or ocular hypertension; to be used with topical miotics. Ocular irritation, dizziness, fatigue, and depression may occur. *Absolute contraindications:* Asthma, AV block, bradycardia, cardiogenic shock, COPD, HF, sick sinus syndrome, sulfite hypersensitivity Pregnancy category: C*
Timolol hemihydrate or maleate, 0.25% or 0.5% ophthalmic solution or gel-forming solution	Sol: A/C: 1 gtt of 0.25% bid, may increase to 1 gtt of 0.5% bid and titrate down to qd Gel: A/C: 1 gtt of 0.25% qd, may increase to 1 gtt of 0.5% qd	Nonselective beta blocker for increased IOP in glaucoma or ocular hypertension. Pregnancy category: C*
CARBONIC ANHYDRASE INHIBITORS		
Acetazolamide	Regular release: A: PO: 250 mg qd-qid; *max:* 1 g/d Extended release: A: PO: 500 mg bid; *max:* 1 g/d A: IV: 500 mg for acute increased IOP or patients unable to take oral dosage; may repeat in 2-4 h Geriatrics: With all formulations, consider dose reduction.	Adjunctive treatment of glaucoma; reduces IOP. Must be administered systemically; penetration is poor when administered topically to the cornea. Volume loss may cause dehydration and postural hypotension. Electrolyte imbalance may occur. Adverse GI effects (e.g., dysgeusia, xerostomia, anorexia) may occur. Drug may be given without regard to food. *Absolute contraindications:* Acidosis, metabolic acidosis, closed-angle glaucoma, adrenal insufficiency, hepatic disease, or renal failure; hyperchloremia, hypokalemia, hyponatremia, anuria Pregnancy category: C*
Brinzolamide, 1% ophthalmic suspension	A: 1 gtt tid	For increased IOP due to ocular hypertension or open-angle glaucoma. Corneal edema may occur with low endothelial cell counts. With ocular administration, drug is absorbed systemically. Must be shaken well prior to each use. *Absolute contraindication:* Sulfonamide hypersensitivity (contains sulfonamide derivative) Pregnancy category: C*
Dorzolamide, 2% ophthalmic solution	A/C/N ≥1 wk: 1 gtt tid	For increased IOP due to ocular hypertension or open-angle glaucoma. It is not recommended to topically administer CAIs concomitantly with oral CAIs. Pregnancy category: C*
COMBINATION DRUGS FOR GLAUCOMA		
Refer to individual drug information for general considerations.		
Timolol maleate/dorzolamide	A/C ≥2 y: 1 gtt bid	Timolol is a nonselective beta blocker and dorzolamide is a carbonic anhydrase II inhibitor. Pregnancy category: C*
Brimonidine/timolol maleate	A/C ≥2 y: 1 gtt q12h	Brimonidine is a selective alpha-agonist and timolol is a nonselective beta blocker. Pregnancy category: C*.
PROSTAGLANDIN ANALOGUES		
Latanoprost, 0.005% ophthalmic solution	See Drug Prototype Chart 44.1.	
Bimatoprost, 0.03% ophthalmic solution	A/C ≥16 y: 1 gtt at bedtime	For increased IOP due to ocular hypertension or open-angle glaucoma. Macular edema, iritis, and cataracts may occur. Pregnancy category: C*

TABLE 44.4 Glaucoma Drugs—cont'd

Generic	Route and Dosage	Uses and Considerations
PROSTAGLANDIN ANALOGUES		
Travoprost, 0.004% ophthalmic solution	A: 1 gtt at bedtime	For increased IOP due to ocular hypertension or open-angle glaucoma. Macular edema or keratitis may occur. Pregnancy category: C*
Tafluprost, 0.0015% ophthalmic solution	A: 1 gtt every evening	For increased IOP due to ocular hypertension or open-angle glaucoma. Drug may cause macular edema or uveitis/iritis. Pregnancy category: C*

*Pregnancy categories have been revised. See http://www.fda.gov/Drugs/DevelopmentApprovalProcess/DevelopmentResources/Labeling/ucm093 307.htm for more information.
A, Adult; *AV,* atrioventricular; *bid,* twice daily; *C,* child; *CAI,* carbonic anhydrase inhibitor; *COPD,* chronic obstructive pulmonary disease; *d,* day; *GI,* gastrointestinal; *gtt,* drop; *h,* hour; *HCl,* hydrochloride; *HF,* heart failure; *IOP,* intraocular pressure; *IV,* intravenously; *max,* maximum; *N,* newborn; *PO,* by mouth; *q,* every; *qid,* four times daily; *Sol,* solution; *Susp,* suspension; *tid,* thrice daily; *wk,* weeks; *y,* year; ≥, greater than or equal to.

Prostaglandin Analogues

Prostaglandin analogues are first-line drugs used primarily in the treatment of open-angle glaucoma and ocular hypertension. These drugs decrease IOP by improving trabecular outflow and by increasing the uveoscleral pathway, which is an alternate pathway of aqueous humor outflow. Examples of prostaglandin analogues include bimatoprost, latanoprost (Prototype Drug Chart 44.1), tafluprost, and travoprost. Prostaglandin analogues are taken at bedtime.

Side Effects and Adverse Reactions. Prostaglandin analogues used for glaucoma have unique side effects. These drugs gradually change the color of the iris by increasing brown pigmentation. This effect is most noticeable in individuals with green-brown and yellow-brown irises, and may be permanent. Darkening of the eyelids may also occur. Another side effect is the development of eyelash hypertrichosis, which is a growth in the number, length, thickness, and pigmentation of eyelashes. Patients may also develop macular edema, blurred vision, redness of the conjunctiva, and itching or stinging of the eye. Systemic effects such as bronchospasm, dizziness, dyspnea, and myalgia are rare. Prostaglandin analogues are generally better tolerated than alternative drugs for glaucoma.

Cholinergic Agents

Ophthalmic cholinergic agents cause miosis, a constriction of the pupil and contraction of the ciliary muscle. These actions result in a widening of the trabecular meshwork to improve outflow of excess aqueous humor. Additionally, as the pupil constricts, it straightens the iris, thus opening or widening the drainage angle to relieve angle-closure glaucoma. The two types of cholinergics are cholinergic agonists and cholinesterase inhibitors. Although their outcomes are similar, cholinergic agonists and cholinesterase inhibitors differ in their mechanism of action.

Cholinergic agonists are direct-acting cholinergics that directly stimulate cholinergic receptors. As a result, these drugs have the same action as the parasympathetic neurotransmitter acetylcholine. Pilocarpine is an example of a cholinergic agonist.

Cholinesterase inhibitors such as echothiophate are indirect-acting cholinergics, which inactivate the enzyme cholinesterase that typically breaks down acetylcholine. By inhibiting enzymatic destruction of acetylcholine, more acetylcholine is available to stimulate cholinergic receptors in the eye.

Side Effects and Adverse Reactions. Systemic absorption of cholinesterase inhibitors through the conjunctiva and lacrimal duct can produce systemic parasympathomimetic effects that include cardiac irregularities, diarrhea, hyperhidrosis, respiratory depression, and urinary incontinence. Other adverse effects from cholinesterase inhibitors include iritis, uveitis, and retinal detachment in addition to common complaints such as ocular irritation and pain, lacrimation, myopia with blurred vision, and paradoxical ocular hypertension. Systemic effects from cholinergic agonists are rare; ocular adverse effects are similar to those of the cholinesterase inhibitors. Cholinergic agonists and cholinesterase inhibitors are contraindicated for use in persons with closed-angle glaucoma.

Figs. 44.1B and C illustrate increased IOP resulting in open-angle and angle-closure glaucoma. Refer to Chapter 16 for more information on cholinergic drugs.

Beta-Adrenergic Blockers

Selective and nonselective beta-adrenergic blockers and beta blockers are first-line drugs used in the treatment of glaucoma. Beta-adrenergic blockers decrease IOP by decreasing the production of aqueous humor. Examples of ophthalmic nonselective beta-adrenergic blockers include carteolol, levobunolol, and timolol (Prototype Drug Chart 44.2). Selective ocular beta blockers include betaxolol.

Side Effects and Adverse Reactions. In the eye, beta-adrenergic blockers (beta blockers) may cause some eye discomfort, which is possible with most eye medications. Some types cause miosis. Because the pupil does not dilate adequately in dark environments, patients taking these drugs may experience vision problems at night.

Although ophthalmic drugs do not typically enter the general circulation in large amounts, it can occur to the extent that systemic effects occur. ⚡ Ophthalmic beta-adrenergic blockers can slow the heart rate, which can worsen bradycardia, atrioventricular (AV) heart block, and heart failure. Also, these drugs can prevent adequate bronchodilation in patients who have asthma and other obstructive pulmonary diseases. See Chapter 15 for more information on beta-adrenergic blockers.

PROTOTYPE DRUG CHART 44.1

Latanoprost

Drug Class	Dosage
Prostaglandin analogue Pregnancy category: C*	1 gtt q evening in affected eye(s)

Contraindications	Drug-Lab-Food Interactions
Latanoprost is indicated only for open-angle glaucoma or ocular hypertension. No absolute contraindications exist, but use caution in patients with a torn or absent lens, intraocular inflammation, or risk of macular edema. Drug is absorbed by soft contact lenses, so advise patients with these to use alternate means of vision correction. *Caution:* Patients with history of diabetic retinopathy who took latanoprost experienced retinal detachment, retinal embolus, and vitreous hemorrhage. This may or may not be related to the latanoprost, but caution is urged.	Drugs: Concomitant administration with eyedrops containing thimerosal causes latanoprost to precipitate out of solution; latanoprost- and thimerosal-containing ophthalmic preparations should be administered at least 5 min apart. Bromfenac ophthalmic solution, an NSAID, may reduce latanoprost's ability to lower IOP. Bimatoprost ophthalmic solution to promote growth of eyelashes may decrease the ability of latanoprost to lower IOP. Combining latanoprost with other prostaglandin analogues is not recommended; combination may decrease the IOP-lowering effects or cause a paradoxical increase in IOP.

Pharmacokinetics	Pharmacodynamics
Absorption: Through the cornea and hydrolyzed to its active form Distribution: 0.16 ± 0.02 L/kg. Primary measurable concentration is in the eye; levels are often undetectable in serum. Metabolism: Hepatic; t½: 17 min Excretion: Primarily in urine (88%)	Onset: 3-4 h Peak: 8-12 h Duration: 24 h

Therapeutic Effects/Uses
Reduction of IOP in open-angle glaucoma or ocular hypertension Mechanism of Action: Prostaglandin FP receptor selective agonist increases aqueous humor outflow.

Side Effects	Adverse Reactions
Ophthalmic effects: Blurred vision, burning/stinging/pruritus/redness, brown pigmentation of iris; increased number/length/thickness and darkening of eyelashes; foreign body sensation, punctate epithelial keratopathy, photophobia, lid edema/erythema/discomfort/crusting	Eye pain, eye infection, loss of vision, dizziness, dyspnea

*Pregnancy categories have been revised. See http://www.fda.gov/Drugs/DevelopmentApprovalProcess/DevelopmentResources/Labeling/ucm093307.htm for more information.
gtt, Drop; *h*, hour; *IOP*, intraocular pressure; *min*, minutes; *NSAID*, nonsteroidal antiinflammatory drug; *q*, every; *t½*, half-life.

Alpha-Adrenergic Agonists

Ophthalmic alpha-adrenergic agonists such as apraclonidine and brimonidine control or prevent elevation of IOP postsurgically by decreasing production and improving outflow of aqueous humor. The major site of action is in the ciliary body.

PROTOTYPE DRUG CHART 44.2

Timolol

Drug Class	Dosage
Nonselective beta blocker Pregnancy category: C*	Sol: 1 gtt of 0.25% bid; may increase to 1 gtt of 0.5% bid and titrate down to once daily dosing. Gel: 1 gtt of 0.25% once daily, may increase to 1 gtt of 0.5% once daily.

Contraindications	Drug-Lab-Food Interactions
Absolute contraindications: COPD and RAD, AV block, bradycardia, cardiogenic shock, and heart failure. Caution against abrupt discontinuation.	Drugs: Ophthalmic timolol can be absorbed systemically, therefore drug-drug interactions are similar to other formulations. See Chapter 15 for more general drug-drug interactions with beta blockers. Some herbal agents may lower vascular resistance (e.g., hawthorn [*Crataegus laevigata*] and ephedra [Ma-huang]).

Pharmacokinetics	Pharmacodynamics
Absorption: Systemic absorption can occur. Distribution: UK Metabolism: Hepatic; t½: 4 h Excretion: Primarily in urine	Onset: 30 min Peak: 1-2 h Duration: <24 h

Therapeutic Effects/Uses
Reduction of IOP in open-angle glaucoma or ocular hypertension Mechanism of Action: Nonselectively antagonizes beta$_1$- and beta$_2$-adrenergic receptors, reducing IOP without affecting visual acuity, pupil size, or accommodation.

Side Effects	Adverse Reactions
Adverse effects for ocular timolol are the same as for the oral drug. See Chapter 15 for more information on timolol and other nonselective beta blockers.	See Chapter 15 for more information on beta blockers.

*Pregnancy categories have been revised. See http://www.fda.gov/Drugs/DevelopmentApprovalProcess/DevelopmentResources/Labeling/ucm093307.htm for more information.
AV, Atrioventricular; *bid*, twice daily; *COPD*, chronic obstructive pulmonary disease; *gtt*, drop; *h*, hour; *IOP*, intraocular pressure; *min*, minute; *RAD*, respiratory airway disease; *Sol*, solution; *t½*, half-life; *UK*, unknown; *<*, less than.

❶ Absolute contraindications for alpha-adrenergic agonists include persons on monoamine oxidase inhibitor (MAOI) therapy. No specific drug interactions with systemic and ophthalmic drugs were noted; however, caution is advised when using these drugs with other alpha blockers, tricyclic antidepressants (TCAs), and CNS depressants.

Side Effects and Adverse Effects. Apraclonidine and brimonidine have minimal, if any, systemic effects. Because of the relative safety of alpha$_2$-adrenergic agonists, they are often used when ophthalmic beta-adrenergic antagonists are contraindicated. The most common effects of topical administration are burning, stinging, blurred vision, and headache. Serious reactions include corneal erosion, keratitis, arrhythmias, and asthma.

Carbonic Anhydrase Inhibitors

Carbonic anhydrase inhibitors (CAIs) decrease IOP by decreasing the production of aqueous humor. These drugs, initially developed as diuretics, are sometimes used for adjunctive treatment of glaucoma. They are indicated for both open-angle and acute closed-angle glaucoma. CAIs are not as effective as other drugs for glaucoma, and they carry a greater risk of adverse effects. For these reasons, they are generally added to a therapeutic regimen only after other treatment options have been exhausted. Both topical (e.g., brinzolamide, dorzolamide) and systemic (e.g., acetazolamide) formulations are available.

Side Effects and Adverse Reactions. Adverse effects of CAIs, particularly with the systemic forms, include CNS effects such as lethargy, drowsiness, headache, seizures, paresthesias, and mental status changes. Gastrointestinal (GI) effects such as nausea, vomiting, diarrhea, dysgeusia, and anorexia may occur. Because CAIs have diuretic effects, polyuria and increased thirst are common, and fluid and electrolyte disturbances may occur as a result. CAIs may promote hyperuricemia, which may precipitate gout attacks, and they may also worsen liver disease, resulting in hepatic encephalopathy and even hepatic necrosis. Because they are sulfonamides, they should not be given to patients who have experienced allergic reactions to other sulfonamide drugs.

 NURSING PROCESS

Patient-Centered Collaborative Care

Glaucoma and Ocular Hypertension Drugs

Assessment
- To avoid drug-drug and drug-supplement interactions, conduct a detailed current medication history that includes prescriptions, over-the-counter medicines, antacids, dietary supplements, vitamins, and herbal supplements.
- Obtain a list of drug and food allergies.
- Obtain baseline information about physical status that includes height, weight, vital signs, cardiopulmonary assessment, intake and output, skin assessment, nutritional status, and any underlying diseases.
- Check baseline visual acuity and intraocular pressure (IOP) measurements.
- ⚡ Assess for contraindications for glaucoma drugs, such as respiratory or cardiac disorders, closed-angle glaucoma, hypertension, acute ocular infection, immunosuppression, and hepatic or renal disorders.

Nursing Diagnoses
- Knowledge, Deficient related to the purpose and administration of therapy
- Sensory Perception (visual), Disturbed related to disease progression and drug-induced visual changes
- Injury, Risk for
- Anxiety related to disease progression and drug-induced visual changes

Planning
- The patient/caregiver will verbalize understanding for the drug therapy and identify when to notify the clinician.
- The patient will take medications in dose and at times prescribed.
- The patient will demonstrate the proper method of ophthalmic drug administration.
- The patient will avoid contaminating the tip of the tube or dropper.
- The patient's IOP will decrease to within the target range.
- The patient will not develop an ocular infection during therapy.
- The patient will verbalize means to allay anxiety.

Nursing Interventions
- Monitor for significant alterations in patient status.
- ⚡ Monitor patients for xerostomia, dehydration, fluid overload, blood dyscrasias, electrolyte imbalances, blurred vision, dyspnea, bradycardia or tachycardia, hypertension, and pulmonary changes.

Patient Teaching
General
- Advise patients to never stop medication suddenly.
- Advise patients to avoid driving or operating machinery while vision is impaired.
- Explain the importance of follow-up appointments for subsequent ophthalmologic examination and reevaluation of IOP.
- Counsel patients with glaucoma to avoid drugs with the potential to increase IOP, such as decongestants, anticholinergics, and corticosteroids.
- If both eyedrops and eye ointment are prescribed, instruct patients to put in eyedrops first.
- If more than one kind of eyedrop is ordered, instruct patients to wait at least 5 minutes before instilling the second medication.
- Teach patients/caregivers not to touch the tip of the tube or eyedropper to the eye, finger, or any other object.
- Explain to patients/caregivers when to notify the clinician (e.g., with fever, wheezing, weight gain, sudden vision changes, or high blood pressure).
- See Chapter 10 for more information on ocular drug administration.

Evaluation
- Evaluate patient and family knowledge of purpose and administration of medications.
- Evaluate effectiveness of drug therapy. IOP should be reduced from baseline measurements.
- Evaluate for alleviation or decrease in adverse effects after interventions targeted to unwanted effects of glaucoma therapy.

Mydriatics and Cycloplegics

Mydriatics dilate the pupils, and cycloplegics paralyze the muscles of accommodation; both are used in diagnostic procedures and ophthalmic surgery. (See the Unit IV opener for a review of the autonomic nervous system and a comprehensive discussion of anticholinergics.)

Anticholinergics actively block acetylcholine from attaching to cholinergic receptors, resulting in both dilation of the pupils and paralysis of the muscles of accommodation. This is accomplished by blocking the response of sphincter muscles that normally constrict the pupil when cholinergic receptors are stimulated. Commonly prescribed anticholinergics for mydriasis and cycloplegic refraction include atropine sulfate, cyclopentolate hydrochloride, homatropine hydrobromide, phenylephrine hydrochloride, and tropicamide. An ophthalmic alpha-receptor antagonist, dapiprazole, is available to reverse drug-induced mydriasis with phenylephrine.

Side Effects and Adverse Reactions. Side effects of topical anticholinergics include xerophthalmia (dry eyes), photophobia (sensitivity to light), and blurred vision. Although uncommon with topical use, systemic effects are typical of all anticholinergic drugs and include xerostomia, cephalgia, and constipation. Serious systemic effects include increased IOP, psychosis, seizures, hypotension, tachycardia, cardiovascular collapse, respiratory depression, and muscle rigidity. These drugs are contraindicated

in patients with angle-closure glaucoma because the paralyzed iris may block the outlet for outflow of aqueous humor (see Fig. 44.1C). Table 44.5 lists selected mydriatics and cycloplegics along with their dosages, uses, and considerations.

PATIENT SAFETY

Do not confuse...
- **Oral** alpha-adrenergic or beta blockers with **ophthalmic** preparations
- **Ocular** with **otic**
- **Prednisone** with **prednisolone** ophthalmic
- **Ophthalmic** solutions with **otic** or other topical solutions of the same name (e.g., Cortisporin *ophthalmic* solution with Cortisporin *otic* solution)

Drugs for Macular Degeneration

Age-related macular degeneration (AMD) is a leading cause of vision loss in older adults. AMD is a deterioration of the macula, which is the part of the eye responsible for sharp central vision; damage to the macula blurs central vision in the affected eye. Two forms of AMD include wet (neovascular or exudative),

TABLE 44.5 Mydriatics and Cycloplegics

Generic	Route and Dosage	Uses and Considerations
Atropine sulfate, 1% ophthalmic solution or ointment	Cycloplegic refraction: A: 1-2 gtt of sol or 0.3-0.5 cm ribbon of oint up to 3 times daily for 14 d; start 1 h prior to procedure. C: 1-2 gtt of sol or 0.3 cm of oint up to 3 times daily for 14 d; start 1-3 d before procedure. Iritis/uveitis: A/C: 1-2 gtt of sol or 0.3-0.5 cm ribbon of oint up to 3 times daily	For cycloplegic refraction, especially in children, and uveitis/iritis. Atropine antagonizes acetylcholine receptors and inhibits cholinergic effects. The most potent cycloplegic, atropine, may cause seizures, arrhythmias, hypotension, respiratory depression, and hallucinations. *Contraindications:* Glaucoma, tachycardia Pregnancy category: C*
Cyclopentolate HCl, 0.5%, 1%, 2% ophthalmic solution	A/C: 1-2 gtt × 1; may repeat × 1 in 5-10 min.	For cycloplegia and mydriasis induction Pregnancy category: C*
Homatropine hydrobromide, 2% and 5% solution	Mydriasis and cycloplegia: A/C: 1-2 gtt before procedure; may repeat x 1 in 5-10 min. Uveitis: A/C: 1-2 gtt q3-4h	For mydriasis and cycloplegia for eye examination and uveitis. Homatropine is similar to atropine, but onset is faster and duration is shorter. Do not use 5% sol in children. Pregnancy category: C*
Phenylephrine HCl, 2.5% and 10% ophthalmic solution	Acute glaucoma: A: 1 gtt. Repeat as necessary. Use with miotic drugs to improve visual acuity. C: 1 gtt of 2.5% sol. Repeat as necessary. Use with miotic drugs to improve visual acuity. Mydriasis induction: A/C: 1 gtt 15-30 min before procedure, may repeat at 3-5 min intervals; *max:* 3 gtt/eye Neonates/infants: 1 gtt of 2.5% sol 15-30 min before procedure; may repeat at 3-5 min intervals; *max:* 3 gtt/eye Uveitis: A: 1 gtt of 2.5% up to 3 times for 2 d or 1 gtt of 10% once a day for up to 2 d C: 1 gtt of 2.5% up to 3 times on same day	For treatment of acute open-angle glaucoma and for mydriasis induction and pupillary dilation in uveitis for examination. Do not use 10% sol in neonates and children. Pregnancy category: C*
Tropicamide	Refraction: A: 1%: 1-2 gtt; repeat in 5 min Fundus examination: 0.5%: 1-2 gtt 15-20 min before examination	Mydriasis and cycloplegia for eye examination Pregnancy category: C*

*Pregnancy categories have been revised. See http://www.fda.gov/Drugs/DevelopmentApprovalProcess/DevelopmentResources/Labeling/ucm093307.htm for more information.

A, Adult; *C,* child; *d,* day; *gtt,* drop; *h,* hour; *HCl,* hydrochloride; *max,* maximum dosage; *min,* minute; *oint,* ointment; *q,* every; *sol,* solution.

which progresses quite rapidly, and dry (atrophic), which slowly destroys vision over a period of years.

Dry AMD is more common and occurs in response to the deposit of extracellular material, called drusen, under the retina. This is coupled with thinning of the macula, which eventually stops functioning properly. Vision loss occurs gradually. Occasionally, dry AMD will progress to wet AMD.

There is no known treatment or medication for dry AMD. An effective drug has not been identified to treat dry AMD, but several drugs are currently in the trial stages. Some studies suggest that antioxidants and zinc supplements may have a role in preventing or slowing progression of dry AMD.

Wet or exudative AMD is associated with the growth of abnormal blood vessels behind the retina. Leakage of fluid from these vessels collects behind the retina and shifts the macula from its normal position. Wet macular degeneration accounts for 10% of AMD cases; however, it causes greater destruction and is responsible for 80% of cases in which patients suffer severe vision loss or become legally blind.

Pharmacologic management of wet AMD targets vascular endothelial growth factor (VEGF), a substance that plays a role in the formation of abnormal vessels in the eye. These VEGF inhibitors are intravitreal drugs that are injected into the eye by an ophthalmologist; trials to evaluate topical agents are in progress. Examples of VEGF inhibitors are ranibizumab, bevacizumab, pegaptanib, and aflibercept. Intravitreal VEGF is contraindicated in persons with ocular infections.

Administration of Eyedrops and Ointments

Techniques for administering eyedrops and ophthalmic ointments are described in Chapter 10. Patients who wear contact lenses should be knowledgeable about products associated with the lenses. Wearing contact lenses is usually discouraged; however, if contact lenses must be worn, patients should wait at least 15 minutes after instilling ocular drugs before reinserting the contact lenses.

Patients With Eye Disorders: General Suggestions for Teaching

- Listen to patient concerns. Eye disorders that carry the possibility of blindness promote high anxiety in patients.
- Provide patient education regarding expected drug effect, dosage, side effects, and when to notify the health care provider.
- Use lay terms rather than medical terminology when providing education.
- Provide written instructions for confused or forgetful patients.
- When developing patient education materials, write them at a fifth- to eighth-grade reading level; use a large, easily read font; and give instructions in the patient's primary language.
- Supplement written instructions with images or pictograms to clarify.
- Instruct patients or family members that one drop of eye medication is the preferred amount with prescriptions written for one to two drops; the conjunctival sac of the lower lid typically holds the volume of one drop without overflowing.

The second drop may cause overflow, greater chance of systemic toxicity, and increased cost of treatment.

- If a second topical medication is ordered to be given at the same time, instruct patients to wait at least 5 minutes before instilling the second medication.
- Instruct patients or family members on proper administration of eyedrops or ointment. Teach them how to maintain sterile technique and prevent dropper contamination.
- Ask patients for a return demonstration of any procedure to ensure their ability to carry it out properly and to determine if additional teaching is needed.
- Advise patients that ointments will diminish vision for a short period due to the film coating the eye. Advise them to avoid potential safety hazards during this time.
- Instruct patients to store drugs away from heat.
- Counsel patients not to stop any medication suddenly without prior approval from the prescribing health care provider.
- Advise patients to check labels on OTC drugs with a pharmacist.
- Instruct patients to carry an identification card or wear a medical alert bracelet at all times if they are allergic to any medications.
- Encourage patients to keep health care appointments. Recommend that patients bring a list of questions about their condition or medications.
- Tailor instructions for patients who wear contact lenses. Notify them of any special procedures that need to be done with use of contact lenses and the various ophthalmic medications. Advise patients to avoid wearing contact lenses in the presence of eye infections.

DRUGS FOR DISORDERS OF THE EAR

Antiinfectives

Common ear conditions that require antibacterial drugs are acute otitis media (AOM) and acute otitis externa (AOE), commonly known as *swimmer's ear*. AOM occurs more often in children, and *Streptococcus pneumoniae* is the most common pathogen, followed by *Haemophilus influenzae* and *Moraxella catarrhalis*. AOM may also be caused by other microorganisms, such as viruses.

Risk factors for the development of AOM include age younger than 2 years, attending day care centers, and exposure to environmental pollutants such as tobacco smoke. A significant decline in AOM has occurred since the pneumococcal conjugate vaccine (PCV) was introduced in 2000. Because it provides immunization against *S. pneumoniae*, families should be urged to have children receive the scheduled PCV13 as a prophylactic measure against AOM as well as against the other more serious conditions that this vaccine prevents.

AOM is usually related to a dysfunction of the eustachian tube, especially after an upper respiratory infection from a virus. The tympanic membrane (TM) is usually bulging, and patients complain of otalgia (ear pain). Other symptoms may include fever and irritability.

Oral amoxicillin is usually the drug of choice when antibiotics are indicated for AOM. The recommended dosage for children 6 months and older is 80 to 90 mg/kg every 12 hours for 7 to 10 days depending on the severity of the condition and the age of the patient. The dosage for adults is 500 to 875 mg every 8 to 12 hours, depending on the severity. Azithromycin and clarithromycin are often ordered if the patient is severely allergic to penicillin. For more mild penicillin allergies, a cephalosporin may be ordered; however, the nurse should be alert to any signs or symptoms of penicillin-cephalosporin cross-sensitivity. For otalgia, topical analgesics such as benzocaine are usually used, especially at bedtime.

Otitis externa (OE) is an infection of the external auditory canal that occurs when excess moisture and breaks in the epithelium allow some pathogen, usually bacterial or fungal, to invade the tissues. The cerumen is lipid rich and hydrophobic (repels water), and it protects the skin from water penetration. However, excessive cerumen can obstruct the canal and can trap water. Trapped moisture in the canal elevates the pH and removes the protective cerumen, allowing pathogens a warm, dark, moist area in which to grow. Like many areas of the body, the external canal contains normal bacterial flora that protect the ear; however, when protective mechanisms fail, a pathogenic flora results. *Pseudomonas aeruginosa* and *Staphylococcus aureus* are the pathogens most often responsible. Fever, otalgia, lymphadenopathy, and swelling can occur. Treatment is usually with topical antibacterial or antifungal drugs, depending on the source of the infection. These are often prescribed as a combination product that contains an antiinflammatory (corticosteroid) drug. An analgesic may also be needed.

If the external ear canal (EAC) becomes so swollen that eardrops cannot reach the inner recesses of the EAC, a wick is usually used (Fig. 44.2). A wick is a thin cylinder composed of highly compressed absorbable material that is inserted into the edematous canal, and eardrops are applied to the exposed tip of the wick. Sufficient drops should be administered to keep the wick moist, which pulls the medication down the length of the wick as the moisture is absorbed, exposing the tissues along the EAC to medication. Wicks should be replaced every 24 to 48 hours. Once the swelling resolves, the wick will fall out, or it can be manually removed.

Oral antibiotics are rarely needed; however, when associated with otitis media or systemic illness, oral drugs are needed. Additionally, if patients are immunosuppressed, oral antibiotics are warranted.

⚡ Patency of the TM presents a special concern when eardrops are used. This is especially true when an edematous EAC prevents adequate visualization of the TM. Topical antibiotics such as neomycin and polymyxin B with hydrocortisone are very effective in treating OE because polymyxin B is effective against *P. aeruginosa*, and neomycin is effective against *S. aureus*. However, if this drug combination is given to a patient with a perforated TM, the risk of ototoxicity is significant. Chloramphenicol is another drug for OE but is contraindicated with a perforated TM. Fluoroquinolones, on the other hand, are effective against both organisms and are safe to use when the TM is incompetent; therefore they are usually the first drug chosen when prescribing treatment for OE. When OE is caused by the growth of fungi, restoring an acidic environment with

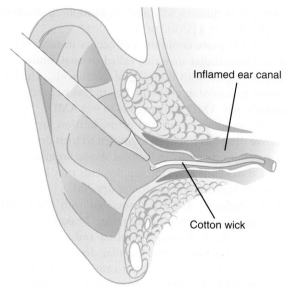

FIG. 44.2 Ear wick inserted into an edematous canal.

an acidifying solution such as acetic acid is usually sufficient. A topical antifungal otic solution such as clotrimazole is typically used if the fungal infection is severe.

Side Effects and Adverse Reactions. The most common side effects of otic antimicrobials are burning and stinging, but ototoxicity can occur with aminoglycoside antibiotics. Chloramphenicol may cause bone marrow suppression and can result in decreased erythrocytes, leukocytes, and platelets. Opportunistic overgrowth of nonsusceptible organisms may occur with any of these drugs. Hypersensitivity is a contraindication.

Table 44.6 lists selected antiinfectives used to treat ear disorders and their dosages, uses, and considerations.

◎ NURSING PROCESS
Patient-Centered Collaborative Care
Topical Antiinfectives: Ear Conditions

Assessment
- Conduct a detailed medication history that includes current prescriptions, OTC medicines, antacids, dietary supplements, vitamins, and herbal supplements.
- Obtain a list of drug and food allergies.
- Obtain baseline information about physical status that includes height, weight, vital signs, cardiopulmonary assessment, intake and output, skin assessment, nutritional status, and any underlying diseases.
- Record otoscopic exam findings for future comparisons.
- Check audiometry and tympanometry, and perform other testing as indicated.
- Assess for conditions in which selected antiinfectives are contraindicated or relatively contraindicated.

Nursing Diagnoses
- Knowledge, Deficient related to drug regimen (purpose, taking medications as ordered, administration of medications)

TABLE 44.6 Otic Antiinfectives

Generic	Route and Dosage	Uses and Considerations
Topical (Otic)		
General considerations: To minimize dizziness upon administration, warm the container between the hands for at least 1 minute prior to use. After administration, maintain patient position for at least 1 minute.		
Acetic acid, 2% otic solution	A/C >3 y: 4-6 gtt q2-3h After administration to affected ear, maintain administration position for 5 min.	For bacterial or fungal infection of the external ear canal (acute diffuse otitis externa). Solution is concentrated and is a highly corrosive irritant; it must be diluted prior to use. Systemic absorption is unlikely. *Absolute contraindications:* Perforated TM Pregnancy category: C*
Ciprofloxacin otic, 0.2% otic solution	OE due to *Pseudomonas aeruginosa* or *Staphylococcus aureus:* A/C: 0.5 mg (one 0.25-mL single-use container): Instill contents q12h for 7 d; *max:* 1 mg/d	For bacterial infection (OE). Use caution treating *Pseudomonas aeruginosa* or *Staphylococcus aureus;* resistant strains have been noted. Otic route should not result in clinically significant plasma concentration. *Absolute contraindication:* Quinolone hypersensitivity Pregnancy category: C*
Ofloxacin 0.3% otic solution	OE: A: 10 gtt once daily for 7 d C 6 mo-13 y: 5 gtt once daily for 7 d Acute OM: C: 5 gtt bid for 10 d Chronic OM: A/C ≥12 y: 10 gtt bid for 14 d	For OE due to *Escherichia coli, P. aeruginosa,* or *S. aureus;* chronic OM with perforated TM due to *P. aeruginosa, S. aureus,* or *Proteus mirabilis;* acute OM with tympanostomy tubes due to *Haemophilus influenzae, Moraxella catarrhalis, P. aeruginosa, S. aureus,* or *Streptococcus pneumoniae.* GI effects (dysgeusia, nausea, vomiting) and otic effects (otalgia, otorrhagia, tinnitus) may occur with otic ofloxacin. Pregnancy category: C*

*Pregnancy categories have been revised. See http://www.fda.gov/Drugs/DevelopmentApprovalProcess/DevelopmentResources/Labeling/ucm093307.htm for more information.
A, Adult; *bid,* twice daily; *C,* child; *d,* day; *GI,* gastrointestinal; *gtt,* drops; *h,* hour; *max,* maximum dosage; *min,* minute; *OE,* otitis externa; *OM,* otitis media; *q,* every; *TM,* tympanic membrane; *y,* year; >, greater than; ≥, greater than or equal to.

- Sensory Perception (Auditory), Disturbed due to inflammation and/or medication
- Pain related to infection
- Injury, Risk for

Planning
- The patient will verbalize understanding of the therapy.
- The patient will be free from ear infection after completion of the drug regimen.
- The patient's pain will be at a tolerable level.
- Adverse effects will be minimized.

Nursing Interventions
- Complete culture and sensitivity testing, if ordered, before starting drug therapy.
- Ensure TM patency before administering eardrops other than fluoroquinolones.
- Provide relief of associated pain, if present.
- Monitor for significant alterations in patient status.
- Assess for the development of superinfections.

Patient Teaching
- Instruct patients to complete the entire course of medication (usually 10 to 14 days) and not to stop medication when the ear feels better.
- If a patient is prone to OE after swimming or showers, give instruction on prevention of OE. The Centers for Disease Control and Prevention recommend the following:

- Keep water out of ears by using custom-fitted ear plugs.
- If water enters the ear, tilt the ear downward to allow water to drain out. Pull the ear in different directions to enhance water drainage.
- Use a portable hair dryer to facilitate drying.
- Instruct the patient to wear a medical alert bracelet at all times if allergic to any medications.
- See Chapter 10 for information on the administration of eardrops.

Evaluation
- Evaluate patient and family knowledge of the drug regimen.
- Determine the effectiveness of the drug therapy.
- Inquire regarding alleviation of side effects.

Antihistamines and Decongestants

For years, antihistamines and decongestants were thought to reduce middle-ear congestion and eustachian tube dysfunction associated with otitis media with effusion (OME), a noninfectious collection of fluid in the middle ear. The rationale was that these drugs would reduce edema of the eustachian tube, which would promote drainage from the middle ear.

In 2006, a landmark Cochrane review of the medical literature concluded that antihistamines and decongestants were not as effective as once assumed and that the risks of adverse effects outweighed the benefits. Shortly thereafter, the American Academy of Pediatrics recommended against their use for ear conditions in young children. A 2012 report by the Agency for Healthcare Research and Quality (AHRQ) states that "the effects on multiple short- and long-term outcomes repeatedly demonstrated no benefit for use of these medications over placebo for treating OME…. The reviewed studies found evidence of increased side effects and harms with use of these medications." Unfortunately, many patients are not aware of these findings and may continue to take these drugs.

The importance of the nurse's role in educating patients regarding this concern cannot be overstated. Numerous OTC antihistamine-decongestant medications are readily available to unknowing patients. Examples of antihistamines include chlorphenamine, clemastine, diphenhydramine, and many others. Examples of decongestants are phenylephrine and pseudoephedrine. (Pseudoephedrine requires a prescription in some states.) Of even greater concern is that most of these are available as combination products that contain both an antihistamine and a decongestant. (See Chapter 35 for a discussion of upper respiratory drugs.)

Ceruminolytics

Cerumen, or earwax, is produced by glands in the outer half of the EAC. Usually cerumen moves to the EAC by itself and is washed away; however, sometimes it accumulates due to overproduction or narrowing of the EAC. In these instances, cerumen can harden in the EAC, creating impaction that can lead to pain, itching, tinnitus, and hearing loss.

Ceruminolytics are topical otic agents that soften or break up the cerumen so that it can be removed. Preparations for ceruminolytics include water-based; oil-based; and non-water, non-oil based products. Water-based products provide hydration to the dried cerumen, allowing it to disintegrate. Oil-based solutions lubricate and soften the cerumen but do not disintegrate it. An example is carbamide peroxide, which is available OTC. Patients may also elect to use regular mineral oil to soften

the wax or prevent cerumen impaction. Generally 2 to 5 drops applied twice a day for 4 days are sufficient.

Administration of Ear Medications

Ear medications are usually contained in a liquid vehicle for ease of administration. Guidelines for the administration of eardrops are provided in Chapter 10.

Sometimes ceruminolytics alone are insufficient. In these instances, ear irrigation can be used to flush the cerumen deposits out of the ear canal. Irrigation is best accomplished when direct visualization of the TM is possible, and it must be done *gently* to avoid damage to the TM. It is also important to warm the water to prevent nausea and vomiting.

Frequently used irrigating solutions include hydrogen peroxide 3% in a 1:1 solution with warm water, normal saline, or acetic acid (vinegar) mixed with warm water. Contraindications to irrigation include perforation of the TM and prior hypersensitivity.

Patients With Ear Disorders: General Suggestions for Teaching

- Instruct patients to not insert any foreign objects into the ear canal.
- Instruct patients to keep drugs away from heat.
- Provide education regarding the expected drug effect, dosage, side effects, and when to notify the health care provider.
- Teach patients about OTC drug concerns, particularly with antihistamines and decongestants. OTC drugs may interact with prescribed drugs and may have risks that outweigh any drug benefit.
- Advise patients to contact their health care provider before using OTC drugs or herbal preparations to treat ear disorders.
- Encourage patients to keep follow-up appointments.

■ CRITICAL THINKING CASE STUDY

MH, a 70-year-old woman with postoperative acute glaucoma, is prescribed one drop of latanoprost 0.005% ophthalmic solution each evening and one drop of timolol 0.25% ophthalmic solution each morning and evening.

1. What is the purpose of giving two different medications to manage MH's glaucoma?
2. What special concerns related to medication timing are important for MH to consider when administering the evening dose of these medications?

3. Although systemic absorption of ophthalmic beta-adrenergic antagonists is usually small, it may potentially create problems for patients with certain conditions. Which conditions create a risk, and how will the nurse monitor for complications?
4. After a few months on these medications, MH notices changes in the appearance of her eyes. Describe the changes that MH is likely experiencing, and explain which drug is responsible.

■ NCLEX STUDY QUESTIONS

1. A patient is taking oral acetazolamide, a carbonic anhydrase inhibitor, to decrease intraocular pressure. When providing drug education, what will the nurse advise the patient to anticipate?
   a. Increased weight
   b. Light sensitivity
   c. Burning or stinging of the eyes
   d. Increased urine output

2. The camp nurse is reviewing the shopping list of supplies needed for the upcoming camping season. Which product will the nurse purchase to prevent and treat cerumen impaction?
   a. Hydrogen peroxide
   b. Rubbing alcohol
   c. Charcoal
   d. Clove oil

3. A patient is about to undergo a diagnostic eye exam. The ophthalmologist asks the nurse to prepare to assist in the administration of tetracaine, fluorescein stain, and atropine. Before assisting in the procedure, it is most important for the nurse to inform the ophthalmologist if the patient has a history of:
   a. Cataracts
   b. Angle-closure glaucoma
   c. Open-angle glaucoma
   d. Macular degeneration

4. The nurse has a patient demonstrate self-administration of eyedrops. Place the steps in the order in which the patient will perform them.
   a. Pull the lower lid away from the eye so that a pouch is formed.
   b. Gently shake the bottle to evenly distribute the drug.
   c. Press a finger against the inner corner of the eye for 2 to 3 minutes.
   d. Remove the cap.
   e. Tilt the head backward, and look upward.
   f. Place the dropper just above the pouch without touching the tip to the eye or finger.
   g. Wash hands.
   h. Gently squeeze one drop of medicine into the pouch.

5. When collecting a medication history from a patient with primary open-angle glaucoma, the nurse identifies several drugs that could exacerbate glaucoma. Which drug poses a priority concern for this particular patient?
   a. Cyclobenzaprine, an antispasmodic
   b. Oxymetazoline, a decongestant
   c. Prednisone, a corticosteroid
   d. Sulfamethoxazole-trimethoprim, a sulfonamide-antibiotic combination

6. The nurse asks a parent to demonstrate administration of eardrops on a toddler. Which steps by the parent indicate the need for additional education? (Select all that apply)
   a. Position with the affected ear upward.
   b. Pull the ear backward and upward.
   c. Instill one drop of medication at a time allowing 3 to 5 minutes between each drop.
   d. Apply gentle pressure to the flap (tragus) over the ear canal.
   e. Keep the ear positioned upward for 5 minutes.

Answers: 1, d; 2, a; 3, b; 4, g, b, d, e, a, f, h, c; 5, c; 6, b, c.

45

Dermatologic Disorders

OBJECTIVES

- Differentiate between acne vulgaris, psoriasis, drug-induced dermatitis, and contact dermatitis.
- Describe nonpharmacologic measures used to treat mild acne vulgaris.
- Describe at least three drugs that can cause drug-induced dermatitis and their characteristic symptoms.
- Compare the topical antibacterial agents used to prevent and treat burn tissue infection.
- Discuss the nursing process, including teaching, related to commonly used drugs for acne vulgaris, psoriasis, and burns.

OUTLINE

KEY TERMS

Numerous skin lesions and eruptions require mild to aggressive drug therapy. Skin disorders include acne vulgaris, psoriasis, eczema dermatitis, contact dermatitis, drug-induced dermatitis, and burn infection. Skin eruptions may result from viruses, such as herpes simplex and zoster; fungi (e.g., tinea pedis [athlete's foot], tinea capitis [ringworm]); and bacteria.

Skin lesions may appear as macules (flat and nonpalpable, usually less than 10 mm in diameter with varying colors), papules (raised and palpable, less than 10 mm in diameter), vesicles (clear, fluid-filled blisters smaller than 10 mm in diameter), or plaques (palpable lesions that are depressed or elevated when compared with the skin surface and greater than 10 mm in diameter). Treatments for skin eruptions include topical creams, ointments, pastes, gels, lotions, and solutions. Selected skin disorders and their drug therapy regimens are discussed separately.

Treatment information can be found at the American Academy of Dermatology (AAD) website: https://www.aad.org.

ACNE VULGARIS

Acne is the most common skin disorder in the United States. Acne is more prevalent among adolescents, but adults and children can also develop acne. Acne vulgaris is the formation of papules, nodules, and cysts on the face, neck, shoulders, and back that results not from dirt but from keratin plugs at the base of the pilosebaceous oil glands near the hair follicles. The keratin plugs trap normal skin flora, including bacteria commonly found on the skin; the primary bacterium is *Propionibacterium acnes*. Bacteria start proliferating, which causes inflammation and irritation. During adolescence, production of androgens and sebum—an oily skin lubricant—are increased. The sebum combines with keratin, a protein that is part of the skin, to form a plug that results in acne. Comedones are types of non-inflammatory acne lesions that may be open (blackheads) or closed (whiteheads). Open comedones are dilated hair follicle openings that allow oxidation of the debris within the follicle; closed comedones are small, plugged hair follicles. As with other forms of acne, comedones are not a result of poor hygiene. All forms of acne should be treated to prevent life-long scars. Acne can be treated nonpharmacologically and pharmacologically. Table 45.1 lists the drugs commonly used to control acne vulgaris along with their dosages, uses, and considerations.

Nonpharmacologic Approach

Nonpharmacologic measures should be tried before drug therapy is initiated. A prescribed or suggested cleansing agent, such as antibacterial soap, is necessary for all types of acne. The skin should be gently cleansed twice daily, but vigorous scrubbing should be avoided. Overscrubbing and overwashing can irritate the skin, worsening the acne and possibly causing an infection. The American Osteopathic College of Dermatology recommends

TABLE 45.1	Drugs for Acne Vulgaris and Psoriasis	
Generic	Route and Dosage	Uses and Considerations
ACNE VULGARIS		
Systemic Preparations		
Tetracycline hydrochloride	A/Adol: PO: Initially, 125-250 mg q6h for 1-2 wk then decrease slowly to 125-500 mg daily or every other day	For moderate to severe inflammatory acne vulgaris concomitantly with topical retinoid and benzoyl peroxide (BP). Best on an empty stomach (1 h before or 2 h after meal/milk). To reduce risk of esophageal irritation or ulceration, take with plenty of water and do not take at bedtime; not for patients with esophageal disorders. Permanent discoloration during tooth development and enamel hypoplasia may occur. See Chapter 26 for other considerations. Pregnancy category: D*
Minocycline hydrochloride	Severe acne: A: IV/PO: 200 mg for 1 dose then 100 mg q12h C ≥8 y: Initially, 4 mg/kg followed by 2 mg/kg q12h; do not exceed adult dose. Nonnodular moderate to severe acne: A/C ≥12 y: PO: 1 mg/kg extended-release capsule/tablets once daily for 12 wk	For adjunctive treatment of moderate to severe inflammatory acne; mono-therapy should be avoided. Drug considerations are similar to those of tetracycline. Pregnancy category: D*
Doxycycline	A/C ≥8 y: weighing ≥45 kg: PO: 100 mg q12h on day 1 then 100 mg once daily C <45 kg: 2.2 mg/kg q12h on day 1 then 2.2 mg/kg/d once daily	Adjunctive treatment for severe acne; monotherapy should be avoided. Drug considerations are similar to those of tetracycline. Pregnancy category: D*
Isotretinoin	A/C ≥12 y: PO: 0.5-1 mg/kg/d in 2 divided doses Take with meals to increase bioavailability. Patient may repeat the course at least 8 wk after completion of the prior course.	For moderate to severe nodular acne unresponsive to conventional treatment, including antibiotics. Vitamin A derivative; reverses sebum production by reducing the size of sebaceous glands. Unlike vitamin A, isotretinoin does not accumulate in the liver. Adverse effects relate to toxicity to cardiovascular, endocrine, hematologic, GI, hepatic, musculo-skeletal, respiratory, ocular, and otic systems. Interacts with tetracycline, vitamin A, methotrexate, contraceptives, and alcohol. Baseline hepatic function, lipid panel, and pregnancy tests must be obtained. Childbearing women must have a pregnancy test every 30 days. Pregnancy category: X*
Amoxicillin	A: PO: 250 mg bid up to 500 mg tid C >3 mo and <40 kg: 25 mg/kg/d q2h or 20 mg/kg/d q8h C >3 mo and >40 kg: 500 mg q12h or 250 mg q8h	Adjunctive treatment for acne, especially during pregnancy. Shake suspension well prior to each administration. Suspension may be added to formula, milk, and other liquids. For other considerations and uses, see Chapter 26. Pregnancy category: B*
Topical Preparations		
General considerations: When using multiple topical products for acne, apply each product at different times throughout the day to decrease skin irritation. Common side effects of topical drugs include xerosis of skin, erythema, and pruritus. Avoid eyes, mouth, and mucous membranes when using topical antiacne preparations.		
Keratolytic Agents		
Azelaic acid	A/C >12 y: Apply a thin layer to the affected area twice daily, morning and evening.	For mild to moderate inflammatory acne; has antimicrobial effect against *Propionibacterium acnes* and *Staphylococcus epidermidis* and an anti-keratinizing effect on the follicular epidermis. May cause hypopigmentation in patients with dark complexions. Pregnancy category: B*

Continued

TABLE 45.1   Drugs for Acne Vulgaris and Psoriasis—cont'd

Generic	Route and Dosage	Uses and Considerations
ACNE VULGARIS		
Benzoyl peroxide	A/C ≥12 y: 2.5%, 5%, or 10% gel, wash, or cream: 1-4 times/d	First-line therapy for mild to moderate inflammatory and noninflammatory acne lesions. Promotes keratolysis, removal of the horny layer of epidermis, resulting in drying and desquamative actions. Can be used concomitantly with other antiacne therapies. Pregnancy category: C*
Salicylic acid	A/C: 0.5%-6% cream, gel, and shampoo 1-3 times/d; if erythema or peeling occurs, reduce application.	For mild to moderate acne; promotes desquamation of the horny layer of skin. Monitor for salicylic toxicity; use of salicylic acid in children with viral infections is not recommended due to increased risk for Reye syndrome. Pregnancy category: C*
Antibiotics General considerations: Antibiotics may be given concurrently with benzoyl peroxide.		
Erythromycin	A: 2% solution, pledget, or gel 1-2 times/d	For mild to moderate inflammatory acne Pregnancy category: B*
Clindamycin	A/C ≥12 y: 1% gel, lotion, solution, or pledget: Apply twice daily to the affected area. 1% foam: Apply once daily	For moderate acne. May cause colitis, dermatitis, folliculitis, pruritus, erythema, dry skin, and peeling. Dispense foam into cap or onto a cool surface to prevent premature melting. Shake other formulations well before use. Can have neuromuscular blocking action; use cautiously with opiate agonists; monitor for any CNS depression (e.g., bradypnea, weakness, paralysis) Pregnancy category: B*
Vitamin A Derivatives General considerations: Topical vitamin A derivatives may be used concurrently with benzoyl peroxide and other antiacne therapies.		
Tretinoin	A/C ≥10 y: Apply a thin layer to the affected area once daily at bedtime.	For mild to moderate acne. Cleanse area first, pat dry, and wait 20-30 min before applying. Wash hands immediately after applying. Caution in patients with fish allergies. Pregnancy category: C*
Adapalene	A/C ≥12 y: 0.1% lotion or gel, 0.3% gel: Apply once daily at bedtime after washing the face with nonmedicated soap.	For mild to moderate acne, adapalene causes less skin irritation than tretinoin. Pregnancy category: C*
Tazarotene	A/C ≥12 y: 0.1% cream, gel, or foam: Apply a thin film once daily in the evening.	For mild to moderate acne; can also be used for psoriasis. Photosensitivity can occur; avoid unnecessary environmental exposures. May use a moisturizer as needed. Pregnancy category: X*
Oral Contraceptives		
Ethinyl estradiol/norethindrone acetate/ferrous fumarate	A/Adol ≥15 y: PO: 1 pill every day at the same time for 21 d followed by 1 wk of no tablets	For the treatment of acne vulgaris. See Chapter 52 for more information on drug uses and considerations. Pregnancy category: X*
Ethinyl estradiol/norgestimate	A/C after menarche: PO: 1 tab at the same time each day	For the treatment of acne vulgaris. See Chapter 52 for more information on drug uses and considerations. Pregnancy category: X*
PSORIASIS		
Systemic Preparations		
Methoxsalen	A: PO: 10-70 mg 2-3 times weekly, according to body weight. Administer 2 h before exposure to therapeutic UV rays.	Systemic antimetabolite for severe psoriasis not responsive to other therapy. Soft and hard gelatin capsules are *not* interchangeable. Separate doses by at least 48 h. Administer with food or milk. Contraindicated in patients with history of or current invasive cutaneous carcinoma or melanoma. Avoid sunlight during drug therapy; sunlight could cause severe burning and blistering. Pregnancy category: C*
Acitretin	A: PO: 25-50 mg/d with main meal. Trials found that 25 mg/d for treatment of psoriasis vulgaris is similar in efficacy to 50 mg/d with fewer and less severe adverse clinical and laboratory events.	Retinoid for recalcitrant psoriasis. May take up to 6 mo for maximal response to treatment. May be given concurrently with phototherapy. Give with food for increased bioavailability. Pregnancy category: X*

TABLE 45.1	**Drugs for Acne Vulgaris and Psoriasis—cont'd**	
Generic	**Route and Dosage**	**Uses and Considerations**
	PSORIASIS	
Topical Preparations		
Anthralin	A: Apply sparingly to lesions once daily and leave on up to 30 min. Rinse thoroughly with cool to lukewarm water, then wash with soap.	For stable plaque psoriasis. May stain clothing, skin, and hair. Pregnancy category: C*
Calcipotriene	A: Apply up to twice daily.	Vitamin D analogue for chronic plaque psoriasis. More effective when used with a topical corticosteroid. Do not exceed 100 g/wk. Excess use may increase serum calcium level. Contraindicated in persons with hypercalcemia. Avoid UV rays. Pregnancy category: C*
Clobetasol propionate	A/C ≥12 y: Cream, gel, foam, or ointment: Apply a thin layer twice daily. A/C ≥16 y: Emollient cream *only.* Apply a thin layer twice daily. A: Spray and lotion: Apply twice daily.	Super–high-potency corticosteroid for moderate to severe plaque psoriasis. ❶ Do not use occlusive dressings. With any formulation, do not exceed 50 g/wk. Reassess lesions after 2 wk of treatment. Contraindicated for application to the axilla, face, or groin. Pregnancy category: C*
Coal tar	A/C ≥2 y: Foam, lotion, suspension, or shampoo: Apply up to 4 times daily, depending on formulation.	For mild to moderate psoriasis. No maximum dosage. Wash affected area to remove loose psoriatic scales for better penetration. Allow skin to air dry after treatment. May stain clothing, skin, and hair. Do not use on inflamed, broken, or infected skin due to increased risk of systemic absorption. UV rays should be avoided for 24 h after treatment. Pregnancy category: C*
Tazarotene	A: Cream: Apply to affected areas once daily in the evening. A/C ≥12 y: Gel: Apply once daily in the evening.	For stable plaque psoriasis. Can also be used for acne vulgaris. May use with skin emollients, but apply at least 1 h before tazarotene. Avoid application to unaffected skin due to increased systemic absorption. Pregnancy category: X* (childbearing women should have a negative pregnancy test within 2 wk of beginning treatment)
❶ Biologic Agents		
General considerations: Prior to initiating therapy, patients must be tested for active infections (e.g., TB, HBV). Rotate injection sites; subsequent injections should be at least 1 inch from previous injection sites. Do not inject in areas that are bruised, red, tender, or hard.		
Adalimumab	Psoriasis: A: Subcut: Start with 80 mg on week 1, then 40 mg on week 2, then 40 mg every other week. Psoriatic arthritis: A: Subcut: 40 mg every other week	A TNF-α MAb for moderate to severe chronic plaque psoriasis and psoriatic arthritis when other systemic therapy is not appropriate. Rotate injections on the front of thighs and abdomen. Subsequent injections should be at least an inch away from previous injection sites. Pregnancy category: B*
Etanercept	Psoriatic arthritis: A: Subcut: 50 mg/wk up to twice weekly Psoriasis: Start with 50 mg twice weekly 3-4 d apart for 3 mo; then 50 mg/wk.	TNF inhibitor for moderate to severe psoriasis. May be administered in an outpatient setting; teach patient or caregiver thoroughly on proper administration. Do not inject directly into scaly patches or lesions. Contraindicated in persons with sepsis. Pregnancy category: B*
Infliximab	A: IV: 5 mg/kg given at weeks 0, 2, and 6 and then every 8 wk.	Chimeric MAb for chronic severe psoriasis and psoriatic arthritis. Infuse over at least 2 h with appropriate filter. *Absolute contraindications:* Heart failure, murine protein hypersensitivity. Black-box warning includes infection (viral, fungal, bacterial) and neoplastic disease. Pregnancy category: B*
Ustekinumab	Based on weight: A >100 kg: Subcut: 90 mg, repeat 4 wk later, then 90 mg q12wk starting at wk 16 A ≤100 kg: Subcut: 45 mg, repeat in 4 wk, then q12wk starting at wk 16	IL-12 and IL-23 antagonists for moderate to severe plaque psoriasis for patients receiving phototherapy or systemic therapy for psoriatic arthritis. Pregnancy category: B*

*Pregnancy categories have been revised. See http://www.fda.gov/Drugs/DevelopmentApprovalProcess/DevelopmentResources/Labeling/ucm093307.htm for more information.

A, Adult; *adol,* adolescent; *bid,* twice daily; *C,* child; *CNS,* central nervous system; *d,* day; *GI,* gastrointestinal; *h,* hour; *HBV,* hepatitis B virus; *IL,* interleukin; *IV,* intravenous; *MAb,* monoclonal antibody; *min,* minutes; *mo,* month; *PO,* by mouth; *q,* every; *Subcut,* subcutaneous; *tab,* tablet; *TB,* tuberculosis; *tid,* three times daily; *TNF,* tumor necrosis factor; *UV,* ultraviolet; *wk,* week; *y,* year; *>,* greater than; *<,* less than; *≥,* greater than or equal to; *≤,* less than or equal to.

not using abrasive cleaners. In addition to facial hygiene, shampooing hair to decrease the oiliness may help with acne. Keeping hair away from the face has also been shown to decrease acne. Cosmetics should be water based because oil-based products can increase the clogging of skin pores. A well-balanced diet that is low in fat and sugar is recommended, and excessive carbohydrates should be avoided. Decreasing emotional stress and increasing emotional support are also suggested. If drug therapy is necessary, nonpharmacologic measures should be maintained as well.

Pharmacologic Treatment

Acne is not curable, but it is manageable. Acne medications may help decrease scar formation related to acne. The best course for patients with acne is to see a dermatologist who can prescribe treatment specific to the individual, therefore the course of therapy will vary according to the severity and extent of the acne.

Topical Antiacne Drugs

Mild acne is generally treated with topical drugs that treat existing acne and prevent new eruptions. Commonly used topical therapies for mild acne include benzoyl peroxide, retinoids, salicylic acid, antibiotics, or combinations of these in addition to gentle cleansing.

Benzoyl peroxide (BP) is an antibacterial agent that kills *P. acnes*, the predominant organism in sebaceous follicles and comedones. BP releases free radical oxygen species that oxidize bacterial proteins. When included as an adjunct to an antibiotic regimen, control of acne is enhanced. Resolution of acne usually occurs within 4 to 6 weeks. BP is applied as a cream, lotion, or gel once or twice a day and can be left on or washed off. Washing BP off may be better tolerated in patients with sensitive skin.

Topical retinoids such as tretinoin, adapalene, and tazarotene are derivatives of vitamin A and are used for mild to moderate acne that alters keratinization. They are the mainstay of topical therapy because of their comedolytic activities, and they also have antiinflammatory actions. Retinoids alter the intracrine and paracrine mediators of cell differentiation and proliferation, apoptosis, and reproduction, thereby modifying gene expression, subsequent protein synthesis, and epithelial cell growth. Retinoids prevent horny cell cohesion, or keratolysis, and increase epithelial cell turnover. They do *not* affect microorganisms in acne and sebum production. Topical retinoids are appropriate for all types of acne when used in combination with other antiacne therapy. They also allow maintenance of acne clearance after discontinuing oral antibiotics. Of the retinoids, tazarotene is contraindicated with pregnancy. Retinoids should *not* be used before or after extended sun exposure or sunburn because they can increase the risk of sunburn and intensify existing sunburn.

Another antiacne topical agent, azelaic acid, has antibacterial, antiinflammatory, and mild comedolytic actions. Azelaic acid is as effective as BP and tretinoin combined. Salicylic acid is also a comedolytic treatment that is available over the counter in various strengths. However, the efficacy of salicylic acid is still unknown. Topical treatments with retinoids, azelaic acid, and salicylic acid can cause burning, pruritus, and erythema after several applications; however, they are less common with azelaic acid.

BOX 45.1 Topical Corticosteroids

Very High Potency
Betamethasone dipropionate, augmented 0.05% (ointment)
Clobetasol propionate 0.05%
Diflorasone diacetate 0.05% (ointment)
Halobetasol propionate 0.05%

High Potency
Amcinonide 0.1%
Betamethasone dipropionate, augmented 0.05% (cream)
Desoximetasone 0.25% (cream, ointment) and 0.05% (gel)
Diflorasone diacetate 0.05% (cream)
Fluocinonide 0.05%
Halcinonide 0.1%
Triamcinolone acetonide 0.5%

Medium Potency
Betamethasone valerate 0.1%
Fluocinolone acetonide 0.025% (cream, ointment)
Flurandrenolide 0.05%
Fluticasone propionate 0.05% (cream) and 0.005% (ointment)
Mometasone furoate 0.1%
Triamcinolone acetonide 0.1% (cream, ointment)

Low-medium Potency
Hydrocortisone butyrate 0.1%
Hydrocortisone probutate 0.1%
Hydrocortisone valerate 0.2%
Prednicarbate 0.1%

Low Potency
Alclometasone dipropionate 0.05%
Fluocinolone acetonide 0.01% (cream, solution)

Lowest Potency
Dexamethasone 0.1%
Hydrocortisone base or acetate 0.25%, 0.5%, 1%

Moderate to severe acne may require a stronger concentration of BP, and topical antibiotics, such as tetracycline, erythromycin, and clindamycin, may be added to the treatment regimen. Erythromycin and clindamycin are the recommended topical antibiotics for acne therapy; however, erythromycin has reduced efficacy when compared with clindamycin. Topical antibiotics accumulate in the hair follicle and have both antiinflammatory and antibacterial effects. Topical antibiotics as monotherapy are *not* recommended due to the development of antibiotic resistance. Severe painful acne may be treated with steroid injection.

Systemic Antiacne Drugs

For severe acne, adjunctive treatment is usually warranted with oral antibiotics (e.g., doxycycline and minocycline [drugs of choice], tetracycline, amoxicillin) in addition to topical corticosteroids (Box 45.1). ❶ Tetracycline antibiotics, however, should not be used among the very young and among pregnant patients; drugs of the tetracycline class may cause dental discoloration to the developing teeth and have teratogenic effects on the fetus. Instead, amoxicillin or another non-tetracycline drug may be given for severe acne. See Chapter 26 for more information on antibacterials.

Isotretinoin, a derivative of vitamin A taken orally, is used for treatment of severe cystic acne that is not responsive to conventional therapy. It decreases sebum formation and secretion and has antiinflammatory and antikeratinizing (keratolytic) effects, decreasing lesions and scars due to acne. Additional benefits of isotretinoin include a decrease in anxiety and depression. The typical patient takes this drug for 4 to 6 months. Adverse reactions may occur that are dose dependent; these include chelitis, dizziness, cephalgia, conjunctivitis, skin irritation, pruritus, epistaxis, myalgia, arthralgia, temporary hair thinning, photosensitivity, depression, and suicidal thoughts. Usually, one course of treatment with isotretinoin is curative of severe acne. Because isotretinoin is a derivative of vitamin A, patients should not take vitamin A concomitantly. Using vitamin A or tetracycline with isotretinoin may increase its adverse effects. Baseline blood tests—liver function tests (LFTs), serum lipid panel, and pregnancy tests among female patients of childbearing age—are required before initiating isotretinoin therapy and at intervals throughout therapy. ❶ Isotretinoin must *not* be used during pregnancy; it is a known teratogen. Additional cautions associated with isotretinoin are to not breastfeed or to give blood during or for 1 month after therapy; patients should not take other medications or herbal products without first consulting their health care provider, drive at night without knowing the effect of isotretinoin on night vision, or have cosmetic procedures to smooth skin. Patient should be instructed to avoid excessively vigorous activity and to contact the health care provider and stop taking isotretinoin if they experience muscle weakness, which may be an indication of serious muscle damage.

❶ Because of isotretinoin's powerful teratogenicity, a risk-management system to prevent isotretinoin-related teratogenicity was implemented. iPLEDGE is the third risk-management program to prevent exposure to isotretinoin during pregnancy. Prior to starting isotretinoin therapy, both males and females must enroll in the iPLEDGE risk-management program and adhere to it. The program was created to ensure patients who receive isotretinoin use two forms of contraception, that no patient is pregnant when treatment is initiated, and that no patient becomes pregnant while taking the drug or for at least 1 month after completing a course of isotretinoin. This comprehensive program also has rules for the health care provider, patient, pharmacist, and wholesaler. Further information can be found at https://www.ipledgeprogram.com.

PSORIASIS

Psoriasis is a multisystem disease with predominant skin and joint disorders. According to the AAD, it affects nearly 2% of the population; of those affected, 80% have mild to moderate disease. A majority of the manifestations are exhibited as chronic skin inflammation that is characterized by scaly, erythematous plaques or scales. These plaques may be painful and are often pruritic, at times causing significant quality-of-life issues. They can appear on the scalp, elbows, palms, knees, and soles of the

TABLE 45.2 Current Treatment Modalities for Psoriasis and Psoriatic Arthritis

TNF Inhibitors	Topical Treatments	Systemic Treatments	Phototherapy and Photochemotherapy
Adalimumab	Anthralin	6-Thioguanine	Broadband and
Etanercept	Coal tar	Azathioprine	narrowband B
Infliximab	Corticosteroids	Cyclosporine	Excimer laser therapy
	Emollients	Fumaric acid	Oral PUVA therapy
	Pimecrolimus	esters	Topical PUVA therapy
	Salicylic acid	Hydroxyurea	
	Tacrolimus	Leflunomide	
	Tazarotene	Methotrexate	
	Vitamin D	Mycophenolate	
	analogues	mofetil	
	Combination	Retinoids	
	therapy of above	Sulfasalazine	
		Tacrolimus	

PUVA, Psoralen and ultraviolet A; TNF, tumor necrosis factor.
Data from American Academy of Dermatology. (2016). Psoriasis clinical guideline. Retrieved from https://www.aad.org/practice-tools/quality-care/clinical-guidelines/psoriasis.

feet. Psoriasis is a chronic disease, and the manifestations wax and wane. Of the different forms of psoriasis, plaque psoriasis is the most common form. Depending on the severity of the disease, recommendations for the treatment of psoriasis include topical and systemic treatments and/or phototherapy. Table 45.1 lists some drugs, dosages, uses, and considerations for psoriasis. Table 45.2 lists current treatment modalities for psoriasis and psoriatic arthritis.

Topical Drugs

Vehicles for topical preparations are many and may include ointments, creams, lotions, solutions, gels, foams, and tape, among others. More than one topical medication may be used concomitantly to increase the effectiveness of each drug. If more than one topical drug is used, patients need to be instructed to apply each drug at separate times throughout the day. Topical drugs for psoriasis include corticosteroids, vitamin D analogues, tazarotene, calcineurin inhibitors (e.g., tacrolimus and pimecrolimus), salicylic acid, anthralin, and coal tar.

Topical corticosteroids are the principal treatment for the majority of patients. Corticosteroids are available in variety of vehicles that are sold over the counter (OTC) or by prescription; differing levels of potency are also available such that the weakest formula (e.g., 1% hydrocortisone) is available OTC, and the strongest (e.g., clobetasol propionate) is by prescription (see Box 45.1). Corticosteroids are classified according to their potency, class 1 to class 7, in which class 1 is the strongest (superpotent). The lower-potency topical steroids are reserved for sensitive skin (e.g., face, intertriginous areas, thin skin areas, in infants and older adults). Patients with thick skin and those with scales or plaques often require the highest-potency steroids. ⚡ The usual length of treatment for most topical steroids is 4 weeks; otherwise, adverse effects that include cutaneous side effects and systemic absorption may occur. Tapering topical steroids after clinical response is recommended by the AAD. Cutaneous side effects include skin atrophy, telangiectasia, striae distensae, acne, folliculitis, and purpura. Other effects include worsening of existing or pre-existing skin conditions (dermatoses) and fungal infections (tineas). Worsening of psoriasis can also occur (rebound effect) with the use of topical corticosteroids. Even though systemic side effects are fewer than cutaneous side effects with topical steroids, these can still occur. Systemic effects usually occur with the highest-potency preparation used over a large surface for a prolonged period. Examples of systemic side effects include Cushing syndrome, cataracts, glaucoma, and suppression of the hypothalamic-pituitary-adrenal (HPA) axis, which can cause growth retardation.

Synthetic vitamin D analogues (e.g., calcipotriene) bind to vitamin D receptors, enhancing the differentiation of keratinocytes while inhibiting their proliferation. Calcipotriene is available in solution, foam, and cream and is usually combined with topical corticosteroids to increase clinical response. Local side effects include burning, pruritus, edema, peeling, dryness, and erythema. Systemic side effects usually occur due to overapplication and include hypercalcemia and suppression of parathyroid hormone. Patients need to be instructed to avoid ultraviolet (UV) light because UVA inactivates calcipotriene.

Topical tazarotene, a retinoid, normalizes abnormal keratinocyte differentiation and decreases hyperproliferation and inflammation. Tazarotene may be used concurrently with moisturizers and topical corticosteroids. Common side effects include local irritation, although tazarotene is a teratogen.

Topical calcineurin inhibitors (CIs) such as tacrolimus and pimecrolimus block the synthesis of proinflammatory cytokines, a major pathogenesis of psoriasis. Common side effects include burning and pruritus of the skin, which appears to increase when applied immediately after bathing. Topical tacrolimus and pimecrolimus are not approved for infants and children younger than 2 years old. Increased susceptibility to infection can occur with the use of topical CIs, including reactivation of latent viral infection. CIs are pregnancy category C.

Other topical preparations include salicylic acid, anthralin, and coal tar. Salicylic acid is a keratolytic agent that loosens psoriatic plaques. Like other salicylate drugs, topical salicylates may be absorbed systemically and cause toxicity; therefore topical salicylic acid should not be used by children due to the risk of Reye syndrome. Anthralin normalizes keratinocyte differentiation and is commonly used for short, contact therapy. Common side effects include skin irritation and staining of adjoining skin, nails, and clothing. Coal tar products are available in shampoos, lotions, creams, and bath solutions. They have an unpleasant odor and can cause burning and stinging, so they are rarely used.

UVA may be used to suppress mitotic (cell division) activity. **Photochemotherapy**, a combination of UV radiation and the psoralen derivative methoxsalen (a photosensitive drug), is used to decrease proliferation of epidermal cells. This type of therapy is called **psoralen and ultraviolet A (PUVA)**, which permits lower doses of methoxsalen and UVA to be given.

Common side effects of PUVA include erythema, pruritus, xerosis, irregular pigmentation, and gastrointestinal (GI) symptoms such as nausea and vomiting. Other toxicities include blisters, melanonychia, hypertrichosis, and squamous cell carcinoma (SCC). PUVA is contraindicated in patients with known lupus erythematosus, xeroderma pigmentosum, and porphyria. A topical preparation of methoxsalen must be administered only by a trained clinician.

Systemic Drugs

Traditional systemic drugs for psoriasis (e.g., methotrexate, cyclosporine, acitretin) are commonly used for refractory psoriasis. Biologic response modifiers (BRMs) also have a role in the treatment of psoriasis without the toxicity of traditional systemic treatment to the liver, kidneys, and bone marrow; furthermore, BRMs are not teratogenic.

A folate antimetabolite, ⊕ methotrexate is a systemic drug that slows high growth fraction. It is prescribed to decrease the acceleration of epidermal cell growth in severe psoriasis. However, methotrexate can cause toxicity to the liver (hepatic fibrosis and cirrhosis), blood (myelosuppression), and lungs (pulmonary fibrosis). Other common adverse effects include nausea, anorexia, stomatitis, and fatigue. It is considered teratogenic and is contraindicated in childbearing women who are trying to conceive. Methotrexate has numerous drug-drug interactions, thereby increasing the risk of methotrexate toxicity (Table 45.3). Before methotrexate administration is initiated, a careful history, physical and laboratory tests (e.g., complete blood count [CBC], creatinine, LFTs, protein status, bilirubin, screening for latent tuberculosis [TB] infections), and chest radiograph must be obtained. During treatment, ongoing studies include CBC and renal and hepatic function tests. Methotrexate has been used in combination with approved BRMs for psoriasis. See Chapter 32 for more nursing considerations with antimetabolites.

Cyclosporine, a cyclic polypeptide immunosuppressive drug, is the most effective systemic preparation for psoriasis. It inhibits T-cell activation and has minimal toxicities in otherwise healthy patients. It must be administered on a consistent

⊕ TABLE 45.3   Methotrexate Drug Interactions

NSAIDs	Antibiotics	Others
Salicylates	Trimethoprim-sulfamethoxazole	Barbiturates
Naproxen	Sulfonamides	Colchicine
Ibuprofen	Penicillins	Dipyridamole
Indomethacin	Minocycline	Ethanol
Phenylbutazone	Ciprofloxacin	Phenytoin
		Sulfonylureas
		Furosemide
		Thiazide diuretics

NSAIDs, Nonsteroidal antiinflammatory drugs.
From American Academy of Dermatology. (2016). Psoriasis: recommendations for methotrexate—toxicity. Retrieved from https://www.aad.org/practice-tools/quality-care/clinical-guidelines/psoriasis/systemic-agents/recommendations-for-methotrexate.

schedule with regard to time of day and in relation to meals to decrease serum level variations. As with other immunosuppressive drugs, patients must be assessed for active infections prior to initiating therapy. Patients must also be monitored for nephrotoxicity and hypertension. Other common side effects include hypertrichosis (darkening of hair), cephalgia, paresthesia, myalgia, arthralgia, asthenia, and fatigue.

Acitretin, a vitamin A derivative, is the least effective drug as monotherapy and is usually used concurrently with phototherapy. It is more effective with pustular psoriasis, and clinical response is dose dependent. Adverse effects include mucocutaneous effects, erythematous scaly patches with superficial fissures, and periungual pyogenic granulomas. Noncutaneous adverse effects include hyperlipidemia, pancreatitis, elevated transaminases, and pseudotumor cerebri–like symptoms. Its use is contraindicated with pregnancy.

High-cost BRMs are helpful in the management of psoriasis in patients who are refractory to ultraviolet B (UVB) phototherapy who need improved control. Agents approved by the U.S. Food and Drug Administration (FDA) include tumor necrosis factor (TNF) inhibitors (e.g., etanercept, infliximab, adalimumab) and interleukin antagonists (e.g., ustekinumab). All TNF inhibitors have a risk of severe opportunistic infection. TB and hepatitis B virus (HBV) testing should be conducted on all patients prior to administering TNF inhibitors. Caution is advised when administering drug to patients with a history of congestive heart failure. These biologic agents are expensive but tend to have fewer side effects with comparable efficacy to traditional systemic treatments. TNF inhibitors are contraindicated in patients with active infections or demyelinating disease (e.g., multiple sclerosis). Adalimumab is the first fully human TNF-inhibitor monoclonal antibody (MAb). Infliximab is a chimeric MAb, and ustekinumab is a human immunoglobulin G (IgG) monoclonal antibody; more information on MAbs can be found in Chapter 33. Etanercept is a soluble recombinant human TNF-α inhibitor. Table 45.1 lists the drugs used to control psoriasis.

NURSING PROCESS
Patient-Centered Collaborative Care
Acne Vulgaris and Psoriasis

Assessment
- Obtain a history from the patient in regard to the onset of skin lesions. Note if there is a familial history.
- Assess the patient's skin eruptions. Describe lesions, locations (body surface area [BSA]), and drainage, if present.
- Obtain cultures of purulent, draining skin lesions.
- Determine baseline vital signs and weight. Report any elevation in temperature.
- Obtain baseline laboratory values (CBC, lipid panel, renal function, and hepatic function).
- Obtain chest radiograph, electrocardiography (ECG), and if applicable, conduct pregnancy, TB, and HBV tests.

- Assess the psychological effects of skin lesions and any changes in perception of body image.
- Assess the effects of skin lesions on quality of life.

Nursing Diagnoses
- Knowledge, Deficient related to management of skin lesions and adverse effects of medications used to treat skin lesions
- Skin Integrity, Risk for Impaired
- Infection, Risk for
- Body Image, Risk for Disturbed

Planning
- The patient will have increased knowledge of management of the skin condition.
- Clinicians will be notified of abnormal diagnostic results.
- The patient will verbalize the need for two methods of contraception during the required period.
- Lesions will be decreased in size or will be absent after drug therapy and skin care.
- The patient will be free from infection during therapy.
- The patient will report improved body image.

Nursing Interventions
- Establish rapport; the patient may be embarrassed.
- Apply topical medications to skin lesions using aseptic technique.
- Monitor vital signs and perform required diagnostic tests. Report abnormal findings.
- During drug therapy, check lesion sites for improvement, and monitor for adverse reactions to drug therapy.
- Listen to the patient's body image concerns and provide community resources if applicable.

Patient Teaching
- Advise patients not to use harsh cleansers. Tell them to gently cleanse the skin several times a day and pat dry. Allow to dry for 20 to 30 minutes before applying product.
- Teach patients to apply topical drugs using clean technique.
- Inform patients about side effects and adverse reactions associated with drugs.
- Advise patients to report abnormal findings immediately.
- Instruct patients to notify their health care provider if pregnant or if there is a possibility of pregnancy. Many agents used to treat acne and psoriasis are teratogenic.
- Advise patients to keep health care appointments and to have diagnostic tests performed as prescribed.

Evaluation
- Evaluate the patient's knowledge of management of the condition.
- Evaluate the effectiveness of drug therapy. If improvement is not apparent, the drug therapy and skin care regimen may need to be changed.
- Be aware of the different time periods for improvement with various drug therapies.

VERRUCA VULGARIS (WARTS)

The common wart is a hard, horny nodule that may appear anywhere on the body, particularly on the hands and feet. Warts occur when the top layer of the skin becomes infected with human papillomavirus (HPV). Warts may be benign lesions, or they may be precursors to cancerous lesions. Warts are contagious and can be spread by contact. Most warts do not require treatment, but they may be removed by cryotherapy (freezing), electrodessication, or surgical excision. Other treatments include using chemical peels with salicylic acid, tretinoin, and glycolic acid; injection of anticancer drugs, such as bleomycin; or immunotherapy, such as diphencyprone (DCP). Salicylic acid promotes desquamation. It can be absorbed through the skin, and salicylism (toxicity) could occur. Podophyllum resin is indicated mainly for venereal warts and is not as effective against the common wart. This drug also can be absorbed through the skin; toxic symptoms such as peripheral neuropathy, blood dyscrasias, and kidney impairment may result if a large area is treated. Podophyllum could cause teratogenic effects, therefore it should not be used during pregnancy. Imiquimod and podofilox may be prescribed as alternative agents for podophyllin, and both may be used for topical treatment of external genital and perianal warts. Bleomycin injections are also used for warts. Side effects of bleomycin injection include nail loss if given for warts on the fingers. Immunotherapy uses the patient's own immune system to fight the warts by causing an allergic reaction to the treated warts, which may cause the warts to disappear.

Cantharidin is used to remove the common wart. For treatment, cantharidin is applied to the wart, allowed to dry, and then the wart is covered with nonporous tape for 24 to 48 hours. Occlusion allows a blister to form beneath the wart, where live viruses are located. A follow-up visit at 2 weeks will allow the hyperkeratosis to be debrided. If verruca is noted after debridement, the procedure may be repeated. Side effects include a tingling or burning sensation at the application site.

Many OTC agents are used to remove warts. The efficacy of some of these is questionable; however, some that contain chemical compounds such as salicylic acid may be effective.

DRUG-INDUCED DERMATITIS

An adverse reaction to drug therapy may result in skin lesions that vary from a rash, urticaria, papules, and vesicles to life-threatening skin eruptions such as erythema multiforme (red blisters over a large portion of the body), Stevens-Johnson syndrome (large blisters in the oral and anogenital mucosa, pharynx, eyes, and viscera), and toxic epidermal necrolysis (widespread detachment of the epidermis from underlying skin layers). A hypersensitive reaction to a drug is caused by the formation of sensitizing lymphocytes. If multiple drug therapy is used, the last drug given may be the cause of the hypersensitivity and skin eruptions. The usual skin reaction is a rash, which may take several hours or a day to appear, and urticaria (hives), which usually takes a few minutes to appear. Certain drugs, such as penicillin, are known to cause hypersensitivity.

Other drug-induced dermatitides include discoid lupus erythematosus and exfoliative dermatitis. Hydralazine hydrochloride (e.g., isoniazid, phenothiazines, anticonvulsants, and antidysrhythmics such as procainamide), may cause lupus-like symptoms. If lupus symptoms occur, the drug should be discontinued. Certain antibacterials and anticonvulsants may cause exfoliative dermatitis, resulting in erythema of the skin, itching, desquamation of large areas of the skin, and loss of body hair (e.g., sulfa antibiotics are one cause of toxic epidermal necrolysis).

CONTACT DERMATITIS

Contact dermatitis is a common form of eczema that results when skin is exposed to irritants (irritant contact dermatitis) or allergens (allergic contact dermatitis). Frequent contact with water (hand washing) can cause irritant contact dermatitis that usually starts with dry, cracked hands that sometimes develop pruritus and bleeding. Lips can also develop irritant contact dermatitis due to continuous licking of the lips. Other irritants include bleach, pepper spray, foods, and soap.

Allergic contact dermatitis is due to exposure to allergens. Examples of such allergens include poison ivy, sumac, and oak; nickel; makeup; jewelry; and latex gloves. Allergic contact dermatitis is considered a delayed hypersensitivity reaction. It may take hours to weeks for skin to develop manifestations, especially if it is a first-time exposure. Manifestations include skin rash with pruritus, swelling, burning, stinging, blistering, oozing, or scaling at the affected skin sites.

Nonpharmacologic treatments include avoiding direct contact with the causative irritant or allergen. Protective gloves or clothing may be necessary if the chemical is associated with work; skin that has been in contact with the irritant should be immediately cleansed and dried. Skin moisturizers, antihistamines (e.g., diphenhydramine), and/or topical corticosteroids may be used, depending on the severity of the dermatitis. Oatmeal baths can also relieve discomfort. Patch testing may be needed to determine the causal factor. Treatment may consist of wet dressings containing Burow's solution (aluminum acetate); lotions that contain zinc oxide, such as calamine; calcium hydroxide solution; and glycerin. Calamine lotion is primarily used for plant irritations. If itching persists, an oral antihistamine (e.g., diphenhydramine) may be used. Topical antipruritics should *not* be applied to open wounds or mucous membranes (e.g., eyes, mouth, or genital area). Other antipruritic treatments include baths of oatmeal and applications of corticosteroid ointments, creams, or gels.

Topical corticosteroids can alleviate dermatitis but can be systemically absorbed into the circulation. The amount and rate of absorption depend on the vehicle (cream, lotion, or ointment), drug concentration, drug composition, and skin area to which the steroid is applied. Absorption is greater where the skin is more permeable, such as the face, scalp, eyelids, neck, axilla, and genital area. Side effects and adverse reactions may occur with prolonged use of the topical drug or if the drug is continuously covered with a dressing. Prolonged use of a topical steroid can cause thinning of the skin with atrophy of the epidermis and dermis and purpura from small-vessel eruptions, therefore prolonged use is discouraged.

IMPETIGO

Impetigo, an infection of the skin that is usually due to *Streptococcus* or *Staphylococcus* species, is most commonly seen in children 2 to 5 years old. Topical agents are used in the treatment of mild and moderate infection, and oral agents are used for severe infection. The two drugs of choice are mupirocin and retapamulin. The lesions should be soaked to facilitate the removal of crusts, and the topical antibiotic should be applied at the base of the lesion. With multiple lesions and ineffective topical therapy, oral antibiotics are needed.

HAIR LOSS AND BALDNESS

Hair loss, or *alopecia*, occurs when the hair shaft is lost and the hair follicle cannot regenerate. Permanent hair loss is associated with a familial history and occurs during the aging process, earlier in some individuals than others. Also known to cause alopecia are some drugs, which includes anticancer agents, sulfonamides, anticonvulsants, aminoglycosides, and some nonsteroidal antiinflammatory drugs (NSAIDs) such as indomethacin. Severe febrile illnesses, pregnancy, myxedema (a condition resulting from hypothyroidism), and cancer therapies are some of the health conditions that contribute to temporary hair loss.

Minoxidil solution has been approved by the FDA for treating hair loss in men and women. A 5% solution is approved for men, 2% for women. The exact mechanism of action to stimulate hair growth is not known. Hair regrowth is usually seen after several months of using; but a few months after discontinuation, hair loss resumes. Minoxidil is available OTC in the form of a solution or foam. Systemic absorption of minoxidil is minimal, so adverse reactions seldom occur. Occasionally, headaches and a slight decrease in systolic blood pressure occur.

Finasteride (1 mg) is an oral drug used for alopecia in males. For growing hair, finasteride is effective in 50% of men. It has been reported that it is relatively ineffective in growing hair in older men, even with an increased dose. Like minoxidil, clinical response is not seen until the drug has been used daily for 3 months or longer; discontinuing the drug leads to hair loss within 12 months. Finasteride is contraindicated in pregnancy and pregnant women should not handle the drug. Side effects include decreased libido, impotence, and ejaculation disorder.

SUNSCREENS

Sunscreens are primarily used to block UV rays that cause sunburn, but they also protect against certain types of keratosis, skin cancer, premature aging, cold sores and fever blisters, and UV photosensitivity reactions. There are two types of sunscreens: chemical blockers and physical blockers. *Chemical blockers* (e.g., oxybenzone and ecamsule) absorb UV radiation and are effective against UVA radiation; and *physical blockers* (e.g., titanium dioxide and zinc oxide) reflect or scatter UV radiation and are effective against both UVA and UVB radiation. UVB radiation is the primary cause of sunburn and skin cancer, whereas UVA is responsible for loss of elasticity (wrinkling) and collagen damage of the skin. UVA radiation also contributes to skin cancer and penetrates the skin at a deeper

TABLE 45.4 Degree and Tissue Depth of Burns

Type	Degree	Depth	Characteristics
Superficial epidermal	First	Outer layer of skin; epidermis (e.g., sunburn without blisters)	Erythema, edema, pain
Partial or full-thickness superficial	Second	Epidermis, upper layers of dermis; blisters may be present.	Partial: Wound is pink and blanches; erythema is present and burn is painful and wet appearing. Full: Blanching is sluggish or absent; burn is red/white and dry in appearance; pain may be present but will be diminished.
Full thickness	Third	All layers extending into the subcutaneous tissues	Skin can appear black or white and dry and is leathery in texture; area will not blanch, and no pain is experienced.

level than UVB, thereby causing damage to deeper skin structures. Broad-spectrum sunscreen protects from both UVA and UVB radiation. The FDA passed a ruling that sunscreen with a sun protection factor (SPF) of less than 15 can denote that it prevents sunburn, and an SPF of 15 and above can reduce the risk of skin cancer and early skin aging if used as directed with other sun-protection measures such as wearing sun-blocking clothing, limiting sun exposure between 10 a.m. and 2 p.m., and reapplying sunscreen at least every 2 hours. Common side effects of sunscreens include cutaneous reactions (e.g., erythema, pruritus, folliculitis, contact dermatitis, and acne vulgaris).

BURNS AND BURN PREPARATIONS

Burns from heat (*thermal burns,* the most common kind of burn injury), electricity (*electrical burns*), and chemical agents (*chemical burns*) can all cause skin lesions. Burns are classified according to degree and depth of the tissue injury (Table 45.4). Burns need immediate attention, regardless of the degree and depth of tissue injury. For minor burns, a cool, wet compress is applied to prevent further tissue damage caused by heat. After the affected area is cooled off, it should be cleansed gently with soap and water; intact blisters should not be opened. After cleaning the area, apply a thin layer of ointment, such as aloe vera or petroleum jelly. A thin layer of antibiotic ointment (e.g., bacitracin, neomycin sulfate, polymyxin B sulfate) can be applied to affected areas one to three times daily to prevent infections of the skin and skin structure.

Persons with burns that involve the dermis and subcutaneous tissue should seek medical help immediately at a

PROTOTYPE DRUG CHART 45.1

Mafenide Acetate

Drug Class	Dosage
Topical antiinfective Pregnancy category: C*	A/C >2 mo: Cream: Apply a layer of 1.6 mm thickness evenly to the affected area once or twice daily; reapply PRN. Be sure burn is covered with cream at all times. A/C ≥3 mo: Sol: Apply to dressing-covered graft site every 4 h or as needed to maintain wet dressing.
Contraindications	**Drug-Lab-Food Interactions**
Hypersensitivity, inhalation injury *Caution:* Renal failure, acid-base imbalance, or hypersensitivity to other sulfonamides/sulfites	No significant drug interactions; caution when using other carbonic anhydrase inhibitors due to increased risk of metabolic acidosis.
Pharmacokinetics	**Pharmacodynamics**
Absorption: Diffuses through devascularized areas with variable systemic absorption Distribution: PB: UK Metabolism: t½: UK Excretion: In urine	Onset: On contact Peak: 2 h Duration: 4 h
Therapeutic Effects/Uses	
Synthetic sulfonamide antibiotics are indicated as an adjunctive treatment for second- and third-degree burns, to prevent organism invasion of burned tissue areas, and to treat burn infections. Mode of Action: Bacteriostatic activity against many gram-negative and gram-positive bacteria, including *Pseudomonas aeruginosa* and other anaerobic strains.	
Side Effects	**Adverse Reactions**
Rash, burning sensation, urticaria, pruritus, swelling, erythema	Metabolic acidosis, respiratory alkalosis, blistering, superinfection (e.g., fungal) *Life threatening:* Bone marrow suppression, fatal hemolytic anemia

*Pregnancy categories have been revised. See http://www.fda.gov/Drugs/DevelopmentApprovalProcess/DevelopmentResources/Labeling/ucm093307.htm for more information.

A, Adult; *C,* child; *h,* hour; *mm,* millimeter; *mo,* month; *PB,* protein binding; *PRN,* as needed; *sol,* solution; *t½,* half-life; *UK,* unknown; *>,* greater than; *≥,* greater than or equal to.

health care facility. Persons with extensive second-degree burns and beyond are at risk of dehydration through interstitial fluid loss and are vulnerable to infection and sepsis. Dehydration can cause hypovolemic shock. Intravenous (IV) fluid therapy should be started immediately, and an analgesic is given for pain. Burn areas are kept clean, and any necrotic tissue is debrided. Broad-spectrum topical antiinfectives effective against many gram-positive and gram-negative organisms and fungi are applied to burn areas to prevent infection. Examples of these antiinfectives include mafenide acetate, silver sulfadiazine, and silver nitrate 0.5% solution. Table 45.5 lists selected topical medications for burns along with their dosages, uses, and considerations. Prototype Drug Chart 45.1 lists the pharmacologic data for the antibacterial agent mafenide acetate.

TABLE 45.5   Topical Antiinfectives: Burns

Generic (Brand)	Route and Dosage	Uses and Considerations
Mafenide acetate	See Prototype Drug Chart 45.1.	
Silver sulfadiazine	A/C: 1% Cream: Apply twice daily to a thickness of 1.6 mm	To prevent and treat infection of second- and third-degree burns. Ten percent of drug is absorbed. Excessive use or extensive application area may cause sulfa crystals (crystalluria). Pregnancy category: C*

*Pregnancy categories have been revised. See http://www.fda.gov/Drugs/DevelopmentApprovalProcess/DevelopmentResources/Labeling/ucm093307.htm for more information.
A, adult; *C,* children; *mm,* millimeter.

Silver Sulfadiazine

Silver sulfadiazine is a common antiinfective used to prevent and treat infections in second- and third-degree burns. It is applied at least twice daily, and it is not absorbed through intact skin. Silver sulfadiazine possesses activity against both gram-negative and gram-positive organisms and fungi. Unlike mafenide, it is not a carbonic anhydrase inhibitor. Sulfadiazine is metabolized by the liver and is excreted in the urine. It is pregnancy category B but is contraindicated in near-term pregnancy and among neonates and infants younger than 2 months old. Side effects and adverse reactions may include photosensitivity, skin discoloration, burning sensation, rashes, erythema multiforme, skin necrosis, and leukopenia.

 NURSING PROCESS

Patient-Centered Collaborative Care

Topical Antiinfectives: Burns

Assessment

- Assess burned tissue for signs of infection such as foul odor, purulent drainage, erythema, and heat.
- Culture the purulent wound.
- Check the patient's vital signs. Report abnormal findings, such as elevated temperature.
- Determine fluid status. Report signs and symptoms of hypovolemia or hypervolemia.

Nursing Diagnoses

- Fluid Volume, Risk for Imbalanced
- Infection, Risk for
- Pain, Acute related to thermal injury
- Knowledge, Deficient related to management of burns

Planning

- The patient will remain free from infection.
- The patient's pain will be decreased or tolerable.
- The patient will remain hydrated.

Nursing Interventions

- Administer prescribed analgesia before treatment, if needed.
- Cleanse burned tissue sites using aseptic technique.
- Apply topical antibacterial drugs and dressings with sterile technique.
- Maintain the patient's fluid balance and renal function.
- Monitor the patient for side effects and adverse reactions to topical drugs.
- ❶ Monitor the patient's vital signs, and be alert for signs of infection or hypovolemic shock.
- Closely monitor the patient's acid-base balance, especially in the presence of pulmonary or renal dysfunction.
- Store drugs in a dry place at room temperature.

Patient Teaching

- Instruct the patient and family about pain management, medications used to treat burns, and signs of complications from burns, such as fluid excess or deficit.
- Teach the patient and family how to apply a topical agent and dressings to burned areas.
- Teach the patient and family about signs and symptoms of infection and to report them promptly to the health care provider.

Evaluation

- Evaluate patient and family knowledge of burn management.
- Evaluate the effectiveness of treatment interventions to burned tissue areas by determining whether healing is proceeding and sites are free from infection.

CRITICAL THINKING CASE STUDY

MG, a 15-year-old patient, complains about blackheads and large, raised acne with surrounding erythema on her face. She seeks help from a health care provider.

1. To assist in identifying her skin problem, what should the health history and assessment include?
2. Which nonpharmacologic measures might the nurse discuss with MG in caring for her skin condition?

MG's skin disorder does not improve. Her health care provider says she has acne vulgaris and has prescribed benzoyl peroxide and oral tetracycline.

3. MG asks the nurse how to use benzoyl peroxide. What should the explanation of the method and frequency for use of benzoyl peroxide include?
4. What should be included in the patient teaching related to the use of oral tetracycline?
5. What other agents for acne might MG use? Explain their uses and side effects.
6. MG asks if she will have to remain on benzoyl peroxide and oral tetracycline for the rest of her life. What is the nurse's best response or course of action? Explain your answer.

NCLEX STUDY QUESTIONS

1. The nurse is reviewing a patient's list of medications. The patient asks, "What do kerolytic agents remove?" What is the nurse's best response?
   a. A horny layer of dermis
   b. A horny layer of epidermis
   c. Erythematous lesions
   d. Hair follicles

2. A male patient is to begin therapy with isotretinoin and asks, "What do I have to remember to do while taking this medicine?" What is the nurse's best response? (Select all that apply.)
   a. Avoid sunlight.
   b. Monitor your weight.
   c. Keep appointments for laboratory tests.
   d. Use two forms of contraceptives.
   e. Always take the drug with food.

3. The nurse is doing health teaching with a patient with psoriasis. Which is a priority nursing implication of a biologic agent such as infliximab for the management of psoriasis?
   a. Monitor weight daily.
   b. Monitor electrolytes.
   c. Monitor urine output.
   d. Monitor complete blood count.

4. A 55-year-old man is concerned about hair loss. The nurse expects that the patient's baldness may be treated with which of the following drugs?
   a. Dexamethasone
   b. Para-aminobenzoic acid
   c. Mupirocin
   d. Finasteride

5. The nurse reviews the patient's medication history. Based on the patient's prolonged use of topical corticosteroids, what could the nursing assessment include? (Select all that apply.)
   a. Weight gain
   b. Thinning of the skin
   c. Erythematous lesions
   d. Purpura
   e. Urinary retention

6. A 20-year-old woman comes to the clinic for follow-up related to isotretinoin use. The nurse reviews the iPLEDGE program, which includes what important information? (Select all that apply.)
   a. One method of contraception must be used throughout treatment.
   b. A review of iPLEDGE educational materials
   c. A negative pregnancy test is required before each monthly refill.
   d. Informed consent is not required.
   e. A prescription for a 60-day supply of drug is to be given.

7. The school nurse prepares a program for junior high school students on sun safety. What is important information to include? (Select all that apply.)
   a. Sunscreen products should contain information about ultraviolet A and B sun protection that includes the sun protection factor.
   b. Ultraviolet B radiation is greatest between 10 a.m. and 2 p.m.
   c. Clouds block radiation, so sunscreen is not needed on cloudy days.
   d. The sun protection factor should be at least 15 in sunscreen products.
   e. Sunscreen is to be applied once daily.

8. A patient is receiving etanercept. Which nursing interventions are appropriate for this patient? (Select all that apply.)
   a. Drug is administered topically.
   b. Tuberculin test is required before the start of therapy.
   c. Monitor for injection site reaction.
   d. Monitor for seizures.
   e. Monitor for heart failure.

9. The nurse is teaching the patient about clobetasol, the medication to be started today. What information needs to be included in the teaching session? (Select all that apply.)
   a. Appropriate treatment is for 6 months' duration.
   b. It can be applied as a lotion to all body parts.
   c. Clobetasol is a super–high-potency corticosteroid.
   d. Maximum dose is 50 g/week.
   e. Occlusive dressing speeds healing.

Answers: 1, b; 2, a, c, d; 3, d; 4, d; 5, b; 6, b, c; 7, a, b, d; 8, b, c, e; 9, c, d.

Endocrine Drugs

The endocrine system consists of ductless glands that secrete hormones into the bloodstream. *Hormones* are chemical substances synthesized from amino acids and cholesterol that act on body tissues and organs and affect cellular activity. They can be divided into two categories: proteins or protein derivatives and steroids. Hormones from the adrenal glands (adrenal cortex) and sex hormones are classified as steroids; all other hormones in the human body are considered proteins or protein derivatives. The major *endocrine glands* include the pituitary (hypophysis), thyroid, parathyroids, adrenals, gonads, and pancreas. The hypothalamus links the endocrine system with the nervous system to maintain homeostasis in the body by producing, releasing, and inhibiting hormones; these hormones control the production of other hormones throughout the body. The action of the glands is mostly regulated by a negative feedback loop. Fig. XV.1 illustrates the regulation of hormones through the negative feedback loop. Fig. XV.2 identifies the location of the major endocrine glands, and Fig. XV.3 correlates the pituitary hormones with their target organs. This unit discusses the hormonal activities of the major endocrine glands.

PITUITARY GLAND

The *pituitary gland,* or *hypophysis,* is located at the base of the brain and has two lobes, the anterior pituitary gland (adenohypophysis) and the posterior pituitary gland (neurohypophysis), connected to the hypothalamus by a pituitary stalk (infundibulum). The pituitary gland is called the *master gland* because it secretes hormones that stimulate the release of most other hormones. The anterior pituitary gland produces and secretes the majority of the pituitary hormones, which then stimulate the production and release of other hormones throughout the body, including the thyroid, adrenals, and gonads. The posterior pituitary gland secretes two neurohormones—antidiuretic hormone (ADH) or vasopressin and oxytocin. These hormones are produced by the hypothalamus and are stored and released by the posterior pituitary. Fig. XV.4 shows the anterior and posterior pituitary glands and their respective hormones secreted.

ANTERIOR PITUITARY GLAND

The anterior pituitary hormones listed in Fig. XV.4 are thyroid-stimulating hormone (TSH), growth hormone (GH), adrenocorticotropic hormone (ACTH), follicle-stimulating hormone (FSH), luteinizing hormone (LH), and prolactin (PRL). TSH, ACTH, FSH, and LH control the synthesis and release of hormones from the thyroid, adrenals, ovaries, and testes, respectively. GH is essential in the early years for development and growth in children; in adults, it promotes healthy bone and muscle mass and affects the distribution of fat. Prolactin is necessary for breast milk production.

The amount of each hormone secreted from the anterior pituitary gland is regulated by a negative

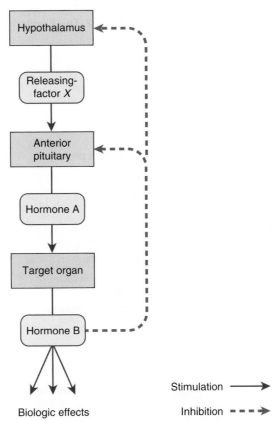

FIG. XV.1 Negative Feedback Loop of Hypothalamus and Pituitary. From Burcham, J., & Rosenthal, L. (2016). *Lehne's pharmacology for nursing care* (9th ed.). St. Louis: Elsevier.

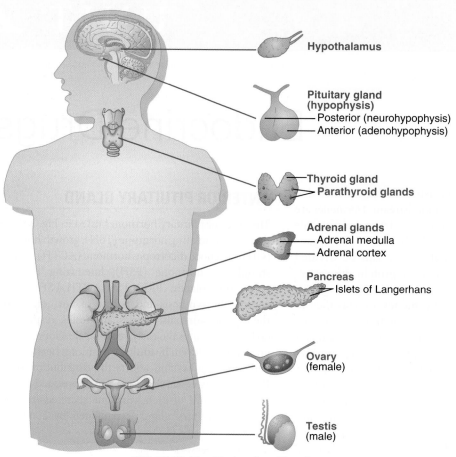

FIG. XV.2 The Endocrine Glands.

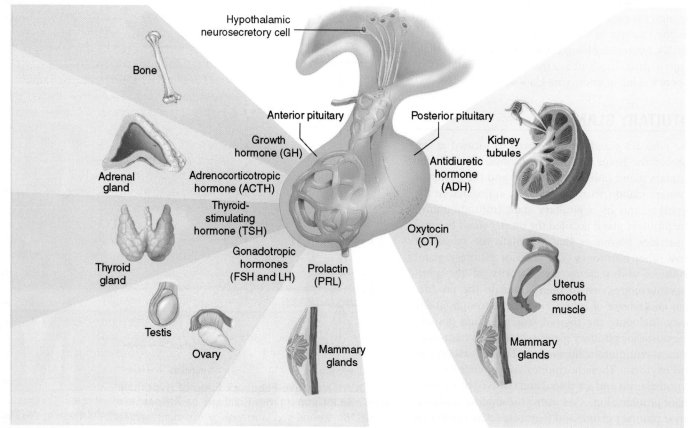

FIG. XV.3 Pituitary Hormones and Their Target Organs. Modified from Patton, K. T., & Thibodeau, G. A. (2016). *Anatomy and physiology* (9th ed.). St. Louis: Elsevier.

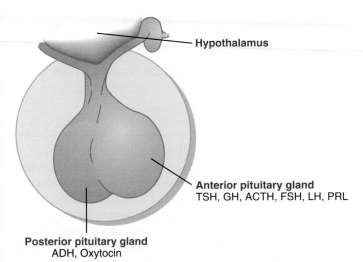

FIG. XV.4 The Anterior and Posterior Pituitary Glands. *ACTH,* Adrenocorticotropic hormone; *ADH,* antidiuretic hormone; *FSH,* follicle-stimulating hormone; *GH,* growth hormone; *LH,* luteinizing hormone; *PRL,* prolactin; *TSH,* thyroid-stimulating hormone.

feedback system. If excess hormone is secreted from the target gland, hormonal release from the anterior pituitary gland is suppressed. If there is a lack of hormone secretion from the target gland, there will be an increase in that particular anterior pituitary hormone (see Fig. XV.1).

THYROID-STIMULATING HORMONE

The anterior pituitary gland secretes TSH in response to thyroid-releasing hormone (TRH) from the hypothalamus. TSH, or thyrotropic hormone, stimulates the release of triiodothyronine (T_3) and thyroxine (T_4) from the thyroid gland. Hypersecretion of TSH can cause hyperthyroidism and thyroid enlargement, and hyposecretion can cause hypothyroidism. Serum TSH levels should be checked to determine whether there is a TSH deficit or excess. TSH and T_4 levels are frequently measured to differentiate pituitary from thyroid dysfunction.

ADRENOCORTICOTROPIC HORMONE

Secretion of ACTH occurs in response to corticotropin-releasing hormone (CRH) from the hypothalamus. ACTH from the anterior pituitary gland stimulates the release of glucocorticoids (cortisol), mineralocorticoids (aldosterone), and androgen from the adrenal cortex (adrenal glands). Elevated serum hormone levels from the adrenal cortex inhibit ACTH and CRH release. When the hormone level is low, ACTH secretion is stimulated, which in turn stimulates the adrenal glands (adrenal cortex and adrenal medulla) to release more of its hormones: cortisol, aldosterone, catecholamines, and androgens (sex hormones). More ACTH is secreted in the morning than in the evening.

GONADOTROPIC HORMONES

The gonadotropic hormones regulate hormone secretion from the ovaries and testes (the gonads). The anterior pituitary gland secretes the gonadotropic hormones FSH, LH, and PRL. FSH promotes the maturation of follicles in the ovaries and initiates sperm production in the testes. LH combines with FSH in follicle maturation and estrogen production and promotes secretion of testosterone from the testes. PRL stimulates milk formation in the glandular breast tissue after childbirth. Estrogen, progesterone, and testosterone are discussed in Unit XVII, Reproductive and Gender-Related Drugs.

GROWTH HORMONE

GH, or somatotropic hormone (STH), acts on all body tissues, particularly the bones and skeletal muscles. The amount of GH secreted is regulated by GH-releasing hormone (GH-RH) and GH-inhibiting hormone (GH-IH, or somatostatin) from the hypothalamus. Sympathomimetics, serotonin, and glucocorticoids can inhibit the secretion of GH.

POSTERIOR PITUITARY GLAND

The posterior pituitary gland (neurohypophysis) secretes ADH (vasopressin) and oxytocin (see Fig. XV.4). Interconnecting nerve fibers (the pituitary stalk) between the hypothalamus and the posterior pituitary gland allow ADH and oxytocin to be synthesized in the hypothalamus and stored in the posterior pituitary gland. ADH increases the reabsorption of water from the renal tubules, returning it to the systemic circulation. Secretion of ADH is regulated by the serum osmolality (concentration of the vascular fluid). An increase in serum osmolality increases the release of ADH from the posterior pituitary gland; more water is then reabsorbed from the renal tubules to dilute the vascular fluid. Excess ADH can cause fluid overload in the vascular system. A decrease in serum osmolality decreases the release of ADH, promoting more water excretion (increased urine formation) from the renal tubules. Oxytocin stimulates contraction of the smooth muscle of the uterus; it is discussed in Unit XVII, Reproductive and Gender-Related Drugs.

THYROID GLAND

Located anterior and to each side of the trachea, the thyroid gland has two lobes that are connected by a bridge of thyroid tissue. The thyroid gland secretes three hormones, triiodothyronine (T_3), thyroxine (T_4), and to a lesser extent calcitonin. T_3 and T_4 affect nearly every tissue and organ by controlling their metabolic rate and activity. Calcitonin helps with the regulation of serum calcium levels. Increased T_3 and T_4 levels result in an increase in cardiac output, oxygen consumption, carbohydrate use, protein synthesis, and breakdown of fat (lipolysis). They also affect body heat regulation and the menstrual cycle. Calcitonin opposes the action of the parathyroid gland. Thyroid hormone levels in the blood are regulated by negative feedback. The anterior pituitary gland secretes TSH, which stimulates the thyroid gland to produce T_3 and T_4 and calcitonin. An increased amount of circulating thyroid hormones suppresses the release of TSH, and a decreased amount increases the release of TSH by the adenohypophysis.

PARATHYROID GLANDS

There are four parathyroid glands (two pairs) that lie on the dorsal surface of the thyroid gland. Parathyroid glands secrete parathormone, or parathyroid hormone (PTH), which regulates calcium levels in the blood. A decrease in serum calcium stimulates the release of PTH, and PTH increases calcium levels by (1) mobilizing calcium from the bone, (2) promoting calcium absorption from the intestine, and (3) promoting calcium reabsorption from the renal tubules. Calcitonin, a hormone produced primarily by the thyroid gland and to a lesser extent by the parathyroid and thymus glands, inhibits calcium reabsorption by bone and increases renal excretion of calcium. Calcitonin counteracts the action of PTH.

ADRENAL GLANDS

The adrenal glands are located at the top of each kidney and consist of two separate sections—the adrenal *medulla,* the inner section, and the adrenal *cortex,* the section that surrounds the adrenal medulla. The adrenal medulla releases the catecholamines, epinephrine and norepinephrine, and is linked with the sympathetic nervous system. The adrenal cortex produces two major types of hormones (corticosteroids), glucocorticoids and mineralocorticoids. The principal *glucocorticoid* is cortisol, and the principal *mineralocorticoid* is aldosterone. The adrenal cortex also produces small amounts of androgen, estrogen, and progestin. Corticosteroids have a profound influence on electrolytes and on the metabolism of carbohydrates, protein, and fat, and corticosteroid deficiencies can result in serious illness and even death.

PANCREAS

The pancreas, located to the left of and behind the stomach, is both an exocrine and an endocrine gland. The exocrine section of the pancreas secretes digestive enzymes into the duodenum; these enzymes are discussed in Unit XIII, Gastrointestinal Drugs. The endocrine section has cell clusters called *islets of Langerhans.* The alpha islet cells produce glucagon, which breaks glycogen down to glucose in the liver, and the beta cells secrete insulin, which regulates glucose metabolism. Insulin, an antidiabetic agent, is used to control diabetes mellitus. Antidiabetic drugs are discussed in Chapter 47.

DRUGS FOR ENDOCRINE DISORDERS

Chapter 46 discusses drugs for disorders of the pituitary, thyroid, parathyroid, and adrenal glands. Chapter 47 discusses the drugs used to diagnose and treat endocrine disorders, and both parenteral and oral antidiabetic drugs (hypoglycemic drugs) are covered.

46

Pituitary, Thyroid, Parathyroid, and Adrenal Disorders

OBJECTIVES

- Compare the hormones secreted from the pituitary, thyroid, parathyroid, and adrenal glands.
- Differentiate among the hormones from the adenohypophysis and the neurohypophysis.
- Differentiate the actions and uses of the hormones from the pituitary, thyroid, parathyroid, and adrenal glands: thyroxine (T_4), triiodothyronine (T_3), calcitonin, parathyroid hormone (PTH), mineralocorticoids, and glucocorticoids.
- Differentiate the side effects of thyroxine (T_4) and triiodothyronine (T_3).
- Apply the nursing process, including patient teaching for drug therapy related to hormonal replacement or hormonal inhibition for the pituitary, thyroid, parathyroid, and adrenal glands.

OUTLINE

Pituitary Gland
Anterior Lobe
Posterior Lobe
Nursing Process: Patient-Centered Collaborative Care—Pituitary Hormones
Thyroid Gland
Hypothyroidism
Hyperthyroidism
Nursing Process: Patient-Centered Collaborative Care—Thyroid Hormone: Replacement and Antithyroid Drugs

Parathyroid Glands
Hypoparathyroidism
Hyperparathyroidism
Nursing Process: Patient-Centered Collaborative Care—Parathyroid Hormone Insufficiencies
Adrenal Glands
Glucocorticoids
Mineralocorticoids
Nursing Process: Patient-Centered Collaborative Care—Adrenal Hormone: Corticosteroids
Critical Thinking Case Study
NCLEX Study Questions

KEY TERMS

acromegaly, p. 670
Addison disease, p. 680
adenohypophysis, p. 670
adrenal glands, p. 680
adrenocorticotropic hormone (ACTH), p. 672
antidiuretic hormone (ADH), p. 673
corticosteroids, p. 670
cretinism, p. 675
Cushing syndrome, p. 680
diabetes insipidus (DI), p. 673
gigantism, p. 670
glucocorticoids, p. 681
Graves disease, p. 676
hyperthyroidism, p. 676

hypophysis, p. 670
hypothyroidism, p. 675
mineralocorticoids, p. 683
myxedema, p. 675
neurohypophysis, p. 673
parathyroid hormone (PTH), p. 678
prolactin (PRL), p. 673
syndrome of inappropriate antidiuretic hormone (SIADH), p. 673
thyroid-stimulating hormone (TSH), p. 670
thyrotoxicosis, p. 676
thyroxine (T_4), p. 675
triiodothyronine (T_3), p. 675

669

This chapter describes drugs used for hormonal replacement and for inhibition of hormonal secretion from the pituitary, thyroid, parathyroid, and adrenal glands. Before reading this chapter, review the introduction to Unit XV, which describes the locations of the endocrine glands and the hormones they secrete. Knowledge of the various endocrine glands and their respective hormones and functions facilitates an understanding of the drugs that act on the endocrine glands.

PITUITARY GLAND

Anterior Lobe

The pituitary gland, or hypophysis, has an anterior and a posterior lobe. The anterior pituitary gland, called the adenohypophysis, secretes hormones that target glands and tissues, including:

- Growth hormone (GH), which stimulates growth in tissue and bone
- Thyroid-stimulating hormone (TSH), which acts on the thyroid gland
- Adrenocorticotropic hormone (ACTH), which stimulates the adrenal gland
- Gonadotropins (follicle-stimulating hormone [FSH] and luteinizing hormone [LH]), which affect the ovaries and testes
- Prolactin (PRL), which primarily affects the breast tissues

Drugs with adenohypophyseal properties used to stimulate or inhibit glandular activity for GH, TSH, ACTH, and PRL are discussed according to their therapeutic use. The negative feedback system that controls the amount of hormonal secretion from the pituitary gland and the target gland is discussed in the introduction to Unit XV.

Growth Hormone

Two hypothalamic hormones regulate growth hormone: (1) GH-releasing hormone (GH-RH; somatropin) and (2) GH-inhibiting hormone (GH-IH; somatostatin). GH does not have a specific target gland. It affects body tissues and bone; GH replacement stimulates linear growth when there are GH deficiencies. Growth hormone drugs cannot be given orally because they are inactivated by gastrointestinal (GI) enzymes. Subcutaneous (subcut) or intramuscular (IM) administration of GH is necessary.

If a child's height is well below the standard for a specified age, GH deficiency may be the cause, and dwarfism can result. Because of the cost, tests are performed to determine whether GH replacement therapy is essential. Since GH acts on newly forming bone, it must be administered before the epiphyses are fused. Administration of GH over several years can increase height by a foot. However, prolonged GH therapy can antagonize insulin secretion, eventually causing diabetes mellitus. Athletes should be advised not to take GH to build muscle and physique because of its effects on blood glucose along with other serious side effects. Table 46.1 lists the drugs used to replace or inhibit GH and gives their dosages, uses, and considerations.

Drug Therapy: Growth Hormone Deficiency. Somatropin is a growth hormone used to treat growth failure in children because of GH deficiency. Somatropin is a product that has the identical amino acid sequence as human growth hormone (HGH); it is contraindicated in pediatric patients who have growth deficiency due to Prader-Willi syndrome and in those who are severely obese or who have severe respiratory impairment because fatalities associated with these risk factors can occur. Corticosteroids can inhibit the effects of somatropin, therefore they should not be taken concurrently. Somatropin can enhance the effects of antidiabetics and can cause hypoglycemia.

Side effects and adverse effects. Somatropin can cause paresthesia, arthralgia, myalgia, peripheral edema, weakness, and cephalgia. Metabolic complications include glucose fluctuations, hypothyroidism, and hematuria. Flulike symptoms and hyperpigmentation of the skin can also occur. Adverse reactions include seizures, intracranial hypertension, and secondary malignancy (e.g., leukemia).

Drug Therapy: Growth Hormone Excess. Gigantism, excessive growth during childhood, and acromegaly, excessive growth after puberty, can occur with GH hypersecretion; these are frequently caused by a pituitary tumor. If the tumor cannot be destroyed by radiation, GH receptor antagonists (e.g., pegvisomant), somatostatin analogues (e.g., lanreotide, octreotide), and dopamine agonists (e.g., bromocriptine) act by either blocking GH receptor sites or by inhibiting secretion of GH.

Pegvisomant blocks GH receptor sites, preventing abnormal growth by normalizing insulin-like growth factor 1 (IGF-1) level, and it is given by injection. Common side effects include hyperhidrosis, cephalgia, and fatigue. Adverse effects include chest pain, hypertension, and elevated hepatic transaminases.

Lanreotide is an analogue of somatostatin that has actions similar to those of endogenous somatostatin. The effects of reduced GH are dose related and have a duration of at least 28 days after a single injection, therefore injections are given every 4 weeks. Lanreotide is available in depot formulation and is administered deep in the subcutaneous layer. Common side effects include mild GI symptoms: diarrhea, abdominal pain, nausea, vomiting, constipation, weight loss, and flatulence.

Octreotide is a synthetic somatostatin-inhibiting secretion of GH. It is available in immediate-release and depot formulations. Immediate-release formulations are given by thrice-daily subcutaneous injection, and depot injection is administered once monthly. Common side effects include GI upsets such as nausea, bloating, and flatus. Adverse effects include cardiac toxicity, such as bradycardia and arrhythmia.

Bromocriptine, a dopamine agonist, inhibits the secretion of GH caused by pituitary adenomas. It is available in oral form and has fewer side effects than other treatments for hyperpituitarism, which include GI symptoms (e.g., nausea, anorexia, dyspepsia, and xerostomia). Adverse effects include cardiac toxicity (e.g., hypertension, myocardial infarction [MI], and angina) and cerebrovascular toxicity (e.g., stroke and seizure). Bromocriptine should be discontinued if hypertension occurs due to pregnancy (e.g., preeclampsia, eclampsia, or pregnancy-induced hypertension).

Thyroid-Stimulating Hormone

The adenohypophysis secretes thyroid-stimulating hormone (TSH) in response to thyroid-releasing hormone (TRH) from

TABLE 46.1 Drug Therapies for Pituitary Disorders

Generic	Route and Dosage	Uses and Considerations
ANTERIOR LOBE		
Growth Hormone (GH-RH)		
Somatropin	C: Subcut/IM: Dosing is based on brand names and is individualized for each patient; review the clinician's orders carefully.	For GH deficiency for adults and growth failure in children. Contraindicated in children with epiphyseal closure, patients with active neoplastic disease, and those with acute critical illness. Do not administer intravenously. Therapy is discontinued when final height is achieved if given for growth failure. Read clinician's orders carefully for the trade name; dosing is *not* interchangeable. Pregnancy category: B* or C*, depending on brand; PB: 20%; t½: 20-30 min
Growth Hormone Suppressant Drugs		
Bromocriptine mesylate	Acromegaly: A: PO: 1.25-2.5 mg/d at bedtime for 3 d; maint: 20-30 mg/d; *max:* 100 mg/d Prolactinemia/pituitary adenoma: A/C ≥16 y: PO: 1.25-2.5 mg/d; titrate dose at 2-7 d intervals as needed; *max:* 30 mg/d C 11-15 y: PO: 1.25-2.5 mg/d, may titrate to 10 mg/d	For acromegaly, pituitary adenoma, and hyperprolactinemia. Also used with pituitary radiation or surgery to decrease GH levels. Decreases lactation and prolactinemia. Pregnancy category: B*; PB: >90%; t½: 3 h
Lanreotide acetate	Acromegaly: A: Subcut: Initially 90 mg q4wk for 3 mo; then adjust dose based on GH, IGF-1, and clinical symptoms q4wk NET: A: Subcut: 120 mg q4wk	For acromegaly and NET. Pregnancy category: C*; PB: 79%-83%; t½: 23-30 d
Octreotide acetate	A: Subcut: 50-200 mcg tid A: IM: 20 mg q4wk for 3 mo, then adjust according to serum GH and IGF-1 levels	For acromegaly. Injectable depot suspension is for IM use only. Pregnancy category: B*; PB: 65%; t½: 1.7 h
Pegvisomant	A: Subcut: Give a 40-mg loading dose, then 10 mg/d; adjust in increments of 5 mg; *max:* 30 mg/d	For acromegaly. IGF-1 concentrations should be measured q4-6wk. Pregnancy category: B*; PB: UK; t½: 6 d
Thyroid-Stimulating Hormone (TSH)		
Thyrotropin	Thyroid cancer: A: IM: 0.9 mg into gluteus maximus, repeat in 24 h for 2 doses; *max:* 0.9 mg/d	For thyroid cancer. Radioiodine study follows last injection. Pregnancy category: C*; PB: UK; t½: 15-35 h
Adrenocorticotropic Hormone (ACTH)		
Corticotropin	Immunosuppressant: A/C: IM/subcut: 40-80 units q24-72h Infantile spasms: C <2 y: IM: 75 units/m² bid for 2 wk Do *not* discontinue abruptly; dose must be tapered. ACTH deficiency diagnosis: A/C: IM/subcut: Up to 80 units MS exacerbations: A: IM: 80-120 units/d in divided doses for 2-3 wk	For ACTH deficiency diagnostic, MS, and infantile spasms. Administer only to patients with adrenal responsiveness. Repository gel must be room temperature before administration. Do not overpressurize vial during withdrawal. Pregnancy category: C*; PB: UK; t½: 15 min
Cosyntropin	A/C >2 y: IM/IV: 0.25 mg over 2 min or slow infusion over 6 h C ≤2 y: IM/IV: 0.125 mg IM or slow infusion over 6 h Term neonates: IM/IV: 0.015 mg/kg	For diagnostic testing to differentiate between pituitary and adrenal cause of adrenal insufficiency. Obtain plasma cortisol level before and 30-60 min after administration. Pregnancy category: C*; PB: UK; t½: 7 min

Continued

TABLE 46.1	Drug Therapies for Pituitary Disorders—cont'd	
Generic	**Route and Dosage**	**Uses and Considerations**
POSTERIOR LOBE		
Antidiuretic Hormone (ADH)		
Desmopressin acetate	DI: A/C: PO: Initial dose 0.05 mg bid; then titrate to response. A: IN: Initial dose is 10 mcg in the evening, then titrate to response. C ≥3 mo: IN: Initial dose 5 mcg in the evening, then titrate to response. A/C ≥12 y: IV/subcut: 2-4 mcg/d given in 2 divided doses daily Hemophilia A or von Willebrand disease: A: IN: One spray in 1-2 nostrils based on weight for 1-2 doses. C ≥11 mo: One 150 mcg spray into 1 nostril; may repeat in 8-24 h A/C ≥ 3 mo: IV/subcut: 0.3 mcg/kg/dose, then titrate to response.	For DI, hemophilia A, and von Willebrand disease. Desmopressin can have a long duration of action (5-21 h). Pregnancy category: B*; PB: UK; t½: 1.5-2.5 h
Vasopressin	A: IM/subcut: 5-10 units q3-4h or 2-3 × daily PRN C: Reduce dose proportionally.	For central DI. Can also be given intranasally. Aspirate IM injections; avoid injection into a blood vessel. Pregnancy category: C*; PB: none; t½: 10-20 min
Demeclocycline	A: PO: 600-1200 mg/d in 3-4 divided doses	For off-label treatment of SIADH. Pregnancy category: C*; PB: 65%-90%; t½: 10-17 h, increases to 42-68 h in patients with severe renal impairment
Conivaptan	A: IV: LD 20 mg over 30 min; *maint:* 20 mg continuous IV over 24 h; then 20 mg/d for 1-3 d; may titrate up to 40 mg/d; *max:* 4 d of therapy	For symptomatic euvolemic hyponatremia associated with SIADH Pregnancy category: C*; PB: 99%; t½: 5-8 h
Tolvaptan	A: PO: Initially 15 mg/d, then 15-30 mg/d; *max:* 60 mg/d for up to 30 d; adjust dose in 24-h increment.	For symptomatic hypervolemic or euvolemic hyponatremia. Avoid fluid restriction during the first 24 h of therapy. Pregnancy category: C*; PB: 99%; t½: 12 h

*Pregnancy categories have been revised. See http://www.fda.gov/Drugs/DevelopmentApprovalProcess/DevelopmentResources/Labeling/ucm093 307.htm for more information.

A, Adult; *bid*, twice daily; *C*, child; *d*, day; *DI*, diabetes insipidus; *GH*, growth hormone; *h*, hour; *IGF*, insulin-like growth factor; *IN*, intranasal; *h*, hour; *IM*, intramuscular; *IN*, intranasal; *IV*, intravenous; *LD*, loading dose; *maint*, maintenance; *max*, maximum dosage; *min*, minute; *mo*, month; *MS*, multiple sclerosis; *NET*, neuroendocrine tumor; *q*, every; *PB*, protein binding; *PO*, by mouth; *PRN*, as needed; *SIADH*, syndrome of inappropriate diuretic hormone; *subcut*, subcutaneous; *t½*, half-life; *tid*, three times daily; *UK*, unknown; *wk*, week; *y*, year; *>*, greater than; *<*, less than; *≥*, greater than or equal to; *≤*, less than or equal to.

the hypothalamus. TSH stimulates the thyroid gland to release thyroxine (T_4) and triiodothyronine (T_3, or liothyronine). Excess TSH secretion can cause hyperthyroidism, and a TSH deficit can cause hypothyroidism. Hypothyroidism may be caused by a thyroid gland disorder (primary cause) or a decrease in TSH secretion (secondary cause). Thyrotropin, a purified extract of TSH for thyroid cancer, is used as a diagnostic agent to differentiate between primary and secondary hypothyroidism. Side effects caused by thyrotropin include symptoms of hyperthyroidism. Other side effects include urticaria, rash, pruritus, and flushing.

Table 46.1 lists the drug used to replace TSH and its dosages, uses, and considerations.

Adrenocorticotropic Hormone

The hypothalamus releases corticotropin-releasing factor (CRF), which stimulates the pituitary corticotrophs to secrete **adrenocorticotropic hormone (ACTH)**, which stimulates the release of glucocorticoids (cortisol), mineralocorticoids (aldosterone), and androgen from the adrenal cortex and catecholamines (epinephrine and norepinephrine) from the adrenal medulla. Usually, ACTH and cortisol secretions follow a diurnal rhythm, in which the ACTH and cortisol secretion is higher in the early morning and then decreases throughout the day. Stresses such as surgery, sepsis, and trauma override the diurnal rhythm, causing an increase in secretions of ACTH and cortisol. Hypocortisolism,

or adrenal insufficiency, can occur and may be due to inadequate secretion of ACTH or dysfunction of the adrenal glands. Cosyntropin (synthetic ACTH) or corticotropin (exogenous ACTH) is administered to establish the endocrine gland responsible for the inadequate serum cortisol. Table 46.1 lists the drugs used to replace ACTH and their dosages, uses, and considerations.

Cosyntropin, a synthetic ACTH, is only approved for diagnostic purposes and is less potent and less allergenic than corticotropin. Cosyntropin stimulates the production and release of cortisol, corticosterone, and androgens from the adrenal cortex. It is administered via IM or intravenous (IV) routes. Plasma cortisol concentrations should be measured just before (basal) and 30 to 60 minutes after administration; normal response is the doubling of the basal cortisol level. Caution is advised when administering cosyntropin in patients receiving diuretics; cosyntropin can increase electrolyte loss. Patients taking estrogens can have an abnormal decreased response to the ACTH stimulation test. Side effects and adverse effects include bradycardia, hypertension, sinus tachycardia, and peripheral edema.

The ACTH drug corticotropin is primarily used to diagnose adrenal gland disorders, treat multiple sclerosis (MS), and treat infantile spasms; it is rarely used for corticosteroid-responsive disorders. Corticotropin is available as repository corticotropin injection (RCI), which is administered via IM or subcut routes. RCI controls the synthesis of ACTH from cholesterol, which stimulates adrenal glands in releasing its

TABLE 46.2	Physiologic Data: Adrenal Hyposecretion and Hypersecretion	
Body System	**Adrenal Hyposecretion (Addison Disease)**	**Adrenal Hypersecretion (Cushing Syndrome)**
Metabolism: Glucose Protein Fat	Hypoglycemia, muscle weakness, weight loss	Hyperglycemia, muscle wasting; thinning of skin; poor wound healing; osteoporosis; fat accumulation in face (moon face), back of neck (buffalo hump), and trunk (protruding abdomen); hyperlipidemia; high cholesterol, weight gain
Central nervous system	Apathy, depression, fatigue, irritability	Increased neural activity, mood elevation, irritability, seizures, weakness, fatigue
Integument	Hyperpigmentation	Easy bruising, striae, plethora, and excess hair growth to face (hirsutism), neck, chest, abdomen, and thighs
Eyes	None	Cataract formation
Cardiovascular	Tachycardia, hypotension, orthostatic hypotension, cardiovascular collapse, syncope, dizziness	Hypertension, edema, heart failure
Gastrointestinal	Nausea, vomiting, diarrhea, abdominal pain, anorexia	Peptic ulcers
Hematology	Anemia	Increased red blood cell count and neutrophils, impaired clotting
Reproductive	Irregular menses or amenorrhea	Amenorrhea, decreased fertility and libido
Fluids and electrolytes	Hypovolemia, hyponatremia, hyperkalemia	Hypervolemia, hypernatremia, hypokalemia

hormones. The effects of RCI are primarily due to the glucocorticoid from the adrenal cortex. RCI decreases the symptoms of MS during its exacerbation phase. ⚡ The drug should be tapered over a 2-week period for infantile spasms to avoid adrenal insufficiency. Corticotropin has numerous drug interactions. Diuretics and anti-*Pseudomonas* penicillins, such as piperacillin, can decrease the serum potassium level (hypokalemia). If the patient is taking a digitalis preparation and hypokalemia is present, digitalis toxicity can result. Phenytoin, rifampin, and barbiturates increase the metabolic rate, which can decrease the effect of the ACTH drug. Persons with diabetes may need increased insulin and oral antidiabetic (hypoglycemic) drugs because ACTH stimulates cortisol secretion, which increases the blood glucose level.

Side effects and adverse effects. Side effects and adverse reactions are due to the activity of the adrenal glands and their hormones. See Table 46.2 for the physiologic data for hypoadrenalism and hyperadrenalism.

Prolactin

The primary function of prolactin (PRL) is stimulation of breast tissue for milk production. PRL deficiency (*hypoprolactinemia*) is generally without symptoms except during breastfeeding, when it can cause lactation disruption. Excess PRL (*hyperprolactinemia*) produces symptoms in both males and females. Males may develop excess breast tissue (*gynecomastia*) and may lactate (*galactorrhea*), and excess PRL decreases sperm production. Females with excess PRL can experience lactation that is not pregnancy related, or they can develop amenorrhea. Excess PRL can be treated with dopamine agonists (e.g., bromocriptine, cabergoline). Cabergoline is better tolerated, has a longer half-life, and offers more convenient dosing than bromocriptine. Dopamine agonists are discussed in Chapter 20.

Posterior Lobe

The posterior pituitary gland, known as the neurohypophysis, secretes antidiuretic hormone (ADH) and oxytocin. ADH and oxytocin are produced by the hypothalamus and travel by way of the hypophysial portal system into the posterior pituitary gland for storage and secretion. (Oxytocin is discussed in Unit XVII.) Table 46.1 lists the drugs used to replace or inhibit ADH and their dosages, uses, and considerations.

ADH promotes water reabsorption from the renal tubules to maintain water balance in the body fluids. When there is a deficiency of ADH, large amounts of water are excreted by the kidneys. This condition, called diabetes insipidus (DI), can lead to severe fluid volume deficit and electrolyte imbalances. Head injury and brain tumors resulting in trauma to the hypothalamus and pituitary gland can also cause DI. Fluid and electrolyte balance must be closely monitored in these patients, and ADH replacement may be needed. The ADH preparations, vasopressin and desmopressin acetate, can be administered intranasally or by injection. Desmopressin is also used in managing patients with bleeding disorders due to hemophilia A or von Willebrand disease type 1. Unlike vasopressin, desmopressin does not induce the release of ACTH, nor does it increase serum cortisol level. It is available as a nasal spray, oral tablet, and in parenteral formulations. ADH is contraindicated in patients with moderate to severe renal disease and in patients with hyponatremia or a history of such. Side effects and adverse reactions include hyponatremia, cephalgia, dyspepsia, diarrhea, nausea, and vomiting. Seizures may occur due to hyponatremia. Hypotension and tachycardia can occur due to hypovolemia.

When secretion of ADH from the posterior pituitary gland is excessive, the most common cause is small cell carcinoma of the lung. Medications, other malignancies, and stressors (e.g., pain, infection, anxiety, trauma) may also be causative factors. These conditions lead to an excessive amount of water retention expanding the intracellular and intravascular volume known as syndrome of inappropriate antidiuretic hormone (SIADH). This increased fluid volume causes enhanced glomerular filtration and decreased tubular sodium reabsorption. Natriuresis, excretion of urinary sodium, can occur and can cause hyponatremia. SIADH can be treated by fluid restrictions, by hypertonic saline, or by drugs such as demeclocycline, conivaptan, and tolvaptan.

Demeclocycline is a tetracycline antibiotic that can induce nephrogenic DI within 5 days of starting treatment that is reversed in 2 to 6 days following cessation of treatment. The most common complaint with demeclocycline is photosensitivity. As with other tetracyclines, dental discoloration and enamel hypoplasia can occur. Fluid and electrolytes must be monitored closely.

Vaptans (e.g., conivaptan and tolvaptan) are vasopressin receptor antagonists and are indicated for the treatment of euvolemic hyponatremia in SIADH. Its effects increase serum sodium and free water clearance. ❶ Conivaptan is contraindicated in patients with corn allergy. Common complications with conivaptan therapy are injection site reactions such as phlebitis, pain, edema, and pruritus; therefore the drug must be administered only in large veins, and infusion sites should be rotated every 24 hours. Other common side effects and adverse reactions include orthostatic hypotension, syncope, hypertension, atrial fibrillation, and electrolyte imbalances.

Tolvaptan is given orally. It has black-box warnings for patients with alcoholism, hepatic disease, and malnutrition; tolvaptan should be avoided in these patients. Common side effects and adverse reactions are related to loss of fluids (e.g., thirst, dry mouth, constipation, hyperglycemia, dizziness, and weakness). Fluid and serum electrolytes must be closely monitored.

Vaptans are contraindicated in patients with hypovolemia. Fluid restrictions should be avoided during therapy to prevent too rapid an increase in serum sodium.

Table 46.1 lists the drugs used for pituitary disorders and their dosages, uses, and considerations.

 NURSING PROCESS
Patient-Centered Collaborative Care

Pituitary Hormones

Assessment
- Obtain baseline vital signs for future comparison. Report abnormal results.
- Assess fluid, hydration, and electrolyte statuses. Report abnormal findings.
- Assess patient for an infectious process. Corticotropin can suppress signs and symptoms of infection.
- Note the patient's physical growth. If a child, compare growth with reported standards. Report findings.

Nursing Diagnoses
- Health Maintenance, Ineffective related to lack of ability to maintain drug regimen
- Growth and Development, Delayed related to deficient stimulation of growth hormone
- Knowledge, Deficient related to inexperience with the medication regimen

Planning
- The patient will be free from any pituitary disorder with the appropriate drug regimen.

Nursing Interventions
Antidiuretic Hormone (ADH)
- Monitor vital signs. Increased heart rate and decreased systolic pressure can indicate fluid volume loss resulting from decreased ADH production. With less ADH secretion, more water is excreted, decreasing vascular fluid (hypovolemia).
- Record urinary output. Increased output can indicate fluid loss caused by a decrease in ADH.
- Obtain daily weight. A liter of fluid weighs approximately 2.2 pounds.

Growth Hormone (GH)
- Monitor blood glucose and electrolyte levels in patients receiving GH. Hyperglycemia can occur with high doses.

Repository Corticotropin
- Monitor the growth and development of a child receiving corticotropin.
- Observe the patient's weight. Check for edema if weight gain occurs. A side effect of repository corticotropin is sodium and water retention.
- Watch carefully for adverse effects when corticotropin is discontinued. Dose should be tapered and not stopped abruptly because adrenal hypofunction may result.
- Check laboratory findings, especially electrolyte levels and glucose. Electrolyte replacement may be necessary, and corticotropin can increase blood glucose.
- Observe for any signs of infection. Corticotropin is an antiinflammatory and can suppress the immune function, increasing the risk for infection.

Patient Teaching
Growth Hormone (GH)
- Advise athletes not to take GH because of side effects. GH can be effective for children whose height is markedly below the expected norm for their age. Because GH acts on newly forming bone, administer before the epiphyses are fused.
- Inform patients with diabetes to closely monitor blood glucose levels. Insulin regulation may be necessary.
- Suggest that the patient or family monitor the patient's growth rate.
- Individuals in some cultural groups may misunderstand the purpose and use of GH. The health care provider must emphasize that these are *not* drugs for building muscles and that they can cause many serious side effects, such as diabetes mellitus, when abused.

Corticotropin
- Advise patients to adhere to the drug regimen. Discontinuation of certain drugs, such as corticotropin, can cause hypofunction of the gland being stimulated.
- Direct patients to decrease salt intake to decrease or avoid edema. Potassium supplementation may be needed.
- Teach patients to report side effects such as muscle weakness, edema, petechiae, ecchymosis, decrease in growth, decreased wound healing, and menstrual irregularities.

Evaluation
- Evaluate effectiveness of drug therapy.

THYROID GLAND

The thyroid gland is an important regulator for many of the bodily functions. The three hormones produced and secreted by the thyroid gland are triiodothyronine (T_3), thyroxine (T_4) that helps with metabolism, and to a lesser extent calcitonin for regulating serum calcium. A majority of thyroid hormone is synthesized as T_4, which is then converted to T_3 to act on target cells. Iodide, an inorganic form of iodine, is needed for the synthesis of T_3 and T_4. These are carried in the blood by thyroxine-binding globulin (TBG) and albumin, which protect the hormones from being degraded. T_3 is more potent than T_4, and only unbound (free) T_3 and T_4 have biologic actions and produce a hormonal response.

Negative feedback mechanisms regulate hormone secretion from the thyroid gland. The hypothalamus releases thyrotropin-releasing hormone (TRH), which stimulates the release of TSH from the pituitary gland. TSH stimulates the synthesis and release of T_3 and T_4 from the thyroid gland. Excess free T_3 and T_4 inhibit the hypothalamus-pituitary-thyroid (HPT) axis, which results in decreased TRH and TSH secretion. Too low of an amount of T_3 and T_4 increases the function of the HPT axis.

For thyroid deficiency (hypothyroidism), synthetic thyroid hormones may be prescribed either alone or in combination. When the thyroid gland secretes an overabundance of thyroid hormone (hyperthyroidism), antithyroid drugs are usually indicated.

Hypothyroidism

Hypothyroidism, a decrease in thyroid hormone secretion, can have a primary cause (thyroid gland disorder); a secondary cause (lack of TSH secretion [pituitary disorder]); or a tertiary cause (lack of TRH [hypothalamus disorder]). Primary hypothyroidism occurs more frequently. Decreased T_4 and elevated TSH levels indicate primary hypothyroidism; the causes of which are acute or chronic inflammation of the thyroid gland, radioiodine therapy, excess intake of antithyroid drugs, or surgical removal of the thyroid gland. Myxedema is severe hypothyroidism in the adult; symptoms include lethargy; apathy; memory impairment; emotional changes; slow speech; a deep, coarse voice; edema of the eyelids and face; dry skin; cold intolerance; slow pulse; constipation; weight gain; and abnormal menses. In children, hypothyroidism can have a congenital onset that can cause delayed physical and mental growth (cretinism) or onset may be prepubertal (juvenile hypothyroidism). Drugs that contain T_3 and T_4, alone or in combination, are used to treat hypothyroidism. ⚡ Exogenous thyroid hormones are contraindicated in patients with thyrotoxicosis, acute myocardial infarction (AMI), and adrenal insufficiency. Because thyroid hormones are catabolized by the hepatic system, drugs with hepatic enzyme–inducing properties (e.g., carbamazepine, hydantoins, rifabutin) should be used with caution. Elevated serum calcium levels could also be related to hypothyroidism; exogenous calcitonin may also be prescribed.

Thyroid Drugs

Levothyroxine sodium is the drug of choice for replacement therapy for the treatment of primary hypothyroidism. It increases the levels of T_4 and metabolically is deiodinated to T_3. Levothyroxine is also used to treat simple goiter and chronic lymphocytic (Hashimoto) thyroiditis. Prototype Drug Chart 46.1 lists the pharmacologic data for levothyroxine sodium.

📄 PROTOTYPE DRUG CHART 46.1

Levothyroxine Sodium

Drug Class	Dosage
Thyroid hormone Pregnancy category: A*	Primary hypothyroidism, with/without goiter, in otherwise healthy persons: A: PO: Initially 25-50 mcg/d; maint: 50-200 mcg/d; increase in increments of 12.5-25 mcg at 6- to 8-wk intervals. C >12 y: PO: 1.7-3 mcg/kg/d; dose dependent on pubescent stage. C ≤12 y: Younger children require higher dosages. Other dosing is also available.

Contraindications	Drug-Lab-Food Interactions
Absolute contraindications: Thyrotoxicosis and myocardial infarction *Caution:* Adrenal insufficiency; cardiovascular disease, including cardiac arrhythmias, hypertension, and angina pectoris; diabetes mellitus; osteoporosis; hypopituitarism; dysphagia	Drug: Many drug-drug interactions exist and may alter the therapeutic effects of thyroid hormone replacement. Increased cardiac insufficiency occurs when levothyroxine is taken with sympathomimetics (e.g., epinephrine); levothyroxine increases the effects of anticoagulants, TCAs, vasopressors, decongestants, corticosteroids; decreases effects of antidiabetics (oral and insulin), digitalis products, beta blockers; decreased absorption of levothyroxine occurs with estrogens, antacids, cholestyramine, colestipol, sucralfate, and simethicone. Ketamines can worsen hypertension and tachycardia. Hepatic inducers (e.g., carbamazepine, barbiturates, hydantoins) increase the metabolism of thyroid hormones. Food: Drug should be taken on an empty stomach at least 30-60 min before breakfast. Tablets may be crushed and mixed in a small amount (5-10 mL) of water; use immediately after mixing. Do not mix with enteral or soy-based feedings. Certain food and beverages inhibit the absorption of thyroid hormones. Herb: Celery seed may reduce thyroid hormones.

Pharmacokinetics	Pharmacodynamics
Absorption: PO: 40%-80% Distribution: PB: 99% Metabolism: t½: 3-10 d depending on initial thyroid state Excretion: Urine (80%) and feces (20%)	PO: Onset: 3-5 d; IV: 6-8 h Peak: 24 h (IV) to several weeks (PO) Duration: Several weeks

Continued

PROTOTYPE DRUG CHART 46.1
Levothyroxine Sodium—cont'd

Therapeutic Effects/Uses

To treat hypothyroidism, myxedema, goiter, and thyroid cancer

Mode of Action: Increases metabolic rate, oxygen consumption, utilization and mobilization of glycogen stores; promotes gluconeogenesis and body growth; stimulates protein synthesis

Side Effects	Adverse Reactions
Nausea, vomiting, anorexia, diarrhea, cramps, tremors, nervousness, irritability, insomnia, headache, weight loss, diaphoresis, and amenorrhea; usually due to undermedication or overmedication	Tachycardia, hypertension, palpitations, osteoporosis, and seizures; usually due to overmedication. Other adverse reactions include urticaria, rash, and alopecia. *Life threatening:* Thyroid crisis, angina pectoris, cardiac dysrhythmias (atrial fibrillation), cardiovascular collapse

*Pregnancy categories have been revised. See http://www.fda.gov/Drugs/DevelopmentApprovalProcess/DevelopmentResources/Labeling/ucm093307.htm for more information.
A, Adult; *C,* child; *d,* day; *h,* hour; *IV,* intravenous; *maint,* maintenance; *min,* minutes; *PB,* protein binding; *PO,* by mouth; *t½,* half-life; *TCA,* tricyclic antidepressant; *wk,* week; *y,* year; >, greater than; ≤, less than or equal to.

Liothyronine is a synthetic T_3 with a biologic half-life of 2.5 days with rapid onset of action (within a few hours). Liothyronine is indicated for use as replacement or supplemental treatment for hypothyroidism of any etiology. Unlike levothyroxine, liothyronine does not need to be deiodinated, which increases the availability for use by the body tissues. Liothyronine is better absorbed from the GI tract (over 95%) than levothyroxine, and because of its rapid onset of action and short half-life, it is frequently used as initial therapy for treating myxedema. Liothyronine is available for oral or IV administration.

Desiccated thyroid is a naturally occurring thyroid hormone from porcine thyroid glands. It contains both levothyroxine and liothyronine. Desiccated thyroid is used to treat hypothyroidism due to thyroid atrophy, thyroid hormone deficiency, and goiter.

Liotrix is a mixture of levothyroxine sodium and liothyronine sodium in a 4-to-1 ratio by weight, respectively. For treating hypothyroidism, there is no significant advantage to using liotrix over levothyroxine sodium alone, because levothyroxine converts T_4 to T_3 in the peripheral tissues.

Table 46.3 lists the natural and synthetic thyroid preparations and their dosages, uses, and considerations.

Hyperthyroidism

Hyperthyroidism is an increase in circulating T_3 and T_4 levels, which usually results from an overactive thyroid gland or excessive output of thyroid hormones from one or more thyroid nodules. Hyperthyroidism may be mild, with few symptoms, or it may be severe, as in thyroid storm, in which death may occur from vascular collapse. **Graves disease,** or **thyrotoxicosis,** is the most common type of hyperthyroidism caused by hyperfunction of the thyroid gland. It is characterized by a rapid pulse (*tachycardia*), palpitations, excessive perspiration (*hyperhidrosis*), heat intolerance, nervousness, irritability, bulging eyes (*exophthalmos*), and weight loss.

Hyperthyroidism can be treated by surgical removal of a portion of the thyroid gland (subtotal thyroidectomy), radioactive iodine therapy, or antithyroid drugs, which inhibit either synthesis or release of thyroid hormone. Any of these treatments can cause hypothyroidism. By blocking beta receptors, propranolol can control cardiac symptoms that result from hyperthyroidism, such as palpitations and tachycardia.

Antithyroid Drugs

The purpose of antithyroid drugs is to reduce the excessive secretion of thyroid hormones by inhibiting thyroid secretion. The use of surgery (subtotal thyroidectomy) and radioiodine therapy frequently leads to permanent hypothyroidism; these patients will need to be on thyroid replacement therapy. Thiourea derivatives (thioamides) are the drugs of choice used to decrease thyroid hormone production. This drug group interferes with synthesis of thyroid hormone. Thiourea derivatives do *not* destroy thyroid tissue, rather they block thyroid action.

Propylthiouracil (PTU) and methimazole are effective thioamide antithyroid drugs. They are used to control overactive thyroid due to Graves disease, toxic nodular goiter, or multinodular goiter; they are also used prior to radioiodine treatment or thyroid surgery. Methimazole does not inhibit peripheral conversion of T_4 to T_3 as does PTU; however, it is 10 times more potent, and it has a longer half-life than PTU and the euthyroid state is achieved in 2 to 4 months. It is the preferred antithyroid because of the less severe side effects. Methimazole is rapidly absorbed from the GI tract. Prolonged use of thioamides may cause goiter because of increased TSH secretion and inhibited T_4 and T_3 synthesis. Minimal doses of thioamides should be given when indicated to avoid goiter formation.

Strong iodide preparations such as potassium iodide have been used to suppress thyroid function for patients who are undergoing subtotal thyroidectomy because of Graves disease. Table 46.3 lists the antithyroid drugs used to treat hyperthyroidism along with their dosages, uses, and considerations.

Drug Interactions

Antithyroid drugs interact with many other drugs. When used with oral anticoagulants (e.g., warfarin), they can cause an increase in the anticoagulation effect. In addition, thyroid drugs decrease the effect of insulin and oral antidiabetics; digoxin and lithium increase the action of thyroid drugs; and phenytoin increases serum T_3 level.

TABLE 46.3 Drug Therapies for Thyroid Disorders

Generic	Route and Dosage	Uses and Considerations
THYROID REPLACEMENTS: HYPOTHYROIDISM		
Desiccated thyroid	A: PO: Initially, 15-30 mg/d; maint: 60-120 mg/d; can increase 15 mg/d q2-3wk C/Adol: Initially, 15-30 mg/d; maint: 1.2-6 mg/kg depending on age	For hypothyroidism and goiter Pregnancy category: A*; PB: >99%; t½: T_3, 2 d; T_4, 6-7 d
Levothyroxine sodium	See Prototype Drug Chart 46.1.	
Liothyronine sodium	A: PO: Initially, 5-100 mcg/d; maint: 25-100 mcg/d C: PO: Initially, 5 mcg/d; increase in 5 mcg increments q3-4d; maint: up to 50 mcg/d; maint: >3 y: 25-100 mcg/d Myxedema coma: A: IV: Initially, 25-50 mcg; subsequent doses based on clinical condition q4-12h to avoid hormone fluctuations	For hypothyroidism, myxedema, thyroiditis, hyperthyroidism diagnosis, cretinism, and goiter. Must be administered with glucocorticoid when treating myxedema coma with IV liothyronine. Pregnancy category: A*; PB: 99%; t½: 2.5 d
Liotrix	A/C ≥6 y: PO: 25-100 mcg T_4/12.5-25 mcg T_3/d C <6 y: PO: 12.5-50 mcg T_4/3.1-12.5 mcg T_3 daily Dosages must be individualized based on clinical response, age, and thyroid levels.	For hypothyroidism, goiter, and hyperthyroidism diagnosis. T_4T_3 drug. Pregnancy category: A*; PB: 99%; t½: T_3, 2.5 d; T_4, 3-10 d
ANTITHYROID DRUGS: HYPERTHYROIDISM		
Thioamides Methimazole	A: PO: 15-60 mg/d in 1-3 divided doses C: PO: 0.2-1 mg/kg/d in 1-3 divided doses	For hyperthyroidism, Graves disease, thyrotoxicosis. Inhibits thyroid hormone synthesis. Dosages greater than 40 mg/d may increase risk of agranulocytosis. Pregnancy category: D*; PB: 0%; t½: 5-9 h
Propylthiouracil	A: PO: 300-900 mg/d divided q8h; then 100-150 mg/d divided q8h C ≥6 y: PO: 50-150 mg/d divided every 8 h; titrate according to clinical response and lab levels	For patients with hyperthyroidism or Graves disease who are intolerant of methimazole and are unable to receive surgery or radioiodine therapy; inhibits conversion of T_4 and T_3 Pregnancy category: D*; PB: 60%-80%; t½: 1 h
IODINE		
Potassium iodide	A/C: PO: 250 mg three times daily for 10-14 d before surgery Dilute drug and administer after meals; sip through a straw to avoid discoloration of teeth.	For hyperthyroidism and thyrotoxicosis to suppress thyroid function prior to surgery. Maximum effect is achieved after 10-15 d. Drug is absorbed from the GI tract as iodinated amino acids and is excreted renally. Pregnancy category: D*; PB: UK; t½: UK

*Pregnancy categories have been revised. See http://www.fda.gov/Drugs/DevelopmentApprovalProcess/DevelopmentResources/Labeling/ucm093 307.htm for more information.

A, Adult; *Adol*, adolescent; *C*, child; *d*, day; *GI*, gastrointestinal; *h*, hour; *IV*, intravenous; *maint*, maintenance; *PB*, protein binding; *PO*, by mouth; *q*, every; *t½*, half-life; *T₄*, thyroxine; *T₃*, triiodothyronine; *UK*, unknown; *wk*, week; *y*, year; >, greater than; <, less than; ≥, greater than or equal to.

◎ NURSING PROCESS
Patient-Centered Collaborative Care

Thyroid Hormone: Replacement and Antithyroid Drugs

Assessment
- Determine baseline vital signs, including weight changes, for future comparisons. Report abnormal results.
- Check serum T_3, T_4, and TSH levels. Report abnormal results.
- Obtain a history of drugs and herbal products the patient is taking.
- ⚡ Assess for signs and symptoms of thyroid crisis (thyroid storm), including tachycardia, cardiac dysrhythmias, fever, heart failure, flushed skin, apathy, confusion, behavioral changes, and later, hypotension and vascular collapse.

Thyroid crisis can result from a thyroidectomy (excess thyroid hormones released), abrupt withdrawal of antithyroid drug, excess ingestion of thyroid hormone, or failure to give antithyroid medication before thyroid surgery.

Nursing Diagnoses
- Activity Intolerance related to imbalanced thyroid hormone
- Health Maintenance, Ineffective related to inability to maintain drug regimen
- Tissue Perfusion, Ineffective Peripheral related to deficient thyroid hormone

Planning
- Activity level will be improved within 1 to 4 weeks of thyroid treatments.

- The signs and symptoms of hypothyroidism will be alleviated within 2 to 4 weeks with prescribed thyroid drug replacement, and the patient will not experience side effects.
- The signs and symptoms of hyperthyroidism will be alleviated in 1 to 3 weeks with prescribed antithyroid drug.

Nursing Interventions
- Record vital signs. With *hypothyroidism,* temperature, heart rate, and blood pressure usually decrease. With *hyperthyroidism,* tachycardia and palpitations usually occur.
- Monitor the patient's weight. Weight gain commonly occurs in patients with hypothyroidism.
- Obtain a pregnancy test, complete blood count (CBC), complete metabolic panel (CMP), liver function test (LFT), and electrocardiograph (ECG).
- Report periodic TSH, T_3, and T_4.

Patient Teaching
- Encourage patients to take drug at the same time each day in relation to meals.
- Teach patients to check warnings on over-the-counter (OTC) drug labels. Avoid OTC drugs that caution against use by persons with heart or thyroid disease.
- Direct patients to report symptoms of hyperthyroidism (tachycardia, chest pain, palpitations, excess sweating) caused by drug accumulation or overdosing.
- Suggest that patients carry a medical alert identification card, tag, or bracelet that shows the health condition and the drug used to treat it.
- Instruct patients that certain foods can interfere with the absorption of thyroid hormones (e.g., soy products [estrogen], cruciferous vegetables [broccoli and cabbage], iodized salt, shellfish [iodine], and coffee).
- Instruct patients to take drugs as instructed; abrupt changes may lead to increased thyroid dysfunction.
- Demonstrate to patients how to take that pulse rate. Instruct patients to monitor pulse rate and to report increases or marked decreases in the rate.
- Teach patients the side effects of antithyroid drugs: skin rash, hives, nausea, alopecia, loss of hair pigment, petechiae or ecchymoses, and weakness.
- Advise patients to contact their health care provider if sore throat and fever occur while taking antithyroid drugs. A serious adverse reaction of antithyroid drugs is agranulocytosis (loss of white blood cells). CBC should be monitored for leukopenia.
- Recognize that members of various cultural groups may need guidance in understanding the disease processes of hypothyroidism or hyperthyroidism. Support patients and family members who may lack knowledge of prescribed drug therapy for management of thyroid conditions. Additional time in explanations and a written plan of care in the native language may be necessary for non–English-speaking persons.

Evaluation
- Evaluate both effectiveness of the treatment and drug compliance.
- Continue monitoring for side effects from drug accumulation or overdosing.
- Evaluate the patient's knowledge of the medication regimen.

PARATHYROID GLANDS

The parathyroid glands secrete parathyroid hormone (PTH), or parathormone, which regulates serum calcium levels in a number of ways:
- It enhances the release of calcium from the bones.
- It enhances calcium reabsorption in the renal tubules.
- It enhances calcium absorption in the intestines by increasing the production of activated vitamin D.

A decrease (negative feedback) in serum calcium stimulates the release of PTH. Calcitonin, one of three thyroid hormones, decreases serum calcium levels by promoting osteoclast activity in bones and calcium excretion by the kidneys and intestines.

For PTH deficiency, PTH analogues are used. Surgical removal (parathyroidectomy) is a common treatment for hyperparathyroidism. Calcimimetic drugs, which mimic calcium in the blood, prevent the parathyroid gland from releasing PTH.

Hypoparathyroidism

Damage to the parathyroid glands is a common cause of hypoparathyroidism. Hypomagnesemia (low serum magnesium) can also cause PTH deficiency. Other causes of hypocalcemia (serum calcium deficit) include vitamin D deficiency, renal impairment, or diuretic therapy; PTH replacement helps correct the calcium deficit. The action of PTH is to promote calcium absorption from the GI tract, promote reabsorption of calcium from the renal tubules, and activate vitamin D. Table 46.4 lists the drugs used to treat hypoparathyroidism and hyperparathyroidism and their dosages, uses, and considerations.

Calcitriol

Calcitriol is a vitamin D analogue that promotes calcium absorption from the GI tract and promotes secretion of calcium from bone to the bloodstream. Prototype Drug Chart 46.2 lists the pharmacologic data for calcitriol.

Hyperparathyroidism

Hyperparathyroidism can be caused by malignancies of the parathyroid glands or ectopic PTH hormone secretion from lung cancer, hyperthyroidism, or prolonged immobility, during which calcium is lost from bone. Partial or full parathyroidectomy is the most common treatment for primary hyperparathyroidism. Calcitonin-salmon, calcimimetics, and bisphosphonates are used to treat patients affected by hyperparathyroidism.

Calcitonin-salmon prevents bone loss and fractures, increases bone density, and alleviates pain due to fractures and bone metastasis. Calcitonin is not as effective as other drugs for hyperparathyroidism. Calcitonin is contraindicated in patients

TABLE 46.4   Drug Therapies for Parathyroid Disorders

Generic	Route and Dosage	Uses and Considerations
HYPOPARATHYROIDISM AND HYPOCALCEMIA: VITAMIN D ANALOGUES		
Calcitriol	See Prototype Drug Chart 46.2.	
Ergocalciferol	Hypoparathyroidism: A/C: PO: 1250-5000 mcg/d with calcium supplements	Prohormone for hypoparathyroidism. Enhances calcium and phosphorus absorption. Long duration of action. Pregnancy category: C*; PB: UK; t½: UK
HYPERPARATHYROIDISM AND HYPERCALCEMIA		
Calcitonin-salmon	Hypercalcemia: A: IM/subcut: 4 IU/kg q12h, can increase to 8 IU/kg q12h; *max:* 8 IU/kg q6h Paget disease: A: IM/subcut: 50-100 IU/1-3 × wk	For hypercalcemia and Paget disease of bone (osteitis deformans). Calcitonin decreases serum calcium by binding at receptor sites on osteoclast. Pregnancy category: C*; PB: UK; t½: 1 h
Cinacalcet	A: PO: Initially 30 mg bid; titrate in 30 mg increments q2-4wk; *max:* 360 mg/d	For hyperparathyroidism and hypercalcemia. Check serum calcium 1 wk after initiating treatment and 2 months thereafter. Administer with food. Pregnancy category: C*; PB: 93%-97%; t½: 30-40 h

*Pregnancy categories have been revised. See http://www.fda.gov/Drugs/DevelopmentApprovalProcess/DevelopmentResources/Labeling/ucm093 307.htm for more information.

A, Adult; *bid*, twice daily; *C*, child; *d*, day; *h*, hour; *IM*, intramuscular; *IU*, international units; *max*, maximum; *PB*, protein binding; *PO*, by mouth; *q*, every; *subcut*, subcutaneous; *t½*, half-life; *UK*, unknown; *wk*, week.

PROTOTYPE DRUG CHART 46.2

Calcitriol

Drug Class	**Dosage**
Vitamin D analogue Pregnancy category: C*	A/C ≥3 y: PO: 0.25-0.5 mcg/d C 1-2 y: PO: 0.01-0.015 mcg/kg/d
Contraindications *Absolute contraindications:* Hypersensitivity, hypercalcemia, hypervitaminosis D *Caution:* Cardiovascular disease, renal calculi, renal failure, hyperphosphatemia, dehydration, excess sunlight exposure, malabsorption syndrome, hypocalcemia	**Drug-Lab-Food Interactions** Drug: Increased cardiac dysrhythmias with digoxin, verapamil; decreased calcitriol absorption with cholestyramine; decreased calcitriol effects with ketoconazole, barbiturates; enhanced calcitriol effects with thiazide diuretics Calcitriol decreases the effects of estrogen. Lab: Increased serum calcium with thiazide diuretics, calcium supplements, calcium-rich foods; decreased serum calcium with low magnesium
Pharmacokinetics Absorption: PO: Well absorbed Distribution: PB: 99% Metabolism: t½: 3-8 h adult; 27 h children Excretion: Feces (50%), urine (16%)	**Pharmacodynamics** PO: Onset: 2-6 h Peak: 3-6 h Duration: 3-5 d
Therapeutic Effects/Uses	
To treat parathyroid disorders (hyperparathyroidism and hypoparathyroidism) and to manage hypocalcemia in chronic renal failure Mode of Action: Calcitriol enhances calcium deposits into bones by the active form of vitamin D's metabolite, calcitriol. Calcitriol reabsorbs calcium by the kidneys; enhances intestinal absorption of dietary calcium; and decreases serum phosphate, bone resorption, and parathyroid hormone levels.	
Side Effects	**Adverse Reactions**
Side effects are generally early signs of hypercalcemia: fatigue, weakness, somnolence, cephalgia, nausea, vomiting, diarrhea, cramps, drowsiness, dizziness, vertigo, metallic taste, lethargy, constipation, and xerostomia.	Adverse effects are late signs of hypercalcemia: anorexia, photophobia, dehydration, cardiac arrhythmias, decreased libido, hypertension, sensory disturbances, hypercalciuria, hypercalcemia, and hyperphosphatemia.

*Pregnancy categories have been revised. See http://www.fda.gov/Drugs/DevelopmentApprovalProcess/DevelopmentResources/Labeling/ucm093307.htm for more information.

A, Adult; *C*, child; *d*, day; *h*, hour; *PB*, protein binding; *PO*, by mouth; *t½*, half-life; *y*, year; ≥, greater than or equal to.

allergic to fish. Common side effects include allergic reactions, GI symptoms (e.g., nausea and vomiting), cephalgia, and hypocalcemia. Adverse reactions due to severe hypocalcemia (e.g., tetany and seizures) can also occur.

Calcimimetics, such as cinacalcet, are used in patients with hyperparathyroidism due to chronic renal disease and parathyroid cancer, and it is also used in those who are unable to undergo parathyroidectomy. Cinacalcet mimics calcium in circulation, increasing the sensitivity of the calcium-sensing receptors of the cells of the parathyroid gland, thereby reducing PTH secretion. This action causes a decrease in serum calcium and slows the progression of bone disease. Because of the hypocalcemic effect, cinacalcet is contraindicated in patients with hypocalcemia. Chapter 12 discusses calcium imbalances more in depth.

Bisphosphonates (e.g., alendronate, etidronate, ibandronate, and risedronate) block osteoclast activities, thereby inhibiting mineralization or resorption of the bone, which may lessen osteoporosis caused by hyperparathyroidism. Prior to treatment with bisphosphonates, bone mineral density measurements should be obtained at baseline and periodically thereafter. Serum calcium concentration should be obtained, and any hypocalcemia must be corrected prior to bisphosphonate therapy. ⚡ Adequate intake of calcium and vitamin D is essential during therapy. Oral bisphosphonates are contraindicated in patients who are unable to sit or stand upright for at least 30 minutes after administration or who have esophageal strictures. During therapy, transient hypocalcemia and hypophosphatemia can occur. Other side effects include abdominal and musculoskeletal pain, GI upsets, hypotension, and fever. Individual bisphosphonates are discussed in Chapter 52.

 NURSING PROCESS
Patient-Centered Collaborative Care
Parathyroid Hormone Insufficiencies

Assessment
- Note serum calcium level, and report abnormal results.
- ❶ Assess for symptoms of tetany in hypocalcemia: twitching of the mouth, tingling and numbness of fingers, carpopedal spasm, spasmodic contractions, and laryngeal spasm.

Nursing Diagnoses
- Diarrhea related to the adverse effects of calcitriol
- Fluid Volume, Deficient related to fluid loss from vomiting, diarrhea, and polyuria
- Knowledge, Deficient related to inexperience with parathyroid medication

Planning
- The patient's serum calcium level will be within the normal range.

Nursing Interventions
- Monitor serum calcium level. The normal reference range is 8 to 10 mg/dL; serum calcium below 8 mg/dL indicates hypocalcemia. Total serum calcium greater than 10.5 mg/dL indicates hypercalcemia.

Patient Teaching
Hypoparathyroidism
- Direct patients to report symptoms of hypocalcemia (e.g., tetany).

Hyperparathyroidism
- Teach patients to report signs and symptoms of hypercalcemia, which include bone pain, anorexia, nausea, vomiting, thirst, constipation, lethargy, bradycardia, and polyuria.
- Advise women to inform their health care provider about pregnancy status before taking calcitonin preparations.
- Encourage patients to check OTC drugs for possible calcium content, especially if the patient has an elevated serum calcium level. Some vitamins and antacids contain calcium. Tell patients to contact their health care provider before taking drugs with calcium.
- Obtain an interpreter when necessary; do not rely on family members, who may not fully disclose because of cultural norms.
- Identify conflicts in values and beliefs, and engage in culturally sensitive patient dialogue and education.

Evaluation
- Monitor effectiveness of drug therapy (e.g., serum calcium level, signs and symptoms of hypercalcemia or hypocalcemia).
- Continue monitoring for signs and symptoms of calcium imbalances.
- Evaluate the patient's knowledge of medication regimen.

ADRENAL GLANDS

The paired adrenal glands consist of the adrenal medulla and adrenal cortex. Hormones secreted from the adrenal medulla are epinephrine and norepinephrine (catecholamines); Unit XVIII further discusses these hormones. The adrenal cortex produces two types of steroid hormones, glucocorticoids (cortisol) and mineralocorticoids (aldosterone), and to a lesser extent the adrenal androgens and estrogens. Steroids are secreted by the adrenal cortex in response to signals from the hypothalamus-pituitary-adrenal (HPA) axis; the levels are regulated by the negative feedback mechanism. A decrease in serum steroid levels (hypocortisolism) increases corticotropin-releasing factor (CRF) and ACTH secretions from the hypothalamus and anterior pituitary gland, respectively; these stimulate the adrenal glands to secrete and release steroids. An increased serum steroid level (hypercortisolism) inhibits the HPA axis, resulting in fewer steroids being released. A decrease in steroid secretion is called *adrenal hyposecretion* (adrenal insufficiency, or Addison disease), and an increase in steroid secretion is called *adrenal hypersecretion* (Cushing syndrome). Additional physiologic functions related to the hormones secreted from the adrenal medulla and adrenal cortex are described in the introduction to Unit XV.

❶ Because of the influences of steroids on electrolytes and on carbohydrate, protein, and fat metabolism, hypocortisolism can result in serious illness or death.

⚡ PATIENT SAFETY

Do not confuse...
- Calcitonin with calcitriol or calcium
- Levothyroxine with liothyronine
- Somatropin with somatostatin or sandostatin

Glucocorticoids

Glucocorticoids are the most potent natural cortisol produced by the body and are influenced by ACTH, which is released from the anterior pituitary gland. Its functions include having an effect on the inflammatory response (see Chapter 24), metabolism, growth, and biorhythms. Glucocorticoids also affect carbohydrate, protein, and fat metabolism and muscle and blood cell activities. Indications for glucocorticoid therapy include trauma, surgery, inflammation, emotional upsets, and anxiety. Table 46.2 lists the physiologic aspects of adrenal hyposecretion (Addison disease) and hypersecretion (Cushing syndrome).

Most of the glucocorticoid drugs, frequently called *cortisone drugs*, are synthetically produced. These drugs have several routes of administration: oral, parenteral (IM or IV), topical (creams, ointments, lotions), and aerosol (inhaler). Drugs administered via the (seldom used) IM route should be administered deep into the muscle; subcutaneous administration is not recommended.

Glucocorticoids are used to treat many diseases and health problems, including inflammatory, allergic, and debilitating conditions. Among the inflammatory conditions that may require glucocorticoids are autoimmune disorders (e.g., MS, rheumatoid arthritis, myasthenia gravis); ulcerative colitis; glomerulonephritis; shock; ocular and vascular inflammation; polyarteritis nodosa; and hepatitis. Allergic conditions include asthma, drug reactions, contact dermatitis, and anaphylaxis. Debilitating conditions are mainly caused by malignancies. Organ transplant recipients may require glucocorticoids to prevent organ rejection.

There are many glucocorticoids, some more potent than others. Dexamethasone has been used to treat severe inflammatory responses that result from head trauma or allergic reactions. An inexpensive glucocorticoid frequently prescribed is prednisone. Prototype Drug Chart 46.3 lists the pharmacologic data for prednisone.

Commonly used glucocorticoid drugs and their dosages, uses, and considerations are listed in Table 46.5. Most of the

📄 PROTOTYPE DRUG CHART 46.3

Prednisone

Drug Class	Dosage
Glucocorticoid/corticosteroid Pregnancy category: C (immediate release) and D (delayed release)*	Dosage is individualized and highly variable depending on the severity of the disease and on patient response. A: PO: 5-60 mg/d in single or divided doses C: PO: 4-5 mg/m² in single or divided doses Delayed-release tablets release drug approximately 4 h after the first dose.

Contraindications	Drug-Lab-Food Interactions
Contraindication: Untreated serious infections, hypersensitivity, varicella *Caution:* Psychosis, diabetes mellitus, renal disease, heart failure, myocardial infarction, hypertension, osteoporosis, cirrhosis, diverticulitis, hypothyroidism, myasthenia gravis, ulcerative colitis, seizures, visual disturbances, GI disorders, ocular herpes simplex	Drug: Additive effects occur with other immunosuppressive drugs when taken concurrently with corticosteroids. Increased corticosteroid levels are seen with estrogens, diltiazem, ketoconazole; decreased levels are seen with barbiturates, phenytoin, and rifampin. Concurrent use of aspirin and NSAIDs increase GI toxicity; concurrent use of diuretics and amphotericin B increases potassium depletion; concurrent use with cardiac glycosides increases risk of dysrhythmias and digitalis toxicity; concurrent use with bupropion lowers seizure threshold Herb: Level is decreased with ephedra (Ma-huang). Lab: Hyperglycemia, false-positive TB test

Pharmacokinetics	Pharmacodynamics
Absorption: PO: Well absorbed Distribution: PB: 65%-91% Metabolism: t½: 2-3 h Excretion: In urine	PO: Onset: UK Peak: 1-2 h Duration: 1 h (plasma); 18-36 h (biologic)

Therapeutic Effects/Uses
Adrenocortical insufficiency, Addison disease
Mode of Action: Suppresses inflammation, immune responses (humoral), and adrenal function; has mild mineralocorticoid activity

Side Effects	Adverse Reactions
Fluid and sodium retention, nausea, diarrhea, abdominal distension, increased appetite, sweating, headache, depression, flushing, mood changes, cataracts, amenorrhea, anorexia, Cushing syndrome, psychosis, immunosuppression, HPA suppression, hypercholesterolemia, elevated hepatic transaminases	Angioedema, cardiac arrhythmia, avascular necrosis, osteoporosis, fractures, cardiac arrest, cardiomyopathy, GI ulceration, exfoliative dermatitis, GI bleeding and perforation, CHF, increased ICP, lupus-like symptoms, pancreatitis, pulmonary edema, ocular disease, CVA, tendon rupture, thromboembolism

*Pregnancy categories have been revised. See http://www.fda.gov/Drugs/DevelopmentApprovalProcess/DevelopmentResources/Labeling/ucm093307.htm for more information.
A, Adult; *C*, child; *CHF*, congestive heart failure; *CVA*, cerebrovascular accident; *d*, day; *GI*, gastrointestinal; *h*, hour; *HPA*, hypothalamic-pituitary-adrenal axis; *ICP*, intracranial pressure; *NSAID*, nonsteroidal antiinflammatory drug; *PB*, protein binding; *PO*, by mouth; *t½*, half-life; *TB*, tuberculosis; *UK*, unknown.

TABLE 46.5 Drug Therapies for Adrenal Disorders

Generic	Route and Dosage	Uses and Considerations
GLUCOCORTICOIDS		
Short Acting		
Cortisone acetate	A: PO: 12-50 mg/d in divided doses to simulate normal diurnal adrenal rhythm	For adrenocortical insufficiency. Give with fludrocortisone (mineralocorticoid). Give oral dose with food to minimize GI irritation. Pregnancy category: D*; PB: 90%; t½: 8-12 h
Hydrocortisone	Primary adrenocortical insufficiency: Hydrocortisone or hydrocortisone *cypionate*: A: PO 20-240 mg/d in 2-4 divided doses. C: PO: 2-8 mg/kg/d or 60-240 mg/m²/d in 3-4 divided doses Hydrocortisone sodium *phosphate*: A: IM/IV/subcut: 15-240 mg/d twice daily (q12h). Hydrocortisone sodium *succinate*: A: IV/IM: 100-500 mg repeated in 2-, 4-, or 6-h intervals C: IV/IM: 186-280 mcg/kg/d or 10-12 mg/m²/d in 3 divided doses Hydrocortisone *acetate* suspension: A: IM: 15-240 mg once daily C: IM: 0.560 mg/kg or 30-37.5 mg/m² once q3d	For adrenocortical insufficiency. Given IV or IM (hydrocortisone sodium succinate) for crisis prophylaxis in ill patients or those undergoing surgery. Hydrocortisone sodium phosphate (subcut/IV/IM), hydrocortisone sodium succinate (IV/IM), and hydrocortisone acetate suspension (IM only) are for acute adrenal insufficiency. Oral hydrocortisone is also available for primary adrenocortical insufficiency. Oral dosages in this table are for primary adrenal insufficiency. Administer with meals to minimize GI irritation. Daily doses should be given in the morning to coincide with the body's normal cortisol secretion. Acetate formulations should never be given intravenously. Pregnancy category: C*; PB: 90%; t½: 1-2 h
Intermediate Acting		
Methylprednisolone	A: PO: 4-48 mg/d in 4 divided doses C: PO: 0.5-1.7 mg/kg or 5-25 mg/m² in divided doses q6-12h Methylprednisolone *acetate*: A: IM: 10-120 mg; subsequent doses determined by clinical response C: IM: 0.5-1.7 mg/kg or 5-25 mg/m² in divided doses q6-12h Methylprednisolone sodium *succinate*: A: IV/IM: 10-40 mg over several minutes; subsequent dosages determined by clinical response C: IV/IM: 0.5-1.7 mg/kg or 5-25 mg/m² in divided doses q6-12h	For adrenocortical insufficiency. Has little to no mineralocorticoid properties. Dosing is highly variable. Administer oral dosages with meals to minimize GI irritation. Acetate formulation should never be given intravenously. Pregnancy category: C*; PB: UK; t½: 3-3.5 h
Prednisolone	A: PO: 5-60 mg/d in 1-2 doses C: PO: 0.14-2 mg/kg/d or 4-60 mg/m²/d in 3-4 divided doses	For parenteral use in primary or secondary adrenocortical insufficiency. Prednisolone is a potent steroid that can be injected into joints and soft tissue. Must be given concomitantly with a mineralocorticoid.. Pregnancy category: C; PB: 70%-90%; t½: 2-4 h
Prednisone	See Prototype Drug Chart 46.3.	
Long Acting		
Betamethasone (PO), betamethasone sodium phosphate/ betamethasone acetate susp (IM)	A/Adol: PO: 0.6-7.2 mg/d in single or divided doses C: PO: 62.5-250 mcg/kg/d in 3-4 divided doses Injectable suspension: A: IM: 0.5-9 mg/d divided q12h C: IM: 17.5 mcg/kg in 3 divided doses q3d Other regimen is available.	Synthetic glucocorticoids with minimal mineralocorticoid properties are used as antiinflammatory or immunosuppressive agents; must be used in conjunction with a mineralocorticoid for primary or secondary adrenocortical insufficiency. Dosing is variable and depends on indications. Should be taken with food. Pregnancy category: C*; PB: 64%; t½: 6.5 h
Dexamethasone	Adrenocortical insufficiency: A: PO: 0.75-9 mg/d in 2-4 divided doses or IV/IM: 0.5-9 mg/d q6-12h. C: PO/IV/IM: 0.03-0.3 mg/kg/d divided in 2-4 doses.	Synthetic glucocorticoids with little or no mineralocorticoid activity. Longest acting corticosteroid. Must use a mineralocorticoid when treating adrenal insufficiency. Higher oral doses are used for dexamethasone suppression test for Cushing syndrome. Give oral dose with food. Pregnancy category: C*; PB: UK; t½: 1.8-3.5 h
MINERALOCORTICOIDS		
Fludrocortisone	A: PO: 0.1-0.2 mg/d. If hypertension occurs due to therapy, decrease dose to 0.05 mg once daily.	For adrenocortical insufficiency (Addison disease). To be used as a supplement to hydrocortisone or cortisone. Circulating drug is bound to protein and transcortin. Only the unbound drugs are active. May be administered without regard to food. Pregnancy category: C*; PB: 42%; t½: 3.5 h

*Pregnancy categories have been revised. See http://www.fda.gov/Drugs/DevelopmentApprovalProcess/DevelopmentResources/Labeling/ucm093 307.htm for more information.

A, Adult; *Adol*, adolescent; *C*, child; *d*, day; *GI*, gastrointestinal; *h*, hour; *IM*, intramuscular; *IV*, intravenous; *PB*, protein binding; *PO*, by mouth; *q*, every; *subcut*, subcutaneous; *susp*, suspension; *t½*, half-life; *UK*, unknown

glucocorticoids are pregnancy category C drugs. Drugs used for adrenocortical insufficiency contain both glucocorticoids and mineralocorticoids, whereas drugs with antiinflammatory or immunosuppressive properties contain mostly glucocorticoids with minimal mineralocorticoid activity.

Side effects and adverse reactions. Side effects and adverse reactions of glucocorticoids that result from high doses or prolonged use include increased blood glucose, abnormal fat deposits in the face and trunk (so-called *moon face* and *buffalo hump*), decreased extremity size, muscle wasting, edema, sodium and water retention, hypertension, euphoria or psychosis, thinned skin with purpura, increased intraocular pressure (glaucoma), peptic ulcers, and growth retardation. Long-term use of glucocorticoid drugs can cause adrenal atrophy (loss of adrenal gland function). ❶ When drug therapy is discontinued, the dose should be tapered to allow the adrenal cortex to produce cortisol and other corticosteroids. Abrupt withdrawal of the drug can result in severe adrenocortical insufficiency.

Drug Interactions

Glucocorticoids increase the potency of drugs taken concurrently, including aspirin and nonsteroidal antiinflammatory drugs (NSAIDs), thus increasing the risk of GI bleeding and ulceration. Use of potassium-wasting diuretics (e.g., furosemide) with glucocorticoids increases potassium loss, resulting in hypokalemia.

Barbiturates, phenytoin, and rifampin decrease the effect of prednisone because they increase glucocorticoid metabolism. Larger doses of glucocorticoids may be required to achieve the desired effect. Prolonged use of glucocorticoids can cause severe muscle weakness.

Dexamethasone, a potent glucocorticoid, interacts with many drugs. Phenytoin, theophylline, rifampin, barbiturates, and antacids decrease the action of dexamethasone, whereas estrogen and NSAIDs such as aspirin increase its action. Dexamethasone decreases the effects of oral antidiabetics. Glucocorticoids can increase blood glucose levels, so insulin or oral antidiabetic drug dosage may need to be increased. When the drug is given with diuretics or anti-*Pseudomonas* penicillin preparations, the serum potassium level may decrease markedly.

Herbal products such as cascara sagrada, yellow dock, and licorice can potentiate the effects of corticosteroids, which can worsen potassium depletion.

Mineralocorticoids

Mineralocorticoids promote sodium retention and potassium and hydrogen excretion in the renal tubules. The primary mineralocorticoid is aldosterone which is controlled by the renin-angiotensin-aldosterone system (RAAS). Mineralocorticoids maintain fluid balance by promoting the reabsorption of sodium from the renal tubules. Sodium attracts water, resulting in water retention. When *hypovolemia* (a decrease in circulating fluid) occurs, more aldosterone is secreted to increase sodium and water retention, thereby restoring fluid balance. With sodium reabsorption, potassium is lost and hypokalemia (potassium deficit) can occur. Some glucocorticoid drugs also contain mineralocorticoid properties; these include cortisone

and hydrocortisone. A severe decrease in the mineralocorticoid leads to hypotension and vascular collapse, as seen in Addison disease. Mineralocorticoid deficiency usually occurs with glucocorticoid deficiency, frequently called *corticosteroid deficiency.*

Fludrocortisone is an oral mineralocorticoid that can be given with a glucocorticoid. Even though fludrocortisone has significant glucocorticoid activity, it is not appreciable at usual therapeutic doses. Fludrocortisone mimics the actions of endogenous aldosterone, facilitating sodium resorption and promoting hydrogen ion and potassium excretion. In larger doses, it can inhibit endogenous hormone secretions of adrenal cortex and pituitary gland, causing a negative nitrogen balance; therefore, a high-protein diet is usually indicated. Because potassium excretion occurs with the use of mineralocorticoids, serum potassium level should be monitored. Other adverse effects include fluid imbalance, fluid overload, and hypertension. These usually indicate overdosage, at which point fludrocortisone should be discontinued then resumed at lower doses. Hypokalemia may cause metabolic alkalosis that can cause GI symptoms (nausea and vomiting), orthostatic hypotension, cardiac rhythm changes, weakness, anorexia, and myalgia. Commonly used mineralocorticoid drugs and their dosages, uses, and considerations are listed in Table 46.5.

◎ NURSING PROCESS
Patient-Centered Collaborative Care
Adrenal Hormone: Corticosteroids

Assessment
- Note baseline vital signs for future comparisons.
- ⚡ Assess laboratory test results, especially serum electrolytes and blood glucose. The serum potassium level usually decreases and blood glucose level increases when a corticosteroid, such as prednisone, is taken over an extended period.
- Obtain the patient's weight and urine output for future comparisons. Corticosteroids can cause fluid retention and weight gain.
- Assess the patient's medical and herbal history. Report if the patient has glaucoma, cataracts, peptic ulcer, psychiatric problems, or diabetes mellitus. Glucocorticoids can intensify these health problems.

Nursing Diagnoses
- Electrolyte Imbalance, Risk for, especially sodium and potassium
- Infection, Risk for
- Knowledge, Deficient of drug regimen related to complicated dosing schedule
- Fluid Volume, Excess related to sodium and fluid retention

Planning
- The patient's inflammatory process will decrease.
- The patient's side effects from glucocorticoid therapy will be minimal.
- The patient will not develop new or worsening infection.
- The patient will have increased knowledge of the medication regimen.

Nursing Interventions

- Determine vital signs. Corticosteroids such as prednisone can increase blood pressure and sodium and water retention.
- Administer corticosteroids only as ordered. Routes of administration include oral, IM (not in deltoid muscle), IV, aerosol, and topical. Apply topical corticosteroids in thin layers (see Chapter 45). Rashes, infection, and purpura should be noted and reported.
- Record weight. Report a weight gain of 5 lb in 2 days; this could indicate water retention due to sodium reabsorption from hyperaldosteronism.
- Monitor laboratory values, especially serum electrolytes and blood glucose. The serum potassium level could decrease to less than 3.5 mEq/L, and serum sodium and glucose could increase.
- Watch for signs and symptoms of hypokalemia: nausea, vomiting, muscular weakness, abdominal distension, paralytic ileus, and irregular heart rate.
- Assess for side effects from corticosteroid drugs when therapy has lasted more than 10 days and drug is taken in high dosages. Cortisone preparations should not be abruptly stopped because adrenal crisis can result.
- Monitor older adults for signs and symptoms of increased osteoporosis. Some corticosteroids promote calcium loss from bone.

Patient Teaching
General

- Advise patients to take drugs as prescribed, and caution patients not to abruptly stop drugs. When the drug is discontinued, the dose is tapered over 1 to 2 weeks.
- Direct patients not to take cortisone preparations (oral or topical) during pregnancy unless necessary and prescribed by the health care provider. Drugs may be harmful to the fetus.

- ⚡ Inform patients that certain herbal laxatives and diuretics may interact with corticosteroid drug therapy and may increase the severity of hypokalemia.
- Teach patients to avoid large crowds and persons with respiratory infections, because corticosteroids can suppress the immune system.
- Teach patients receiving corticosteroids to inform other health care providers of all drugs taken.
- Encourage patients to carry a medical alert identification card, tag, or bracelet stating that corticosteroids are taken.
- Teach patients proper use of the drug.
- Teach patients to report signs and symptoms of Cushing syndrome: moon face, puffy eyelids, edema in the feet, increased bruising, dizziness, bleeding, and menstrual irregularity.
- Counsel patients to take cortisone preparations at mealtime or with food to prevent irritation of gastric mucosa.
- Advise patients to eat foods rich in potassium, such as fresh and dried fruits, vegetables, meats, and nuts. Some corticosteroid preparations promote potassium loss.
- Recognize that members of various cultural groups may need guidance in understanding disease processes. Explain to the family that the patient is not "dumb" or "uninterested" but has an adrenal problem. Explain that symptoms do not go away and may be progressive if prescribed therapy is not followed.

Evaluation

- Evaluate effectiveness of corticosteroid therapy. If clinical manifestations have not improved, a change in drug therapy may be necessary.
- Continue monitoring for side effects, especially when a patient is receiving high doses of corticosteroids.
- Evaluate the patient's knowledge of the therapy.

▌ CRITICAL THINKING CASE STUDY

MP, a 68-year-old woman, had a severe allergic reaction to shellfish and was taken to the emergency department. She presented with angioedema and anaphylactic shock. A single dose of dexamethasone 100 mg IV (direct IV over 30 seconds) was ordered. MP weighs 65 kg.

1. Why is MP receiving dexamethasone intravenously? Is the dosage of dexamethasone within the safe therapeutic range? Explain your answer.
2. Describe the various ways dexamethasone can be given intravenously. Which IV fluid is compatible with dexamethasone? Describe other routes by which dexamethasone can be administered.
3. What additional health information and assessment may aid the health care provider in treating MP's condition?

Twenty-one tablets of prednisone, 5 mg each, were prescribed to be taken over 5 days, with tapering daily doses. The dosage is as follows: Day 1, take 10 mg four times a day; day 2, take 10 mg

three times a day; day 3, take 10 mg twice a day; day 4, take 10 mg once a day; and day 5, take 5 mg once a day.

4. Why was prednisone ordered for MP and not oral dexamethasone? Explain your answer.
5. What is the purpose for tapering prednisone doses? Explain your answer.
6. Is the drug dose within the safe therapeutic range? Explain your answer.
7. Should MP have side effects such as peripheral edema caused by water and sodium retention as a result of tapered prednisone doses? Explain your answer.
8. What is the difference between prednisone and prednisolone?
9. What are the adverse reactions from prolonged use of prednisone?
10. What are the nursing interventions and patient teaching for MP and for patients who take prednisone?

NCLEX STUDY QUESTIONS

1. A patient is receiving the drug somatropin. The nurse understands that the action of this drug is to do what?
   a. Act as an antiinflammatory agent
   b. Increase metabolic rate and oxygen consumption
   c. Stimulate growth in long bones at epiphyseal plates
   d. Promote water reabsorption from the renal tubules
2. A patient is given desmopressin acetate. The nurse knows that this drug is used to treat which of the following conditions?
   a. Gigantism
   b. Diabetes mellitus
   c. Diabetes insipidus
   d. Adrenal insufficiency
3. A patient is taking levothyroxine. For which adverse effect would the nurse monitor?
   a. Tachycardia
   b. Drowsiness
   c. Constipation
   d. Weight gain
4. A patient has just begun taking calcitriol. Which is a nursing implication of this drug?
   a. Monitor the patient's weight.
   b. Monitor serum calcium levels.
   c. Teach side effects of alopecia and petechiae.
   d. Instruct the patient to avoid persons with respiratory infections.
5. A patient is given corticotropin. The nurse knows to monitor the patient for which condition?
   a. Weight gain
   b. Hyperkalemia
   c. Hypoglycemia
   d. Dehydration

6. A nurse is administering prednisone to a newly admitted patient who is taking multiple other drugs. The nurse should consider which drug interactions with prednisone? (Select all that apply.)
   a. Cardiac and central nervous system actions are increased when drug is taken with an adrenergic agent.
   b. Potassium-wasting diuretics increase potassium loss, resulting in hypokalemia.
   c. Risk for gastrointestinal bleeding and ulceration increases when drug is taken with aspirin or other nonsteroidal antiinflammatory drugs (NSAIDs).
   d. The action of prednisone is decreased when taken with phenytoin because phenytoin increases glucocorticoid metabolism.
   e. Risk for dysrhythmias and digitalis toxicity increase when drug is taken with cardiac glycosides.
   f. Dosage of antidiabetic agents may need to be decreased when taken concurrently with glucocorticoids.
7. The nurse is administering vasopressin to a patient. Which of the following nursing interventions are indicated when administering vasopressin? (Select all that apply.)
   a. Record urinary output.
   b. Observe the patient's weight, and note edema.
   c. Monitor the patient for decreased blood pressure.
   d. Closely monitor the patient's blood glucose levels.
   e. Monitor the patient's pulse for increased heart rate.
   f. Record the patient's daily calcium levels.

Answers: 1, c; 2, c; 3, a; 4, b; 5, a; 6, b, c, d, e; 7, a, b, c, e.

47

Antidiabetics

OBJECTIVES

- Compare type 1 and type 2 diabetes mellitus.
- Describe the symptoms of diabetes mellitus.
- Differentiate symptoms of hypoglycemic reaction and hyperglycemia.
- Compare onset, peak, and duration of rapid-acting, short-acting, intermediate-acting, and long-acting insulins.
- Compare the action of oral antidiabetic drugs and their side effects.
- Differentiate between the actions of insulin, oral antidiabetic agents, and glucagon.
- Apply the nursing process to the patient taking insulin and oral antidiabetic agents.

OUTLINE

Diabetes Mellitus

Insulin

Nursing Process: Patient-Centered Collaborative Care—
Antidiabetics: Insulin

Oral Antidiabetic (Hypoglycemic) Drugs

Nursing Process: Patient-Centered Collaborative Care—
Oral Antidiabetics

Other Antidiabetic Agents

Hyperglycemic Drugs

Critical Thinking Case Study

NCLEX Study Questions

KEY TERMS

diabetes mellitus, p. 686
hypoglycemic reaction, p. 690
insulin, p. 686
insulin shock, p. 690
ketoacidosis, p. 691
lipodystrophy, p. 688
oral antidiabetic drugs, p. 686

oral hypoglycemic drugs, p. 686
polydipsia, p. 686
polyphagia, p. 686
polyuria, p. 686
type 1 diabetes mellitus, p. 686
type 2 diabetes mellitus, p. 686

Antidiabetic drugs are used primarily to control diabetes mellitus, a chronic disease that affects carbohydrate metabolism. The two groups of antidiabetic agents are insulin and oral hypoglycemic (antidiabetic) drugs. **Insulin**, a protein secreted from the beta cells of the pancreas, is necessary for carbohydrate metabolism and plays an important role in protein and fat metabolism. The beta cells make up 75% of the pancreas, and the alpha cells that secrete glucagons—a hyperglycemic substance—occupy approximately 20% of the pancreas. **Oral hypoglycemic drugs**, also known as **oral antidiabetic drugs** (to avoid confusion with the term *hypoglycemic reaction*), are synthetic preparations that stimulate insulin release or otherwise alter the metabolic response to hyperglycemia.

DIABETES MELLITUS

Diabetes mellitus, a chronic disease that results from deficient glucose metabolism, is caused by insufficient insulin secretion

from the beta cells. This results in high blood glucose (*hyperglycemia*). Diabetes mellitus is characterized by the three *p*'s: **polyuria** (increased urine output), **polydipsia** (increased thirst), and **polyphagia** (increased hunger). Diabetes *mellitus* is a disorder of the pancreas, whereas diabetes *insipidus* is a disorder of the posterior pituitary gland, discussed in detail in Chapter 46.

The four types of diabetes are presented in Table 47.1. Viral infections, environmental conditions, and genetic factors contribute to the onset of **type 1 diabetes mellitus**. **Type 2 diabetes mellitus** is the most common type of diabetes. Some sources suggest that heredity and obesity are the major factors that cause type 2 diabetes. With type 2 diabetes, there is some beta-cell function with varying amounts of insulin secretion. Hyperglycemia may be controlled for some type 2 diabetes patients with oral antidiabetic (*hypoglycemic*) drugs and a diet prescribed by the American Diabetic Association (ADA); however, about one third of patients with type 2 diabetes need insulin. Patients with

686

TABLE 47.1 Types and Occurrences of Diabetes Mellitus

Types of Diabetes Mellitus	Percentage of Occurrences
Type 1	10%-12%
Type 2	85%-90%
Secondary diabetes (medications, hormonal changes)	2%-3%
Gestational diabetes mellitus	1% (2%-5% of all pregnancies)

type 2 diabetes who use one or two oral antidiabetic drugs may become insulin dependent years later.

Certain drugs increase blood glucose and can cause hyperglycemia in prediabetic persons. These include glucocorticoids (cortisone, prednisone), thiazide diuretics (hydrochlorothiazide), and epinephrine. Usually the blood glucose level returns to normal after the drug is discontinued.

During the second and third trimesters of pregnancy, the levels of the hormones progesterone, cortisol, and human placental lactogen (hPL) increase. These increased hormone levels can inhibit insulin usage. This is a contributing factor for the occurrence of gestational diabetes mellitus (GDM). Glucose is then mobilized from the tissue and from lipid storage sites. After pregnancy, the blood glucose level may decrease; however, some patients may develop diabetes mellitus, whereas others may develop type 2 diabetes in later years.

Insulin

Insulin is released from the beta cells of the islets of Langerhans in response to an increase in blood glucose. Oral glucose load is more effective in raising the serum insulin level than an intravenous (IV) glucose load. Insulin promotes the uptake of glucose, amino acids, and fatty acids and converts them to substances that are stored in body cells. Glucose is converted to glycogen in the liver and muscle for future glucose needs, thereby lowering the blood glucose level. The normal range for fasting blood glucose is 70 to 99 mg/dL. When the blood glucose level is greater than 180 mg/dL, glycosuria—glucose in the urine—can occur. Increased blood glucose acts as an osmotic diuretic, causing polyuria. When blood glucose remains elevated (>200 mg/dL), diabetes mellitus occurs.

Hemoglobin A1c (HbA1c), a derivative of the interaction of glucose with hemoglobin in red blood cells (RBCs), is used for the diagnosis of diabetes as recommended by the ADA. Because RBCs have a life span of approximately 120 days, the HbA1c level reflects the average glucose level for up to 3 months. In monitoring treatment, the goal is to keep the diabetic patient's HbA1c below 7%. For diagnostic purposes, an HbA1c level of 5% or less indicates that the patient does *not* have diabetes, 5.7% to 6.4% indicates prediabetes, and 6.5% or greater indicates a diagnosis of diabetes mellitus.

Beta-Cell Secretion of Insulin

The beta cells in the pancreas secrete approximately 0.2 to 0.5 units/kg/day of insulin. A patient who weighs 70 kg (154 pounds) secretes 14 to 35 units of insulin per day, although more insulin secretion may occur if the person consumes more calories. A patient with diabetes mellitus may require 0.2 to 1 units/kg/day. The higher range may be because of obesity, stress, or tissue insulin resistance.

❶ Commercially Prepared Insulin

Early insulin preparations utilized pancreas tissue extracted from animals—either pigs or cattle. Pork insulin is structurally closer to human insulin than beef insulin. Today, insulins are currently manufactured biosynthetically using recombinant DNA technology. *Human insulin* duplicates insulin produced by the pancreas of the human body; examples of human insulin include Humulin R and Novolin N. The use of human insulin has a low incidence of both allergic effects and insulin resistance. *Human insulin analogues* are modifications of human insulin with alterations in onset and duration of action. Insulin lispro and insulin aspart are examples of human insulin analogues.

Insulins are usually administered subcutaneously. Abdominal injections of insulin are absorbed faster than those at other body sites and have been found to be more consistent. Newly diagnosed patients with insulin-dependent diabetes are usually prescribed human insulin. In addition, patients in whom hyperglycemia develops during pregnancy or who already have diabetes and become pregnant are usually prescribed human insulin.

The concentration of insulin is 100 units/mL or 500 units/mL (U100/mL or U500/mL, respectively), and the insulin is packaged in a 10-mL vial. Insulin in 500 units/mL is only available in short-acting regular insulin. Insulin in 500 units/mL is seldom used except in emergencies and for patients with serious insulin resistance (>200 U/day). Insulin in 40 units/mL is no longer used in the United States, although it is still used in other countries. Insulin syringes are typically marked in units of 100 U/mL or 50 U/0.5 mL for insulin U100. Insulin syringes must be used for accurate dosing. To prevent dosage errors, the nurse must be certain that there is a match of the insulin concentration with the calibration of units on the insulin syringe. Before use, the patient or nurse must roll—not shake—cloudy insulin bottles to ensure that the insulin and its ingredients are well mixed. Shaking a bottle of insulin can cause bubbles, which can lead to an inaccurate dose. Insulin requirements vary; usually less insulin is needed with increased exercise, and more insulin is needed with infections and high fever.

Administration of Insulin

Insulin is a protein and cannot be administered orally because gastrointestinal (GI) secretions destroy the insulin structure. It is administered subcutaneously at a 45- to 90-degree angle. The 90-degree angle is made by raising the skin and fatty tissue, and the insulin is injected into the pocket between the fat and the muscle. In a thin person with little fatty tissue, the 45- to 60-degree angle is used. Regular insulin is the *only* type that can be administered intravenously.

The site and depth of insulin injection affect absorption. Insulin absorption is greater when given in the abdomen than when given in the thigh or buttocks. Heat and massage could

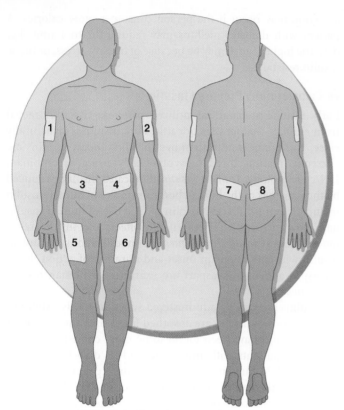

FIG. 47.1 Sites for insulin injection.

increase subcutaneous absorption, and cooling the subcutaneous area can decrease absorption.

Insulin is usually given in the morning before breakfast, and it can be given several times a day. Insulin injection sites should be rotated to prevent **lipodystrophy**, tissue atrophy or hypertrophy, which can interfere with insulin absorption. *Lipoatrophy*, tissue atrophy, is a depression under the skin surface that primarily occurs in women and children; *lipohypertrophy*, tissue hypertrophy, is a raised lump or knot on the skin surface that is more common in men. It is frequently caused by repeated injections into the same site. The patient needs to develop a "site rotation pattern" to avoid lipodystrophy and to promote insulin absorption. There are various insulin rotation programs, such as an 8-day rotation schedule in which insulin is given at a different site each day. The ADA suggests that insulin be injected daily at a chosen site for 1 week. Injections should be 1.5 inches (a knuckle length) apart each day. When a patient requires two insulin injections a day, morning and evening, one site should be chosen on the right side (morning) and one on the left side (evening). Fig. 47.1 illustrates the sites for insulin injections. A record of injection area sites and dates administered should be kept.

Illness and stress increase the need for insulin, so doses should *not* be withheld during illness, including infections and stress. Hyperglycemia and ketoacidosis may result from insufficient insulin.

Types of Insulin

Several standard types of insulin are available that include rapid-, short-, intermediate-, or long-acting types and combinations of these. *Rapid- and short-acting insulins* are in a clear solution without any added substance to prolong insulin action. *Intermediate-acting insulins* are cloudy and may contain protamine, a protein that prolongs the action of insulin, or zinc, which also slows the onset of action and prolongs the duration of activity.

Rapid-acting insulins include insulin lispro (human analogue), human insulin aspart (recombinant DNA [rDNA] origin), insulin glulisine, and human oral inhalation insulin. Insulin lispro is formed by reversing two amino acids in human regular insulin. Insulin aspart (rDNA origin) is another human insulin analogue in which a single amino acid (proline) has been substituted with aspartic acid to help prevent the molecules from clumping together to allow quicker entry into blood circulation. Insulin lispro, insulin aspart, insulin glulisine, and human oral inhalation insulin act faster than regular insulin, so they must be administered within 10 to 15 minutes before mealtime (food should be present before administering these insulins). Patients who are insulin dependent and take rapid-acting insulin usually require intermediate-acting insulin as well.

Short-acting insulin has an onset of action of 30 minutes. The peak action occurs in 2.5 to 5 hours, and the duration of action is 4 to 12 hours. Regular (unmodified, crystalline) insulin is short-acting insulin that can be administered intravenously or subcutaneously. Regular insulin is generally given 30 to 60 minutes before meals.

Intermediate-acting insulins include neutral protamine Hagedorn (NPH). Isophane insulins like NPH contain protamine, a protein that prolongs the action of insulin. The onset of intermediate-acting insulin is 1 to 2 hours, peak action occurs in 4 to 12 hours, and the duration of action is 14 to 24 hours.

Insulin glargine is long-acting insulin with an onset of 1 to 1.5 hours. It is evenly distributed over a 24-hour duration of action; thus it is administered once a day, usually at bedtime. The incidence of nocturnal hypoglycemia is not as common as with other insulins because of its continuous sustained release. Insulin detemir is another long-acting insulin that peaks in 6 to 8 hours and lasts for 24 hours, and insulin degludec, a *long-acting insulin,* has an onset of 1 hour, peaks at 12 hours, and lasts for 42 hours; these insulins are analogues of human insulin. Glargine was the first long-acting rDNA-origin human insulin for patients with types 1 and 2 diabetes. Glargine, detemir, and degludec are available in a prefilled cartridge for the OptiPen insulin pen device. Some patients complain of more pain at the injection site with the administration of glargine than with NPH insulin.

Combination insulins are commercially premixed. These include NPH 70/regular 30 and NPH 50/regular 50. These combinations are widely used. The NPH 70/regular 30 is available in vials or as prefilled disposable pens. The exterior of an insulin pen resembles a fountain pen. It can be stored at room temperature for up to 10 days. With these combinations of insulin, the patient does not have to mix regular and NPH insulins as long as one of these combinations is effective. However, some patients need less than 25% or 30% regular insulin and more intermediate-acting insulin. These patients need to mix the two insulins in the prescribed proportions.

PROTOTYPE DRUG CHART 47.1

⚠ Insulins

Drug Class	Dosage
Antidiabetic: Insulin Lispro, rapid acting Regular, short acting NPH, intermediate acting Glargine, long acting Pregnancy category: B*, C*	Must be individualized and varies according to patient's blood glucose and health status

Contraindications	Drug-Lab-Food Interactions
Hypersensitivity, hypoglycemia, rosiglitazone use *Caution:* Hypokalemia, fever, surgery or trauma, vomiting, pioglitazone use, renal or hepatic impairment	Drug: Increased hypoglycemic effect with aspirin, oral anticoagulants, alcohol, oral hypoglycemics, beta blockers, ACE inhibitors, ARBs, TCAs, MAOIs, and tetracycline; decreased hypoglycemic effect with thiazides, glucocorticoids, oral contraceptives, thyroid drugs, furosemide, bumetamide, phenytoin, fluoroquinolones, smoking, and green tea

Pharmacokinetics	Pharmacodynamics
Absorption: Lispro and regular, rapidly absorbed from subcut injection site; NPH is absorbed at a slower rate; glargine is absorbed at a slow, evenly distributed rate. Distribution: PB: UK Metabolism: t½: Varies with type of insulin Excretion: Mostly in urine	Lispro: Subcut: Onset: 15-30 min Peak: 30-90 min Duration: 3-5 h Regular: Subcut: Onset: 30 min Peak: 2.5-5 h Duration: 4-12 h NPH: Subcut: Onset: 1-2 h Peak: 4-12 h Duration: 14-24 h Glargine: Subcut: Onset: 1-1.5 h Peak: None Duration: 24 h

Therapeutic Effects/Uses
To control diabetes mellitus, to lower blood glucose Mode of Action: Promotes use of glucose by body cells

Side Effects	Adverse Reactions
Confusion, agitation, tremors, headache, flushing, hunger, UTI, weakness, lethargy, fatigue, urticaria, redness, diarrhea, flulike symptoms, weight gain, irritation or swelling at injection site	Tachycardia, palpitations, hypoglycemic reaction, rebound hyperglycemia (Somogyi effect), lipodystrophy, hypokalemia *Life threatening:* Shock, anaphylaxis, ketoacidosis

*Pregnancy categories have been revised. See http://www.fda.gov/Drugs/DevelopmentApprovalProcess/DevelopmentResources/Labeling/ucm093307.htm for more information.
ACE, Angiotensin-converting enzyme; *ARB,* angiotensin II–receptor blocker; *h,* hour; *MAOI,* monoamine oxidase inhibitor; *min,* minute; *NPH,* neutral protamine Hagedorn; *PB,* protein binding; *subcut,* subcutaneous; *t½,* half-life; *TCA,* tricyclic antidepressant; *UK,* unknown; *UTI,* urinary tract infection.

Regular insulin can be mixed with other insulin in the same syringe. However, mixing insulin can alter the absorption rate.

Insulin Resistance

Antibodies develop over time in persons taking animal insulin. This can slow the onset of insulin action and extend its duration of action. Antibody development can cause insulin resistance and insulin allergy, and obesity can also be a causative factor for insulin resistance. Skin tests with different insulin preparations may be performed to determine whether an allergic effect is present. Human and regular insulins produce fewer allergens.

Storage of Insulin

Unopened insulin vials are refrigerated until needed. Once an insulin vial has been opened, it may be kept at room temperature for 1 month or in the refrigerator for 3 months; insulin is less irritating to the tissues when injected at room temperature. Insulin vials should not be put in the freezer, nor should they be placed in direct sunlight or in a high-temperature area. Prefilled syringes should be stored in the refrigerator and should be used within 1 to 2 weeks. Opened insulin vials lose their strength after approximately 3 months.

Prototype Drug Chart 47.1 lists the pharmacologic data for the different types of insulin.

Pharmacokinetics All insulins can be administered subcutaneously, but only regular insulin can be given intravenously. The half-life varies. Insulin is metabolized by the liver and muscle and is excreted in the urine.

Pharmacodynamics Insulin lowers blood glucose by promoting the use of glucose by the body's cells. Insulin is also active in the storage of glucose as glycogen in muscles. The onset of action of rapid-acting insulin given subcutaneously is approximately 10 to 30 minutes. The onset of action of regular insulin is 30 minutes given subcutaneously and 15 minutes given intravenously. The onset of action of intermediate-acting insulin is 1.5 hours. The peak action of insulins is important because of the possibility of a hypoglycemic reaction (insulin shock) occurring during that time. The peak action for rapid-acting insulin is approximately 30 to 90 minutes. The peak time for regular insulin is 1.5 to 3.5 hours; for intermediate-acting insulin, the peak time is 4 to 12 hours. The nurse needs to assess for signs and symptoms of hypoglycemic reaction, such as nervousness, tremors, confusion, sweating, and increased pulse rate. Orange juice, sugar-sweetened beverages, or hard candy should be kept available to be given if a reaction occurs. If the patient is unable to ingest fast-acting carbohydrates, glucagon may be given. Glucagon promotes the breakdown of glycogen in the liver and raises blood glucose within 10 minutes.

Regular insulin can be given several times a day, especially during the regulation of insulin dosage. Intermediate- and long-acting insulins are usually administered once a day. Regular insulin can be mixed with intermediate-acting NPH insulin, especially if rapid onset of action is needed. When switching from one type of insulin to another, the patient may require a dose adjustment because human insulin has a shorter duration of action.

Sliding-Scale Insulin Coverage

Insulin may be administered in adjusted doses that depend on individual blood glucose test results. When the diabetic patient has extreme variances in insulin requirements—such as with stress from hospitalization, surgery, illness, or infection—adjusted dosing or sliding-scale insulin coverage provides a more constant blood glucose level. Blood glucose testing is performed several times a day at specified intervals, usually before meals. A preset scale usually involves directions for the administration of rapid- or short-acting insulin.

Drug Interactions. Drugs such as thiazide diuretics, glucocorticoids (cortisone preparations), thyroid agents, and estrogen increase blood glucose, therefore the insulin dosage may need adjustment. Drugs that decrease insulin needs are tricyclic antidepressants (TCAs), monoamine oxidase inhibitors (MAOIs), aspirin products, and oral anticoagulants.

Table 47.2 lists the rapid-, short-, intermediate-, and long-acting insulins with their dosages, uses, and considerations.

Side Effects and Adverse Reactions: Hypoglycemic Reactions and Ketoacidosis. When more insulin is administered than is needed for glucose metabolism, a hypoglycemic reaction, or insulin shock, occurs. The person may exhibit nervousness, trembling, and lack of coordination; have cold and clammy skin; and complain of a headache. Some patients become combative and incoherent. Giving sugar orally or intravenously increases the use of insulin, and the symptoms disappear immediately.

In response to an excessive dose of insulin, diabetic patients may develop what is known as the *Somogyi effect,* a hypoglycemic condition that usually occurs in the predawn hours of 2:00 am to 4:00 am wherein a rapid decrease in blood glucose during the nighttime hours stimulates a release of hormones (cortisol, glucagon, and epinephrine) to increase blood glucose by lipolysis, gluconeogenesis, and glycogenolysis. Management of the Somogyi effect involves monitoring blood glucose between 2:00 am and 4:00 am and reducing the bedtime insulin dosage.

！ TABLE 47.2　Antidiabetics: Insulins

Drug	Pregnancy Category	Half-Life	ACTION		
			Onset	Peak	Duration
Rapid-Acting Insulins					
Insulin lispro	B*	1 h	15-30 min	30-90 min	3-5 h
Insulin aspart	B*	1.5 h	10-20 min	40-50 min	3-5 h
Insulin glulisine	C*	5-6 min	20-30 min	55 min	1-2.5 h
Oral inhalation insulin	C*	28-39 min	12-15 min	53 min	2.5 h
Short-Acting Insulins					
Insulin regular	B*	1.5 h	Subcut: 30 min IV: 15 min	Subcut: 2.5-5 h IV: 15-30 min	Subcut: 4-12 h IV: 30-60 min
Intermediate-Acting Insulins					
Insulin isophane NPH	B*	5-6 min	1-2 h	4-12 h	14-24 h
Long-Acting Insulins					
Insulin glargine	C*	5-6 min	1-1.5 h	None	24 h
Insulin detemir	B*	5-6 min	1-2 h	6-8 h	24 h
Insulin degludec	C*	25 h	1 h	12 h	42 h

*Pregnancy categories have been revised. See http://www.fda.gov/Drugs/DevelopmentApprovalProcess/DevelopmentResources/Labeling/ucm093 307.htm for more information.

h, Hour; *IV,* intravenous; *min,* minute; *NPH,* neutral protamine Hagedorn; *subcut,* subcutaneous.

Hyperglycemia on awakening is known as the *dawn phenomenon*. The patient usually awakens with a headache and reports night sweats and nightmares. Management of the dawn phenomenon involves increasing the bedtime dose of insulin.

With an inadequate amount of insulin, sugar cannot be metabolized, and fat catabolism occurs. The use of fatty acids (ketones) for energy causes ketoacidosis (diabetic acidosis or diabetic coma). Table 47.3 lists the signs and symptoms of hypoglycemic reaction and ketoacidosis.

Insulin Pen Injectors

An insulin pen resembles a fountain pen but contains a disposable needle and a disposable insulin-filled cartridge. Insulin pens come in two types, prefilled and reusable, and are considered to deliver a more accurate dose than the traditional 100-unit syringe and vial.

To operate the insulin pen, the insulin dose is obtained by turning the dial to the number of insulin units needed. The capacity of these prefilled and reusable insulin pens is 150 to 300 units, or 1.5 to 3 mL; the 1.5-mL replaceable cartridges for insulin pens are being phased out. Insulin pens available on the market include the NovoLog FlexPen (Novo Nordisk), Humalog KwikPen (Lilly), Apidra SoloSTAR (Sanofi-Aventis), Lantus SoloSTAR (Sanofi), and Levemir FlexPen (Novo Nordisk). Insulin pens tend to be more expensive than other delivery systems, but their advantages may outweigh the extra cost.

The use of insulin pens increases the patient's compliance with the insulin regimen. The convenience of the pen is most appealing, and patients may choose to use the insulin pen for its portability; it can be used at work or while traveling, whereas the traditional method for administering insulin may be used at other times. The cost of insulin in vials is somewhat less than the prefilled pens, but most patients state that less injection pain is associated with insulin pens than with the traditional insulin syringe.

TABLE 47.3 Hypoglycemic Reaction and Diabetic Ketoacidosis

Reaction	Signs and Symptoms
Hypoglycemic reaction (insulin shock)	Headache, lightheadedness Nervousness, apprehension Tremor Excess perspiration; cold, clammy skin Tachycardia Slurred speech Memory lapse, confusion, seizures Blood glucose <60 mg/dL
Diabetic ketoacidosis (hyperglycemic reaction)	Extreme thirst Polyuria Fruity breath odor Kussmaul breathing (deep, rapid, labored, distressed, dyspneac) Rapid, thready pulse Dry mucous membranes, poor skin turgor Blood glucose >250 mg/dL

>, Greater than; <, less than.

Insulin Pumps

Insulin pumps are an alternative to daily insulin injections used in association with blood glucose monitoring and carbohydrate counting. These computerized devices have an insulin reservoir and programming capacity to deliver continuous rapid-acting insulin in varying amounts at different times throughout a 24-hour period. These pumps are smaller than most mobile phones, and the types of insulin pumps include implantable and portable. The *implantable insulin pump* is surgically implanted in the abdomen and delivers both basal infusion (continuous release of a small amount of insulin) and bolus (additional) doses with meals. It is administered intraperitoneally. With the use of implantable insulin pumps, fewer hypoglycemic reactions occur, and blood glucose levels are controlled. Long-term effectiveness of the pump is currently under study.

External or *portable insulin pumps,* also called *continuous subcutaneous insulin infusion* (CSII), may have a tube or infusion set placed under the skin. The needle is inserted into the abdomen, upper thigh, or upper arm. This type of pump is worn outside the body and is placed in a pocket or bra. The external tubeless pump lies directly on the skin and injects insulin through the skin without tubes. The external insulin pump keeps blood glucose levels as close to normal as possible. This insulin pump is a battery-operated device that uses rapid-acting insulin, which is stored in a reservoir syringe placed inside the device. It delivers both basal insulin infusion and bolus doses with meals. Infusions are programmed by the patient. About three basal rates are programmed per day; however, the patient can adjust the rate according to changes in activity. The patient pushes a button to deliver a bolus dose at meals. Only rapid-acting insulin is used; modified (NPH) insulins are not used because of unpredictable control of blood glucose. The pump delivers exactly as much insulin as the patient programs.

The ongoing insulin delivery therapy helps decrease the risk of severe hypoglycemic reaction and maintains tight glucose (glycemic) control. Glucose levels should be monitored at least four times daily with an insulin pump. The patient must count carbohydrates and bolus doses prior to meals.

Most insulin pumps have a (time and day) memory of the last 24 boluses. An alarm sounds so the patient can take appropriate action when insulin is not delivered or when there is an oncoming low or high. Newer pumps have an automatic shutoff for 1 to 2 hours during periods of low blood glucose. This feature is designed for patients who may not hear the alarm and for those in whom blood glucose is allowed to elevate. The pump can be disconnected from the insertion site for bathing, swimming, and other activities; however, it is recommended that it not be discontinued for longer than 1 to 2 hours.

Success of insulin pump therapy depends on the individual's knowledge and compliance related to insulin use and the diabetic state. The person with type 1 diabetes mellitus may benefit most from the use of insulin pump therapy. This insulin delivery method is considered more effective than the use of multiple injections of regular and modified types of insulins, and it lessens the long-term diabetic complications. Studies have shown that myocardial infarction, renal disease, nerve damage, eye damage, and death have all been greatly reduced by tight blood glucose control. Also, HbA1c levels, neuropathy pain, and sexual performance have improved with the use of insulin pump control.

Insulin Jet Injectors

Insulin jet injectors shoot insulin, without a needle, directly through the skin into the fatty tissue. Because the insulin is delivered under high pressure, stinging, pain, burning, and bruising may occur. This method of insulin insertion is not indicated for children or older adults. This type of device is also expensive, costing approximately 2 to 10 times as much as the subcutaneous dose.

 NURSING PROCESS
Patient-Centered Collaborative Care

Antidiabetics: Insulin

Assessment

- Identify the drugs a patient currently takes. Certain drugs such as alcohol, aspirin, oral anticoagulants, oral antidiabetics, beta blockers, TCAs, MAOIs, and tetracycline increase the hypoglycemic effect when taken with insulin. Note that thiazides, glucocorticoids, oral contraceptives, thyroid drugs, and smoking can increase blood glucose.
- Assess the type of insulin and dosage. Note whether it is given once or multiple times a day.
- Note blood pressure (BP), heart rate, and blood glucose levels. Tachycardia and heart palpitations may occur with hypoglycemia, and hypotension may occur with hyperglycemia. Report abnormal findings.
- Determine the patient's knowledge of diabetes mellitus and use of insulins.
- Check for signs and symptoms of hypoglycemic reaction (insulin shock), hyperglycemia, or ketoacidosis.

Nursing Diagnoses

- Skin Integrity, Risk for Impaired
- Nutrition, Readiness for Enhanced related to excessive intake associated with metabolic need
- Injury, Risk for
- Knowledge, Deficient related to inexperience with insulin therapy

Planning

- The patient's blood glucose will be within normal values (70 to 99 mg/dL).
- The patient will self-administer insulin correctly.

Nursing Interventions

- Monitor vital signs. Tachycardia can occur during insulin reaction.
- Determine blood glucose levels (70 to 99 mg/dL) and report changes.
- Monitor the patient's HbA1c to provide feedback of diabetic control.

- Prepare a teaching plan based on the patient's knowledge of the health problem, diet, and drug therapy.

Patient Teaching
General

- ⚡ Teach patients to recognize and immediately report symptoms of *hypoglycemic* (insulin) reaction—such as headache, nervousness, sweating, tremors, rapid pulse—and those of *hyperglycemic* reaction (diabetic acidosis): thirst, increased urine output, and a sweet, fruity breath odor.
- Advise patients that hypoglycemic reactions are more likely to occur during peak action time. Most diabetic patients know whether they are having a hypoglycemic reaction, but some have a higher tolerance to low blood glucose and can have a severe reaction without realizing it.
- Explain that orange juice, sugar-containing drinks, and hard candy may be used when a hypoglycemic reaction begins.
- Teach family members to administer glucagon by injection if a patient has a hypoglycemic reaction and cannot drink sugar-containing fluid.
- Inform patients that certain herbs may interact with insulin and oral antidiabetic drugs. A hypoglycemic or hyperglycemic effect might occur (Complementary and Alternative Therapies 47.1).
- Teach patients about the necessity of compliance with prescribed insulin therapy and diet. HbA1c provides the most accurate picture of optimal diabetic control.
- ⚡ Advise patients to carry a MedicAlert card, tag, or bracelet that indicates the health problem and the insulin dosage.

Self-Administration

- Instruct patients on how to check blood glucose with a glucometer (OneTouch AccuSure, GlucoSure, Accu-Chek).
- Teach patients about the care of insulin containers and syringes. Inform patients taking NPH insulin with regular insulin that regular insulin is drawn up before NPH insulin.

Diet

- Advise patients taking insulin to eat the prescribed diet on a consistent schedule. Diet information may be obtained from the ADA or from a nutritionist.

🌐 *Cultural Considerations*

- Provide additional instructions about insulin action, administration, reactions, and possible complications in the language the patient speaks and reads most easily.
- Determine whether follow-up by a community health nurse is needed to assist with a patient's compliance with insulin use and the prescribed diet and exercise regimen.

Evaluation

- Evaluate the effectiveness of insulin therapy by noting whether the blood glucose level is within the accepted range.
- Establish the patient's ability to perform self-care.
- Determine the patient's knowledge of the signs and symptoms of hypoglycemic or hyperglycemic reaction.

Oral Antidiabetic (Hypoglycemic) Drugs

First- and Second-Generation Sulfonylureas

Oral antidiabetic drugs, also called *oral hypoglycemics*, should be used by those with type 2 diabetes; persons with type 1 diabetes should not use them. Patients with type 2 diabetes have some degree of insulin secretion by the pancreas. The sulfonylureas, a group of antidiabetics chemically related to sulfonamides but lacking antibacterial activity, stimulate pancreatic beta cells to secrete more insulin. This increases the insulin cell receptors, which increases the ability of the cells to bind insulin for glucose metabolism.

The sulfonylureas are classified as first- and second-generation drugs. First-generation sulfonylureas are divided into short-, intermediate-, and long-acting antidiabetics. Tolbutamide is a first-generation, short-acting sulfonylurea; tolazamide is a first-generation, intermediate-acting sulfonylurea; and chlorpropamide is a first-generation, long-acting sulfonylurea.

Second-generation sulfonylureas increase the tissue response to insulin and decrease glucose production by the liver. They have greater hypoglycemic potency than the first-generation sulfonylureas. Effective doses for the second-generation drugs are lower than for the first-generation drugs; the second-generation drugs also have a longer duration of action and cause fewer side effects. The second-generation drugs also have less displacement potential from protein-binding sites by other highly protein-bound drugs, such as salicylates and warfarin, than do first-generation drugs. Second-generation sulfonylureas should *not* be used when liver or kidney dysfunction is present. A hypoglycemic reaction is more likely to occur in older adults.

Second-generation sulfonylureas include glimepiride and glipizide, which directly stimulate the beta cells to secrete insulin, thus decreasing the blood glucose level. Glimepiride improves postprandial glucose levels and may be used in combination with insulin in persons with type 2 diabetes. Side effects include GI disturbances such as nausea, vomiting, diarrhea, and abdominal pain.

Table 47.4 lists the sulfonylureas and their dosages, uses, and considerations. Prototype Drug Chart 47.2 lists the pharmacologic data for the second-generation sulfonylurea glipizide.

Pharmacokinetics Glipizide is well absorbed from the GI tract and is highly protein bound. Glipizide is metabolized by the liver. The primary metabolites are inactive and are excreted mainly in urine.

Pharmacodynamics Glipizide is the most common sulfonylurea drug prescribed for type 2 diabetes mellitus. It lowers blood glucose by stimulating pancreatic beta cells to secrete insulin. The onset of action usually occurs within 90 minutes, and the peak action time is between 2 and 3 hours. Glipizide is normally given once a day in the morning because of its long duration of action of 24 hours.

Side Effects, Adverse Reactions, and Contraindications. The side effects of most oral antidiabetic drugs are similar to those of insulin. Taking antidiabetic drugs without adequate food can lead to an insulin reaction with signs and symptoms such as nervousness, tremors, and confusion. Adverse reactions include hematologic disorders such as aplastic anemia, leukopenia, and thrombocytopenia. Weight gain, seizures, and coma may also occur. Sulfonylureas are contraindicated in type 1 diabetes (no functioning beta cells), diabetic ketoacidosis, pregnancy, and lactation and during stress, surgery, or severe infection.

The major side effect of sulfonylureas is hypoglycemia. Acarbose does *not* cause hypoglycemia unless it is taken with a sulfonylurea or insulin, but it can cause increased flatulence (gas), diarrhea, and abdominal distension.

Drug Interactions. Aspirin, oral anticoagulants, MAOIs, sulfonamides, cimetidine, and some nonsteroidal antiinflammatory drugs (NSAIDs) can increase the action of sulfonylureas, especially first-generation ones, by binding to plasma proteins and displacing sulfonylureas. Because this causes increased free sulfonylurea, an insulin reaction can result. The action of sulfonylureas is decreased by concurrent administration of thiazide diuretics, isoniazid, phenytoin, and corticosteroids. Patients should be alerted not to drink alcohol while taking sulfonylureas because alcohol increases the half-life, and a hypoglycemic reaction can result.

Nonsulfonylureas

Expanding knowledge of glucose metabolism has revealed new mechanisms for the management of type 2 diabetes. The drugs metformin and acarbose use different methods to control serum glucose levels following a meal. Unlike the sulfonylureas, which enhance insulin release and receptor interaction, these drugs affect the hepatic and GI production of glucose.

Biguanides: Metformin

Metformin is a biguanide compound that acts by decreasing hepatic production of glucose from stored glycogen. This diminishes the increase in serum glucose following a meal and blunts the degree of postprandial hyperglycemia. Metformin also decreases the absorption of glucose from the small intestine, and there is evidence that it increases insulin receptor sensitivity as well as peripheral glucose uptake at the cellular level. Unlike sulfonylureas, metformin does *not* produce hypoglycemia or hyperglycemia, although it can cause GI disturbances.

Metformin is 51% to 60% bioavailable and is absorbed primarily from the small intestine. It does not undergo hepatic

! TABLE 47.4   Antidiabetics

Drug	Route and Dosage	Uses and Considerations
First-Generation Sulfonylureas: Short Acting		
Tolbutamide	A: PO: Initially 1-2 g/d; maint: 250-2000 mg/d in 1-3 divided doses; *max:* 3000 g/d	For managing type 2 diabetes mellitus. May cause headache, dysgeusia, pyrosis, hypoglycemia, weight gain, weakness, dizziness, fatigue, and blurred vision. Pregnancy category: C*; PB: 98%; t½: 4.5-6.5 h
First-Generation Sulfonylureas: Intermediate Acting		
Tolazamide	A: PO: Initially 100-250 mg/d with breakfast; *max:* 1 g/d	For managing type 2 diabetes. May cause weakness, fatigue, dizziness, headache, blurred vision, weight gain, and hypoglycemia. Pregnancy category: C*; PB: 94%; t½: 7 h
First-Generation Sulfonylureas: Long Acting		
Chlorpropamide	A: PO: Initially 250 mg/d; *max:* 750 mg/d	For managing type 2 diabetes. Avoid administration to older adults. May cause headache, dizziness, blurred vision, hypoglycemia, and weight gain. Pregnancy category: C*; PB: 60%-90%; t½: 25-60 h
Second-Generation Sulfonylureas		
Glipizide	See Prototype Drug Chart 47.2.	
Glyburide	A: PO: Initially 2.5-5 mg/d conventional form, 1.5-3 mg/d micronized; maint: 1.25-20 mg/d conventional, 0.75-12 mg/d micronized; *max:* 20 mg/d for conventional, 12 mg/d for micronized	For managing type 2 diabetes. May cause dizziness, hypoglycemia, weight gain, blurred vision, and diarrhea. Pregnancy category: C*; PB: 99%; t½: 10 h
Glimepiride	A: PO: Initially 1-2 mg/d with breakfast; maint: 1-4 mg/d ac; *max:* 8 mg/d	For managing type 2 diabetes. May cause dizziness, weakness, headache, blurred vision, hypoglycemia, and nausea. Pregnancy category: C*; PB: 99.5%; t½: 5-9 h
Nonsulfonylureas		
Biguanides		
Metformin	See Prototype Drug Chart 47.3.	
Alpha-Glucosidase Inhibitors		
Acarbose	A: PO: Initially 25 mg tid with first bite of each meal; maint: 50-100 mg tid; *max:* 150 mg/d if <60 kg, 300 mg/d if >60 kg	For managing type 2 diabetes mellitus. May cause flatulence, elevated hepatic enzymes, diarrhea, and abdominal pain. Pregnancy category: B*; PB: UK; t½: 2 h
Miglitol	A: PO: Initially 25 mg tid with first bite of each meal; *max:* 100 mg tid	For managing type 2 diabetes. May cause flatulence, diarrhea, and abdominal pain. Pregnancy category: B*; PB: <4%; t½: 2 h
Thiazolidinediones (Insulin-Enhancing Agents)		
Pioglitazone hydrochloride	A: PO: 15-30 mg/d; *max:* 45 mg/d	For managing type 2 diabetes. Contraindicated for patients with class III and IV CHF. May cause headache, blurred vision, dizziness, infection, fluid retention, peripheral edema, HF, weight gain, flatulence, diarrhea, URI, and UTI. Pregnancy category: C*; PB: 99%; t½: 3-7 h
Rosiglitazone	A: PO: Initially 4 mg/d; *max:* 8 mg/d	For managing type 2 diabetes. Contraindicated for patients with class III and IV CHF. May cause headache, blurred vision, dizziness, weight gain, pulmonary and peripheral edema, HF, abdominal pain, nausea, diarrhea, bone fractures, and infection. Pregnancy category: C*; PB: 99.8%; t½: 3-4 h
Meglitinides		
Repaglinide	A: PO: Initially 0.5-2 mg ac tid/qid; *max:* 16 mg/d	For managing type 2 diabetes. May cause headache, hypoglycemia, infection, diarrhea, and back pain. Pregnancy category: C*; PB: 98%; t½: 1 h
Nateglinide	A: PO: 60-120 mg tid ac; *max:* 360 mg/d	For managing type 2 diabetes. May cause dizziness, infection, peripheral edema, back pain, elevated hepatic enzymes, diarrhea, and hypoglycemia. Pregnancy category: C*; PB: 98%; t½: 1.5 h
Dipeptidyl Peptidase 4 Inhibitors		
Sitagliptin phosphate	A: PO: 100 mg/d; *max:* 100 mg/d	For managing type 2 diabetes. May cause headache, nasopharyngitis, infection, and peripheral edema. Pregnancy category: B*; PB: 38%; t½: 12.4 h
Saxagliptin	A: PO: 2.5-5 mg/d; *max:* 5 mg/d	For managing type 2 diabetes. May cause headache, hypoglycemia, nasopharyngitis, infection, and oral ulceration. Pregnancy category: B*; PB: 0%; t½: 2.5 h
Linagliptin	A: PO: 5 mg/d; *max:* 5 mg/d	For managing type 2 diabetes. May cause headache, hypoglycemia, diarrhea, nasopharyngitis, and arthralgia. Pregnancy category: B*; PB: 70%-80%; t½: 12 h

! TABLE 47.4   Antidiabetics—cont'd

Drug	Route and Dosage	Uses and Considerations
Alogliptin	A: PO: 25 mg/d; *max*: 25 mg/d	For managing type 2 diabetes. May cause headache, hypoglycemia, nasopharyngitis, diarrhea, elevated hepatic enzymes, and HF. Pregnancy category: B*; PB: 20%; t½: 21 h
Selective Sodium-Glucose Transporter 2		
Canagliflozin	A: PO: 100 mg/d before first meal; *max:* 300 mg/d	For managing type 2 diabetes. May cause infections, candidiasis, hyperkalemia, hyperlipidemia, diuresis, cystitis, and vaginitis. Pregnancy category: C*; PB: 99%; t½: 10.6-13.1 h
Dapagliflozin	A: PO: 5 mg/d in the morning; *max*: 10 mg/d	For managing type 2 diabetes. May cause nasopharyngitis, candidiasis, cystitis, and hypoglycemia. Pregnancy category: C*; PB: 91%; t½: 12.9 h
Empagliflozin	A: PO: 10 mg/d in the morning; *max*: 25 mg/d	For managing type 2 diabetes. May cause infection, candidiasis, cystitis, vaginitis, hypercholesterolemia, and hypoglycemia. Pregnancy category: C*; PB: 86.2%; t½: 12.4 h
Amylin Analogue		
Pramlintide	Type 1: A: Subcut: Initially 15 mcg ac, then 30-60 mcg; *max*: 120 mcg/dose Type 2: A: Subcut: Initially 60 mcg ac, then 60-120 mcg; *max*: 120 mcg/dose	For managing types 1 and 2 diabetes as an adjunct to insulin therapy. Decreases postmeal glucagon and glucose. Give subcutaneously in abdomen and thigh immediately before each major meal. Never administer in the arm; absorption is unpredictable. May cause headache, dizziness, fatigue, pharyngitis, anorexia, nausea, vomiting, abdominal pain, and hypoglycemia. Pregnancy category: C*; PB: 40%; t½: 48 min
Glucagon-Like Peptide 1 Agonists		
Exenatide	Regular release: A: Subcut: 5 mcg bid within 60 min before morning and evening meals; *max*: 20 mcg/d Extended release: A: Subcut: 2 mg/wk	For managing type 2 diabetes. Exenatide suppresses glucagon secretion. May be given in the abdomen, arm, or thigh. May cause headache, restlessness, fatigue, GI distress, constipation, hypoglycemia, and injection site reaction. Pregnancy category: C*; PB: UK; t½: 2.4 h
Liraglutide	A: Subcut: 0.6 mg/d for 1 wk, then 1.2-1.8 mg/d	For managing type 2 diabetes and obesity. Monitor patients closely for thyroid C-cell tumors. May cause injection site reaction, headache, fatigue, hypoglycemia, GI distress, constipation, and tachycardia. Pregnancy category: C*; PB: 98%; t½: 12-13 h
Dulaglutide	A: Subcut: 0.75 mg/wk; *max*: 1.5 mg/wk	For managing type 2 diabetes. May cause GI distress, fatigue, tachycardia, and hypoglycemia. Pregnancy category: C*; PB: UK; t½: 5 d
Albiglutide	A: Subcut: 30 mg/wk; *max*: 50 mg/wk	For managing type 2 diabetes. May cause infection, dyspepsia, diarrhea, injection site reaction, arthralgia, back pain, and hypoglycemia. Pregnancy category: C*; PB: UK; t½: 5 d
Fixed-Combination Oral Antidiabetic Drugs		
Glyburide-metformin	A: PO: Initially 1.25/250 mg (glyburide/metformin) once daily or bid ac; increase dose at 2-wk intervals; maint: 2.5/510 mg/d or 5/510 mg/d or bid ac; *max:* 20/2000 mg/d	For managing type 2 diabetes. May be used when glucose is not controlled with either drug alone. Contraindicated for patients with renal insufficiency because of risk for lactic acidosis. May cause GI distress and hypoglycemia. Pregnancy category: B*; PB: 0%-99%; t½: 6.2-17.6 h
Sitagliptin-metformin	A: PO: Initially sitagliptin 50 mg, metformin 500 mg bid; *max*: sitagliptin 100 mg, metformin 2000 mg/d	For managing type 2 diabetes. May cause headache, metallic taste, dyspepsia, nasopharyngitis, infection, peripheral edema, and weight loss. Pregnancy category: B*; PB: 0%-38%; t½: 6.2-17 6 h
Linagliptin-metformin	A: PO: Initially linagliptin 2.5 mg/metformin 500 mg bid with meals; *max*: 5 mg linagliptin, 2000 mg metformin	For managing type 2 diabetes. May cause dizziness, dyspepsia, diarrhea, flushing, nasopharyngitis, and vitamin B12 deficiency. Pregnancy category: B*; PB: 0%-80%; t½: 6.2-17.2 h
Dapagliflozin-metformin	A: PO: Initially 5 mg dapagliflozin, 500 mg metformin/d; *max*: 10 mg dapagliflozin, 2000 mg metformin	For managing type 2 diabetes. May cause headache, metallic taste, GI distress, infection, candidiasis, dyspnea, myalgia, nasopharyngitis, and vitamin B12 deficiency. Pregnancy category: C*; PB: 0%-91%; t½: 6.2-17.6 h
Empagliflozin-metformin	A: PO: Individualize doses bid with meals; *max*: 25 mg empagliflozin, 2000 mg metformin	For managing type 2 diabetes. May cause GI distress, candidiasis, UTI, hypercholesterolemia, and vitamin B12 deficiency. Pregnancy category: C*; PB: 0%-86.2%; t½: 6.2-17.6 h

*Pregnancy categories have been revised. See http://www.fda.gov/Drugs/DevelopmentApprovalProcess/DevelopmentResources/Labeling/ucm093 307.htm for more information.

A, Adult; *ac,* before meals; *bid,* twice a day; *CHF,* congestive heart failure; *d,* day; *GI,* gastrointestinal; *h,* hour; *HF,* heart failure; *maint,* maintenance; *max,* maximum; *min,* minute; *PB,* protein binding; *PO,* by mouth; *qid,* four times a day; *subcut,* subcutaneous; *t½,* half-life; *tid,* three times a day; *UK,* unknown; *URI,* upper respiratory infection; *UTI,* urinary tract infection; *wk,* week; *>,* greater than; *<,* less than.

PROTOTYPE DRUG CHART 47.2
❶ Glipizide

Drug Class	Dosage
Glipizide: Sulfonylurea, second generation Pregnancy category: C*	Regular release: A: PO: Initially 2.5-5 mg/d ac; maint: 10-15 mg/d; *max:* 40 mg/d Extended release: A: PO: 5-10 mg/d; *max:* 20 mg/d
Contraindications	**Drug-Lab-Food Interactions**
Diabetic ketoacidosis, sulfonamide hypersensitivity *Caution:* Hepatic or renal dysfunction, older adults, debilitated or mal- nourished patients, adrenal or pituitary insufficiency, type 1 diabetes, trauma, infection	Drug: Alcohol may produce disulfiram-like reaction (flushing, headache, sweating, nausea, violent vomiting, weakness). Beta blockers, systemic azole antifungals, clarithromycin, oral anticoagu- lants, MAOIs, atypical antipsychotics, salicylates, probenecid, sulfonamides, antacids, cimeti- dine, clofibrate, and phenylbutazone may potentiate hypoglycemia. Oral contraceptives, thiazide diuretics, glucocorticoids, phenothiazines, and anticonvulsants may enhance hyperglycemia. Lab: Altered liver function tests Food: Green tea may potentiate hypoglycemia.
Pharmacokinetics	**Pharmacodynamics**
Absorption: Rapidly absorbed from GI tract Distribution: PB: 99% Metabolism: t½: 2-4 h Excretion: Primarily in urine	Regular release: PO: Onset: 90 min Peak: 2-3 h Duration: 12-24 h Extended release: PO: Onset: UK Peak: 6-12 h Duration: UK

Therapeutic Effects/Uses
To control hyperglycemia in type 2 diabetes mellitus
Mode of Action: Directly stimulates beta cells in the pancreas to secrete insulin; indirectly alters sensitivity of peripheral insulin receptors, allowing increased insulin
binding

Side Effects	Adverse Reactions
Drowsiness, dizziness, headache, confusion, blurred vision, anxiety, hyperhidrosis, dyspepsia, flatulence, nausea, vomiting, constipa- tion, diarrhea, disulfiram-like reaction, tremor, weight gain	Hypoglycemia, hyponatremia *Life threatening:* Agranulocytosis, leukopenia, thrombocytopenia

*Pregnancy categories have been revised. See http://www.fda.gov/Drugs/DevelopmentApprovalProcess/DevelopmentResources/Labeling/ucm093307.htm for more information.
A, Adult; *ac,* before meals; *d,* day; *GI,* gastrointestinal; *h,* hour; *maint,* maintenance; *MAOI,* monoamine oxidase inhibitor; *max,* maximum; *min,* minute; *PB,* protein binding; *PO,* by mouth; *t½,* half-life; *UK,* unknown.

metabolism and is eliminated unchanged in the urine. It is not recommended for patients with renal impairment. Monotherapy with metformin is effective; however, when combined with a sulfonylurea, the drug is useful in cases that are resistant to oral antidiabetics (hypoglycemics). Metformin therapy should be withheld for 48 hours before and after administration of IV contrast because lactic acidosis or acute renal failure may develop.

Alpha-Glucosidase Inhibitors: Acarbose and Miglitol
Acarbose acts by inhibiting the digestive enzyme in the small intestine that is responsible for the release of glucose from complex carbohydrates in the diet. By inhibiting alpha glucosidase, absorption of complex carbohydrates is delayed. Acarbose has no demonstrated systemic effects and is not absorbed into the body in significant amounts. It does not cause a hypoglycemic reaction. Acarbose is intended for use in patients who do not achieve results with diet alone. Miglitol, like acarbose, inhibits alpha glucosides. Miglitol is absorbed from the GI tract. This drug will not cause hypoglycemia, but if taken with a sulfonylurea or insulin, hypoglycemia could occur.

Thiazolidinediones
Pioglitazone and rosiglitazone are examples of thiazolidinedione drugs. Both drugs are contraindicated in class III and IV heart failure due to dose-related fluid retention. These two drugs can be prescribed as monotherapy or combined with other oral antidiabetic drugs. Pioglitazone can be taken in combination with sulfonylurea or insulin, and rosiglitazone may be combined with metformin (Prototype Drug Chart 47.3). These drugs do not induce hypoglycemic reactions if taken alone; they decrease insulin resistance and improve blood glucose control.

Meglitinides
Repaglinide and nateglinide are classified as meglitinide oral antidiabetic agents. They stimulate the beta cells to release insulin. The action of repaglinide and nateglinide is similar to that of sulfonylureas. These agents can be used alone or in combination with metformin for patients with type 2 diabetes mellitus; they are short-acting antidiabetic drugs. Repaglinide and nateglinide should *not* be prescribed for patients with liver dysfunction because of a possible decreased liver metabolism rate; more of the drug could remain in the body, which could cause a hypoglycemic reaction.

PROTOTYPE DRUG CHART 47.3

 Metformin

Drug Class	Dosage
Metformin: Biguanide Pregnancy category: B*	Regular release: A: PO: Initially 500 mg bid or 850 mg/d with meals; increase dose gradually; *max:* 2550 mg/d Extended release: A: PO: 500 mg/d with evening meal; *max:* 2500 mg/d
Contraindications Hypersensitivity, diabetic ketoacidosis, radiographic contrast administration, renal dysfunction *Caution:* Pregnancy, lactation, children, concurrent infection, hepatic dysfunction, cardiopulmonary insufficiency, alcoholism	**Drug-Lab-Food Interactions** Drug: ACE inhibitors, ARBs, calcium channel blockers, beta blockers, procainamide, quinidine, digoxin, MAOIs, furosemide, alcohol, cimetidine, ranitidine, oral contraceptives, sulfonamides, azole antifungals, trimethoprim, vancomycin, and quinine may potentiate hypoglycemia. Nicotine, triamterene, thiazide diuretics, niacin, phenytoin, phenothiazines, and atypical antipsychotics may cause hyperglycemia. Lab: Altered liver function tests Food: Green tea may lead to hypoglycemia.
Pharmacokinetics Absorption: 51%-60% absorbed Distribution: PB: 0% Metabolism: t½: 6.2-17.6 h Excretion: Primarily in urine	**Pharmacodynamics** PO: Onset: UK Peak: Regular release 2.5 h; extended release 4-8 h Duration: UK
Therapeutic Effects/Uses To control hyperglycemia in type 2 diabetes mellitus Mode of Action: Increases binding of insulin to receptors, improves tissue sensitivity to insulin, increases glucose transport to skeletal muscles and fatty tissues, decreases glucose production in the liver by reducing gluconeogenesis, and reduces glucose absorption from intestines	
Side Effects Dizziness, headache, flushing, metallic taste, hyperhidrosis, weakness, dyspepsia, nausea, vomiting, flatulence, diarrhea, weight loss	**Adverse Reactions** Lactic acidosis; vitamin B12 deficiency, palpitations, hypoglycemia, elevated liver enzymes, infection *Life threatening:* Lactic acidosis

*Pregnancy categories have been revised. See http://www.fda.gov/Drugs/DevelopmentApprovalProcess/DevelopmentResources/Labeling/ucm093307.htm for more information.
A, Adult; *ACE*, angiotensin-converting enzyme; *ARB*, angiotensin II–receptor blocker; *bid*, twice daily; *d*, day; *h*, hour; *MAOI*, monoamine oxidase inhibitor; *max*, maximum; *PB*, protein binding; *PO*, by mouth; *t½*, half-life; *UK*, unknown.

Incretin Modifier

The oral antidiabetics sitagliptin phosphate and saxagliptin are classified as *incretin modifiers*, also called *dipeptidyl peptidase 4 (DPP-4) inhibitors* and *gliptins*, for treatment of type 2 diabetes mellitus. The action of DPP-4 inhibitors is to increase the level of incretin hormones, increase insulin secretion, and decrease glucagon secretion to reduce glucose production. This incretin modifier is used as an adjunct treatment with exercise and diet to reduce both fasting and postprandial plasma glucose levels.

Guidelines for Oral Antidiabetic (Hypoglycemic) Therapy for Type 2 Diabetes

The following are criteria for the use of oral antidiabetic drugs:

- Onset of diabetes mellitus at age 40 years or older
- Diagnosis of diabetes within the past 5 years
- Normal weight or overweight
- Fasting blood glucose of 200 mg/dL or less
- Fewer than 40 units of insulin required per day
- Normal renal and hepatic function

NURSING PROCESS
Patient-Centered Collaborative Care
Oral Antidiabetics

Assessment

- Identify drugs the patient currently takes. Aspirin, alcohol, sulfonamides, oral contraceptives, and monoamine oxidase inhibitors (MAOIs) increase the hypoglycemic effect; a decrease in oral antidiabetic drug may be needed. Glucocorticoids (cortisone), thiazide diuretics, and estrogen increase blood glucose.
- Note vital signs and blood glucose levels, and report abnormal findings.
- Determine the patient's knowledge of diabetes mellitus and use of oral antidiabetics.

Nursing Diagnoses

- Injury, Risk for
- Nutrition, Readiness for Enhanced related to excessive food intake

- Knowledge, Deficient related to lack of exposure to teaching about taking adequate food with oral antidiabetics

Planning

- The patient's blood glucose will be within normal serum levels (70 to 110 mg/dL).
- The patient will adhere to a prescribed diet, blood testing, and drug regimen.
- The patient will demonstrate knowledge of oral hypoglycemics and their importance.

Nursing Interventions

- Determine vital signs. Oral antidiabetics increase cardiac function and oxygen consumption, which can lead to cardiac dysrhythmias.
- Administer oral antidiabetics with food to minimize gastric upset.
- Monitor blood glucose levels, and report changes. Reference value is 60 to 100 mg/dL for blood glucose and 70 to 110 mg/dL for serum glucose.
- Prepare a teaching plan based on the patient's knowledge of health problems, diet, and drug therapy.

Patient Teaching
General

- Advise patients that a hypoglycemic (insulin) reaction can occur when taking an oral hypoglycemic drug, especially sulfonylureas. Such drugs stimulate the release of insulin from beta cells of the pancreas. Oral antidiabetics are not insulin. Normally, patients with diabetes mellitus type 1 do not have functioning beta cells and should not take oral antidiabetics, only insulin. Sulfonylureas are prescribed for patients with diabetes mellitus type 2.
- ⚡ Teach patients to recognize symptoms of a hypoglycemic reaction—headache, nervousness, sweating, tremors, and rapid pulse—and hyperglycemic reaction, which includes thirst; increased urine output; and a sweet, fruity breath odor.
- Explain that insulin might be needed instead of an oral antidiabetic drug during stress, surgery, or serious infection. Blood glucose levels are usually elevated during stressful times.
- Tell patients about the necessity for compliance with a diet and drug regimen.
- ⚡ Advise patients to carry a MedicAlert card, tag, or bracelet that indicates their health problem and the antidiabetic dosage.

Self-Administration

- Teach patients how to check blood glucose levels with a glucometer. Patients should record and report abnormal results.

Side Effects

- Advise patients to report side effects such as vomiting, diarrhea, and rash.

Diet

- ⚡ Caution patients not to ingest alcohol with antidiabetic drugs to avoid a hypoglycemic reaction.
- Advise patients taking oral antidiabetics to eat the prescribed diet on schedule. Delaying or missing a meal can cause hypoglycemia.
- Explain the use of orange juice, sugar-containing drinks, or hard candy when a hypoglycemic reaction begins. Explain the importance of reporting such problems to a health care provider.
- Direct patients to take oral antidiabetics with food to decrease gastric irritation.

🌐 Cultural Considerations

- Respect patients' cultural beliefs and alternative methods for treating diabetes and elevated blood glucose levels. Discuss the safety of methods and use of oral antidiabetic drugs to correct the problem (an interpreter may be necessary). If a patient takes an oral antidiabetic drug to decrease the blood glucose level, emphasize the importance of checking levels daily or as indicated. A hypoglycemic reaction can result from increased doses of oral antidiabetic agents and insufficient dietary intake.

Evaluation

- Evaluate the effectiveness of drug therapy by noting whether blood glucose levels are within the accepted range.
- Determine the patient's knowledge of the diabetic regimen.

Other Antidiabetic Agents

Exenatide and liraglutide are in a classification of antidiabetic drugs known as *incretin mimetics,* also called *glucagon-like peptide 1 (GLP-1) agonists.* These drugs improve beta-cell responsiveness, which improves glucose control in people with type 2 diabetes mellitus. The actions of exenatide and liraglutide are to enhance insulin secretion, increase beta-cell responsiveness, suppress glucagon secretion, slow gastric emptying, and reduce food intake. Exenatide and liraglutide are not a substitute for insulin and should not be administered to patients with type 1 diabetes mellitus, diabetic ketoacidosis, severe renal dysfunction, or severe GI disease. Common adverse effects that occur with exenatide include headache, dizziness, jitteriness, nausea, vomiting, and diarrhea. Exenatide is administered by injectable prefilled pens in twice-a-day dosing and has significantly improved HbA1c levels and weight loss in many patients. Liraglutide is given subcutaneously once a day.

Pramlintide acetate is another antidiabetic agent in a classification called *amylin analogues,* approved by the U.S. Food and Drug Association (FDA) for adults with type 1 and type 2 diabetes mellitus. The primary purpose of pramlintide is to improve postprandial glucose control in diabetic patients who are using insulin but are unable to achieve and maintain glucose control. The actions of pramlintide are to suppress glucagon secretion, slow gastric emptying, and modulate appetite by inducing satiety. Suppression of glucagon secretion reduces postprandial hepatic glucose for approximately 3 hours. By slowing gastric emptying, the absorption rate of glucose is reduced; satiety promotes reduced food intake. Common adverse effects include dizziness, anorexia, nausea, vomiting, and fatigue. Pramlintide is administered by subcutaneous injection before meals in the abdomen or thigh; it is never given in the arm.

Hyperglycemic Drugs
Glucagon
Glucagon is a hyperglycemic hormone secreted by alpha cells of the islets of Langerhans in the pancreas. Glucagon increases blood glucose by stimulating glycogenolysis (glycogen breakdown) in the liver. It protects the body cells, especially those in the brain and retina, by providing the nutrients and energy needed to maintain body function.

Glucagon is available for parenteral use (subcutaneous, intramuscular [IM], and IV). It is used to treat insulin-induced hypoglycemia when other methods of providing glucose are not available. For example, the patient may be semiconscious or unconscious and unable to ingest sugar-containing products. Patients with diabetes who are prone to severe hypoglycemic reactions (insulin shock) should keep glucagon in the home, and family members should be taught how to administer subcutaneous or IM injections during an emergency hypoglycemic reaction. The blood glucose level begins to increase within 10 minutes after administration.

Diazoxide
Oral diazoxide, which is chemically related to thiazide diuretics, increases blood glucose by inhibiting insulin release from the beta cells and stimulating release of epinephrine from the adrenal medulla. This drug is *not* indicated for hypoglycemic reaction, rather it is used to treat hypoglycemia caused by hyperinsulinism.

Diazoxide has a long half-life and is highly protein bound. Its onset of action is 1 hour, and the duration of action is 8 hours. Most of the drug is excreted unchanged in urine.

CRITICAL THINKING CASE STUDY

TC, a 32-year-old patient, was diagnosed with diabetes mellitus after the birth of her first child; her blood glucose level was 180 mg/dL. Her serum glucose level has been maintained within the normal range with metformin 500 mg/day.

1. Why was TC, at 32 years of age, taking an oral antidiabetic drug instead of insulin?
2. Metformin is indicated for what type of diabetes mellitus? When should metformin not be taken?
3. Why should TC monitor her blood glucose using a home glucometer?

Two years later, TC became pregnant again. Metformin was discontinued, and NPH insulin 25 units was prescribed.

Since the birth of her second child, she has remained on NPH 25 units/day.

4. Give a possible reason why the health care provider changed the antidiabetic drug to insulin when TC became pregnant.
5. What are examples of human insulin and what are its advantages?
6. How should insulin be administered?
7. What is NPH and what are the pros and cons for TC to receive NPH 70/regular 30 insulin?
8. What are the signs and symptoms of hypoglycemic reaction?
9. What should be included in patient teaching?

NCLEX STUDY QUESTIONS

1. A patient is diagnosed with type 2 diabetes mellitus. The nurse is aware that which statement is true about this patient?
   a. The patient is most likely a teenager.
   b. The patient is most likely a child younger than 10 years.
   c. Heredity and obesity are major causative factors.
   d. Viral infections contribute most to disease development.
2. Antidiabetic drugs are designed to control signs and symptoms of diabetes mellitus. The nurse primarily expects a decrease in which?
   a. Blood glucose
   b. Fat metabolism
   c. Glycogen storage
   d. Protein mobilization

3. A patient is to receive insulin before breakfast, and the time of breakfast tray delivery is variable. The nurse knows that which insulin should not be administered until the breakfast tray has arrived and the patient is ready to eat?
   a. NPH
   b. Lispro
   c. Glargine
   d. Regular
4. A patient is receiving a daily dose of NPH insulin at 7:30 am. The nurse expects the peak effect of this drug to occur at what time?
   a. 8:15 am
   b. 10:30 am
   c. 5:00 pm
   d. 11:00 pm

5. A patient is prescribed glipizide. The nurse knows that which side effects and adverse effects may be expected? (Select all that apply.)
   a. Tachypnea
   b. Tachycardia
   c. Increased alertness
   d. Increased weight gain
   e. Visual disturbances
   f. Hunger

6. A nurse is teaching a patient how to recognize symptoms of hypoglycemia. Which symptoms should be included in the teaching? (Select all that apply.)
   a. Headache
   b. Nervousness
   c. Bradycardia
   d. Sweating
   e. Thirst
   f. Sweet breath odor

7. A patient is newly diagnosed with type 1 diabetes mellitus and requires daily insulin injections. Which instructions should the nurse include in the teaching of insulin administration?
   a. Teach family members how to administer glucagon by injection when the patient has a hyperglycemic reaction.
   b. Instruct the patient about the necessity for compliance with prescribed insulin therapy.
   c. Teach the patient that hypoglycemic reactions are more likely to occur at the onset of action time.
   d. Instruct the patient in the care and handling of the insulin container and syringe.

Answers: 1, c; 2, a; 3, b; 4, c; 5, b, e, f; 6, a, b, d; 7, b, d.

Renal and Urologic Drugs

Unit XVI discusses agents prescribed to combat disease-producing microorganisms. Included in this unit are antiseptics, antibacterials, analgesics, stimulants, antispasmodics, antimuscarinics, anticholinergics, and other drugs for urinary tract disorders. Common disorders of the urinary tract are presented in this unit. Urinary tract infections, acute cystitis, and pyelonephritis are focused upon.

Disease-producing organisms may be gram-positive or gram-negative bacteria, viruses, or fungi. The degree to which they are pathogenic depends on the microorganism and its virulence. Chapter 48 addresses drugs for urinary tract disorders.

Fig. XVI.1 illustrates the various sites of infection in the upper and lower urinary tracts. Fig. XVI.2 illustrates the female and male urethra showing the female urethra being the shortest.

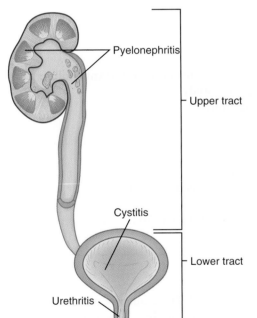

FIG. XVI.1 Sites of infectious processes in the upper and lower urinary tracts. From Lewis, S. L., Dirksen, S. R., Heitkemper, M. M., & Bucher, L. (2014). *Medical-surgical nursing: Assessment and management of clinical problems* (9th ed.). St. Louis: Elsevier.

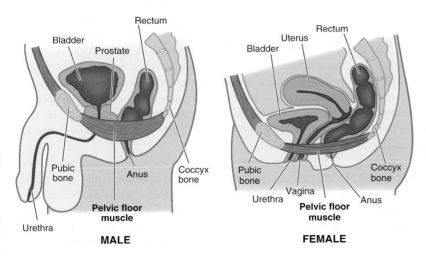

FIG. XVI.2 Shorter urethra in the female than in the male. From Lewis, S. L., Dirksen, S. R., Heitkemper, M. M., & Bucher, L. (2014). *Medical-surgical nursing: Assessment and management of clinical problems* (9th ed.). St. Louis: Elsevier.

48

Urinary Disorders

Ⓔ http://evolve.elsevier.com/McCuistion/pharmacology

OBJECTIVES

- Compare the groups of drugs that are urinary antiseptics and antiinfectives.
- Describe the side effects and adverse reactions to urinary antiseptics and antiinfectives.
- Differentiate the uses for a urinary analgesic, a urinary stimulant, and a urinary antispasmodic/antimuscarinic/anticholinergic.

- Apply the nursing process, including teaching, to nursing care of the patient receiving urinary antiseptic/antiinfective drugs.

OUTLINE

Urinary Antiseptics/Antiinfectives and Antibiotics
Nitrofurantoin
Nursing Process: Patient-Centered Collaborative Care—
    Urinary Antiinfective: Nitrofurantoin
Methenamine
Trimethoprim and Trimethoprim-Sulfamethoxazole
Fluoroquinolones (Quinolones)

Drug-Drug Interactions
Urinary Analgesics
Phenazopyridine
Urinary Stimulants
Urinary Antispasmodics/Antimuscarinics/Anticholinergics
Critical Thinking Case Study
NCLEX Study Questions

KEY TERMS

acute cystitis, p. 702
acute pyelonephritis, p. 702
antimuscarinics, p. 706
antispasmodics, p. 706
bactericidal, p. 702
bacteriostatic, p. 702

micturition, p. 706
urinary analgesics, p. 702
urinary antiseptics/antiinfectives, p. 702
urinary stimulants, p. 702
urinary tract infections (UTIs), p. 702

The largest number of urinary tract disorders is caused by **urinary tract infections (UTIs)**, microbial infections of any part of the urinary tract. The infection may be referred to as an *upper UTI*, such as pyelonephritis, or a *lower UTI*, such as cystitis, urethritis, or prostatitis. A group of drugs called **urinary antiseptics/antiinfectives** prevents bacterial growth in the kidneys and bladder, but these drugs are not effective for systemic infections. When given in lower dosages, urinary antiseptics/antiinfectives have a **bacteriostatic** effect—that is, they inhibit bacterial growth. When given in higher dosages, they also have a **bactericidal** (bacteria killing) effect. Urinary antiseptics/antiinfectives are presented in this chapter, along with **urinary analgesics**, which relieve pain and burning in the urinary tract; **urinary stimulants**, agents that increase the tone of urinary muscles; and urinary antispasmodics/antimuscarinics. Chapter 26 presents further discussions of antibiotics used to treat UTIs, such as fluoroquinolones and sulfonamides. Diuretics are discussed in Chapter 38.

Acute cystitis, a lower UTI, frequently occurs in female patients because of the short urethra. It is more common in women of childbearing age, older women, and young girls. Acute cystitis is commonly caused by *Escherichia coli* (also called *E. coli*). Other bacterial causes include the gram-positive *Staphylococcus saprophyticus* and gram-negative *Klebsiella*, *Proteus*, and *Pseudomonas* species. Symptoms of cystitis include pain and burning on urination and urinary frequency and urgency. A urine culture is usually obtained before the start of any antiinfective/antibiotic drug therapy. In male patients, a lower UTI is most likely prostatitis with symptoms similar to cystitis.

Acute pyelonephritis, an upper UTI, is commonly seen in women of childbearing age, older women, and young girls. *E. coli* is the most common organism to cause pyelonephritis. Symptoms include chills, high fever, flank pain, pain during urination, urinary frequency and urgency, and pyuria. The bacterial count in the urine is greater than 100,000 bacteria/

702

mL. In severe cases, the patient may be hospitalized and may receive intravenous (IV) antibiotics (e.g., an aminoglycoside or piperacillin-tazobactam).

The most commonly used agents for treating UTIs are nitrofurantoin and trimethoprim-sulfamethoxazole. Treatment may consist of a single double-strength dose of the chosen drug, a 3-day course, or the traditional method of 7 to 14 days of drug dosing. Fosfomycin tromethamine, a nitrofurantoin prototype drug, is effective for UTIs as a single-dose treatment. Other agents used to treat UTIs include third-generation cephalosporins (cefixime, cefpodoxime proxetil, or ceftibuten), fourth-generation cephalosporins (cefepime), fifth-generation cephalosporins (ceftolozane-tazobactam), and fluoroquinolones, such as ofloxacin, ciprofloxacin, and levofloxacin. For uncomplicated UTIs, fluoroquinolones, especially levofloxacin, may be used only when other options are not available. With severe UTIs, IV drug therapy followed by oral drug therapy is usually recommended.

URINARY ANTISEPTICS/ANTIINFECTIVES AND ANTIBIOTICS

Urinary antiseptics/antiinfectives are limited to the treatment of UTIs. Drug action occurs in the renal tubule and bladder, where it is effective in reducing bacterial growth. A urinalysis, as well as a culture and sensitivity test, is usually performed before the initiation of drug therapy. As bactericidal agents, these drugs have the potential to cause superinfections. The urinary antiseptics/antiinfectives are fosfomycin tromethamine, nitrofurantoin, methenamine hippurate, trimethoprim, ertapenem, and the fluoroquinolones.

Nitrofurantoin

Nitrofurantoin was first prescribed to treat UTIs in 1953. It is bacteriostatic or bactericidal, depending on the drug dosage, and it is effective against many gram-positive and gram-negative organisms, especially *E. coli*. It is used to treat cystitis and UTIs.

Pharmacokinetics Nitrofurantoin is well absorbed from the gastrointestinal (GI) tract. The drug is usually taken with food to decrease GI distress, which includes anorexia, nausea, vomiting, abdominal pain, and diarrhea. Decreased absorption occurs when the drug is taken with antacids. Nitrofurantoin is moderately protein bound. With normal renal function, the drug is rapidly eliminated because of its short half-life of 20 minutes; however, it accumulates in the serum with urinary dysfunction.

Pharmacodynamics When nitrofurantoin is given in low doses for prophylactic use, the drug has a bacteriostatic effect. However, higher concentrations of nitrofurantoin cause a bactericidal effect, and it is effective against many gram-positive and gram-negative organisms such as *E. coli*, *Staphylococcus aureus*, streptococci, and *Neisseria* and *Klebsiella* species. The onset and duration of action are unknown. Peak action occurs 30 minutes after absorption. If sudden onset of dyspnea, chest pain, cough, fever, and chills develops, the patient should contact the health care provider. Symptoms resolve after discontinuing the drug.

The nursing process for nitrofurantoin is applicable to the other urinary antiseptics/antiinfectives.

◎ NURSING PROCESS
Patient-Centered Collaborative Care
Urinary Antiinfective: Nitrofurantoin

Assessment
- Obtain a history from the patient of clinical problems with UTI, incontinence, or other urinary tract disorders.
- Assess the patient for signs and symptoms of UTI: pain or burning sensation on urination and frequency and urgency of urination.
- Monitor complete blood count (CBC) regularly in patients on long-term therapy.
- Monitor urine culture and sensitivity results.
- Assess renal and hepatic function.
- Determine urine pH. A pH of 5.5 is desired, but alkalinization of the urine is not recommended.

Nursing Diagnoses
- Pain, Acute related to inflammation in the urinary tract
- Infection, Risk for

Planning
- The patient will be free of signs and symptoms of UTI within 10 days.

Nursing Interventions
- Monitor urinary output and urine specific gravity. Careful attention to output is required when administering urinary antiseptics to patients with anuria and oliguria. Report promptly any decrease in urine output.
- Obtain urine culture to identify infecting organism before initiation of drug therapy to treat UTI.
- Observe the patient for side effects and adverse reactions to urinary antiseptic drugs. Peripheral neuropathy (tingling, numbness of extremities) may result from renal insufficiency (inability to excrete drug) or long-term use of nitrofurantoin. Peripheral neuropathy may be irreversible.

Patient Teaching
General
- Teach patients not to crush tablets or open capsules.
- Advise patients to rinse the mouth thoroughly after taking oral nitrofurantoin. The drug can stain teeth.
- Encourage patients to avoid antacids because they interfere with drug absorption.
- Teach patients to shake suspensions well before administration and to protect them from freezing.
- ⚡ Warn patients not to drive a motor vehicle or operate dangerous machinery; the drug may cause drowsiness.
- Advise female patients to immediately report pregnancy to their health care provider.

Diet
- Inform patients to increase fluids and take the drug with food to minimize GI upset.

Side Effects
- Advise the patient to drink an adequate amount of fluids.

- Encourage the patient to report any signs of secondary fungal or bacterial infection (superinfection) such as stomatitis or anogenital discharge or itching.

Nitrofurantoin
- Alert the patient that urine may turn a harmless brown color.
- Direct the patient to report a sudden onset of dyspnea, chest pain, cough, fever, and chills to health care provider.

Methenamine
- Educate patients to drink cranberry juice, eat plums, or take vitamin C (with approval of the health care provider) to keep urine acidic. Foods that are alkaline, such as milk and some vegetables, may increase urine pH. Urine pH should be less than 5.5 for the antiseptic to be effective.

Fluoroquinolones
- ⚡ Warn patients to avoid operating hazardous machinery or driving a car while taking the drug, especially if dizziness is present.
- Encourage patients to take the drug with food and to avoid antacids because they interfere with drug absorption.
- Direct patients to report any signs of superinfection or secondary fungal or bacterial infection.

Trimethoprim and Trimethoprim-Sulfamethoxazole
- Tell patients to avoid excessive exposure to sunlight when taking nitrofurantoin.

🌐 *Cultural Considerations*
- Alleviate fears or concerns of patients from different cultural backgrounds. Use culturally consistent communication when explaining the treatment regimen for a UTI. An interpreter may be necessary. The use of pamphlets in the language the patient reads or speaks most easily can facilitate patient understanding.

Evaluation
- Evaluate the effectiveness of the urinary antiinfectives in alleviating UTI. The patient should be free of side effects and adverse reactions to the drug.

Methenamine

Methenamine produces a bactericidal effect when the urine pH is less than 5.5. It is effective against gram-positive and gram-negative organisms, especially *E. coli, Enterococcus* and *Proteus* species, and *Pseudomonas aeruginosa*. It is used for chronic UTIs. Methenamine should not be taken with sulfonamides because crystalluria is likely to occur. Methenamine is absorbed readily from the GI tract, and approximately 90% of the drug is excreted in the urine unchanged. Methenamine forms ammonia and formaldehyde in acid urine, therefore the urine needs to be acidified to exert a bactericidal action. Cranberry juice (several 8-ounce glasses per day), ascorbic acid, and ammonium chloride can be taken to decrease the urine pH.

Trimethoprim and Trimethoprim-Sulfamethoxazole

Trimethoprim can be used alone for the treatment of UTIs, but it is usually used in combination with a sulfonamide, sulfamethoxazole (the combined generic preparation is called *TMP-SMZ*), to prevent the occurrence of trimethoprim-resistant organisms. This drug combination produces slow-acting bactericidal effects against most gram-positive and gram-negative organisms, especially strains of *S. aureus,* including methicillin-resistant *S. aureus* (MRSA), and also *Shigella* and *Proteus* species. TMP-SMZ is discussed further in Chapter 26 and it is used in the treatment and prevention of acute and chronic UTIs. The amount of TMP-SMZ in the prostatic fluid is about two to three times greater than the amount in the vascular fluid. The half-life of TMP-SMZ is normally 6 to 12 hours, but it is longer in patients with renal dysfunction.

Fluoroquinolones (Quinolones)

Fluoroquinolones are one of the groups of urinary antibacterials that are effective against strains of *Acinetobacter, Chlamydia, Clostridium, Klebsiella, Staphylococcus,* and *Streptococcus* species that cause lower UTIs; they include ciprofloxacin, ofloxacin, and levofloxacin. Fluoroquinolones should be reserved for patients who have no alternative treatment options due to their harsh adverse reactions of tendon rupture, peripheral neuropathy, central nervous system effects, and exacerbation of myasthenia gravis. The drug dosage must be decreased when renal dysfunction is present. The half-lives of these drugs are ordinarily 2 to 8 hours, but half-lives are prolonged in patients with renal dysfunction. Table 48.1 lists the urinary antiseptics/antiinfectives and their dosages, uses, and considerations. Due to the serious adverse reactions of fluoroquinolones, they are used with caution for complicated UTIs and acute pylonephritis and levofloxacin is only used for uncomplicated UTIs when no other options are available. Levofloxacin is illustrated in Prototype Drug Chart 26.6.

Side Effects and Adverse Reactions

Nitrofurantoin. Side effects of nitrofurantoin include GI disturbances such as anorexia, nausea, vomiting, diarrhea, and abdominal pain and pulmonary reactions such as dyspnea, chest pain, and cough.

Methenamine. Methenamine has side effects that include nausea, dysuria, hematuria, and crystalluria.

Trimethoprim-Sulfamethoxazole. GI symptoms such as anorexia, nausea, and vomiting and skin problems such as rash and pruritus can accompany trimethoprim-sulfamethoxazole use.

Fluoroquinolones. Side effects of ciprofloxacin and ofloxacin include headaches, photosensitivity, dizziness, nausea, vomiting, diarrhea, visual impairment, rash, and pruritus. Serious adverse reactions include peripheral neuropathy, tendinitis, and tendon rupture. Fluoroquinolones may exacerbate muscle weakness in patients with myasthenia gravis. Direct patients to stop taking fluoroquinolones immediately if experiencing serious adverse reactions and notify health care provider.

Drug-Drug Interactions

The following drug-drug interactions can occur with the use of urinary antiseptics/antiinfectives:
- Antacids decrease nitrofurantoin absorption.
- Sodium bicarbonate inhibits the action of methenamine.
- Methenamine taken with sulfonamides increases the risk of crystalluria.
- Most urinary antiseptics cause false-positive Clinitest (glucose urine test) results.

TABLE 48.1 Antiseptics and Urinary Antiinfectives

Generic Name	Route and Dosage	Uses and Considerations
Fosfomycin tromethamine	A/Females: PO: 3-g packet dissolved in 4 oz water as a single dose	For cystitis and UTIs in females. May cause headache, vaginitis, nausea, and diarrhea. Pregnancy category: B*; PB: 0%; t½: 2.9-8.5 h
Methenamine hippurate	A/Adol: PO: 1 g qid pc and at bedtime; *max:* 2 g/d Adol/C 6-12 y: PO: 0.5 g qid; *max:* 2 g/d	For cystitis and UTIs. May cause crystalluria, rash, nausea, vomiting, hematuria, urinary frequency, and elevated hepatic enzymes. Encourage fluids. Pregnancy category: C*; PB: UK; t½: 4 h
Nitrofurantoin	A: PO: 50-100 mg q6h with meals and at bedtime for 3-7 d; *max:* 7 mg/kg/d Adol/C/infants >1 mo: PO: 5-7 mg/kg/d in 4 divided doses; *max:* 7 mg/kg/d	For cystitis and UTIs. May cause GI distress, chest pain, dyspnea, cough, peripheral neuropathy, rust or brown urine discoloration, dizziness, headache, and *Clostridium difficile*–associated diarrhea. Pregnancy category: B*; PB: 20%-60%; t½: 20 min
Trimethoprim	UTIs: A: PO: 100 mg q12h or 200 mg/d for 10-14 d; *max:* 20 mg/kg/d	For cystitis, UTIs, and otitis media. May cause hyperkalemia, hyponatremia, rash, pruritus, GI distress, crystalluria, fatigue, photosensitivity, and *Clostridium difficile*-associated diarrhea. Pregnancy category: C*; PB: 45%; t½: 8-10 h
Ertapenem	UTIs: A/Adol: IM/IV: 1 g/d for 10-14 d; *max:* 1 g/d C/infants >3 mo: IM/IV: 15 mg/kg bid for 7-14 d; *max:* 30 mg/kg/d	For UTIs; community-acquired pneumonia; and intraabdominal, skin, and diabetic foot infections. May cause headache, drowsiness, confusion, agitation, GI distress, anemia, and elevated hepatic enzymes. Pregnancy category: B*; PB: 95%; t½: 4.5 h
SULFONAMIDES		
Trimethoprim sulfa-methoxazole (TMP-SMZ)	UTIs: A: PO: TMP 160 mg, SMZ 800 mg q12h for 3-14 d; *max:* 20 mg/kg/d A/Adol/C 2 mo-17 y: IV: 8-10 mg/kg/d in 2-4 divided doses for 7-14 d; *max:* 960 mg/d TMP and 4800 mg/d SMZ See Prototype Drug Chart 26-7.	For cystitis, UTIs, bronchitis, otitis media, pneumonia, and gastroenteritis. May cause hypersensitivity, rash, pruritus, headache, insomnia, dizziness, nervousness, photosensitivity, seizures, hyperkalemia, GI distress, elevated hepatic enzymes, crystalluria, fatigue, myalgia, *Clostridium difficile*-associated diarrhea, and torsades de pointes. Pregnancy category: C/D*; PB: TMP, 44%; SMZ, 70%; t½: TMP, 8-10 h; SMZ, 6-12 h
QUINOLONES (FLUOROQUINOLONES)		
Ciprofloxacin	UTIs: Regular release: A/Females: PO: 250 mg q12h for 3 d; *max:* 1.5 g/d Extended release: A females: PO: 500-1000 mg/d for 3 d; *max:* 1 g/d A: IV: 200-400 mg q12h for 7-14 d; *max:* 1.2 g/d	For respiratory, urinary, skin, bone, joint, and anthrax infections. May cause headache, dizziness, corneal deposits, visual impairment, peripheral neuropathy, injection site reaction, tendinitis, tendon rupture, arthralgia, bone pain, myalgia, elevated hepatic enzymes, dysgeusia, GI distress, *Clostridium difficile*-associated diarrhea, seizures, and photosensitivity. Use with caution in patients with seizure disorders and dysrhythmias. Can be taken without food; antacids inhibit drug absorption. Avoid excessive exposure to sunlight. Pregnancy category: C*; PB: 20%-40%; t½: 4 h
Ofloxacin	UTIs: A: PO: 200 mg q12h for 3-10 d; *max:* 800 mg/d	For respiratory, urinary, and skin infections. May cause headaches, dizziness, dysgeusia, GI distress, *Clostridium difficile*-associated diarrhea, visual impairment, rash, pruritus, insomnia, peripheral neuropathy, tendinitis, and tendon rupture. Pregnancy category: C; PB: UK; t½: 4-8 h
OTHER		
Aztreonam	A: IM/IV: 500 mg to 1 g q8-12h; *max:* 8 g/d Adol/C/infants >9 mo: IM/IV: 30 mg/kg q6-8h; *max:* 120 mg/kg/d	For septicemia and intraabdominal, respiratory, skin, gynecologic, and urinary tract infections. May cause injection site reaction, neutropenia, elevated hepatic enzymes, fever, cough, wheezing, and nasal congestion. Pregnancy category: B*; PB: 56%-65%; t½: 1.7 h
Imipenem and cilastatin sodium	A: IV: 250-500 mg q6h; *max:* 4 g/d or 50 mg/kg/d, whichever is less	For respiratory, bone, intraabdominal, urinary, and joint infections; septicemia; and endocarditis. May cause nausea, diarrhea, seizures, thrombocytosis, eosinophilia, and elevated hepatic enzymes. Pregnancy category: C*; PB: imipenem, 20%; cilastatin, 40%; t½: 1 h
Polymyxin B sulfate	A/C: IV: 15,000-25,000 units/kg/d in divided doses q12h or as a continuous infusion; *max:* 25,000 units/kg/d A: IM: 25,000-30,000 units/kg/d; *max:* 2 million units/d	For meningitis; bacteremia; and ophthalmic, skin and urinary tract infections. May cause dizziness, drowsiness, weakness, blurred vision, headache, paresthesias, and renal impairment. Monitor renal function (BUN, serum creatinine). Pregnancy category: B*; PB: UK; t½: 4-6 h
Ceftazidime and avibactam	UTIs: A: IV: 2.5 g (ceftazidime 2 g and avibactam 500 mg) q8h over 2 h for 7-14 d; *max:* 7.5 g/d (6 g ceftazidime + 1.5 g avibactam)	For intraabdominal infections and UTIs. May cause nausea, constipation, abdominal pain, anxiety, dizziness, and renal impairment. Pregnancy category: B*; PB: ceftazidime, 10%; avibactam, 5%-8%; t½: ceftazidime, 1.5-2 h; avibactam, 2 h
Ceftolozane and tazobactam	UTIs: A: IV: 1.5 g (1 g ceftolozane and 0.5 g tazobactam) q8h for 7 d; *max:* 4.5 g/d (3 g ceftolozane and 1.5 g tazobactam)	For intraabdominal infections and UTIs. May cause headache, nausea, vomiting, diarrhea, and fever. Pregnancy category: B*; PB: ceftolozane, 16%-21%; tazobactam, 30%; t½: 1-3 h

*Pregnancy categories have been revised. See http://www.fda.gov/Drugs/DevelopmentApprovalProcess/DevelopmentResources/Labeling/ucm093307.htm for more information.

A, Adult; *Adol,* adolescent; *bid,* twice a day; *BUN,* blood urea nitrogen; *C,* child; *d,* day; *GI,* gastrointestinal; *h,* hour; *IM,* intramuscular; *IV,* intravenous; *max,* maximum dosage; *min,* minute; *mo,* month; *PB,* protein binding; *pc,* after meals; *PO,* by mouth; *q,* every; *qid,* four times a day; *t½,* half-life; *UK,* unknown; *UTI,* urinary tract infection; *y,* year; *>,* greater than.

URINARY ANALGESICS

Phenazopyridine

Phenazopyridine hydrochloride, an azo dye, and dimethyl sulfoxide (also called DMSO) are urinary analgesics that are used to relieve the urinary pain, burning sensation, frequency, and urgency of urination that are symptomatic of cystitis. Phenazopyridine can cause GI disturbances such as abdominal cramps, hemolytic anemia, and renal and hepatic dysfunction. The urine becomes a harmless reddish orange because of the phenazopyridine dye. Phenazopyridine can alter the glucose urine test (Clinitest), therefore a blood test should be used to monitor glucose levels. Dimethyl sulfoxide may cause a garlic-like taste and skin hyperpigmentation.

URINARY STIMULANTS

When bladder function is decreased or lost as a result of (1) a neurogenic bladder (a dysfunction caused by a lesion of the nervous system), (2) a spinal cord injury (paraplegia, hemiplegia), or (3) a severe head injury, a parasympathomimetic may be used to stimulate micturition (urination). The drug of choice, bethanechol chloride, is a urinary stimulant also known as a *direct-acting parasympathomimetic*. The drug action is to increase bladder tone by increasing tone of the detrusor urinal muscle, which produces a contraction strong enough to stimulate urination. Bethanechol is discussed in detail in Chapter 16.

URINARY ANTISPASMODICS/ANTIMUSCARINICS/ANTICHOLINERGICS

Urinary tract spasms resulting from infection or injury can be relieved with antispasmodics that have a direct action on the smooth muscles of the urinary tract. This group of drugs—mirabegron, oxybutynin, and flavoxate—is contraindicated for use if urinary or GI obstruction is present or if the patient has glaucoma. Antispasmodics have the same effects as antimuscarinics, agents that block parasympathetic nerve impulses; parasympatholytics; and anticholinergics (see Chapter 16). Tolterodine tartrate, trospium chloride, and solifenacin succinate are antimuscarinic/anticholinergic drugs used to control an overactive bladder, which causes frequency in urination. These drugs also decrease urgency and urinary incontinence. Antispasmodics/antimuscarinics/anticholinergics frequently have side effects including blurred vision, headache, dizziness, dry mouth, constipation, and tachycardia. The patient taking these drugs should be taught to report urinary retention, severe dizziness, blurred vision, palpitations, and confusion. Table 48.2 lists drugs that are urinary analgesics, stimulants, and antispasmodics/antimuscarinics/anticholinergics.

TABLE 48.2	**Urinary Analgesics, Stimulants, and Antispasmodics**	
Generic	**Route and Dosage**	**Uses and Considerations**
URINARY ANALGESICS		
Phenazopyridine hydrochloride	A: PO: 200 mg tid pc; *max:* 600 mg/d	For cystitis, dysuria, and urgency. May cause headache, contact lens discoloration, reddish orange urine, renal and hepatic dysfunction, and hemolytic anemia. Do not use long term for undiagnosed urinary tract pain. Pregnancy category: B*; PB: UK; t½: UK
Dimethyl sulfoxide	Bladder instillation: 50 mL of 50% sol retained for 15 min; repeat q2wk until relief	For cystitis. May cause bladder discomfort and spasm, dysgeusia, skin hyperpigmentation, and anaphylactoid reactions. Pregnancy category: C*; PB: UK; t½: UK
URINARY STIMULANTS		
Bethanechol chloride	A: PO: 10-50 mg tid/qid 1 h ac or 2 h pc; *max:* 200 mg/d A: Subcut: 5 mg tid/qid PRN; *max:* 40 mg/d	For urinary retention and neurogenic bladder. Do not take if peptic ulcer is present. May cause GI distress, headache, dizziness, nephrotoxicity, and hepatotoxicity. Pregnancy category: C*; PB: UK; t½: UK
URINARY ANTISPASMODICS		
Flavoxate hydrochloride	A/Adol/C >12 y: PO: 100-200 mg tid/qid	For urinary urgency and incontinence, dysuria, and overactive bladder. Avoid in patients with glaucoma. Use with caution in older adults. May cause headache, nausea, vomiting, dry mouth, drowsiness, blurred vision, and tachycardia. Pregnancy category: B*; PB: UK; t½: UK
Oxybutynin chloride	A/Adol: PO: 5 mg bid/qid; *max:* 5 mg qid Older adults: PO: 2.5 mg bid/tid; *max:* 5 mg tid C >5 y: PO: 5 mg bid; *max:* 5 mg tid Extended release: A: PO: 5-10 mg/d; *max:* 30 mg/d C >6 y/Adol: 5 mg/d; *max:* 20 mg/d	For urinary incontinence, and neurogenic and overactive bladder. May cause drowsiness, dizziness, headache, insomnia, tachycardia, blurred vision, dry mouth, GI distress, and constipation. Cautious use for patients with GERD; cardiac, renal, hepatic, and prostate hypertrophy; and those who smoke tobacco or wear contact lenses. Pregnancy category: B*; PB: UK; t½: 2-5 h
Mirabegron	Extended release: A: PO: 25 mg/d; *max:* 50 mg/d	For urinary incontinence and overactive bladder. May cause headache, dizziness, dry mouth, nasopharyngitis, constipation, tachycardia, and hypertension. Pregnancy category: C*; PB: 71%; t½: 50 h

TABLE 48.2 Urinary Analgesics, Stimulants, and Antispasmodics—cont'd

Generic	Route and Dosage	Uses and Considerations
	ANTIMUSCARINICS/ANTICHOLINERGICS	
Tolterodine tartrate	A: PO: 1-2 mg bid; max: 4 mg/d Extended release: A: PO: 4 mg/d; max: 4 mg/d	For overactive bladder, and urinary urgency and incontinence. May cause headache, dizziness, confusion, blurred vision, dry mouth, diarrhea, constipation, and abdominal pain. Contraindicated in narrow-angle glaucoma and hepatic impairment. Pregnancy category: C*; PB: 96%; t½: regular release, 2-4 h; extended release, 6.9-18 h
Trospium chloride	A: PO: 20 mg bid; max: 60 mg/d Extended release: A: PO: 60 mg/d in the morning	For overactive bladder, urinary incontinence, and neurogenic bladder. May cause headache, blurred vision, dry mouth, and constipation. Pregnancy category: C*; PB: 48%-85%; t½: regular release, 20 h; extended release, 35 h
Solifenacin succinate	See Prototype Drug Chart 48.1.	
Darifenacin hydrobromide	Extended release: A: PO: Initially 7.5 mg/d, then in 2 wk 15 mg/d; max: 15 mg/d	For overactive bladder and urinary incontinence. May cause headache, dry mouth, dyspepsia, vomiting, and constipation. Pregnancy category: C*; PB: 98%; t½: 13-19 h

*Pregnancy categories have been revised. See http://www.fda.gov/Drugs/DevelopmentApprovalProcess/DevelopmentResources/Labeling/ucm093 307.htm for more information.
A, Adult; *ac,* before meals; *Adol,* adolescent; *bid,* twice a day; *C,* child; *d,* day; *GERD,* gastroesophageal reflux disease; *GI,* gastrointestinal; *h,* hour; *max,* maximum; *min,* minute; *PB,* protein binding; *pc,* after meals; *PO,* by mouth; *PRN,* as needed; *q,* every; *qid,* four times a day; *sol,* solution; *subcut,* subcutaneous; *t½,* half-life; *tid,* three times a day; *UK,* unknown; *wk,* week; *y,* year; *>,* greater than.

PROTOTYPE DRUG CHART 48.1

Solifenacin Succinate

Drug Class	**Dosage**
Urinary antimuscarinic, anticholinergic, bladder antispasmodic Pregnancy category: C*	A: PO: Initially 5 mg/d, then up to 10 mg/d; max: 10 mg/d
Contraindications	**Drug-Lab-Food Interactions**
Hypersensitivity, glaucoma, gastroparesis, GI obstruction, urinary retention *Caution:* Alcoholism, angioedema, bradycardia, dysrhythmias, CAD, diabetes mellitus, GERD, heart failure, hypertension, breastfeeding, contact lenses	Drug: Antagonizes action of cisapride and metoclopramide; potentiates dysrhythmias and torsades de pointes with fluconazole, chlorpromazine, citalopram, droperidol, haloperidol, risperidone, azithromycin, and fluoroquinolones
Pharmacokinetics	**Pharmacodynamics**
Absorption: Well absorbed Distribution: PB: 98% Metabolism: t½: 55 h Excretion: Urine, feces	PO: Onset: UK Peak: 5 h Duration: UK
Therapeutic Effects/Uses	
To treat overactive bladder and urinary incontinence Mode of Action: Exerts selective muscarinic receptor antagonist effect on all muscarinic receptors; depresses voluntary and involuntary bladder contractions, salivary gland secretion, gastric ciliary muscle, and CNS	
Side Effects	**Adverse Reactions**
Blurred vision, dizziness, cough, pharyngitis, dry mouth, dysphonia, GI distress, constipation, urinary retention, peripheral edema	Palpitations, elevated hepatic enzymes, ocular hypertension *Life threatening:* Dysrhythmias, hyperkalemia

*Pregnancy categories have been revised. See http://www.fda.gov/Drugs/DevelopmentApprovalProcess/DevelopmentResources/Labeling/ucm093307.htm for more information.
A, Adult; *CAD,* coronary artery disease; *CNS,* central nervous system; *d,* day; *GERD,* gastroesophageal reflux disease; *GI,* gastrointestinal; *h,* hours; *max,* maximum dosage; *PB,* protein binding; *PO,* by mouth; *t½,* half-life; *UK,* unknown.

CRITICAL THINKING CASE STUDY

FL, a 29-year-old woman, has complained to her health care provider of painful urinary frequency and urgency. The patient has an elevated temperature. A urine specimen indicates that FL has a urinary tract infection (UTI). The health care provider prescribes trimethoprim-sulfamethoxazole (TMP-SMZ) double-strength tablets (trimethoprim 160 mg, sulfamethoxazole 800 mg) twice a day for 14 days.

1. What other information should the health care provider obtain from the patient?

2. Why was TMP-SMZ prescribed? Explain your answer.
3. What should the health care provider discuss with the patient in regard to taking the drug and its possible side effects? What other information should FL receive?
4. What is the recommended time for follow-up care for FL?
5. What other drugs might be used instead of TMP-SMZ? Would one urinary antiinfective drug be more effective than another? Explain your answer.

NCLEX STUDY QUESTIONS

1. A patient is taking nitrofurantoin. What will the nurse teach the patient?
   a. Expect the urine to turn blue.
   b. Keep the urine acidic by drinking milk.
   c. Rinse the mouth after taking oral nitrofurantoin to avoid staining teeth.
   d. Take an antacid with oral nitrofurantoin to avoid gastrointestinal distress.

2. A patient complains about a burning sensation and pain when urinating. Which urinary analgesic does the nurse suspect will be ordered?
   a. Tolterodine
   b. Oxybutynin
   c. Bethanechol
   d. Phenazopyridine

3. A patient is taking the urinary antiseptic methenamine for a urinary tract infection (UTI). The nurse understands that this drug should *not* be given concurrently with which other drug to avoid crystalluria?
   a. Ertapenem
   b. Ciprofloxacin
   c. Fosfomycin
   d. Trimethoprim-sulfamethoxazole

4. A patient is receiving solifenacin succinate. The nurse knows that this drug is used to treat which condition?
   a. Chronic cystitis
   b. Urinary tract stones
   c. Urinary tract infection
   d. Overactive bladder

5. The patient is taking tolterodine. The nurse plans to teach the patient to report which condition?
   a. Alkaline urine
   b. Urinary retention
   c. Excessive tearing
   d. Reddish orange urine

6. The nurse is caring for a patient who is taking nitrofurantoin. Which nursing interventions are appropriate for this patient? (Select all that apply.)
   a. Monitor urinary output and urine specific gravity.
   b. Monitor the patient for peripheral neuropathy.
   c. Advise the patient to take the medication on an empty stomach to enhance absorption.
   d. Warn the patient to avoid excess exposure to sunlight.
   e. Inform the patient that urine may turn a harmless brown color.

Answers: 1, c; 2, d; 3, d; 4, d; 5, b; 6, a, b, e.

Reproductive and Gender-Related Drugs

This unit comprises six chapters that focus on reproductive and gender-related drugs. Chapters 49 through 54 address pharmacologic treatments specifically associated with female health and disorders. Drugs used throughout the female reproductive cycle, which includes pregnancy and preterm labor, are comprehensively discussed in Chapter 49, Pregnancy and Preterm Labor. Chapter 50—Labor, Delivery, and Postpartum—provides pharmacologic treatments used before, during, and after delivery. Chapter 51, Neonatal and Newborn, focuses on the pharmacology available for infants. Chapter 52, Women's Reproductive Health, details the variety of oral contraceptive products and the drugs used to treat menopausal discomforts. Chapter 53, Men's Reproductive Health, describes androgens and anabolic steroids, antiandrogens, and other drugs related to male reproductive health and disorders. Chapter 54, Sexually Transmitted Infections, concludes this unit with a discussion of drugs used to treat specific reproductive health issues, including endometriosis, premenstrual syndrome, infertility, and sexually transmitted infections.

FEMALE REPRODUCTIVE PROCESSES

The uterus is a pear-shaped, hollow, highly muscular organ located in the pelvic cavity between the rectum and the bladder; it is connected to the vagina by the cervix (Fig. XVII.1). Three distinct layers compose the uterine wall: (1) the outer layer (perimetrium), (2) the muscular middle layer (myometrium), and (3) the inner mucosal layer (endometrium).

The myometrium is a network of involuntary (smooth) muscles divided into three layers; the muscles of each layer are configured in different patterns. For example, the outer muscles are arranged longitudinally to assist with cervical effacement (thinning and shortening) and to expel the fetus at the time of delivery. Muscles in the middle layer are arranged in a figure-8 design. These muscles are extremely important in the control of bleeding (hemostasis). Blood vessels are threaded throughout these muscles;

during uterine contractions, the vessels are compressed, creating a hemostatic effect. Circular muscle fibers are found in the area of the internal os and help control its sphincter. These circular muscles keep the fetus contained in the uterus for the normal gestational period. It is these muscles that stretch (dilate) the cervix to a diameter of 10 cm during labor. When all three muscle layers work together during labor, contractions cause cervical dilation and descent and delivery of the infant.

The Menstrual Cycle

The reproductive cycle is hormonally controlled by interactions between the endocrine and reproductive systems. The hypothalamus secretes gonadotropin-releasing hormone (Gn-RH), which stimulates the anterior pituitary gland to synthesize and release follicle-stimulating hormone (FSH) and luteinizing hormone (LH). These gonadotropins stimulate the ovaries to produce estrogen and progesterone, respectively.

In most women, the menstrual cycle lasts 28 days (range: 22 to 34 days). The ovarian hormones estrogen and progesterone regulate the cycle, which has three ovarian phases: (1) follicular, (2) ovulatory, and (3) luteal. Endometrial phases occur simultaneously with these ovarian phases.

The *follicular phase* occurs during days 1 to 14 of the cycle. Days 1 to 6 of this period constitute the *menstrual phase,* and days 7 to 14 constitute the *proliferative phase.* During the total 14-day period, FSH increases and follicles begin to mature within the ovary. One graafian follicle from the group matures and swells by days 10 to 13, ruptures on day 14, and releases the ovum to the fallopian tube. The *ovulatory phase* occurs around day 14 when the ovum is released. The *luteal phase* occurs around days 15 to 28 and includes the secretory phase of the endometrial cycle. During this period, estrogen and progesterone are produced by the ovarian corpus luteum (the ruptured graafian follicle), reaching peak levels 8 days into the phase. Changes occur in the endometrium for optimal implantation of a fertilized ovum. FSH and LH levels decrease, mediated by dopamine, norepinephrine, and serotonin. Estrogen and progesterone are withdrawn immediately before menstruation, and the endometrial prostaglandin level increases. The cycle begins anew with the follicular phase. In cycles that are nonovulatory, hormonal secretion of estrogen, FSH, and LH is erratic; there is also an alteration in the usual amount of progesterone. These physiologic alterations become the basis for planning and implementing pharmacologic interventions.

MALE REPRODUCTIVE PROCESSES

There are three male reproductive processes: (1) spermatogenesis, or sperm production; (2) regulation of male sexual functioning; and (3) sexual intercourse.

Male Reproductive Anatomy and Physiology

The anatomy of the male sexual organs is depicted in Fig. XVII.2. The external reproductive organs include the penis, scrotum,

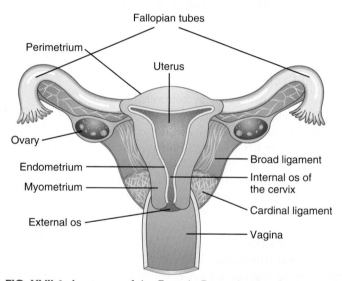

FIG. XVII.1 Anatomy of the Female Reproductive System.

and testes. The penis consists of three cylindrical bodies of erectile tissue: two corpora cavernosa and the corpus spongiosum. With sexual excitement, the vascular spaces fill with blood to produce an erection (Fig. XVII.3).

The scrotum has two compartments, each of which holds a testis, epididymis, and spermatic cord. The spermatic cord supports the testis and includes the vas deferens, blood vessels, nerves, and muscle fibers. Each testis contains seminiferous tubules in which spermatogenesis occurs; sperm then move into the epididymis, which leads into the vas deferens, the source of about 20% of ejaculate (semen). On either side of the prostate gland, a seminal vesicle empties seminal fluid into the ampulla. Seminal fluid contains prostaglandins, fibrinogen, fructose to provide energy for the sperm, and a sperm-activating factor.

The contents of the ampulla and the seminal vesicles empty into an ejaculatory duct that leads through the body of the prostate to empty into the urethra. Prostatic fluid, which constitutes about 20% of semen, empties from the prostate gland into the ejaculatory duct. The urethra carries semen to its distal end. The urethral glands along the length of the urethra and the bulbourethral glands near the prostatic end of the urethra supply the urethra with mucus. The bulbourethral glands secrete alkaline preejaculatory fluid to protect sperm from the acidity of the urethra.

Hormonal Regulation of Male Reproductive Functioning and Spermatogenesis

Gn-RH from the hypothalamus stimulates the anterior pituitary gland to secrete two major gonadotropins, LH and FSH, in both men and women. LH stimulates the interstitial Leydig cells of the testes to mature and produce testosterone. A direct relationship exists between the amount of circulating LH and the amount of testosterone produced. Testosterone is also produced to a lesser extent in the adrenal cortex and in the ovaries of women.

In men, FSH stimulates the Sertoli cells to begin conversion of spermatids into mature sperm. In addition, the Sertoli cells are stimulated to secrete estrogens, which may promote spermatogenesis. For spermatogenesis to be complete, testosterone

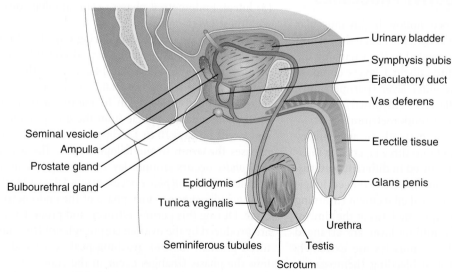

FIG. XVII.2 Anatomy of the Male Reproductive System.

must be secreted simultaneously by the Leydig cells and diffused into the seminiferous tubules.

Testosterone is the precursor of two classes of sex steroids: 5-alpha–reduced androgens and estrogens. The net effect of endogenous androgens is the sum of the effects of the 5-alpha–reduced metabolite dihydrotestosterone (DHT) and its estrogen derivative, estradiol. Most testosterone is loosely bound by plasma protein and circulates for 15 to 30 minutes before it is fixed to target tissues or metabolized. Most testosterone fixed to target cells is then converted to its active form, DHT.

The rate of testosterone production is controlled by a negative feedback loop. With increased testosterone, the hypothalamus decreases production of Gn-RH (Fig. XVII.4). With sperm production, the Sertoli cells release a hormone called *inhibin,* which suppresses FSH production by the anterior pituitary gland to maintain a constant rate of spermatogenesis. It is not known how the brain stimulates the hypothalamus before puberty to begin Gn-RH secretion, but if the brain is not intact, this may not occur.

Sexual Function

The human sexual response cycle consists of five phases: 1) desire, 2) excitement, 3) plateau, 4) orgasm, and 5) resolution. Sexual desire is the stimulus that causes an individual to initiate or be receptive to sexual activity. During the excitement phase, the man experiences penile erection; men are incapable of engaging in sexual intercourse without this arousal. The plateau

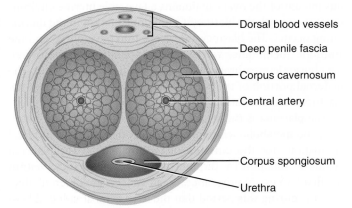

FIG. XVII.3 Erectile Tissue of the Penis.

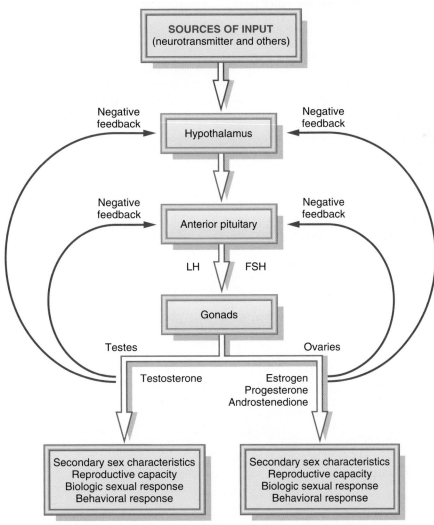

FIG. XVII.4 Hypothalamic-Pituitary-Gonadal Feedback Loops.

phase is characterized by genital enlargement, mucous secretion, generalized muscle tension, hyperventilation, tachycardia, and increased blood pressure. During the orgasmic phase, the vas deferens, seminal vesicles, ejaculatory duct, and penile urethra undergo multiple contractions over few seconds, which causes ejaculation. During resolution, there is a refractory period in which pelvic vasocongestion declines and generalized muscle relaxation takes place.

PROCESS OF FERTILIZATION

Fertilization, or conception, occurs when a sperm penetrates an ovum, usually in the distal third of the fallopian tube.

In a single ejaculation, between 200 and 400 million spermatozoa are deposited in the vagina. Sperm move up the female reproductive tract using the flagellar motion of their tails. It takes an average of 4 to 6 hours for the sperm to reach the distal fallopian tube. Semen contains prostaglandins that may enhance uterine motility to facilitate sperm migration. The ciliary action of the fallopian tubes enhances migration of the ovum to the uterus and of sperm toward the ovary.

Uterine enzymes capacitate the sperm by altering their glycoprotein coat. In an acrosomal reaction, the sperm release the enzyme hyaluronidase, which breaks through the outer layer of the ovum. The moment one sperm penetrates the ovum, a chemical reaction occurs that blocks other sperm from entering. Cellular division begins immediately in what is now called the *zygote,* or fertilized egg.

After 3 days, the zygote enters the uterus. It has now differentiated into an inner solid mass of cells, the blastocyst, and an outer layer, the trophoblast. Progesterone secreted by the corpus luteum of the ovary maintains a favorable uterine environment to nourish the blastocyst until implantation in the uterine lining occurs. The blastocyst develops into the embryo and the amniotic membrane, whereas the trophoblast develops into the chorionic membrane and the fetal side of the placenta. The maternal portion of the placenta develops under the site of the blastocyst's implantation.

The placenta is the structure through which oxygen, nutrients, and metabolic wastes pass between the maternal and fetal circulations for the duration of the pregnancy. The placenta begins to function by the fourth week of pregnancy. Within the first 8 weeks of pregnancy, organ systems are differentiated, and it is during this period that the fetus is most vulnerable to teratogens. Growth of the fetus throughout pregnancy depends on adequate oxygenation and nutrition, the metabolic environment, freedom from infection, and integrity of the mother's reproductive tract.

49

Pregnancy and Preterm Labor

http://evolve.elsevier.com/McCuistion/pharmacology/

OBJECTIVES

- Explain potential health-promoting and detrimental effects of substances ingested during pregnancy.
- Describe the drugs that alter uterine muscle contractility.
- Discuss drug therapy used during preterm labor to decrease the incidence or severity of neonatal respiratory dysfunction.
- Compare systemic and regional medications for pain control during labor.
- Describe the drugs used in gestational hypertension.
- Describe the nursing process, including patient teaching, associated with drugs used during pregnancy and preterm labor.

OUTLINE

KEY TERMS

PHYSIOLOGY OF PREGNANCY

Because pregnancy elicits many changes in the normal physiology of the body, the normal and expected pharmacokinetics and pharmacodynamics of drugs are also changed during pregnancy. Changes in drug action during pregnancy include the (1) effect of circulating steroid hormones on the liver's metabolism of drugs; (2) reduced gastrointestinal (GI) motility and increased gastric pH; (3) increased glomerular filtration rate and increased renal perfusion, resulting in more rapid renal excretion of drugs; (4) expanded maternal circulating blood volume, resulting in dilution of drugs; and (5) alteration in the clearance of drugs in later pregnancy, resulting in a decrease in serum and tissue concentrations of drugs. Because of alterations in the normal physiology of the body,

drugs should not be ordered in lower doses with longer intervals between doses because of the possibility of subtherapeutic serum concentrations.

Other factors, such as late pregnancy and labor, can alter the half-lives of some drugs. Antibiotics and barbiturates are examples of drugs that have shorter half-lives during pregnancy. In contrast to later pregnancy, labor can actually increase the half-life of some drugs (e.g., analgesics, hypnotics, antibiotics); it is believed that drug clearance decreases as a result of transient reduced blood flow associated with uterine contractions when the patient is in a supine position. There is also concern about the effects of certain disease states on medication usage during pregnancy. Disorders such as diabetes mellitus and gestational hypertension may result in decreased renal perfusion and subsequent drug accumulation.

The placenta plays an important role in drug use and metabolism. It was once thought that the placenta played a barrier role, but it is now known that the placenta has an important function as the organ of exchange for numerous substances, including drugs. It allows some substances to transfer quickly or slowly between mother and fetus, depending on variables such as (1) maternal and fetal blood flow; (2) molecular weight of the substance (low–molecular-weight substances cross more readily than do high–molecular-weight substances; most drugs have a low molecular weight, so they readily cross the placenta); (3) degree of ionization of the drug molecule (the more ionized the molecule, the less readily it crosses the placenta); (4) degree of protein binding (highly bound drugs do not cross readily); (5) metabolic activity of the placenta (the metabolic activity can biotransform molecules into active metabolites that can affect the fetus); and (6) maternal dose.

Guidelines for drug administration during pregnancy must include determination that the benefits of prescribing a drug outweigh potential short- or long-term risks to the maternal-fetal system. Careful selection and monitoring for the minimum effective dose for the shortest interval in the therapeutic range are required. Consideration must be given to alterations related to the physiologic changes of pregnancy.

Liver metabolism of drugs is much slower in the fetus as a result of immaturity of the liver, which can cause more evident or longer drug effects on the fetus than on the mother. The degree of fetal exposure to a drug and its breakdown products are more important to fetal outcome than the rate at which the drug is transported to the fetus.

The mechanisms by which drugs cross the placenta are analogous to the way in which drugs infiltrate breast tissue. Lactation results in increased blood flow to the breasts, and drugs accumulate in adipose breast tissue through simple diffusion. Long-term effects on infants from drugs in breast milk are unknown, but drugs that accumulate in breast milk are known, and the breastfeeding patient should be alerted to the potential accumulation.

Despite prenatal education, public service announcements, and information conveyed through the media, use of legal and illicit drugs by pregnant patients continues. Additionally, health care providers may prescribe drugs for maternal disorders that indirectly affect the fetus. It is estimated that half the drugs taken by pregnant patients are over-the-counter (OTC) drugs. The drugs most commonly ingested during pregnancy are iron supplements, vitamins, antiemetics, antacids, stool softeners, nasal decongestants, mild analgesics, and antibiotics. Although many drugs required by pregnant patients can be used safely, pregnant patients should be discouraged from using OTC drugs until they consult with their health care provider.

Drugs conclusively determined to be safe for the embryo are limited in number. Clinical trials can be resources for reliable drug information; however, it is unethical to test for the safety and efficacy of drugs in pregnant patients. Animal studies are required during drug testing, but the information obtained from such studies is difficult to extrapolate to humans. The U.S. Food and Drug Administration (FDA) recently changed its pregnancy category system to assist with safe prescribing for pregnant patients who require drugs. See http://www.fda.gov/Drugs/DevelopmentApprovalProcess/DevelopmentResources/Labeling/ucm093307.htm for more information.

There are many known **teratogens**, substances that cause developmental abnormalities. Timing, dose, and duration of exposure are crucial in determining the teratogenicity of a given drug. In humans, the teratogenic period begins 2 weeks after conception, before which the embryo is not susceptible to teratogenesis. After this 2-week point in fetal development, however, exposure to teratogens may result in either death of the embryo or minor cellular damage without congenital birth defects. Gestational week 2 through week 12 (first trimester) is the period of organogenesis, in which major structures and organs develop.

Table 49.1 shows adverse effects of selected illicit substances commonly used during pregnancy.

THERAPEUTIC DRUGS AND USE OF HERBS IN PREGNANCY

The most common indications for use of drugs during pregnancy are to supplement nutrition with iron, vitamins, and minerals and to treat nausea and vomiting, gastric acidity, and mild discomforts; however, caution must be exercised (Complementary and Alternative Therapies 49.1).

Iron

During pregnancy, approximately twice the normal amount of iron is needed to meet fetal and maternal daily requirements: 27 mg/day during pregnancy compared with 18 mg/day for nonpregnant women 19 to 30 years of age. Supplementation with iron is not generally necessary until the second trimester, when the fetus begins to store iron; the goal is to prevent maternal iron-deficiency anemia, *not* to supply the fetus. The fetus is adequately supplied through the placenta even though the mother is deficient. The greatest iron demand occurs in the third trimester: 22.4 mg/day, compared with 6.4 mg/day in the first trimester and 18.8 mg/day in the second trimester.

Although a normal diet generally provides the 18-mg recommended daily allowance (RDA) of iron for nonpregnant patients, pregnant patients at risk for anemia are usually instructed to supplement with 60 to 120 mg of elemental iron per day. The elemental iron content of the most common iron salts includes ferrous sulfate 20% (300 mg of ferrous sulfate is equivalent to 60 mg elemental iron), exsiccated ferrous sulfate 30%, ferrous gluconate 12%, and ferrous fumarate 33%. The estimated net iron cost of pregnancy is approximately 600 to 800 mg. This iron cost is due to the iron use by the fetus, placenta, and increased red blood cell (RBC) volume. Patients are advised to continue supplements for 6 weeks postpartum.

Pregnant patients generally have decreased hematocrit early in the third trimester. Those with levels below 30% will have their supplemental iron dosages increased, and a complete blood count (CBC) with platelet and ferritin will be measured. In those with true iron-deficiency anemia, response to iron supplementation is usually noted in 5 to 7 days with a modest

TABLE 49.1 General Adverse Effects of Substances Commonly Abused During Pregnancy

Substance	Maternal Effects	Fetal and Neonatal Effects*
Alcohol	1 oz twice a week increased risk for spontaneous abortion.	Fetal alcohol syndrome (FAS): mild to moderate mental retardation, altered facial features, growth retardation, low birthweight, small head circumference, hypotonia, and poor motor coordination. Full FAS seen only in some children; others display only fetal alcohol effect (FAE). Pregnancy category: There is no known safe amount of alcohol use during pregnancy†.
Caffeine	2 cups increase epinephrine concentrations after 30 min and decrease intervillous blood flow with potential for spontaneous abortion (dependent on amount and gestational period).	Excess consumption (>6-8 cups/d) likely toxic to embryo. Pregnancy category: C†
Cocaine	Clearance via urine is 72 h. Incidence of spontaneous abortion is increased in the first trimester. Continued use or sporadic use *is* related to premature delivery and abruptio placentae secondary to placental vasoconstriction and hyperextension.	In a newborn, renal clearance is 4-5 d because of liver immaturity and lack of cholinesterase. IUGR, decreased head circumference, and intrauterine cerebral infarction are also risks. Increased irritability, hyperreflexia, and tremulousness may occur along with deficient organization and interactive abilities. By month 4, the infant is still hypertonic, tremulous, and has impaired motor development. Studies suggest that subtle cognitive and behavioral impairments occur from the neonatal stage to adolescence. Pregnancy category: C†
Heroin	Heroin can cause first-trimester spontaneous abortion, premature delivery, and inadequate maternal caloric and protein intake.	Neonatal meconium aspiration syndrome; decreased weight and length through postnatal month 9, smaller head circumference at birth and during childhood development, impaired interactive abilities (hard to engage and console); inconsistent behavioral responses; increased tremulousness and irritability Pregnancy category: UK†
Cannabis	Studies show that women who use *Cannabis* during pregnancy are more likely to experience placental complications and to give birth to babies with lower birthweights.	Adverse fetal outcomes related to *Cannabis* use in pregnancy remain unclear. Incidence of meconium passage during labor is higher. Pregnancy category: X†.
Tobacco/nicotine	Degenerative placental lesions with areas of poor oxygen exchange; higher incidence of abruptio placentae and placenta previa; vaginal bleeding during pregnancy; possible PROM and possible amnionitis; less likely to choose to breastfeed	Short stature, smaller head and arm circumferences; no increase in mortality rate or congenital anomalies but some evidence of increased oral clefts; respiratory infections beyond the perinatal period were increased. Pregnancy category: C/D†
Methadone	Detoxification should be avoided during first trimester due to risk of spontaneous abortion and in the third trimester due to fetal stress and preterm labor.	Smaller weight and length through postnatal month 9 (catch up on weight and length occurs by 1 y); smaller head circumference (no catch-up); withdrawal-induced fetal distress occurs if the mother detoxifies after 32 weeks gestation. Pregnancy category: C†
Barbiturates	CNS depression; lethargy; sleepiness; mood alterations; impaired judgment; decreased fine motor skills. When taken during labor, drug may reduce the force and frequency of contractions, prolonging labor and delaying delivery. Selective anticonvulsant activity without anesthesia effects may warrant use in pregnancy for seizure disorders. Contraindicated with active labor and imminent delivery because no antagonist drug is available.	Rapidly cross placenta; with excessive use. High doses cause CNS depression, respiratory depression, hyperactivity, and decreased sucking reflex. Pregnancy category: D†
Tranquilizers	Effects are dose-dependent. Toxic reactions include ataxia, syncope, vertigo, and drowsiness. Tranquilizers are used to control acute eclamptic seizures during labor.	Benzodiazepine use in third trimester or labor in high doses is associated with hyperbilirubinemia, hypotonia, hypothermia, and poor sucking reflex. Effects may be enhanced if mother receives systemic analgesia. Fetal effects are prolonged. Pregnancy category: D†

*Children with prenatal drug exposure scored significantly lower on measures of language, school readiness skills, impulse control, and visual attention span/sequencing at age 5 years when compared with non–drug-exposed children from a comparable environment.
†Pregnancy categories have been revised. See http://www.fda.gov/Drugs/DevelopmentApprovalProcess/DevelopmentResources/Labeling/ucm093 307.htm for more information.
CNS, Central nervous system; *d,* day; *h,* hour; *IUGR,* intrauterine growth restriction; *min,* minute; *PROM,* premature rupture of fetal membranes; *UK,* unknown; *y,* year; *>,* greater than.

reticulocytosis and an increase in hemoglobin in 3 weeks. No teratogenic effects have been reported with physiologic doses. In contrast, increasing evidence has associated prenatal iron supplementation with glucose impairment and hypertension in midpregnancy. Many OTC and prescription iron products (Table 49.2) are available in varying dosages, which differ in the amount of elemental iron contained in the form of iron salts.

Adverse Reactions

Common side effects of iron supplements include nausea, constipation, black tarry stools, GI irritation, epigastric pain, vomiting, discoloration of urine, and diarrhea.

Nursing Implications

Liquid forms can cause temporary tooth discoloration and therefore should be diluted and administered through a straw. Iron supplements are best absorbed when administered with water or juice on an empty stomach. Vitamin C increases the absorption of iron. If gastric irritation does occur, administer the iron with food. Iron supplementation may inhibit the absorption of several drugs, and appropriate separation of doses should be followed (e.g., iron supplementation should be administered 2 hours before or 4 hours after antacids). Additional examples of drugs that may require separation in dose include levodopa, levothyroxine, methyldopa, penicillins, quinolones, and tetracyclines. For the same reasons, do not administer iron with milk, cereal, tea, coffee, or eggs.

Folic Acid

Folic acid supplementation as part of preconception planning improves the outcome of pregnancy. During pregnancy, folic acid (vitamin B9, folate) is needed in increased amounts. Folic acid deficiency early in pregnancy can result in spontaneous abortion or birth defects, especially neural tube defects; a failure of the embryonic neural tube to close properly can lead to spina bifida or skull and brain malformations. Deficiency of folic acid may also contribute to premature birth, low birthweight, and premature separation of the placenta (abruptio placentae). In the United States, approximately 4000 pregnancies a year are affected by neural tube defects (NTDs). Controlled clinical trials have demonstrated that folic acid supplementation can reduce this incidence by as much as 50%.

Normally, the RDA for folic acid is 180 mcg, but the U.S. Preventive Services Task Force recommends that women who are planning pregnancy take a supplement containing 0.4 mg to 0.8 mg of folic acid 1 month before and for the first 2 to 3 months after conception. The American Congress of Obstetricians and Gynecologists (ACOG) recommends that all women of childbearing age ingest 400 mcg of folic acid daily for birth defect prevention (during pregnancy, the RDA rises to 600 mcg). The reasoning behind the ACOG recommendation is the high incidence of unplanned and unrecognized pregnancies.

The neural tube closes within the first 4 weeks of pregnancy (18 to 26 days after conception), therefore it is important that women consume the recommended amounts of folic acid every day. For patients who have had a pregnancy that was affected by an NTD, higher doses of folic acid are recommended: 4 mg starting 1 to 3 months before conception.

The recommended amount should be ingested from folate-rich foods, such as dark green leafy vegetables, asparagus, papaya, strawberries, and oranges; from folate-enriched foods, such

COMPLEMENTARY AND ALTERNATIVE THERAPIES 49.1

Pregnancy

Herbal preparations are not generally recommended during pregnancy. In particular, the following herbs should be avoided:
- Feverfew and sage are emmenagogues that stimulate blood flow in the uterus.
- Kava decreases platelets.
- Dong-quai, garlic, and gingko biloba increase bleeding when used with anticoagulants.
- Ginseng may decrease the action of anticoagulants.
- St. John's wort has mutagenic effects on the cells of the developing embryo and fetus.
- Pennyroyal taken by mouth or applied to skin can be abortifacant.

TABLE 49.2   Iron Products

Generic	Route and Dosage	Uses and Considerations
Iron salts (ferrous sulfate, ferrous gluconate, ferrous fumarate) *Caution*: Read the label carefully. The amount of elemental iron differs according to the formulation.	PO: 27-100 mg/d of elemental iron Dose dependent on prepregnancy iron stores.	Hematinic for iron-deficiency anemia and prophylaxis for iron deficiency in pregnancy. Replaces iron stores needed for RBC development. Absorption PO is 5%-30% in intestines, therefore GI side effects may occur. Toxic reactions include pallor, hematemesis, shock, cardiovascular collapse, and metabolic acidosis. Contraindicated in patients with hypersensitivity or peptic ulcer. Decreased absorption of zinc, tetracycline and penicillamine and increased absorption with ascorbic acid, such as orange juice; decreased absorption with antacids, eggs, milk, coffee, and tea. Take at bedtime to avoid GI upset. Use straw for elixir to prevent staining of teeth, swallow tab/cap whole with full glass of water or juice, preferably on an empty stomach. Sit upright 30 min after dose to decrease reflux. Increase fluids, activity, and dietary bulk. Keep out of reach of children. Peak reticulocytosis: 5-10 d; hemoglobin values increase in 2-4 wk Pregnancy category A*; PB: UK; t½: UK; onset: 3-10 d; duration: 3-4 mo

*Pregnancy categories have been revised. See http://www.fda.gov/Drugs/DevelopmentApprovalProcess/DevelopmentResources/Labeling/ucm093307.htm for more information.

cap, Capsule; *d,* day; *GI,* gastrointestinal; *min,* minutes; *mo,* months; *PB,* protein binding; *PO,* by mouth; *RBC,* red blood cell; *t½,* half-life; *tab,* tablet; *UK,* unknown; *wk,* weeks.

as bread, rice, cornmeal, pasta, and cereal; and from supplementation because the amount of naturally occurring folic acid ingested in foods varies from day to day, and the folic acid from these sources is not well absorbed.

Adverse Reactions

Side effects of folic acid supplementation are uncommon but include allergic bronchospasm, rash, pruritus, erythema, and general malaise. Patients should be aware that folic acid supplementation may cause urine to turn more intensely yellow.

Multiple Vitamins

Prenatal vitamin preparations are routinely recommended for pregnant women. These preparations generally supply vitamins A, B-complex, B12, C, calcium, D, E, iron, and other minerals.

Inadequate nutrition cannot be rectified through supplements alone; vitamins are used most effectively by the body when taken with meals, and calories and protein are not supplied by supplements.

Large doses of vitamins and minerals above the recommended amounts do not improve health and may cause harm to the pregnant patient and fetus. Some vitamins and minerals can be teratogenic or toxic when taken in large amounts.

Drugs for Minor Discomforts of Pregnancy

Many complaints associated with pregnancy are related to the GI tract and include nausea and vomiting, heartburn, and constipation. The etiology of nausea and vomiting is unclear, although research suggests that it is probably related to an increase in human chorionic gonadotropin (hCG) levels during pregnancy. Increased progesterone during pregnancy, which relaxes smooth muscle, contributes to heartburn and constipation. The elevation in female sex hormones during pregnancy changes the motility of the GI tract, and the enlarging uterus displaces the bowel.

Nausea and Vomiting

Nausea and vomiting ("morning sickness") during early pregnancy are major complaints for about 88% of pregnant patients, but hyperemesis gravidarum—severe nausea and vomiting that may require hospitalization for hydration and nutrition—occurs with a much lower incidence (1% to 3%). Nonpharmacologic measures to decrease nausea and vomiting include (1) eating crackers, dry toast, or other carbohydrates before rising; (2) avoiding high-fat or highly seasoned foods; (3) eating small, frequent meals; (4) drinking fluids between, rather than with, meals; (5) drinking apple juice or flat soda between meals; (6) eating a high-protein bedtime snack; (7) stopping smoking; and (8) taking an iron supplement at bedtime. These measures work well for most patients, but if vomiting is severe, fluid replacement and pharmacologic measures may be necessary.

The FDA has approved pyridoxine hydrochloride and doxylamine succinate for treatment of morning sickness. Table 49.3 lists drugs used for management of nausea and vomiting during pregnancy with their dosages, uses, and considerations.

Many patients use ginger to help treat the nausea and vomiting associated with pregnancy. Studies suggest that ginger can be safely used in moderation, but as with all drugs and herbal supplements, encourage the pregnant patient to discuss use of ginger with her health care provider. Ginger can increase the risk for bleeding, particularly if the patient has a history of bleeding disorder.

Iron supplementation during pregnancy may add to the problems of nausea and vomiting. Taking these supplements with

TABLE 49.3 Drugs for Management of Nausea and Vomiting During Pregnancy*

Generic	Route and Dosage	Uses and Considerations
VITAMIN		
Pyridoxine (B6) (Also available as combination drug with doxylamine)	PO: Up to 25 mg tid	In the United States, B6 is the drug of choice for nausea and vomiting in pregnancy; it is a coenzyme for various metabolic functions, including metabolism of proteins, carbohydrates, and fats. Side effects are rare and include headache, nausea, somnolence, and sensory neuropathy. Pregnancy category: A[†]; absorbed in the jejunum, metabolized in the liver, excreted in urine. Peak plasma time: 5-6 h (pyridoxine); t½: 15-20 d
ANTIHISTAMINE PLUS VITAMIN B6 ANALOGUE		
Doxylamine succinate (10 mg)/ pyridoxine 10 mg	PO: 2 tabs at bedtime	Mechanism of Action: Competes with histamine for H₁ receptor sites on effector cells. Side effects include CNS depression, which may impair physical or mental ability. Patients must be cautioned about performing tasks that require mental alertness, like driving or operating machinery. Effects may be potentiated when used with other sedative drugs. Contraindicated in women with known hypersensitivity to doxylamine succinate or any other component of the drug. MAOIs intensify and prolong the adverse CNS effects. Has anticholinergic properties and should be used with caution in women with asthma, increased intraocular pressure, narrow-angle glaucoma, stenosing peptic ulcer, pyloroduodenal obstruction, and urinary bladder–neck obstruction. Not for use by nursing mothers. Pregnancy category: A[†]; primarily metabolized in the liver; excreted in the kidney; peak: 2-4 h; t½: 10-12 h

Continued

TABLE 49.3	Drugs for Management of Nausea and Vomiting During Pregnancy*—cont'd	
Generic	**Route and Dosage**	**Uses and Considerations**
	**PHENOTHIAZINES**	
Promethazine	PO/IV/IM/PR: 12.5-25 mg q4-6h PRN *Black Box Warning:* Regardless of route of administration, promethazine injections can cause severe tissue injury, including gangrene, necrosis, abscess, erythema, edema, severe spasms of distal vessels, phlebitis, sensory loss, and paralysis.	Blocks postsynaptic mesolimbic dopaminergic receptors in the brain; exhibits a strong α-adrenergic blocking effect and depresses release of hypothalamic and hypophyseal hormones; competes with histamine for H$_1$ receptor. Side effects include dizziness, drowsiness, excitation, fatigue, insomnia, photosensitivity reactions, nausea, vomiting, and constipation. Contraindicated in patients with CNS depression, or hypersensitivity to the drug or any component. Use caution in patients with cardiovascular disease; not recommended for subcut or intraarterial administration; injection may contain sulfites, which may cause allergic reaction. Pregnancy category: C[†]; t½: 9-16 h; onset: IM, 20 min; IV, 3-5 min; duration: 4-6 h, but may have effects up to 12 h

	**ANTICHOLINERGICS**	
Scopolamine	IM/IV/subcut: 0.32-0.65 mg 3-4 times/d	Antagonizes histamine and serotonin Side effects include confusion, drowsiness, headache, fatigue, dry skin, constipation, vomiting, and bloated feeling. Cardiovascular side effects include orthostatic hypotension, ventricular fibrillation, tachycardia, and palpitations. Contraindicated in patients with hypersensitivity to the drug or any component and those with narrow-angle glaucoma, acute hemorrhage, GI or GU obstruction, tachycardia secondary to cardiac insufficiency, and myasthenia gravis. Use with caution in patients with hepatic or renal impairment. Pregnancy category: C[†]; onset: IM, 0.5-1 h; duration, 4-6 h
	**PROKINETIC AGENTS**	
Metoclopramide	PO: 5-10 mg q8h	Blocks dopamine receptors in the CTZ; causes enhanced motility and accelerated gastric emptying without stimulating secretions Side effects include restlessness, drowsiness, diarrhea, weakness, insomnia, depression, and tardive dyskinesia. Contraindicated in patients with hypersensitivity to the drug or any component; GI obstruction, perforation, or hemorrhage; pheochromocytoma; or history of seizure disorder Pregnancy category: B[†]; onset: 0.5-1 h; duration: 1-2 h; t½: 4-7 h
	**OTHER**	
Trimethobenzamide	PO: 300 q6-8h PRN IM: 200 mg q6-8h	Inhibits medullary CTZ by blocking emetic impulses to the vomiting center. Contraindicated in patients with cardiac dysrhythmias, narrow-angle glaucoma, asthma, and pyloro-duodenal obstruction. Rectal doses of drug are more unpredictable. Side effects include drowsiness, headache, blurred vision, diarrhea, depression, hypotension, muscle cramps, allergic reaction, extrapyramidal symptoms, and blood dyscrasias. Contraindicated with benzocaine and in patients with hypersensitivity to trimethobenzamide. *Caution:* Do not use in patients with acute emesis to avoid masking symptoms. Drug interactions occur with phenothiazines, barbiturates, and belladonna. Pregnancy category: C [†]; onset: PO, 45 min; IM, 30 min; duration 3-4 h; t½: 7-9 h
Ondansetron	PO/IV: 4-8 mg 2-3 times/d It is recommended that ondansetron is only reserved for severe hyperemesis gravidarum or when conventional treatments are not effective (ACOG, 2004).	Antiemetic; selective 5-HT$_3$ receptor antagonist that blocks serotonin both peripherally on vagal nerve terminals and centrally in the CTZ. Side effects include headache, constipation, diarrhea, and malaise/fatigue. Contraindicated in patients with hypersensitivity to the drug or other selective 5-HT$_3$ antagonists *Caution:* Use as scheduled, not PRN. Use with caution in patients who have congenital/medical conditions that cause prolonged QT interval or who take medications that prolong QT interval. Drug interactions: Drugs that alter the activity of liver enzymes Pregnancy category: B[†]; onset: 30 min; duration: 4-8 h; t½: 3-6 h

*Recommendation not implied.

[†]Pregnancy categories have been revised. See http://www.fda.gov/Drugs/DevelopmentApprovalProcess/DevelopmentResources/Labeling/ucm093 307.htm for more information.

ACOG, American Congress of Obstetricians and Gynecologists; *CNS,* central nervous system; *CTZ,* chemoreceptor trigger zone; *d,* day; *GI,* gastro-intestinal; *GU,* genitourinary; *H$_1$,* histamine$_1$; *h,* hour; *IM,* intramuscular; *IV,* intravenous; *MAOI,* monoamine oxidase inhibitor; *min,* minute; *PO,* by mouth; *PR,* by rectum; *PRN,* as needed; *qid,* four times a day; *subcut,* subcutaneously; *t½,* half-life; *tabs,* tablets; *tid,* three times a day.

food or at bedtime may help decrease gastric distress. Prenatal vitamins should be taken at the time of day the patient is least likely to experience emesis because a high incidence of nausea and vomiting is associated with prenatal vitamins. For patients with continued iron-induced gastric distress, many health care providers recommend taking two children's chewable multivitamins with iron. Salting food to taste may help replace vomited chloride; foods rich in potassium and magnesium may also help replace lost nutrients.

Patients whose symptoms persist and who experience weight loss and dehydration may require intravenous (IV) rehydration, including replacement of electrolytes and vitamins. Antiemetic therapy (probably with phenothiazines) may be used, and ondansetron may be administered only in severe cases of hyperemesis gravidarum.

Heartburn

Heartburn, or *pyrosis,* is a burning sensation in the epigastric and sternal regions that occurs with reflux of acidic stomach contents, which occurs in approximately 80% of pregnant patients. *The normal increase in the hormone progesterone causes decreased motility of the GI tract during pregnancy.* Progesterone also relaxes the cardiac sphincter—the sphincter that leads into the stomach from the esophagus, also called the *lower esophageal sphincter*—making reflux activity, or *reverse peristalsis,* more likely. During pregnancy, digestion and gastric emptying are slower than in the nonpregnant state. Heartburn is common when a pregnant patient sits or lies down soon after eating a normal meal, only to have her gravid uterus exert upward pressure on her stomach, causing increased reflux activity and the perception of hyperacidity. Heartburn is a disorder of the second and third trimesters of pregnancy.

Nonpharmacologic measures are preferred in the management of heartburn. These include (1) limiting the size of meals; (2) avoiding highly seasoned or greasy foods; (3) avoiding gas-forming foods (e.g., cabbage, onions); (4) eating slowly and chewing thoroughly; (5) avoiding citrus juices; (6) drinking adequate fluids, but not with meals; and (7) avoiding reclining immediately after eating.

Antacids should be considered first-line therapy if the patient does not respond to nonpharmacologic therapy. The antacids of choice for the pregnant patient include nonsystemic low-sodium products (those considered dietetically sodium free) that contain aluminum and magnesium (in the form of hydroxide) in combination. Discourage long-term use or large doses of magnesium antacids because fetal renal, respiratory, cardiovascular, and muscle problems may result. Sucralfate is likely safe during pregnancy because the drug is not systemically absorbed. Calcium carbonate antacid preparations may be avoided in pregnancy because of the rebound effect following acid neutralization. Chewable calcium carbonate tablets are frequently taken by pregnant patients for heartburn, but because they are calcium based, excessive use may contribute to constipation.

Most patients do not realize that remedies commonly used by nonpregnant patients (e.g., baking soda, sodium bicarbonate) can be harmful during pregnancy. Selection of the wrong antacid can result in diarrhea, constipation, or electrolyte imbalance. A combination of nonpharmacologic measures and minimal use of safe antacids should effectively meet the pregnant patient's needs.

Liquid antacids are the preparations most commonly used in pregnancy because of their uniform dissolution, rapid action, and greater activity. Tablets are also acceptable, particularly for convenience, provided they are thoroughly chewed and the patient maintains adequate fluid intake.

Histamine$_2$ (H$_2$)-receptor antagonists can be used during pregnancy, but only if their use is recommended by a health care provider and initial treatment with antacids has failed. The teratogenicity of these medications is unknown. H$_2$-receptor antagonists work by competitively and reversibly binding to the histamine receptors of the parietal cells, causing a reduction in gastric acid secretion. The onset of action is generally in 1 hour and can persist for 6 to 12 hours.

There is even less experience with the use of proton pump inhibitors. These medications work to suppress gastric acid secretion by inhibiting the proton pump on the surface of the parietal cells. With the release of OTC omeprazole, pregnant patients may wonder about its use for heartburn during pregnancy. Encourage patients to discuss the options with their health care provider. Currently, the use of omeprazole in pregnancy is limited to cases in which the benefits of therapy far outweigh the risks.

Table 49.4 presents medications for heartburn commonly used during pregnancy.

Constipation

Constipation is a frequent occurrence during pregnancy. Its cause may be related to hormonal changes—specifically progesterone, which decreases GI motility. As with heartburn, nonpharmacologic treatments for constipation should be tried first. These include (1) increased fluid intake, (2) increased dietary fiber intake, and (3) moderate physical exercise. If these methods do not work, treatment is indicated, and the safest agents are bulk-forming preparations that contain fiber because they are not systemically absorbed. Also, docusate sodium, a stool softener, would be appropriate as first-line treatment during pregnancy. Agents that should be reserved for occasional use include milk of magnesia, magnesium citrate, lactulose, sorbitol, bisacodyl, and senna.

Castor oil should be avoided during pregnancy because it can stimulate uterine contractions. Mineral oil should also be avoided because it can reduce the absorption of fat-soluble vitamins such as vitamin K. Low levels of vitamin K in the neonate can result in hemorrhage.

Pain

Through week 26 of pregnancy, headaches that result from hormonally induced body changes, sinus congestion, or eye strain are quite common. It is not unusual for the pregnant patient to experience backaches, joint pains, round ligament pain (resulting in mild abdominal aches and twinges), and pain from minor injuries. Nonpharmacologic pain-relief measures should be tried initially, including rest; a calming environment; relaxation

TABLE 49.4   Over-the-Counter Antacids Commonly Used in Pregnancy

Generic	Route and Dosage	Uses and Considerations
Aluminum hydroxide	PO: As directed* Recommended dose is 600 mg 5-6 times/d	Contains 320 mg of aluminum hydroxide gel per 300-mg tab or per 5 mL; ANC 8 contains saccharin and sorbitol. OTC preparation for heartburn secondary to reflux, it neutralizes gastric acidity. Side effects include constipation; adverse reactions include dehydration, hypophosphatemia (long-term use), GI obstruction. Effects are decreased with tetracycline, phenothiazine, benzodiazepines, isoniazid, and digoxin; follow dose with water. Pregnancy category: Not assigned†; PB: UK; onset: 15-30 min; peak: 0.5 h; duration: 1-3 h; t½: UK
Magnesium hydroxide and aluminum hydroxide with Simethicone	PO: Multiple formulations available OTC – take as directed*	Antiflatulant and neutralizes gastric acid. Liquid: Each 5 mL contains 400 mg aluminum hydroxide; 400 mg magnesium hydroxide; 40 mg simethicone, parabens, saccharin, and sorbitol; and 2 mg sodium. Tablets: Each contains 200 mg aluminum hydroxide, 200 mg magnesium hydroxide, and 20 mg simethicone. Tabs must be chewed thoroughly. Adverse effects include acid rebound. Aluminum-based antacids may cause constipation, whereas magnesium-based antacids have a laxative effect. Aluminum and magnesium–based combination antacids are given to balance the constipation and laxative effects. Do not administer magnesium-based antacids to patients with renal disease. Drug interactions: Concurrent administration with digoxin, indomethacin, or iron salts may decrease absorption of these drugs. Decreased pharmacologic effect with antacids and benzodiazepines, captopril, corticosteroids, fluoroquinolones, H₂ antagonists, hydantoins, ketoconazole, penicillamine, phenothiazines, salicylates, and ticlopidine. Increased pharmacologic effect with levodopa, sulfonylureas, and valproic acid. Pregnancy category C†; PB: UK; t½: UK

*Dosage recommendations for antacid preparations should be clarified by the health care provider; however, as a general rule, no more than 12 tablets or 12 tsp should be taken in a 24-h period, depending on the strength of the product. Major side effects are changes in bowel habits (diarrhea or constipation), nausea, vomiting, alkalosis, and hypermagnesemia. Antacids figure in numerous drug interactions because of their increased action on gastric pH and their propensity to bind with other drugs to form poorly absorbed complexes. Antacids should not be taken within 2 h of taking iron, digitalis products, tetracycline, or phenothiazine.

†Pregnancy categories have been revised. See http://www.fda.gov/Drugs/DevelopmentApprovalProcess/DevelopmentResources/Labeling/ucm093307.htm for more information.

ANC, acid-neutralizing capacity (per tablet or 5 mL); d, day; GI, gastrointestinal; h, hour; H₂, histamine 2; min, minute; OTC, over-the-counter; PB, protein binding; PO, by mouth; t½, half-life; tab, tablet; tsp, teaspoon; UK, unknown.

exercises; alteration in routine; mental imagery; ice packs; warm, moist heat; postural changes; correct body mechanics; and changes in footwear.

Acetaminophen. Acetaminophen, a para-aminophenol analgesic, is the most commonly ingested nonprescription drug during pregnancy. Acetaminophen may be used during all trimesters of pregnancy in therapeutic doses on a short-term basis for its analgesic and antipyretic effects. The drug is a weak prostaglandin inhibitor and does not have significant antiinflammatory effects. See Prototype Drug Chart 25.1 for the pharmacologic data for acetaminophen.

Pharmacokinetics The rate of absorption of acetaminophen is dependent on the rate of gastric emptying. Acetaminophen is 10% to 25% protein bound and crosses the placenta during pregnancy; it is also found in low concentrations in breast milk. Acetaminophen is partially hepatically metabolized into inactive metabolites; however, a highly active metabolite (N-acetyl-p-benzoquinone) produced when the drug is taken in large doses can have potential liver and kidney toxicity. The half-life is 2 to 3 hours. There is no concrete evidence of fetal anomalies associated with the use of acetaminophen, and no adverse effects have been noted in breastfed infants of patients who used the drug while pregnant or breastfeeding.

Pharmacodynamics The maximum daily dose of acetaminophen is 3000 mg per day, and the use of acetaminophen during pregnancy should not exceed 12 tablets per 24 hours of a 325-mg formulation (regular strength) or 8 tablets per 24 hours of a 500-mg (extra strength) formulation because of the potential

for kidney and liver toxicity. The drug should be taken at 4- to 6-hour intervals. Onset of effects after oral ingestion is within 10 to 30 minutes, peak action occurs at 1 to 2 hours, and duration is from 3 to 5 hours.

Manufacturers of OTC products that contain acetaminophen have lowered the maximum daily dose recommendation to 3000 mg due to the frequency of overdose with acetaminophen. One reason for the high frequency of overdose is that patients may take multiple OTC products that contain acetaminophen.

Most patients without preexisting renal or hepatic disease tolerate acetaminophen well. Patients with hypersensitivity to the compound should not use it. Acetaminophen should be used cautiously in patients who are at risk for infection because of the possibility of masking signs and symptoms. The most frequent adverse reactions are skin eruptions, urticaria, unusual bruising, erythema, hypoglycemia, jaundice, hemolytic anemia, neutropenia, leukopenia, pancytopenia, and thrombocytopenia.

Aspirin and Ibuprofen. Aspirin, a salicylate, is classified as a mild analgesic. It is a prostaglandin synthetase inhibitor with antipyretic, analgesic, and antiinflammatory properties.

Aspirin can inhibit the initiation of labor and may actually prolong labor through its effects on uterine contractility, therefore its use is not recommended during pregnancy. Aspirin use late in pregnancy is also associated with greater maternal blood loss at delivery, and there may be increased risk for anemia in pregnancy and of antepartum hemorrhage. Hemostasis is affected in the newborn whose mother ingested aspirin during the last 2 months of pregnancy even without use during the week of delivery. Platelets are unable to aggregate to form clots, and it appears that this is *not* a reversible effect after delivery; the infant must wait for its own bone marrow to produce new platelets. Ibuprofen is a prostaglandin synthetase inhibitor with antipyretic, analgesic, and antiinflammatory properties. Bleeding risks are similar to those reported with aspirin, although ibuprofen causes less inhibition of platelet aggregation than aspirin formulations. If taken late in pregnancy, ibuprofen may cause premature closure of the ductus arteriosus, therefore ibuprofen use is contraindicated during the third trimester and during labor and delivery.

Antidepressant Drugs

Depressive disorders and exposure to antidepressant drugs have been associated with adverse birth outcomes. Adverse outcomes have included low birthweight (LBW), infants born small for gestational age (SGA), preterm delivery, and increased neonatal irritability and decreased attentiveness. Use of selective serotonin reuptake inhibitors (SSRIs) in pregnancy is associated with LBW and SGA infants. Preterm delivery (before 37 weeks) is significantly higher in patients taking SSRIs and tricyclic antidepressants (TCAs). Although TCA use in pregnancy has not been associated with structural malformations, in utero exposure has been linked to neonatal jitteriness and irritability. *Poor neonatal adaptation*—a term for transient symptoms such as tachypnea, irritability, hypoglycemia, and weak cry—has been reported in neonates exposed to SSRIs in late pregnancy. Options for treatment for pregnant patients include psychotherapy alone or in conjunction with pharmacologic therapy as determined by the health care provider.

 NURSING PROCESS
Patient-Centered Collaborative Care

Antepartum Drugs

Assessment
- Gather comprehensive medical and drug history to include illicit, herbal, and pharmacologic formulations, and nonpharmacologic interventions, such as acupuncture.
- Obtain baseline vital signs.
- Identify patients at risk for substance abuse, and collaborate with other professionals to plan strategies to minimize risks.
- Assess drug history to determine whether antacid use will interfere with absorption of the drug.
- Review history of aspirin use when admitting a patient in labor. If aspirin has been used, alert staff and monitor for increased bleeding.
- Ascertain any medical history of alcoholism, liver disease, viral infection, or renal deficiencies. Acetaminophen should be used cautiously in these patients.
- Assess group B *Streptococcus* colonization in pregnancy for treatment and neonatal prevention.

Nursing Diagnoses
- Knowledge, Deficient related to health maintenance needs during pregnancy

- Knowledge, Deficient related to potential adverse fetal outcomes from exposure to teratogens

Planning
- The patient will use or avoid various drugs during pregnancy as advised.
- The patient will discuss drugs and herbal supplements with a health care provider or pharmacist before use.

Nursing Interventions
General
- Be cognizant that drug use may be part of multiple-substance abuse and may also involve maternal-neonatal infections.
- Stress the importance of prenatal care, and discuss the patient's fears about health care professionals and concerns about legal action in the event of substance abuse.

Specific
- Advise on nonpharmacologic and pharmacologic measures to relieve common pregnancy discomforts.
- Refer patients to tobacco, alcohol, or drug treatment programs if appropriate.
- Counsel patients on nutritional and therapeutic supplements needed during pregnancy.
- Monitor hemoglobin/hematocrit of prenatal patients per agency protocol.

Iron
- Question patients about nausea, constipation, and bowel habit changes if they are taking iron preparations.
- Give diluted liquid iron preparations through a plastic straw to prevent discoloration of teeth. Giving iron with orange juice, which is high in ascorbic acid, enhances absorption.
- Store iron in a light-resistant container.
- Recognize that a false-positive result of occult blood in the stool can occur in patients taking iron.

Patient Teaching
General
- Advise patients that tobacco, alcohol, and heavy caffeine use may have adverse effects on the fetus.
- Encourage patients to speak with their health care provider before taking drugs—illicit, OTC, or prescribed—because of their teratogenic potential.
- Counsel patients planning to breastfeed to discuss drugs—illicit, OTC, and prescribed—with their health care provider.

Aspirin, Acetaminophen, and Ibuprofen
- Advise patients to take acetaminophen, rather than aspirin, during pregnancy; aspirin and ibuprofen are particularly contraindicated during the third trimester.
- Counsel patients against ingesting multiple OTC pain or cough/cold preparations because many OTC products contain acetaminophen.

Antepartum Drugs
- Advise patients not to take nonsteroidal antiinflammatory drugs (NSAIDs) with acetaminophen.

- Advise patients not to take NSAIDS after the second trimester.

Caffeine, Alcohol, and Nicotine

- Advise patients to limit coffee ingestion to 1 cup per day and to limit other sources of caffeine (tea, soda, chocolate, certain drugs).
- If caffeine is allowed by the health care provider, encourage patients to space limited caffeine intake evenly throughout the day, because caffeine passes readily to the fetus, who cannot metabolize it. Caffeine can decrease intervillous placental blood flow.
- Advise patients to use decaffeinated products or to dilute caffeinated products.
- Suggest that patients discuss use of herbal products with their health care provider (see Complementary and Alternative Therapies 49.1).
- If the patient plans to breastfeed, explain that 1% of caffeine consumed will appear in breast milk within 15 minutes. Therefore although one cup of coffee is fine, it is not wise to drink several cups of coffee in succession; excess caffeine will accumulate in the infant's tissues because it lacks the enzymes to adequately clear the caffeine for 7 to 9 months after birth.
- Advise pregnant patients not to drink alcohol because no safe level has been determined; emphasize that even *minimal* exposure can result in fetal alcohol effect (FAE), and moderate/excessive exposure may result in fetal alcohol syndrome (FAS).
- Advise patients that smoking can cause loss of nutrients such as vitamins A and C, folic acid, cobalamin, and calcium. Tobacco use may contribute to shortened gestation and low-birthweight infants.

Antacids

- Advise patients that antacids should not be taken within 1 hour of taking an enteric-coated tablet because the acid-resistant coating may dissolve in the increased alkaline condition of the stomach, and the medication will not be released in the intestine as intended. Stomach upset may result.
- Instruct patients to store antacid liquid suspensions at room temperature or to place them under refrigeration to improve palatability; advise that suspensions should not be frozen and that the bottle must be shaken well before ingesting.

Iron

- Advise patients about dietary sources of iron, including red meat, nuts and seeds, wheat germ, spinach, broccoli, prunes, and iron-fortified cereal.
- Explain to patients that if supplemental iron is taken between meals, increased absorption—and increased side effects—may result. Taking iron 1 hour before meals is suggested. Give with orange juice or water but not with milk or antacids.

Self-Administration of Iron and Antacids

- Advise patients to swallow iron tablets whole, not crush them. Liquid iron preparations are taken with a plastic straw to avoid staining teeth.

- Caution patients not to take antacids with iron; antacids impair absorption and are generally discouraged during pregnancy. Iron and antacids should be taken 2 hours apart if both are prescribed.

Side Effects of Iron and Antacids

- Advise patients to keep iron tablets away from children. Iron tablets look like candy, and death has been reported in small children. Iron is a leading cause of fatal poisoning in children.
- Advise patients that there may be a change in bowel habits when taking antacids. Aluminum and calcium carbonate products can cause constipation, whereas magnesium products can cause diarrhea. Many antacids contain a combination of ingredients to reduce adverse effects.

🌐 Cultural Considerations

- Consider cultural food practices and beliefs in regard to the use of prenatal vitamins. For example, in Mexico, some may view vitamins as a "hot food" that should not be ingested during pregnancy.

Evaluation

- Evaluate effectiveness of prescribed drug therapy. Report side effects.
- Evaluate the patient's understanding of possible effects on the fetus from maternal use of drugs (prescribed, OTC, and illicit) and tobacco or alcohol.

DRUGS THAT DECREASE UTERINE MUSCLE CONTRACTILITY

Preterm Labor

Preterm labor (PTL) is defined as cervical changes and uterine contractions that occur between 20 and 37 weeks of pregnancy. *Preterm birth* is any birth that occurs before the completion of 37 weeks of pregnancy, regardless of birthweight. Complications related to preterm birth account for more newborn and infant deaths than any other cause (Simhan, Iams, & Romero, 2012). PTL occurs in 12% of pregnancies.

Although PTL has no single known cause, certain risk factors have been identified: maternal age younger than 18 years or older than 40 years, low socioeconomic status, previous history of preterm delivery (17% to 37% chance of recurrence), intrauterine infections (e.g., bacterial vaginosis), polyhydramnios, multiple gestation, uterine anomalies, antepartum hemorrhage, smoking, drug use, urinary tract infections, and incompetent cervix. Attempts to arrest PTL are contraindicated in (1) pregnancy of less than 20 weeks gestation (confirmed by ultrasound), (2) bulging or premature rupture of membranes (PROM), (3) confirmed fetal death or anomalies incompatible with life, (4) maternal hemorrhage and evidence of severe fetal compromise, and (5) chorioamnionitis.

Nonpharmacologic treatment measures for PTL include bed rest, hydration (ingestion of 6 to 8 glasses of fluids daily or more, IV fluid bolus), pelvic rest (no sexual intercourse or douching), and screening for intrauterine and urinary tract infections. Patient assessment includes uterine activity (frequency, duration, and intensity), vaginal bleeding or discharge, and fetal monitoring.

Tocolytic Therapy

When patients in true PTL (with cervical change) have no contraindications, they become candidates for tocolytic therapy—drug therapy to decrease uterine muscle contractions—using β_2-adrenergic receptor agonists (e.g., terbutaline) or, more commonly, the calcium antagonist magnesium sulfate. Other tocolytics used are calcium channel blockers (nifedipine) and prostaglandin inhibitors (indomethacin). Prostaglandin inhibitors work by limiting the available calcium for uterine contractions. With concerns regarding the safety profiles of β-sympathomimetics and magnesium sulfate comes an increased interest in the latter two drug categories for tocolysis. No medication has been approved by the FDA as a tocolytic, and these are considered "off label" uses of drugs approved for other functions, such as treatment of asthma and hypertension. The goals in tocolytic therapy are to (1) interrupt or inhibit uterine contractions to create additional time for fetal maturation in utero, (2) delay delivery so antenatal corticosteroids can be delivered to facilitate fetal lung maturation, and (3) allow safe transport of the patient to an appropriate facility if required. Table 49.5 lists the drugs used to decrease preterm uterine contractions and their dosages, uses, and considerations.

Beta-Sympathomimetic Drugs

Beta-sympathomimetic drugs act by stimulating β_2-receptors on uterine smooth muscle. The frequency and intensity of uterine contractions decrease as the muscle relaxes. Terbutaline is used in the late second and early third trimesters, more commonly limited to a single-dose therapy as an acute tocolytic. Terbutaline can effectively decrease uterine contractions; however, use of terbutaline in the United States has decreased with increased awareness of its effects on maternal and fetal cardiovascular systems and free placental passage. The FDA is recommending that *injectable* terbutaline should not be used in pregnant women for prevention of PTL or prolonged treatment (beyond 48 to 72 hours) secondary to the risk of maternal cardiac problems and death (see http://www.fda.gov/drugs/drugsafety/ucm243539.htm).

⚡ PATIENT SAFETY

Do not confuse...

- **Methylergonovine,** used to *stimulate* uterine contractions in the prevention and treatment of postpartum hemorrhage, with **terbutaline sulfate,** used to *decrease* uterine contractions in preterm labor. These drugs have the same packaging but opposite actions. Both are amber ampules with amber plastic packaging and colored neckbands wrapped in foil. Do not store together. Manufacturers of terbutaline are now packaging this drug in vials, but some ampules may still be in circulation.

Pharmacokinetics Patients with contractions may be initially given subcutaneous terbutaline 0.25 mg every 20 minutes to 6 hours if the maternal pulse is less than 120 beats/min. Less commonly, health care providers administer continuous subcutaneous infusions 50 to 100 mcg/hour. Patients are monitored to determine whether and when contractions diminish or cease. Terbutaline is minimally protein bound (25%) and is metabolized via the liver to inactive metabolites. Its half-life is 11 to 16 hours.

Pharmacodynamics IV and subcutaneous terbutaline have an onset of action of 6 to 15 minutes, a peak serum concentration level in 30 to 60 minutes, and a duration of action of 1.5 to 4 hours subcutaneously.

Adverse Reactions. Maternal side effects include tremors, dizziness, nervousness, tachycardia, hypotension, chest pain, palpitations, nausea, vomiting, hyperglycemia, and hypokalemia. Many

---

TABLE 49.5 Drugs Used to Decrease Uterine Contractility

Generic	Route and Dosage	Uses and Considerations
	BETA-ADRENERGIC AGENTS	
Terbutaline	Subcut; 0.25 mg q20min-6h; hold for pulse >120 beats/min. Subcut cont infusion: 50-100 mcg/h, adjust to fetal response; *max.* 17.5-30 mcg/min (use with caution) Follow agency protocol for specific directives plus individual health care provider's orders. See black-box warning.*	Relaxes bronchial and uterine smooth muscle by acting on β_2-receptors. Partially metabolized in liver, excreted in urine and feces. Drug rapidly crosses the placenta, increases maternal pulse and FHR; monitor MHR. Breastfeeding is *not* contraindicated because of short half-life. Additive effect with CNS depressants (narcotics, sedative-hypnotics) and neuromuscular blocking agents *Contraindication:* Hypersensitivity to terbutaline, sympathomimetic amines, or any component of the formulation. Pregnancy category: C†; onset: 6-15 min; PB: 25%; peak: 30-60 min; duration: 1.5-4 h; t½: 11-16 h
	CALCIUM ANTAGONISTS	
Magnesium sulfate	See Table 49.8: Drugs used in severe preeclampsia	

Black-Box Warning: The United States Food and Drug Administration has concluded that the risk of serious adverse events outweighs any potential benefit to pregnant women receiving prolonged tocolytic treatment beyond 48-72 hours.

†Pregnancy categories have been revised. See http://www.fda.gov/Drugs/DevelopmentApprovalProcess/DevelopmentResources/Labeling/ucm093307.htm for more information.

CNS, Central nervous system; *cont,* continuous; *FHR,* fetal heart rate; *h,* hour; *max,* maximum; *MHR,* maternal heart rate; *min,* minutes; *PB,* protein binding; *q,* every; *Subcut,* subcutaneously; *t½,* half-life; *>,* greater than.

of these effects are associated with terbutaline's cross-reactivity with β$_1$-adrenergic receptors. More serious adverse reactions include pulmonary edema, dysrhythmias, ketoacidosis, and anaphylactic shock. Fetal side effects include tachycardia and potential hypoglycemia resulting from fetal hyperinsulinemia caused by maternal hyperglycemia. Terbutaline is contraindicated in patients with cardiac disease and in those with poorly controlled hyperthyroidism or diabetes mellitus.

Drug Interactions. The increased effects of general anesthetics can produce additive hypotension. Pulmonary edema can occur with concurrent use of corticosteroids. Cardiovascular effects may be additive with other sympathomimetic drugs, such as epinephrine, albuterol, and isoproterenol. Beta-adrenergic blocking agents—such as propranolol hydrochloride (HCl), nadolol, pindolol, timolol maleate, and metoprolol tartrate antagonize β-sympathomimetics.

Magnesium Sulfate

Parenteral magnesium sulfate, a calcium antagonist and central nervous system (CNS) depressant, relaxes the smooth muscle of the uterus through calcium displacement and is more commonly given as a tocolytic. Administered intravenously, the drug has a direct depressant effect on uterine muscle contractility; it also increases uterine perfusion, which has a therapeutic effect on the fetus. Magnesium sulfate may be safer to use than the β-sympathomimetics because it has fewer adverse effects, and it can be used when β-sympathomimetics are contraindicated (e.g., in patients with diabetes and cardiovascular disease). The drug is excreted by the kidneys and crosses the placenta. Magnesium sulfate is administered as a 4 to 6 g IV loading dose over 20 to 30 minutes followed by a 2 to 4 g/hour continuous infusion for 12 to 24 hours after contractions ceased. Continuous infusion should not exceed 5 to 7 days or a maximum of 40 g/24 hours. The maintenance dose must be titrated to keep uterine contractions under control, and magnesium levels are drawn based on clinical response of the patient. Magnesium sulfate therapy is contraindicated in patients who have myasthenia gravis, and impaired kidney function or recent myocardial infarction (MI) are relative contraindications. Patients with renal impairment may require adjusted dosages.

Adverse Reactions. Dosage-related side effects in the patient include flushing, feelings of increased warmth, perspiration, dizziness, nausea, headache, lethargy, slurred speech, sluggishness, nasal congestion, heavy eyelids, blurred vision, decreased GI action, increased pulse rate, and hypotension. Increased severity is evidenced by depressed reflexes, confusion, and magnesium toxicity (respiratory depression and arrest, circulatory collapse, cardiac arrest). Decreased fetal heart rate (FHR) variability is one side effect, and side effects in the neonate are respiratory depression, slight hypotonia with diminished reflexes, and lethargy for 24 to 48 hours. If maternal neurologic, respiratory, or cardiac depression is evidenced, the antidote is calcium gluconate (1 g IV push over 3 minutes).

Nursing Interventions During Tocolytic Therapy

- Monitor vital signs, FHR, fetal activity, and uterine activity as ordered. Report respirations of fewer than 12 per minute, which may indicate magnesium sulfate toxicity.

- Monitor intake and output (I&O). Report urinary output below 30 mL/hour.
- Assess breath and bowel sounds as ordered or at least every 4 hours.
- Assess deep tendon reflexes (DTRs) and clonus before initiation of therapy and as ordered. Notify the health care provider of changes in DTRs (areflexia or hyporeflexia) and clonus.
- Assess pain and uterine contractions.
- Weigh daily at the same time.
- Monitor serum magnesium levels as ordered (therapeutic level is 4 to 7 mg/dL).
- Have calcium gluconate (1 g given IV over 3 minutes) available as an antidote.
- Observe the newborn for 24 to 48 hours for magnesium effects if drug was given to the mother before delivery.

 NURSING PROCESS
Patient-Centered Collaborative Care
Beta$_2$-Adrenergic Agonists: Terbutaline

Assessment
- Identify risks for PTL early in pregnancy.
- When a patient has preterm uterine contractions, obtain a history, complete physical assessment, vital signs, FHR, and urine specimen for screening for intrauterine infection and urinary tract infection.

Nursing Diagnoses
- Anxiety related to potential for early labor and birth and pregnancy loss.
- Knowledge, Deficient related to etiology and nonpharmacologic and pharmacologic interventions for PTL
- Health Management, Ineffective related to nonpharmacologic and pharmacologic interventions for PTL and long-term implications for patient and fetus or infant
- Activity Intolerance, Risk for

Planning
- The patient's preterm uterine contractions will cease by resting in a left side-lying position, increasing fluid intake, assuming pelvic rest, and following tocolytic therapy as directed.
- The patient has no progressive cervical change.

Nursing Interventions
- Monitor and assess uterine activity and FHR.
- Maintain the patient in a left lateral position as much as possible to facilitate uteroplacental perfusion.
- Monitor vital signs per unit protocol, specifically maternal pulse. Report maternal heart rate (MHR) greater than 130 beats/min.
- Report auscultated cardiac dysrhythmias. An electrocardiograph (ECG) may be ordered.
- Auscultate breath sounds anteriorly, posteriorly, and bilaterally every 4 hours. Notify the health care provider if

respirations are more than 30 per minute or if the breath quality changes (e.g., wheezes, rales, coughing).

- Monitor daily weight at the same time every day to assess fluid overload; implement strict I&O measurement.
- Report baseline FHR over 180 beats/min or any significant increase in uterine contractions from pretreatment baseline.
- Report persistence of uterine contractions despite tocolytic therapy.
- Report leakage of amniotic fluid, vaginal bleeding or discharge, and complaints of rectal pressure.
- Be alert to the presence of maternal hyperglycemia and hypokalemia and hypoglycemia in the newborn delivered within 5 hours of discontinued β-sympathomimetic drugs.

Patient Teaching
General
- Advise the patient of signs and symptoms of PTL: menstrual-type cramps, sensations of pelvic pressure, low backache, increased vaginal discharge, and abdominal discomfort.
- Instruct the patient that if she experiences PTL contractions, her initial action should be to void, recline on her left side to increase uterine blood flow, and drink extra fluids. Emphasize that she should notify her health care provider if uterine contractions do not cease or if they increase in frequency.
- Explain side effects of β-sympathomimetic drugs. Report heart palpitations or dizziness to the health care provider.
- Advise the patient to contact her health care provider before taking any other drugs while on tocolytic drug therapy.

🌐 Cultural Considerations
- Provide an interpreter with the same ethnic background as the patient if possible, especially when dealing with sensitive topics or stressful situations.

Evaluation
- Evaluate effectiveness of the tocolytic drug by noting six or fewer uterine contractions in 1 hour or per the health care provider's order.
- Evaluate the patient's understanding of nonpharmacologic measures for decreasing preterm contractions: bed rest, increasing oral fluid intake, pelvic rest, and lying on the left side.
- Continue monitoring the patient's vital signs, FHR, and uterine activity. Report any change immediately.

CORTICOSTEROID THERAPY IN PRETERM LABOR

The desired outcome of tocolytic therapy is to delay birth long enough to allow time for corticosteroids to reach maximum benefit. Patients at risk for preterm delivery (24 to 34 weeks gestation) should receive antenatal corticosteroid therapy with betamethasone or dexamethasone. An off-label use, administration of antenatal corticosteroids accelerates lung maturation and lung surfactant development in the fetus in utero, decreasing the incidence and severity of respiratory distress syndrome (RDS) and increasing survival of preterm infants. Antenatal therapy decreases infant mortality, RDS, and intraventricular bleeds in neonates born between 24 and 34 gestational weeks. The effects and benefits of corticosteroid administration are believed to begin 24 hours after administration, and they last for up to 1 week. The goal is to delay delivery by 48 hours to maximize the effect of the glucocorticoids.

Surfactant is made up of two major phospholipids: sphingomyelin and lecithin. Sphingomyelin initially develops in greater quantity than lecithin from about the 24th week. However, by the 33rd to 35th weeks of gestation, lecithin production peaks, making the ratio of the two substances about 2:1 in favor of lecithin. This lecithin/sphingomyelin (L/S) ratio is measured in the amniotic fluid and is a predictor of fetal lung maturity and risk for neonatal RDS.

Patients with gestational hypertension, PROM, placental insufficiency, or some types of diabetes, and those who abuse narcotics may have amniotic fluid with higher-than-expected L/S ratios for the gestational date because of a stress-induced increase in endogenous corticosteroid production.

Betamethasone

When PTL occurs before the 32nd week of gestation, corticosteroid therapy with betamethasone may be prescribed. The usual dose is 12 mg intramuscularly (IM) every 24 hours for 2 doses.

Adverse Reactions. Side effects of betamethasone are rare but include seizures, headache, vertigo, edema, hypertension, increased sweating, petechiae, ecchymoses, and facial erythema.

Dexamethasone

In clinical controlled trials, evidence is insufficient to recommend betamethasone over dexamethasone, because the two have not been directly compared. Investigations have noted a trend of decreased risk of neonatal cystic periventricular leukomalacia and intraventricular hemorrhage with exposure to betamethasone over dexamethasone. Dexamethasone has a rapid onset of action and a shorter duration of action, therefore it must be prescribed in a shorter frequency compared with betamethasone. The recommended antepartum regimen for dexamethasone is 6 mg IM every 12 hours for 4 doses.

⚡ PATIENT SAFETY

Do not confuse…
- **Dexamethasone,** a corticosteroid used to accelerate fetal lung maturity during weeks 24 to 34 of gestation, with **desoximetasone**, which is used to treat inflammation from corticosteroid-responsive dermatoses.

Adverse Reactions. The potential adverse reactions associated with dexamethasone therapy include insomnia, nervousness, increased appetite, headache, hypersensitivity reactions, and arthralgias. Table 49.6 lists the prenatal drugs used for surfactant development and their dosages, uses, and considerations.

NURSING PROCESS
Patient-Centered Collaborative Care

Betamethasone

Assessment
- Assess for history of hypersensitivity.
- Assess vital signs; report abnormal findings.
- Assess FHR.

Nursing Diagnoses
- Anxiety related to potential for preterm labor and birth with uncertain fetal outcome secondary to fetal immaturity
- Knowledge, Deficient related to use of antenatal corticosteroids for promotion of fetal lung maturity in preterm delivery

Planning
- The patient will not deliver within 24 hours of receiving betamethasone.

Nursing Interventions
- Shake the suspension well. Avoid exposing it to excessive heat or light.
- To avoid local muscle atrophy, inject drug into a large muscle, not the deltoid.
- Monitor maternal vital signs.
- Maintain accurate I&O measurements.
- Check blood glucose in patients with diabetes mellitus.

Cultural Considerations
- Provide an interpreter with the same ethnic background as the patient if possible, especially when dealing with sensitive topics or stressful situations.

Evaluation
- Continue monitoring patient vital signs. Report changes.
- Continue monitoring FHR. Report any changes.
- Monitor the neonate for hypoglycemia and presence of neonatal sepsis.

DRUGS FOR GESTATIONAL HYPERTENSION

Gestational hypertension, elevated blood pressure (BP) without proteinuria after 20 gestational weeks in patients normotensive before pregnancy, is the most common serious complication of pregnancy and can have devastating maternal and fetal effects. Gestational hypertension has replaced the term *pregnancy-induced hypertension,* still commonly used in clinical discussions but no longer correct. With proper management of gestational hypertension, the prognosis for both patient and infant is good. Hypertensive disorders are reported in 10% to 20% of all pregnant patients, with 5% to 8% of all pregnancies reflecting the incidence of preeclampsia (gestational hypertension with proteinuria). The condition is most often observed after 20 weeks gestation, intrapartum, and during the first 72 hours postpartum; however, late postpartum preeclampsia-eclampsia may present more than 48 hours but less than 4 weeks postpartum.

The cause of preeclampsia remains unknown, although numerous hypotheses exist. The pathophysiology of preeclampsia and eclampsia, new-onset grand mal seizures in a patient with preeclampsia, is believed to be related to decreased levels of vasodilating prostaglandins with resulting vasospasm. The major predisposing risk factors for the development of preeclampsia are listed in Box 49.1.

The two categories of gestational hypertension, preeclampsia and eclampsia, are based on clinical manifestations. Preeclampsia is the presence of hypertension (systolic BP >140 mm Hg or diastolic BP >90 mm Hg) and proteinuria (≥300 mg in a 24-hour urine collection) in a normotensive pregnant patient after 20 weeks gestation. Preeclampsia is subdivided into *mild* and *severe* preeclampsia (Table 49.7).

About 5% of preeclamptic patients, notably those without adequate prenatal care, progress to eclampsia, in which seizure activity occurs; the maternal mortality rate is about 10% to 15% in low- and middle-income countries. Early diagnosis of preeclampsia with appropriate treatment keeps most preeclamptic patients from progressing to this stage. Approximately 13% to 16% of eclampsia occurs postpartum.

One severe sequela of preeclampsia is defined by its symptoms—*h*emolysis, *e*levated *l*iver enzymes, and *l*ow *p*latelet

TABLE 49.6	Prenatal Therapy for Surfactant Development	
Generic	**Route and Dosage**	**Uses and Considerations**
Betamethasone	IM: 12 mg q24h × 2 doses	Corticosteroid. Given to prevent RDS in preterm infants by injecting the mother before delivery to stimulate surfactant production in fetal lung. Not effective in treating preterm infant after delivery. Most effective if given at least 24 h (preferably 48-72 h) but less than 7 d before delivery in week 33 or before. Contraindicated in severe gestational hypertension and in systemic fungal infection. Simultaneous use with terbutaline may enhance risk for pulmonary edema. Not usually given with ruptured membranes; may mask signs of chorioamnionitis. Metabolized in liver and excreted by kidneys; crosses placenta; enters breast milk. Therapy less effective with multifetal birth and with male infants. Pregnancy category: C*; PB: 64%; onset: 1-3 h; peak: IV: 10-36 min; duration: 7-14 d; t½: 6.5 h
Dexamethasone	IM: 6 mg q12h × 4 doses	Same as betamethasone but shorter half-life and more significant variation in circulating serum levels. Pregnancy category: C*

*Pregnancy categories have been revised. See http://www.fda.gov/Drugs/DevelopmentApprovalProcess/DevelopmentResources/Labeling/ucm093307.htm for more information.

d, Days; *h,* hours; *IM,* intramuscular; *IV,* intravenous; *min,* minutes; *PB,* protein binding; *q,* every; *RDS,* respiratory distress syndrome; *t½,* half-life.

count—and is therefore known as HELLP syndrome, which occurs in about 2% to 12% of patients with gestational hypertension. Patients who manifest severe preeclampsia are most likely to also have HELLP syndrome.

In addition to delivery of an uncompromised fetus and psychological support for the patient and family, two primary treatment goals in preeclampsia are reduction of vasospasm and prevention of seizures.

Delivery of the infant and placenta (products of conception) is the only known cure for preeclampsia. Vaginal delivery is preferred so that anesthesia and surgical risks will not be added. Labor induction via cervical ripening may be initiated to facilitate labor. For a vaginal delivery, epidural anesthesia or combined epidural and spinal anesthesia is frequently performed for pain management while promoting uteroplacental circulation.

Maternal hypotension is a significant concern for hypertensive patients who have epidurals. In contrast, parturients with worsening preeclampsia or fetal distress may be delivered via cesarean section. Patients with HELLP syndrome may have their labor induced for a vaginal delivery at 32 or more weeks gestation. For patients with HELLP syndrome who are at less than 32 weeks gestation, cesarean delivery may be considered.

If HELLP syndrome progresses to the point of eclampsia (maternal seizure), delivery is generally postponed for 1 to 3 hours if fetal status allows. The labor induction or cesarean delivery is an additional stressor for the patient who exhibits acidosis and hypoxia resulting from seizure. Ideally, once vital signs are stabilized with improved urinary output and decreased acidosis/hypoxia, delivery is pursued.

Nonpharmacologic treatments for preeclampsia include activity reduction; lying on the left side; eating a nutritious, balanced diet; and drinking six to eight 8-ounce glasses of water a day. Studies have shown that nonpharmacologic treatments have not had clinically beneficial effects, therefore drug therapy is commonly used for treatment.

Methyldopa, Hydralazine, Magnesium Sulfate, and Labetalol

Methyldopa, hydralazine, and labetalol are considered first-line therapies for mild preeclampsia because they have been most widely used in pregnant patients and their safety and efficacy have been established. Additional alternatives include the beta blocker prazosin, the calcium channel blocker nifedipine, and the centrally acting alpha agonist clonidine. Beta blockers are generally considered safe, but there is potential for impaired fetal growth if used early in pregnancy. Nifedipine has been used with no major problems. Patients should avoid diuretics

---

BOX 49.1   Predisposing Factors for Preeclampsia

- African American
- Obesity
- Primigravida (first pregnancy)
- History of preeclampsia
- Younger than 20 years or older than 35 years (especially primigravida)
- Multifetal gestation
- Family history of preeclampsia
- Maternal infection/inflammation in current pregnancy
- Pregestational diabetes mellitus
- Preexisting hypertensive, vascular, or renal disease
- Antiphospholipid antibody syndrome
- Connective tissue disease
- Paternal history (partner previously fathered a preeclamptic pregnancy in another woman)

TABLE 49.7   Comparison of Mild and Severe Preeclampsia and Eclampsia

Mild Preeclampsia	Severe Preeclampsia	Eclampsia
Blood pressure increase to >140 systolic and/or >90 diastolic but <160 systolic × 2 at least 4-6 h apart but within 1-week period	Blood pressure of >160/110 on two occasions at least 6 h apart (patient on bed rest)	Signs and symptoms of mild or severe preeclampsia and one grand mal seizure
Proteinuria >300 mg in 24 h or +1 or more on two random urine samples collected at lease 4-6 h apart	Proteinuria >5 g in 24 h or 3+ or greater in two random samples 4 h apart; edema generalized; found in face (periorbital, coarse features), hands, lower extremities (ankles), abdomen, and dependent areas	
Edema noted in hands and feet; not generalized	Edema generalized; found in face (periorbital, coarse features), hands, lower extremities (ankles), abdomen, and dependent areas	
Deep tendon reflexes in arms and legs only slightly increased (0: no response; 1+: sluggish/low; 2+: normal active; 3+: more brisk then expected; slightly hyperactive)	Deep tendon reflexes in arms and legs hyperactive (4+: brisk, hyperactive with intermittent or transient clonus; 5+: brisk, clonus sustained)	
Adequate urinary output: >25-30 mL/h	Oliguria present (<500 mL per 24 h)	
No major cerebral or visual symptoms; may have mild frontal headache	Cerebral or visual symptoms, particularly blurred vision, spots, flashing lights; persistent or severe headache	
Pulmonary edema absent, thrombocytopenia absent	Pulmonary edema, cyanosis, or thrombocytopenia	
No epigastric pain; irritability or changes in affect that may be transient	Epigastric pain, severe irritability or changes in affect	

h, Hour; >, greater than; <, less than.

because of the potential alteration in plasma volume. Patients in the second and third trimesters should avoid taking angiotensin-converting enzyme (ACE) inhibitors because of the potential for fetal renal toxicity. Magnesium sulfate is used for severe preeclampsia for the prevention of eclampsia. Table 49.8 lists the commonly used drugs for treating preeclampsia, along with their dosages, uses, and considerations.

Adverse Reactions of Methyldopa

Observe the patient for peripheral edema, anxiety, nightmares, drowsiness, headache, dry mouth, drug-induced fever, and mental depression. These are the most common potential adverse reactions.

Adverse Reactions of Hydralazine

Observe the patient for headache, nausea, vomiting, nasal congestion, dizziness, tachycardia, palpitations, and angina pectoris. Avoid a sudden decrease in maternal BP, which may cause fetal hypoxia. Hydralazine has no known direct adverse effects on the fetus.

Adverse Reactions of Magnesium Sulfate

Early signs of increased magnesium levels include lethargy, flushing, feelings of increased warmth, perspiration, thirst, sedation, heavy eyelids, slurred speech, hypotension, DTR, and decreased muscle tone. Therapeutic magnesium levels are 4 to 7 mEq/L. Loss of patellar reflexes is often the first sign of magnesium toxicity and may be seen at 8 to 10 mEq/L. Respiratory

TABLE 49.8 Drugs Used in Severe Preeclampsia

Generic	Route and Dosage	Uses and Considerations
Magnesium sulfate	IV: 4-6 g loading dose in 20 min; followed by 2-4 g/h continuous infusion for at least 24 h.	Prevention and treatment of seizures related to preeclampsia. Calcium antagonist and CNS depressant. Decreases acetylcholine from motor nerves, which blocks neuromuscular transmission and decreases incidence of seizures. Secondary effect is reduction in BP as magnesium sulfate relaxes smooth muscle. Secondarily affects peripheral vascular system with increased uterine blood flow caused by vasodilation and some transient BP decrease during the first hour; also inhibits uterine contractions. Depresses DTRs and respiration; maintenance dose depends on reflexes, respiratory rate, urinary output, and magnesium level. Main risk is production of abnormally high serum magnesium levels. Therapeutic levels range from 4-7 mEq/L; effective in preventing seizures. Patient at risk if respiratory rate <12/min, urinary output <30 mL/h, DTR absent or hyporeflexic. Patellar reflexes disappear with serum magnesium levels of 8-10 mEq/L. Maternal respiratory depression may occur with levels >10-15 mEq/L; cardiac arrest occurs with levels >20-25 mEq/L. Notify health care provider if any of the above occur. Can be given IV or IM (infrequent). Do not give parenterally to patients with heart block or myocardial damage. Use with caution in patients with renal impairment. Absorbed magnesium is excreted by kidneys; excreted in breast milk, but breastfeeding is not contraindicated. Contraindicated in patients with myasthenia gravis. Relative contraindications: myocardial damage or heart block. Antidote: Calcium gluconate 1 g slow IV push over 3 min. IV use for preeclampsia/eclampsia is not recommended during 2 h prior to delivery. Pregnancy category: D*; PB: UK; onset: IV, immediate; IM, 1 h; duration: IV, 30 min; IM, 3-4 h; t½: UK
Hydralazine hydrochloride	IV: 5-10 mg q20min; *max cumulative total:* 20 mg or until BP is controlled. After initial dose, may initiate a continuous infusion of 0.5-10 mg/h instead of intermittent dosing (ACOG, 2015).	Antihypertensive agent. Causes arteriolar vasodilation. Usually lowers diastolic BP more than systolic BP. Objective is to maintain diastolic BP of 90-110 mm Hg. Usually well tolerated; maternal tachycardia and increased cardiac output and oxygen consumption may occur. Usually not given to pregnant preeclamptic patients with diastolic BP >105 mm Hg because of risk for reduced intervillous blood flow. Patients with impaired renal function may require lower doses. Pregnancy category: C*; Parenteral: Onset, 5-20 min; peak, 10-80 min; duration, 1-4 h
Methyldopa	IV: 250-500 mg q6-8h; *max:* 4 g/d. PO: 250 mg bid, *max:* 3 g/d	Stimulates central α-adrenergic receptors, resulting in decreased sympathetic outflow to heart, kidneys, and peripheral vasculature. *Contraindication:* Hypersensitivity to drug or any component, active hepatic disease, liver disorders previously associated with use of methyldopa, concurrent use of MAOIs. *Caution:* Sedation is usually transient during initial treatment and during dosage increases. Pregnancy category: B*; onset: 3-6 h; peak: 2-4 h; duration: 10-16 h (multiple doses: 24-48 h)
Labetalol	IV: 20 mg, followed by 40 mg, then 80 mg, and then 80 mg every 10 min until BP is controlled or max cumulative dose of 300 mg is given. After the initial dose, may initiate a continuous infusion of 1-2 mg/min	Blocks α-, β1-, and β2-adrenergic receptor sites. Monitor BP frequently. Adverse effects: orthostatic hypotension; dizziness; ventricular arrhythmia. Pregnancy category: C*; onset: 2-5 min; peak: 5-15 min; duration: 2-18 h (dose dependent); t½: 5.5 h

*Pregnancy categories have been revised. See http://www.fda.gov/Drugs/DevelopmentApprovalProcess/DevelopmentResources/Labeling/ucm093 307.htm for more information.
ACOG, American Congress of Obstetricians and Gynecologists; *bid,* twice daily; *BP,* blood pressure; *CNS,* central nervous system; *d,* day; *DTR,* deep tendon reflex; *h,* hour; *IM,* intramuscular; *IV,* intravenous; *MAOI,* monoamine oxidase inhibitor; *max,* maximum; *min,* minutes; *PB,* protein binding; *PO,* by mouth; *q,* every; *t½,* half-life; *UK,* unknown; >, greater than; <, less than.

depression may manifest at levels greater than 10 to 15 mEq/L, and cardiac arrest may manifest at levels greater than 20 to 25 mEq/L.

Decreased variability is commonly seen on the FHR tracing. If the patient received magnesium sulfate close to the time of delivery, the neonate may exhibit low Apgar scores, hypotonia, lethargy, weakness, and potential respiratory distress. The fetal level of magnesium generally reaches more than 90% of maternal levels within 3 hours of administration, but the greater risk to the fetus is from maternal preeclampsia with resulting decreased placental blood flow and intrauterine growth retardation.

 NURSING PROCESS
Patient-Centered Collaborative Care

Gestational Hypertension

Assessment
- Review baseline vital signs from early pregnancy and BP readings during prenatal visits.
- Identify patient history that may predispose the patient to preeclampsia.

Nursing Diagnoses
- Knowledge, Deficient related to preeclampsia, diagnosis, treatment modalities, and common outcomes for the patient and infant
- Renal Perfusion, Risk for Ineffective with risk to fetal well-being secondary to vasospasm
- Tissue Perfusion, Risk for Ineffective Cerebral with risk to fetal well-being secondary to vasospasm
- Tissue Perfusion, Risk for Ineffective Peripheral with risk to fetal well-being secondary to vasospasm
- Anxiety related to possible preterm hospitalization and delivery with possible adverse fetal or maternal outcomes
- Injury, Risk for
- Fluid Volume, Deficient related to the shift of intravascular fluid to the extravascular space as an outcome of vasospasm with subsequent elevated arterial hypertension

Planning
- The patient's BP will be maintained within acceptable ranges.
- The patient will verbalize understanding of preeclampsia and its etiology, signs and symptoms, and nonpharmacologic and pharmacologic treatment measures.
- The patient will understand and comply with the planned preeclampsia treatment regimen.
- The fetus will tolerate impaired uteroplacental perfusion and subsequent delivery without injury.
- Therapeutic magnesium levels will be maintained.
- A magnesium sulfate infusion will be planned for at least 24 hours postpartum.

Nursing Interventions
Magnesium Sulfate
- Provide continuous electronic fetal monitoring.

- Monitor for maternal toxicity. Lethargy and weakness result from blocking of neuromuscular transmission. Diaphoresis, flushing, feelings of warmth, and nasal congestion are results of vasodilation from relaxation of smooth muscle.
- Have airway suction, resuscitation equipment, and emergency drugs available.
- Have the antidote available: calcium gluconate 1 g IV given over 3 minutes.
- Maintain the patient in a left lateral recumbent position in a low-stimulation environment. Provide close observation.
- For IM administration, use the Z-track technique and rotate sites (drug is painful and irritating). Rarely is magnesium sulfate administered IM.
- Monitor BP, pulse, and respiratory rate per agency protocol; monitor DTRs, clonus, and I&O every hour. Some health care providers will request manual BP measurements.
- Monitor temperature, breath sounds, and bowel sounds every 4 hours.
- Check urine for protein every hour.
- Assess for epigastric pain, headache, visual symptoms (blurred vision and scotoma), sensory changes, edema, level of consciousness, and seizure activity on an ongoing basis.
- Monitor serum magnesium levels according to agency protocol for a range between 4 and 7 mEq/L.
- Notify the health care provider if you observe a decreased or changed level of consciousness; fewer than 12 respirations per minute; absence of DTR; urinary output below 30 mL/hour; systolic BP of 160 mm Hg or more, unless ordered otherwise; magnesium level greater than 7 mEq/L; absent bowel sounds or altered breath sounds; epigastric pain or right upper quadrant pain (associated with hepatic edema causing stretching of the liver capsule); headache; visual symptoms (blurred vision and scotoma); sensory changes; change in affect or level of consciousness; or seizure activity.
- Monitor laboratory reports for low platelet count, elevated liver enzymes (aspartate aminotransferase [AST], lactate dehydrogenase [LDH]), and bilirubin levels. Observe for evidence of excessive bleeding.
- Monitor fetal status. FHR baseline should remain at 110 to 160 beats/min.
- Monitor 24-hour urinary protein laboratory results if ordered (≥300 mg/day is abnormal).
- Monitor the patient for magnesium toxicity.
- Monitor the newborn for effects of placental exposure to excess magnesium sulfate. Although infrequent, newborn side effects include lethargy, neurologic or respiratory depression, and muscle hypotonia.

Hydralazine
- Monitor blood pressure frequently with an electronic BP monitoring device during drug administration.
- Observe for maintenance of diastolic BP between 90 and 110 mm Hg or as ordered.
- Observe for changes in level of consciousness and headache.

- Monitor I&O to avoid hypotensive episodes or overload.
- Monitor FHR.

Patient Teaching
General
- Explain preeclampsia and its implications for the patient, fetus, and newborn.
- Provide information about nonpharmacologic and pharmacologic treatment measures for preeclampsia.
- Advise avoiding exposure to the common cold, flu, and other infectious diseases.
- Remind patients with diabetes to check their glucose level as ordered.

Side Effects
- Advise patients to report immediately any breathing difficulty, weakness, or dizziness.
- Advise patients to report changes in stool, easy bruising, bleeding, blurred vision, unusual weight gain, and emotional changes.

Safety
- Advise patients to lie in the left lateral recumbent position, and explain the rationale.
- Educate patients on the signs and symptoms of progressive preeclampsia and when to seek medical assistance.
- Explain to the patient that fetal well-being will be assessed through biophysical profile (BPP), nonstress test (NST), or contraction stress test (CST) at frequent intervals, depending on the health care provider and preeclampsia severity (e.g., NST and/or BPP 1 to 2 times per week until delivery).
- Educate the family regarding the possibility of seizures and appropriate actions if seizure occurs.

Diet
- Provide nutritional counseling regarding a nutritious, balanced diet.
- Discuss the importance of adequate fluid intake.

Magnesium Sulfate
- Explain to the patient why she will have an indwelling catheter, infusion pump, continuous fetal monitoring, and assessment of DTRs and clonus. Explain that therapy will extend into the postpartum period 24 to 48 hours, depending on the agency and health care provider.
- Explain to the patient about visitor restrictions and the need for a low-stimulation environment.
- Advise the patient that she will likely experience a flushing, warm sensation and possibly nausea and vomiting during the initial loading dose.
- Advise the patient that evidence of magnesium levels within the therapeutic range includes decreased appetite, some speech slurring, double vision, and weakness.

Hydralazine
- Explain to the patient that nurses will be monitoring pulse and BP almost constantly, until they become stable after administration, then every 15 minutes thereafter. Explain that an electronic BP monitor may be used to obtain constant readings. Some health care providers will request manual BP measurements.
- Explain to the patient the need for careful measuring of I&O.
- Inform the patient that she may experience headache as a side effect of the drug.

🌐 Cultural Considerations
- Provide an interpreter with the same ethnic background and sex as the patient if possible, especially when dealing with sensitive topics or stressful situations.

Evaluation
- Evaluate effectiveness of therapy to reduce BP.
- Continue monitoring vital signs. Report any changes.
- Document effect of teaching and learning opportunities on patient's knowledge deficit about preeclampsia treatment modalities and outcomes.
- Note fetal well-being secondary to treatment with drugs as evidenced by fetal monitoring and fetal movement assessment.
- Monitor maternal physiologic changes in relation to magnesium sulfate levels.
- Continue monitoring FHR. Report changes.

▌ CRITICAL THINKING CASE STUDY

TA (gravida 3, para 0) has a history of spontaneous abortion at 10 weeks gestation and a preterm delivery and demise of a neonate at 21 weeks gestation. At her 28-week prenatal visit, she reports increased clear vaginal discharge and feelings of pelvic pressure. Examination of her cervix reveals 2-cm dilation and a presenting fetal part low in the pelvis. TA is admitted to the hospital, and uterine activity is documented. Magnesium sulfate therapy is ordered for treatment of preterm labor. The nurse prepares for IV magnesium sulfate administration.

1. How will magnesium sulfate therapy be initiated? What intervals and dosages should be anticipated?
2. What maternal and fetal side effects will the nurse expect to observe?
3. What should TA be told about the drug effects she will experience?
4. How would the nurse respond to TA's questions about the risks of preterm delivery?

After 24 hours of magnesium sulfate therapy, uterine contractions have been reduced to two to three per hour. TA is to be discharged home, and the nurse is preparing TA's discharge teaching.

5. What instructions should the nurse give TA about her activity and diet?
6. TA asks whether the side effects of magnesium sulfate will continue. What is an appropriate nursing response?
7. What signs and symptoms should TA be advised to report?

NCLEX STUDY QUESTIONS

1. A patient in her first trimester of pregnancy calls the nurse to ask for suggestions on decreasing nausea in the morning when she wakes. Which nonpharmacologic measures are used to decrease nausea and vomiting: (Select all that apply.)
   a. Eating crackers, dry toast, or other carbohydrate before rising
   b. Eating small frequent meals
   c. Eating a high-protein bedtime snack
   d. Eating high fat or seasoned foods

2. A patient is complaining of continued constipation after nonpharmacologic constipation treatment was attempted without success. Which drug would be a first-line treatment for constipation during pregnancy?
   a. Docusate sodium
   b. Magnesium citrate
   c. Castor oil
   d. Mineral oil

3. The nurse is teaching a pregnant patient how to decrease the gastrointestinal distress she experiences with prenatal vitamins. The nurse instructs the patient to do what?
   a. Take her vitamins between meals
   b. Eat when she takes her vitamins
   c. Drink orange juice when she takes her vitamins
   d. Drink milk when she takes her vitamins

4. The nurse at an infertility clinic is working with a preconceptional couple. The nurse advises the woman to take which supplement for at least 3 months before becoming pregnant?
   a. Iron
   b. Ginger
   c. Folic acid
   d. Vitamin B6

5. The nurse at a prenatal clinic is reviewing messages to be returned to patients that afternoon. Which patient will the nurse call first?
   a. Primigravida, 10 gestational weeks, with nausea and vomiting who requests information about ginger
   b. Gravida 2, 35 gestational weeks, with Braxton-Hicks contractions who requests information about caffeine
   c. Gravida 2, 32 gestational weeks, with gestational diabetes and a blood glucose of 132 who requests information about her insulin
   d. Primigravida, 28 gestational weeks, with preeclampsia who requests information about taking ibuprofen for headache

6. A patient with severe preeclampsia is on magnesium sulfate. The laboratory report shows a magnesium sulfate level of 7 mEq/L. Which of these is the most appropriate initial nursing intervention?
   a. Continue to monitor the patient because this level is therapeutic.
   b. Contact the health care provider and report the level.
   c. Prepare to administer 1 g of calcium gluconate.
   d. Turn the patient on her left side, and administer 10 L of oxygen by nasal cannula.

7. The nurse is assessing a patient in preterm labor who is receiving magnesium sulfate. What is the finding of most concern?
   a. Lethargy
   b. Feelings of warmth
   c. Loss of patellar reflexes
   d. Positive clonus +2 bilaterally

8. The patient has been receiving magnesium sulfate IV for 24 hours to treat severe preeclampsia. On assessment, the nurse finds a temperature of 37.3°C (99°F), pulse of 88, respirations at 14, blood pressure of 138/76, 21 patellar reflexes, and negative ankle clonus. What is the priority nursing intervention?
   a. Obtain a stat magnesium sulfate level.
   b. Discontinue magnesium sulfate.
   c. Contact the health care provider.
   d. Continue to monitor the patient.

9. A primigravida patient, 8 gestational weeks, is at the prenatal clinic for her first examination. She complains of nausea and vomiting "every morning." Which comment made by the patient would indicate the need for further instruction?
   a. My friend gave me ginger cookies to eat.
   b. I have been eating dry crackers before I get up.
   c. I have tried to avoid foods with strong smells.
   d. I have been drinking chamomile tea every day.

10. The nurse in labor and delivery is reviewing messages to be returned to patients. Which patient statement alerts the nurse to call that patient first?
    a. "I'm 32 weeks pregnant and taking calcium carbonate for my heartburn. Is there anything else I can take?"
    b. "I'm 38 weeks pregnant and taking ibuprofen for my backache. Should I take aspirin too?"
    c. "I'm 8 weeks pregnant and taking folic acid. Will it hurt me or the baby if I stop?"
    d. "I checked my blood glucose with a friend's machine and it was 120 mg. I'm not diabetic. Is that normal?"

11. A young adolescent—gravida 1, para 0—is admitted to labor and delivery with preterm labor at 29 weeks gestation. Which nursing interventions should the nurse include? (Select all that apply.)
    a. Administration of antenatal glucocorticoid
    b. Liver function tests
    c. Bed rest in the left lateral position
    d. Administration of bolus intravenous fluids
    e. Administration of tocolytics
    f. Administration of an antihypertensive

12. A patient is planning to become pregnant. Which actions should the nurse counsel the patient to initiate before she stops taking her oral contraceptive? (Select all that apply.)
    a. Stop smoking.
    b. Take omega-6 fatty acids every day.
    c. Take a multivitamin every day.
    d. Stop taking over-the-counter acetaminophen.
    e. See her health care provider.

Answers: 1, a, b, c; 2, a; 3, b; 4, c; 5, d; 6, a; 7, c; 8, d; 9, d; 10, b; 11, a, c, d, e; 12, a, c, e.

50

Labor, Delivery, and Postpartum

http://evolve.elsevier.com/McCuistion/pharmacology

OBJECTIVES

- Critique systemic and regional medications for their action, pain control during labor, side effects, and nursing implications.
- Describe the nursing process associated with the drugs used during labor and delivery, and include patient teaching.
- Compare drugs used to enhance uterine contractility during labor and after placental expulsion along with their action, side effects, and nursing implications.
- Discuss the purpose, action, side effects, and nursing implications of the drugs commonly administered during the postpartum period.
- Describe the nursing process related to drugs used during the postpartum period immediately after delivery, and include patient teaching.

OUTLINE

Drugs for Pain Control During Labor
Analgesia and Sedation
Nursing Process: Patient-Centered Collaborative Care—Pain-Control Drugs
Anesthesia
Regional Anesthesia
Nursing Process: Patient-Centered Collaborative Care—Regional Anesthetics
Drugs That Enhance Uterine Muscle Contractility
Oxytocin
Nursing Process: Patient-Centered Collaborative Care—Enhancement of Uterine Contractility: Oxytocin
Other Drugs That Enhance Uterine Contractions: Ergot Alkaloids
Nursing Process: Patient-Centered Collaborative Care—Other Oxytocics: Ergonovine and Methylergonovine
Drugs Used During the Postpartum Period

Pain Relief for Uterine Contractions
Pain Relief for Perineal Wounds and Hemorrhoids
Nursing Process: Patient-Centered Collaborative Care—Pain Relief for Perineal Wounds and Hemorrhoids
Lactation Suppression
Promotion of Bowel Function
Nursing Process: Patient-Centered Collaborative Care—Laxatives
Immunizations
$Rh_0(D)$ Immune Globulin
Nursing Process: Patient-Centered Collaborative Care—$Rh_0(D)$ Immune Globulin
Rubella Vaccine
Nursing Process: Patient-Centered Collaborative Care—Measles-Mumps-Rubella Vaccine
Critical Thinking Case Study
NCLEX Study Questions

KEY TERMS

antiflatulents, p. 750
Bishop score, p. 742
cervical ripening, p. 742
congenital rubella syndrome, p. 752
episiotomy, p. 747
ergot alkaloids, p. 744
ergotism, p. 744
flatus, p. 750
folliculitis, p. 748
labor augmentation, p. 742

labor induction, p. 741
lactation, p. 745
necrosis, p. 748
occlusive, p. 748
puerperium, p. 745
Rh sensitization, p. 751
$Rh_0(D)$ immune globulin, p. 751
urticaria, p. 752
uterine contractility, p. 742
uterine inertia, p. 742

DRUGS FOR PAIN CONTROL DURING LABOR

Labor and delivery are divided into four stages. During the first stage, the *dilating stage,* cervical effacement and dilation occur; the cervix thins and becomes fully dilated at 10 cm. The first stage consists of three phases categorized by cervical dilation: the *latent phase* (0 to 4 cm), the *active phase* (4 to 7 cm), and the *transition phase* (8 to 10 cm). The second stage of labor, the *pelvic stage,* begins with complete cervical dilation and ends with delivery of the newborn (Fig. 50.1). During the third stage of labor, *placental separation and expulsion,* the placenta separates from the uterine wall and is delivered. The fourth stage of labor, *early postpartum,* comprises the first 4 hours after the delivery of the placenta, and is a period of physiologic stabilization for the mother and initiation of familial attachment.

During the first stage of labor, uterine contractions produce progressive cervical effacement and dilation. As the first stage of labor progresses, uterine contractions become stronger, longer, and more frequent, and discomfort increases. Pain and discomfort in labor are caused by uterine contraction, cervical dilation and effacement, hypoxia of the contracting myometrium, and perineal pressure from the presenting part. Pain perception is influenced by physiologic, psychological, social, and cultural factors—in particular, the woman's past experiences with pain, anticipation of pain, fear and anxiety, knowledge deficit of the labor and delivery process, and involvement of support persons.

Before administering pharmacologic treatment, nonpharmacologic measures should be initiated. Nonpharmacologic measures for pain relief during labor include (1) ambulation, (2) effleurage and counterpressure, (3) touch and massage, (4) changing positions and rocking, (5) engaging support persons, (6) breathing and relaxation techniques, (7) transcutaneous electrical nerve stimulation, (8) application of heat and cold, (9) aromatherapy, and (10) hydrotherapy (warm-water baths or showers).

Other nonpharmacologic measures include alternative and complementary drugs. Of particular concern is the use of herbal supplements by the pregnant patient later in pregnancy to stimulate labor. For example, some women ingest pregnancy toner tea, which includes raspberry, nettle, dandelion, alfalfa, and peppermint leaf. Other herbal supplements used include blue cohosh, castor oil, and evening primrose oil. Pregnant patients may self-administer, or the practice may be part of their traditional beliefs and framework of health. Concerns with herbal supplements are related to the often numerous physiologically active components of the herbs, adulterants, inconsistent dosing, and lack of proven efficacy. Herbs taken in late pregnancy may contribute to preterm labor or increased bleeding during delivery. Nurses must be culturally sensitive to the use of herbal supplements and health practices during pregnancy, specifically in the later gestational weeks.

When pharmacologic intervention is needed for pain relief, drugs are used as an adjunct to nonpharmacologic measures.

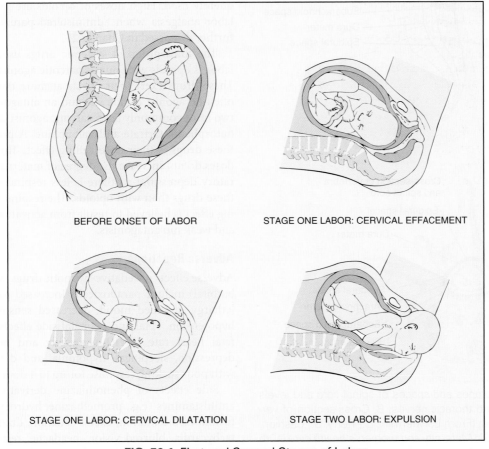

BEFORE ONSET OF LABOR

STAGE ONE LABOR: CERVICAL EFFACEMENT

STAGE ONE LABOR: CERVICAL DILATATION

STAGE TWO LABOR: EXPULSION

FIG. 50.1 First and Second Stages of Labor.

Drugs should be selected not only to decrease the patient's pain but also to minimize side effects for the patient and the fetus or neonate. Pain relief in labor can be obtained with systemic analgesics and regional anesthesia, injection of drug near the nerves or spinal canal to numb a specific area of the body (Fig. 50.2). Analgesics alter the patient's perception and sensation of pain without producing unconsciousness.

Analgesia and Sedation

Systemic drugs used during labor include sedative-hypnotics, narcotic agonists, and mixed narcotic agonist-antagonists. Seco-barbital, a sedative-hypnotic, is administered orally, whereas hydroxyzine is administered orally or intramuscularly. Intrave-nous (IV) use is considered contraindicated because hydroxyzine is a vesicant. Because of variable response and blood levels with intramuscular (IM) administration, pentobarbital is primarily given intravenously. These drugs should be administered at the onset of the uterine contraction because parenteral administra-tion at the onset decreases neonatal drug exposure because blood flow is decreased to the uterus and fetus.

Table 50.1 lists the analgesics and sedatives commonly used during labor, delivery, and postpartum and their dosages, uses, and considerations.

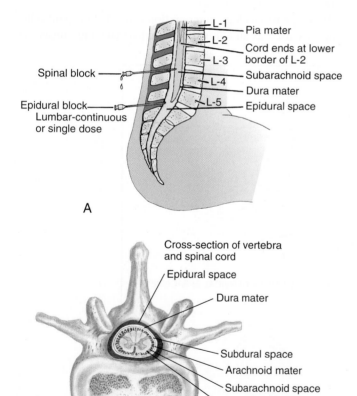

FIG. 50.2 A, Membranes and spaces of spinal cord and levels of sacral, lumbar, and thoracic nerves. B, Cross-section of ver-tebra and spinal cord. (From Lowdermilk, D., Perry, S., Cashion, C., & Alden, K. [2012]. *Maternity and women's health care* (10th ed.). St. Louis: Mosby.)

The sedative-tranquilizer drugs are most commonly given for false or latent labor or with ruptured membranes without true labor. These drugs may also be administered to minimize maternal anxiety and fear, and although they promote rest and relaxation, they do not provide pain relief. The sedative drugs most commonly used are barbiturates or hypnotics (e.g., seco-barbital sodium and pentobarbital sodium). Other drugs, such as hydroxyzine, can be given alone during early labor or in combination with narcotic agonists when the patient is in active labor. In addition to decreasing anxiety and apprehension, hydroxyzine potentiates the analgesic action of the opioids and minimizes emesis. Promethazine, also a phenothiazine deriva-tive, has been noted in studies to impair the analgesic efficacy of opioids and is now only labeled for nausea and vomiting.

The second group of drugs given for active labor is the nar-cotic agonists. These drugs may be administered parenterally or via regional blocks. When administered with neuraxial anesthe-sia, a lower dose of anesthetic is required for effective pain relief, thereby minimizing side effects. These drugs interfere with pain impulses at the subcortical level of the brain. To effect pain relief, opioids interact with mu and kappa receptors; for exam-ple, morphine sulfate activates both mu and kappa receptors.

Of the narcotic agonists, meperidine is the most commonly prescribed synthetic opioid for pain control during labor. A sec-ond narcotic agonist used for pain relief during labor is fentanyl, a short-acting synthetic opioid best administered intravenously because of its short duration of action. Morphine sulfate may also be used for pain control in active labor, but it is less fre-quently used. High doses of opioids are required for effective labor analgesia when administered parenterally. Opioids are further discussed in Chapter 25.

The third group of systemic drugs used for pain relief in labor is opioids with mixed narcotic agonist-antagonist effects. These drugs exert their effects at more than one site and are often an agonist at one site and an antagonist at another. The two most commonly used narcotic agonist-antagonist drugs are butorphanol tartrate and nalbuphine. A primary advantage of these drugs is their dose-ceiling effect. This means additional doses do not increase the degree of maternal or neonatal respi-ratory depression, so there is less respiratory depression with these drugs than with opioids. The respiratory depression ceil-ing effect is believed to result from activation of kappa agonists and weak mu antagonists.

Adverse Reactions

Adverse effects of sedative-hypnotic drugs (secobarbital, pento-barbital) include paradoxically increased pain and excitability, lethargy, subdued mood, decreased sensory perception, and hypotension. Fetal and neonatal side effects include decreased fetal heart rate (FHR) variability and neonatal respiratory depression, sleepiness, hypotonia, and delayed breastfeeding with poor sucking response for up to 4 days.

Side effects of phenothiazine derivatives and antiemetic antihistamines (e.g., promethazine, hydroxyzine) include con-fusion, disorientation, excess sedation, dizziness, hypotension, tachycardia, blurred vision, headache, restlessness, weakness, and urinary retention with promethazine; drowsiness, dry

TABLE 50.1   Analgesics Used During Labor, Delivery, and Postpartum

Drug	Route and Dosage	Uses and Considerations
SEDATIVE-HYPNOTICS		
Secobarbital	PO: 100 mg x 1 dose	To decrease anxiety during the latent phase of labor; does not affect uterine tone or contractility; rapidly crosses placenta; can cause decreased variability in FHR because of decreased CNS control over heart rate. No antagonist exists for barbiturates, so secobarbital is administered only if delivery is not expected for 24-48 h. Onset: 15-30 min; peak: 15-30 min; duration: 1-4 h. Pregnancy category D*; PB: 45%-60%; t½: 15-40 h
Pentobarbital	IV: Initial: 100 mg then in increments of 25-50 mg as indicated	Short-acting barbiturate and sedative for latent phase of labor. Onset: Immediate (5 min). Pregnancy category D*; PB: Varies based upon lipid solubility; t½: 15-50 h
Promethazine, promethazine hydrochloride	IM/IV: 12.5-50 mg; may repeat q4h; *max:* 100 mg/24 h	A phenothiazine antihistamine and antiemetic often given with opioids to increase sedation and reduce nausea and vomiting in labor. Do not give subcutaneously. ❶ *Black-box warning:* Severe tissue damage has been seen with injections and extravasation, which can result in necrosis and gangrene; use the Z-track method for IM injection to prevent or reduce complications, and dilute IV doses and give over 10-15 min. Instruct patients to report signs of pain and burning with administration. Onset: IM: 20 min; IV: 3-5 min. Pregnancy category C*; PB: 35%-55%; t½: 22 h
Hydroxyzine	Anxiety: PO: 25-100 mg qid PRN Preoperative sedation: PO: 50-100 mg as a single dose	Anxiolytic antiemetic antihistamine used as a preoperative and postoperative adjunct for sedation. Onset: 15-30 min; peak: 2 h; duration: 2-36 h. Pregnancy category C*; PB: UK; t½: 3-7 h
NARCOTIC AGONISTS		
Fentanyl citrate	IM/IV: 50-100 mcg Give IV over 1-2 min, may repeat q1-2h PRN; muscle rigidity may occur when IV administration is too rapid. Regional anesthesia: Initial 50-100 mcg bolus, then 10-15 mL/h of bupivacaine and fentanyl cont. infusion.	❶ A synthetic opiate that is 50 to 100 times as potent as morphine; provides mild to moderate sedation and pain relief during labor; also used as an adjunct to regional anesthesia. Drug crosses the placenta and is excreted in breast milk, so watch for respiratory depression in neonates of mothers who receive this drug in labor; withdrawal symptoms may occur in the neonate if the mother was a regular opioid user during pregnancy. Use is contraindicated in patients with severe asthma. Onset: IV, 1-2 min; IM, 7-15 min. Peak: IV, 3-5 min; IM, 20-30 min. Duration: IV, 30-60 min; IM, 1-2 h. Pregnancy category C*; PB: UK; t½: 2-4 h
Morphine sulfate	IM/IV/Subcut: 2-10 mg q3-4h PRN When giving IV, dilute in 4-5 mL of sterile water and administer slowly (15 mg over 3-5 min). Can also be given via epidural at 1/10th of the IV dose.	An opioid that binds to CNS opiate receptors and inhibits ascending pain pathways; used for relief of moderate to severe pain, for preoperative medication, and as a supplement to anesthesia. Monitor for CNS and respiratory depression. Have naloxone available as antidote. Onset: IM, 20-30 min; IV, 3-10 min. Peak: IM, 0.5-1 h; IV, 20 min. Duration: IM, 3-4 h; IV, 3-5 h. Pregnancy category C*; PB: 30%-35%; t½: 2-4 h
MIXED NARCOTIC AGONIST-ANTAGONISTS		
Butorphanol tartrate	IM/IV: 1-2 mg q4h PRN	Mixed opioid agonist-antagonist used for relief of moderate to severe pain. Used in pregnancies >37 wk with no fetal distress. Use alternative analgesic if delivery is anticipated in 4 h or less. Onset: 5-10 min; peak: 4-5 min; duration: 3-4 h. Pregnancy category C*; PB: 80%; t½: 2.5-4 h
Nalbuphine hydrochloride	IV: 10 mg q3-6h PRN	Mixed opioid agonist-antagonist narcotic Onset: 2-3 min; peak: 2-3 min; duration: 3-6 h. Pregnancy category B*; PB: UK; t½: 5 h
POSTPARTUM PERINEAL WOUNDS AND HEMORRHOIDS		
Benzocaine, aerosol 20%	Spray liberally tid/qid 6-12 inches from the perineum following perineal cleansing.	A local anesthetic that inhibits impulses from sensory nerves by decreasing permeability of the cell membrane to sodium ions; it is hydrolyzed in plasma and liver (to a lesser extent) by cholinesterase and is eliminated as metabolites in urine. Drug is well absorbed from mucous membranes and traumatized skin and is contraindicated in patients with secondary bacterial infection of tissue and known hypersensitivity. Peak: 1 min; duration: 30-60 min. Pregnancy category C*; PB: UK; t½: UK

Continued

TABLE 50.1	Analgesics Used During Labor, Delivery, and Postpartum—cont'd	
Drug	**Route and Dosage**	**Uses and Considerations**
POSTPARTUM PERINEAL WOUNDS AND HEMORRHOIDS		
Witch hazel or pramoxine premedicated pads	Apply premoistened pads up to 6 times daily, especially after bowel movements.	Precipitates protein, causing tissue to contract. May be refrigerated in the original container for additional comfort. If liquid, pour over ice and dip absorbent pads into solution; change when diluted. Medical intervention should be sought if rectal bleeding is present. Side effect: local irritation (discontinue use) Pregnancy category UK*; PB: UK; t½: UK
Hydrocortisone acetate 10 mg	Insert 1 suppository bid rectally for 2 wk. Wear gloves to administer.	Acts as an antiinflammatory agent to relieve pain and itching from irritated anorectal tissue. Contraindicated in patients with known hypersensitivity. Discontinue if tissue infection occurs. If anorectal symptoms do not improve in 7 days or if bleeding, protrusion, or seepage occurs, inform the health care provider. Do not use if fourth-degree perineal laceration is present. It is unknown whether drug is excreted in breast milk; use cautiously. Onset, peak, and duration are unknown. Pregnancy category C*
Dibucaine ointment, USP 1%	Apply to cleansed rectum 3-4 times daily, using no more than 30 g in 24 h	Topical anesthetic with the same action as benzocaine. Do not use near eyes or over denuded surfaces or blistered areas or if rectal bleeding is present. Do not use with known hypersensitivity to amide-type anesthetics. Side effects include burning, tenderness, irritation, inflammation, contact dermatitis, urticaria, cutaneous lesions, and edema. Onset: Within 15 min; peak: UK; duration: 2-4 h. Pregnancy category C*

*Pregnancy categories have been revised. See http://www.fda.gov/Drugs/DevelopmentApprovalProcess/DevelopmentResources/Labeling/ucm093 307.htm for more information.

bid, Twice daily; *CNS*, central nervous system; *cont.*, continuous; *FHR*, fetal heart rate; *h*, hour; *IM*, intramuscular; *IV*, intravenous; *max*, maximum; *min*, minute; *PB*, protein binding; *PO*, by mouth; *PRN*, as needed; *q*, every; *qid*, four times daily; *subcut*, subcutaneously; *t½*, half-life; *tid*, three times daily; *UK*, unknown; *USP*, U.S. Pharmacopeia; *wk*, weeks; *>*, greater than.

mouth, dizziness, headache, blurred vision, dysuria, urinary retention, and constipation with hydroxyzine. Decreased FHR variability can occur, and the neonate can experience moderate central nervous system (CNS) depression, hypotonia, lethargy, poor feeding, and hypothermia.

The adverse effects of opioids depend on the responses activated by the mu and kappa receptors. Activation of mu receptors results in analgesia, sedation, euphoria, decreased gastrointestinal (GI) motility, respiratory depression, and physiologic dependence. Activation of kappa receptors results in analgesia, decreased GI motility, miosis, and sedation. When parenterally administered, the side effects of opioids include nausea, vomiting, sedation, orthostatic hypotension, pruritus, and maternal and neonatal respiratory depression. The associated nausea and vomiting result from stimulation of the chemoreceptor trigger zone in the medulla. Motor block is another concern; mothers may not walk after delivery until they are able to maintain a straight leg raise against downward pressure applied by the practitioner. Fetal and neonatal effects include decreased FHR variability, depression of neonatal respirations, and depression of neonatal neurobehavior. For example, neonatal respiratory depression occurs within 2 to 3 hours after administering meperidine and may require reversal by administration of naloxone. Through inhibition of both mu and kappa receptors, naloxone may reverse the effects of opioids. It is important to note that with maternal administration of naloxone, there will be a subsequent increase in pain.

Narcotic agonist drugs (e.g., morphine, fentanyl) can cause orthostatic hypotension, nausea, vomiting, headache, sedation, hypotension, and confusion. Decreased FHR variability and neonatal CNS depression can occur with meperidine.

Mixed narcotic agonist-antagonist drugs (e.g., butorphanol tartrate, nalbuphine) can cause nausea, clamminess, sweating, sedation, respiratory depression, vertigo, lethargy, headache, and flush. Side effects in the fetus and neonate include decreased FHR variability, moderate CNS depression, hypotonia at birth, and mild behavioral depression.

 NURSING PROCESS
Patient-Centered Collaborative Care

Pain-Control Drugs

Assessment
- Assess the patient's level of pain.
- Assess the patient's cultural framework to determine beliefs regarding labor and cultural expectations related to pain experiences.
- Assess for use of complementary and alternative medicine (CAM), including supplements, at any point during the pregnancy.
- Screen for drug history to ascertain the potential for drug-drug interactions.
- Before administering analgesic, obtain vital signs (blood pressure [BP], heart rate [HR]), respiratory status, quality of uterine contractions, degree of effacement and dilation, and FHR; monitor the effectiveness of pain management.
- Assess the laboring patient's behavior for relaxation and progress of labor in relation to expected norms.
- Assess the patient's verbal and nonverbal behavior for data supportive or nonsupportive of coping with labor.

Nursing Diagnoses
- Anxiety related to uncertainty about the labor experience and coping ability
- Pain, Acute related to processes of labor and birth
- Fear related to deficient knowledge of processes and birth and expected sensations with analgesic interventions

Planning
- The patient will verbalize the desired amount of pain relief during labor.
- The patient will demonstrate minimal to no side effects from pain-control drugs during labor.
- The patient will verbalize a decrease in pain on a scale of 1 to 10 or per the agency's pain scale.

Nursing Interventions
- Offer analgesia appropriate for the stage and phase of labor and anticipated method of delivery. Encourage the patient and her support persons to participate in decision making about analgesia.
- Document the administration of drugs per agency protocol.
- Provide appropriate safety measures after administration of drugs.
- ⚡ Check a compatibility chart for any mixing of drugs.
- Verify that correct antidote drugs are available.
- Within agency protocol, safe obstetric practice, and patient preferences, administer drugs before pain and anxiety reach maximum intensity.
- Assess the patient's level of pain using an agency-appropriate pain scale 30 to 60 minutes after analgesic administration.

Sedative-Hypnotics: Barbiturates
- Do not give if active labor is imminent.
- Monitor FHR and expect decreased variability.

Phenothiazine Derivatives
Promethazine
- If administered intravenously, give at the onset of uterine contractions. Administer at a rate not to exceed 25 mg/min.
- Monitor the amount of promethazine the patient receives in 24 hours, and monitor maternal heart rate after administration.
Hydroxyzine
- Administer deep IM only (Z-track technique). Do not give subcutaneously or intravenously.

Narcotic Agonists and Mixed Narcotic Agonist-Antagonists
- Assess patient parity, obstetric delivery history, and anticipated time until delivery.
- Because of risk of neonatal respiratory depression, do not administer when delivery is likely within 2 hours.
- Monitor urine output.
- Monitor FHR, assessing for fetal well-being before and during drug administration.

Fentanyl
- Fentanyl is not generally given before active labor. Have neonatal and maternal naloxone available as an antidote.
- If drug is administered intravenously, give slowly at the beginning of a contraction and over several minutes to decrease the amount of drug perfused to the fetus via the placenta.
- Assess respirations. They must be greater than 12 per minute before administration.
- Provide a restful environment as adjunctive therapy.
- Keep bed rails up when the patient is nonambulatory, and have the patient solicit assistance with ambulation.
- Monitor FHR, assessing for fetal well-being before and during drug administration.

Butorphanol Tartrate
- Have naloxone available.
- Monitor for signs of narcotic withdrawal in narcotic-dependent patients.
- Monitor for maternal and neonatal respiratory depression.
- Assess respirations. They must be greater than 12 per minute before administration.
- When drug is given intramuscularly, inject deep into the muscle; when given intravenously, administer slowly at the onset of a contraction. Do not administer subcutaneously.
- Provide a restful environment as adjunctive therapy.
- Monitor the FHR tracing, assessing for fetal well-being before and during drug administration.
- Keep bed rails up when the patient is nonambulatory, and have the patient solicit assistance with ambulation.

Patient Teaching
General
- Advise the patient concerning (1) drugs ordered, (2) route of administration and reason, (3) expected effects of the drug on labor, and (4) potential drug effects on the mother and the fetus or neonate.
- Inform the patient that most drugs used for pain relief in labor and delivery are not given by mouth because the GI tract functions more slowly during labor, and drug absorption is decreased, making the oral route ineffective.
- Counsel the patient about safety precautions to be used while receiving the drug, including (1) positioning in bed, (2) use of side rails, and (3) assistance with ambulation.

🌐 Cultural Considerations
- Acknowledge and incorporate the patient's cultural belief framework into nursing care.
- Assess the patient's use of CAM, including herbal supplements, during pregnancy and labor.
- Recognize cultural influences on the patient's expression of discomfort and pain.
- Provide an interpreter as appropriate.

Evaluation
- Evaluate effectiveness of the drug in alleviating pain.
- Evaluate fear and anxiety in regard to pain and the ability to cope with labor.

- Monitor maternal respirations, heart rate, BP, uterine contractions, dilation and effacement, and FHR for alterations from baseline. Report deviations beyond those expected with normally progressing labor.
- Document findings using agency protocol and obstetric nursing standards of care.

Anesthesia

Anesthesia in labor and delivery represents the loss of painful sensations with or without loss of consciousness. Two types of pain are experienced in childbirth, visceral and somatic. *Visceral pain* from the cervix and uterus is carried by sympathetic fibers and enters the neuraxis at the thoracic (T10-T12) and lumbar (L1) spinal levels, and early labor pain is transmitted to T11 and T12 with later progression to T10 and L1. *Somatic pain* is caused by pressure of the presenting part and by stretching of the perineum and vagina. This is the pain of the transition phase and the second stage of labor, and it is transmitted to the sacral (S2-S4)

areas by the pudendal nerve. Table 50.2 lists the anesthetics used during labor and delivery and their dosages, uses, and considerations.

Regional Anesthesia

Regional anesthesia achieves pain relief during labor and delivery without loss of consciousness. Injected local anesthetic agents temporarily block conduction of painful impulses along sensory nerve pathways to the brain. Regional anesthesia allows the patient to experience labor and childbirth with relief from discomfort in the blocked area while maintaining consciousness. The two primary types of anesthesia are *local anesthetics* for local infiltration (e.g., episiotomy) and *regional blocks* (e.g., epidural, spinal). The most common types of peridural anesthesia are spinal, epidural, and combined spinal-epidural blocks. Other less commonly administered regional blocks include caudal, paracervical, and pudendal blocks. The anesthesiologist or nurse anesthetist is responsible for administering regional anesthesia. Nurses may assist with administration of anesthesia, and

TABLE 50.2 Anesthetic Used in Obstetrics†

Drug	Route and Dosage	Uses and Considerations
Chloroprocaine	Lumbar epidural block: 2% or 3%, 2 to 2.5 mL per segment; usual start volume is 15-25 mL; *max:* single dose (with epinephrine 1:200,000), 14 mg/kg; total dose, 750 mg	An ester-type local anesthetic that stabilizes the neuronal membranes and prevents initiation and transmission of nerve impulses, affecting local anesthetic actions (local or pudendal block) Duration: Up to 60 min. Pregnancy category C*; PB: UK; t½: 21-25 sec
Tetracaine 0.2%, 0.3%	Spinal anesthesia: Lower abd: 9-12 mg of 0.3% Perineum: 3-6 mg of 0.3% Saddle block: 2-4 mg of 0.2%; *max:* 15 mg Other anesthesia dosages available.	An ester-type local anesthetic that blocks both initiation and conduction of nerve impulses by decreasing neuronal membrane permeability to sodium ions; a low spinal block or spinal anesthesia for cesarean delivery Pregnancy category C*; PB: UK; t½: UK
Lidocaine injectable	50-75 mg of 5% solution; *max:* 4 mg/kg/dose or 300 mg per procedure when used without epinephrine	Suppresses automaticity of conduction tissue by increasing the electrical stimulation threshold of the ventricle; blocks both initiation and conduction of nerve impulses by decreasing neuronal membrane permeability to sodium ions Onset: 45-90 s; duration: 10-20 min. Pregnancy category B*; PB 60%-80%; t½: 1.5-2 h
Bupivacaine	Epidural block: 3-4 mL increments IV or intrathecal administration of 10-20 mL of 0.25% or 0.5% The 0.75% concentration is not recommended for obstetric anesthesia; reports of cardiac arrest with difficult resuscitation and death have been reported.	Epidural or spinal for labor and cesarean delivery; blocks both initiation and conduction of nerve impulses by decreasing neuronal membrane permeability to sodium ions Onset: Up to 17 min; duration: epidural, 2-7.7 h; spinal, 1.5-2.5 h. Pregnancy category C*; PB: 84%-95%; t½: 2.7 h
Ropivacaine	Lumbar epidural block for cesarean section: 20-30 mL dose of 0.5% solution or 15-20 mL of 0.75% solution in incremental doses Doses available for vaginal obstetric anesthesia as incremental administration or continuous infusion.	Epidural for cesarean delivery; blocks both initiation and conduction of nerve impulses by decreasing neuronal membrane permeability to sodium ions Onset: 3-15 min; duration: 3-15 h. Pregnancy category C*; PB: UK; t½: 5-7 h

*Pregnancy categories have been revised. See http://www.fda.gov/Drugs/DevelopmentApprovalProcess/DevelopmentResources/Labeling/ucm093307.htm for more information.
†The following nursing considerations apply to all types of epidurals: Use a test dose (3 mL of lidocaine 1.5% with 1:200,000 epinephrine) to confirm correct catheter placement. If a local anesthetic is injected into a vein, the patient may experience dizziness, ringing in the ears, numbness, a metallic taste in the mouth, or a toxic response. Maternal lateral positioning is done to prevent aortocaval compression. Maternal diastolic blood pressure (BP) should be less than 110 mm Hg before initiating the epidural. When maternal hypotension occurs, place the patient on her left side, infuse IV fluids rapidly, and administer ephedrine 5 to 10 mg IV or 100 mcg phenylephrine IV. Repeat as necessary. Monitor BP every 1 to 2 min for the first 10 min, then every 10 to 30 min until the block wears off. Assess the level of analgesia. After administration of the anesthetic, assess motor strength prior to ambulation.
abd, Abdomen; *h,* hour; *IV,* intravenous; *max,* maximum dosage; *min,* minute; *PB,* protein binding; *t½,* half-life; *UK,* unknown.

they monitor the patient for drug effectiveness and side effects during and after administration.

Women receiving parenteral analgesic for labor and delivery may require more focused anesthesia for episiotomies and repair of perineal lacerations. Local anesthetic drugs may be administered alone, and the anesthetic drug primarily administered is lidocaine. Burning at the site of injection is the most common side effect.

Spinal anesthesia, also known as a *saddle block,* is injected in the subarachnoid space at the T10 to S5 dermatome. This anesthesia may be administered as a single dose or as a combined spinal-epidural block. Spinal anesthesia is administered immediately before delivery or late in the second stage, when the fetal head is on the perineal floor. Drugs frequently administered either alone or in combination with the local anesthetic for a vaginal delivery include bupivacaine with fentanyl. Dosages vary depending on whether administration of the anesthetic agent is plain or with epinephrine. Bupivacaine 0.75% concentration is *not* recommended for obstetric anesthesia due to reports of cardiac arrest with difficult resuscitation or death. Spinal anesthesia has a rapid onset, requires less local anesthetic, and may be used with high-risk patients. Postdural puncture headache is a primary concern and occurs 6 to 48 hours after dural puncture; it may also occur after accidental dural puncture with epidural anesthesia. Treatment for postdural headache includes analgesics, increased fluids, and bed rest. An epidural blood patch is the most effective means to treat postdural headache.

Lumbar epidurals may be administered as a single injection, by intermittent injection, as continuous patient-controlled epidural anesthesia (PCEA), or as a combined spinal-epidural block. Epidurals may be administered as a single anesthetic drug or with opioids or epinephrine. Most frequently, patients now receive a continuous epidural infusion, which provides more consistent drug levels and more effective pain relief. Rescue doses are given as necessary to achieve pain relief.

Opioids are administered with the local anesthetic to more effectively control the somatic pain of transition and second-stage labor. The opioids most frequently used in combination with the local anesthetic (bupivacaine, ropivacaine) are fentanyl or sufentanil, *lipophilic opioids* commonly used with continuous or patient-controlled epidural; these opioids offer rapid analgesia and fewer side effects than hydrophilic opioids. In contrast, morphine sulfate and hydromorphone are *hydrophilic opioids,* which have a slower onset of action, variable duration, and increased side effects, specifically respiratory depression (Table 50.2).

Another additive to the local anesthetic is epinephrine, which increases the duration of the local anesthetic, decreases its uptake and clearance from the cerebrospinal fluid (CSF), and enhances the intensity of the neural blockade. Single and intermittent injections have wide variations in drug levels and provide less effective control of pain. A continuous lumbar epidural allows a more evenly spaced drug level; less anesthetic is required to provide more effective pain control. Continuous-infusion PCEA gives the patient better control of her anesthesia Often single and intermittent injections and PCEA will require rescue doses to improve analgesia.

Lastly, combined spinal-epidural analgesia couples the rapid analgesia and specificity of catheter placement of spinal anesthesia with the continuous infusion via catheter of epidural anesthesia, providing pain relief for later labor.

Controversy exists regarding the effect of regional analgesia, specifically epidurals, on the progress of labor. Some studies indicate no significant effect on labor, whereas other research has demonstrated a decreased maternal urge to push and increased length of labor.

Anesthesia for cesarean delivery may be general, spinal, or epidural. General anesthesia, although rarely used, may be necessary for emergency deliveries, when spinal or epidural anesthesia are contraindicated. It allows for rapid anesthesia induction and control of the airway. Before the administration of general anesthesia, antacids or other drugs that reduce gastric secretions are given to decrease gastric acidity. See Unit XIII: Gastrointestinal Drugs for more information on acid reducers. More commonly, spinal or epidural anesthesia is administered for cesarean births. Spinal anesthesia is the more common choice for cesarean delivery because of rapid onset, increased reliability, and improvement in spinal needle design (smaller gauge and shape [Sprotte needle]) with subsequent reduction in postdural headaches. With spinal anesthesia, the local anesthetic most commonly administered is bupivacaine with fentanyl; pain relief begins in 5 minutes and lasts for approximately 2 hours. Sufentanil or morphine may also be administered. With the additives, spinal anesthesia provides 18 to 24 hours of pain relief. For epidural inductions, the test dose of lidocaine with epinephrine—followed by administration of local anesthetics— is given. This is followed by a bolus or maintenance infusion with anesthetics with or without opioids and/or epinephrine to maintain maternal comfort. The nurse should assess the level of analgesia and motor block at least hourly. Monitor for complications, such as cardiovascular or central nervous system toxicity, postdural puncture headache, fetal bradycardia, or respiratory depression.

◎ NURSING PROCESS
Patient-Centered Collaborative Care
Regional Anesthetics

Assessment
- Check the patient's history for drug sensitivity to local anesthetic agents.
- Assess the patient's labor plan with expectations for coping with labor and beliefs about use of analgesia and anesthesia.
- Assess the patient's knowledge about regional anesthesia.
- Assess cervical dilation and effacement and labor progress.
- Monitor fetal status.
- Review the patient's history for contraindications to regional anesthesia; notify the anesthesia provider.

Nursing Diagnoses
- Fear related to deficient knowledge of regional anesthesia/analgesia and expected sensations
- Pain, Acute related to processes of labor and delivery

- Gas Exchange, Risk for Impaired (fetal)
- Tissue Perfusion, Ineffective (maternal/fetal) related to the effects of analgesia/anesthesia and maternal position
- Mobility, Impaired related to paresthesia secondary to regional anesthesia
- Urinary Retention, Risk for

Planning
- The patient will verbalize the desired amount of pain relief during labor.
- The patient will remain normotensive and will maintain a normal pulse rate; FHR will remain within normal parameters.
- The patient will not experience bladder distension.
- The patient will be able to discuss use of regional anesthesia for labor and delivery pain control.

Nursing Interventions
General
- ⚡ Assess hydration status before regional anesthesia is given; monitor for anesthetic hypotensive effects. Provide bolus IV fluids as ordered, usually 500 to 1000 mL before regional anesthesia administration.
- Insert an indwelling urinary catheter before administration to monitor maternal fluid status.
- Position and support the patient on her left side or as instructed by the anesthesia provider.
- Monitor labor progress for any decrease in frequency or intensity of uterine contractions.
- ⚡ Monitor maternal vital signs and FHR.
- ⚡ Have oxygen and emergency drugs, including ephedrine and antihistamines, available along with resuscitation equipment.
- Be aware of how to place a patient in Trendelenburg position (supine on a surface inclined 45 degrees, head at the lower end and legs flexed over the upper end) if necessary.
- Monitor for postdural puncture headache; notify the anesthesia provider.

Spinal
- Assess uterine contractions; anesthetic drugs must be given immediately after a contraction.
- ⚡ Monitor BP for hypotensive effects per agency protocol; this is generally a decrease in systolic BP greater than 20% to 30% of baseline or below 100 mm Hg.
- ⚡ Have oxygen with positive-pressure ventilation equipment readily available.
- Assess level of analgesia following administration and sensory and motor status following delivery.
- Document procedures per agency protocol.

Epidural
- ⚡ Ensure that the patient has 500 to 1000 mL IV bolus of an isotonic solution before the procedure to increase circulatory volume and prevent maternal hypotension.
- Monitor FHR and progress of labor, and keep in mind that anesthetic can inhibit fetal descent.
- ⚡ Monitor BP for hypotensive effects per agency protocol.
- Assess the level of analgesia following administration.

- ⚡ If maternal hypotension occurs, maintain the patient on her left side and increase the rate of IV fluids per agency protocol. Notify the health care provider immediately.
- Assess for bladder distension. If voiding cues are unsuccessful (e.g., placement in semi-Fowler position, privacy, running water over the perineum, running water over the hand), catheterize the patient.
- Before allowing the patient to ambulate after delivery, assess sensory and motor status.
- ⚡ Conduct ongoing pain assessment. If the nature of the patient's pain changes, contact the anesthesia provider to evaluate anesthesia needs.
- Document procedures per agency protocol.

Caudal
- Place the patient in the position requested by the anesthesia provider for administration.

Paracervical Block
- Maintain continuous FHR monitoring for fetal bradycardia after administration.
- Monitor maternal BP.

Patient Teaching
General
- Discuss technique, potential benefits, and side effects of the patient's particular method of anesthesia.

Side Effects
- Instruct the patient that regional anesthetics may slow labor and that she may need a drug to enhance uterine contractions.
- ⚡ Assess the patient for postdural puncture headache after spinal anesthesia or after accidental dural puncture with epidural anesthesia. Advise the patient that bed rest, oral analgesics, caffeine, or an autologous blood patch may be used for headache pain relief.

Skill
- Teach the patient how to curl into position for epidural administration.
- Advise the patient that forceps or vacuum extraction may be needed for delivery because of reduction of the "urge to push" sensation.
- Teach the patient how to assume the left lateral or other position as requested by the anesthesia provider for caudal anesthesia.
- ⚡ Advise a patient receiving epidural anesthesia that she will have an IV and close monitoring of FHR and uterine contractions secondary to anesthesia.

Evaluation
- Evaluate BP compared with preprocedure baseline; evaluate FHR for alterations in variability and for decelerations.
- Evaluate effectiveness of anesthetic in relieving discomfort. Evaluate for uniformity of anesthesia; if there is lateralization or if it is "patchy," notify the anesthesia provider.
- Assess for bladder distension. If voiding cues are unsuccessful, catheterize the patient.
- Before allowing the patient to ambulate after delivery, assess sensory and motor status.
- Evaluate the uterine fundus for firmness.

Absolute Contraindications to Regional Anesthesia

- Severe gestational hypertension (increased risk of profound hypotension associated with the underlying disease state)
- Coagulation disorders and risk of bleeding secondary to decreased platelets (The patient should have a normal partial thromboplastin time and platelet count.)
- Generalized sepsis or local infection at the needle insertion site

DRUGS THAT ENHANCE UTERINE MUSCLE CONTRACTILITY

Uterotropic drugs enhance uterine contractility by stimulating the smooth muscle of the uterus. Oxytocin, the ergot alkaloids, and some prostaglandins constitute the uterotropics.

Oxytocin is synthesized in the hypothalamus and is transported to nerve endings in the posterior pituitary gland. The hormone is released by the nerve endings under appropriate stimulation; capillaries absorb the substance and carry it into the general circulation, where it facilitates uterine smooth muscle contraction. Table 50.3 lists drugs commonly used for cervical ripening and uterine contraction.

In the presence of adequate estrogen levels, those normally achieved by the third trimester, IV oxytocin stimulates uterine contraction. Oxytocin prepared in a synthetic form is approved by the U.S. Food and Drug Administration (FDA) for **labor induction**, the process of causing or initiating labor, and also for labor augmentation. Box 50.1 presents common medical indications for labor induction.

TABLE 50.3	Cervical Ripening and Uterine Contractions	
Drug	**Route and Dosage**	**Uses and Considerations**
	CERVICAL RIPENING	
Dinoprostone cervical gel, 0.5 mg	Contains 0.5 mg of dinoprostone in 2.5 mL of gel for intracervical use. Repeat in 6-12 h if negative cervical or uterine response. *Max.* 1.5 mg/24 h. Before beginning oxytocin after dinoprostone cervical gel administration, there should be a 6- to 12-h delay.	Naturally occurring form of prostaglandin E_2 (PGE_2). Used to ripen an unfavorable cervix at or near term in women needing labor induction. Must be at room temperature before administration and is administered by sterile technique. Patient is to remain recumbent 15-30 min following administration of gel and 2 h after insert. Pregnancy category C*; PB: UK; t½: UK; onset: 10-60 min; peak: UK; duration: 12 h
Dinoprostone vaginal inserts, 10 mg	Contains 10 mg of dinoprostone in a timed-release insert that supplies 0.3 mg/h. Insert is left in place for 12 h. Oxytocin may be started 30-60 min after removal of an insert. In contrast to gel, inserts may be removed with FHR decelerations or uterine hyperstimulation. Ripening an unfavorable cervix: 10 mg over 12 h; remove 12 h after insertion or at onset of active labor.	Assess cervical dilation and effacement at time of insertion. After administration, patient remains in a lying position for 30 min to 2 h. Monitor FHR and uterine stimulation. Have medication available for frequent GI side effects of abdominal cramping, diarrhea, nausea, and vomiting. If uterine hyperstimulation occurs, remove the insert and have oxygen or beta-adrenergic drugs to treat. Onset: UK; peak: UK; duration: up to 2-3 h. Pregnancy category C*; PB: UK; t½: UK
	UTERINE CONTRACTION	
Oxytocin	See Prototype Drug Chart 50.1.	
Carboprost tromethamine	IM: Initially, 0.25 mg; repeat every 15-90 min as needed; *max:* 4 doses if hypertensive, otherwise 2 mg	Naturally occurring prostaglandin F2-alpha. Direct stimulation of uterine smooth muscle. Treatment of postpartum hemorrhage secondary to uterine atony. Give deep IM and aspirate prior to injection. Contraindicated before delivery of placenta. Use with caution in patients with acute renal disease, cardiac disease, hypertension, PID, and asthma. *Adverse reactions:* Diarrhea, nausea, vomiting, fever, and abdominal pain with cramps. Pregnancy category C*; PB: UK; t½: 8 min
Methylergonovine maleate	PO: 0.2 mg 3-4 times daily in the puerperium for up to 7 d IM: 0.2 mg after delivery of anterior shoulder (if full obstetric supervision), after delivery of placenta, or postpartum; repeat q2-4h. Oral doses may follow parenteral administration. IV: Same as for IM but slowly over 1 min with careful monitoring of BP (IV route for acute emergencies only [e.g., bleeding])	Prevention and treatment of postpartum hemorrhage, subinvolution, and postabortion hemorrhage. Exhibits similar smooth-muscle action to ergotamine but primarily affects smooth muscle, producing sustained contractions and shortening the third stage of labor. Not routinely administered IV because of possible sudden hypertensive and cerebrovascular accidents; limit use in patients with hypertension (especially IV). Contraindicated with maternal sepsis, labor induction, threatened spontaneous abortion. ❶ Do *not* use with vasodepressors, other ergot alkaloids, or vasoconstrictors. Appears in breast milk, but interference with breastfeeding is less than with ergonovine. *Adverse reactions:* Transient hypertension, diaphoresis, palpitations, dizziness, headache, nausea, vomiting, tinnitus, transient chest pain, dyspnea. Pregnancy category C*; PB: UK; t½: (biphasic) initial: 1-5 min; terminal: 30 min-2 h

*Pregnancy categories have been revised. See http://www.fda.gov/Drugs/DevelopmentApprovalProcess/DevelopmentResources/Labeling/ucm093307.htm for more information.

BP, Blood pressure; *d,* day; *FHR,* fetal heart rate; *GI,* gastrointestinal; *h,* hour; *IM,* intramuscular; *IV,* intravenous; *max,* maximum; *min,* minute; *PB,* protein binding; *PID,* pelvic inflammatory disease; *PO,* by mouth; *q,* every; *t½,* half-life; *UK,* unknown.

Before labor induction begins, risks and benefits and the status of the mother and fetus must be assessed, and informed consent for induction must be obtained. The gestational age of the fetus must be considered, together with the position of the fetus (head down and deep in the pelvis) and the size of the fetus in relation to the mother's pelvis. Cervical ripening, or softening of the cervix, is also assessed; the cervix is ripe and thus ready for induction when it is soft and progressing in effacement and partial dilation. An objective measurement called the Bishop score assists in predicting whether labor induction may be successful, and it is used to assess readiness for induction. Elements assessed in the modified Bishop scoring system are (1) dilation, (2) effacement, (3) station, (4) cervical consistency, and (5) cervical position. Modified Bishop scores of 8 or greater are associated with a successful labor induction.

Some patients are not suitable candidates for labor induction because the risks of the procedure outweigh the potential benefits. Box 50.2 presents some major contraindications to labor induction.

In pregnant women at or near term with a medical or obstetric indication for labor induction, two approaches are used to ripen and efface the cervix and begin cervical dilation: mechanical methods and prostaglandins.

BOX 50.1   Indications for Labor Induction

- Gestational hypertension
- Chronic hypertension
- Membrane rupture >24 hours
- Chorioamnionitis
- Postdates (>42 weeks' gestation)
- Intrauterine growth retardation
- Positive contraction stress test
- Maternal diabetes mellitus (classes B through F)
- Maternal renal disease
- Isoimmunization
- Intrauterine fetal death

BOX 50.2   Contraindications to Labor Induction

- Disproportion between fetal head and maternal pelvis (cephalopelvic disproportion)
- Unfavorable fetal presentation (transverse or breech)
- Documented fetal intolerance of uterine contractions
- Prematurity
- Placenta previa or suspected abruptio placentae
- Severe gestational hypertension
- Multiparity (six or more)
- Multifetal gestation
- History of uterine trauma
- Previous major surgery in the area of the cervix or uterus
- Prior classical uterine incision
- Active genital herpes infection
- Umbilical cord prolapse
- Excessive amniotic fluid causing an overdistended uterus

One mechanical method involves insertion of a 36-French indwelling catheter through an undilated cervix and internal os with subsequent inflation of the 30-mL balloon. The indwelling catheter bulb provides mechanical stimulation similar to stripping of the membranes. When the catheter falls out, the patient is started on IV oxytocin. A second mechanical method is insertion of an extra amniotic saline infusion with a balloon catheter into the space between the internal cervical os and the placental membrane to induce labor. A third mechanical method is membrane stripping, with which there is release of prostaglandin F_2 from the decidua or prostaglandin E_2 (PGE_2) from the cervix. Spontaneous labor has been induced within 72 hours of membrane stripping with no increase in infection rates. Amniotomy, artificial rupture of the membranes, is commonly performed in patients with a partially dilated and effaced cervix. When done at 5 cm, dilated spontaneous labor is shortened by 1 to 4 hours without an increase in maternal or fetal complications. With rupture of the membranes, nursing care includes assessment of FHR and umbilical cord prolapse. Chorioamnionitis and cord compression have been reported.

The second approach to labor induction uses administration of dinoprostone, the naturally occurring form of PGE_2. It is thought that intracervically or intravaginally administered PGE_2 acts to create cervical effacement and softening through a combination of contraction-inducing and cervical-ripening properties, possibly secondary to an increased submucosal water content and collagen degradation resulting from collagenase secretion in response to PGE_2. One approach uses prefilled syringes of commercially prepared dinoprostone cervical gel, 0.5 mg, which is introduced just inside the cervical os. A second approach is the placement in the posterior vaginal fornix of a vaginal insert of dinoprostone containing 10 mg of controlled-release dinoprostone at 0.3 mg/h.

Misoprostol (PGE_1) is also effective in stimulating cervical ripening, although administration represents an off-label use. PGE_1 is administered intravaginally into the posterior vaginal fomix. Dosing ranges from 25 to 100 mcg every 3 to 6 hours.

Side effects associated with the use of prostaglandins include uterine hyperstimulation, which can be treated with terbutaline sulfate. Uncommonly, some patients experience chills, fever, vomiting, and diarrhea. Contraindications to the use of prostaglandins include active vaginal bleeding and known allergies to prostaglandins. With hepatic or renal disease, cautious use of PGE_2 is recommended; use of PGE_2 is contraindicated in patients with glaucoma. Contraindications for PGE_1 include a previous cesarean delivery or hysterotomy.

Table 50.3 lists the dosages, uses, and considerations for administration of dinoprostone for cervical ripening.

Oxytocin

In addition to labor induction, IV oxytocin can also be used for labor augmentation, stimulation of effective uterine contractions once labor has begun. It facilitates smooth-muscle contraction in the uterus of a patient already in labor but experiencing inadequate uterine contractility, tightening and shortening of uterine muscles. The patient with uterine inertia, uterine inactivity or hypotonic contractions, may be more responsive to oxytocin than the patient who has not begun labor, therefore a lower starting dose will be needed.

In both labor induction and labor augmentation, oxytocin is infused at a prescribed individualized dosage rate, and this rate is increased, decreased, or maintained at fixed intervals based on uterine and fetal response. The objective is to establish an adequate contraction pattern that promotes labor progress, generally represented by contractions every 2 to 3 minutes that last for 50 to 60 seconds with moderate intensity. It is important that the patient receiving oxytocin *not* experience uterine hyperstimulation, which causes markedly increased pain and compromised FHR patterns secondary to impaired placental perfusion. Continuous nursing observation during labor induction or augmentation is critical. The need for an accurate infusion rate requires the use of an infusion pump with oxytocin as an IV piggyback line. Once cervical dilation has reached 5 to 6 cm and an adequate contraction pattern is evident, the rate of oxytocin infusion can often be slowed or stopped.

After delivery, oxytocin 10 to 40 units is usually added to an existing IV solution to help the uterus stay contracted and close the uterine sinuses at the placental site. The maximum concentration should be 40 units per 1000 mL IV fluid. Prototype Drug Chart 50.1 lists the pharmacologic data for oxytocin.

Oxytocin is well absorbed from the nasal mucosa when administered intranasally for milk letdown. The protein-binding

PROTOTYPE DRUG CHART 50.1

Oxytocin

Drug Class
Oxytocic agent
Used to induce labor during pregnancy, to control postpartum hemorrhage, and to prevent uterine atony postdelivery
Pregnancy category C*

Dosage
For induction or augmentation of labor:
Dilute 10 units (1 amp) of oxytocin in 1000 mL lactated Ringer's solution for10 milliunits/mL
Connect to primary IV line close to needle site as a piggyback line.
IV: Low-dose regimen: Start with 0.5-2 milliunits/min; gradually increase dose in increments of 1-2 milliunits/min q15-60min until desired contraction pattern is established. Dose may be decreased by similar increments after desired frequency of contractions is reached and cervix is 5-6 cm dilated. Infuse up to 6 milliunits/min. Provides oxytocin levels similar to those of spontaneous labor; rates >9 milliunits/min are rarely required.
High-dose regimen: Start with 6 milliunits/min; may increase 6 milliunits/min q15-60min until desired contraction pattern is established. If uterine hyperstimulation, decrease dose to 3 milliunits/min; may be further decreased to 1 milliunits/min.
For reduction and control of postpartum hemorrhage and postdelivery uterine contractions:
IV: 10-40 units added to 1000 mL compatible IV solution; infuse at a rate to prevent uterine atony.
IM: 3-10 units after delivery of the placenta

Contraindications
Proven cephalopelvic disproportion, fetal intolerance of labor, hypersensitivity, anticipated nonvaginal delivery; intranasal spray is contraindicated in pregnancy.
Black-box warning: To be used for medical, rather than elective, induction of labor

Drug-Lab-Food Interactions
Drug: Hypertension can occur with vasopressors, and hypotension and/or bradycardia can occur with cyclopropane anesthetics.
Herbals: Black cohosh, cottonroot, squaw vine, and cinnamon can have a synergistic effect to oxytocin

Pharmacokinetics
Absorption: Not well absorbed PO; intranasal and IM absorption is very rapid.
Distribution: Low PB; widely distributed in extracellular fluid; minute amounts in fetal circulation
Metabolism: t½: 1-9 min; rapidly metabolized in liver
Excretion: In urine

Pharmacodynamics
IM:
Onset: 3-5 min; peak: 40 min; duration: 2-3 h
IV:
Onset: Within 1 min; peak: UK; duration: 1 h
Intranasal:
Onset: Minutes; peak: UK; duration: UK

Therapeutic Effects/Uses
To induce or augment labor contractions, to treat uterine atony, to stimulate milk letdown (intranasal spray)
Mechanism of Action: Oxytocin promotes uterine contractions by increasing intracellular concentrations of calcium in uterine myometrial tissue, thereby increasing the activity of the calcium-dependent phosphorylating enzyme myosin light-chain kinase. The nasal spray works by forcing milk into larger ducts and sinuses, which occurs because oxytocin promotes milk ejection by causing contraction of the smooth muscle fibers that surround the breast alveoli and lactiferous ducts.

Side Effects
Maternal effects with undiluted IV use include hypertension, dysrhythmias, uterine hyperstimulation (contractions lasting at least 2 min or 5 or more contractions in a 10-min window), and tachysystole (6 or more uterine contractions in a 20-min window).

Adverse Reactions
Seizures; water intoxication can occur if given in electrolyte-free solution or at a rate greater than 20 milliunits/min. (Water intoxication is manifested by nausea, vomiting, hypotension, tachycardia, and cardiac arrhythmias.)
Life threatening: Maternal intracranial hemorrhage, cardiac dysrhythmias, asphyxia; fetal jaundice, hypoxia

*Pregnancy categories have been revised. See http://www.fda.gov/Drugs/DevelopmentApprovalProcess/DevelopmentResources/Labeling/ucm093307.htm for more information.
amp, Ampule; *h,* hour; *IM,* intramuscular; *IV,* intravenous; *min,* minute; *PB,* protein binding; *PO,* by mouth; *q,* every; *t½,* half-life; *UK,* unknown; *>,* greater than.

percentage is low, and the half-life is 1 to 9 minutes. It is rapidly metabolized and excreted by the liver.

The peak concentration time is unknown for all methods of administration, but the onset of action of IM oxytocin is 3 to 5 minutes, and the duration of action is 2 to 3 hours; the onset of action of IV oxytocin is immediate, and the duration of action is 1 hour; the onset of action of intranasally administered oxytocin is a few minutes, and the duration of action is 20 minutes.

The medication is diluted and administered by IV piggyback for induction or augmentation of labor. Oxytocin is diluted in a variety of ways and is administered via infusion pump in milliunits-per-minute dosing with the volume determined by the dilution. IV administration of undiluted oxytocin is not recommended because of the risk of a sudden acute hypotensive response.

Concurrent use of vasopressors can result in severe hypertension, whereas hypotension can occur with concurrent use of cyclopropane anesthesia and with undiluted IV push administration. The Institute for Safe Medication Practices (ISMP) includes oxytocin on its list of high-alert medications because of its heightened risk of causing significant harm when used in error.

 NURSING PROCESS
Patient-Centered Collaborative Care

Enhancement of Uterine Contractility: Oxytocin

Assessment
- Confirm term gestation before inducing or augmenting labor, and obtain the patient's informed consent.
- Collect accurate baseline data before beginning infusion, including maternal pulse and BP, uterine history, uterine activity, and FHR pattern.
- Interview the patient and review the history to ascertain that no contraindications exist.

Nursing Diagnosis
- Knowledge, Deficient related to drugs used to promote uterine contractility

Planning
- Oxytocin will enhance uterine contractions without adverse maternal or fetal effects.
- The patient's vital signs will be within acceptable ranges throughout labor, delivery, and the postpartum period.
- FHR will demonstrate a normal rate, pattern, and variability throughout labor and delivery.

Nursing Interventions
- ⚡ Have tocolytic drugs, such as terbutaline, and oxygen readily available.
- Monitor intake and output.
- ⚡ Monitor maternal pulse and BP, uterine activity, and FHR during oxytocin infusion.
- Maintain the patient in a sitting or lateral recumbent position to promote placental infusion.

- ⚡ Monitor for signs of uterine rupture, which include FHR decelerations, sudden increased pain, loss of uterine contractions, hemorrhage, and rapidly developing hypovolemic shock.
- ⚡ Use an IV pump to administer drug.

Patient Teaching
- Inform the patient that drug is given intravenously and that dosage is adjusted in response to the uterine contraction pattern.
- For milk letdown, teach the patient the timing and method of nasal administration.

Evaluation
- Evaluate for effective labor progress.
- Monitor maternal vital signs every 30 to 60 minutes and with every increment in dose, and monitor FHR every 15 minutes and with every increment in dose during the first stage of labor and every 5 minutes in the second stage of labor. Report changes in vital signs and FHR, specifically late decelerations, and report any vaginal bleeding.

Other Drugs That Enhance Uterine Contractions: Ergot Alkaloids

The ergot alkaloids, one of a large group of alkaloids derived from fungi, act by direct smooth muscle cell–receptor stimulation. These drugs are *not* used during labor because they can cause sustained uterine contractions (tetanic contractions), which would result in fetal hypoxia and could rupture the uterus. In addition, the uterus becomes more sensitive to these drugs. After delivery, however, sustained contractions are effective to prevent or control postpartum hemorrhage and to promote uterine involution.

The most commonly used ergot derivative is methylergonovine maleate, which can be given by mouth but is most frequently administered intramuscularly. IV administration is not recommended and is used only in emergency situations. If IV methylergonovine maleate is given, administer 0.2 mg over 1 minute. Transient significant elevations in BP can occur, particularly after IV infusion. Patients with preexisting or gestational hypertension or peripheral vascular diseases should *not* receive ergot derivatives. Table 50.3 lists commonly used uterotonic drugs and their dosages, uses, and considerations.

Side Effects and Adverse Reactions

Side effects of ergot alkaloids include uterine cramping, nausea and vomiting, dizziness, hypertension with IV administration, sweating, tinnitus, chest pain, dyspnea, itching, and sudden severe headache. Signs of ergot toxicity, also called ergotism, include pain in the arms, legs, and lower back; numbness; cold hands and feet; muscular weakness; diarrhea; hallucinations; seizures; and blood hypercoagulability.

NURSING PROCESS
Patient-Centered Collaborative Care

Other Oxytocics: Ergonovine and Methylergonovine

Assessment
- Assess lochia and uterine tone before giving ergonovine or methylergonovine.
- Assess effectiveness of uterine massage and oxytocin administration on local flow and uterine tone.
- Recognize that these two drugs have a vasoconstrictive effect that may cause hypertension. Ergonovine is more vasoconstrictive than methylergonovine.
- Obtain baseline BP before administration.

Nursing Diagnoses
- Cardiovascular Function, Risk for Impaired
- Pain related to an increase in uterine contractions

Planning
- The patient's BP will remain within normal limits.

Nursing Interventions
- ⚡ Monitor the patient's BP per agency protocol.
- Protect drugs from exposure to light.
- ⚡ Monitor for side effects or symptoms of ergot toxicity (ergotism). Notify the health care provider if systolic BP increases by 25 mm Hg or diastolic BP increases by 20 mm Hg over baseline.

Patient Teaching
- Advise the patient that she will feel more intense uterine cramps after receiving the drug but may receive analgesics for pain.
- Encourage the patient to avoid smoking. Nicotine increases vasoconstrictive properties of these drugs.

Side Effects
- If the patient is breastfeeding, explain that the drug lowers serum prolactin levels and has the potential to inhibit postpartum lactation. Ergonovine has greater potential to inhibit lactation than methylergonovine.

 Cultural Considerations
- Recognize cultural influences on a patient's expression or lack of expression of discomfort or pain.
- Provide an interpreter as appropriate.

Evaluation
- Evaluate effectiveness of the drug by assessment of lochia and uterine tone. Count and weigh perineal pads as appropriate.
- Continue monitoring maternal vital signs, specifically pulse and BP. Report changes in maternal vital signs, continued excessive vaginal bleeding, or uterine atony.

DRUGS USED DURING THE POSTPARTUM PERIOD

During the puerperium, the period from delivery until 6 weeks postpartum, the mother's body physically recovers from antepartal and intrapartal stressors and returns to its prepregnant state.

Pharmacologic and nonpharmacologic measures commonly used during the postpartum period have five primary purposes: (1) to prevent uterine atony and postpartum hemorrhage; (2) to relieve pain from uterine contractions, perineal wounds, and hemorrhoids; (3) to enhance or suppress lactation, production and release of milk by the mammary glands; (4) to promote bowel function; and (5) to enhance immunity (Tables 50.4 and 50.5).

Whenever possible, nonpharmacologic measures are preferred to the use of drugs or are used in conjunction with drugs (Complementary and Alternative Therapies 50.1). Postpartum nursing care ideally occurs as a partnership between the nurse and the new family. To enhance health and wellness, the nurse collaborates with the mother and family to strengthen the new mother's self-confidence and ability to handle her own health challenges. The nurse's role in this system is threefold:
- To assess and discuss postpartal physical changes and pain management with the patient and determine healing progress within a standard and effectiveness of medications
- To teach the patient and administer postpartal medications
- To teach the patient and administer narcotic analgesics as prescribed when pain control by nonnarcotics is ineffective

Pain Relief for Uterine Contractions

Afterbirth pains may occur during the first few days postpartum, when uterine tissue experiences ischemia during contractions, particularly in multiparous patients and when breastfeeding. Nonsteroidal agents may be used to control postpartal discomfort and pain; narcotic agents are reserved for more severe pain, such as that experienced by the patient after cesarean delivery, tubal ligation, or extensive perineal laceration. Table 50.1 lists systemic analgesics commonly used during the postpartum period.

Because some systemic analgesics (e.g., codeine, meperidine) can cause decreased alertness, it is important for the nurse to observe the patient as she cares for her newborn to ensure safety. Patients who receive opioids such as morphine sulfate or codeine sulfate should be assessed for bowel function and respirations.

COMPLEMENTARY AND ALTERNATIVE THERAPIES 50.1

Herbal Supplements and Lactation

Because little is known about the safety of herbal supplements, they are not generally recommended during lactation. Breastfeeding patients should be advised to check with their health care provider before taking any herbal supplements; those contraindicated for breastfeeding patients include aloe, belladonna, black tea, bromelain, buckthorn bark, burdock, cat's claw, chondroitin, comfrey, echinachea, ephedra (Ma-huang), eucalyptus, flaxseed, kava kava, lavender, licorice, milk thistle, pennyroyal, and saw palmetto. This list is not exhaustive. Again, it is important to check with the health care provider on all complementary and alternative therapies used during lactation.

TABLE 50.4　Nonpharmacologic Measures for Common Postpartum Needs

Indication	Intervention
Uterine contractions	Patient is positioned on the abdomen with a pillow under the abdomen for 20-30 min for 3-4 d. Distraction, breathing techniques, therapeutic touch, relaxation, guided imagery, and ambulation may be used. No heat should be applied to the abdomen because of the risk of uterine relaxation and increased bleeding.
Perineal wound resulting from episiotomy or laceration	Ice packs made with a nonlatex glove filled with crushed ice and covered in a thin, absorbent material to protect tissue are applied for 6-8 h after delivery. The patient is positioned on her side as much as possible with a pillow between the legs; early and frequent ambulation and perineal exercises (Kegels) are encouraged. A cool sitz bath should be taken 2-3 h after delivery along with warm sitz baths 12-24 h after delivery two to three times daily. The perineum is cleansed front to back using a peri-spray squeeze bottle or cleansing shower. Patient is advised to tighten the buttocks or squeeze them together before sitting and to sit tall and flat, not rolled back onto the coccyx. No tampons, douches, or feminine hygiene sprays should be used until advised by the health care provider. Advise no intercourse until after lochia has ceased or as advised by the health care provider.
Hemorrhoids	As above but particularly: 　Ice 　Sims position to help increase venous return 　Warm, moist heat or sitz bath 　Witch hazel pads (e.g., Tucks)
Lactation suppression	Tight bra worn continuously for 10-14 d Normal fluid intake No manipulation or stimulation of breasts Pyridoxine (vitamin B6) 200 mg for 5 d
Engorgement	Same as for lactation suppression above plus ice to the axillary area of the breasts if bottle feeding or warm compresses if breast-feeding; cold cabbage leaves placed inside the bra may also be helpful. If breastfeeding, express a small amount of colostrum or milk by hand before putting the infant to the breast to facilitate latching on.
Sore or cracked nipples	Wear absorbent breast pads to keep moisture away from nipples. Do not use soap on nipples. Air-dry nipples after nursing. After nursing, express a small amount of breast milk on nipples to use as a protective lubricant. After nursing, apply hypoallergenic purified lanolin to nipples as a protective lubricant to promote healing. For cracked nipples, use comfort gel pads (hydrogel pads). Do not use nipple shields because they can promote chafing. Do not limit the infant's nursing time; if the milk ducts are not emptied, increased pressure can occur. Ensure proper positioning for feeding, and initiate nursing on the less sore nipple. After feeding, the infant may instinctively suck during attempts to disengage: break the suction with your little finger to prevent pulling on the nipple.

d, Day; *h,* hour; *min,* minute.

TABLE 50.5　Promote Postpartum Bowel Function

Generic	Route and Dosage	Uses and Considerations
Docusate sodium, docusate calcium (various dosages available)	50-360 mg/d PO in 1-4 divided doses; *max.* 360 mg/d for docusate sodium; 240 mg/d for docusate calcium	Reduces surface tension of the oil-water interface of the stool, resulting in enhanced incorporation of water and fat and subsequent stool softening. Docusate salts are interchangeable (Na, Ca, or K is clinically insignificant). Do not use concomitantly with mineral oil. Do not use for more than 1 wk. Prolonged, frequent, or excessive use may cause bowel dependence or electrolyte imbalance. Contraindicated in patients with intestinal obstruction, acute abdominal pain, nausea, or vomiting. Compatible with breastfeeding. Side effect is rash. Onset: 12-72 h. Pregnancy category C*; PB: NA; t½: NA
Sennosides 8.6 mg tab or 8.8 mg/5 mL	PO: 1-2 tabs bid; take with a full glass of water or 10-15 mL at bedtime	A stimulant laxative that acts on the colon as a local irritant to promote peristalsis and bowel evacuation; also increases moisture content of stool by accumulating fluids in the intestine. Metabolized in liver, eliminated in feces (viable) and urine. Drug interactions may occur with MAOIs, disulfiram, metronidazole, and procarbazine. May discolor urine or feces. May create laxative dependence and loss of bowel function with prolonged use. Contraindicated in patients with fluid and electrolyte disturbances, abdominal pain, and nausea and vomiting; excreted in breast milk. Onset: 8-12 h but may require up to 24 h. Pregnancy category C*; PB: NA; t½: NA

TABLE 50.5 Promote Postpartum Bowel Function—cont'd

Generic	Route and Dosage	Uses and Considerations
Bisacodyl (10 mg supp or 5 mg tab)	PO: 1-3 tabs as a single dose PR: 1 supp as a single dose *Max.* PO: 15 mg/d; PR 10 mg/d	Stimulant laxative; irritates smooth muscle of the intestine and possibly the colon and intramural plexus; alters water and electrolyte secretion, increasing intestinal fluid and producing a laxative effect. Following oral or rectal administration, 5% absorbed systemically; metabolized in the liver to conjugated metabolites; excreted in breast milk, bile, and urine. Do not crush tablets or give within 1 h of milk or antacid because enteric coating may dissolve, resulting in abdominal cramping and vomiting. Side effects include abdominal cramps, nausea, vomiting, rectal burning, electrolyte and fluid acidosis or alkalosis, and hypocalcemia. Onset: PO, 6-10 h; PR, 15 min-1 h. Pregnancy category C*
Magnesium hydroxide Magnesium concentrate is three times as potent as regular-strength product.	PO: 15-60 mL reg susp or 15-30 mL conc susp per d, preferably at bedtime; may be taken in divided doses Tab: 6-8 tab/d, preferably at bedtime; may be taken in divided doses.	A laxative that acts by increasing and retaining water in the intestinal lumen, causing distension that stimulates peristalsis and bowel elimination. Absorbed drug is excreted in kidneys; unabsorbed drug is excreted in feces. Drug poses a risk to patients with renal failure because 15%-30% of the magnesium is systemically absorbed. Use with caution in patients with impaired renal function; hypermagnesemia and toxicity may occur as a result of decreased renal clearance of absorbed magnesium. Contraindicated in patients with colostomy, ileostomy, abdominal pain, nausea, vomiting, fecal impaction, and renal failure. Drug interactions may occur with tetracyclines, digoxin, indomethacin, iron salts, or isoniazid. Side effects are abdominal cramps and nausea. Adverse reactions include hypotension, hypermagnesemia, muscle weakness, and respiratory depression. Onset: 4-8 h. Pregnancy category B*
Mineral oil	PO: 30-90 mL/d; doses may be divided.	A lubricant laxative that eases passage of stool by decreasing water absorption and lubricating the intestine; may impair absorption of fat-soluble vitamins (A, D, E, K), oral contraceptives, coumarin, and sulfonamides. Avoid bedtime doses because of risk of aspiration (lipid pneumonitis), and do not give with food or meals because of risk of aspiration and decreased fat-soluble vitamin absorption. Contraindicated in patients with ileostomy, colostomy, appendicitis, ulcerative colitis, and diverticulitis. Best administered on an empty stomach. Side effects include nausea, vomiting, diarrhea, and abdominal cramps. Onset: 6-8 h; peak, duration: UK. Pregnancy category C*; PB: NA; t½: NA
Simethicone	PO: 40-125 mg qid after meals and at bedtime. *Max:* 500 mg/d	An antiflatulent that acts by dispersing and preventing formation of mucus-surrounded gas pockets in the GI tract; drug changes the surface tension of gas bubbles and allows them to coalesce, making them easier to eliminate as belching and rectal flatus. Tablets must be chewed thoroughly before swallowing; follow with a full glass of water. Drug is excreted unchanged in feces; may interfere with results of guaiac tests of gastric aspirates, but no other side effects are known. Do *not* take double doses to make up for missed doses. Store below 104°F (40°C) in a well-closed container. Onset: UK. Pregnancy category C*; t½: UK

*Pregnancy categories have been revised. See http://www.fda.gov/Drugs/DevelopmentApprovalProcess/DevelopmentResources/Labeling/ucm093 307.htm for more information.

bid, Twice daily; *Ca,* calcium; *conc,* concentration; *d,* day; *GI,* gastrointestinal; *h,* hour; *K,* potassium; *MAOI,* monoamine oxidase inhibitor; *max,* maximum dosage; *min,* minute; *Na,* sodium; *NA,* not applicable; *PB,* protein binding; *PO,* by mouth; *PR,* per rectum; *qid,* four times a day; *reg,* regular; *supp,* suppository; *susp,* suspension; *t½,* half-life; *tab,* tablet; *UK,* unknown; *wk,* week.

With continued opioid use, patient assessment of bowel history is necessary because these drugs can exacerbate the constipation of pregnancy. During the intrapartum period, women are NPO (nothing by mouth) or ingest limited liquids and are not ambulatory, all factors that contribute to decreased bowel activity. In addition, respiratory assessment is important for patients receiving opioids because respiratory depression may occur. Frequently, nonsteroidal agents like ibuprofen and ketorolac tromethamine are used to control postpartum discomfort and pain. Nonsteroidal antiinflammatory drugs (NSAIDs) inhibit the enzyme cyclooxygenase (COX), of which there are two isoenzymes, COX-1 and COX-2; both decrease prostaglandin synthesis. These drugs are effective in relieving mild to moderate pain caused by postpartum uterine contractions, episiotomy, hemorrhoids, and perineal wounds. NSAIDs commonly cause GI irritation, and it is recommended that patients take them with a full glass of water or with food to minimize GI distress. With administration of NSAIDs, a lower narcotic dosage may control pain as a result of the additive analgesic effect. The use of NSAIDs requires ongoing assessment for GI bleeding. These drugs inhibit platelet synthesis and may prolong bleeding time. Patient teaching with this category of drugs is important because some NSAIDs may be purchased over the counter (OTC). Patient teaching includes avoidance of these drugs while pregnant if symptoms of GI bleeding occur (dark, tarry stools; blood in urine; coffee-ground emesis) and avoidance of the concurrent use of alcohol, aspirin, and corticosteroids, which may increase the risk for GI toxicity.

Pain Relief for Perineal Wounds and Hemorrhoids

Pregnancy and the delivery process increase the pressure on perineal soft tissue causing it to become ecchymotic or edematous. Increased edema, ecchymosis, and pain may occur if an **episiotomy,** incision made to enlarge the vaginal opening to facilitate newborn delivery, or perineal laceration is present. The perineum is assessed for *r*edness, *e*cchymosis, *e*dema, *d*ischarge, and *a*pproximation (REEDA). In addition, hemorrhoids that developed during pregnancy may be exacerbated by the pushing during labor. Comfort measures—ice packs immediately after birth, tightening of the buttocks before sitting, use of peri-bottles, and cool or warm sitz baths—and selected topical agents such as witch hazel and dibucaine ointment may relieve pain and minimize discomfort (see Table 50.1). Note that rectal suppositories should *not* be used by women with fourth-degree perineal lacerations.

Side Effects and Adverse Reactions

The most commonly reported side effects of topical or local agents include burning, stinging, tenderness, edema, rash, tissue irritation, and sloughing in addition to tissue **necrosis**, tissue death caused by disease or injury. The most commonly reported side effects of hydrocortisone local or topical drugs include burning, pruritus, irritation, dryness, **folliculitis** (skin inflammation resulting from contact with an irritating substance or allergen), allergic contact dermatitis, and secondary infection. These side effects are more likely to occur when **occlusive** (i.e., obstructive) dressings are used.

 NURSING PROCESS
Patient-Centered Collaborative Care
Pain Relief for Perineal Wounds and Hemorrhoids

Assessment
- Assess the patient's cultural framework for health.
- Assess the patient's pain using an agency pain scale. Assess the perineal area for wounds and hemorrhoids (size, color, location, pain scale, REEDA [redness, ecchymosis, edema, discharge, and approximation]).
- Check expiration dates on topical spray cans, bottles, and ointment tubes.
- Assess for presence of infection at the perineal site; avoid use of benzocaine on infected perineal tissue.

Nursing Diagnoses
- Knowledge, Deficient of causes of pain and discomfort; inexperience with treatment measures, nonpharmacologic and pharmacologic
- Pain, Acute related to episiotomy, perineal laceration, or hemorrhoids

Planning
- The patient's perineal discomfort will be alleviated by use of topical sprays, compresses, sitz baths, and ointments.

Nursing Interventions
- Teach patients about use of the peri-bottle. Use warm, direct water on the perineum from front to back (clean to dirty).
- Do not use benzocaine spray when perineal infection is present.

- Shake the spray can and administer benzocaine 6 to 12 inches from the perineum with the patient lying on her side, top leg up and forward, to provide maximum exposure. This can also be done with one foot on the toilet seat.
- Use witch hazel compresses (glycerin and witch hazel or witch hazel solution) with an ice pack and a peri-pad to apply cold to the affected area in addition to the active agent.
- Store pramoxine and zinc oxide topical or hydrocortisone acetate suppositories below 86°F (30°C), but protect them from freezing. Use gloves for administration. If a patient is breastfeeding, assess to determine whether the patient is ready to switch to a preparation without hydrocortisone (the goal is to discontinue use of suppositories as quickly as possible).
- Check lot numbers and expiration dates.
- Use of pramoxine hydrochloride (HCl) must be explained carefully; directions instruct the patient to place the agent inside the anus, which is not generally done with obstetric patients because they may have perineal wounds that extend into the anus. Rectal suppositories should not be used by patients with fourth-degree perineal laceration.

Patient Teaching
General
- Describe the process of perineal wound healing.
- Explain the expected action and side effects. With witch hazel, a cooling, soothing sensation will provide relief. Ointment and suppositories will soothe, lubricate, and coat mucous membranes. Pramoxine HCl is not chemically related to the "-caine" type of local anesthetics, and there is a decreased chance of cross-sensitivity reactions in patients who are allergic to other local anesthetics.
- Advise patients that the drug is not for prolonged use (no more than 7 days) or for application to a large area.
- Explain that topical analgesia lasts for several hours after use.
- Advise patients to store suppositories below 86°F (30°C) so they do not melt, and do not freeze. Counsel the patient with bleeding hemorrhoids to use the drug carefully and to keep their health care provider informed if the condition exacerbates or does not improve within 7 days.

Self-Administration: Perineal Wounds—Topical Spray Containing Benzocaine
- Apply three to four times daily or as directed.
- Apply without touching sensitive areas.
- Hold the can 6 to 12 inches from the affected area. Teach the patient to administer the spray by either lying on her side in bed while spraying from behind or by standing with one foot on a chair or toilet seat.
- Avoid contact of medication with eyes.
- Assess use of CAM, including herbal supplements.
- Teach the patient not to use a perineal heat lamp after application because this could cause tissue burns.
- If the condition exacerbates or symptoms recur within a few days, notify the health care provider and discontinue use until directed.

- Keep medication out of children's reach in the postpartum unit and later in the home. If ingested, contact a poison control center immediately.
- Store below 120°F (49°C). Dispose of empty cans without puncturing or incinerating.

Self-Administration: Hemorrhoids and Perineal Wounds—Witch Hazel Compresses

- Pour liquid witch hazel over chipped ice; place soft, clean, absorbent squares in the solution; squeeze each square to eliminate excess moisture, and fold and place the moist square against the episiotomy site or hemorrhoids.
- If using commercial medicated pads, the entire container may be placed in the refrigerator.
- Avoid touching the surface of the pad placed next to the perineal wound.
- Teach the patient when to change the compress and how to place the ice bag and peri-pad over the compress.
- Do not insert medicated pads into the rectum.
- Keep products out of children's reach.
- Do not use if rectal bleeding is present.
- Discontinue use if local irritation occurs.

Self-Administration: Hemorrhoids—Ointment and Suppositories

- Apply ointment externally in the postpartum period.
- Place the suppository in the lower portion of the anal canal. Caution must be used because products usually are not inserted rectally if fourth-degree lacerations are present.
- Apply a small quantity of ointment onto a 2-inch square gauze pad; place inside the peri-pad against the swollen anorectal tissue approximately five times per day.
- If a suppository is ordered, tell the patient to keep it refrigerated but not frozen. Remove the wrapper before inserting the suppository in the rectum (hold the suppository upright, and peel evenly down the sides). Do not hold the suppository for a prolonged period; it will melt. If a suppository softens before use, hold it in the foil wrapper under cold water for 2 to 3 minutes.
- Ascertain patient hypersensitivity to any components of the ointment (e.g., pramoxine HCl, mineral oil, zinc oxide).
- Avoid contact of medication with eyes.
- Ointment may occasionally cause a burning sensation in some patients, especially if anal tissue is not intact.
- If erythema, irritation, edema, or pain develops or increases, discontinue use and consult the health care provider.
- Notify the health care provider if bleeding occurs.

Self-Administration: Hydrocortisone and Pramoxine and Pramoxine Hydrochloride

- Advise the patient that the product is for anal or perianal use only and is not to be inserted into the rectum.
- Shake the can vigorously before use.
- Fully extend the applicator plunger; hold the can upright to fill the applicator.
- Express the contents of the applicator onto a 2-inch square gauze pad, and place it inside the peri-pad and against the rectum.
- Use two to three times daily and after bowel movements.

- Take the applicator apart after each use, and wash it with warm water.
- Keep the aerosol container out of children's reach in the postpartum unit and later in the home.
- Store below 120°F (49°C).
- Dispose of the aerosol container without puncturing or incinerating it.
- Avoid contact of medication with eyes.
- Advise the patient that it is unknown whether topical administration of corticosteroids results in sufficient systemic absorption to produce detectable quantities in breast milk. Burning, itching, irritation, dryness, and folliculitis may occur, especially if occlusive dressings are used.

Self-Administration: Dibucaine Ointment, 1%

- Express ointment from the applicator on a tissue or 2-inch square gauze pad, and place it against the anus. Do not insert the applicator into the rectum. Effects should occur within 15 minutes and should last for 2 to 4 hours. Ointment is poorly absorbed through intact skin but is well absorbed through mucous membranes and excoriated skin.
- Do not use near eyes, over denuded surfaces or blistered areas, or if there is rectal bleeding.
- Do not use more than one tube (30-g size) in 24 hours.
- Keep medication out of children's reach.
- Ask the patient if they have any known hypersensitivity to amide-type anesthetics; if so, dibucaine ointment is contraindicated.
- Local effects may include burning, tenderness, irritation, inflammation, and contact dermatitis; inform the health care provider if these occur.
- Other side effects may include edema, cutaneous lesions, and urticaria.

⊕ Cultural Considerations

- Provide an interpreter of the same sex and ethnic background if possible, especially with sensitive topics.

Evaluation

- Reevaluate the patient's perception of pain after use of nonpharmacologic and pharmacologic measures. Identify the need for additional patient teaching.
- Reassess perineal and anal tissues for integrity, healing, and side effects.

Lactation Suppression

Due to severe side effects such as thrombophlebitis and potential carcinogenic effects, medications that were once prescribed for lactation suppression are no longer used. Nonpharmacologic measures are currently recommended for lactation suppression, such as wearing a well-fitted support bra or breast binder continuously for 72 hours after giving birth and avoiding breast stimulation, including running warm water over the breast and expressing milk.

If breast engorgement occurs while trying to suppress lactation, ice packs to the breasts (15 min on and 45 min off each hour) can help decrease the discomfort and swelling. The use of cabbage leaves is often recommended to help decrease engorgement. It is recommended that the woman wear a cold cabbage leaf over each breast inside of her bra and replace the leaves each time they wilt. A mild analgesic can help decrease discomfort during this time (see Table 50.1).

Promotion of Bowel Function

Constipation is common during the postpartum period. The residual effects of progesterone on smooth muscle decrease peristalsis. This decrease in peristalsis—added to decreased liquid intake during labor, decreased activity, and relaxation of the abdominal muscles—amplifies the problem. Patients who deliver by cesarean are even more likely to experience constipation and flatus (intestinal gas). Nonpharmacologic measures such as high-fiber foods, early ambulation, drinking at least 64 ounces of fluids per day, and promptly responding to the defecation urge are generally instituted after delivery.

Pharmacologic measures include the use of stool softeners, laxative stimulants, and for the postcesarean patient, antiflatulents to treat excessive gas in the stomach and intestines (see Table 50.5).

Side Effects and Adverse Reactions

The following side effects have been reported:
- Docusate sodium: Bitter taste, throat irritation, rash
- Sennosides: Nausea, abdominal cramping, diarrhea, rash; can also cause diarrhea in breastfed infants
- Bisacodyl: Proctitis and inflammation
- Magnesium hydroxide: Abdominal cramps, nausea
- Mineral oil: Nausea, vomiting, diarrhea, abdominal cramps; if aspirated, lipid pneumonitis

◎ NURSING PROCESS
Patient-Centered Collaborative Care
Laxatives

Assessment
- Note time of delivery, predelivery food and fluid intake, ambulation and activity, and predelivery bowel habits. Obtain a history of bowel problems.
- Assess bowel sounds in all four quadrants, particularly after cesarean delivery, and note abdominal distension.
- Assess the perineal area for wounds, hemorrhoids, and episiotomy (REEDA).

Nursing Diagnoses
- Constipation, Risk for
- Pain, Acute (fear of) related to first postdelivery bowel movement secondary to episiotomy, hemorrhoids, or perineal wounds

Planning
- The patient will have a bowel movement by 2 to 4 days postpartum.
- The patient will resume a normal bowel elimination pattern within 4 to 6 weeks.

Nursing Interventions
Docusate Sodium and Sennosides
- Store at room temperature.
- If a liquid preparation is ordered, give with milk or fruit juice to mask the bitter taste.
- Take with a full glass of water.
- Assess for a history of laxative dependence.
- Drug interaction may occur with mineral oil, phenolphthalein, or aspirin.

Bisacodyl
- Store tablets and suppositories below 77°F (25°C), and avoid excess humidity.
- Do not crush tablets.
- Do not administer within 1 to 2 hours of milk or antacid because enteric coating may dissolve, resulting in abdominal cramping and vomiting.
- Take with a full glass of water.

Mineral Oil
- Do not give with or immediately after meals.
- Give with fruit juice or a carbonated drink to disguise the taste.

Magnesium Hydroxide
- Shake the container well.
- Do not give 1 to 2 hours before or after oral drugs because of the effects on absorption.
- Take with a full glass of water.
- Note that milk of magnesia concentrate is three times as potent as the regular-strength product.
- Give laxatives 1 hour before or 1 hour after any oral antibiotic.

Senna
- Protect senna from light and heat.

Simethicone
- Administer after meals and at bedtime.
- If chewable tablets are ordered, instruct the patient to chew tablets thoroughly before swallowing and to follow with a full glass of water.

Patient Teaching
General
- Advise patients that stool softeners are given to enable bowel movement without straining.
- Advise patients that measures to prevent and treat constipation include drinking 6 to 8 glasses of fluid per day, ingesting foods high in fiber (bran, fruits, vegetables), and increasing daily ambulation and activity. Instruct patients to avoid or minimize ingestion of gas-forming foods (beans, cabbage, onions) and to increase ambulation and other activity.
- Advise patients regarding temperature and storage requirements for particular drugs.
- Caution patients that prolonged, frequent, or excessive use may result in electrolyte imbalance or dependence on the drug.
- Advise patients that many laxatives contain sodium. Instruct them to check with their health care provider or pharmacist before using any laxative if they are on a low-sodium diet.

Docusate Sodium and Sennosides With Docusate Sodium
- Advise patients to drink at least six 8-oz glasses of liquid daily and to drink one glass of fluid with each dose. Patients should not take the drug if they are already taking mineral oil or having acute abdominal pain, nausea, vomiting, or signs of intestinal obstruction. Patients should not use products for longer than 1 week, and they should report skin rash or stomach or intestinal cramping that does not diminish.
- Senna: Instruct patients that senna may change urine and feces to a yellow-green color; advise discontinuation of senna if abdominal pain, nausea, or vomiting occurs; also, remind patients that the syrup form is 7% alcohol.
- Mineral oil: Instruct patients not to take other laxatives (e.g., docusate products) if they are already taking mineral oil. Advise taking the oil on an empty stomach, not with food or meals, because of risk of aspiration and decreased fat-soluble vitamin absorption. Caution patients to avoid bedtime doses because of risk of aspiration, and instruct them to report nausea, vomiting, diarrhea, or abdominal cramping.

Magnesium Hydroxide
- Advise patients that laxative action generally occurs in 4 to 8 hours. Instruct them to take magnesium hydroxide with a full glass of water.
- Caution patients to note whether the drug is in regular or concentrated form; the concentrate is three times more potent than the regular-strength product.
- Advise patients that the drug may interact with tetracyclines, digoxin, indomethacin, iron salts, and isoniazid. Instruct them to notify their health care provider if any of these drugs are used.
- Instruct patients to report any muscular weakness, diarrhea, or abdominal cramps.

Simethicone
- Advise patients that simethicone will help relieve flatus and associated pain and that it should be taken after meals; if chewable tablets are ordered, instruct patients to chew tablets thoroughly and to drink a full glass of water afterward. If a dose is missed, the patient should take it as soon as possible but should not take double doses.

🌐 *Cultural Considerations*
- In some cultures, pregnancy is considered a "cold" state, so warm foods and activities are encouraged to balance the body; it is believed that failure to do so may contribute to later poor health. For example, women of Mexican ethnicity may wish to avoid chilling and exposure to drafts and may not accept perineal cold compresses.
- Provide an interpreter of the same sex and ethnic background if possible, especially with sensitive topics.
- Be cognizant that different cultures discuss elimination in different ways. Be aware of cultural beliefs and practices.

Evaluation
- Evaluate for the return of regular bowel function.

IMMUNIZATIONS

Rh$_0$(D) Immune Globulin

A patient who lacks the Rhesus (Rh) factor in her own blood (a Rh-negative mother) may carry a fetus who is either Rh negative or Rh positive. During pregnancy, minimal amounts of fetal blood can cross the placenta. Also, abortion, either spontaneous, therapeutic, or induced; amniocentesis; ectopic pregnancy; and placenta previa or abruption can result in some mixing of maternal and fetal blood. Subsequently, anti-D antibodies develop in an Rh-negative mother with an Rh-positive fetus; with the development of these antibodies, the mother becomes sensitized against the Rh factor. If mother and fetus are both Rh negative, no incompatibility exists to trigger this maternal antibody response; but if the fetus is Rh positive, the Rh-negative mother is at risk for Rh sensitization (i.e., development of protective antibodies against incompatible Rh-positive blood). Initially, immune globulin M (IgM) is formed and does not cross the placenta. Later, IgD antibodies develop, which may cross the placenta with isoimmunization to the D antigen with subsequent hemolysis of fetal red blood cells (RBCs). Prenatal IgD isoimmunization occurs in approximately 1% to 2% of Rh-negative women. In later exposure, as with subsequent pregnancies, there is a more rapid IgG (secondary) immune response and an increased potential for fetal hemolysis in an Rh-positive fetus. Once formed, the protective antibodies remain throughout life and may result in hemolytic difficulties for fetuses in subsequent pregnancies. Maternal blood is assessed for the anti-D antibody at the initial prenatal laboratory evaluation and at 26 to 28 gestational weeks. Rh$_0$(D) immune globulin is routinely administered to women with maternal/fetal blood mixing, such as after abortion or with threatened abortion at any stage of gestation with continuation of the pregnancy, obstetric manipulation or trauma, or ectopic pregnancy. If abortion occurs up to and including 12 weeks' gestation, the microdose is administered if less than 2.5 mL of Rh-incompatible RBCs were administered. During the postpartum period, Rh$_0$(D) immune globulin should be administered within 72 hours, therefore one full dose (300 mcg) is given postpartum if the newborn is Rh positive, as antepartum prophylaxis at 26 to 28 weeks' gestation, and after amniocentesis, chorionic villus sampling, and percutaneous umbilical blood sampling. For women with abruption, previa, cesarean births, or manual placental removal, a Kleihauer-Betke analysis (serum test) should be done because more than 15 mL of fetal-maternal hemorrhage of Rh-positive RBCs may have occurred, necessitating an increased dose of Rh$_0$(D) immune globulin. When 15 mL or more of Rh-positive RBCs are suspected, a fetal RBC count should be performed to determine the appropriate dose of Rh$_0$(D) immune globulin.

The Rh-sensitization process can be prevented through the administration of Rh$_0$(D) immune globulin to unsensitized Rh-negative women after each actual or potential exposure to Rh-positive blood.

Adverse Reactions

Adverse reactions to Rh$_0$(D) immune globulin include hypotension, chills, dizziness, fever, headache, pruritus, rash, abdominal pain, diarrhea, and injection site reactions (discomfort, mild pain, redness, swelling).

 NURSING PROCESS

Patient-Centered Collaborative Care

$Rh_0(D)$ Immune Globulin

Assessment

- Determine blood type and Rh status of all prenatal patients.
- Assess the patient for understanding of both her own and her partner's Rh status.
- Ask the patient about previous pregnancies and outcomes; ask whether she has ever received $Rh_0(D)$ immune globulin.
- Follow agency policy for Rh blood testing for patients and infants at the time of delivery.
- Postpartum, assess data about the neonate's Rh type. If the infant is Rh negative, drug is not needed. If the infant is Rh positive and the Rh-negative mother is not sensitized (negative indirect Coombs test) and the infant has a negative direct Coombs test, the mother is a candidate to receive the injection to prevent antibody production or "sensitization."
- Obtain the patient's written consent before administration. Some agencies require a refusal form if the drug is declined.
- Assess for a history of allergy to immune globulin products.

Nursing Diagnoses

- Knowledge, Deficient related to maternal/fetal Rh incompatibility and sensitization
- Knowledge, Deficient related to the purpose, action, and side effects of $Rh_0(D)$ immune globulin

Planning

- The patient will receive $Rh_0(D)$ immune globulin as indicated within 72 hours after delivery or abortion.
- The patient will be able to discuss Rh sensitization and actions indicated during subsequent pregnancies.

Nursing Interventions

- Document Rh workup and eligibility of the patient to receive the drug. Convey information in a verbal report and in the patient's record according to agency policy.
- Check lot numbers on vials and laboratory slips for agreement before administration; check expiration dates. Check the identification band and laboratory slip for matching numbers. Return required slips to the laboratory or blood bank.
- Administer $Rh_0(D)$ immune globulin, and dose (microdose/standard dose) according to gestational weeks, exposure and route, provider orders, and agency protocol. Administer intramuscularly, normally in the deltoid, within 72 hours after delivery. If more than 72 hours have passed, administer as soon as possible up to 28 days, although a lesser degree of protection may result.
- IV administration of $Rh_0(D)$ immune globulin is possible but infrequent. Check provider orders and dosage. For IV

administration, reconstitute with normal saline. Store at 36° to 46°F (2° to 8°C).
- Have epinephrine available to treat anaphylaxis.

Patient Teaching

General

- Explain the action, purpose, and side effects of prescribed drugs.
- Advise patients to avoid live virus vaccines for 3 months after administration.
- Provide written documentation of the date of administration for the patient's personal health record.

 Cultural Considerations

- Provide an interpreter of the same sex and ethnic background if possible, especially with sensitive topics.
- Assess the patient's religious beliefs. Some patients may refuse $Rh_0(D)$ immune globulin, considering it to be a blood product.

Evaluation

- Evaluate the patient's understanding of the need for $Rh_0(D)$ immune globulin.

Rubella Vaccine

Maternal rubella, also called *German measles,* is a potentially devastating infection for the fetus, depending on gestational age. If an unimmunized woman (rubella titer <1:10 or negative titer) contracts the virus during the first trimester, a high rate of abortion and neurologic and developmental sequelae associated with **congenital rubella syndrome** (transmission of the rubella virus to the fetus via the placenta) may result. Cataracts, glaucoma, deafness, heart defects, and mental retardation are seen with this syndrome. When infection occurs after the first trimester, there is less risk of fetal damage because of the developmental stage of the fetus. There is no treatment for maternal or congenital rubella infection. The goals are immunization and prevention of rubella in patients of childbearing age.

Adverse Reactions

Side effects of the rubella vaccine are generally mild and temporary. Burning or stinging at the injection site is caused by the acidic pH of the vaccine. Regional lymphadenopathy, **urticaria** (skin rash caused by an allergic reaction), rash, malaise, sore throat, fever, headache, polyneuritis, arthralgia, and moderate fever are occasionally seen.

 NURSING PROCESS

Patient-Centered Collaborative Care

Measles-Mumps-Rubella Vaccine

Assessment

- Review history and laboratory results to determine the need for measles-mumps-rubella (MMR) vaccination.

- A rubella titer of less than 1:8/1:10 (agency laboratory), negative, or not immunized indicates the need for MMR vaccine administration.
- MMR vaccine is contraindicated if the patient verbalizes, or if medical record review indicates, any of the following conditions, and the presence of any of these factors should be documented:
  - Pregnancy
  - Receipt of whole-blood transfusions, plasma transfusion, or human immune serum globulin within the past 3 months
  - History of anaphylactic or anaphylactoid reactions to neomycin, gelatin, or gelatin-containing products
  - Cannot be given within 1 month before or after other virus vaccines
  - Immunosuppression, radiation therapy, or untreated active tuberculosis (TB), AIDS, or symptomatic HIV
  - Blood dyscrasias, leukemia, lymphomas of any type, or other malignant neoplasms that affect bone marrow or the lymphatic system
  - Any febrile or respiratory illness or other acute illness
- Determine whether the patient is also a candidate to receive $Rh_0(D)$ immune globulin. Administration of both drugs may result in suppression of rubella antibodies with the need to recheck rubella titers in approximately 3 months.

Nursing Diagnoses
- Knowledge, Deficient related to risk for rubella infection and benefit of prevention in patients of childbearing age
- Fetal Injury, Risk for

Planning
- The patient will receive the MMR vaccine to protect against rubella.
- The patient will plan to prevent pregnancy for 4 weeks after subcutaneous injection.

Nursing Interventions
- Protect vaccine from light, and store at 35.6°F to 46.4°F (2°C to 8°C) before reconstitution.
- Reconstitute with the diluent provided, and administer within 8 hours. Administer 0.5-mL vaccine subcutaneously in the upper outer arm. Do not administer intravenously.
- If a tuberculin skin test (TST) is to be done, administer it before or simultaneously with the rubella vaccine (temporary depression in tuberculin skin sensitivity may result). If MMR was given before the TST, postpone the TST until 4 to 6 weeks after MMR administration. If giving both simultaneously, use the Mantoux test.

Skill: Reconstitution
- Single-dose vial: Withdraw the full amount of diluent into the syringe.
- Inject the full volume into the vial of lyophilized vaccine, and agitate to mix thoroughly.

- Withdraw the entire contents into the syringe, and inject the total volume of restored vaccine.
- Have epinephrine readily available in case of anaphylactic reaction.
- Clearly convey in a verbal report and in documentation that vaccination has occurred.
- Record the date of administration, lot number, manufacturer, name, and title to comply with agency policy.

Patient Teaching
General
- Discuss with the patient the importance of immunity to rubella, and help her understand the need to obtain titers to determine immune status.
- Discuss the importance of effective contraception for 4 weeks after vaccination. Identify the contraceptive method of choice, and document instructions.
- Reassure the patient that there is no risk to her from being near small children who received the injection, even if she is pregnant and not immune.
- Advise the patient regarding vaccine action, purpose, and side effects.
- Recommend that the patient have her titer rechecked in 3 months if she also received $Rh_0(D)$ immune globulin.

Side Effects
- The most common side effect is burning or stinging at the injection site; some also experience malaise, fever, headache, and a slight rash about 2 to 4 weeks after injection. About 1 to 10 weeks after injection, some may experience joint pain that lasts 1 to 3 days.

⊕ Cultural Considerations
- Some cultures are opposed to vaccinations. Clarify with the family their desires regarding vaccinations. Explore the legal requirements for vaccinations in your state.

Evaluation
- Evaluate the need for the MMR vaccine and administration to patients with a negative titer or a titer less than 1:8/1:10 (agency laboratory) and those not immunized.

⚡ PATIENT SAFETY

Do not confuse...
- **Fentanyl citrate,** used as an adjunct to general or regional anesthesia or for persistent moderate to severe postoperative pain, with **sufentanil,** an agent used to induce anesthesia in combination with other drugs or as the sole anesthetic agent.

CRITICAL THINKING CASE STUDY

TA (gravida 3, para 0) is at 42 weeks' gestation. At her prenatal visit, her health care provider notes signs and symptoms of pregnancy-induced hypertension and advises TA about a plan to induce labor after administration of prostaglandin gel. TA asks the nurse, "Can you help me understand all of this?"

1. What objective tool (scoring system) can be used to predict the extent to which TA's cervix is "ripe" and therefore favorable for successful induction?

TA's health care provider orders dinoprostone gel for use in the cervix.

2. What will be accomplished with use of the gel?
3. Who will administer the gel?
4. How often can the gel be administered?
5. How long after the last dose of gel can the IV oxytocic medication be started to induce labor?
6. Why is there a waiting period before starting the oxytocin?
7. Further questioning reveals that TA has been ingesting a pregnancy tonic that includes herbal supplements since 36 weeks' gestation. List three concerns specific to pregnancy.

It is 16 hours since TA first had the gel applied. Responding to her call light, the nurse finds TA in the bathroom, upset because she feels nauseated and is occasionally vomiting a little stomach fluid and complaining that her stool is watery. "Is something wrong?" TA asks.

8. Analysis of the data about TA's symptoms supports what conclusion?
9. What nursing actions might be taken to support TA?
10. When TA returns to bed and the external fetal monitor is reapplied, what data should the nurse collect, record, and report to the obstetric provider? It is 24 hours since TA had the first gel instillation and 6 hours since her last insertion.

A vaginal examination reveals that TA's cervix is soft, 50% effaced, and 3 cm dilated and that the presenting part is at 2 station. Contractions are 5 minutes apart and mild, and the health care provider elects to begin an oxytocin infusion.

11. TA asks how "a medicine running into my arm is able to make my uterus contract." How should the nurse explain the mode of action of oxytocin to TA?
12. Why is the oxytocin infusion run through a secondary line attached as a piggyback to the primary line? At which port along the primary line is the piggyback inserted and why?
13. Why is oxytocin administered via infusion pump? What is the measurement for dosing?
14. In regard to the IV equipment setup, what actions should be taken as safety measures before starting the oxytocin?
15. What drugs should be nearby in the event of an emergency with the oxytocin?
16. What information should be recorded during the infusion?
17. While setting up the oxytocin infusion, a new nurse being precepted to labor and delivery asks what criteria are used to know when to slow the rate or stop the infusion. The nurse correctly responds that contractions should be _____ minutes apart with _____ intensity, and the cervix would be dilated at least _____ cm.
18. If uterine hyperstimulation occurs, explain how to handle the situation. Address the following:
    Position TA; rationale: _____
    IV fluids; rationale: _____
    Oxygen; rationale: _____
19. TA asks what side effects can occur if she receives a continuous lumbar epidural. What is the appropriate response?

NCLEX STUDY QUESTIONS

1. A patient (gravida 3, para 2, at 40.6 weeks' gestation) asks, "Is there anything we can do to start labor besides medication? I'm so ready to have this baby." What is the nurse's best response?
   a. There is nothing we can do until you go into labor.
   b. Amniocentesis should be done to be sure the lungs are mature before we start labor.
   c. Some women have sex or ride in a car on a bumpy road to start labor.
   d. Some health care providers may place a balloon catheter or strip the membranes if the cervix is ripe.

2. A patient is to receive 10 mg nalbuphine by slow intravenous push for pain relief during labor. When will the nurse plan to administer nalbuphine?
   a. During the uterine contraction
   b. At the end of the uterine contraction
   c. Between uterine contractions
   d. At any time during the contraction

3. A patient received butorphanol 2 mg intravenously 10 minutes before delivery. Which of these is important nursing care for this patient?
   a. Subcutaneous administration
   b. Having naloxone available
   c. Intravenous fluid bolus to the mother
   d. Oxygen 10 L by nasal cannula to the mother

4. A patient is to have lumbar epidural anesthesia. Based on this health care provider order, what would the nurse prepare to administer?
   a. Citric acid/sodium citrate
   b. Promethazine
   c. A bolus of 500 to 1000 mL of a crystalloid intravenous solution
   d. A $Rh_0(D)$ immune globulin injection

5. A 33-year-old patient in active labor is experiencing "back labor" with intense pain in her lower back. What is the most effective nursing intervention?
   a. Counterpressure against the sacrum
   b. Pant-blow breathing techniques
   c. Effleurage
   d. Conscious relaxation or guided imagery

6. A patient has an epidural for pain control during labor. During the assessment, the nurse notes a drop in the patient's blood pressure. What is the priority nursing intervention?
   a. Administer low-flow oxygen.
   b. Turn her on her left side.
   c. Assess her urinary output.
   d. Monitor her vaginal bleeding.
7. A patient is to have an emergency cesarean delivery due to late fetal decelerations. Before surgery, the nurse administers an antacid, citric acid/sodium citrate. What patient response would indicate effective patient teaching regarding this drug?
   a. Citric acid/sodium citrate will prevent infection after the cesarean section.
   b. The drug will neutralize the contents in my stomach.
   c. The citric acid/sodium citrate will reduce the need to use pain drug after the cesarean delivery.
   d. This drug is administered to prevent vomiting after the cesarean section.
8. Spinal anesthesia with morphine is administered to a patient for pain relief during cesarean section. The patient complains of itching. The nurse prepares to administer which drug?
   a. Diphenhydramine
   b. Ephedrine sulfate
   c. Butorphanol tartrate
   d. Lidocaine
   e. None; this is a normal transient finding that should be documented.

9. A patient (gravida 2, para 1) is admitted to labor and delivery at 39.6 weeks' gestation in active labor. The health care provider performs an amniotomy. What is the nurse's priority intervention?
   a. Monitor uterine contraction frequency and intensity
   b. Check fetal heart rate
   c. Assess for cervical dilation and effacement
   d. Check for umbilical cord compression
10. A patient in labor is to have an epidural administered. Which nursing interventions should the nurse perform before the epidural is administered? (Select all that apply.)
    a. Infuse 500 to 1000 mL of the ordered intravenous fluids.
    b. Check maternal blood pressure.
    c. Assess fetal heart rate.
    d. Have the patient empty her bladder.
    e. Position the patient in a lithotomy position.
    f. Administer 2 L/min of oxygen via nasal cannula.

Answers: 1, d; 2, a; 3, b; 4, c; 5, a; 6, b; 7, b; 8, a; 9, b; 10, a, b, c, d.

51

Neonatal and Newborn

http://evolve.elsevier.com/McCuistion/pharmacology

OBJECTIVES

- Discuss the purposes, actions, side effects, and nursing implications of drugs administered to the newborn.

- Describe the nursing process, including parent teaching, for medications and immunizations administered to the newborn.

OUTLINE

KEY TERMS

This chapter focuses on drugs commonly administered to the neonate, which includes late preterm newborns immediately after delivery.

As discussed in Chapter 49, A thorough medical history, such as acquired immunodeficiency syndrome (AIDS), Group B *streptococcal* infection, and viral hepatitis B or hepatitis C should be conducted. Labor is determined to be preterm if it commences before 37 weeks of pregnancy. If there are no contraindications to halting preterm labor, **tocolytic** therapy is administered to delay birth (see Chapter 49 for more information on pregnancy and preterm labor drugs). However, when preterm labor is not arrested, premature delivery of the neonate occurs, which puts the newborn at risk for health problems. Premature neonates are at risk for respiratory distress, hypothermia, hypoglycemia, and hyperbilirubinemia, and they may have feeding difficulties.

DRUG ADMINISTERED TO PRETERM NEONATES

Synthetic Surfactant

Respiratory distress syndrome (RDS) can occur because of immature lung development and breathing control and decreased airway muscle tone and surfactant level. **Surfactant**, a lipoprotein, is necessary to decrease the surface tension of the **alveoli** (air sacs) to allow the lungs to fill with air and prevent the alveoli from

deflating. Immature lungs have lower than normal levels of surfactant; the more premature the neonate is, the higher the chance of RDS. One approach used to minimize respiratory difficulties in the preterm neonate is surfactant replacement. Supplementing the amount of endogenous surfactant available to maintain distension of the alveolar sacs is the focus of this therapy.

The U.S. Food and Drug Administration (FDA) has approved the use of beractant, calfactant, and poractant alfa. Beractant intratracheal suspension, a natural bovine lung extract, contains phospholipids, neutral lipids, fatty acids, and surfactant-associated proteins to which colfosceril palmitate (dipalmitoylphosphatidylcholine, or DPPC), palmitic acid, and tripalmitin are added. Beractant does not require reconstitution. Calfactant also does not require reconstitution, nor does it need to be warmed at room temperature prior to use, unlike beractant and poractant. Poractant alfa is porcine lung surfactant and is indicated for rescue treatment, whereas beractant and calfactant are approved for prophylaxis and rescue treatment. Poractant should be slowly warmed to room temperature and also does not need reconstitution. Each of these products defines *prophylactic* and *rescue* use differently and has different dosing and administration requirements. Table 51.1 lists the surfactant drugs used for prevention and treatment of RDS along with their dosages, uses, and considerations.

TABLE 51.1   Exogenous Surfactant Therapy for Prevention and Treatment of Respiratory Distress Syndrome

Generic	Route and Dosage	Uses and Considerations
Beractant	PN: IT: 4 mL/kg per dose divided into four equal amounts; administer each quarter amount followed by repositioning and extra ventilation; repeat q6h.	Bovine-derived surfactant to be administered IT for prophylaxis and treatment of RDS in premature infants <1250 g birthweight or with evidence of surfactant deficiency within 15 min of birth or neonate with confirmed RDS requiring ET intubation by 8 h. Drug must be given by health care personnel experienced with using ventilators for prevention or rescue in treatment of RDS. Administer through a 5-French end-hole catheter as a dosing catheter inserted into an ET tube; *do not shake*; warm 20 min at room temperature or in the hand for at least 8 min. Reposition infant to distribute drug followed by ventilation for 20 s after each quarter dose. Does not affect the CYP450 isoenzymes.
Calfactant	PN: IT: 3 mL/kg per dose divided in two equal amounts; administer each half amount over a total of 20-30 breaths during the inspiratory phase followed by repositioning and monitoring respiratory status; repeat q12h.	Calf-derived surfactant to be administered IT for prophylaxis and treatment of RDS in premature infants <29 wk of gestational age at risk for RDS or ≤72 h of age with RDS requiring ET intubation. Drug must be given by health care personnel experienced with ventilators and RDS. Gently swirl the vial to ensure a uniform suspension; avoid foaming. Draw dose with a 20-gauge needle; do *not* filter or dilute; administer via a 5-French end-hole catheter inserted into the proximal end of the ET tube.
Poractant alfa	PN: IT: 2.5 mL/kg per dose divided in two equal amounts; administer each half amount to each main bronchus followed by repositioning and monitoring respiratory status; repeat q12h.	Porcine-derived surfactant to be administered IT for the treatment of RDS in premature infants within 15 h of birth. Drug must be given by health care personnel experienced with ventilators and RDS. Warm to room temperature; gently invert to obtain uniform suspension. Draw dose with a 20-gauge or larger needle; do *not* filter or dilute; administer via a 5-French end-hole catheter inserted into the proximal end of the ET tube.

CYP450, Cytochrome P450; *ET,* endotracheal; *h,* hour; *IT,* intratracheally; *min,* minute; *PN,* premature neonate; *q,* every; *RDS,* respiratory distress syndrome; *s,* second; *wk,* weeks; <, less than; ≤, less than or equal to.

All exogenous surfactants require a patent endotracheal (ET) tube for administration and specified alterations in positioning the infant throughout the procedure to ensure even drug dispersion. These precise position changes allow gravity to assist in the distribution of the product in the lungs, particularly at the alveolar surface.

Crackles and moist breath sounds may be a transient finding after administration of these products, particularly with beractant. Exogenous surfactant can cause postadministration complications such as hyperoxia (excessive oxygenation) and hypocarbia (decreased carbon dioxide [CO_2]). Additionally, transient endotracheal reflux can obstruct the ET tube and lead to oxygen desaturation, cyanosis, bradycardia, and apnea. These issues do not usually lead to serious long-term complications when properly managed. Unless obvious signs of airway obstruction are noted, suctioning should not be performed immediately after administration of supplemental surfactant. Dosing is slowed or halted if the infant (1) becomes dusky colored, (2) becomes agitated, (3) experiences transient bradycardia, (4) has oxygen saturation increases of more than 95%, (5) experiences improved chest expansion, or (6) has arterial or transcutaneous CO_2 levels below 30 mm Hg. Suctioning before dosing decreases the chance for ET tube blockage during dosing. No long-term complications or sequelae of synthetic surfactant therapy have been reported. Surfactant replacement therapy has been found effective in reducing the severity of RDS; rapid improvements in lung compliance and oxygenation may require immediate decreases in ventilator settings to prevent lung overdistension and pulmonary air leak.

 NURSING PROCESS

Patient-Centered Collaborative Care

Drug Administered to Preterm Neonate: Synthetic Surfactant

Assessment
- Obtain informed consent. Separate consents are needed for multifetal births.
- Assess the infant's vital signs, perform a physical examination, and monitor arterial blood gases (ABGs).

Nursing Diagnoses
- Gas Exchange, Impaired related to inadequate lung surfactant secondary to fetal immaturity
- Knowledge, Deficient (parents) related to treatment needs of the infant

Planning
- The infant's oxygen requirement and respiratory effort will decrease.
- The infant's need for mechanical ventilation will be quickly reduced.
- The infant will experience no respiratory distress after surfactant administration.

Nursing Interventions
- Maintain a patent airway.
- Continuously monitor the infant's vital signs before, during, and after surfactant therapy. Ventilation-perfusion

TABLE 51.2   Drugs Administered to Newborns

Generic	Route and Dosage	Uses and Considerations
Erythromycin ophthalmic ointment	Within 1 h of delivery and without touching the tip of the tube to the eye, fingertips, or any other surface, place a 1-cm ribbon of ointment in the lower conjunctival sac of each eye, beginning at the inner canthus.	Prevention of ophthalmia neonatorum, an eye infection among newborns, and protection against gonococcal and chlamydial conjunctivitis. Most states mandate erythromycin ophthalmic ointment, but consult your facility's policy.
Hepatitis B immune globulin (HBIG)	IM: 0.5 mL within 12 h after birth into the anterolateral thigh (vastus lateralis)	For newborns of mothers positive for HBsAg for passive immunity; obtain consents from parents. Initiate recombinant HB as a separate injection at different sites; aspiration is not required.
Phytonadione	0.5-1 mg into the anterolateral thigh (vastus lateralis) within 1 h after birth; check health care provider or agency standing orders for dosage.	An anticoagulant antagonist for prevention of hemorrhagic disease of the newborn. Drug is readily absorbed after IM administration.
Recombinant hepatitis B	IM/Subcut: 0.5 mL (5 mcg) within 12 h after birth (first dose); subsequent doses at 1 and 6 mo of age into anterolateral thigh (vastus lateralis)	Stimulates the immune system to produce anti–HBsAg antibodies without the risk of developing active infection. Because hepatitis D occurs only in persons infected with hepatitis B, recombinant HB protects against hepatitis D. Protection usually occurs 1 mo after the third dose.

h, Hour; *HB,* hepatitis B; *HBsAg,* hepatitis B surface antigen; *IM,* intramuscularly; *mo,* month; *Subcut,* subcutaneous.

matching can occur rapidly after administering surfactant. Anticipate the need to alter ventilator settings.
- Maintain adequate respiratory status.
- Have a multidisciplinary team at the bedside.
- Monitor ABGs and obtain a chest radiography study.
- Prepare and administer drug according to the manufacturer's drug insert.
- Do not perform ET suction immediately after administration of surfactant unless signs of airway obstruction are present.
- Position and reposition the infant as needed for equal distribution of surfactant throughout the lungs.
- Support and educate parents.
- Acknowledge the parents' concerns regarding the well-being of the newborn.

Patient Teaching
- Explain to parents what RDS is and how surfactant helps the neonate.
- Explain to parents the purpose of multiple monitoring devices to reduce unrealistic fears about the neonate's condition.
- Ensure informed consent for drug usage.
- Encourage parents to verbalize their understanding about risks associated with use of the drug.

Cultural Considerations
- Provide an interpreter with same ethnic background and gender if possible, especially with sensitive topics.
- Provide health information written in the patient's primary language.

Evaluation
- Evaluate preadministration breath sounds, ABGs, respiratory status, and ventilator pressure readings to compare with postadministration findings.
- Evaluate the effectiveness of teaching to parents.

DRUGS ADMINISTERED TO FULL-TERM, HEALTHY NEONATES

According to the World Health Organization (WHO, 2016), newborns should receive eye care (e.g., erythromycin ophthalmic ointment), phytonadione, and immunizations for hepatitis B. Additionally, an antiinfective agent (e.g., chlorhexidine) may be applied to the cord stump during the first few hours after birth and for up to 1 week for at-risk newborns and newborns born in homes.

Erythromycin Ophthalmic Ointment

A common antiinfective administered to a newborn's eyes within the first hour of birth is erythromycin ophthalmic ointment. It is given as a prophylaxis against eye infections; side effects include chemical conjunctivitis in about 20% of neonates, manifesting as edema and inflammation that lasts about 24 to 48 hours. It may interfere slightly with eye-to-eye contact between parents and the neonate.

Phytonadione

Phytonadione, a synthetic vitamin K, is a fat-soluble vitamin given to newborns to prevent vitamin K–deficiency bleeding (VKDB). It is administered as a single-dose injection. Side effects include pain and edema at the injection site. Some allergic reactions, manifested by urticaria and rash, have been reported. Neonates who receive larger doses may exhibit hyperbilirubinemia and jaundice resulting from competition for binding sites.

Table 51.2 covers erythromycin and phytonadione and their dosages, uses, and considerations.

Immunizations

The American Academy of Pediatrics and the Centers for Disease Control and Prevention (CDC) have recommended that immunization against hepatitis B virus (HBV) begin in the newborn period. HBV infection may result in serious long-term liver disease, cancer, and death in adulthood. The goal of immunization is to reduce the number of chronic carriers of the virus in the population, thus decreasing the prevalence of HBV infection.

In pregnancy, HBV transmission occurs vertically—that is, by **perinatal transmission**—primarily at the time of delivery. Hepatitis B **immune globulin** (HBIG) is given to infants born to mothers who are positive for hepatitis B surface antigen (HBsAg). HBIG provides the newborn passive protection against HBV. Adverse effects of the injection include pain, tenderness, and erythema at the injection site. Hypotension, erythematous rash, and anaphylaxis after receiving HBIG can also occur.

A three-dose series vaccine for hepatitis B, **recombinant hepatitis B**, is indicated for HBV prophylaxis in infants; the first injection is given at birth. Recombinant hepatitis B (HB) can provide active immunity against HBV by stimulating the immune system to produce antibodies against hepatitis B (anti–hepatitis B antigen), and it can be given concurrently with HBIG if the infant is born to an HBsAg-positive mother. Recombinant HB is given as separate injection administered to separate sites. Adverse effects from recombinant HB are generally mild and include pain, tenderness, pruritus, erythema, swelling, and induration at the injection site.

Table 51.2 lists HBIG and recombinant HB and their dosages, uses, and considerations.

 NURSING PROCESS
Patient-Centered Collaborative Care

Drugs Administered to Full-Term, Healthy Neonates

Assessment
- Assess the newborn for signs of distress such as cyanosis, bleeding, ecchymosis, apnea, fever, and hypotension.
- Assess the mother's HB status.
- Assess the parents' knowledge of treatments (e.g., medications and immunizations) given to their newborn.

Nursing Diagnoses
- Injury, Risk for neonatal
- Knowledge, Deficient parental related to immunization misinformation

Planning
- The neonate will experience minimal or no side effects from drugs routinely administered after delivery.
- Parents will express understanding of medications and immunizations given to their newborn.

Nursing Interventions
- Obtain parental consents for immunizations.

- Do not delay skin-to-skin contact between mother and infant while preparing medications and immunizations. Skin-to-skin contact in the first hour of birth prevents hypothermia and promotes breastfeeding.
- Wear gloves for administration of medications and immunizations.
- If the mother is HBsAg positive, prepare to administer HBIG to the infant.
- Prepare and administer drugs and immunizations according to the manufacturer's instructions while the infant maintains contact with the mother's skin.
- Administer erythromycin ophthalmic ointment *before* administration of phytonadione and hepatitis B injections. The infant may cry after injections, making administration of ophthalmic ointment more difficult.
- Monitor for any reactions, such as redness and swelling in and around the eye from the eye ointment or redness, swelling, or ecchymosis at injection sites. Monitor for any respiratory distress (e.g., grunting, apnea, nasal flaring).
- Acknowledge parent concerns about immunizations.
- Provide printed literature on hepatitis B and other immunizations.

Patient Teaching
- Instruct parents regarding the action, purpose, and side effects of medications and immunizations.
- Inform parents that any edema around the eyes usually disappears within 24 to 48 hours.
- Explain to parents the difference between HBIG and recombinant HB injections.
- Instruct parents regarding childhood immunizations as recommended by current immunization schedules, and inform them when repeat doses should be given. Give parents written information regarding the infant's immunization record and vaccination schedule. Document administration of hepatitis B vaccine on the infant's immunization record.
- Instruct parents on the signs and symptoms of adverse effects and when to notify the nurse.

🌐 *Cultural Considerations*
- Cultural values influence infant care. It is important for nurses to be culturally sensitive to the family's cultural belief framework and to try to include this framework, as appropriate, in provision of care and establishing rapport with the patient and family members.

Evaluation
- Evaluate for newborn bleeding, particularly on days 2 and 3 after administration of phytonadione.
- Evaluate for drug hypersensitivity or side effects.
- Evaluate parents' understanding about medications administered to their newborn.

CRITICAL THINKING CASE STUDY

TA, an older adolescent, was admitted to the hospital for labor induction/augmentation with signs and symptoms of gestational hypertension at 42 weeks' gestation (gravida 4, para 1). TA's mother arrived at the hospital when TA was dilated 8 cm and in time for the late stages of TA's labor. Her mother remained as TA's support person throughout the delivery, which occurred at 6:00 AM by vacuum extraction. TA had a continuous epidural for her labor and delivery. An episiotomy was performed at the time of delivery, and a fourth-degree laceration occurred. A cluster of hemorrhoids was evident. Baby JA, weighing 8 lb 7 oz, had Apgar scores of 7 and 9. The infant is alert and active.

TA lives with her parents and has been going to high school while working part time in an automotive parts store. She wants to keep her infant and to breastfeed "for at least 3 months." She plans to finish school and return to work in 6 weeks.

Immediately after the delivery, the nurse conducts an assessment of TA, analyzes the data, and determines and prioritizes TA's nursing care needs. The same is done for the newborn.

1. Within the standard, how should bonding be promoted—including eye contact between mother and infant—while eye prophylaxis is being administered?
2. Including safety for the nurse administering the ointment, what steps should the nurse follow to instill ointment into the infant's eyes?
3. What should TA be taught about the side effects of eye prophylaxis?
4. How should the nurse explain the reason for the vitamin K injection for the infant in terms TA can understand?
5. Which newborns are eligible to receive the hepatitis B vaccine?
6. How many doses constitute the total series, and what is the duration for these?
7. Why is this vaccine given to newborns? Why is it important?

NCLEX STUDY QUESTIONS

1. A patient asks the nurse why her baby is receiving a vitamin K injection. The nurse's best response is based on what knowledge?
   a. Vitamin K causes an increase in newborn platelets.
   b. A newborn's liver is too immature to produce vitamin K.
   c. A newborn lacks appropriate intestinal flora to synthesize vitamin K.
   d. Vitamin K is not produced in bone marrow until an infant is 8 days old.
2. It is mandatory to have maternal signed consent before administering which newborn drug?
   a. Erythromycin ophthalmic ointment
   b. Phytonadione
   c. Hepatitis B vaccine
   d. Betamethasone
3. The nurse is mentoring a new graduate who is preparing to administer the phytonadione injection to a newborn. Which muscle sites selected by the new graduate would indicate the need for further teaching? (Select all that apply.)
   a. Anterolateral thigh
   b. Gluteus maximus
   c. Rectus femoris
   d. Vastus lateralis
   e. Vastus medialis
4. The nurse is preparing to administer an ophthalmic drug to a newborn. Education for the parents includes which fact about the drug?
   a. Infants of mothers who test positive for syphilis receive this medication.
   b. Eye ointments are administered in the bottom of the eye from the inner to the outer eye.
   c. This drug will prevent congenital cataracts.
   d. Infants with a negative direct Coombs test receive this drug.
5. A newborn is admitted to the nursery, and the nurse reviews the maternal history. It is important that the nurse assess the mother's status specific to which infectious process(es)? (Select all that apply.)
   a. Rubeola
   b. Hepatitis A
   c. Hepatitis B
   d. HIV/AIDS
   e. Group B *Streptococcus*
6. A neonate whose mother is positive for the hepatitis B surface antigen (HBsAg) is admitted to the nursery. Which immunizations are appropriate for this neonate? (Select all that apply.)
   a. Hepatitis B immune globulin (HBIG)
   b. Recombinant hepatitis B (HB)
   c. *Haemophilus influenzae* type B
   d. Hepatitis A
   e. Phytonadione

Answers: 1, c; 2, c; 3, a, d; 4, b; 5, c, d, e; 6, a, b, e.

Women's Reproductive Health

OBJECTIVES

- Recognize that successful contraception is essential to the health and well-being of women.
- Describe methods of contraception commonly prescribed, patient selection, mechanisms of action, and possible side effects.
- Identify specific nursing actions that will enhance successful contraception for women and their partners.
- Describe the nursing process, including teaching and risk-benefit–alternative education associated with drugs used for contraception and family planning.
- Explain the pathophysiology of women's health conditions, pharmacologic therapies, and expected outcomes of pharmacologic therapies.
- Understand pharmacologic interventions used in the treatment of female infertility.

- Describe the mechanism of action for ovulatory stimulation therapy.
- Identify drug therapies used for common gynecologic conditions, such as dysfunctional uterine bleeding, endometriosis, dysmenorrhea, and premenstrual syndrome.
- Describe the nursing process, including teaching, related to drugs used in women's health and infertility.
- Provide information for nonpharmacologic and pharmacologic interventions for women experiencing menopausal symptoms.
- Differentiate among types of drugs used for osteoporosis.
- Describe the nursing process, including teaching and risk-benefit–alternative education associated with drugs used for menopausal symptoms.

OUTLINE

KEY TERMS

Women have specific health care needs throughout their reproductive and postreproductive life cycle. A woman's reproductive life cycle begins with menarche, the start of spontaneous menstruation, and continues through menopause, the permanent cessation of menstruation. Successful contraception is essential to the health and well-being of sexually active women of reproductive age. During the reproductive years, many disorders can occur in women's health. These gynecologic conditions interfere with a woman's overall health and well-being and may impede her ability to become pregnant.

Successful adaptation to menopause, control of menopausal symptoms, and continued sexual health is essential to the well-being of older women. This chapter reviews pharmacologic products that may be used throughout the reproductive and menopausal life cycle of women as well as typical drug regimens used for disorders in women's health. Drugs for female infertility are also addressed with an emphasis on drugs that stimulate ovulation.

Under the Affordable Care Act, contraception is classified as a preventive health service. All plans in the Health Insurance Marketplace must cover contraceptive methods approved by the U.S. Food and Drug Administration (FDA) (e.g., barrier methods, hormonal methods, implanted devices, emergency contraception and sterilization) and related counseling for women. These services are provided without copay or coinsurance, thus reducing the cost of contraception and improving access to health care.

COMBINED HORMONAL CONTRACEPTIVES

All combined hormonal contraceptives (CHCs) contain a synthetic version of *estrogen* and a compound known as *progestin*. Ethinyl estradiol (EE) is the most commonly used synthetic estrogen found in CHCs; however, a new CHC contains estradiol valerate. Progestins are natural or synthetic hormones that have *progesterone-like* effects. *Progesterone* is the naturally occurring sex hormone produced in the ovaries of women; *progestogen* refers to any synthetically produced progesterone compound. Almost all progestins are derivatives of testosterone, a steroid

hormone classified under the androgen group that binds to and activates the progesterone receptors. The term *progestin* will be used to describe the compound used in CHC products. Not only do progestins have contraceptive properties, they serve to balance out the effects of estrogen.

One of eight different types of progestins is used in CHC products. Norethindrone, norethindrone acetate, and ethynodiol diacetate are first-generation progestin compounds (estrane family) and were the earliest progestin formulations to be used in oral contraceptives (OCs). Second-generation progestins (gonane family) include norgestrel and levonorgestrel (LNG). Third-generation progestins include desogestrel, and norgestimate. The new-generation progestins have a higher efficacy rating and fewer effects on lipid and carbohydrate metabolism compared with their earlier counterparts. They also have fewer androgenic side effects, which are described later in this chapter.

Drospirenone (DRSP) is a fourth-generation progestin. It is an analogue of spironolactone. As with spironolactone, a potassium-sparing diuretic, DRSP can increase serum potassium levels in women taking DRSP-containing OCs, altering water and electrolyte balance.

One of the newer progestins, dienogest, is considered a hybrid progestin, as it is derived from the estrane family and is an analog of spironolactone. Like DRSP, dienogest can alter fluid and electrolyte balance.

The amount of estrogen and type of progestin determine bioactivity and possible side effects of CHC products. The combination of estrogen and progestin causes the products to have estrogen-like, or *estrogenic*, activity; progesterone-like, or *progestational*, activity; and androgen-like, or *androgenic*, activity. The combination of estrogen and the selected progestin also has an effect on the uterine endometrium, therefore the lowest effective dose that successfully prevents conception should be used.

Mechanism of Action

The estrogen component of CHC products inhibits ovulation by preventing the formation of a dominant follicle. When a dominant follicle does not mature, estrogen remains at a consistent level and is unable to reach the peak level needed to stimulate the luteinizing hormone (LH) surge. The progestin component also suppresses the LH surge. When the LH surge is suppressed, ovulation is prevented, and pregnancy does not occur. Any cycle in which ovulation does not occur, whether induced by drugs or naturally occurring, is called an anovulatory cycle. CHCs produce drug-induced anovulatory cycles. The estrogen component of CHC products also stabilizes the uterine endometrium, inhibiting proliferation and secretory changes and decreasing the occurrence of irregular or heavy bleeding. The progestational effects of progestin change the endometrium to make it less favorable for implantation of a fertilized ovum. In addition, progestins have an effect on the quantity and viscosity of the cervical mucus, making it thick and hostile to sperm penetration. Progestins alter the motility of both the muscles of the fallopian tube and the cilia within the tube, impeding the movement of the ovum through the tube.

Route of Delivery

There are several routes of administration for CHC products. Most women are familiar with oral contraception, in which a pill is ingested daily that is absorbed by the gastrointestinal (GI) tract and metabolized by the liver. However, CHC products can also be administered through transvaginal and transdermal routes. The advantage of these alternative sites is avoiding GI absorption and the initial metabolism by the liver, or the *first-pass effect*. Theoretically, side effects such as nausea and vomiting, heart and circulatory risks, and nonadherence with a daily dosage regimen can be avoided. Intramuscular (IM) and subcutaneous (subcut) routes of administration for CHCs are not available in the United States.

Combined Hormonal Contraceptives

Combined hormonal contraceptives are one of the most commonly used methods of reversible contraception in the world because of their ease of use, high degree of effectiveness, and relative safety. The theoretic effective rate (absolute correct use) for CHCs is 99.3%, whereas the typical use effective rate (accounting for patient error) is around 92%. This means that CHCs are 92% to 99.3% effective for contraception. When the pill was approved for use by the FDA in 1960, little was known about the best combination of estrogen and progestin or their optimum effective doses. In the 1970s, research provided evidence that the adverse side effects, particularly heart and circulatory effects, were directly related to the dose of estrogen in OCs. The higher dose of estrogen increased risk for venous thromboembolism (VTE), myocardial infarction (MI), and stroke. Subsequently, low-dose OCs and, more recently, ultra-low-dose OCs have been introduced. Low-dose CHCs greatly reduce the risk for dangerous side effects. A low-dose CHC contains 35 mcg or less of ethinyl estradiol and a progestin, whereas ultra-low-dose CHC pills contain 20 mcg or less of EE and a progestin. Research continues to focus on actual and potential short- and long-term benefits and risks associated with use of low-dose oral contraceptives, particularly in the areas of heart and circulatory risks as well as carcinogenesis.

Clinical studies also continue to investigate the venous circulatory effects of new-generation progestins.

CHC formulations are differentiated based on the strength of the estrogen component, the type of progestin used, and whether estrogen or progesterone (and androgen) activity predominates. Increased estrogenic activity may include side effects such as cyclic breast changes, dysmenorrhea (painful periods), menorrhagia (heavy periods), chloasma (hyperpigmentation of the skin), and VTE, whereas decreased estrogenic activity can cause amenorrhea (absence of periods) or spotting at certain points in the cycle. Increased progestational activity can cause weight gain, depression, fatigue, and decreased libido, and a lack of progestational activity may cause breakthrough bleeding (BTB) and headaches. BTB is an episode of bleeding that occurs during the active pill cycle of CHCs. It is more common at the start of CHC use, when a woman changes the type of pill she is taking, and with progestin-only preparations of contraception. There is no evidence that an episode of BTB is associated with a decrease in the CHC's effectiveness as long as the patient continues to take the pill on a daily basis as prescribed. Increased androgenic activity may cause acne, hirsutism, edema, and cholestatic jaundice. The estrogens and progestins in OC pills also have an effect on the uterine endometrium, which may cause changes in the patient's periods that can include irregular bleeding, heavy or light periods, or spotting between periods. The undesirable side effects of hormonal contraception products are discussed later in this chapter.

Most women on CHC products experience shorter, lighter periods. Other advantages with CHCs are decreased blood loss and uterine cramps, elimination of mittelschmerz (mid-cycle pain usually associated with ovulation), reduction of symptoms in many forms of benign breast disorders, and prevention of physiologic ovarian cysts. CHC products also reduce the incidence of pelvic inflammatory disease (PID), ectopic pregnancy, endometrial and ovarian cancer risk, and deaths from colorectal cancer. CHC products do *not* reduce the incidence of sexually transmitted infections (STIs; see Chapter 54 for further discussion of STIs.)

The goal of therapy is to identify the product that offers the best contraceptive protection while producing the fewest unwanted side effects as a result of either the estrogen or the progestin component. It is important to note that the effectiveness of oral contraceptives can also be compromised by concurrent use of some drugs (e.g., antibiotics) or herbal products (Complementary and Alternative Therapies 52.1).

COMPLEMENTARY AND ALTERNATIVE THERAPIES 52.1

St. John's Wort

- St. John's wort may decrease the level of contraceptive hormones in the bloodstream, reducing the effectiveness of combined hormonal contraceptives (CHCs). This may result in breakthrough bleeding and/or spontaneous ovulation.
- Chasteberry extract should be used with caution with CHCs or hormone therapy, as it may alter contraceptive hormone levels in the body and can make them less effective.
- Other herbal remedies that may alter the effectiveness of contraceptive hormones include Dong-quai, black cohosh, and red clover.

TABLE 52.1   Oral Combined Hormonal Contraceptives

Drug	Route and Dosage	Uses and Considerations
Combination products containing norethindrone and ethinyl estradiol	Oral: 1 tablet PO daily from the 21-tablet package: 1 tablet daily for 21 consecutive days followed by 7 days off. A new course begins on the eighth day after a tablet is taken. 28-tablet package: 1 tablet daily without interruption taken at the same time each day	Estrogen and progestin combination used for contraception and for treatment of moderate acne vulgaris in females 15 years and older who have achieved menarche, are unresponsive to topical treatments, have no contraindications to CHC use, and plan to stay on therapy for 6 months or longer. *Contraindications:* History of or current thrombophlebitis, DVT, PE, CVA, CAD, valve disease, hypertension, diabetes mellitus with vascular involvement, migraines in women >35 y, cancers, neoplasms, and tumors. Cardiovascular side effects are increased in women who smoke, especially those >35 y and in those who use CHCs. Pregnancy category: X* PB: >95%; t½: 19-24 h
Combination products containing levonorgestrel (LNG) and ethinyl estradiol (EE)	Same as above	Estrogen and progestin combination used for contraception. Contraindications and black-box warnings are same as above; use with caution in patients with depression, and monitor patients on thyroid replacement therapy, who may require higher doses of thyroid hormone while receiving estrogens. Pregnancy category: X*; PB: 95%-99%; t½: EE, 12-23 h; LNG, 22-49 h
Combination products containing norgestrel and EE	Same	Same
Combination products containing ethynodiol diacetate and EE	Same	Same
Combination products containing norethindrone and mestranol	Same	Same
Combination products containing desogestrel and EE	Same	Same
Combination products containing DRSP and EE	Same	Estrogen and progestin combination used for contraception, for acne treatment in adults, and for PMDD Same contraindications and black-box warnings as above Pregnancy category: X*; PB: 97%-98%; t½: 24-30 h
Combination products containing norgestimate and EE	Same	Estrogen and progestin combination used for contraception and for acne treatment in adults Same contraindications and black-box warnings as above Pregnancy category: X*; PB: 97%-99%; t½: 16-38 h
Combination with folate in the form of EE–DRSP–levomefolate calcium	Same	Estrogen and progestin combination used for contraception, acne, and PMDD Same contraindications and black-box warnings as above Pregnancy category: X*; PB: 97%-99%; t½: DRSP, 31 h; EE, 24 h (approx.); levomefolate calcium, 4-5 h (approx.)

*Pregnancy categories have been revised. See http://www.fda.gov/Drugs/DevelopmentApprovalProcess/DevelopmentResources/Labeling/ucm093 307.htm for more information.

CAD, Coronary artery disease; *CHC,* combined hormonal contraceptive; *CVA,* cerebrovascular accident; *DRSP,* drospirenone; *DVT,* deep venous thrombosis; *EE,* ethinyl estradiol; *h,* hours; *LNG,* levonorgestrel; *PB,* protein binding; *PE,* pulmonary embolus; *PMDD,* premenstrual dysphoric disorder; *PO,* by mouth; *t½,* half-life; *y,* year; *>,* greater than.

Types of Combined Hormonal Contraceptives

Combination pills are classified as either monophasic or multiphasic (biphasic, triphasic, or four-phasic). The *monophasics* provide a fixed ratio of estrogen to progestin throughout the menstrual cycle. In *biphasics,* the amount of estrogen is fixed throughout the cycle, but the amount of progestin varies; it is reduced in the first half to provide for some proliferation of the endometrium and is increased in the second half to promote secretory development of the endometrium. This simulates the normal physiologic process of menstruation while still inhibiting ovulation. The *triphasics* deliver low doses of both hormones with minimal side effects, including BTB. With triphasics, the amount of either estrogen or progesterone varies throughout the cycle in different ratios during the phases (Table 52.1). The newest CHC is a *four-phasic* drug where each phase has varying doses of estradiol valerate (1, 2, or 3 mg) and dienogest (0, 2, or 3 mg). Each pill pack contains 26 pills with hormones and 2 without.

One monophasic combination pill contains 30 mcg of ethinyl estradiol and 3 mg of DRSP. Whereas the progestin found in other CHCs is structurally similar to androgens, DRSP is an analog of spironolactone, which is structurally similar to progesterone. As noted, use of DRSP may increase serum potassium, which can alter water and electrolyte balances in women using this product. Consequently, this drug is contraindicated in women with kidney, liver, or adrenal insufficiency and in women who require daily long-term treatment with drugs such as nonsteroidal antiinflammatory drugs (NSAIDs; e.g., ibuprofen) taken long-term daily for arthritis or other diseases or conditions, potassium-sparing diuretics (e.g., spironolactone), potassium supplementation, angiotensin-converting enzyme (ACE) inhibitors, angiotensin II–receptor antagonists, and heparin.

Withdrawal Bleeding

Most of the monophasic, biphasic, and triphasic CHC products are packaged in both 21- and 28-day tablet packs. In the 21-day tablet packs, 21 days of active pills that contain estrogen and progestin are followed by a 7-day "pill-free" period. A new pack of pills is started after the 7-day pill-free period. In the 28-day tablet pack, 21 days of active pills are followed by 7 days of inert pills, called *counters*. The patient takes one pill daily and begins a new pack the day after the last counter is taken. During the hormone-free period (counters) or the 7-day pill-free period, the level of estrogen and progestin decreases to allow for a breakdown of the endometrial lining. This causes a pseudomenstruation known as withdrawal bleeding or *withdrawal menses*. The withdrawal bleeding is not a true menstrual period, and the bleeding experienced by a woman can vary in amount and duration.

There are CHCs that provide ferrous fumarate, an iron compound, or folic acid, a B vitamin, during the hormone-free period. Ferrous fumarate provides supplementation during the phase of withdrawal bleeding, promoting healthy iron stores in women and protecting against menstrual-associated iron-deficiency anemia. Folic acid reduces the risk of neural tube defect should the woman become pregnant on OCs or shortly after OCs are discontinued.

Withdrawal bleeding periods are scheduled monthly to mimic a normal 28-day menstrual cycle; however, researchers have established that a monthly episode of withdrawal bleeding is not necessary to maintain a healthy uterus. CHCs are available that (1) decrease the number of withdrawal menses per year by having 81 to 84 continuous days of active pills and 7 days of less-active pills, resulting in four withdrawal menses per year; or (2) eliminate withdrawal bleeding altogether by continuous oral administration of active pills.

Extended-Use Combined Hormonal Contraceptives

A continuous-dosing CHC pill that contains EE and LNG is a 91-day regimen of pills. This regimen includes 84 days of active pills and 7 days of inert pills. This drug causes withdrawal bleeding to occur just four times per year. The active hormone pills contain 30 mcg of EE and 0.15 mg of LNG.

Another combination is still a 91-day regimen, but it contains 30 mcg of EE and 0.15 mg of LNG and is followed with 7 days of tablets that contain 10 mcg EE, instead of 7 days of inactive pills. During the 7 days of low-dose estrogen pills, women usually experience withdrawal menses. However, by adding very low levels of estrogen in the 7-day "break" period, instead of inert pills, this combination provides additional benefits such

as a reduction in breakthrough bleeding. Users of extended-use birth control pills are more likely to experience bleeding or spotting between periods. The continued progestin dose causes extreme atrophy of the endometrial lining; the atrophic endometrium subsequently breaks down, and the patient experiences uterine bleeding in an irregular pattern.

Continuous-Use Combined Hormonal Contraceptives

The first continuous-dose CHC to be FDA approved comes in a 28-day pack and contains 20 mcg of EE and 90 mcg of LNG. This drug is taken daily and continuously without interruption for withdrawal menses.

Although these products are more commonly known for their contraceptive value, women with menstrual disorders such as menorrhagia (heavy periods), metrorrhagia (irregular bleeding between periods, usually heavy), endometriosis, dysmenorrhea, premenstrual syndrome (PMS), and physiologic ovarian cyst formation may benefit from continuous-cycle CHC products because of their ability to suppress ovarian function and limit uterine bleeding.

Ethinyl Estradiol and Norelgestromin Transdermal Patch

This is a weekly form of CHC patch that delivers either 20 mcg EE and 150 mcg norelgestromin every 24 hours or 35 mcg EE and 150 mcg norelgestromin every 24 hours through a transdermal system. The system is a thin plastic patch placed on the skin of the buttocks, stomach, upper outer arm, or upper torso. The patch is placed once a week for 3 weeks in a row. The fourth week is patch-free to allow for withdrawal bleeding. The patch should be placed on clean, dry skin; placement on or near the breasts should be avoided because of the estrogen component, and the site of the patch placement should be rotated to avoid skin irritation. If the patch partially or completely detaches from the skin, a new patch should be placed. When used correctly, the patch protects against pregnancy on a monthly basis. The theoretic and typical use effective rate for the patch is 99.3% and 92%, respectively, making it 92% to 99.3% effective at preventing pregnancy.

The patch works in a similar manner to CHC pills by inhibiting ovulation, thickening cervical mucus to prevent sperm penetration, and preventing a fertilized egg from implanting in the uterus. The patch avoids the first-pass effect (through the liver). Advantages include not having to remember to take a pill daily. As with CHC products, the ability to become pregnant returns quickly when the pill is discontinued. Menstrual flow, cramping, acne, iron-deficiency anemia, excess body hair, premenstrual symptoms, and vaginal dryness are all lessened with the patch. As with CHC pills, the patch reduces the risk for ovarian and endometrial cancers, PID, breast and ovarian cysts, and osteoporosis (loss of bone mass) that predisposes women to fractures. With the patch, occurrences of ectopic pregnancy are also reduced.

Disadvantages of the patch include skin reaction at the site of application, menstrual cramps, and a change in vision or the inability to wear contact lenses; it is not as effective for women who weigh more than 198 lb. The EE and norelgestromin transdermal patch carries a boxed warning stating that it exposes women to higher levels of estrogen, thereby increasing the risk for VTE. With OCs, peak serum estrogen levels are reached rapidly after ingestion and then steadily decline. With the patch, peak serum estrogen levels are 25% less than in women taking the pill; however, these peak levels remain fairly constant throughout the week the patch is in place and then decline, exposing women to 60% more estrogen than with OCs. Ongoing research is necessary to demonstrate the exact risk for VTE, as well as other cardiovascular complications (particularly heart attack and stroke), in women using the transdermal patch. Women being prescribed the transdermal route of CHCs should be notified of potential risks, and the patch should be used with extreme caution in any patient with increased risk for VTE. Women who are older than 35 years and smoke should not use the transdermal patch. Other side effects include temporary irregular bleeding, weight gain or loss, breast tenderness, and nausea.

Ethinyl Estradiol and Etonogestrel Transvaginal Contraception

The ethinyl estradiol and etonogestrel transvaginal ring is a 2-inch flexible indwelling ring that is inserted into the vagina. It is nonbiodegradable, transparent, and colorless. This ring releases 15 mcg of EE and 120 mcg of the progestin etonogestrel daily, similar to the quantities of estrogen and progestin found in lower-dose CHC products. Etonogestrel is a biologically active metabolite of desogestrel and is a third-generation progestin, which may be associated with an increased risk for VTE. The transvaginal ring remains in place for 3 weeks. As with the transdermal patch, this may expose the patient to higher levels of estrogen. Studies have been inconclusive, therefore the FDA has placed no additional warnings on the transvaginal ring.

Theoretic effectiveness and typical effectiveness rates are 98% and 92%, respectively, which reflects a rate similar to that of other leading CHCs. The patient inserts the ring during the first 5 days of the menstrual cycle and removes the ring after 3 weeks, remains "ring-free" for 1 week (for withdrawal menses), and then inserts a new ring. Backup contraception is recommended during the first 7 days after the first ring is placed. During this time, the hormones reach an appropriate protective level. After this, contraceptive effects are expected to be continuous provided the ring is correctly inserted. Correct insertion involves placing the ring into the middle or upper third of the vagina. Unlike the diaphragm, it does not need to be placed near or over the cervix. It is the close proximity of the ring to the vaginal mucosa that causes absorption of steroid hormones to occur. The ring remains in place during intercourse, tampon use, or administration of intravaginal drugs. If the ring slips out, it can be rinsed with lukewarm water and reinserted into the vagina. It should be reinserted within 3 hours after becoming dislodged; if the ring remains out for more than 3 hours, additional contraception is required until the ring has been in place for 7 days. Possible side effects include vaginal discharge, irritation, or infection. Other associated risks are the same as for low-dose CHCs and are increased in patients who smoke.

PROGESTIN CONTRACEPTIVES

Progestin contraceptives do not contain estrogen. The estrogen component of contraceptives increases the risk of circulatory disorders, therefore these products allow contraception to be available for women who cannot take CHCs. Advantages of progestin contraceptive include relative safety, ease of use, spontaneity of sexual intercourse, and reversibility. However, because the estrogen component is missing, these products have a higher incidence of irregular bleeding and spotting as well as the possibility of depression, mood changes, decreased libido, fatigue, and weight gain. Progestin contraceptives do not protect women against STIs. Women who cannot take estrogen but may be candidates for progestin contraceptives include patients with a personal or strong family history of VTE or heart disease, breastfeeding patients, smokers older than 35 years of age, and women with uncontrolled hypertension. Women who have an untoward response to estrogenic effects such as chloasma, migraine headaches, or changes in lipid profiles may also be candidates for progestin contraceptives. Progestin contraceptives are available in oral, IM, subcut, and implantable routes of delivery.

Progestin-Only Oral Contraceptive Pills

The progestin-only oral contraceptive pill (POP), called the *minipill*, has four mechanisms of action: (1) it alters cervical mucus, making it thick and viscous, which blocks sperm penetration; (2) it interferes with the endometrial lining, which makes implantation difficult; (3) it decreases peristalsis in the fallopian tubes, slowing the transport of ovum; and (4) in approximately 50% of cycles, it interferes with the LH surge and thereby inhibits ovulation.

POPs contain 0.35 mg of norethindrone. The minipill is taken continuously, without a break for withdrawal bleeding. Patients should be instructed to take the minipill daily within a 3-hour window.

The theoretic and typical use effective rates for the first year of use are similar to those of CHC products even though patient adherence to the dosage schedule with POPs is more specific. It takes 4 to 6 hours for the progestin to thicken the cervical mucus to prevent sperm penetration, and the duration of the effect of the progestin on cervical mucus lasts just over 24 hours. Risk for pregnancy will increase if a patient misses a pill because POPs do not suppress the release of follicle-stimulating hormone (FSH) and LH to the same degree as CHC products. If the minipill is taken more than 3 hours late, a back-up contraceptive method should be used for 48 hours. There are no placebo pills in a pack of progestin-only pills. All 28 pills contain active hormones, so the patient continuously takes one active pill daily. Because the endometrial lining is altered, an increase in the amount of irregular bleeding is noted.

Depot Medroxyprogesterone Acetate

Depot medroxyprogesterone acetate (DMPA) is a highly effective, long-acting injectable progestin with theoretic and typical use efficacy rates of 99% and 97%, respectively. This makes DMPA one of the most effective hormonal methods of contraception. It appeals to women because it is discreet and has a convenient dosing schedule; DMPA is popular with adolescents for these same reasons. Injectable progestin is administered in a flexible dosing schedule every 11 to 13 weeks. The mechanism of action of DMPA relies on the progestational activities: thickening of the cervical mucus, thinning of the uterine endometrium, and a decrease in fallopian tube motility. Because the progestin in DMPA reaches a higher circulating level than with POPs, DMPA inhibits both FSH and LH secretion from the anterior pituitary gland. This results in both anovulation (lack of ovulation) and amenorrhea. Because FSH and LH secretion is inhibited, formation of a dominant follicle is inhibited, and the production of estrogen in the body is greatly decreased. However, the patient experiences a hypoestrogen state, which can affect bone mineral density (BMD).

The DMPA vial or prefilled syringe should be vigorously shaken just prior to administration to ensure a uniform drug suspension. DMPA 150 mg/1 mL is given by deep IM injection into the ventral gluteus or deltoid muscle. The site should *not* be massaged after injection, and the injection site must be documented so that sites can be rotated. The patient is given a personalized calendar for subsequent doses and should return for another injection within 13 weeks. If the patient is late for her injection (e.g., 13 weeks and *1 day*), pregnancy should be ruled out before she receives another injection.

As with oral contraceptives, DMPA does not protect against STIs. Due to the hypoestrogenic state produced by DMPA, bone resorption exceeds bone formation. This results in a reduction of BMD, greatest during the first 1 to 2 years of DMPA use. Following discontinuation of DMPA, BMD substantially improves (more so at the spine than hips), but may not be completely reversible. Based on this data, the FDA issued a boxed warning recommending DMPA be discontinued after 2 years of continuous use, unless other methods of contraception are inadequate. Many professional provider organizations agree that the concerns of the 2-consecutive-year limit given by the FDA and the BMD effects of DMPA should not prevent the practitioner from considering the benefit-risk ratio for each individual patient. The American Congress of Obstetricians and Gynecologists (ACOG) states in a committee opinion that "the possible adverse effects of DMPA must be carefully balanced against the significant personal and public health impact of unintended pregnancy." The benefits, risks, and alternatives and the prevention of BMD loss while taking DMPA must be discussed with the patient before administration of the product.

Women taking DMPA should be instructed to increase calcium and vitamin D intake to the daily recommended allowance for their age and to participate in regular weight-bearing exercises. DMPA is safe to receive immediately postpartum, and women can breastfeed while using this contraceptive without affecting milk supply. The most common side effects include initially irregular uterine bleeding or spotting. Menstruation may cease about 1 year after starting. In addition, DMPA has been shown to cause progressive weight gain in some women. Other side effects include breast tenderness and an increase in depression. The drug is contraindicated in cases of undiagnosed vaginal bleeding and known or suspected pregnancy. Caution should be used in giving DMPA postpartum in women who are at risk for or have a history of postpartum depression.

Depot medroxyprogesterone acetate formulated for subcutaneous injection is available as an injectable suspension of 104 mg/0.65 mL. It is administered to women every 11 to 13 weeks. This drug has the same mechanism of action, benefits, and risks as DMPA for intramuscular injection, and women should be counseled about the potential loss of BMD. Women taking DMPA have a slower return to fertility than those using other hormonal methods of contraception.

Progestin Implant

A progestin implant is a single-rod device that contains 68 mg of etonogestrel; it is implanted in the inner side of the upper nondominant arm. It needs to be removed no later than 3 years after the date of insertion; it may be replaced with a new implant at the time of removal. The progestin implant contains barium, a radiopaque substance that can help locate the device on two-dimensional radiography, ultrasound, magnetic resonance imaging (MRI), and computed tomography (CT) scanning if necessary. Also, the device comes in a preloaded application system that reduces insertion errors. The progestin implant may not be as effective in women who have a body mass index (BMI) greater than 30 (obese) or who are on drugs that induce liver enzymes. Theoretic and typical effectiveness rates for implantable progestins are the same, at 99.6%.

Pharmacokinetics: Combined Hormonal Contraceptives Ethinyl estradiol is rapidly absorbed orally and reaches peak serum concentration in 1 to 2 hours. It undergoes significant first-pass metabolism resulting in 40% bioavailability. Ethinyl estradiol is 98.5% protein bound. It is excreted as metabolites, via feces and urine. It undergoes some enterohepatic circulation.

The steroid hormones in the transvaginal ring are rapidly absorbed through the vaginal mucosa. Etonogestrel in the transvaginal ring has a bioavailability of 100%; bioavailability of EE is 55%. The transdermal patch also bypasses the hepatic portal system. Avoiding first-pass metabolism through the liver has the potential to decrease adverse drug interactions. The norelgestromin in the patch binds to albumin. Levels of serum steroid hormones in the patch reach constant levels of contraceptive efficacy within 48 hours. Serum hormone levels are rapidly reached, and blood levels do not fluctuate as much as is seen with oral contraceptive products.

Pharmacokinetics: Progestin Contraceptives Progestin contraceptives are well absorbed from the GI tract. Peak plasma levels occur 1 to 2 hours after ingestion, depending on the particular compound. Norethynodrel and ethynodiol diacetate are converted to norethindrone. LNG is 100% bioavailable and does not undergo first-pass liver metabolism; norethindrone undergoes first-pass metabolism and is 65% available. The progestins are bound to plasma proteins and to sex-hormone–binding globulin. The half-life of norethindrone varies from 5 to 14 hours; the half-life of LNG is 11 to 45 hours.

DMPA provides higher peak levels of progestin than POPs and implantable progestins. Once injected, the levels of DMPA increase for 3 weeks, remain stable for a few days, then begin to decline. DMPA is undetectable in the blood between 120 and 200 days after injection. The formulation for subcutaneous administration of DMPA provides a slower and more sustained absorption than IM, permitting a lower dose. DMPA is 90% protein bound, metabolized in the liver, and excreted primarily in the urine.

A progestin implant is a sustained-release system that releases progestin at a level of 60 to 70 mcg/day during the first 6 weeks after insertion, declining to 35 to 45 mcg/day during the first year. This decreases to 30 to 40 mcg/day after 2 years of implantation and 25 to 30 mcg/day by the end of the third year. Bioavailability remains constant at 95%. Once the rod is inserted, effective contraceptive levels are reached within 8 hours.

Start Date and Dosing Schedule

There are three ways to implement the start of hormonal contraception products unless otherwise indicated by the manufacturer. With the *first-day start method,* the contraception product is initiated on the first day a women experiences bleeding; the first day of bleeding is day 1 of the menstrual cycle. Days are then counted 2, 3, 4, 5, 6, and so on until the first-day bleeding begins again, usually around day 28. Most methods of contraception can be safely started on day 1 through day 5 of the menstrual cycle, when it is less likely that the patient has an early undiagnosed pregnancy. No back-up method of contraception is needed when the product is started on the first through fifth day of menstruation. (A back-up method is a second method of contraception that is used until the primary method reaches its peak level of contraceptive effectiveness; usually this is a barrier method, such as a condom or diaphragm.)

Many products require a *Sunday start,* meaning the patient starts the tablets or patch on the Sunday after the first day of menstruation. If menstruation actually starts on Sunday, the patient starts her tablet or patch on that day. The Sunday start aids a woman in remembering the first day of her contraception cycle. If a patient starts the contraception later than day 5 of her menstrual cycle, a back-up form of contraception should be used for 7 days.

The *quick-start method* of initiating contraception starts on the day the patient receives the prescription regardless of where she might be in her menstrual cycle. This method increases patient adherence and resolves the risk for becoming pregnant while waiting for a menstrual period to begin to start the contraceptive. Pregnancy should be ruled out prior to the quick-start method, but there is a risk that the patient could have an early pregnancy undetectable by screening. A back-up method of contraception must be used for 7 days if the quick-start method is used after the first 5 days of the menstrual cycle. Both estrogen-progestin and progestin-only contraception methods are contraindicated in pregnancy (formerly category X). *Nonetheless, there is no evidence of fetal risks associated with these drugs when inadvertently used in pregnancy.* If withdrawal menses does not occur when planned, a pregnancy test is administered.

BOX 52.1   Guidelines for Missed Doses of Oral Contraceptives

Combined Hormonal Contraceptives
One Tablet
Take the tablet as soon as the missed dose is realized.
Take the next tablet as scheduled.

Two Tablets
Take 2 tablets as soon as the missed dose is realized and 2 tablets the next day. Use a back-up method of contraception for the rest of the cycle.

Three Tablets
Discontinue the present pack and allow for withdrawal bleeding. Start a new package of tablets 7 days after the last tablet is taken. Use another form of contraception until tablets have been taken for 7 consecutive days.

Progestin-Only Pills
One or More Tablets
Take the tablet as soon as the missed dose is realized, and follow with the next tablet at the regular time *plus* use a back-up method of contraception for 48 hours.

Special Considerations

DMPA and the transvaginal ring should be started within the first 5 days of the menstrual cycle. (Sunday start and quick-start methods are off label.) The continuous-dosing CHC products use a Sunday start only. If the patient is on a 21-day CHC regimen, the next pack should be started following the 7-day break whether bleeding has stopped or not. With 28-day packs, a pill is taken daily without stopping regardless of the bleeding pattern. Usually, withdrawal menses occur in a cyclic fashion. In multiphasic preparations, the day 1 pill is clearly marked, and the tablets are taken in the order noted. A difference in the color of the tablets delineates the change in the dose of estrogen or progestin through the phases. With the POP, a pill is taken daily without a break. To increase effectiveness, all OCs should be taken at the same time daily. With the POP, women should strictly adhere to this instruction.

Missed Doses

Box 52.1 provides guidelines for patients on how to handle missing a dose of their OC.

Contraindications

Not every patient is a candidate for use of CHCs. Box 52.2 lists contraindications to CHC use.

Drug Interactions

The effectiveness of some drugs is impaired by CHC products; other drugs impair the effectiveness of CHCs and progestin contraceptives. Box 52.3 shows drugs that may have interactive effects with CHCs. Patients receiving low-dose formulations of oral contraceptives need to be particularly cautious about potential interactions. If a patient is taking a drug that affects estrogen absorption or metabolism, a CHC with a higher dose of EE may be prescribed.

BOX 52.2 Contraindications for Combined Hormonal Contraceptives

Absolute Contraindications
Pregnancy (known or suspected)
Venous thrombosis history or risk factors
Vascular disease, including coronary artery disease and cerebrovascular accident (CVA) and past or current history of deep venous thrombosis (DVT) or pulmonary embolism
Liver disease, including cirrhosis, viral hepatitis, and benign or malignant liver tumors
Undiagnosed vaginal bleeding or known or suspected endometrial cancer
Breast cancer
Tobacco use of more than 15 cigarettes per day in a patient older than 35 years of age

Cautious Use
Hypertension with associated vascular disease
Hypertension with blood pressure greater than 160/100
Hyperlipidemia
Diabetes mellitus complicated by neuropathy, retinopathy, nephropathy, or vascular disease
Diabetes mellitus for more than 20 years' duration
Postpartum fewer than 3 weeks
Lactation fewer than 6 weeks
Age greater than 35 years and smoking fewer than 15 cigarettes per day
Hypercoagulation disorders
Prolonged immobility
Use of drugs that affect liver enzymes (e.g., anticonvulsants, rifampin)

BOX 52.3 Drugs That Interact With Combined Hormonal Contraceptives

Drugs That Decrease the Effectiveness of Combined Hormonal Contraceptives
Use a higher-dose pill or an alternative form of contraception (if the drug is continuous).
Use a back-up method for the duration of treatment plus 7 days (if drug is short term).

Anticonvulsant Drugs
Carbamazepine
Hydantoins (ethotoin, mephenytoin, phenytoin)
Succinimide anticonvulsants (ethosuximide)

Antituberculin Drugs
Rifampin

Antifungal Drugs
Griseofulvin

Antibiotics
Amoxicillin
Ampicillin
Doxycycline
Metronidazole
Minocycline
Neomycin
Nitrofurantoin
Penicillin
Tetracycline

Barbiturates
Phenobarbital
Primidone

Hypnotics and Sedatives
Benzodiazepines

Migraine Drugs
Topiramate

Drugs That May Increase Combined Hormonal Contraceptive Activity
Acetaminophen
Ascorbic acid
Fluconazole

Other Drug Interactions
An alternative method of contraception is necessary.
Anticoagulants: CHCs increase clotting factors and decrease the effectiveness of anticoagulants.
Anticonvulsants: CHCs may increase the risk for seizure.

CHC, Combined hormonal contraceptive.

Potential Side Effects and Adverse Reactions

It is accepted by health care providers that the risks associated with hormonal contraception are much less than the risks associated with pregnancy. This is especially true if the patient does not have any of the contraindications listed in Box 52.2. In most cases, the benefits of any contraceptive method usually outweigh the risks when using a benefit-risk ratio to determine patient eligibility.

Benefit-risk ratio is partially determined by the risk related to the particular contraceptive method compared with the risk pregnancy poses for the patient. Also included in the benefit-risk ratio is consideration of age, smoking status, allergies and drugs, health histories and physical assessments, and patient lifestyle patterns and changes. These considerations determine patient selection or nonselection for the method as well as continuing or discontinuing a method of contraception.

Most of the untoward side effects are related to differences in the estrogen-progestin ratio of the products and the patient's response to these differences. Side effects primarily caused by an excess of estrogen include nausea, vomiting, dizziness, fluid retention, edema, bloating, breast enlargement, breast tenderness, **chloasma** (slightly more in dark-skinned patients on higher-dose tablets who are exposed to sunlight), leg cramps, decreased tearing, corneal curvature alteration, visual changes, vascular headache, and hypertension (in about 1% to 5% of previously normotensive patients within the first few months).

Side effects primarily caused by estrogen deficiency include vaginal bleeding (BTB, especially in the first few cycles after starting therapy) that lasts several days, usually during days 1 to 14; **oligomenorrhea** (very scant periods), especially after long-term use; nervousness; and **dyspareunia** (painful sexual intercourse) secondary to atrophic vaginitis.

Side effects primarily caused by an excess of progestin include increased appetite, weight gain, oily skin and scalp, acne, depression, vulvovaginal candidiasis (vaginitis from the yeast microbe *Candida*), excess hair growth, decreased breast size, and amenorrhea after cessation of use (1% to 2% of patients).

Side effects primarily caused by progestin deficiency include dysmenorrhea, bleeding late in the cycle (days 15 to 21), heavy menstrual flow with clots, or amenorrhea. There may also be changes in laboratory values, including thyroid and liver function, blood glucose, and triglycerides.

CHCs may increase the vascularity of the cervical epithelium, extend the area of cervical ectopy, and alter certain immune parameters. Advise pill users to use male or female latex or polyurethane condoms unless they are confident that both partners are free of human immunodeficiency virus (HIV) and other STIs.

Adverse reactions of a more severe nature include cardiovascular and carcinogenetic risks.

Cardiovascular. There is an increased risk for hypertension (usually seen within 3 months after initiating CHCs in women with preexisting risk) and arterial blood clot complications such as MI, pulmonary embolus, and cerebrovascular accident (CVA) in women using CHCs compared with women who are not using CHCs. However, in terms of absolute risk for adolescents and women, the rate of dangerous complications from hormonal methods of contraception is extremely low because women younger than 50 years rarely experience heart attack or stroke. The risk for hypertension in women younger than 35 years is also low. Hormonal methods of contraception that contain DRSP or etonogestrel may double a woman's risk for venous thromboembolic events. Cardiovascular risks are increased in women older than 35 years who smoke, women older than 45 years, and women with hypertension that is undiagnosed or uncontrolled by drugs.

Carcinogenesis. Long-term use of CHCs may increase the risk for breast cancer in younger women, but the risk is minimal. Breast cancer risk returns to normal 10 years or more after discontinuing CHCs. There is also an increased risk for benign liver tumors. Risk for cervical cancer is slightly increased, which is thought to be because CHCs change cervical epithelium, making it more susceptible to the high-risk pathogenic strains of human papillomavirus (HPV) and because condoms may be used less frequently in prevention of STIs. Women who use hormonal methods of contraception have a greatly reduced risk for ovarian and endometrial cancers, and the protective effect is directly related to the duration of time the method is used.

 NURSING PROCESS
Patient-Centered Collaborative Care
Combined Hormonal Contraceptives

Assessment
- Obtain a record of the patient's drug, supplement, and complementary and alternative medicine (CAM) use.
- Obtain baseline vital signs that include temperature, pulse, and respirations; blood pressure (BP); weight; and height. Calculate BMI, and report any abnormal findings.

- Obtain a complete menstrual history that includes age at menarche, menstrual pattern, cycle length, duration, and amount of bleeding and the first day of the last menstrual period (LMP). A detailed history of the menstrual cycle in reproductive-age and climacteric women should be considered as another vital sign.
- Determine pregnancy status.
- Obtain a family medical history specific to contraindications for CHCs and progestin contraceptives.
- Obtain a family history of premenopausal breast cancer.
- Assess for domestic violence, intimate partner violence, and past or recent sexual abuse/assault.
- Obtain a medical history, assessing for history of allergies to drugs, smoking, hypertension, and the contraindications to CHCs listed in Box 52.2.
- Obtain a complete obstetric and gynecologic history that includes gravida, parity, abortion (spontaneous, therapeutic, or elective); age at first and last pregnancy; time frame between pregnancies; complications during pregnancy, delivery, and postpartum; genetic anomalies and health of children; time since the last Papanicolaou (Pap) test; history of abnormal Pap testing; history of gynecologic and/or sexual infections; gynecologic problems and/or surgeries; and gynecologic anomalies.
- Obtain a complete sexual history that includes sexual expression and sexual risk practices, history of STIs and treatment, and past or present sexual abuse and/or assault.
- Recognize the need for periodic reassessment of baseline data and side effects. Most patients should be seen 1 to 3 months after beginning a contraceptive regimen.

Nursing Diagnoses
- Knowledge, Deficient regarding reproduction, reproductive health, and self-care
- Decisional Conflict related to contraception methods
- Decisional Conflict with the partner regarding the contraceptive method choice and/or family planning
- Knowledge, Deficient regarding contraceptive method(s) and appropriate use
- Fear related to contraceptive method side effects
- Infection, Risk for
- Decisional Conflict related to a discrepancy between cultural and/or religious beliefs and the choice of contraception

Planning
- Patients with contraindications to hormonal contraception will be determined by evaluation of risk-benefit.
- The patient will understand the difference between combined hormonal contraceptives and progestin contraceptives and their various routes of administration.
- The patient will verbalize understanding of the bleeding patterns associated with both types of contraceptives by reporting menstrual changes that occur.
- The patient will choose a contraceptive method suitable for her lifestyle and health status.

- The patient will understand the benefits, risks, and alternatives to the method chosen through the BRAIDED method: discuss *benefits* (advantages, positive aspects, and both theoretic and actual effective rates of the method), *risks* (dangers, complications, disadvantages, and failure rates), *alternatives* (other contraception options available), *inquiries* (opportunity for the patient to ask questions about options proposed), *decision* (deciding on a method with opportunity to change the decision as needed), *explanation* (health care teaching specific to the method chosen), and *documentation*.
- Starting method, dosing schedule, and use of contraceptive method chosen will be explained at the patient's level of understanding.
- For reporting symptoms of dangerous cardiovascular side effects to the health care provider, explain the ACHES acronym: *abdominal pain* (severe); *chest pain* or shortness of breath; *headaches* (severe), dizziness, weakness, numbness, or speech difficulties; *eye disorders,* which includes blurring or loss of vision; and *severe* leg pain or swelling in the calf or thigh.
- The patient will take oral contraceptives as prescribed and will report side effects that occur.
- The patient will place the contraceptive patch as prescribed and will report adverse side effects that occur.
- The patient will demonstrate and report comfort with placement of the transvaginal ring and will report adverse side effects that occur.
- The patient will be aware of the specific scheduling needed for progestin-only pills.
- The patient will understand initiation and scheduling of DMPA injections and the need for weight-bearing exercises and calcium supplementation.
- The patient will be given time to ask questions related to reproductive health, method choice, benefits and risks, alternatives, and use of the method.
- Follow-up appointments will be scheduled as needed.

Nursing Interventions
- Separate personal views from those of the patient regarding contraception and use of specific products.
- Address the patient's misconceptions and provide factual, evidence-based information.
- Encourage informed consent for the contraceptive method through the BRAIDED method.
- Use health teaching to encourage effective use of the chosen contraceptive method.
- Ensure that the patient understands the start date, continuation of drug, and appropriate follow-up.
- Recognize that a percentage of patients on hormonal contraceptives will abandon the method within 1 year; plan to provide the patient with alternatives, and encourage the patient to seek care with a qualified health care provider before discontinuing any method of contraception.
- Nonnursing mothers can begin CHCs 4 to 6 weeks postpartum, regardless of whether menstruation has

spontaneously occurred. Some sources indicate that a CHC method can be initiated as early as 3 weeks postpartum.
- Nonnursing and nursing mothers can begin DMPA immediately postpartum if there is no increased risk for postpartum depression. POPs can be started at 4 to 6 weeks postpartum.
- Recognize that combined hormonal contraceptives may decrease milk production in patients who are breastfeeding. CHCs can be used by breastfeeding mothers, but these methods should be initiated after breastfeeding is well established. This is usually 2 to 3 months after the birth, although some sources state that 6 weeks is sufficient.

Patient Teaching
General
- Remind patients that these drugs should be used only under the direction of a qualified health care provider.
- Advise patients that concurrent use of some drugs and herbal products decreases the effectiveness of hormonal contraceptives. Patients should use a second form of contraception during use of these drugs and herbal supplements and possibly as long as 7 days after discontinuing counteracting drugs.
- Patients will understand that hormonal methods of contraception do *not* prevent transmission of STIs or the pathogen that causes HIV infection and AIDS. If a patient is at risk for STI or HIV infection, condoms should be used concurrently with the CHC method, and safe-sex practices should be discussed. Inform patients regarding proper condom use.

Safety
- ⚡ Counsel patients not to smoke tobacco because of increased cardiovascular risks.
- Advise patients to use a barrier method of contraception as needed during the first 7 days of contraception use if the method is started 5 days or more after the first day of the menstrual period. Instruct patients on how to use barrier methods properly.
- Teach patients about how to manage missed pills. Provide instruction for missed POPs and on patch, ring, and injection methods. Review instructions for emergency contraception.
- Advise patients to report any effects from hormonal contraception to their provider so therapy can be adjusted to suit patient needs. Encourage patients not to discontinue use of the method until an adequate trial time frame has been completed, which should be at least 3 to 6 months.
- ⚡ Counsel patients that health care professionals should be advised of CHC use before surgery in which immobilization for an extended period may be needed.
- Encourage patients to report any irregular bleeding or BTB. A change in dose or type of hormonal contraceptive method may be advised.
- Advise patients to always report use of hormonal contraceptives when seeing a health care provider because of possible synergistic or antagonistic responses to other drugs and therapies.

- Advise nursing mothers that the use of CHCs may decrease the quantity and quality of breast milk.

Side Effects

- ⚡ Advise patients that rare but serious side effects can occur, including VTE, MI, CVA, and retinal vein thrombosis.
- ⚡ Teach patients the ACHES acronym for reporting symptoms of dangerous cardiovascular side effects to their health care provider.
- Encourage patients to notify their health care provider immediately if any of these symptoms occur.
- Advise patients that menstrual flow may be less in amount and duration because of thinning of the endometrial lining with CHCs and progestin contraceptives.
- Advise patients of menstrual changes that can occur at the start of combined estrogen-progestin contraception use, when changing types of hormonal contraception products, and with progestin contraceptives.
- Determine whether the patient wears contact lenses, and discuss how to handle alterations in the shape of the cornea and dry eyes caused by decreased tearing.
- Counsel patients who experiences post-CHC amenorrhea that 95% of women have regular periods within 12 to 18 months. Advise her that those who participate in endurance fitness activities may have increased post-CHC amenorrhea.
- Advise patients of a possible decrease in libido caused by an alteration in vaginal secretions and decreased levels of testosterone.
- Ensure that patients understand the ability to return to fertility after discontinuing a hormonal contraception product and the time frame in which pregnancy can be expected.
- Ensure a safe transition between contraceptive methods if a change in method is desired.

Skill

- Teach patients breast health awareness and self-examination.
- Teach patients how to inspect genitalia for abnormalities and note changes in vaginal secretions.
- Show patients the packet of pills, and discuss how to recognize start dates and follow the sequential pill dosing. Demonstrate how to remove the pill from the pill packet.
- Teach patients how to place and remove transdermal contraception patches.
- Teach patients how to place and remove transvaginal contraception rings.
- Teach patients how to use a calendar to record placement and removal of transvaginal rings or transdermal patches.
- Advise patients to return for a DMPA injection within the 13-week time frame.

Diet

- Counsel patients to moderate caffeine intake because elimination of caffeine may be decreased as a result of prescribed CHC products.
- Tell patients to take OCs with a snack or after meals to help eliminate nausea.
- Advise patients using DMPA to increase calcium and vitamin D intake and to do 15 to 30 minutes of weight-bearing exercises 3 to 4 times per week.
- Discuss foods that increase iron and iron absorption.

🌐 *Cultural Considerations*

- Be aware of different cultures' contraception practices. For example, in some cultures, methods that involve touching the vagina may be difficult for a woman to use.
- Consider religious and spiritual beliefs with regard to contraceptive choices. Be accepting and supportive of beliefs or practices that are not consistent with personal beliefs—yours or the patient's.

Evaluation

- Encourage the patient in planning follow-up evaluations.
- Evaluate the patient's adherence with the hormonal contraceptive regimen; assess for changes in sexual partners and/or health status that may compromise the method.

OTHER METHODS OF CONTRACEPTION

Spermicides

Spermicides are chemical agents that inactivate sperm before they can travel through the cervix and into the upper genital tract. The most common spermicide is nonoxynol-9, which is infused into carrying agents—jellies and creams, foams, suppositories, and films—and is also impregnated into over-the-counter (OTC) sponges used for birth control. Some of the carrying agents contain a short-acting spermicide, whereas others adhere to the vaginal mucosa to provide extended spermicidal action. When combined with barrier methods such as a condom or diaphragm, spermicides increase protection against pregnancy. Spermicide can cause vulvovaginal abrasions and altered vaginal flora, which can increase susceptibility to pathogens.

Barrier Methods

Both male and female condoms are available over the counter. The female condom is a polyurethane (plastic) pouch with flexible rings at each end. It is inserted deep into the vagina like a diaphragm. The ring at the closed end holds the pouch in the vagina, and the ring at the open end stays outside the vulva. Male condoms are available in latex, lambskin, and polyurethane. Latex condoms offer excellent protection against STIs and HIV. (See Chapter 54 for further discussion.) Other barrier methods include the cervical cap and diaphragm, which require a medical visit for proper fitting. Barrier methods are more effective at preventing pregnancy when paired with a spermicide. Appropriate health care teaching for the use of these methods is essential to enhance pregnancy prevention. Patients with latex allergies need to avoid products that contain latex.

Intrauterine Contraception

Intrauterine devices (IUDs) and intrauterine systems (IUSs) are safe methods of contraception with high patient satisfaction rates. Although intrauterine contraception methods are used more widely outside the United States, IUDs and IUSs have the highest effectiveness rates of reversible forms of contraception. Both the expected and the typical efficacy rate is 99.9%. Patient selection for IUD and IUS use should consider menstrual factors, known or suspected uterine anomalies and fibroids, risk factors for STIs, and history of PID—an infection of the upper genital tract, usually the uterine endometrium, fallopian tubes, or ovaries. (PID and STIs are further discussed in Chapter 54.) After insertion, the device's filamentous strings protrude through the cervix and into the vagina. The strings ensure that the device remains in place, and they aid in removal when needed. It was previously thought that the strings can act as a wick, a mechanism by which microbes can ascend into the endometrial cavity. However, studies show that the risk of upper genital tract infections is related to insertion; thus PID incidence is minimal after 20 days of insertion.

If a woman contracts an STI while the device is inserted, in most cases the STI can be treated without removing the device. If the patient contracts PID during IUD/IUS insertion, health care providers will remove the IUD/IUS. Age and parity are not significant factors in patient selection for IUD or IUS use, and these methods do *not* increase the risk for ectopic pregnancy.

Currently, two IUDs are on the market in the United States. The copper IUD releases copper, which primarily interferes with the contractions within the uterus, impeding sperm migration. A secondary effect is an inflammation of the endometrium, which also obstructs sperm motility and prevents implantation in the rare case that conception should occur. The copper IUD can increase blood loss during menstruation by 35% and may also increase uterine cramping and blood clots in menstrual flow. The use of NSAIDs helps decrease both menorrhagia and dysmenorrhea caused by this IUD. The copper IUD may be inserted up to day 7 of the menstrual cycle, and it can remain in place for up to 10 years.

The levonorgestrel-releasing intrauterine system (LNG-IUS) causes cervical mucus to become thicker so sperm cannot enter the upper reproductive tract or reach the ovum. Changes in uterotubal fluid also impair sperm migration. Alterations in the endometrium prevent implantation in the rare case that conception occurs with the device in place. The LNG-IUS may also suppress ovulation. Unlike the copper IUD, menorrhagia is improved by 90% with the LNG-IUS; this makes the LNG-IUS an effective treatment for heavy menstrual bleeding caused by hormonal dysfunction, uterine fibroids (as long as the fibroid is not located in the uterine cavity), or endometriosis. The LNG-IUS can also be used to decrease perimenopausal bleeding. Dysmenorrhea is also improved. There is a 20% chance of amenorrhea by 1 year of use, which increases to 60% within 5 years. The LNG-IUS is as effective as female sterilization, decreases a woman's risk of PID by 60%, and may also decrease the risk for ectopic pregnancy. The LNG-IUS should be inserted within 7 days of the start of menstruation. During this time the cervical canal is slightly open, making the insertion of the device easier for the provider. The LNG-IUS is effective for 5 years.

Both the copper IUD and the LNG-IUS can be inserted as early as 6 weeks postpartum. There are no contraindications with breastfeeding women and intrauterine contraception. Contraindications to the LNG-IUS are known or suspected pregnancy, uterine anomalies, and risk for acquiring an STI. The LNG-IUS may be effective at preventing endometrial cancer and invasive cervical cancer. The copper IUD should not be placed in women with a small intrauterine cavity (<6 cm) or a large intrauterine cavity (>9 cm). The expulsion risk is 5%, but this rate is slightly higher in women younger than 20 years of age and when the device is inserted immediately postpartum. Perforation of the uterus is a rare complication of insertion.

Women who choose the IUD or IUS for contraception should be taught how to feel for the string from the device, which extends beyond the cervix. The string check is done monthly after the menstrual cycle and ensures that the device has remained in place. Removal of the device is done at the end of the prescribed time frame, when pregnancy is desired, or at the patient's request. The patient should also be advised that she can become pregnant immediately after removal of the device. The device is also removed in the rare event that a pregnancy has occurred with the device intact. The patient should be advised that removal of the device with an intrauterine pregnancy could possibly end in miscarriage. Both types of IUDs can be located on pelvic and transvaginal ultrasound, should any question arise as to proper placement or with the occurrence of full or partial expulsion of the device. The patient should be instructed to use a back-up method of contraception until the device is found to be correctly placed. The device should be removed by the provider if it is found to be incorrectly placed or if partial expulsion has occurred. Reinsertion of a new device or an alternative method of contraception should be prescribed if the patient does not want to become pregnant. Fertility returns immediately after removing the device.

Emergency Contraception

Emergency contraception (EC) can prevent pregnancy after unprotected sex. There are several options:

- Under the supervision of a health care provider, taking 2 to 5 CHCs at one time
- Using Plan B One-Step, an over-the-counter progestin-only EC taken as a single pill, within 72 hours;
- Using Next Choice, an over-the-counter progestin-only EC taken in two doses (12 hours apart), within 72 hours
- Using ulipristal acetate, a prescription-only drug taken as a single tablet within 5 days of unprotected sex
- Inserting a copper-releasing IUD to prevent implantation of a fertilized egg within 5 to 7 days of unprotected sex

EC is intended to be used one time in the event that a condom breaks, a diaphragm or a cervical cap is displaced, or doses of a hormonal contraception method are missed. EC is indicated in the event of sexual assault. The only documented contraindication to EC is an established pregnancy. Women should be instructed that EC is most effective when taken within 24 hours after unprotected sex.

⚡ PATIENT SAFETY

Do not confuse...

- **Mifepristone** with **misoprostol** or **methotrexate:** *Mifepristone* is used for early pregnancy termination by blocking progesterone; lack of progesterone causes the uterine lining to shed and ends the pregnancy. *Misoprostol* causes the uterus to contract and is used for early pregnancy termination or for cervical ripening at any gestational age. It can also be used to control postpartum hemorrhage. *Methotrexate* is a folate antagonist used to manage ectopic pregnancy.

CHCs can be used to prevent fertilization after an incidence of unprotected vaginal intercourse or failure of a contraceptive method. The method involves taking 2 to 5 OC pills at one time. This raises both estrogen and progestin levels to delay or prevent ovulation; it interferes with tubal transport of the embryo, egg, or sperm; and it changes the hormones necessary for the preparation of the uterine lining. Using this method decreases the risk for pregnancy by 75% for each act of sexual intercourse. The major side effect is nausea; to prevent this, an OTC antinausea medicine should be taken 1 hour before CHC administration. Antihistamines are the most commonly used OTC drug for nausea, and some are marketed specifically for this purpose. Antihistamines include diphenhydramine, dimenhydrinate, and meclizine. Irregular menstrual bleeding is another side effect. If a woman does not begin menstruation within a few days of the expected time, a pregnancy test should be performed. Patients who are unable to take estrogen should *not* take CHCs as emergency contraception.

Family planning agencies and women's health organizations provide a full list of CHC pills along with the dosage and administration regimen for these products when used for EC. Treatment should be initiated within 72 hours of intercourse. The sooner a plan is initiated, the more effective it will be at preventing pregnancy.

The first EC pill available in the United States was approved in 1999; it was known as Plan B (levonorgestrel, a progestin-only pill). In 2006, the FDA approved this drug without a prescription for women aged 18 years or older. In 2009, the FDA stated that both men and women can obtain this drug without a prescription if they are older than 17 years. Those younger than 17 years need a prescription.

The EC pill should be taken within 72 hours after intercourse, but it is still effective 120 hours afterward. If taken within 24 hours of intercourse, EC reduces the risk of pregnancy by 95%. Just 12 hours after the initial 24-hour postcoital period, the effectiveness rate of EC decreases to approximately 60%. In Plan B One-Step, one 1.5 mg levonorgestrel tablet is taken. If Next Choice is used, one 0.75 mg tablet is taken, followed by another 12 hours later. If vomiting occurs within 3 hours, the dose should be repeated. Less nausea is associated with this drug than with estrogen-containing EC methods.

Ulipristal is an EC product that is FDA approved for up to 120 hours after unprotected intercourse. Patients of all ages need a prescription to obtain ulipristal. This EC contains 30 mg of ulipristal acetate, a selective progesterone receptor agonist/antagonist. This drug inhibits or delays ovulation and alters the endometrium, possibly preventing implantation. Pregnancy must be excluded before taking ulipristal because this drug was designated pregnancy category X and is considered to be teratogenic and fetotoxic. It is reported that the manufacturers of ulipristal want to maintain its use as an EC option and not promote off-label use as a product for medical abortion.

Hormonal methods of EC are not considered a method of contraception and should not be promoted as such. CHC products, barrier methods, and IUD/IUS devices are more reliable and effective at preventing pregnancy. Women should be instructed that their next menstrual period could be delayed after a dose of EC. With the exception of ulipristal, if pregnancy is already established or if implantation occurred since the episode of sexual intercourse, the pregnancy is not disrupted, and studies indicate that there are no untoward effects on the fetus. However, with ulipristal, if pregnancy has been established when the method is administered, the pregnancy *can* be disrupted and teratogenic fetal effects may occur. Side effects of ulipristal include headaches, nausea, abdominal pain, dysmenorrhea, and dizziness. Breastfeeding mothers should not use this drug.

Copper Intrauterine Device

A copper IUD may be inserted within 5 days of unprotected intercourse as a method of postcoital contraception. The device can be removed after the woman's next menstrual period, or it may remain in place as a method of contraception for up to 10 years. The mechanism of action is interruption of sperm migration and penetration of the ovum.

MEDICAL ABORTION

Medical abortion ends a pregnancy that is less than 63 days from the first day of the LMP, or less than 9 weeks' gestation. Medical abortion uses drugs to disrupt an established pregnancy. (*Surgical abortion* refers to procedures used to remove the products of conception from the uterus.) Mifepristone is a drug that stops the pregnancy in the uterus. It may also be used to treat an *early* ectopic pregnancy that is encapsulated and less than 3 cm in size. Mifepristone is an antiprogestin that blocks the hormone progesterone. Without progesterone, the lining of the uterus breaks down, ending support for the embryo. The hormone human chorionic gonadotropin (hCG) is decreased. The placenta produces hCG, and it is the hormone tested to confirm pregnancy; decreasing levels of hCG signify that the pregnancy has been disrupted. Misoprostol is then given to cause the uterus to contract and expel the products of conception.

DRUGS USED TO TREAT DISORDERS IN WOMEN'S HEALTH

Common reasons women seek gynecologic health care include alterations in menstrual cycle, menstrual or pelvic pain, and changes in vaginal secretions. Included within these broad categories are irregular uterine bleeding, dysmenorrhea, and PMS. This section describes common disorders in women's health and presents current pharmacologic approaches to management.

Irregular or Abnormal Uterine Bleeding

Irregular uterine bleeding is a term that describes many different medical conditions or pathologies related to the menstrual cycle. Irregular uterine bleeding, also known as *abnormal uterine bleeding* (AUB), is a common reason women seek gynecologic care. AUB encompasses a wide range of variable bleeding patterns in women, such as amenorrhea, menorrhagia, metrorrhagia, meno-metrorrhagia, intramenstrual bleeding, and dysfunctional uterine bleeding (DUB).

Amenorrhea

Amenorrhea is the absence of menses. *Primary amenorrhea* is defined as no menses by age 14 years *without* secondary sex characteristics or no menses by age 16 years *with* secondary sex characteristics. Primary amenorrhea may be caused by abnormalities in the structures of the female reproductive tract, chromosomal alterations, or endocrine disorders. Many times the cause is just a physiologic delay in the onset of menstruation. *Secondary amenorrhea* is the absence of a spontaneous menstrual period for 6 consecutive months in women who have experienced menstrual cycles in the past. Pregnancy is the most common reason a patient may experience amenorrhea, and breastfeeding or menopausal patients also may not menstruate, therefore secondary amenorrhea is a *symptom* of these normal physiologic processes. Other causes of secondary amenorrhea include anovulatory cycles (cycles without ovulation), hypothyroidism or hyperthyroidism, and hyperprolactinemia (high levels of the hormone prolactin, which stimulates lactation). Extreme weight loss and anorexia can also cause amenorrhea.

After assessment of the patient's health history and a physical examination; after laboratory testing to include FSH, serum prolactin (PRL), thyroid-stimulating hormone (TSH), and serum estradiol (ES); and after pregnancy has been ruled out, a *progestin withdrawal test* may be administered to determine the underlying cause of amenorrhea. This test uses an oral progestin administered for a limited time to confirm that the hypothalamic-pituitary-ovarian (HPO) responses—that is, the hormonal system that mediates the menstrual cycle—are intact.

With the progestin withdrawal test, a patient is given medroxyprogesterone 10 mg for 10 days. The progestational activity thickens the endometrial lining and increases secretory activity. When the drug is discontinued, progesterone levels decrease, resulting in a breakdown of the endometrial lining and withdrawal bleeding. Withdrawal bleeding should occur within 7 to 10 days after completing the drug and indicates that the HPO axis (the menstrual cycle) is functioning in providing the hormones necessary to regulate the menstrual cycle. Even the smallest amount of bleeding, such as one incidence of scant spotting, is considered a positive test. However, if no withdrawal bleeding occurs, other pathophysiologic problems may exist, and further evaluation and diagnostic testing by the health care provider are needed.

Polycystic Ovarian Syndrome

Another common cause of secondary amenorrhea is polycystic ovarian syndrome (PCOS), a disorder in the metabolism of androgens and estrogen. PCOS may be caused by dysfunction of the HPO axis. Women with PCOS experience menstrual dysfunction, anovulation, hyperandrogenism, hirsutism, infertility, obesity, metabolic syndrome, diabetes, and obstructive sleep apnea.

Diet and exercise are first-line treatment for PCOS. Weight loss of 5% to 10% has been shown to improve overall metabolic status and reduce serum androgen concentrations. Pharmacologic treatment of PCOS is used to treat anovulation, hirsutism, and menstrual irregularities. To manage menstrual irregularities, low-dose CHCs are prescribed. With the addition of the progestin in the CHC product and a cycling of a monthly withdrawal menses (or four times per year, depending on the product), the risks of unopposed estrogen on the endometrium are significantly reduced.

For women who are attempting to conceive and unable to lose weight, clomiphene citrate is first-line treatment; it is described in the section *Drugs Used to Promote Fertility*. Metformin may be added to inhibit the production of glucose in the liver and increase peripheral cell sensitivity to insulin, effectively treating insulin resistance and decreasing androgen levels.

Abnormal Uterine Bleeding Patterns

The normal menstrual cycle occurs every 25 to 35 days and lasts 2 to 7 days, with an estimated blood loss of no more than 80 mL. Menorrhagia is *regular* uterine bleeding greater than 80 mL or lasting more than 7 days. Women with menorrhagia may describe their periods as very heavy or state the need to change a tampon or sanitary pad frequently. Metrorrhagia is *irregular* uterine bleeding greater than 80 mL or lasting more than 7 days. Women with metrorrhagia describe their periods as irregular and heavy. They may state that they have no idea when bleeding will occur and that when it does happen, it will soak through sanitary products or clothing. Menometrorrhagia is a combination of these two. *Intramenstrual bleeding* is an episode of bleeding, usually light, that occurs between menstrual periods.

A common complaint that brings a woman into the gynecologic health care setting is that she is having menstrual cycles that are suddenly different from the pattern she usually experiences. In women of reproductive age, pregnancy should always be considered first as the possible cause of AUB. However, AUB can result from physiologic processes such as stress, severe dieting and weight loss, eating disorders, or excessive exercise. Irregular bleeding patterns are a sign of decreasing ovarian function or approach of menopause in older women. AUB can also be caused by pathologic processes such as endocrine disorders, thyroid disease, leiomyomata (benign tumors in the uterus), ovarian cysts, infections of the genital tract, or cancer. If a woman is pregnant, uterine bleeding may indicate ectopic pregnancy or impending miscarriage. Some pharmacologic drugs, substances, and herbal preparations can also cause irregular bleeding, including anticoagulants, antipsychotics, benzodiazepines, hormone therapy, ginkgo, ginseng, and soy products. Once physiologic, pathologic, and pharmaceutic causes have been ruled out, the patient may be diagnosed with DUB.

Dysfunctional Uterine Bleeding

DUB is the most common classification of irregular bleeding. Diagnosis of DUB is made when no organic pathology can be determined to cause the irregular bleeding. Pharmacologic treatment of DUB primarily involves normalizing the bleeding pattern and correcting anemia that may have resulted from chronic or acute blood loss. In the normal physiologic menstrual cycle, estrogen and progesterone levels are low during menstruation. Once estrogen levels start to rise with the formation of a dominant follicle, uterine bleeding is effectively stopped, ending menstruation. Increasing levels of estrogen by administration of an estrogen drug product is usually effective in stopping prolonged DUB.

Because estrogen is *never* used alone in treatment, because of the detrimental effects of unopposed estrogen on the uterine endometrium and the risk for endometrial cancer, estrogen-progestin combination products are used. Progestins alone are not as effective as estrogen in reducing an episode of acute bleeding; however, because *prolonged* progestin administration causes atrophy of the endometrial lining, progestins can be very effective if long-term control is needed. DMPA by IM injection or an LNG-IUS inserted into the uterus are the products used for extended progestin therapy.

Pharmacologic Management of Irregular Bleeding

NSAIDs can be used for the treatment of menorrhagia, reducing bleeding by 25% to 35%. NSAIDs block the production of prostaglandin, which decreases both excessive bleeding and uterine cramps. Common NSAIDs used for menorrhagia are mefenamic acid, ibuprofen, and naproxen sodium. Only mefenamic acid has FDA approval for menorrhagia. Although approved for the treatment of dysmenorrhea, ibuprofen and naproxen sodium are used by providers as off-label options in the treatment of menorrhagia. The correct dosage of mefenamic acid is 500 mg by mouth (PO) once, followed by 250 mg PO every 6 hours as needed for 2 to 3 days. Mefenamic acid should be taken with food to avoid gastric upset. Tranexamic acid may also be given at 1300 mg three times a day for a maximum of 5 days. Tranexamic acid inhibits plasminogen binding sites, thus decreasing plasmin formation and fibrinolysis, reducing blood loss by 40% to 60%.

CHCs can be used to decrease and regulate DUB. The increase in estrogen suppresses endometrial development, restores predictable bleeding, and reduces menstrual flow. Reduction in flow should be seen within 24 hours. If a heavy flow continues for more than 48 hours, the patient should be reevaluated. Benefits, risks, and patient instructions are the same as if the product were being used for contraception. Women who are not candidates for estrogen therapy or CHCs should be excluded. Women using a CHC product for DUB should see their periods normalize within the first 3 months of use. Patients can continue the method for contraception, or they can discontinue use in 6 to 9 months, depending on the effectiveness in controlling bleeding.

Progestins are not as effective as estrogens at reducing episodes of irregular bleeding. However, progestins are effective in the long-term treatment of AUB and may be the method of choice in women who have contraindications to estrogen use. Progestins are given cyclically (e.g., norethindrone acetate 2.5

to 5 mg PO daily for 21 days or medroxyprogesterone 10 mg/day for 21 days) to produce a monthly withdrawal bleeding. DMPA and the LNG-IUS are also used for treatment of DUB. Long-term use of progesterone has an atrophic effect on the uterine endometrium, consequently decreasing incidences of irregular bleeding. Women using DMPA or the LNG-IUS for DUB should see heavy bleeding patterns decrease within 3 to 6 months.

Dysmenorrhea

Dysmenorrhea, also called *cyclic pelvic pain* (CPP), is pelvic pain associated with the menstrual cycle. Other symptoms that may occur with the menstrual cycle are uterine cramping, lower back pain, abdominal cramps, changes in bowel patterns, increased bowel movements, and nausea and vomiting. Dysmenorrhea is experienced by approximately 80% of women in their late teens and early twenties, when it is more prevalent. It is the most common reason young women miss school or work. Dysmenorrhea is classified as either primary dysmenorrhea or secondary dysmenorrhea, depending on whether there is a known etiology for the menstrual pain. *Primary dysmenorrhea* is diagnosed when there is no apparent underlying pathology. It is caused by larger-than-normal amounts of prostaglandins at the start of the menstrual period. Prostaglandins cause arterioles in the uterus to contract, decreasing blood flow to the endometrium. All of these mechanisms are necessary for breakdown of the endometrial lining and for menstruation to occur. However, this process causes increased pain in some women.

In *secondary dysmenorrhea,* there is an underlying cause for the pelvic pain. Conditions that may cause secondary dysmenorrhea are urinary tract infections (UTIs), PID, irritable bowel syndrome (IBS), uterine leiomyomata (fibroids), and endometriosis.

Pharmacologic Management of Dysmenorrhea

Nonsteroidal Antiinflammatory Drugs. NSAIDs block pain by preventing synthesis of prostaglandins. The mechanism of drug action is the inhibition of cyclooxygenase (COX). The COX enzyme converts arachidonic acid into prostaglandins, which cause constriction of the uterine arterioles, necrosis of the endometrial lining, uterine contractions, and menstrual pain. Usually nonselective and COX-2 inhibitors are used. The most commonly used NSAIDs for relief of pain associated with dysmenorrhea include naproxen sodium, diclofenac potassium, ibuprofen, naproxen, celecoxib, and mefenamic acid. Many NSAIDs can be purchased over the counter, so the nurse should include health information about the benefits, risks, and alternatives as well as specific dosage amounts, drug interactions, and administration instructions. Some drugs (diclofenac potassium, celecoxib, and mefenamic acid) are by prescription only. Patients must understand the differences in these drugs and avoid them if they have allergies to, or side effects from, any of the ingredients. Patients should avoid taking two different NSAID drugs at the same time. GI upset is a common side effect of NSAIDs, so most drugs in this category should be taken with food and water. NSAIDs can also be taken with an antacid or calcium supplement to prevent GI upset. NSAIDs should not be taken for more than 10 days.

Combined Hormonal Contraceptives. CHCs are effective in the treatment of dysmenorrhea. CHCs reduce the thickness of the uterine endometrium. The 24/4 day CHCs shorten withdrawal bleeding periods, and the extended-use CHCs decrease the number of withdrawal menses per year or eliminate them altogether. DMPA, progestin implants, and the LNG-IUS decrease dysmenorrhea in patients who are candidates for these methods. Long-term progestin-only products cause atrophy of the uterine lining, limiting the occurrence of dysmenorrhea and the amount of bleeding during menstruation.

Endometriosis

Endometriosis is the abnormal location of endometrial tissue outside the uterus. The tissue is known as *ectopic endometrial implants*. It is a common cause of dysmenorrhea, chronic pelvic pain, and infertility. The ectopic endometrial implants can be found affixed to the ovaries, the posterior surface of the uterus, the uterosacral ligaments, the broad ligaments, or the bowel. They also can be found on other organs within the pelvic or thoracic cavity. The ectopic endometrial implants respond to hormonal control, particularly estrogen, in the same way as the normal endometrial tissue located inside the uterus. Thus when menstruation occurs, the ectopic endometrial implants proliferate and then bleed. As the number of menstrual cycles increases, inflammation of surrounding organ tissue, scar tissue formation, and adhesions result, causing pelvic pain.

Diagnosis of endometriosis is based on laparoscopic evidence of endometrial tissue, or implants, outside the uterus. The most common symptoms of endometriosis are dysmenorrhea and pelvic pain, sometimes including chronic pelvic pain, which lasts more than 6 months and is not associated specifically with menstruation. The patient may experience back pain; painful, sometimes bloody bowel movements; and dyspareunia (painful sexual intercourse). An increased number of women with endometriosis experience primary or secondary infertility; although a specific cause linking the two has not been established, it is theorized that the ectopic endometrial implants or the resultant scar tissue and adhesions obstruct or affect the motility of the fallopian tubes or other reproductive organs. Affected women have an increased risk for ectopic pregnancy.

Pharmacologic Management of Endometriosis

Pharmaceutic treatment strategies for endometriosis include drugs that decrease the amounts of circulating estrogen and limit or eliminate menstruation. This interrupts internal bleeding and irritation associated with the ectopic endometrial implants and may even cause them to recede.

Combined Hormonal Contraceptives. These drugs suppress gonadotropin-releasing hormone (GnRH) release, prevent ovulation, and cause atrophy of the uterine lining, actions thought to relieve pelvic pain by causing a regression of the endometrial implants. CHCs relieve the pain of endometriosis in approximately 75% of women. Extended-use CHCs can also manage endometriosis by causing fewer cycles per year or eliminating withdrawal menses altogether.

Progestin Therapy

These drugs suppress ovulation and cause long-term endometrial atrophy. They also inhibit GnRH release, similar to CHCs. Over time, progestins can shrink or eliminate endometrial implants. The most commonly used progestin is DMPA, with which 70% to 90% of patients' experience relief of symptoms associated with endometriosis. This effect may last months after discontinuing the drug. Benefits and risks are the same as if using DMPA for contraception, so concerns for BMD loss and prevention, irregular bleeding or amenorrhea, possible weight gain, and mood changes should be discussed with the patient. The injection is given every 11 to 13 weeks.

Alternatively, norethindrone acetate may be taken at 5 mg PO daily for 2 weeks, then increasing the dose by 2.5 mg every 2 weeks until a dose of 15 mg per day is reached and continued for 6 to 9 months.

Gonadotropin-Releasing–Hormone Agonists. In women who experience severe symptoms and who NSAIDs, CHCs, or progestins do not help, GnRH agonists may be used. GnRH agonists are potent drugs that inhibit GnRH release and create a hypoestrogenic environment. The side effects are menopause-like and include hot flashes, atrophic vaginitis, vaginal dryness, decreased sex drive, and potential for bone loss. Leuprolide is administered either 3.75 mg IM monthly or 11.25 mg IM every 3 months. Leuprolide should be initiated in the first 3 days of the menstrual cycle because it is pregnancy category X. Women may be able to become pregnant on leuprolide, so a barrier method of contraception should be used. Oral norethindrone acetate 5 mg daily is prescribed concurrently to minimize the hypoestrogenic side effects of GnRH agonist; this is referred to as "add-back therapy."

Alternatively, nafarelin nasal spray is administered in a divided 400-mcg daily dose, with 1 spray (200 mcg) into one nostril in the morning and 1 spray (200 mcg) into the other nostril in the evening for up to 6 months. Other GnRH agonists are available (e.g., buserelin, goserelin, and triptorelin); drug selection is based on availability and cost. Use of these drugs past 6 months, as well as retreatment, can cause irreversible adverse changes in BMD. Approximately 90% of women experience relief of symptoms with gonadotropin inhibitors and GnRH agonists.

Studies investigating DMPA preparations compared with GnRH inhibitors/agonists report that DMPA is as effective as leuprolide in reducing symptoms of endometriosis and shrinking or eliminating endometrial implants. DMPA preparations are much less expensive for the patient than leuprolide, which causes an increased hypoestrogen state compared to DMPA. In studies, DMPA caused irregular bleeding, including menorrhagia, in addition to weight gain and prolonged time returning to menstruation after the treatment was discontinued. DMPA also causes BMD changes, and preventive measures must be reviewed with the patient before initiating treatment.

Premenstrual Syndrome

Premenstrual syndrome (PMS) comprises a collection of cyclic physical symptoms and perimenopausal mood alterations. Symptoms increase in the 2 weeks before menstruation and subside after menses begins. These physical, emotional, and behavioral symptoms interfere to varying degrees with a woman's ability to function.

PMS can result in decreased work effectiveness and distressing mood variations. PMS affects as many as 80% of all adult women, with 3% to 8% meeting diagnostic criteria for premenstrual dysphoric disorder (PMDD) as defined in the *Diagnostic and Statistical Manual of Mental Disorders*, Fifth Edition (DSM-5). The hallmark of PMS and PMDD is that symptoms occur in a repetitive pattern during the luteal phase (days 15 to 28) of the menstrual cycle and decrease significantly in the early follicular phase (days 1 to 14).

There is no universal agreement about the definition, etiology, symptoms, or treatment of PMS. Researchers theorize that the etiology of PMS could be hormonal excess or deficits, fluid or sodium retention, or nutritional deficiencies. It is also proposed that an imbalance exists in the HPO axis function. Other hypotheses center on the neuroregulatory effects of estrogen and progesterone on the release or uptake of serotonin.

A patient can help with the diagnosis of PMS by recording three variables on a perimenstrual assessment calendar: (1) group of symptoms, (2) severity of symptoms, and (3) impact on function (degree of distress). Diagnosis of PMS can be made when the patient's symptoms consistently occur in a cyclic pattern at least 1 week before the menstruation cycle and decrease significantly after menses begins. Symptoms usually have a negative impact on the ability to function effectively. Other endocrine abnormalities must be ruled out. Also, it should be noted that not every symptom associated with the menstrual cycle is indicative of PMS.

Physical Symptoms of Premenstrual Syndrome

Physical symptoms that can be related to PMS include weight gain, edema, bloating in the lower abdomen, breast soreness, fatigue, backaches, acne flareups, joint pain, constipation, headache, and insomnia or alterations in sleep patterns.

Emotional Symptoms of Premenstrual Syndrome

Emotional symptoms that can be seen with PMS include anger, anxiety, agitation, feelings of being out of control, labile emotions and rapid mood alterations, tension, difficulty concentrating, irritability, tearfulness, depression, and suicidal thoughts.

Behavioral Symptoms of Premenstrual Syndrome

Some behavioral symptoms that may be seen in PMS include increased or decreased sexual desire, impulsive behavior, acting out aggression or emotional alterations, increased appetite, craving for foods high in sugar or salt, and a sudden increase or decrease in anxiety.

Pharmacologic Treatment of Premenstrual Syndrome

Pharmacologic treatment of PMS should consider evidence-based recommendations that are appropriate in treating the patient's specific symptoms. A number of treatments have been identified that will be discussed here.

Nonpharmacologic Treatment. Nonpharmacologic treatment modalities are very important in treating women with PMS. Therapies include expression of empathy, support from family and friends, correction of knowledge deficits about PMS, exercise, and dietary changes. Aerobic exercise improves general health, heightens endorphin levels, and may facilitate an overall sense of well-being. Dietary changes include limiting salty foods, alcohol, caffeine, and concentrated sweets. Eating four to six small, high-carbohydrate, low-fat meals may also help relieve some symptoms. Stress-reduction exercises are also helpful. These measures may help the patient feel proactive regarding her diagnosis of PMS.

Antidepressant Drugs. PMS is improved with selective serotonin reuptake inhibitors (SSRIs). Symptom relief includes a decrease in irritability, mood swings, fatigue, tension, and breast tenderness. SSRIs block the reuptake of serotonin into nerve terminals in the central nervous system (CNS), regulating serotonin use by the brain. The most commonly used SSRIs are fluoxetine and sertraline, paroxetine, citalopram, and escitalopram. Venlafaxine, a serotonin norepinephrine reuptake inhibitor (SNRI) has also demonstrated relief in patients with severe PMS symptoms, but is not considered a first-line agent (see Chapter 23 for further information on antidepressants). SSRIs may be taken continuously, during the luteal phase only (drug is started on day 14 of the cycle and discontinued with menses), or as intermittent therapy beginning with symptom onset and discontinuing after the first few days of menses. Determining a treatment regimen depends on history and physical, patient preference, and predictability of symptoms.

Hormonal Therapy. Long-term suppression of ovulation has been shown to decrease cyclic physical discomforts and to normalize mood variations in some women. CHCs, such as OCs containing the progestin drospirenone along with a shorter (4-day) pill-free interval or transdermal and transvaginal hormone therapy can be used in this manner. Caution should be used with progestin-only products because they may exacerbate symptoms of depression.

DRUGS USED TO PROMOTE FERTILITY

Infertility is defined as the inability to conceive a child after 12 months of unprotected sexual intercourse. Women older than 35 years may be considered infertile after 6 months of attempting pregnancy. Infertility is considered *primary infertility* if a couple has never conceived or has never carried a pregnancy to term. *Secondary infertility* describes a couple who has conceived and brought a pregnancy to term but is unable to conceive afterward. Approximately 15% to 20% of couples in the United States experience infertility. Fertility rates decrease in both men and women as they get older; however, the risk for infertility increases more abruptly in women than in men as women reach the end of the reproductive life cycle. The monthly chance of achieving pregnancy decreases to 5% after age 40 years.

Assessing the Infertile Couple

Causes of infertility are numerous. Infertility can be attributed to a female factor, a male factor, and many times, a combination of both. (Male infertility is discussed in depth in Chapter 53.) In the female partner, the most common causes for infertility are alterations in ovarian function and anatomic disorders. Alterations in ovarian function are categorized as *ovulatory dysfunction disorders*. Any process, whether a disease state or the normal biologic process of aging, that causes anovulation or a decrease in ovulation cycles will affect the process of conception. Many of these women present with irregular menstrual periods. Causes of ovulatory dysfunction include alterations in the HPO axis, such as metabolic disorders (most commonly PCOS), and age approaching the end of the reproductive spectrum. Fertility declines sharply in women after age 35 years, and infertility becomes a factor from age 38 to 40 years. Endocrine disorders such as hyperprolactinemia (increase in circulating prolactin, the hormone that promotes breastfeeding) or thyroid disorders (hypothyroidism or hyperthyroidism) can also cause anovulatory cycles. Ovulation can be disrupted by eating disorders (anorexia and bulimia) and by stress.

The most common anatomic disorder is blocked fallopian tubes. Blocked tubes can be the result of a history of STI or PID. STIs, treated or undiagnosed, and PID can lead to scarring within the tubes, impeding sperm or ovum transport. A previous ectopic pregnancy or other tubal surgery can also result in infertility. Other causes include endometriosis, uterine leiomyomata (fibroids), or scarring within the uterine endometrium. (See Chapter 53 for male infertility discussion.)

Treatment of infertility depends on the cause. A general health assessment of the infertile couple includes (1) complete health history, including nutritional, reproductive, and social histories; drugs; herbal and illicit drug use; and gynecologic, menstrual, obstetric, and sexual histories as they pertain to each partner; (2) complete physical examinations with breast and pelvic examinations of the female partner and examination of male genitalia and function; (3) Pap testing, HPV testing, collections of cultures for STI testing; and (4) laboratory tests and other diagnostic tests. Semen evaluation is also necessary.

The leading cause of infertility in women is ovulatory dysfunction (most often, PCOS). The first line of pharmacologic treatment for ovulatory dysfunction is usually induction of ovulation by oral drug therapy.

Induction of Ovulation

Clomiphene citrate (CC) is a selective estrogen receptor modulator (SERM) that competes for estrogen receptors within the hypothalamus. With the binding of CC to the estrogen receptors, the hypothalamus receives a signal that circulating estrogen levels are low. This sets the hypothalamus in motion to secrete more GnRH, thus stimulating the HPO axis. The GnRH instructs the anterior pituitary gland to release FSH and LH to initiate a response from the ovarian follicles. Estrogen levels increase in response to FSH and LH, and a follicle becomes dominant, producing the level of estrogen needed for the LH surge. The LH surge causes release of an ovum from the dominant follicle. It is important for LH to reach a level high enough to produce an ovulatory cycle and that the timing of the LH surge be at the height of follicle formation, which is mid-cycle.

PROTOTYPE DRUG CHART 52.1

Clomiphene Citrate

Drug Class	Route and Dosage
Clomiphene citrate (CC)	A: PO: 50-150 mg/d for days 5-9 of the cycle
Uses and considerations: Ovulation stimulant	If ovulation does not occur with 50 mg/d, increase the next course to 100 mg/d; *max*: 150 mg/d; maximum sequential cycles is three. Under strict supervision by physicians specializing in infertility, as much as 250 mg/d may be used.

Contraindications	Drug-Lab-Food Interactions
Pregnancy, undiagnosed vaginal bleeding, depression, fibroids, hepatic dysfunction, thrombophlebitis, primary pituitary or ovarian failure	Drug: None are significant; danazol may inhibit response; drug decreases effects of ethinyl estradiol. Lab: Increases serum thyroxine

Pharmacokinetics	Pharmacodynamics
Absorption: Readily absorbed from GI tract	PO: Onset: 5-14 d
Distribution: PB: UK	Peak: UK
Metabolism: t½: 5-8 d	Duration: UK
Excretion: In feces	Pregnancy category X*

Therapeutic Effects/Uses
To stimulate ovarian follicle growth
Mode of Action: Stimulates release of follicle-stimulating hormone and luteinizing hormone

Side Effects	Adverse Reactions
Breast discomfort, fatigue, dizziness, depression, anxiety, nausea, vomiting, constipation, increased appetite, headache, flatulence, multiple gestation, hot flashes, fluid retention	Visual disturbances, abdominal pain, weight gain, hair loss, ovarian hyperstimulation, anxiety, ovarian cysts, ectopic pregnancy

*Pregnancy categories have been revised. See http://www.fda.gov/Drugs/DevelopmentApprovalProcess/DevelopmentResources/Labeling/ucm093307.htm for more information.
A, Adult; *d*, day; *GI*, gastrointestinal; *max*, maximum dosage; *PB*, protein binding; *PO*, by mouth; *t½*, half-life; *UK*, unknown.

CC is the most commonly used ovulation stimulant (Prototype Drug Chart 52.1). Women with PCOS may need concurrent treatment for hyperinsulinemia with metformin. While metformin is known to help regulate the menstrual cycle and promote ovulation, it should not be used specifically for ovulation induction.

CC is given in a 50-mg oral dose on days 5 through 9 of the menstrual cycle. If ovulation does not occur, the dose can be increased to 100 mg. It may be repeated up to 6 cycles. Women are at an increased risk for multiple gestation; twin gestation is experienced by 6.9% to 9% of women with induced ovulation by clomiphene.

In women with PCOS who have not responded to CC or other therapies, gonadotropin therapy may be an option. Recombinant human menopausal gonadotropin (hMG) and FSH are available. Recombinant hMG and FSH work directly on ovarian function to stimulate follicle maturation and promote

TABLE 52.2   Ovulatory Stimulants and Ovulation Control

Drug	Route and Dosage	Use and Considerations
Clomiphene citrate	See Prototype Drug Chart 52.1.	
GnRH analogues Agonists: nafarelin Antagonists: cetrorelix, ganirelix	Nafarelin: Spray up to 800 mcg/d (200 mcg per nostril bid) Cetrorelix: 0.25 mg in a single dose subcut daily on stimulation day 5 or day 7, or 3 mg subcut in a single dose on stimulation day 7 (to control day of LH surge) Ganirelix: 250 mcg subcut once daily after initiating FSH, during mid to late follicular stage	Enhances ovulation stimulation for IVF cycles by suppression of a spontaneous LH surge and controls the fertility cycle, improving pregnancy outcomes. Pregnancy category X*; PB: 86%; t½: 11-23 h
Human menopausal gonadotropin (hMG)	IM/subcut: 150 units once daily for the first 5 d of treatment; max: 450 units/d Adjustments should not be made more frequently than once every 2 d and should not exceed 75-150 units per adjustment based on ultrasound monitoring of ovarian response and/or measurement of serum estradiol.	Possesses the same activities as FSH and LH; will induce ovulation in women with hypothalamic amenorrhea. Risks include ovarian hyperstimulation and multiple gestation. Pregnancy category X*; PB: UK; t½: 54-59 h
Recombinant FSH, follitropin alpha, recombinant LH, hCG, or recombinant hCG	Recombinant FSH: Subcut or IM injection; dosage individualized for each patient, usually 75-150 units/d, early follicular phase continuing for 10-14 d Recombinant LH: Subcut 75 units given along with an FSH or recombinant FSH Recombinant hCG 250 mcg prefilled syringe; subcut injection given 1 d after last dose of gonadotropin (FSH and/or LH) 5000-10,000 units IM 1 d after last dose of gonadotropin (FSH and/or LH)	Recombinant FSH possesses the same hormonal activities as FSH. Ovarian hyperstimulation remains a risk, although minimal, with recombinant products. Multiple gestation is a risk, which is reduced by careful monitoring. Avoid use with herbal supplements that contain black or blue cohosh. Pregnancy category X*; PB: UK; t½: IM, 23-77 h; subcut, 13-35 h

*Pregnancy categories have been revised. See http://www.fda.gov/Drugs/DevelopmentApprovalProcess/DevelopmentResources/Labeling/ucm093307.htm for more information.

bid, Twice daily; *d*, day; *FSH*, follicle-stimulating hormone; *GnRH*, gonadotropin-releasing hormone; *h*, hour; *hCG*, human chorionic gonadotropin; *hMG*, human menopausal gonadotropin; *IM*, intramuscular; *IVF*, in vitro fertilization; *LH*, luteinizing hormone; *max*, maximum dosage; *PB*, protein binding; *subcut*, subcutaneously; *t½*, half-life; *UK*, unknown.

ovulation. FSH is less likely than hMG to result in ovarian hyperstimulation syndrome (OHSS), a medical emergency presenting with acute abdominal pain and distension, nausea, vomiting, diarrhea, and weight gain, along with gross ovarian enlargement, ascites, dyspnea, oliguria, and pleural effusion. OHSS may result in death.

These therapies supply women with exogenous hormones to enhance the normal physiologic process of the menstrual cycle, promoting ovulation and increasing the probability of conception; the use of another gonadotropin, human chorionic gonadotropin (hCG), triggers ovulation when ovarian follicles are mature (as determined by ultrasonography). The corpus luteum provides for adequate levels of both estrogen and, more importantly, progesterone to maintain the uterine endometrium and a pregnancy, should one occur. These drugs are more potent than CC and have an increased risk for multiple births (up to 36%). Further details are listed in Table 52.2.

Pharmacokinetics Clomiphene citrate is readily absorbed from the GI tract. It is partially metabolized in the liver and is primarily excreted in the feces via biliary elimination. CC has a half-life of about 5 days.

Pharmacodynamics The mechanism of action of CC is unknown, but it is hypothesized that it competes with estrogen at receptor sites. The perception of decreased circulating estrogen by the hypothalamus and pituitary gland triggers the negative feedback response that increases secretion of FSH and LH. The results are ovarian stimulation, maturation

of the ovarian follicle, ovulation, and development of the corpus luteum.

Side Effects. Side effects of CC include breast discomfort, fatigue, dizziness, depression, nausea, increased appetite, dermatitis, urticaria, anxiety, weakness, heavier menses, vasomotor flushing, and abdominal bloating or pain. Antiestrogenic effects include interference with endometrial maturation and cervical mucus production. Paradoxically, this may interfere with fertilization or implantation.

Adverse reactions. Adverse reactions include bloating and stomach or pelvic pain, photophobia, diplopia, and decreased visual acuity. Patients may also experience hot flashes, breast discomfort, dizziness, headache, heavy menstrual periods, depression, nausea or vomiting, and fatigue. OHSS may occur.

Postmarket surveillance of CC has revealed the following fetal/neonatal abnormalities: delayed development, mental retardation, abnormal bone development, tissue malformation, abnormal organ development (including anencephaly), dwarfism, chromosomal disorders, and neural tube defects.

Contraindications. Contraindications for treatment with CC include undiagnosed vaginal bleeding, pregnancy, uterine fibroids, clinical depression, history of hepatic dysfunction or thromboembolic disease, and primary pituitary or ovarian failure. CC may cause existing ovarian cysts to enlarge. Contraindications to the use of other ovulatory stimulants are listed in Table 52.2.

Drug interactions. There are no known significant drug interactions with CC. Danazol may inhibit patient response to CC, and CC may suppress response to ethinyl estradiol. There are no known drug interactions with hMG or hCG.

Other Drug Treatments

Endocrine disorders include hyperprolactinemia and thyroid disorders. In women with hyperprolactinemia, an elevated level of prolactin is the causative factor of infertility. Prolactin is a hormone secreted by the anterior pituitary gland and elevated during pregnancy and postpartum to support milk production. Breastfeeding causes a natural rise in prolactin, and hyperprolactinemia can be seen in women who are or have recently discontinued breastfeeding.

Drug therapies such as haloperidol, metoclopramide, methyldopa, reserpine, and long-term CHC use have been known to cause hyperprolactinemia. The most common cause of pathologic hyperprolactinemia is a small, benign pituitary tumor called a *pituitary adenoma.* Regardless of the cause of hyperprolactinemia, most women can be treated with the ergot derivative bromocriptine, which binds to dopamine receptors in the pituitary gland and inhibits prolactin secretion. Treatment continues until pregnancy is confirmed. Clomiphene can be introduced if needed after 2 months.

In addition, hypothyroidism or hyperthyroidism and adrenal dysfunction must be assessed and managed to attain euthyroid levels. Endometriosis can be treated with a course of leuprolide or DMPA to suppress gonadotropin output.

NURSING PROCESS
Patient-Centered Collaborative Care

Infertility

Assessment
- Assess the general health history, including drug and herbal product use. Physical examination, including speculum and bimanual exam, are required. Assess patients' reproductive and sexual histories, with attention to history of abnormal Pap testing and treatment, history of vaginal infections and STIs and treatment, past use of contraception methods, pelvic surgery and past and present gynecologic abnormalities, and pregnancy and birth history and complications.
- Assess the complete menstrual history, including menarche; LMP; length, duration, and flow of bleeding; and any signs or symptoms related to the menstrual cycle.
- Assess sexual practices to include the use of lubricants and timing and technique of intercourse.
- Assess the couple's mental health status, and refer to a support group or counseling as needed. Infertility can be isolating because many couples may have several peers who are pregnant or already have children.
- The couple will undergo an exhaustive battery of diagnostic tests to evaluate the cause of infertility. Once this is determined, conditions that contraindicate the treatment of choice are ruled out.

- It is particularly important that the couple's interpretation of their infertility be explored, along with its impact on their relationship. The nurse should help the couple discuss their feelings in a safe, supportive environment.

Nursing Diagnoses
- Knowledge, Deficient related to the menstrual cycle, ovulation, conception, causes of infertility, prognosis, and assisted reproductive technologies
- Knowledge, Deficient related to treatment regimens and outcomes
- Sexuality Pattern, Ineffective related to infertility
- Sexual Dysfunction, related to vulnerability, deficient knowledge and disease or physiologic processes
- Body Image, Disturbed related to the inability to conceive
- Self-Esteem, Situational Low related to infertility
- Anxiety related to infertility and treatment drug and procedures
- Powerlessness related to infertility diagnosis
- Decisional Conflict related to discrepancy between cultural and/or religious beliefs and assisted reproductive therapies
- Grieving related to loss of the plan to have a biologic child

Planning
- The patient will understand the normal physiologic process of conception.
- The patient will identify basic concepts that increase fertility.
- The patient will adhere to the medical regimen with minimal adverse effects physically, psychologically, emotionally, and spiritually.
- The patient will report adverse effects of treatment or pharmacologic therapy.
- The long-term goal is a successful pregnancy. If pregnancy cannot be achieved, the patient will be able to consider alternatives and make the transition with confidence, with the relationship and sense of self-worth intact.
- The patient will recognize that many treatment regimens for infertility must be repeated before successful conception is attained.

Nursing Interventions
General
- Initiate teaching to assist the patient and her partner in understanding the menstrual cycle, patterns and symptoms of ovulation, temperature changes with ovulation, specific physiologic signs of ovulation, use of ovulation predictor kits, and timing of sexual intercourse.
- Help the patient to understand the interrelationships among the menstrual cycle, ovulation, and coitus as they relate to conception.
- Advise the patient on the sexual techniques that enhance fertilization: placement of a pillow under the woman's hips during coitus and placement of the woman in a supine position with the hips elevated for about 30 minutes after her partner ejaculates.

- Initiate drug treatment regimens as prescribed by the provider. The patient and partner(s) will understand the treatment regimen and the expected outcomes of the treatment regimen.
- Provide the patient and her partner psychological counseling and support.

Specific

- ⚡ Counsel the patient to report adverse effects such as abdominal pain or visual disturbances to her infertility specialist at once and to be cautious with tasks that require alertness. If she misses a dose of her drug, she should call her infertility specialist.
- Advise the patient that treatment increases the chance of multiple births.
- ⚡ Ensure that the patient understands the risks, benefits, and alternatives to pharmacologic therapy.

Patient Teaching

- Teach couples how to evaluate and record on a chart the woman's basal body temperature and changes in the cervical mucus. The first day of menses is day 1 of the cycle. Ovulation is predicted by a 0.5°F drop in basal body temperature, followed by a 1°F rise. OTC diagnostic kits for assessing ovulatory status can also be used to time coitus. The couple is advised to engage in coitus frequently from 4 days before to 3 days after ovulation.
- Advise the female partner to take the drug at the same time each day to maintain steady blood levels.
- Encourage the patient and her partner to verbalize concerns and express feelings about treatment successes and failures.

🌐 *Cultural Considerations*

- A number of churches and religions do not support the use of reproductive technologies. Some couples may opt for adoption instead of reproductive assistance, whereas others may suffer additional anxiety if they go against their religious or cultural traditions and use reproductive technology.
- Some women may prefer to be examined only by a female health care provider. These women should remain covered as much as is possible and appropriate. Some patients combine traditional practices with conventional medicine, therefore a complete history of nonpharmacologic therapy is needed.
- Use of a certified medical interpreter is necessary for individuals who have limited English skills; one of the same sex and culture is preferred for sensitive topics.

Evaluation

- Successful outcomes of fertility treatment include avoidance of ovarian hyperstimulation and other untoward effects. Pregnancy that results in the birth of a live infant fulfills the objectives of treatment. If pregnancy is not achieved, intervention is aimed at helping the couple consider alternatives to childbearing without any adverse impact on their self-esteem or harm to their relationship.

MENOPAUSE

The transitional process experienced by women as they move from the reproductive years into the nonreproductive stage of life is called *menopause,* a naturally occurring event and part of the normal life cycle of women. It occurs for most women between their mid-forties and mid-fifties but may start as early as the late thirties. The menopause has three stages: perimenopause or premenopause, menopause, and postmenopause, during which certain physiologic events occur. As women go through menopause, providers do not treat the cessation of menses but rather address the symptoms that may occur with the menopausal passage.

Perimenopause

The perimenopausal period includes the years before the natural cessation of spontaneous menstruation. During this period, menstrual variations become evident. Women may experience short cycles (<25 days), long cycles (>35 days), heavy bleeding, light bleeding, or periods of longer or shorter duration. Women may start to skip periods or abruptly stop menstruating altogether. Oligomenorrhea, very scant periods, and menorrhagia are common. Symptoms experienced during perimenopause are similar to those during menopause, with the exception that perimenopausal women continue to have some type of cyclic bleeding. The most common symptoms are hot flashes caused by a surge in LH levels and vaginal dryness caused by estrogen withdrawal. Other symptoms include insomnia, headaches, irritability or anxiety or other variations in mood, cognitive difficulties, memory lapses, joint aches, and decreased libido. These unpredictable changes may last a short period of time, or they may last for several years.

There are a set number of follicles in the ovaries at birth. They are dormant throughout childhood and become active with puberty. Ovarian follicles are high in number during puberty and until age 35 years, but the number of follicles steadily declines after age 35 years, and the decline is more rapid after age 40 years. During the menstrual cycle, these follicles provide high levels of estrogen in the form of estradiol. The highest level of estradiol production in women occurs from puberty until the early thirties. Follicular growth, and therefore the secretion of estradiol, is under the influence of FSH and, to a lesser degree, LH, both of which are released by the anterior pituitary gland.

During the perimenopausal period, ovarian follicles become depleted, causing estrogen levels to diminish. The decrease in estrogen is gradual and allows for fluctuating levels of FSH and LH. Subsequently, menstrual cycles become anovulatory and therefore irregular. The onset of menstrual irregularity is one of the early indications of perimenopause. Symptoms are thought to be related to hormone fluctuations, particularly estrogen withdrawal, and increased levels of LH and FSH. Serum FSH testing is used as a marker of follicular activity, and an elevated level of FSH can be an indication of decreased ovarian function.

Menopause

Menopause is the permanent end of spontaneous menstruation caused by cessation of ovarian function. This natural event is documented as having occurred once a woman has stopped menstruating for 1 year. The triggering event is not known. Women who experience menopause before 40 years of age are said to have premature ovarian failure. Menopause can also occur abruptly as a secondary effect of oophorectomy (surgical removal of the ovaries), radiologic procedures in which ovarian function is destroyed, severe infection, ovarian tumors, or as a temporarily induced state for treatment of conditions such as endometriosis. During this transitional period, and with any episodes of menstrual changes or irregularities caused by perimenopause, women should use contraception until menstruation has ceased for 1 year if they do not want to become pregnant.

Postmenopause

Postmenopause is the stage when the body adapts to a new hormonal environment. The production of estrogen and progesterone from the ovaries decreases during the late premenopausal and early postmenopausal periods. The ovaries continue to secrete androgens (testosterone) in varying amounts as a result of the influence of increased LH levels. This surge in LH causes hot flashes: transient sensations of intense heat with or without sweating, tachycardia, and sleep disruption. During postmenopause, androstenedione—the main androgen secreted by the ovaries and adrenal cortex, which is present in reduced amounts after menopause—is converted into estrone, a naturally occurring estrogen formed in extraglandular tissues of the brain, liver, kidney, and adipose tissue. This represents the main source of available estrogen once the ovaries lose the ability to produce estradiol.

⚡ PATIENT SAFETY

Do not confuse…
- **Premarin** with **Prempro** or **Premphase:** Premarin is estrogen only for hormone replacement therapy. Both *Prempro* and *Premphase* have combined estrogen and progesterone for use by women with an intact uterus to prevent uterine hyperplasia when estrogen is used.

Hormone therapy (HT) significantly improves vasomotor symptoms and vaginal dryness, two frequently encountered symptoms of menopause. Vasomotor symptoms have the potential to disrupt sleep quality and to exacerbate irritability, mood swings, depression, and problems with concentration. Decreases in systemic estrogen cause vaginal dryness and atrophic vaginitis, leading to dyspareunia and sexual dysfunction. Decreased estrogen also has an effect on libido, sexual arousal, and the achievement of orgasm, and it has an untoward effect on urinary health. Current guidelines do not support the use of HT for the prevention of cardiovascular disease, osteoporosis, or dementia.

The FDA has issued a boxed warning that states that HT should be used only for the treatment of menopausal symptoms, at the lowest dose possible, for the shortest duration possible, usually fewer than 5 years (Box 52.4). Most health care providers adhere to this practice when prescribing HT. Health

---

BOX 52.4 FDA Boxed Warnings for Combined Hormonal Contraceptives (CHCs) and Hormone Therapy Products

CHCs: "Cigarette smoking increases the risk of serious cardiovascular side effects from oral contraceptive use. This risk increases with age and with heavy smoking (15 or more cigarettes per day) and is quite marked in women over 35 years of age. Women who use oral contraceptives should be strongly advised not to smoke."

Ethinyl estradiol and norelgestromin transdermal patch: "Do not use this transdermal patch if you smoke cigarettes and are over 35 years old. Smoking increases your risk of serious cardiovascular side effects (heart and blood vessel problems) from hormonal contraceptives, including death from heart attack, blood clots, or stroke. The risk increases with age and the number of cigarettes you smoke."

Ethinyl estradiol and etonogestrel transvaginal ring: "Cigarette smoking increases the risk of serious cardiovascular side effects from combination oral contraceptive use. This risk increases with age and with heavy smoking (15 or more cigarettes per day) and is quite marked in women over 35 years of age. Women who use combination hormonal contraceptives, including the transvaginal ring, should be strongly advised not to smoke."

Hormone replacement therapies with estrogen and estrogen plus progesterone: "Warning: Cardiovascular disorders, breast cancer, endometrial cancer and probable dementia [can occur]. … Estrogens, with or without progestins, should be prescribed at the lowest effective doses and for the shortest duration consistent with treatment goals and risks for the individual woman."

---

teaching must be done with menopausal women to ensure that they are aware of the risks and benefits of hormone replacement therapy.

Pharmacologic Therapy for Perimenopausal and Menopausal Symptoms

Hormone Therapy

HT is used only for the relief of symptoms related to menopause, most commonly hot flashes, vaginal dryness, and associated sleep disorders. HT includes estrogen-progestin therapy (EPT) for use with women who have an intact uterus and estrogen therapy (ET) for use with women who have had a hysterectomy, surgical removal of the uterus. Hysterectomy is performed for a variety of gynecologic problems including cancer, fibroids (benign uterine tumors), uterine prolapse, chronic pelvic pain, and heavy or abnormal uterine bleeding. The nurse should determine whether the patient has had a hysterectomy in the past prior to administration of HT. It is the estrogen component in HT that relieves the symptoms of menopause. The progestin is added to protect the uterine endometrium from hyperplasia, an abnormal proliferation or overgrowth of tissue. When the uterus is exposed to unopposed estrogen—that is, estrogen without concurrent progestins—the endometrium becomes hyperplastic, potentiating the development of endometrial cancer. Estrogen alone can be used with women who have had a hysterectomy. With women who still have their uterus, estrogen—most commonly in the form of conjugated equine estrogens (CEEs)—is taken together with the synthetic progestin. The progestin, however, has the potential to cause unpredictable uterine bleeding.

PATIENT SAFETY

Do not confuse...
- **CHC products** with **HT products**. Oral, transdermal, and vaginal ring preparations for contraception and HT are dispensed in packages and boxes that are very similar. Once opened, CHC products and HT products may have the same disc-dispensing systems and splintered packaging and may have similar-appearing skin patches and vaginal rings.

HT is available in oral preparations, transdermal applications, and vaginal preparations. Vaginal preparations are creams, suppositories, or rings. All vaginal preparations contain estrogen only and are very effective in treating vaginal dryness. FDA-approved estrogens used in HT are derived from natural sources and synthetic sources.

CEEs are mixtures of natural estrogens isolated from the urine of pregnant mares. Although CEEs are derived from nonhuman sources, they are naturally occurring estrogens. Synthetic estrogens include ethinyl estradiol (EE), which is the same estrogen found in CHC products. Conjugated equine estrogens, the most frequently used estrogen, is presented in Prototype Drug Chart 52.2.

Dosage Forms. The oral route is most commonly used because it is well tolerated by most patients and relatively easy to administer. It requires daily dosing. Some patients experience GI upsets, particularly nausea and vomiting. A patient with GI disorders such as colitis, irritable bowel syndrome, peptic ulcer, or a malabsorption disorder may receive inconsistent doses with oral administration, necessitating the use of another route. Oral estrogens have a particularly beneficial effect on lipids by increasing high-density lipoproteins. Although the oral route does result in complete absorption from the GI tract, there is greater impact on liver proteins. In women with an intact uterus, oral estrogen is combined with a progesterone or progestin, completing the combined therapy. This can be given in a separate estrogen tablet combined with a separate progestin tablet (two oral pills taken daily) or in a combined estrogen-progestin tablet (one oral pill taken daily). Oral estrogens are typically used continuously. Common HT products include CEE, estradiol, synthetic conjugated estrogen, and esterified estrogen.

The transdermal skin patch is a convenient method to deliver HT because it does not require daily dosing. The patch is applied to intact skin in the prescribed dosage. Generally, the lower abdomen is used, but other sites may also be used. As with the transdermal patch used for contraception, the HT patch should not be placed on or near the breasts. The patch allows for absorption of the estrogen directly into the bloodstream through a membrane that limits the absorption rate. All types of transdermal patches, both estrogen-only and estrogen-progestin combination patches, contain plant-derived 17-β estradiol; many women prefer to take an estrogen derived from a plant source. The advantage is the same as the first-pass avoidance in CHC products using the transdermal route: the GI tract and liver are bypassed initially, which results in less nausea and vomiting and less impact on the hepatic system. Transdermal patches are changed twice a week or weekly, depending on the product, and they are used continuously. A progestin should be taken concurrently with the estrogen patch in women with an intact uterus.

HT is also available in topical gels, emulsions, and sprays; synthetic plant-based transdermal estradiol gels are applied once daily

PROTOTYPE DRUG CHART 52.2
Conjugated Estrogens

Drug	Route and Dosage
Estrogen replacement Pregnancy category: X*	A: PO: 0.3, 0.45, 0.625, 0.9, and 1.25 mg/d or cyclically (with or without progestins)
Contraindications	**Drug-Lab-Food Interactions**
Undiagnosed vaginal bleeding, pregnancy, lactation, severe liver disease, venous thrombosis, personal history of breast cancer *Caution:* Cardiovascular disease, severe renal disease, diabetes mellitus	Drug: Increased effects with corticosteroids; decreases effects of anticoagulants and oral hypoglycemics; decreased effects with rifampin, anticonvulsants, and barbiturates; toxicity with tricyclic antidepressants
Pharmacokinetics	**Pharmacodynamics**
Absorption: PO: Well absorbed Distribution: PB: Largely bound to sex hormone–binding globulin (SHBG) and albumin. Widely distributed; crosses placenta and enters breast milk Metabolism: t½: UK Excretion: In urine and bile	PO/IV: Onset: Rapid Peak: UK Duration: UK IM: Onset: Delayed
Therapeutic Effects/Uses	
For moderate to severe vasomotor symptoms of menopause and vaginal dryness/atrophy Mode of Action: Develops and maintains female genital system, breast, and secondary sex characteristics; increases synthesis of protein	
Side Effects	**Adverse Reactions**
Nausea, vomiting, fluid retention, breast tenderness, leg cramps, breakthrough bleeding, chloasma	Jaundice, thromboembolic disorders, depression, hypercalcemia, gallbladder disease *Life threatening:* Thromboembolism, CVA, PE, MI, endometrial cancer

*Pregnancy categories have been revised. See http://www.fda.gov/Drugs/DevelopmentApprovalProcess/DevelopmentResources/Labeling/ucm093307.htm for more information.
A, Adult; *CVA,* cerebrovascular accident; *d,* day; *IM,* intramuscular; *IV,* intravenous; *MI,* myocardial infarction; *PB,* protein binding; *PE,* pulmonary embolism; *PO,* by mouth; *t½,* half-life; *UK,* unknown.

for the treatment of moderate to severe vasomotor symptoms. A thin film is applied to one arm from the shoulder to the wrist; the gel dries in 2 to 5 minutes. The dosage regimen is designed to deliver a specific amount of estradiol with each application.

With the topical HT products listed previously, a progestin should be taken concurrently in women who have an intact uterus. Medroxyprogesterone acetate (MPA) is the oral progestin most often administered in combination with estrogen. Other available products are norethindrone acetate and micronized progesterone. Combination products contain both estrogen and a progestin, which offers the added convenience of not having to take two pills daily. Combination products have the same adverse effects as estrogen-only and progestin-only HT.

Two combination transdermal products contain estrogen and progestin combinations to treat menopausal symptoms such as hot flashes. The transdermal patch allows for continuous delivery of hormones at much lower doses than in oral HT. This route avoids first-pass metabolism by the liver and may be better tolerated. Patients should be treated with the lowest effective dose and for the shortest duration consistent with treatment goals.

Vaginal cream preparations are used in the treatment of vaginal atrophy, which causes painful intercourse and urinary difficulties. There is estradiol cream and conjugated equine topical cream, which is an estrogen derivative. Both preparations are rapidly absorbed into the bloodstream via the mucous membranes that line the vagina. Vaginal creams may be used in conjunction with another method, such as tablets or the transdermal patch. However, vaginal creams do *not* need a progestin counter because they do not affect the uterine endometrium to the extent that oral and transdermal products will. Conjugated estrogen vaginal cream is usually delivered in a dose of 0.5 to 2 g/day intravaginally for 2 weeks; then the dosing is decreased to twice weekly, three weeks out of each month.

One estradiol vaginal ring is a low-dose estradiol-releasing ring containing 2 mg of estradiol per 90-day ring (7.5 mcg/24 hours). This ring is inserted into the upper portion of the vagina, where it releases the estradiol, providing a consistent low dose of estrogen for 3 months. It may be left in place during intercourse and during treatment for vaginal infections. It is used to treat local symptoms of urogenital atrophy, which affects 20% to 40% of postmenopausal women.

Another estradiol vaginal ring consists of a low-dose estradiol-acetate releasing ring, made from silicone elastomer. This vaginal ring is available in two dosage strengths: 0.05 mg/day or 0.1 mg/day. This ring is inserted into the upper portion of the vagina, where it releases the estradiol, providing a consistent low dose of estrogen for 3 months. The lowest effective dose should be used. In women with an intact uterus, consideration should be given to adding progestin 10 to 14 days out of a 4-week menstrual cycle.

Vaginal estrogen tablets that contain estradiol can be inserted intravaginally once daily for 2 weeks. The dose is one 10-mcg tablet to be inserted once daily, and then the dose is decreased to one 10-mcg tablet twice weekly. Consideration should be given to adding progestin for 10 to 14 days out of a 4-week menstrual cycle if the woman's uterus is intact.

Contraindications. Contraindications to HT include pregnancy, history of endometrial cancer (when treatment for early endometrial cancer has been completed, it is no longer a contraindication to HT), personal history of breast cancer, history of thromboembolic disorders, acute liver disease or chronic impaired liver function, active gallbladder or pancreatic disease, coronary artery disease (CAD), undiagnosed vaginal bleeding, and endometriosis. Lifestyle factors such as smoking, known to enhance the risk of thromboembolism, should be considered in the treatment decision. The patient with a history of fibroid tumors is not started on HT for a full year after the last menstruation, because estrogen would likely result in tumor growth. The hypoestrogenic state associated with natural menopause usually causes existing fibroids to shrink. The presence of fibrocystic breast disease or diabetes may require extra caution.

Pharmacokinetics Conjugated equine estrogens are water soluble and well absorbed from the GI tract following tablet disintegration. Tablets are designed to release conjugated estrogens slowly over several hours. The estrogens are widely distributed in the body and circulate in the blood largely bound to sex hormone–binding globulin (SHBG) and albumin. Exogenous estrogens are metabolized in the liver, converted to metabolites, and excreted in the urine. Estrogens undergo enterohepatic recirculation.

Other Drugs for Menopausal Symptoms

Women who are not candidates for HT—more specifically, women with contraindications and breast cancer survivors—can be prescribed other drugs.

Selective Serotonin Reuptake Inhibitors and Serotonin Norepinephrine Reuptake Inhibitors. SSRIs and SNRIs reduce the number and severity of vasomotor symptoms in women. SSRIs also have the added benefit of reducing depression, which may relieve the irritability and mood changes associated with menopause. SSRIs and SNRIs can be gradually tapered in most postmenopausal women after 1 to 2 years of therapy.

Gabapentin. Gabapentin is an antiseizure drug that reduces the number and severity of nocturnal vasomotor symptoms in menopausal women. It should be administered in a single dose at bedtime. Gabapentin should be limited to those women who cannot take HT drugs and who have vasomotor symptoms that are affecting their quality of life. Gabapentin can cause drowsiness and should not be used concurrently with other drugs with similar precautions or if the patient's activities of daily living include those that would be affected or even dangerous if sleepiness, dizziness, or syncope should occur.

Clonidine. Clonidine, a drug used for hypertension, also reduces the number and severity of vasomotor symptoms in women. It is used for this purpose, however infrequently due to its side effect profile, for women in whom HT is contraindicated. Blood pressure must be monitored at regular intervals, and the drug is discontinued if hypotension occurs.

Osteoporosis

Osteoporosis is a progressive, debilitating skeletal disease that affects older men and women. Women older than 50 years are at greatest risk because the loss of estrogen during menopause is directly related to loss in BMD. Bone mass is at its highest density at age 30 years and then steadily declines. Osteoporosis occurs through an imbalance of osteoblasts (bone-building cells) and osteoclasts (cells that break down bone), which causes bone reabsorption to accelerate. This imbalance causes both deterioration of the microstructure within the bone and a decrease bone density. The loss of bone structure and "porous bone" fragility lead to an increased risk for fractures. Osteoporosis has significant morbidity and mortality in the United States. The most serious fracture site is the hip, and hip fracture is the second most common reason for older women to be placed in nursing homes, exceeded only by Alzheimer disease. Women who experience hip or vertebral fracture may have long-term, progressive, and debilitating health problems that can eventually lead to death. More than half of American women older than 50 years have some degree of osteopenia (low BMD) or osteoporosis (a severe decline in BMD).

Diagnosis of osteopenia and osteoporosis is made by axial skeletal measurements of bone density in the lumbar spine and hip through a dual-energy X-ray absorptiometry (DXA) scan. The World Health Organization (WHO) defines osteopenia and osteoporosis by translating the results of the DXA scan into a T score. Normal BMD is a T score of −1 or greater. Osteopenia is defined by a T score of −1 to −2.5, and osteoporosis is defined by a T score of −2.5 or less.

HT is no longer recommended for the *treatment* of osteoporosis; however, it may be considered as a *preventive* measure in postmenopausal women who are at risk, although not as first-line therapy. Women who have used HT for 5 years or more have been shown to have a 35% reduction in hip and vertebral fractures. Other drugs can manage osteoporosis and prevent fractures without the concerns raised by HT. These include bisphosphonates, which can reduce the breakdown of bone microstructure, and selective estrogen receptor modulators (SERMs). SERMs are a new class of synthetic estrogens that act like estrogens in certain parts of the body, such as the bones, while leaving other parts unaffected. Contraindications to SERM therapy include past history of or risk for VTE and pregnancy. Caution is used in women with heart disease, risk of MI or stroke, and hepatic or renal insufficiency.

The side effects of oral bisphosphonates include nausea, abdominal or stomach pain, difficulty swallowing, esophageal inflammation, reflux, and ulcers. Injectable bisphosphonates do not have the GI side effects, and it can be easier for the patient to schedule a quarterly or yearly injection than to remember to take a daily or weekly pill. A rare complication of bisphosphonates is full or partial spontaneous femur fractures. Oral bisphosphonates should not be taken with aspirin, NSAIDs, or antacids. Contraindications to bisphosphonates include esophageal abnormalities or delayed emptying of the esophagus, inability to sit or stand for 30 minutes after oral ingestion, and hypocalcemia.

Nursing Interventions

Prevention of osteoporosis includes sufficient intake of calcium and vitamin D throughout the lifespan by either dietary intake or supplementation. The recommended daily requirement of calcium for women aged 19 to 50 years is 1000 mg/day, whereas women older than 50 years need 1200 mg/day.

Calcium should be taken in divided doses and with adequate vitamin D to enhance absorption. The recommended daily allowance of vitamin D is 600 IU/day for women aged 19 to 70 years and 800 IU/day for women older than 70 years. All calcium preparations, with the exception of calcium citrate, should be taken with food. Smoking cessation should be encouraged because smoking interferes with vitamin D absorption. Alcohol consumption should be limited to one drink per day because alcohol reduces GI absorption of calcium. Weight-bearing exercise includes walking, jogging, low-impact aerobics, weight training, and yoga; these strengthen the bones, increase muscle strength, and enhance balance. Caution should be used in patients who are prescribed drugs that cause hypotension or dizziness. The patient should be assessed for fall risk, and the prevention of falls should be part of the nurse's health care teaching.

Drugs

Alendronate is a bisphosphonate used to treat osteopenia and osteoporosis. It is available in a daily or weekly dose. For prevention of osteoporosis, the oral weekly dose is 35 mg. For treatment, the oral weekly dose is 70 mg. Alendronate must be taken with 8 ounces of water 30 minutes before ingesting any food, liquids, or drug, and the patient must remain upright for 30 minutes. Once-a-week dosing has made this a first-line therapy. Common side effects include abdominal pain and acid reflux. Alendronate is also available with added vitamin D for enhanced absorption of calcium.

Ibandronate is a once-a-month bisphosphonate indicated for the treatment and prevention of osteoporosis in postmenopausal women. It comes in both oral and intravenous (IV) formulations. The oral dose has the same directions for use and side effects as the other bisphosphonates. Ibandronate can be administered as 150-mg once-monthly tablets, or 3 mg every 3 months administered IV over 15 to 30 seconds.

Risedronate is also available in a daily or weekly dose. It has similar directions for use and side effects similar to the bisphosphonates. The dosing schedule is a 5-mg tablet once daily or a 35-mg tablet once weekly and should be taken immediately following breakfast with at least 4 ounces of water.

Zoledronic acid is a bisphosphonate that is administered IV in a 5-mg dose yearly for the treatment of osteoporosis; the dose should be administered over 15 minutes. Zoledronic acid can be given in a 5-mg dose every 2 years for prevention of osteoporosis.

Kidney failure is a rare but serious condition that may be associated with the use of bisphosphonates in patients with underlying renal disease or renal impairment. These drugs should not be used in patients with chronic kidney disease (CKD) and a glomerular filtration rate (GFR) lower than 30 to 35 mL/minute.

Nurses should teach patients to advise their health care provider of any increased thigh or groin pain, which can be symptoms of rare, atypical femur fractures.

Studies suggest that some patients may be able to discontinue the use of these drugs after 3 to 5 years and still benefit from using bisphosphonates. It is recommended that the DXA of the hip and spine be repeated after 2 years. Health care providers should reassess patients on an individual basis every 5 years to determine whether continued therapy is beneficial. It has been determined that bisphosphonates do work to improve osteoporosis; however, the time frame for safe use of these drugs needs to be investigated. Research is ongoing to determine whether the use of bisphosphonates increases the risk for esophageal cancer, which is extremely rare in women.

Raloxifene is a SERM that increases BMD, decreases bone turnover, and reduces vertebral fractures. A secondary analysis of osteoporotic women treated with raloxifene showed a decrease in the risk for breast cancer. Side effects include hot flashes and increased risk for deep venous thrombosis (DVT). Raloxifene is taken orally once a day in a 60-mg tablet. Patients need to take calcium and vitamin D to prevent or treat hypocalcemia while taking this drug.

Teriparatide is a parathyroid hormone used for treatment of postmenopausal osteoporosis, and it is administered 20 mcg subcutaneously on a daily basis for 2 years. It can be used by both men and women who have had a fracture related to osteoporosis or who have multiple risk factors for fracture and cannot use other osteoporosis treatments. The patient can be taught self-administration.

Calcitonin-salmon is composed of calcitonin, a naturally occurring hormone that regulates calcium in the body and promotes bone metabolism. It is administered 100 units subcutaneously or IM every day to every other day. Another delivery option is via intranasal spray in a 200-IU dose administered daily.

Denosumab is a monoclonal antibody and bone-modifying agent used in women who are at a high risk for osteoporotic fracture, who have had a fracture, or who have not had improvement in T score after using the bisphosphonates for osteoporosis. A 60-mg dose is given subcutaneously every 6 months. Patients need to take calcium and vitamin D to prevent or treat hypocalcemia while taking this drug.

NURSING PROCESS
Patient-Centered Collaborative Care
Management of Symptomatic Menopausal Women

Assessment
- Obtain a record of the patient's drug, supplement, and CAM use.
- Obtain baseline vital signs that include temperature, pulse, respirations, BP, and weight and height. Report abnormal findings.
- Obtain a family history to assess for risk factors regarding osteoporosis and osteoporotic fractures; cardiovascular risks, including CAD, ischemic and hemorrhagic stroke, and VTE; cognitive disorders; and cancers that affect women.
- Obtain a history of allergies to drugs, foods, and supplements.
- Obtain a medical-surgical history, asking about present or past hypertension; falls and fractures; cardiovascular disease; cerebral vascular disorders; hepatic, renal, and urinary tract disorders and infections; GI problems; neurologic disorders; and past systemic infections. Assess for past and present history of cancer. Ask about previous surgeries, in particular, gynecologic or pelvic surgery. Assess for smoking, alcohol,

and illicit drug use. Assess risk for falls and fractures, self-care concerns, and ability to take drugs.
- Obtain a complete menstrual history including age at menarche and age at menopause. If the patient is perimenopausal, assess menstrual pattern; cycle length, duration, and amount of bleeding; first day of LMP; and method used for contraception. If the patient is in menopause, assess past and present menopausal symptoms along with their effects on quality of life. Assess for any incidence of postmenopausal bleeding.
- Obtain a full gynecologic history, including the last Pap testing results, history of abnormal Pap testing and colposcopy, and gynecologic problems, disorders, and surgeries.
- Obtain a complete sexual history, including sexual expression and sexual risk practices, menopausal symptoms and effects on sexual expression, and past or present sexual abuse and/or assault.
- Assess the patient's perception of menopause and knowledge of nonpharmacologic and pharmacologic hormone therapies.

Nursing Diagnoses
- Knowledge, Deficient regarding perimenopause and menopause
- Decisional Conflict related to starting or continuing HT
- Knowledge, Deficient related to HT method(s) and appropriate use of the method
- Fear related to the potential side effects of HT
- Infection, Risk for
- Falls, Risk for and/or osteoporotic fracture
- Body Image, Disturbed related to menopausal changes
- Sleep Pattern, Disturbed related to perimenopause or menopause

Planning
- The risks and benefits associated with HT will be evaluated on an individual basis.
- The patient will verbalize menopausal symptoms and will understand nonpharmacologic and pharmacologic measures that may aid in alleviating symptoms.
- If a patient elects HT, she will choose the route of administration that is best suited for her lifestyle and will increase safety and effective use of the product.
- The patient will understand the difference between EPT and ET.
- The patient will report side effects that occur.
- The patient will self-administer oral, transdermal, topical, or vaginal drugs as prescribed.
- The patient will place the patch as directed and will report any adverse side effects that occur.
- The patient will be comfortable with vaginal placement of drugs.
- The patient will report abnormal uterine bleeding and other side effects associated with HT.
- Explain dosing schedule, risks, benefits, and alternatives to the patient.
- The patient will schedule follow-up appointments as needed.

Nursing Interventions

- ⚡ Teach patients about the nature of menopause, its potential effects, and the benefits, risks, and alternatives of both nonpharmacologic and pharmacologic treatment modalities.
- Determine the patient's misconceptions about HT and provide factual, research-based information.
- Use the BRAIDED method in assisting the patient who is choosing an HT method.
- Use health teaching to encourage effective use of HT.
- Place current educational materials in health and community sites.

Patient Teaching
General

- ⚡ Review risks, benefits, and alternatives for use of HT.
- Review contraindications to HT.
- Advise patients to have breast and pelvic examinations and a Pap test before starting HT.
- Tell patients that warm weather and stress exacerbate hot flashes.
- Advise patients to use a fan, drink cool liquids, and decrease intake of caffeine and spicy foods.
- ⚡ Encourage patients on HT to have a medical follow-up every 6 to 12 months, including a BP check and a clinical breast and pelvic examination.
- Stress the need to use a method of contraception until 1 year after cessation of spontaneous menstruation.
- Suggest to patients the use of a water-soluble vaginal lubricant to reduce painful intercourse (dyspareunia) and prevent trauma.
- Advise patients to decrease use of antihistamines and decongestants if experiencing vaginal dryness.
- Advise patients to wear cotton underwear and pantyhose with a cotton liner and to avoid douches and feminine hygiene products.
- Suggest that patients take HT oral drugs after meals to avoid nausea and vomiting.
- Advise patients that they may experience some vaginal bleeding that should stop 3 to 6 months after starting HT.
- Suggest that patients carry sanitary pads or tampons for breakthrough bleeding or irregular menstruation.

- Advise patients to report any heavy bleeding or irregular bleeding patterns and to have hematocrit and hemoglobin evaluated.
- Advise patients that after HT is discontinued, there may be a recurrence of menopausal signs and symptoms such as hot flashes.
- Tell patients wanting to stop HT that it should be done with guidance by the health care provider.

Self-Administration

- Teach patients about breast health, and teach them to perform regular breast self-examination.
- Teach patients to perform regular genital inspections.
- Advise patients when Pap screening is due.
- If a patient uses vaginal cream, review the application procedure and suggest that she wear minipads.
- If a patient uses the transdermal patch, teach her to open the package and apply it immediately and to hold it in place for about 10 seconds; check edges to ensure adequate contact; use the abdomen (except the waistline) for the patch; rotate sites with at least 1 week before reuse of a site; do not use the breast area as a site; do not put the patch on an irritated or oily area; do not reapply the patch if it loosens, and do not apply a new one; and advise her to follow the same cycle schedule.
- Advise patients about appropriate use of gels, sprays, and mists.

Balanced Diet and Exercise

- Teach patients about osteoporosis prevention and encourage (1) weight-bearing exercise; (2) a well-balanced diet high in fiber, vegetables, fruits, whole grains, and plant proteins and low in animal proteins and sugar; (3) supplementation with 1000 mg/day of calcium (if <50 years old) or 1200 mg/day (if >50 years old) and vitamin D 600 IU/day if <70 years old; (4) smoking cessation and reduced alcohol consumption.

Evaluation

- Evaluate the effectiveness of nonpharmacologic or pharmacologic measures for premenopausal symptoms.
- Determine whether side effects occur. Plan alternative measures to control menopausal symptoms with the patient.
- Plan follow-up appointments and health care screenings.

CRITICAL THINKING CASE STUDY

TA (gravida 3, para 1) is ready to leave the hospital after delivery of a healthy baby. TA had developed gestational hypertension during her pregnancy, but she had no prior history of hypertension. TA plans to breastfeed for 3 months; she desires contraception and asks about hormonal contraceptive methods.

1. TA asks whether she can take OCs while breastfeeding. What are the nursing diagnoses for TA based on her communication? Are other CHC methods available for TA besides the pill? What CHC start method is best for TA?
2. The nurse tells TA that she may breastfeed and can start using CHCs in about 6 weeks when her milk flow is established. Is

this information correct or incorrect? Why? What further information will TA need?
3. What other methods of oral contraception are available for TA that would not affect quantity and quality of breast milk? What nursing health teaching should be stressed with the initiation of these products?
4. TA asks if there are any advantages to using oral contraceptives rather than an LNG-IUS. What are four advantages and four disadvantages the nurse could include in the discussion? What health teaching would the nurse provide for TA to ensure that she will use CHC pills correctly?

NCLEX STUDY QUESTIONS

1. The nurse is preparing a teaching plan for combined hormonal contraceptive use. Which information should the nurse include in the teaching plan? (Select all that apply.)
   a. The patient should report abdominal pain, chest pain, headaches, blurred vision and visual disturbances, and severe leg pain.
   b. Combined hormonal contraceptives are safe for smokers older than 35 years who smoke fewer than 20 cigarettes per day.
   c. Combined hormonal contraceptive use will not protect patients from sexually transmitted infections.
   d. The pills can be missed but not for more than 12 hours.
   e. Vaginal spotting after starting combined hormonal contraceptives is a sign that the method is not effective in preventing pregnancy.

2. A 54-year-old menopausal patient comes into the gynecology office and is interested in hormone therapy. Which are indications for prescribing hormone therapy? (Select all that apply.)
   a. Relief of hot flashes
   b. Prevention of breast cancer
   c. Prevention of cardiovascular disease
   d. Prevention of osteoporosis in a high-risk patient
   e. Relief of vaginal dryness

3. A 24-year-old patient tells the nurse that she would like to use the progestin-only pill for contraception. Nursing evaluation of this patient as a candidate for the progestin-only pill includes what?
   a. Obtaining an obstetric history to make sure that the patient has given birth in the past
   b. Obtaining a gynecologic history to ensure that the patient has regular periods
   c. Assessing patient reliability in taking an oral pill daily
   d. Interviewing the patient about past smoking habits

4. A 39-year-old patient who smokes one pack of cigarettes (20) per day asks about a contraception method that is best for her. She is normotensive and has used combined hormonal contraceptives in the past. She is in a monogamous relationship and has had two children with no complications during pregnancy. She is not planning any more pregnancies. The nurse determines that which method would be best for this patient?
   a. Combined hormonal contraceptives
   b. A levonorgestrel intrauterine system
   c. Progestin-only pills
   d. Levonorgestrel (systemic) progestin

5. An 18-year-old woman calls the clinic office and tells the triage nurse that she had sex last night and the condom broke. She is concerned about unintended pregnancy. Which statement made by the triage nurse is the best advice for this patient?
   a. Levonorgestrel (systemic) progestin is available over the counter.
   b. You should make an appointment with the provider for a prescription of ulipristal acetate.
   c. You have time to wait a few days to make a decision.
   d. The provider can insert an intrauterine device. I will make an appointment for you.

6. The nurse is instructing a patient on the use of depot medroxyprogesterone acetate. Which statements are correct? (Select all that apply.)
   a. Patients who use depot medroxyprogesterone acetate usually do not have any changes in their periods.
   b. You should increase your intake of calcium.
   c. You can expect some irregular bleeding at first.
   d. You can use depot medroxyprogesterone acetate if you are breastfeeding.
   e. Depot medroxyprogesterone acetate also helps with postpartum depression.

7. The nurse is counseling a 62-year-old patient with a T score of −2.0 after her dual-energy X-ray absorptiometry scan. What is the best advice for this patient?
   a. The patient should take a daily calcium supplement, 1200 to 1500 mg orally in the morning.
   b. The patient should increase weight-bearing exercises like swimming and cycling.
   c. The patient most likely will be prescribed a drug of the bisphosphonate classification by the health care provider.
   d. The patient should supplement her diet with 1200 mg of calcium with vitamin D 600 IU orally once daily.

8. A 48-year-old patient arrives at the clinic to discuss her perimenopausal symptoms. She states that her last menstrual period was 8 months ago, and before that, her periods had been irregular. What is the most important nursing advice to give this patient?
   a. Hormone therapy is only used for hot flashes and vaginal dryness.
   b. The patient should be using some form of contraception to avoid pregnancy.
   c. The patient should have a dual-energy X-ray absorptiometry scan to test for osteopenia.
   d. At this time, herbal supplementation is probably best to relieve her perimenopausal symptoms.

9. A patient has been prescribed clomiphene citrate therapy by her doctor. The patient asks the nurse, "How does my new medicine work?" What can the nurse say to convey the mechanism of action of clomiphene citrate therapy to this patient? (Select all that apply.)
   a. This drug works by stimulating the ovaries, increasing the chance of ovulation.
   b. This drug increases circulating progesterone levels.
   c. This drug usually does not work on the first cycle.
   d. This drug helps the ovaries form multiple follicles.

Answers: 1, a, c, e; 2, a, d, e; 3, c; 4, b; 5, a; 6, b, c, d; 7, d; 8, b; 9, a, b, d.

53

Men's Health and Reproductive Disorders

http://evolve.elsevier.com/McCuistion/pharmacology/

Reproductive health requires the production of adequate quantities of various hypothalamic, pituitary, and gonadal hormones as well as the appropriate hormone receptors. It requires normal development and patency of the reproductive tract. In addition, reproductive health implies that men and women at developmentally appropriate life stages are fertile (i.e., able to produce gametes [sperm or eggs]). Finally, reproductive health entails the ability to engage in sexual intercourse with ejaculation by the male.

Alterations in male reproductive health reflect a wide range of developmental, endocrine, infectious, inflammatory, hypertrophic, malignant, and psychoemotional processes. Review the introduction to this unit to gain a better understanding of ways in which reproductive health

is affected, including anatomy and physiology, sperm production, regulation of male sexual functioning, and sexual intercourse.

The drug family most clearly associated with male reproductive processes is the androgens. Because synthetic anabolic steroids and antiandrogens affect male reproduction, they are also discussed.

DRUGS RELATED TO MALE REPRODUCTIVE DISORDERS

Androgens

Androgens, or male sex hormones, control the development and maintenance of sexual processes, accessory sexual organs,

TABLE 53.1 Testosterone Levels by Age

Age	T Level (ng/dL)
0-5 months	75-400
6 mos.-9 yrs.	<7-20
10-11 yrs.	<7-130
12-13 yrs.	<7-800
14 yrs.	<7-1,200
15-16 yrs.	100-1,200
17-18 yrs.	300-1,200
19+ yrs.	240-950
Avg. Adult Male	270-1,070
30+ yrs.	-1% per year

From: http://www.mayomedicallaboratories.com/test-catalog/Clinical+
and+Interpretive/83686

cellular metabolism, and bone and muscle growth. **Testosterone**, an anabolic steroid, is the principal male sex hormone. It is the prototype of the androgen hormones, synthesized primarily in the testes and, to a lesser extent, in the adrenal cortex. In women, the ovaries synthesize small amounts of testosterone. In adult males, normal plasma concentrations of testosterone are 270 to 1070 ng/dL, with a slow decline of 1% per year after the age of 30 (Table 53.1). Prototype Drug Chart 53.1 lists the natural and synthetic androgens and their dosages, uses, and considerations.

Pharmacokinetics Testosterone secretion is greater in men than in women in most stages of life. About 98% of circulating testosterone is bound to both sex hormone–binding globulin (SHBG) and albumin protein, leaving about 2% unbound, or circulating free in the plasma; this unbound portion is biologically active. Estrogen elevates the production of SHBG, resulting in more protein-bound testosterone in women than in men. The half-life of endogenous, or naturally occurring, free testosterone in the blood is 10 to 20 minutes.

Because as much as 50% of testosterone is metabolized on its first pass through the hepatic circulation when taken orally, oral testosterone is not available for prescription in the United States. Testosterone can be combined with esters to form esterified testosterone in an oil base for intramuscular (IM) injection.

Ninety percent of testosterone is excreted in the urine as glucuronic and sulfuric acid conjugates and its metabolites. About 6% of the hormone is excreted unconjugated in the feces. Synthetic androgens may be excreted as unaltered hormone or as metabolites. In some tissues the action of testosterone depends on its reduction to 5-alpha-dihydrotestosterone (DHT), whereas in other tissues testosterone itself is the active hormone. In the central nervous system, the metabolite estradiol affects hormonal action.

Pharmacodynamics Testosterone is responsible for the development of male sex characteristics. The biologic effects of testosterone may be mediated directly by testosterone or by its metabolites. Testosterone and dihydrotestosterone act as androgens by way of a single androgen receptor officially designated NR3A. The hormones bind to sites on certain responsive genes, causing a change to take place in the target cell. The

PROTOTYPE DRUG CHART 53.1

⚡ Testosterone

Drug Class	Dosage
Androgen	Androgen replacement:
Testosterone cypionate	IM: 50-400 mg q2-4wk
Pregnancy category: X*	
CSS III	

Contraindications	Drug-Food Interactions
Pregnancy, nephrosis, hypercalcemia, pituitary insufficiency, hepatic dysfunction, benign prostatic hyperplasia, prostatic cancer, history of myocardial infarction, prepubertal status, non–estrogen-dependent breast cancer *Caution:* Hypertension, hypercholesterolemia, coronary artery disease, gynecomastia, renal disease, seizure disorders; prepubescent patients, older adults	Drug: Increases effects of anticoagulants; decreases effect with barbiturates, phenytoin, phenylbutazone; antagonizes calcitonin and parathyroid; corticosteroids exacerbate edema.

Pharmacokinetics	Pharmacodynamics
Absorption: IM: Well absorbed Distribution: PB: 98% Metabolism: t½: 10-100 min Excretion: In urine and bile	IM: Onset: UK Peak: UK Duration: Cypionate/enanthate: 2-4 wk

Therapeutic Effects/Uses
Develops and maintains male sex organs and secondary sex characteristics Mode of Action: Binds to androgen receptors, producing multiple anabolic and androgenic effects.

Side Effects	Adverse Reactions
Abdominal pain, nausea, diarrhea, constipation, hives, irritation at injection site, increased salivation, mouth soreness, increased or decreased libido, insomnia, aggressive behavior, weakness, dizziness, pruritus	Acne, masculinization, irregular menses, urinary urgency, gynecomastia, priapism, red skin, jaundice, sodium and water retention, allergic reaction, depression, habituation *Life threatening:* Hepatic necrosis, hepatitis, hepatic tumors, respiratory distress

*Pregnancy categories have been revised. See http://www.fda.gov/Drugs/DevelopmentApprovalProcess/DevelopmentResources/Labeling/ucm093307.htm for more information.
CSS, Controlled Substances Schedule; *IM,* intramuscular; *min,* minute; *PB,* protein binding; *q,* every; *t½,* half-life; *UK,* unknown; *wk,* week.

effects of the testosterone depend on which receptor it activates and the tissues in which these effects occur. The manufacture of protein within the target cells results in the buildup of cellular tissue (anabolism), especially in muscles. This leads to development of secondary sex characteristics such as pubic hair growth, beard and body hair growth, baldness, deepening of the male voice, thickening of the skin, sebaceous gland activity, increased musculature, bone development, and red blood cell formation.

Fetal testes begin to produce testosterone during the first 3 months in utero. After birth until just before puberty, production is negligible. During puberty, production increases rapidly and continues until later adulthood. As men age, the number of Leydig cells decreases, sperm production declines, and

TABLE 53.2   Androgens (Controlled Substance, Schedule III)

Drug	Route and Dosage	Uses and Considerations
NATURAL ANDROGENS		
Testosterone		
Testosterone nasal	Nasal: 5.5 mg per gel pump actuation; 1 pump actuation in each nostril 3 times/d	For primary hypogonadism, male and hypogonadotropic hypogonadism, male.
Transdermal testosterone patch	Transdermal patch: 2 mg/24 h or 4 mg/24 h patch; apply to nongenital skin; avoid bony areas	Drug is started at the full dose and adjusted according to tolerance and therapeutic response.
Testosterone topical gel	1% Gel: 50-100 mg once daily	Less skin irritation occurs with the gel than with the patch.
	2% Gel: 40-70 mg once daily	Pregnancy category: X*; PB: 98%; t½: 10-100 min
Buccal testosterone	Buccal: 30 mg twice daily	
Testosterone pellet	Subcut implantable 75-mg pellets: implant two 75-mg pellets for each 25 mg testosterone propionate required weekly. Replace every 4 to 6 mo.	
Testosterone cypionate	IM: 200-400 mg q3-4wk	For androgen replacement and delayed puberty; therapy generally lasts 3-4 y. Pregnancy category: X*; PB: 98%; t½: 8 d
SYNTHETIC ANDROGENS		
Fluoxymesterone	PO: 5 mg 1-4 times/d	For androgen deficiency and palliative treatment of carcinoma of the breast. Pregnancy category: X*; PB: 98%; t½: 29.2 h
Methyltestosterone	PO: 10-50 mg/d in divided doses initially; reduced for maintenance	For androgen deficiency and palliative treatment of carcinoma of the breast. Pregnancy category: X*; PB: UK; t½: 2.5-3.5 h

*Pregnancy categories have been revised. See http://www.fda.gov/Drugs/DevelopmentApprovalProcess/DevelopmentResources/Labeling/ucm093 307.htm for more information.

d, Day; *h,* hour; *IM,* intramuscular; *min,* minute; *mo,* month; *PB,* protein binding; *PO,* by mouth; *q,* every; *subcut,* subcutaneous; *t½,* half-life; *UK,* unknown; *wk,* week; *y,* year.

luteinizing hormone (LH) and follicle-stimulating hormone (FSH) levels rise. Levels of unbound testosterone are reduced in older men to one third to one fifth the peak value. If men experience osteoporosis and anemia, and if their testosterone levels are 300 ng/dL or less, testosterone replacement therapy should be considered.

Indications for Androgen Therapy

Table 53.2 lists the natural and synthetic androgens with their dosages, uses, and considerations. Androgen therapy is approved for use in androgen deficiency in males, specifically hypogonadism; replacement therapy for testicular failure in adult males; and delayed puberty in adolescents.

Hypogonadism. The clearest indication for exogenous androgen therapy is hypogonadism. Male hypogonadism is a defect of the reproductive system that results in failure of the testes to produce testosterone, sperm, or both. Deficiency of sex hormones can result in defective primary or secondary sexual development, and defective sperm development can result in infertility. Hypogonadism is either *primary,* reflecting testicular abnormality, or *secondary,* reflecting hypothalamic or pituitary failure. A combination of disorders can also occur. Inadequate pituitary function will severely affect young boys and results in infertility and a lack of secondary sex characteristics. Adult men may experience testicular atrophy, impotence, decreased libido, decreased bone density, loss of muscle mass, hair loss, gynecomastia, fatigue, difficulty concentrating, or vasomotor flushing.

The timing and extent of treatment depend on the clinical manifestations. Because accelerated bone maturation can lead to premature closure of bone epiphyses and short stature, androgen therapy should be used cautiously in children and only by specialists aware of the adverse effects on bone maturation. Skeletal maturation must be monitored every 6 months by radiography of the hand and wrist. Artificial induction of puberty is undertaken only after boys reach age 15 to 17 years and after hypothalamic and pituitary function has been assessed. A 4- to 6-month trial of androgen therapy is implemented, followed by a similar period of rest for reevaluation. If prolonged therapy is required, testosterone cypionate is used, 50 to 400 mg IM every 2 to 4 weeks. It should be given deep in the IM. Inspect vials visually for particulate matter and discoloration before administration, and warm and shake the vial to dissolve any crystals that may have formed during storage. It takes 3 or 4 years for sexual development to occur, and plasma testosterone levels should be monitored and dosages adjusted as needed to maintain normal levels; if the serum testosterone level is below the normal range, the provider will adjust the dose upward. Therapy may be lifelong.

Testosterone may be administered buccally, nasally, transdermally, or parenterally. Drug selection depends on the balance of growth and sexual maturation desired and on the preferred route of administration. A buccal mucoadhesive system is available that provides a 30-mg dose every 12 hours. Advise the patient to place the rounded surface of the system against the gum above an incisor tooth and hold it firmly in place with finger over the lip and against the product for 30 seconds. To remove, slide gently downward toward the tooth to avoid scratching the gums. Sites must be rotated with each application. If the product falls off within the 12-hour dosing interval, or if it falls out of position within 4 hours before next dose, remove it and apply a new system. The patient should not chew or swallow the system. Advise the patient to regularly inspect gums where the system has been applied. Testosterones are considered Schedule III controlled substances.

Transdermal testosterone (TT) patches achieve adequate serum concentrations when applied to the arm, back, or upper buttocks. TT patches can be applied to any healthy skin site other than the scrotum or bony areas. Daily application of one to two TT 2 mg/24 h or 4 mg/24 h skin patches at 10 PM results in serum testosterone concentrations approaching those of healthy young men. The first day of dosing results in morning serum testosterone concentrations within the normal range. There is no testosterone accumulation with continued use. After removal of TT patches, hypogonadal status returns within 24 hours. Keep testosterone gel out of reach of children.

Testosterone gel is applied to clean dry skin of shoulders or upper arms. It should not be applied to the genitals. Hands should be thoroughly washed with soap and water following application. Testosterone gel carries a boxed warning, as it can be transferred to others through personal contact with skin or clothing. Children should avoid contact with unwashed application sites or application sites not covered by clothing. Children can experience virilization from secondary exposure. Caution is advised. ⚡

Side Effects. Hypogonadal men on androgen therapy may experience frequent erections or priapism (painful, continuous erection), gynecomastia (mammary gland enlargement in men), or urinary urgency. Continued use of androgens by normal men can halt spermatogenesis (formation of spermatozoa). The sperm count may be low (oligospermia) for 3 or more months after therapy is stopped.

Other side effects of androgen therapy include abdominal pain, nausea, insomnia, diarrhea or constipation, hives or redness at the injection site, increased salivation, mouth soreness, and increased or decreased sexual desire. Advise the patient to notify the health care provider if side effects persist, worsen, or are bothersome.

Adverse Reactions. Androgen therapy may cause hypercalcemia by stimulating bone resorption in immobilized patients and those with breast cancer. The drug should be discontinued and appropriate measures instituted if signs of hypercalcemia occur; signs include nausea and vomiting, lethargy, decreased muscle tone, polyuria, and increased urine and serum calcium.

Virilization refers to the development of male secondary sex characteristics in women or hypogonadal males. Such characteristics include growth of facial hair, acne and skin oiliness, and vocal huskiness. Menstrual irregularities or amenorrhea, suppressed ovulation or lactation, baldness or increased hair growth (hirsutism), and hypertrophy of the clitoris may develop in women undergoing androgen therapy. Although most adverse effects slowly reverse themselves after short-term therapy is completed, vocal changes may be permanent. With long-term therapy, as in the treatment of breast cancer, adverse effects may be irreversible.

Children may experience profound virilization as well as impaired bone growth. During pregnancy, androgens can cross the placenta and cause masculinization of the fetus. Virilization can occur in those secondarily exposed to testosterone gel and may cause teratogenic effects in fetuses. Women and children should not handle the gel and should avoid contact with application sites in men using testosterone gel.

Less frequent adverse effects include dizziness, weakness, changes in skin color, frequent headaches, confusion, respiratory distress, depression, pruritus, allergic skin rash, edema of the lower extremities, jaundice, bleeding, paresthesias, chills, polycythemia, muscle cramps, and sodium and water retention. Hepatocellular carcinoma can occur in patients who have received selected androgens for long-term therapy and in cases of abuse of androgenic hormones by athletes.

Serum cholesterol may become elevated during androgen therapy. Other alterations in laboratory tests include increased hematocrit, altered thyroid and liver function tests, and elevated urine 17-ketosteroids (a by-product of the breakdown of androgens). Rare complications of long-term therapy include hepatic necrosis, hepatic peliosis (blood-filled cysts), hepatic tumors, and leukopenia.

Contraindications. Androgen therapy is contraindicated during pregnancy and in individuals with nephrosis or those in the nephrotic phase of nephritis; it is also contraindicated in patients with hypercalcemia, pituitary insufficiency, hepatic dysfunction, benign prostatic hyperplasia (BPH), prostate cancer, or history of myocardial infarction. Men with breast cancer are not treated with androgens, nor are women whose breast cancer is not estrogen dependent.

Caution must be exercised when using androgen therapy in individuals with hypertension, hypercholesterolemia, coronary artery disease, renal disease, or seizure disorder. It is used with caution in infants and prepubertal children because of the potential for growth disturbances and in older men because of their increased risk for BPH and prostate cancer.

Drug Interactions. Androgens potentiate the effects of oral anticoagulants, necessitating a decrease in anticoagulant dosage. Androgens antagonize calcitonin and parathyroid hormones. Because androgens can decrease blood glucose in patients with diabetes, dosages of insulin or other antidiabetic agents may need to be reduced. Concurrent use of corticosteroids exacerbates the edema that can occur with androgen therapy. Barbiturates, phenytoin, and phenylbutazone decrease the effects of androgens.

Anabolic Steroids

Anabolic steroids, or anabolic-androgenic steroids (AASs), are a class of steroid hormones related to the hormone testosterone. They increase protein synthesis within cells, which results in the buildup of cellular tissue (anabolism), especially in muscles. Anabolic steroids also have androgenic and virilizing properties, including the development and maintenance of masculine characteristics such as the growth of the vocal cords and body hair. While the American College of Sports Medicine notes that AASs, combined with sufficient diet and exercise, can contribute to increased lean body mass in some individuals, they also note it is in the best interest of all sports to eradicate the use of AASs by athletes, due to the risk of serious harm or death in those who use AASs. See Chapter 7, Drugs in Substance Use Disorder, for further information.

Testosterone precursors available as nutritional supplements include androstenediol, androstenedione, and dehydroepiandrosterone (DHEA). Older teens are the heaviest users, but more than one-half million junior high school students also use them. Marketed as "sport supplements" or "teen formulas," they can be purchased without a prescription in stores and on the Internet. A sudden dramatic increase in weight and body size, increased acne, and changes in mood and behavior can be signs of exogenous anabolic steroid use. Individuals using anabolic steroids may become more aggressive and physical, and health risks can result from long-term use or excessive intake of anabolic steroids; these effects include increased low-density lipoprotein (bad) cholesterol and decreased high-density lipoprotein (good) cholesterol, acne, high blood pressure, liver damage, and dangerous changes in the structure of the left ventricle of the heart. Adverse effects may not be recognized until years later. See Chapter 7, Drugs in Substance Use Disorder, for further information.

Two other steroids that have gained popularity, especially with athletes, are human chorionic gonadotropin (hCG) and tetrahydrogestrinone (THG); hCG is a hormone used to treat infertility and stimulate testosterone production, and THG is a potent androgen developed to escape detection on urine drug screens, although tests have since been developed for rapid screening. It is not approved by the U.S. Food and Drug Administration (FDA) and is not legally marketed. All major athletic organizations prohibit the use of anabolic steroids, but their continued use despite bans has led to "antidoping" investigations and punitive action.

NURSING PROCESS
Patient-Centered Collaborative Care
Androgens

Assessment
- Assess the reason for androgen therapy and the patient's perception of it. If delayed puberty is the indication, assess patient and family attitudes about the condition.
- Monitor weight, blood pressure, liver and thyroid function, hemoglobin and hematocrit, creatinine, clotting factors, glucose tolerance, serum lipids and electrolytes, and blood count before and throughout treatment. Note the presence of liver or endocrine dysfunction and any elevation in blood pressure.
- Note concomitant anticoagulant therapy.
- When a prepubertal child is treated, obtain hand and wrist radiographs before, every 6 months during, and after treatment to monitor growth.
- Appraise the patient's expressive affect during therapy, particularly aggressiveness in patients taking large doses. Self-concept is an important consideration in the patient on androgen therapy, particularly in children with delayed puberty and in women.

Nursing Diagnoses
- Body Image, Disturbed related to altered hormonal function
- Self-esteem, Situational Low related to growth delay and/or virilizing effects of androgen therapy
- Sexual Dysfunction related to androgen deficiency
- Sleep Pattern, Disturbed related to altered hormonal function
- Knowledge, Deficient related to diagnosis and treatment androgen deficiency

Planning
- Through collaboration the patient agrees to (1) adhere to the prescribed regimen for taking drug and for monitoring, (2) use drug appropriately, (3) report adverse effects immediately, and (4) maintain a positive self-concept during long-term treatment.

Patient Teaching
General
- Collaborate with the patient and family on proper administration of drugs, their reasons for use, and potential undesired effects. Review which effects warrant prompt medical attention (e.g., urinary problems, priapism, respiratory distress).
- Advise patients that an intermittent approach to treatment allows for monitoring of endocrine status between courses of androgen therapy. Explain the need to return to the health care facility for monitoring, and confirm the patient's ability to do so. Arrange social service referrals if necessary.
- Counsel the family pursuing treatment for a child with delayed puberty about the range of normal development.
- Encourage patients to monitor muscle strength during treatment.

Self-Administration
- Instruct patients to administer androgens as directed.

Side Effects
- Coach patients about good skin hygiene to decrease the severity of acne.
- Urge men undergoing androgen therapy to report priapism promptly so the drug dosage can be reduced to avoid subsequent erectile dysfunction (ED).
- Instruct men to report decreased urinary stream promptly so they can be evaluated for prostatic hypertrophy.

Diet
- Assess and review the nutritional intake to ensure adequate intake of essential nutrients.
- Counsel patients to record body weight several times per week. Restrict sodium if edema develops.
- Advise patients with elevated serum calcium of the need to drink 2 L per day or more of fluid to prevent kidney stones. Individuals on bed rest need range-of-motion exercises, whereas ambulatory patients need to engage in active weight bearing. Hypercalcemia requires prompt medical attention because it can lead to cardiac arrest.

- Assess how the patient's cultural group regards expressions of sexuality.
- Ascertain any culturally defined expectations about male-female or male-male relationships, including health care relationships.
- Ask if the patient has restrictions related to sexuality, exposure of body parts, or discussion of sexual functioning.

Evaluation
- Monitor the patient's ability to adhere to a treatment regimen and response to prescribed drugs. The ability to adhere to a treatment plan and discuss treatment and effects knowledgeably suggests that teaching has been effective and that the patient accepts the treatment.
- Ask the patient about therapeutic and adverse drug effects on follow-up visits. Monitoring of weight, blood pressure, and laboratory tests will continue throughout therapy with alterations in the plan of care as needed.
- Periodically assess children and women who experience virilizing effects or acne for the ability to cope with these changes and to maintain a positive self-concept.
- Assess sexual function when appropriate.

Antiandrogens

Antiandrogens, or androgen antagonists, block the synthesis or action of androgens (Table 53.3). These drugs are used in the treatment of BPH, advanced prostatic cancer, and as hormonal therapy in the treatment of endometriosis. They may also be used to treat male-pattern baldness (MPB), acne, hirsutism, virilization syndrome in women, and precocious puberty in boys, although their effectiveness is not well established.

Gonadotropin-releasing hormone (GnRH), or a synthetic analogue such as leuprolide, is the most effective inhibitor of testosterone synthesis. When such agents are given over time, LH and testosterone levels fall. Normally, GnRH is released in a pulsatile fashion, but the sustained activity of leuprolide leads to decreased production of FSH and LH. In the male, this activity stops testosterone production in the testis. In the female, it stops estrogen production in the ovaries. This drug should not be used in combination with herbal or dietary supplements such as black cohosh, chasteberry, or DHEA.

Ketoconazole, an antifungal drug, has testosterone-suppressing effects similar to those of GnRH analogues when given at doses higher than those required for antifungal activity (400 mg orally every 8 hours as opposed to 200 to 400 mg daily for the treatment of fungal infections). The mechanism of action of this non–GnRH drug is unclear. GnRH analogues act directly through their impact on testosterone production for the treatment of prostate cancer. Ketoconazole as treatment of prostate cancer is an off-label use.

Flutamide is an oral nonsteroidal antiandrogen drug used as an antihormonal agent in the treatment of metastatic prostate cancer. It is most effective when used simultaneously with luteinizing hormone–releasing hormone (LHRH) analogues such as leuprolide acetate. When used alone, the best response

TABLE 53.3 Antiandrogens

Mechanism	Drugs
Elevates gonadotropin-releasing hormone (GnRH) level	Goserelin acetate Leuprolide acetate
Inhibits testosterone synthesis	*Ketoconazole
Blocks conversion of testosterone to dihydrotestosterone	Finasteride
Receptor inhibitors	Flutamide Bicalutamide **Spironolactone

*Off-label use for prostate cancer
**Off-label use for acne vulgaris

is seen in untreated patients. Flutamide is not effective in treating other hormonally dependent diseases such as breast cancer or BPH. Flutamide competes with androgens at androgen receptor sites in the prostate gland, blocking the conversion of testosterone to dihydrotestosterone; by doing so, it prevents the androgens from stimulating the prostate cancer cells to grow. Men receiving flutamide show elevations in plasma LH and testosterone levels. Bicalutamide is structurally related to flutamide but has a long plasma half-life that allows once-daily dosing, compared with thrice-daily dosing for flutamide. In addition, bicalutamide is more selective for the peripheral androgen receptor and has less activity at the central androgen receptor on the hypothalamic-pituitary axis.

Spironolactone is a weak potassium-sparing diuretic used primarily to treat high blood pressure, heart failure, and ascites in patients with liver disease. Although not FDA approved for these indications, spironolactone has also been used to treat acne vulgaris and idiopathic hirsutism. Dosage ranges from 25 to 200 mg/day in divided doses with a maximum adult dose of 400 mg/day.

Finasteride, a synthetic compound, inhibits conversion of testosterone to DHT. This orally active agent decreases the concentration of dihydrotestosterone in plasma and in the prostate without elevated plasma concentrations of LH or testosterone. Finasteride is used to treat BPH and MPB. The recommended 5-mg daily dose of finasteride for BPH needs to be reevaluated at 6 months and periodically thereafter. The 1-mg dose of finasteride for MPB is taken once a day for 12 months, and continued treatment is recommended for sustained results. Following discontinuation of therapy, reversal of effect is typically seen within 1 year. Adverse reactions include impotence, decreased libido, and decreased ejaculate. Women of childbearing age must not use finasteride and should not handle crushed or broken tablets because the active ingredient may cause abnormalities of a male fetus's sex organs.

Drugs Used in Other Male Reproductive Disorders
Delayed Puberty

Puberty is considered to be delayed when testicle enlargement, followed by penile growth and pubic hair development, has not begun by age 14. Delay in growth may be a normal part of the maturation process, but the cause could also be androgen deficiency or a deficiency of growth hormone. Secretion of

GnRH, LH, or FSH is insufficient in up to 5% of cases of **delayed puberty**. Treatment is only begun after 14 years of age, following a full evaluation, including serum LH, FSH, thyroid-stimulating hormone (TSH), and testosterone levels. Therapy with testosterone cyprionate 50 mg IM every month, for 3 to 6 months or less before epiphyseal closure, may result in linear growth without adverse permanent effects on hypothalamic, pituitary, or gonadal maturation.

Pituitary, Thyroid, and Adrenal Disorders

Inadequate pituitary function can be another cause of hypogonadism. Menotropins are purified combination preparations of the human pituitary gonadotropins FSH and LH. These drugs are indicated when both LH and FSH levels are low. When given in combination with hCG, the drug stimulates testosterone production in men to encourage spermatogenesis when injected three times a week for 4 to 9 months to ensure adequate spermatozoa production. One ampule of a menotropin contains 75 international units each of LH and FSH. The initial dose is 75 to 150 international units subcutaneously (subcut) or 3 times per week. Subsequent doses are adjusted according to individual response but not exceeding 75 to 150 international units per adjustment; the maximum dose is 300 units 3 times per week. Use the lower abdomen (alternating sides) for subcut administration. Menotropin must be used immediately after reconstitution and must be protected from light. Advise patients to discard unused drug. Adverse effects include nausea, vomiting, diarrhea, gynecomastia, and fever.

Inadequate thyroid and adrenal gland function can also affect sexuality. **Hypothyroidism**, a deficiency in thyroid hormone, can be the result of insufficient thyroid hormone production or resistance to its effects at the target organs. The problem can be congenital or acquired. It can cause **inhibited sexual desire**, a lack of or decreased interest in sexual activity, and ED. In **Addison disease**, there is a deficit of both cortisol and the mineralocorticoid aldosterone. Men with Addison disease may experience inhibited sexual desire, ED, or diminished fertility. Both hypothyroidism and Addison disease are highly responsive to replacement therapy with the appropriate hormones. (Refer to Chapter 46 for a discussion of Addison disease.)

Sexual Dysfunction

Sexual dysfunction is the inability to experience sexual desire, erection, ejaculation, and/or detumescence—the four phases of the sexual response cycle in men. Inhibited sexual desire can result from androgen deficiency, an affective disorder, or discord in the sexual relationship. Many drugs can also cause sexual dysfunction (Table 53.4).

Ejaculatory dysfunction, impaired ejection of seminal fluid from the male urethra, can be psychogenic or a result of drug therapy, androgen deficiency, or sympathetic degeneration. Failure of detumescence (reduction of penile engorgement) is most commonly caused by penile disease, systemic disease, trauma, or adverse effects of drugs. Individuals who experience premature ejaculation related to excessive anxiety about sexual intercourse may be helped by treatment with one of the many antidepressants alone or in conjunction with psychotherapy.

TABLE 53.4	**Drugs That Cause Sexual Dysfunction in Males**
Drug Category	**Drugs or Drug Families**
Anticholinergics	Atropine Scopolamine Benztropine Trihexyphenidyl
Antidepressants	Tricyclic antidepressants Monoamine oxidase inhibitors Selective serotonin reuptake inhibitors
Antihistamines	Diphenhydramine Hydroxyzine
Antihypertensives	Centrally acting alpha$_2$ agonists Alpha- and beta-receptor blockers Diuretics Angiotensin-converting enzyme inhibitors
Antipsychotics	Phenothiazines Thioxanthenes Butyrophenone
Antiulcer drugs	Cimetidine Ranitidine Famotidine
Sedatives and recreational drugs	Alcohol Barbiturates Diazepam Chlordiazepoxide *Cannabis* Cocaine Opiates Methadone
Others	Aminocaproic acid Baclofen Steroids Ethionamide Digoxin Chemotherapeutic agents Lithium

Erectile dysfunction (ED) is the inability to achieve or maintain an erection satisfactory for sexual performance. ED happens when not enough blood flows to the penis during sexual stimulation. This may be caused by psychoemotional problems, diabetes, hypertension, lower urinary tract symptoms, pelvic surgery, vascular insufficiency, neurologic disorders, androgen deficiency or resistance, or diseases of the penis. ED caused by vascular insufficiency is occasionally treated on a short-term basis by local vasoactive drugs, including papaverine, phentolamine, prostaglandin E, and nitroglycerin. Other drug options for the treatment of ED include oral drugs, drugs injected into the penis, intraurethral alprostadil, or testosterone.

A class of drugs called *phosphodiesterase inhibitors* facilitate erection by enhancing blood flow to the penis. Phosphodiesterase-5 (PDE-5) inhibitors are currently the most commonly used medical treatment for ED. These drugs have a high success rate, are easy to use, and often result in erection during sexual stimulation. The PDE-5 inhibitors currently approved by the

TABLE 53.5 **Phosphodiesterase-5 Inhibitors for Erectile Dysfunction**			
Generic	**Onset/Duration**	**Side Effects**	**Drug Interactions**
Avanafil 50-200 mg; not affected by food	Onset: 15-30 min Duration: 4-6 h Use once in 24 h.	• Abdominal symptoms such as diarrhea, heartburn, and upset stomach • Abnormal vision such as blurring and sensitivity to light and blue-green color tint • Dizziness • Flushing • Headache • Nasal congestion	• Nitrates: Isosorbide, nitroglycerin, amyl nitrate, butyl nitrate • Alpha blockers: Alfuzosin, doxazosin, prazosin, tamsulosin, terazosin, amiodarone • Antiinfective agents: Fluconazole, itraconazole, ketoconazole, clarithromycin, moxifloxacin, erythromycin • Cardiac drugs: Disopyramide, procainamide, quinidine, sotalol, thioridazine, verapamil • HIV protease inhibitors: Atazanavir, indinavir, ritonavir, saquinavir • Other drugs: Methadone, pimozide, haloperidol
Sildenafil 20 mg; works best on an empty stomach	Onset: 30-60 min Duration: 4 h		
Tadalafil 5-20 mg; not affected by food	Onset: 15-60 min Duration: 24-36 h		
Vardenafil 10 mg; less effective with a high-fat meal	Onset: 25-30 min Duration: 4-5 h Use once in 24 h.		

h, Hour; *HIV*, human immunodeficiency virus; *min*, minute.

FDA are sildenafil, tadalafil, vardenafil, and avanafil. PDE-5 inhibitors are taken before sexual activity with variations in effective start time and duration of benefit (Table 53.5).

Nitroglycerin and other nitrate drugs used to treat heart disease can cause a significant decrease in blood pressure when taken with PDE-5 inhibitors, therefore this class of drugs is contraindicated for use by any patient using organic nitrates in *any* form. Patients with a prescription for as-needed (PRN) sublingual nitroglycerin can take PDE-5 inhibitors but should still be cautioned about taking them concomitantly. Organic nitrates include nitroglycerin, isosorbide mononitrate, isosorbide nitrate, isosorbide dinitrate/phenobarbital, pentaerythritol tetranitrate, erythritol tetranitrate, and illicit substances (amyl nitrate/nitrite, butyl nitrate). Sildenafil is contraindicated in patients with significant cardiovascular disease and in individuals who have anatomic deformities or conditions that predispose them to priapism.

Studies have shown that vardenafil and tadalafil are safer for patients with heart failure or a history of myocardial infarctions. Like sildenafil, they are contraindicated if the patient is taking nitrate-containing drugs. Common side effects of these drugs are headache (most common), dyspepsia, nasal congestion, and nasopharyngitis. Other rare side effects can also occur, and the patient should be taught about them; these effects include blurred vision, photosensitivity, changes in color perception (especially blue and green), hearing loss, seizures, priapism and urinary tract symptoms such as frequent or painful urination and cloudy or bloody urine. Patients are instructed to notify their health care provider of any side effects they experience.

The PDE-5 inhibitors interact with grapefruit juice and grapefruit products by increasing the amount of the PDE-5 inhibitor absorbed, thereby increasing the risk of side effects. Many drugs interact with PDE-5 inhibitors, so be sure to obtain a complete list of drugs taken by the patient.

Certain drugs are often abused by individuals seeking a heightened sexual experience. Amyl nitrate is commonly believed to be an aphrodisiac. Sudden death, myocardial infarction, and methemoglobinemia have been reported with its use. Cantharides (Spanish fly) causes bladder and urethral irritation, accounting for its use as a sexual stimulant. Permanent penile damage has been reported with its use.

> ### ⚡ PATIENT SAFETY
>
> **Do not confuse...**
> - **Lupron Depot-3 Month** with **Lupron Depot-Ped**
> - **Anabolic steroids** with **corticosteroids**

Complementary and Alternative Medicine. To self-treat sexual problems or to enhance sexual performance, consumers use a wide variety of herbs and plant-derived compounds (phytochemicals). Despite new science-based therapies, men are attracted to phytochemicals because they are easy to obtain and may be cheaper than prescription drugs and therapies, procedures, or surgeries not covered by insurance. Consumers may mistakenly perceive natural products as providing health benefits beyond sexual performance because they can be purchased at nutrition centers or health food stores. Common herbs used for sexual health and performance include *Pausinystalia yohimbine, Panax quinquefolius*, ginkgo biloba, saw palmetto, muira puama, *Lepidium meyenii, Mandia whitei,* and *Tribulus terrestris*. Limited studies have been conducted on these products; all studies have yielded mixed results. As such, there is insufficient evidence to recommend any complementary or alternative medicine (CAM). Its benefits appear to reflect popular or cultural beliefs. Reports in health magazines and advertising are anecdotal and based on a small number of users. However, it is important for the nurse to be aware of CAM, as ED affects 50% of men between the ages of 50 and 70, but only 10% seek medical attention. These statistics indicate men may be choosing to use CAM to avoid the discomfort of discussing this sensitive topic with their health care provider.

Non–Sexually Transmitted Infections

Drugs used to treat acute or chronic prostatitis, orchitis, or epididymitis are the same as those used to treat urinary tract infections (see Chapter 48).

Benign Prostatic Hyperplasia. As a man ages, the glandular units in the prostate gland begin to undergo tissue hyperplasia, an abnormal increase in the number of cells, which results in prostatic hypertrophy, or enlargement of the gland. The

TABLE 53.6   Drugs Used for Treatment of Benign Prostatic Hyperplasia

Drug	Route and Dosage	Side Effects
5-ALPHA-REDUCTASE INHIBITORS		
Finasteride	PO: 5 mg daily	Decreased libido, erectile dysfunction, orthostatic
Dutasteride	PO: 0.5 mg daily	hypotension, gynecomastia

SAFETY IN ADMINISTRATION

Women of childbearing age must not handle crushed or broken tablets due to possible absorption and potential risk to male fetuses; immediately wash contact area with soap and water if contact occurs. Inform patients of an increase in high-grade prostate cancer in men treated with 5-alpha-reductase inhibitors indicated for BPH treatment. Inform patients that the volume of ejaculate may be decreased and that impotence or decreased libido may occur. Instruct patients to promptly report to their physician any changes in breasts (lumps, pain, or nipple discharge).

Drug	Route and Dosage	Side Effects
ALPHA-ADRENERGIC BLOCKING AGENTS		
Tamsulosin	PO: 0.4 mg/d 30 min after a meal; titrate up to 0.8 mg/d	Postural hypotension, dizziness, fatigue, headache,
Doxazosin	PO: Start 1 mg/d at bedtime; titrate up to 8 mg/d	edema, rhinitis, dyspnea, palpitations, blurred
Terazosin	A: PO: Start 1 mg/d at bedtime; titrate up to 10 mg/d *max:* 20 mg/d	vision, polyuria.
Alfuzosin	PO: 10 mg/d after a meal	
Silodosin	PO: 8 mg/d with a meal	

SAFETY IN ADMINISTRATION

Alpha-adrenergic blocking agents are also used to control blood pressure. To avoid hypotensive episodes, advise using at bedtime, and reconcile all drugs taken before adding another antihypertensive drug.

Instruct patients to take these drugs with food. Counsel about possible symptoms of postural hypotension (dizziness); caution patients about driving, operating machinery, or performing hazardous tasks while using these drugs. Inform patients that orgasm with reduced or no semen does not pose a safety concern and is reversible when the drug is stopped. Advise patients to notify their ophthalmologist about use before cataract surgery or other eye procedures.

Drug	Route and Dosage	Side Effects
PHOSPHODIESTERASE-5 INHIBITORS		
Tadalafil	PO: 5 mg	See Table 53.5.

SAFETY IN ADMINISTRATION

Tadalafil should not be used by patients taking nitrates such as nitroglycerin because the combination may trigger an unsafe drop in blood pressure. Tadalafil should not be used with alpha blockers for the treatment of BPH because the combo therapy has not been adequately studied and may increase the risk of lowering blood pressure.

A, Adult; *BPH,* benign prostatic hyperplasia; *d,* day; *max,* maximum; *min,* minute; *PO,* by mouth.

exact cause of BPH is unknown, but its development is almost universal in older men. The enlarged prostate gland contributes to overall lower urinary tract symptoms either through direct bladder outlet obstruction or from resistance within the enlarged gland itself. The man experiences storage and/or voiding disturbances, such as a sensation of bladder fullness, frequency, nocturia, hesitation when trying to begin urinating, dribbling of urine, and erectile dysfunction. Although BPH is not a life-threatening condition, the impact of symptoms on quality of life can be significant. Because these are the same symptoms that prostate cancer may cause, the patient should have a prostate-specific antigen (PSA) blood test and may undergo a prostate biopsy to make sure no cancer is present. Traditionally, the primary goal of treatment has been to alleviate bothersome symptoms. More recently, treatment has also been focused on the alteration of disease progression and prevention of complications. Drugs from several pharmacologic classes are used; they include alpha-adrenergic antagonists (alpha blockers), 5-alpha-reductase inhibitors (5-ARIs), anticholinergics (only used in men without large post-void residuals), and the PDE-5 inhibitor tadalafil. Choosing the correct medical treatment for BPH is complex (Table 53.6). The

American Urological Association 2010 Guidelines are a useful reference on the effective evidence-based management of lower urinary tract symptoms caused by BPH. The guidelines advise a discussion of benefits and risks of each recommended treatment alternative (e.g., watchful waiting; medical, surgical, or minimally invasive surgical treatments). The choice of treatment is reached in a shared decision-making process between provider and patient.

With initiation of drug therapy, the patient should be followed every 1 to 3 months, depending on the class of drug chosen, to assess success and inquire about side effects. The patient with an enlarged prostate should avoid drugs that can cause urinary retention, such as anticholinergics, antihistamines, and decongestants.

Malignant Tumors. Prostatic cancer accounts for about 10% of all cancer deaths among American men. Most prostatic cancers are adenocarcinomas. Metastasis to lymph nodes, bone, lungs, liver, and adrenal glands is common. Prostatic cancer is often asymptomatic, but urinary obstruction is commonly the first sign. Treatment may include a combination of surgical resection, cryotherapy, antiandrogen administration, radiation therapy, chemotherapy, and pain management.

Testicular tumors peak in early adulthood. They include malignant germinal cell tumors and benign Leydig or Sertoli cell tumors. Treatment depends on the type and stage of the tumor. Surgical excision, radiation therapy, and chemotherapy are used alone or in combination.

Approximately 1% of breast cancer cases occur in men, most commonly after the age of 60 years. Treatment is similar for men and women and entails surgery, radiation therapy, chemotherapy, and endocrine therapy. Carcinoma of the penis represents less than 1% of all malignancies among men. In situ, treatment entails local excision, radiation therapy, and local application of 5-fluorouracil cream or solution. Invasive carcinoma is treated by surgical resection of the penis and the involved nodes. Radiation and chemotherapy follow as needed.

CRITICAL THINKING CASE STUDY

MT, age 16 years, is a high school junior who is 59.3 inches tall and weighs 126 pounds. He is having increased feelings of discomfort about not fitting in with the other students at school because he has not yet begun sexual maturation. He is a good student and an accomplished violinist in the school orchestra. His father states that he also was a "late bloomer," but both parents are concerned about MT's increasing social withdrawal and seem determined to seek medical intervention for him. The nurse at the clinic assesses the needs and status of MT and his parents.

1. What is the patient's primary complaint?
2. What is concerning MT's parents?
3. What information must be included in the history and physical examination?
4. What education should the nurse prepare before the parents decide whether to start their son on androgen therapy? The decision is made to prescribe testosterone 30 mg every 12 hours by buccal tablet (held inside the cheek until it dissolves). MT will be on this regimen for 4 months, during which time he is to come to the clinic at monthly intervals.
5. MT asks why he will be treated for 4 months. What will the nurse reply?
6. About what adverse effects do MT and his parents need to be educated?
7. What physical and psychosocial parameters will be assessed at MT's monthly visits?
8. What special hygiene needs does MT have while on this regimen?
9. When should MT have x-rays taken? Explain your answer.
10. During a clinical visit, MT mentions that he heard that the use of anabolic steroids might improve his chances of making the wrestling team. What should he be told about the safety and efficacy of anabolic steroid use?

NCLEX STUDY QUESTIONS

1. A young male patient is referred to the nurse for initiation of intramuscular androgen therapy for hypogonadism. What information should the nurse give this patient? (Select all that apply.)
   a. A 4- to 6-month trial of androgen therapy will be followed by a period of rest for reevaluation.
   b. Sexual development will begin to occur immediately.
   c. Dosages may be adjusted based on periodic plasma testosterone levels.
   d. Growth will be monitored periodically by radiography.
   e. The patient should not consume alcohol.

2. A married man with two daughters is taking finasteride to treat benign prostatic hyperplasia. Which nursing assessment data are most critical in developing a care plan? (Select all that apply.)
   a. His spouse and children should not handle the drug.
   b. The drug may cause decreased libido and urinary retention.
   c. The dose needs to be reevaluated periodically.
   d. This drug may also cause his hair to grow.
   e. Using finasteride will not increase his risk for developing prostate cancer.

3. The nurse is discussing androgen therapy with a patient. Which statements will the nurse include in the patient education? (Select all that apply.)
   a. Lower extremity edema associated with androgen therapy can be increased by corticosteroids.
   b. Only men are prescribed androgen replacement therapy.
   c. Androgen therapy is safe in pregnancy.
   d. Androgen therapy can affect glucose levels, cholesterol, and thyroid and liver functioning.
   e. Androgen therapy may cause seizures.

4. During his annual physical examination, a patient tells the nurse he is in a new relationship and having some problems with erectile dysfunction. He is interested in nutrition and natural therapies. Which are the most appropriate responses by the nurse? (Select all that apply.)
   a. Herbal therapies are commonly used by men to enhance sexual performance.
   b. Side effects from using some herbal therapies include increased anxiety, frequent headaches, and trouble sleeping.
   c. Phytochemicals have been widely researched and are safe to use.
   d. Men who have cardiovascular, neurologic, or psychological problems should not use some of the herbal products.
   e. It is a good idea to increase intake of dietary vitamins.

5. The nurse is interviewing a man with erectile dysfunction who is interested in one of the phosphodiesterase inhibitors. Which response by the nurse is best for this patient?
   a. The onset of action varies among the different drugs in this class.
   b. These drugs should not be used if you take nitroglycerine for angina.
   c. Common side effects include headache, blurred vision, photosensitivity, changes in color perception, and urinary tract symptoms.
   d. There are many causes of sexual dysfunction in men, so a complete history and physical is the first step in treatment.

6. A 17-year-old is brought to the health care provider by his father because he has been taking nutritional supplements sold at the gym. Which assessment data are most critical in developing a care plan for this patient? (Select all that apply.)
   a. His blood pressure is low.
   b. His acne is worsening.
   c. He has been in several fistfights with other teenagers.
   d. He has gained 60 pounds.
   e. His liver function tests are abnormal.

7. A male patient presents with complaints of lower urinary tract symptoms, getting up three times at night to urinate, dribbling after urination, and feeling pressure throughout the day. Recent screening laboratory tests are normal. The provider starts him on doxazosin 1 mg at bedtime. What advice can the nurse give this patient? (Select all that apply.)
   a. Advise the patient about signs and symptoms of low blood pressure.
   b. Tell the patient to notify his ophthalmologist about the doxazosin use before cataract surgery.
   c. Caution the patient that he should not allow his wife to handle the medicine.
   d. Advise the patient to immediately report problematic prolonged erection.
   e. Instruct the patient to take the drug on an empty stomach.

Answers: 1. a, c, d; 2. a, b, c, d; 3. a, d; 4. a, b, d; 5. d; 6. b, c, d, e; 7. a, b, d.

54

Sexually Transmitted Infections

ⓔ http://evolve.elsevier.com/McCuistion/pharmacology

OBJECTIVES

- Describe the pharmacologic intervention for sexually transmitted infections (STIs) caused by bacterial and viral agents, parasites, and other pathogens.

- Describe the nursing process, including teaching, related to the prevention of STIs.

OUTLINE

KEY TERMS

Each day, over 1 million new cases of sexually transmitted infection (STI) occur worldwide. The incidence of STIs has been increasing since 2013. Young adults are at risk, particularly young women, but infections among men are also rising. Over 30 bacteria, viruses, and parasites can cause STIs. The most common bacterial pathogens are *Chlamydia, Neisseria gonorrhoeae,* and *Treponema pallidum* (syphilis); *Trichomonas* is a common parasite; and the most common viral pathogens are hepatitis B virus (HBV), herpes simplex virus (HSV), human immunodeficiency virus (HIV), and human papillomavirus (HPV). The majority of persons with STIs experience few or no symptoms, making it difficult to diagnose and treat to stop the spread of infections. STIs are spread through sexual contact, via blood or blood products, and through mother-to-child transmission during pregnancy and childbirth.

SEXUALLY TRANSMITTED INFECTIONS

Sexual transmission of pathogens can occur through breaks in the vaginal or cervical mucosa or in the skin covering the shaft or glans of the penis. Each act of coitus results in tiny, friction-induced fissures on these surfaces. Seminal fluid, spermatozoa, vaginal secretions, blood, and other body fluids can carry pathogens. Skin and mucosal lesions can be penetrated by microorganisms, and skin and mucosa can shed microorganisms.

Sexual contact can involve transmission of pathogens through the skin or mouth and via oral-genital, oral-anal, or hand-anal transmission of pathogens through breaks in the skin or mucosal surfaces or from inoculation by infectious body fluids. Anal penetration is particularly risky because of the likelihood of tissue trauma that results in the partner's exposure to enteric microorganisms. The risk for contracting an STI increases with substance abuse, imprisonment, sexual activity with a partner who has been imprisoned, sexual activity with individuals being paid for sex acts, and rape or sexual assault.

Patients who engage in sexual activity with multiple partners are at high risk for transmission of STIs, particularly HIV. The Centers for Disease Control and Prevention (CDC) reports the risk for getting STIs is markedly increased among individuals who have more than one sexual partner per year versus those who have fewer partners. It should be noted that 5.2% of men between the ages of 15 and 44 report having 5 or more partners in a 12-month period, and 2% of women report the same. Additionally, 21.8% of men between the ages of 15 and 44 report having had 15 or more sexual partners, and 10.6% of women report the same.

Other high-risk practices are anal or vaginal intercourse without a condom, hand-anal contact, contact with menstrual blood during sexual activity, use of an enema before anal intercourse, and urination on broken skin or inside the body. Refer to Fig. 54.1 for guidelines provided by the CDC on the prevention of STIs.

STIs are often manifested as multiple infections. Individuals undergoing treatment for one STI should be assessed for others,

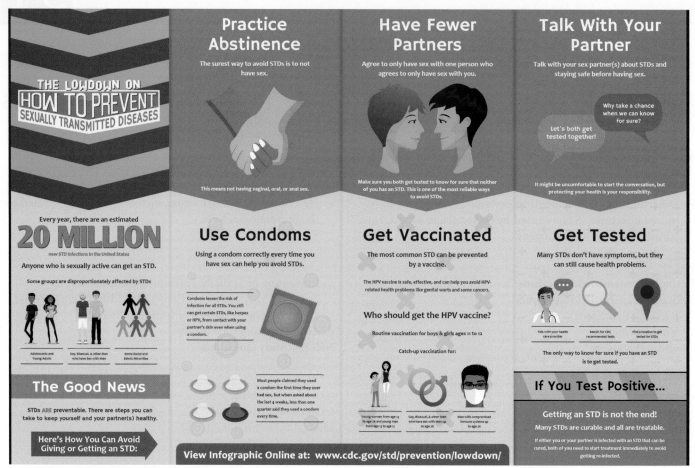

FIG. 54.1 How to Prevent Sexually Transmitted Infections. From Centers for Disease Control and Prevention. (2016). How you can prevent sexually transmitted diseases. Retrieved from www.cdc.gov/std/prevention

including HIV. This is especially true if genital or perianal ulcerations are present.

Vertical transmission is the passage of infecting organisms from mother to neonate. Microbes can travel up the reproductive tract from the vagina or cervix and enter the intrauterine environment. Organisms that are of little consequence to healthy adults can be devastating to a fetus. Transmission can also occur through contact with the mother's blood at birth or through breast milk, as in the case of HIV and HBV. Many STIs, such as syphilis, are transmitted through the placenta and membranes. Others, such as the herpes simplex virus type 2 (HSV-2), require actual contact by the infant with microorganisms in the birth canal. Because of the risk for blindness caused by *Chlamydia trachomatis* and *N. gonorrhoeae*, erythromycin ointment is routinely administered in the eyes of neonates as prophylaxis. This is usually done within the first hour after birth.

CDC guidelines for the primary treatment of some STI pathogens are listed in Table 54.1; the most common pathogens are discussed in the following section. All sexual contacts of an infected individual should be informed of the exposure so they can be treated. Partners should refrain from sexual activity until each is clear of infection on follow-up evaluation or, at the very least, condoms should be used until each is clear of infection.

SEXUALLY TRANSMITTED PATHOGENS

The information in this chapter comes directly from the 2015 treatment guidelines for sexually transmitted infections, available at www.cdc.gov/std/tg2015/default.htm.

Bacterial Pathogens

Sexually transmitted bacterial pathogens can be effectively treated with antibiotic therapy. When present, common symptoms include vaginal discharge, urethral discharge or burning (in men), genital ulcers, and abdominal pain.

Bacterial Vaginosis

Bacterial vaginosis (BV) causes a large amount of homogenous, thin, white vaginal discharge with a strong fishy odor. In BV, normal, healthy bacteria in the vagina—lactobacilli—are replaced with anaerobic bacteria, most commonly *Gardnerella vaginalis, Mycoplasma hominis, Ureaplasma urealyticum,* or *Prevotella, Porphyromonas, Bacteroides, Peptostreptococcus, and Mobiluncus* species. BV can be transmitted via sexual contact but is not considered an STI; however, having BV can increase a woman's risk for getting an STI due to the imbalance in vaginal bacteria.

BV is treated with metronidazole 500 mg by mouth (PO) twice a day for 7 days. Because metronidazole can cause

TABLE 54.1   Current Guidelines for Other Sexually Transmitted Infections

Pathogen	Primary Therapy	Notes
Haemophilus ducreyi (chancroid)	Azithromycin PO: 1 g, single dose *or* Ceftriaxone IM: 250 mg, single dose *or* Ciprofloxacin PO: 500 mg bid for 3 d *or* Erythromycin base PO: 500 mg tid for 7 d Data suggest ciprofloxacin presents a low risk to the fetus during pregnancy with a potential for toxicity during breastfeeding, therefore alternate drugs should be used during pregnancy and lactation.	Regardless of whether symptoms of the disease are present, sex partners of patients who have chancroid should be examined and treated if they had sexual contact with the patient during the 10 days preceding the patient's onset of symptoms. Chancroid is a risk factor in the transmission and acquisition of HIV infection.
Klebsiella granulomatis (granuloma inguinale)	Recommended regimen: Azithromycin PO: 1 g/wk or 500 mg/d for at least 3 wk and until all lesions have completely healed Alternative regimens: Doxycycline PO: 100 mg bid for at least 3 wk and until all lesions have completely healed *or* Ciprofloxacin PO: 750 mg bid for at least 3 wk and until all lesions have completely healed *or* Erythromycin base PO: 500 mg four times a day for at least 3 wk and until all lesions have completely healed *or* Trimethoprim-sulfamethoxazole PO: One double-strength (160 mg/800 mg) tablet bid for at least 3 wk and until all lesions have completely healed	All persons who receive a diagnosis of granuloma inguinale should be tested for HIV. Persons who have had sexual contact with a patient who has granuloma inguinale within the 60 days before onset of the patient's symptoms should be examined and offered therapy. Doxycycline should be avoided in the second and third trimester of pregnancy because of the risk for discoloration of teeth and bones, but it is compatible with breastfeeding. Data suggest that ciprofloxacin presents a low risk to the fetus during pregnancy. Alternate drugs should be used during pregnancy and lactation.
Hepatitis A virus (HAV)	Patients with acute HAV usually require only supportive care, with no restrictions in diet or activity. Hospitalization might be necessary for patients who become dehydrated because of nausea and vomiting and is critical for patients with signs or symptoms of acute liver failure.	Vaccination is the most effective means of preventing HAV transmission among persons at risk for infection (see Chapter 31 for a discussion on vaccines).
Hepatitis B virus (HBV)	No specific therapy is available for persons with acute hepatitis B; treatment is supportive.	Two products have been approved for hepatitis B prevention: hepatitis B immune globulin (HBIG; recommended dose is 0.06 mL/kg IM x one) for postexposure prophylaxis and hepatitis B vaccine (see Chapter 31 for a discussion on vaccines).
Hepatitis C virus (HCV)	The treatment of HCV is constantly changing; please see www.hcvguidelines.org for the latest recommendations.	No vaccine for hepatitis C is available, and prophylaxis with immune globulin is not effective in preventing HCV infection after exposure.
Chlamydia trachomatis serovars (lymphogranuloma venereum [LGV])	Recommended regimen: Doxycycline PO: 100 mg bid for 21 d Alternative regimen: Erythromycin base PO: 500 mg four times a day for 21 d Pregnant and lactating women should be treated with erythromycin. Doxycycline should be avoided in the second and third trimester of pregnancy because of risk for discoloration of teeth and bones, but it is compatible with breastfeeding.	Persons who have had sexual contact with a patient who has LGV within the 60 days before onset of the patient's symptoms should be examined and tested for urethral, cervical, or rectal chlamydial infection depending on anatomic site of exposure. They should be presumptively treated with an antichlamydial regimen (azithromycin 1 g PO single dose or doxycycline 100 mg PO bid for 7 d).

Continued

Pathogen	Primary Therapy	Notes
Molluscum contagiosum virus	Molluscum contagiosum is self-limited in healthy individuals, so treatment may be unnecessary. Treatment is usually recommended if lesions are in the genital area (on or near the penis, vulva, vagina, or anus). *Physical removal:* Cryotherapy (freezing the lesion with liquid nitrogen), curettage (the piercing of the core and scraping of caseous [cheesy] material), and laser therapy may be effective. *Oral therapy:* Drug therapy may result in the gradual disappearance of lesions and is often desirable for pediatric patients because it is generally less painful and can be administered by the parents at home (i.e., a less threatening environment). Oral cimetidine has been used as an alternative treatment for small children. *Topical therapy:* Podophyllotoxin cream (0.5%) is reliable as a home therapy for men but is not recommended for pregnant women because of presumed toxicity to the fetus. Each lesion must be treated individually because the therapeutic effect is localized. Other topical options include iodine and salicylic acid, potassium hydroxide, tretinoin, cantharidin (a blistering agent usually applied in an office setting), and imiquimod (a T-cell modifier).	If all lesions are not eradicated, infection may recur.
Zika virus	*Treat the symptoms:* Get plenty of rest. Drink fluids to prevent dehydration. Take medicine such as acetaminophen or paracetamol to reduce fever and pain. To reduce the risk of bleeding, do not take aspirin or other NSAIDS until dengue can be ruled out.	There is no vaccine to prevent or medicine to treat Zika virus.

TABLE 54.1   Current Guidelines for Other Sexually Transmitted Infections—cont'd

bid, Twice daily; *d,* day; *HIV,* human immunodeficiency virus; *IM,* intramuscularly; *NSAID,* nonsteroidal antiinflammatory drug; *PO,* by mouth; *tid,* three times daily; *wk,* weeks.
From Centers for Disease Control and Prevention. (2015). 2015 Sexually transmitted diseases treatment guidelines. Retrieved from https://www.cdc.gov/std/tg2015/default.htm

stomach upset, it should be taken with food or a full glass of water or milk. Alcohol causes severe nausea and vomiting when ingested with metronidazole, so patients should be instructed not to drink alcoholic beverages or use products that contain alcohol, such as mouthwash, for the duration of drug therapy and for 48 hours after treatment.

Vaginal preparations are also effective in treating BV, such as metronidazole gel 0.75%, one 5-g applicator intravaginally at bedtime for 5 nights; clindamycin cream 2%, one 5-g applicator intravaginally at bedtime for 5 days; or clindamycin ovules, 100 mg intravaginally at bedtime for 3 days.

Oral drugs that are alternatives to metronidazole include tinidazole, either 2 g orally once a day for 2 days or 1 g orally once a day for 5 days, or clindamycin 300 mg orally twice a day for 7 days. Tinidazole has the same precautions with alcohol as metronidazole and should be taken with food. Tinidazole causes slightly less gastrointestinal (GI) upset than metronidazole. Patients taking clindamycin should be instructed to notify their health care provider if diarrhea develops because it may be an indication of *Clostridium difficile*–associated diarrhea (CDAD). Treating BV is especially important for pregnant women because of the risk of spontaneous abortion, delivery of premature or low-birthweight babies, or pelvic infection developing after delivery. Metronidazole (oral or intravaginal) or clindamycin (oral) are the drugs of choice in pregnancy, and tinidazole should *not* be used during the first trimester of pregnancy. *None* of the drugs should be used by nursing mothers because these drugs are excreted in breast milk.

Chlamydia

Chlamydia trachomatis is the most common STI in the United States in young adults. This infection is most often asymptomatic. Women who contract the infection are at risk for developing pelvic inflammatory disease (PID), ectopic pregnancies, and infertility. Because of this, it is recommended that all sexually active women under the age of 25 be screened annually for *C. trachomatis* and that all women over 25 be screened based on risk factors.

The CDC recommends azithromycin 1 g orally in a single dose as treatment for *C. trachomatis* infections or doxycycline 100 mg orally twice a day for 7 days. Alternatively, erythromycin base 500 mg orally four times a day for 7 days, erythromycin ethylsuccinate 800 mg orally four times a day for 7 days, levofloxacin 500 mg orally once daily for 7 days, or ofloxacin 300 mg orally twice a day for 7 days may be given.

Doxycycline is contraindicated in the second and third trimesters of pregnancy. In the case of a chlamydial infection during pregnancy, azithromycin 1 g orally in a single dose is the treatment of choice. Alternatively, amoxicillin 500 mg orally three times a day for 7 days may be given. If neither azithromycin nor amoxicillin is an option, erythromycin may be used.

Neonates may contract *C. trachomatis* from exposure to the mother's infected cervix during delivery. It most frequently presents as conjunctivitis that develops 5 to 12 days after delivery; however, *C. trachomatis* can also cause pneumonia in infants between 1 and 3 months old. Prenatal screening and treatment is the best means of prevention. Erythromycin ophthalmic ointment, administered to prevent gonococcal ophthalmia, may also prevent conjunctivitis caused by *C. trachomatis*.

Persons treated for *Chlamydia* infection should be instructed to abstain from sexual intercourse for 7 days after single-dose therapy or until a 7-day regimen is completed. Partners should be treated if they had sexual contact during the 60 days preceding the onset of symptoms or diagnosis.

Gonorrhea

In the United States, gonorrhea is the second most common communicable disease. In men, infection by *N. gonorrhoeae* causes a greenish yellow or whitish discharge from the penis, accompanied by burning with urination. These symptoms usually prompt them to seek evaluation and treatment but often not until they have spread the infection to others. In women, *N. gonorrhoeae* is frequently asymptomatic. Left untreated, women with *N. gonorrhoeae* infections develop PID, which can cause tubal scarring that leads to ectopic pregnancies and infertility. Oral infections caused by *N. gonorrhoeae* cause sore throat and trouble swallowing; on examination, the pharynx resembles strep throat.

Because of the development of resistant *N. gonorrhoeae*, dual drug therapy is recommended with ceftriaxone 250 mg given intramuscularly (IM) in a single dose plus azithromycin 1 g orally in a single dose for uncomplicated urogenital infections or oral infections. If ceftriaxone is not available, cefixime 400 mg orally in a single dose plus azithromycin 1 g orally in a single dose may be given. Use of two drugs improves treatment efficacy and slows the development of drug resistance.

For those who are allergic to cephalosporins, gemifloxacin 320 mg orally in a single dose plus azithromycin 2 g orally in a single dose may be used; or, alternatively, gentamicin 240 mg IM in a single dose plus azithromycin 2 g orally in a single dose may be used. Women who are diagnosed with *N. gonorrhoeae* while pregnant should be treated with ceftriaxone 250 mg in a single IM dose and azithromycin 1 g orally as a single dose. Children under 45 kg should receive 25 to 50 mg/kg intravenously (IV) or IM, not to exceed 125 mg IM in a single dose.

Neonates may contract *N. gonorrhoeae* from exposure to the mother's infected cervix during delivery. The infection most frequently presents as an acute illness that develops 2 to 5 days after delivery. Prenatal screening and treatment is the best means of prevention, and most states require neonates to be administered erythromycin (0.5%) ophthalmic ointment in each eye in a single application at birth to prevent conjunctivitis caused by *N. gonorrhoeae*.

Persons receiving treatment for gonorrhea should be instructed to abstain from sexual activity for 7 days after treatment. Persons diagnosed with gonorrhea should also be tested for *Chlamydia*, syphilis, and HIV. Partners should be treated if they had sexual contact during the 60 days preceding the onset of symptoms or diagnosis.

Syphilis

Syphilis is caused by the bacteria *Treponema pallidum*; if not treated early in the infectious process, it produces systemic disease that can be fatal. The disease is divided into three stages: primary, secondary, and tertiary.

Primary syphilis infections present with a sore, or **chancre**, at the site where the infection entered the body—typically, the penis in men and outer genitals or inner vagina in women. It is usually painless. The chancre develops about 3 weeks after exposure and resolves in 3 to 6 weeks without treatment. During this stage, the person is very contagious, even after the chancre has resolved.

Secondary syphilis is characterized by a skin rash that appears 2 to 8 weeks after the chancre. It may occur anywhere on the body, commonly on the hands and soles of the feet; the rash usually does not itch. Mucocutaneous lesions, fever, fatigue, sore throat, and lymphadenopathy may occur as well. The rash usually resolves in about 2 months. During this stage, the person remains very contagious, even after the rash has resolved. After the rash has resolved, a period that lasts anywhere from 1 year to 20 years goes by without any symptoms. This is called the **latent stage**, and it occurs in persons who have gone untreated. A person may remain contagious during the latent period, and diagnosis can only be made through blood testing.

Tertiary syphilis may occur as early as 1 year after infection or at any time during an untreated person's lifetime. Large sores inside the body or on the skin occur in the tertiary stage, along with cardiovascular and ocular syphilis and neurosyphilis. Examination of the cerebral spinal fluid (CSF) should be done in persons in the tertiary stage to determine neurologic involvement, even in the absence of clinical neurologic findings.

To diagnose syphilis, two types of serologic testing are necessary to avoid false positives. One test should be a nontreponemal antibody test (e.g., Rapid Plasma Reagin [RPR] or Venereal Disease Research Laboratory [VDRL]) that tests for antibodies produced when a person has syphilis, although it may be produced in other diseases as well (e.g., Lyme disease or malaria). The other test should be a treponemal antibody test (e.g., fluorescent treponemal antibody absorption [FTA-ABS] or *T. pallidum* particle agglutination assay [TP-PA]), a test for antibodies that specifically target *T. pallidum*.

Treatment for primary and secondary syphilis is benzathine penicillin G, 2.4 million units given IM in one dose. Infants and children should be treated with benzathine penicillin G 50,000 units/kg IM up to the adult dose of 2.4 million units in a single dose, and these patients should be followed by a pediatric infectious disease specialist.

Adults with early latent syphilis should be treated with benzathine penicillin G 2.4 million units IM in a single dose; those with late latent syphilis or latent syphilis of unknown duration should receive benzathine penicillin G 7.2 million units total, administered as three doses of 2.4 million units IM each at 1-week intervals. Infants and children with early latent syphilis should be treated with benzathine penicillin G 50,000 units/kg IM, up to the adult dose of 2.4 million units in a single dose; those with late latent syphilis should receive benzathine penicillin G 50,000 units/kg IM, up to the adult dose of 2.4 million units, administered as three doses at 1-week intervals (total 150,000 units/kg up to the adult total dose of 7.2 million units). Infants and children should be managed by a pediatric infectious disease specialist.

Persons with tertiary syphilis should receive CSF analysis before initiating treatment. Those with normal CSF should receive benzathine penicillin G 7.2 million units total, administered as three doses of 2.4 million units IM each at 1-week intervals. Those with neurosyphilis or ocular syphilis should receive aqueous crystalline penicillin G 18 to 24 million units per day, administered as 3 to 4 million units IV every 4 hours or as a continuous infusion for 10 to 14 days. Alternatively, persons with neurosyphilis or ocular syphilis may be treated with procaine penicillin G 2.4 million units IM once daily plus probenecid 500 mg orally four times a day, both for 10 to 14 days. This alternative treatment should only be given to persons whose adherence can be ensured.

Pregnant women can pass syphilis to their fetus, with potentially fatal consequences. Benzathine penicillin G is the only treatment for syphilis during pregnancy. Pregnant women with syphilis in any stage who report they are allergic to penicillin should undergo penicillin allergy skin testing and desensitization, and then should be treated with penicillin.

Partners should be treated if they had sexual contact during the 90 days preceding the diagnosis of primary, secondary, or early latent syphilis even if serologic testing is negative. If greater than 90 days, treatment should be initiated if serologic testing is positive or if testing is not available. All persons with syphilis at any stage should be tested for HIV.

Viral Pathogens

Infection caused by viral pathogens is not curable, although medication therapy is palliative. These include herpes simplex virus 1 (HSV-1; cross-contaminated from oral to genital) and HSV-2, HPV, and HIV.

Herpes Simplex Virus

Genital herpes is a life-long viral infection. Two types of HSV can cause genital herpes: HSV-1 and HSV-2. Most cases of recurrent genital herpes are caused by HSV-2. Approximately 50 million people in the United States are infected with genital herpes. However, an increasing number of herpes infections are caused by HSV-1. Both types of the virus cause lesions that look like blisters, which crust over and scab. They may last for 2 to 4 weeks. The lesions may be accompanied by fever, lymphadenopathy, headache, and painful urination. Most HSV-2 cases go undiagnosed and are transmitted by people unaware that they have the infection or who are asymptomatic when transmission occurs.

Antiviral drugs are beneficial to most symptomatic patients and are the mainstay of management. It is imperative that nurses counsel patients with herpes regarding sexual and perinatal transmission and methods to reduce transmission.

Systemic antiviral drugs can control some of the signs and symptoms of genital herpes during initial and recurrent episodes or when used for daily suppressive therapy. However, these do not cure herpes or reduce the frequency and severity of recurrent episodes following drug discontinuation. Three antiviral drugs are used in the management of genital herpes: (1) acyclovir, (2) valacyclovir, and (3) famciclovir.

Recommendations for drug therapy of initial genital herpes infections is recommended using acyclovir 400 mg orally three times a day for 7 to 10 days, acyclovir 200 mg orally five times a day for 7 to 10 days, valacyclovir 1 g orally twice a day for 7 to 10 days, or famciclovir 250 mg orally three times a day for 7 to 10 days. Treatment can be extended if healing is incomplete after 10 days of therapy.

Suppressive therapy reduces the frequency of genital herpes recurrences by 70% to 80% in patients who have frequent recurrences. Recommended regimens are acyclovir 400 mg orally twice a day, valacyclovir 500 mg orally once a day, valacyclovir 1 g orally once a day, or famciclovir 250 mg orally twice a day. Valacyclovir 500 mg once a day might be less effective than other valacyclovir or acyclovir dosing regimens in persons who have 10 episodes or more per year.

For episodic treatment to be effective, treatment should begin within 1 day of lesion onset or during the prodrome (e.g., burning, itching, or tingling) that occurs anywhere from 30 minutes to a couple of days before some outbreaks. Patients should be provided with a prescription for the drug with instructions to initiate treatment immediately when symptoms begin. The recommended regimens for episodic therapy are acyclovir 400 mg orally three times a day for 5 days, acyclovir 800 mg orally twice a day for 5 days, acyclovir 800 mg orally three times a day for 2 days, valacyclovir 500 mg orally twice a day for 3 days, valacyclovir 1 g orally once a day for 5 days, famciclovir 125 mg orally twice daily for 5 days, famciclovir 1 g orally twice daily for 1 day, or famciclovir 500 mg once, followed by 250 mg twice daily for 2 days.

Sexual partners should be evaluated, treated if symptomatic, and counseled. Asymptomatic sex partners should be questioned about a history of genital lesions and offered serologic testing for HSV infection.

The risk of vertical transmission is high (30% to 50%) among women who become infected near the time of delivery and low (<1%) among women with a prenatal history of herpes or those who become infected early in the pregnancy. Prevention of vertical transmission depends on both preventing infection during late pregnancy and avoiding exposure to viral shedding during delivery. The recommended drug regimen for suppressive therapy of pregnant women with recurrent genital herpes is acyclovir 400 mg orally three times a day or valacyclovir 500 mg orally twice a day with treatment recommended starting at 36 weeks of gestation.

Human Immunodeficiency Virus

Two to four weeks after exposure, HIV infection typically presents with an acute flulike syndrome that includes fever, fatigue, rash, pharyngitis, and lymphadenopathy. HIV is a chronic illness that progressively depletes CD4 T lymphocytes and ends with symptomatic acquired immunodeficiency syndrome (AIDS). Early diagnosis and treatment is essential to reduce the risk of transmitting HIV to others and to maintain quality of life.

Persons with acute HIV infection are at high risk for transmitting HIV to their partner because the concentration of virus in blood and genital secretions is extremely elevated. Antiretroviral therapy (ART) during acute HIV infection is recommended because it substantially reduces transmission to others. See Chapter 29 for drugs used to treat HIV.

Partners (sexual partners and those with whom needles and syringes are shared) should be notified concerning possible exposure to HIV. Early diagnosis and treatment reduces the risk for further HIV transmission. Partner notification for HIV infection should be confidential.

All pregnant women should be tested for HIV infection during the first prenatal visit. A second test during the third trimester, preferably at less than 36 weeks' gestation, is recommended for those known to be at high risk for HIV.

Human Papillomavirus

Of the roughly 100 types of HPV infection that have been identified, nearly 40 infect the genital area. Most HPV infections are self-limited and asymptomatic, and most sexually active persons will become infected with HPV at some point in their lifetime. High-risk HPV infections (e.g., HPV types 16 and 18) cause most cervical, penile, vulvar, vaginal, anal, and oropharyngeal cancers. Low-risk HPV infection (e.g., HPV types 6 and 11) cause genital warts and recurrent respiratory papillomatosis. Screening with the Papanicolaou ("Pap") test can detect cervical dysplasia, which can be a precursor to cervical cancer if left untreated. Whereas the Pap test can determine whether the cervical cells are abnormal, an HPV test specifically looks for high-risk HPV in cervical cells.

There are several HPV vaccines approved for use in the United States: a bivalent vaccine that prevents infection with HPV types 16 and 18, which cause 66% of all cervical cancers; a quadrivalent vaccine that prevents infection with HPV types 6, 11, 16, and 18, which cause 90% of all genital warts; and a 9-valent vaccine that prevents infection with HPV types 6, 11, 16, 18, 31, 33, 45, 52, and 58. See Chapter 31 for a discussion on vaccines.

Because most HPV infections do no harm, they do not require treatment and tend to resolve on their own. Because of this, antiviral therapy is not recommended. Treatment is aimed at removal of genital warts and precancerous lesions and treatment of cervical cancer and includes cryotherapy (freezing) or a loop electrosurgical excision procedure (LEEP) to cut away abnormal tissue.

Condom use can lower the risk of transmitting and developing HPV infections. Limiting the number of sex partners can also reduce the risk for HPV. However, abstaining from sexual activity is the most reliable method for preventing HPV infection.

Other Pathogens

Pediculosis Pubis

Persons with pediculosis pubis, a parasitic infection caused by *Phthirus pubis,* usually seek treatment because of extreme pruritus of the body part or area where the lice are moving and laying egg cases. Infected persons may also notice lice or nits on their pubic hair. Pediculosis pubis is usually transmitted by sexual contact.

Recommended treatment is with a permethrin 1% cream rinse applied to affected areas and washed off after 10 minutes, or pyrethrins with piperonyl butoxide are applied to the affected area and washed off after 10 minutes. Alternatively, malathion 0.5% lotion can be applied to affected areas and washed off after 8 to 12 hours, or ivermectin 250 mcg/kg can be given orally and repeated in 2 weeks.

Sexual partners within the previous month should be treated, and bedding and clothing must be decontaminated. Sexual contact should be avoided until treatment is complete. Pregnant and lactating women should be treated with either permethrin or pyrethrins with piperonyl butoxide.

Scabies

Infection with *Sarcoptes scabiei* causes pruritus, which takes up to several weeks to develop. Scabies in adults frequently is sexually acquired, although scabies in children usually is not.

Treatment consists of permethrin 5% cream applied to all areas of the body from the neck down and washed off after 8 to 14 hours or ivermectin 200 mcg/kg orally, repeated in 2 weeks. Permethrin is the treatment of choice for infants and young children. Alternatively, lindane 1%—either 1 oz of lotion or 30 g of cream—applied in a thin layer to all areas of the body from the neck down and thoroughly washed off after 8 hours may be used; however, pregnant women, infants, and children under the age of 10 years should *not* be treated with lindane.

Bedding and clothing should be decontaminated by either machine washing, machine drying using the hottest cycle, or dry cleaning; alternatively, bedding and clothing should be removed from body contact for at least 72 hours. Persons who have had sexual, close personal, or household contact with the patient within the month preceding scabies infestation should be examined and treated if infected.

Ivermectin likely poses a low risk to pregnant women and is likely compatible with breastfeeding; however, because of limited data regarding ivermectin use in pregnant and lactating women, permethrin is the preferred treatment

Trichomoniasis

The protozoan parasite *Trichomonas vaginalis* is the most common curable STI in the United States. Nearly 7.5 million cases occur annually. Most people with *T. vaginalis* (70% to 85%) have minimal or no symptoms. Men may develop urethritis, epididymitis, or prostatitis. Some infected women may develop a diffuse vaginal discharge that is malodorous and yellow green, with or without vulvar irritation.

The nitroimidazoles are the only class of antimicrobials effective against *T. vaginalis*. Metronidazole and tinidazole are approved for oral or parenteral treatment of trichomoniasis. The recommended regimen is metronidazole 2 g orally in a single dose or tinidazole 2 g orally in a single dose. Alternatively, metronidazole 500 mg orally twice a day for 7 days may be used.

Alcohol should be avoided during treatment with nitroimidazoles to prevent the likelihood of a disulfiram-like reaction. Abstinence from alcohol use should continue for 24 hours after completion of metronidazole or 72 hours after completion of tinidazole. Concurrent treatment of all sex partners is critical to prevent transmission and reinfection.

T. vaginalis is readily passed between sex partners. The best way to prevent infection is through consistent and correct use of condoms. Partners of men who have been circumcised might have a somewhat reduced risk of *T. vaginalis* infection.

T. vaginalis infection in pregnant women is associated with premature rupture of membranes, preterm delivery, and delivery of a low-birthweight infant. The recommended treatment regimen in pregnant women is metronidazole 2 g orally in a single dose.

Vulvovaginal Candidiasis

Vulvovaginal candidiasis (VVC) is usually caused by *Candida albicans* but may also be caused by other *Candida* species. Typical symptoms of VVC include pruritus, vaginal soreness, dyspareunia, external dysuria, and abnormal vaginal discharge. Signs include vulvar edema, fissures, excoriations, and a thick, curdy vaginal discharge.

Treatment with topically applied azole drugs results in symptomatic relief and negative cultures in 80% to 90% of patients who complete therapy. A variety of over-the-counter (OTC) and prescription drugs may be used to treat VVC. Treatment regimens include OTC and prescription intravaginal agents.

Over-the-Counter Intravaginal Agents. Clotrimazole 1% cream 5 g intravaginally daily for 7 to 14 days, clotrimazole 2% cream 5 g intravaginally daily for 3 days, miconazole 2% cream 5 g intravaginally daily for 7 days, miconazole 4% cream 5 g intravaginally daily for 3 days, one miconazole 100-mg vaginal suppository daily for 7 days, one miconazole 200-mg vaginal suppository daily for 3 days, one miconazole 1200 mg vaginal suppository, or tioconazole 6.5% ointment 5 g intravaginally in a single application.

Prescription Intravaginal Agents. Butoconazole 2% cream (single-dose bioadhesive product) 5 g intravaginally in a single application, terconazole 0.4% cream 5 g intravaginally daily for 7 days, terconazole 0.8% cream 5 g intravaginally daily for 3 days, or one terconazole 80 mg vaginal suppository daily for 3 days. Alternatively, an oral drug—fluconazole 150 mg orally in a single dose—may be used.

Topical agents usually cause no systemic side effects, although local burning or irritation might occur. Oral azoles occasionally cause nausea, abdominal pain, and headache.

VVC occurs frequently during pregnancy. Only topical azole therapies, applied for 7 days, are recommended for use among pregnant women. Uncomplicated VVC is not usually acquired through sexual intercourse, thus treatment of sexual partners is not necessary.

Prevention of Sexually Transmitted Infections

Because STIs can threaten reproductive health, neonatal health, fertility, and even life, early diagnosis and treatment are crucial but are less effective than prevention. Please review the information in Box 54.1 and in the Nursing Process box that discusses STI prevention.

BOX 54.1   Special Topic: Sexually Transmitted Infections in the Older Adult

The rates of *Chlamydia*, gonorrhea, and syphilis have more than doubled in adults over the age of 50 in recent years. Over 15% of newly diagnosed cases of HIV occur in adults over the age of 50. This spike in sexually transmitted infections (STIs) is felt to be related to a combination of factors:

- We are living longer and have higher divorce rates than past generations, leading to increased numbers of older adults entering the dating scene.
- Postmenopausal changes in women (e.g., decreased vaginal lubrication) put them at increased risk for infection.
- The availability of drugs for erectile dysfunction makes sex possible for an increased number of older men.
- Rates of condom use are low because condoms were used to prevent pregnancy in previous generations, not to prevent STIs.

Nurses must discuss the risks for developing STIs with their older adult patients and should provide information on prevention. Nurses should not make the faulty assumption that older adults do not engage in sexual activity. Among men, 85% report that sex is important in their relationships; 61% of women report that sex is important in their relationships. Among older adults, 28% have sex at least once a week. However, only 12% of men and 32% of women use condoms.

 ### NURSING PROCESS
Patient-Centered Collaborative Care

Preventing Sexually Transmitted Infections

Assessment

- Assess use of barrier methods and the patient's ability to obtain them.
- Assess patient history before gathering physical data. Address less sensitive issues before more personal ones so trust can first be established. Use the term *partner* when discussing sexual activity, rather than judgment-laden terms such as *wife* or *boyfriend*. Include the following questions for all patients, regardless of gender or sexual orientation: "Do you have sex with women?" and "Do you have sex with men?" Include information regarding the number of sexual partners.
- Assess history of drug use.
- Assess history of STIs.
- Assess support systems.
- Complete a review of body systems and obtain a general health history and a gynecologic history that includes reproductive history; also review lifestyle and social habits, and identify known allergies.
- Physical examination includes inspection and palpation of the mouth, oropharynx, throat and lymph nodes, abdomen, and inguinal lymph systems. Also perform a physical

examination of the genitalia and other points of potential inoculation.

Nursing Diagnoses
- Health Maintenance, Ineffective related to deficient knowledge regarding transmission, symptoms, and treatment of STIs
- Infection, Risk for
- Injury, Risk for

Planning
- The patient will adopt risk-reducing sexual behaviors.
- The patient will remain free of STIs.
- The patient will verbalize five ways to prevent STIs.

Nursing Interventions
- Advise patients to plan periodic health checkups.
- Discuss condom use negotiation.
- Refer to Fig. 54.1.
- Counsel patients on effective use of both male and female condoms.
  - See Fig. 54.2 for the right way to use a male condom.
  - See Fig. 54.3 for the right way to use a female condom.
- Review modes of transmission of STIs, the relationship of all STIs to HIV infection, and how HIV risk is avoided.

🌐 *Cultural Considerations*
- In male-dominated cultures, male patients may be unwilling to undergo testing or treatment.
- Some women prefer to be examined only by a female health care provider.
- Use a certified medical interpreter of the same sex and culture, especially for sensitive topics.

Evaluation
- Intervention has been successful if patients and their partners remain free of infection.
- The patient is able to avoid sexual practices that carry risk for acquiring STIs, including intercourse without the use of a condom.

The Right Way To Use A Male Condom

Condom Dos and Don'ts

- DO use a condom every time you have sex.
- DO put on a condom before having sex.
- DO read the package and check the expiration date.
- DO make sure there are no tears or defects.
- DO store condoms in a cool, dry place.
- DO use latex or polyurethane condoms.
- DO use water or silicone-based lubricant to prevent breakage.
- DO remember that condoms come in many sizes and thicknesses, so find a brand that works best for you and your partner.

- DON'T store condoms in a car or keep them in your wallet.
- DON'T use nonoxynol-9 (a spermicide), as this can cause irritation.
- DON'T use oil-based products like baby oil, lotion, petroleum jelly, or cooking oil because they will cause the condom to break.
- DON'T use more than one condom at a time.
- DON'T reuse a condom.
- DON'T flush condoms as they may clog the toilet.

How To Put On and Take Off a Male Condom

Carefully open and remove condom from wrapper.

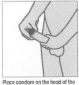
Place condom on the head of the erect, hard penis. If uncircumcised, pull back the foreskin first.

Pinch air out of the tip of the condom.

Unroll condom all the way down the penis.

After sex but before pulling out, hold the condom at the base and withdraw the penis.

Carefully remove the condom and throw it in the trash.

For more information please visit
www.cdc.gov/condomeffectiveness

FIG. 54.2 How to Use a Male Condom. From Centers for Disease Control and Prevention. (2016). The right way to use a male condom. Retrieved from www.cdc.gov/condomeffectiveness/male-condom-use.html

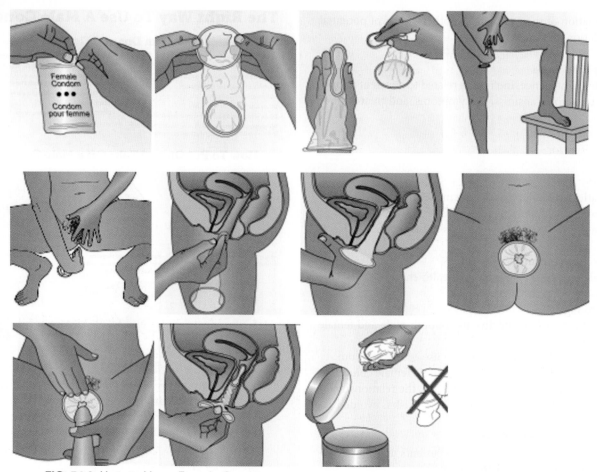

FIG. 54.3 How to Use a Female Condom.
1. Before using the female condom for the first time during sex, you should practice placing the condom in your vagina a couple of times. Inserting the condom becomes easier once you get the hang of it.
2. When you are ready to have intercourse, but before you become intimate, check the expiration date on the package to make sure that you can still use it. Then open the package and spread lubricant or spermicide on the outside of the closed end.
3. When you are ready to insert the female condom, you will need to find a comfortable position that works for you. Try squatting down, lying down, or placing one foot on a chair while standing.
4. Using your thumb and forefinger, squeeze the sides of the inner ring together. The condom may be a bit slippery, so make sure you have a firm grip before attempting to insert it into your vagina.
5. Using your forefinger as a guide, insert the inner ring much like you would a tampon, and push it up toward your cervix with your finger.
6. Once you have reached the cervix, the condom will expand naturally, and you will no longer be able to feel it. If you can still feel it, you have not placed it far enough inside.
7. Gently remove your finger and make sure that at least one inch of the condom is hanging outside of the vagina. Anything more than that indicates it has not been inserted far enough, and you'll need to check that the inner ring is positioned correctly.
8. When you are ready to have intercourse, have your partner insert his penis in the outer ring and into the condom. You may want to help him, making sure that his penis is actually entering the condom and not just pushing it to one side.
From New Health Advisor. (2016). How to use a female condom: Pictures and instructions. Retrieved from www.newhealthadvisor.com/How-to-Use-Female-Condom-Picture.html

CRITICAL THINKING CASE STUDY

A 16-year-old Caucasian female is seen in your office for evaluation of a possible STI. She states that her partner has noted a whitish penile discharge and has burning with urination. When questioned, she states she's been sexually active, both orally and vaginally, for 2 years and has had four partners. When questioned, she denies using any barrier methods to avoid infection, admits to having a sore throat, and denies vaginal symptoms.

1. What is the presumptive diagnosis?
2. Based on this diagnosis, what is the most appropriate treatment for your patient?
3. Why are two drugs recommended for treatment?
4. Should your patient's partner be treated? What about past partners?
5. What is the best way to avoid reinfection?

NCLEX STUDY QUESTIONS

1. A patient at the sexually transmitted infection clinic asks why he was not prescribed antibiotics. He has been diagnosed with herpes simplex virus type 2. The nurse's best response is based on what knowledge? (Select all that apply.)
   a. Antibiotics will not lessen the symptoms of herpes simplex virus.
   b. Herpes simplex virus can be cured with antiviral medications only.
   c. Antibiotics are used to successfully treat viral infections.
   d. Herpes simplex virus symptoms may be relieved with palliative antiviral medications.
   e. Antibiotics combined with antiviral medications are the best treatment for herpes simplex virus type 2 infections.
2. The nurse is teaching a group of junior high school students about preventing sexually transmitted infections if they are sexually active. Which of the following are the best methods of prevention? (Select all that apply).
   a. Douching after intercourse
   b. Monogamy
   c. Vaccination
   d. Consistent condom use
   e. Use of spermicidal creams
3. The nurse prepares a class for high school students. What best describes why ulcerative sexually transmitted infections increase an individual's risk for human immunodeficiency virus infection?
   a. Ulcerative sexually transmitted infections decrease the amount of lubrication.
   b. Sexually transmitted infections are commonly associated with other high-risk behaviors.
   c. Sexually transmitted infections are only found in individuals with multiple sexual partners.
   d. A break in the skin increases the transmission of pathogens.
4. The nurse is reviewing a patient's medications with her. The nurse knows that effective pharmacologic treatment for vulvovaginal candidiasis includes which drug?
   a. Metronidazole
   b. Fluconazole
   c. Metformin
   d. Ibuprofen

5. A patient has been diagnosed with primary syphilis. When assessing the patient, which of these findings will the health care provider anticipate?
   a. A painless genital ulcer
   b. Rash on the palms and the soles of feet
   c. Pharyngitis and lymphadenopathy
   d. Fatigue and visual changes
6. When teaching a group of students about *Chlamydia*, which of the following should the health care provider emphasize? (Select all that apply).
   a. Most people who have *Chlamydia* have no symptoms.
   b. Good handwashing technique is the best way to prevent chlamydial infections.
   c. *Chlamydia* is the least common of all the major sexually transmitted infections.
   d. Burning and pain with urination may be a symptom of chlamydial infections.
7. A patient diagnosed with trichomoniasis is being treated with a nitroimidazole. When teaching the patient about this medication, which of the following is the most important for the nurse to include?
   a. Call our office if you experience any tendon pain or tenderness.
   b. You should avoid milk or dairy products during therapy.
   c. Do not drink alcohol while you are taking this medication.
   d. Report the occurrence of pain in your upper abdomen immediately.
8. Your patient diagnosed with infection from *Trichomonas vaginalis* did not return for the 3-month follow-up. When called, she reported that she stopped taking the oral metronidazole that was prescribed because her symptoms resolved and she wanted to drink at her best friend's bridal shower. As her nurse, what is your best response?
   a. No serious complications can happen from untreated *T. vaginalis,* so don't worry.
   b. Without treatment, the organism remains in your body, and you remain contagious.
   c. Because your symptoms are gone, there is no need to complete the course of metronidazole.
   d. If symptoms return, come back.

Answers: 1, a, d; 2, b, c, d; 3, d; 4, b; 5, a; 6, a, d; 7, c; 8, b.

UNIT XVIII

Emergency Drugs

This final unit focuses on adult and pediatric first-line emergency drugs. Chapter 55 considers oxygen as an emergency drug and discusses pharmacologic treatment for five categories of emergency situations: (1) cardiac disorders, (2) intracranial hypertension, (3) poisoning, (4) shock, and (5) hypertensive crises and pulmonary edema. Specific drug protocols and dosages for the pediatric patient are included.

Drugs for cardiac disorders include treatments for angina, myocardial infarction (MI), cardiac arrhythmias, and cardiopulmonary arrest. Mannitol is described for the treatment of increased intracranial pressure. Treatment for poisonings may include opiate antagonists, benzodiazepine reversal agents, or activated charcoal. Treatment for shock is to improve cardiac performance, which includes the administration of fluids for hypovolemic shock. Hypertensive crises are generally treated with adrenergic blockers and/or drugs that inhibit the effects of the sympathetic and parasympathetic nervous systems. Diuretics, especially loop diuretics, and opiates such as morphine can be used for the management of pulmonary edema.

55

Adult and Pediatric Emergency Drugs

ⓔ http://evolve.elsevier.com/McCuistion/pharmacology/

OBJECTIVES

- Describe indications for the emergency drugs listed in this chapter.
- Define the basic mechanism of action for each emergency drug.
- Discuss pertinent nursing considerations and actions specific for each drug.
- Explain how to properly administer emergency drugs.
- Describe significant adverse effects of each drug.

OUTLINE

KEY TERMS

The drugs described in this chapter are first-line agents used to treat various medical emergencies. Nurses must have knowledge of the indications and actions of these drugs because medical and surgical emergencies can occur in virtually any area of nursing practice. Learning key nursing implications *before* a crisis situation enables the nurse to function at the highest possible level when the patient requires life-saving intervention.

At the end of the discussion of each group of emergency drugs is a summary prototype drug chart that contains dosages and indications. Common adult dosages are listed in the drug charts; pediatric dosages may vary widely depending on the child's age and weight. For the purpose of drug dosing, advanced life support (ALS) guidelines consider adults to be older than 8 years and children to be 8 years or younger; infants are younger than 1 year. The drug charts list only the most common indications and dosages for the emergency drugs discussed; they do *not* describe all possible uses and dosing regimens for each drug.

OXYGEN AS AN EMERGENCY DRUG

Oxygen can be classified as a drug because it can have both beneficial and adverse effects on the body based on the amount and manner in which it is administered. Oxygen is essential to life—without it, brain death begins within 6 minutes. Inadequate oxygenation produces hypoxemia, inadequate oxygen in the blood, and leads to significant physiologic sequelae to all body systems; therefore oxygen is a first-line drug for all emergency situations in which hypoxemia poses a physiologic threat. Depending on the circumstances, adequate oxygenation may be all that is necessary to effectively treat physiologic disturbances that arise from hypoxemia, such as chest pain, bradycardia, and cardiac dysrhythmias. Oxygen also acts as a potent pulmonary vasodilator and may be beneficial for patients in heart failure.

Before the other pharmacologic drugs discussed in this chapter are administered, ensure that the patient's airway and breathing are addressed to promote normoxemia, oxygen saturation between 94% and 99%. Giving a drug to treat a disorder brought on by hypoxemia without effectively correcting the cause of the hypoxemia is ineffective and ultimately does not produce the desired outcome. Pulse oximetry, which provides a digital display of oxygen saturation, is an essential monitoring tool that should be used in emergency situations to assess the adequacy of oxygenation and guide further interventions. Ideally oxygen saturation should be kept in a range between 94% and 99%. It is important to recognize, however, that certain pathophysiologic states can make pulse oximetry readings inaccurate. These conditions include vasoconstriction, severe anemia, hypothermia, carbon monoxide poisoning, and shock.

The ambient room air contains approximately 21% oxygen. When patients breathe room air, the oxygen they inspire constitutes 21% of the total volume of gas they take in with each breath. This measure is termed the fraction of inspired oxygen (FiO_2). Patients with hypoxemia due to severe physiologic stress from shock states, major traumatic injury, acute myocardial infarction (AMI) with hemodynamic instability, and cardiac arrest initially require supplemental oxygen in high concentrations (i.e., an FiO_2 close to 100%). The initial emergency oxygen delivery devices of choice for these conditions include a nonrebreather mask with an oxygen reservoir (oxygen flow rate set at 10 to 15 L/min) for spontaneously breathing patients and a bag-valve-mask device attached to an oxygen source at a flow rate of 15 L/min for patients who require assisted ventilation until definitive airway management and a mechanical ventilator are available.

Although caution must be exercised for patients with chronic obstructive pulmonary disease (COPD), who may lose their hypoxic respiratory drive when given oxygen in high concentration, oxygen should never be denied to a patient who needs it. In the case of COPD, the nurse should be prepared to ventilate the patient manually with a bag-valve-mask if respiratory depression or arrest occurs. Some patients in respiratory distress as a result of obstructive pulmonary disease or acute cardiogenic pulmonary edema may also benefit from oxygen therapy delivered through noninvasive mask ventilation via a continuous positive airway pressure (CPAP) or bilevel positive airway pressure (BiPAP) circuit; these devices deliver oxygen via a positive-pressure mechanism.

Whatever the underlying injury or disease process, as the patient's condition stabilizes, the oxygen concentration should be decreased to achieve an arterial oxygen saturation between 94% and 99%. An FiO_2 above 50% for a prolonged period can lead to oxygen toxicity and other detrimental effects in both adults and children.

For situations that do not involve severe physiologic stress (e.g., angina, dysrhythmias, pulmonary disease), supplemental oxygen delivered by nasal cannula at 1 to 6 L/min or by simple face mask at 6 to 10 L/min may be considered. Young children may better tolerate a face tent with a high oxygen flow of 10 to 15 L than a face mask. Current evidence suggests that oxygen administration to hemodynamically stable patients without heart failure who are normoxemic may offer no therapeutic benefit and should be avoided.

EMERGENCY DRUGS FOR CARDIAC DISORDERS

Drugs described in this section are indicated for cardiac emergencies such as angina, myocardial infarction ([MI] heart attack), disturbances of cardiac rate or rhythm, and cardiac arrest. In a resuscitation situation, the foundation of patient therapy is based upon proper oxygenation and ventilation, performance of optimal cardiopulmonary resuscitation (CPR), and application of electrical therapy (cardioversion and defibrillation) according to established treatment algorithms and standards. Pharmacologic drugs are used as adjuncts in synchrony with these efforts when indicated to enhance the likelihood of a successful outcome. These drugs often must be prepared and administered rapidly. A sound knowledge base and easy access to the drugs and necessary equipments are essential for the best patient response in a cardiac emergency. Usually in an emergency, detailed personal, medical, drug, and herbal histories are unavailable (Complementary and Alternative Therapies 55.1). Treatment is based on patient presentation.

Herbs and Emergency Medications

In emergency situations, a detailed personal health history is often not available; therefore treatment is based on patient presentation. Herbal products with anticoagulation properties or those that interact with catecholamines, which may cause hypertensive crisis, could adversely influence the effectiveness of medications used to treat emergency conditions.

Aspirin

The nonenteric form of aspirin is a first-line emergency drug used to decrease platelet aggregation in the management of acute coronary syndromes and MI. It is best administered immediately upon the onset of chest pain in doses of 162 to 325 mg orally. The patient should be asked to chew the tablet to speed absorption of the drug instead of swallowing the tablet whole. For patients experiencing nausea and vomiting, an aspirin rectal suppository in a dose of 300 mg can be given as an alternative. Aspirin is also indicated in the initial treatment algorithm for patients suffering from acute ischemic stroke who are not candidates for fibrinolytic therapy. Contraindications to aspirin administration include a true drug allergy, presence of cerebral hemorrhage on computed tomography (CT) scan, and recent gastrointestinal (GI) bleeding.

Nitroglycerin

Nitroglycerin dilates coronary arteries and improves blood flow to an ischemic myocardium. It is therefore the treatment of choice for angina pectoris (chest pain) and MI. Nitroglycerin is also considered a first-line drug in the management of patients with acute cardiogenic pulmonary edema due to its ability to decrease both preload and afterload. A focused prescription drug history is essential prior to administration, even in emergency situations, because nitroglycerin in combination with drugs for erectile dysfunction (i.e., sildenafil, vardenafil, tadalafil) causes profound hypotension that may be refractory to treatment when taken within a 24- to 48-hour period. This combination is contraindicated. Nitroglycerin is available in sublingual, translingual aerosol spray, oral, topical, and intravenous (IV) forms. Only the sublingual, translingual aerosol spray, and IV preparations are discussed.

Sublingual nitroglycerin (0.3 to 0.8 mg) and the translingual aerosol spray (0.4-mg metered dose) preparations are indicated for patients experiencing an acute anginal attack who have a systolic blood pressure above 90 mm Hg. The patient is taught to sit or lie down and moisten 1 sublingual nitroglycerin tablet with saliva and then place it under the tongue to allow it to dissolve slowly. If the chest pain is not relieved, sublingual nitroglycerin may be repeated at 3- to 5-minute intervals—as long as the patient's systolic blood pressure remains above 90 mm Hg—until a total of 3 tablets have been taken. Patients prescribed the translingual aerosol preparation should be reminded that the spray should not be inhaled. Instead, it should be sprayed onto or under the tongue. The patient should be instructed not to swallow for approximately 10 seconds to allow absorption of the drug. As with sublingual nitroglycerin, up to 3 doses may be taken within 15 minutes. If pain persists despite 3 doses of the sublingual or aerosol forms, further interventions are necessary in an emergency or critical care setting. An ambulance should be called if the patient is outside the hospital, and blood pressure and heart rate must be monitored closely. Hypotension is a common adverse effect, especially the first time a patient takes nitroglycerin. Tachycardia, an abnormally high heart rate in adults (>100 beats/min), or uncommonly bradycardia, a slow heart rate, also may occur. Patients who take sublingual or translingual aerosol spray nitroglycerin while wearing a nitroglycerin patch may be at higher risk for hypotension. This situation warrants caution. However, individuals who take daily nitroglycerin can develop tolerance to the drug, which can provide some protection against hypotension. If hypotension persists or worsens, the nitroglycerin patch may need to be removed. To prevent arcing and the potential for skin burns, the nitroglycerin patch must be removed prior to cardioversion or defibrillation.

IV nitroglycerin is reserved for patients with unstable angina or AMI. A continuous infusion is usually initiated at a rate of 5 mcg/min and titrated by 5 mcg/min every 3 to 5 minutes based on chest pain and blood pressure response. Maximum rate of titration is 20 mcg/min every 3 to 5 minutes. Continuous blood pressure and heart monitoring are required because hypotension is a common adverse effect. Hypotension usually is treated by reducing or discontinuing the nitroglycerin infusion (see Chapter 37) and by placing the patient in a supine position with legs elevated if tolerated.

Morphine Sulfate

Morphine sulfate, a narcotic analgesic, is used to treat the chest pain associated with ST-segment elevation myocardial infarction (STEMI). It also is indicated for acute cardiogenic pulmonary edema. Morphine relieves pain, dilates venous vessels, and reduces the workload on the heart. The standard dosage of morphine sulfate is 1 to 4 mg IV over 1 to 5 minutes, repeated every 5 to 30 minutes until chest pain is relieved. Because respiratory depression and hypotension are common adverse effects, the drug must be administered slowly and must be carefully titrated to achieve the desired therapeutic effects. Close patient monitoring is essential. It is important to realize that although morphine can produce respiratory depression, this drug can relieve the dyspnea caused by pulmonary edema. In this situation, respiratory distress is not a contraindication to morphine administration. The narcotic antagonist naloxone may be ordered to reverse the action of morphine if adverse effects pose a significant risk to the patient. The dose is 0.4 to 2 mg every 2 minutes as indicated (see Chapter 25).

Atropine Sulfate

Atropine sulfate is the primary drug indicated for the treatment of hemodynamically significant bradycardia and some types of heart block (e.g., atrioventricular [AV] block at the nodal level). Atropine acts to increase heart rate by inhibiting the action of the vagus nerve (parasympatholytic effect). Atropine sulfate is also used as an emergency drug to reverse the toxic effects of organophosphate pesticide and nerve agent exposure, which includes bradycardia and excessive secretions.

In symptomatic bradycardia, atropine is administered IV in 0.5-mg doses at 3- to 5-minute intervals until the desired heart rate is achieved or until 0.04 mg/kg (not more than 3 mg) is given. Dosing in this manner may be repeated every 3 to 5 minutes up to a limit of 0.04 mg/kg (usually not more than 3 mg IV).

The adult IV atropine dose should never be less than 0.5 mg. Doses below 0.5 mg may produce a paradoxical bradycardia; at doses of 0.04 mg/kg or greater, vagal activity is considered completely blocked, and further atropine administration may have no benefit. However, in the case of organophosphate insecticide or nerve agent poisoning, *very high* doses of atropine may be necessary to counteract the pathophysiologic effects of these toxins. Therefore the typical dosing range and limits do not apply under these circumstances.

If venous access is not available in an emergency situation, atropine sulfate should be administered through the intraosseous (IO) route. As a last resort, atropine may be given via the endotracheal tube (ETT) route if venous or IO access cannot be achieved. The dose for endotracheal administration is 2 to 2.5 times the venous dose, diluted with normal saline or sterile water. Accordingly, 2 to 3 mg of atropine would be diluted in 10 mL of normal saline or sterile water and instilled deep into the ETT via a feeding tube attached to a syringe. After endotracheal administration, the patient should be ventilated vigorously with a bag-valve device to enhance absorption of the drug.

Continuous cardiac and blood pressure monitoring is essential for the patient who receives atropine sulfate. Significant adverse effects include cardiac dysrhythmias, tachycardia, myocardial ischemia, restlessness, anxiety, mydriasis, thirst, and urinary retention. See Chapter 16 for more information on atropine and other anticholinergics.

Pediatric Implications

The definition of bradycardia is variable and age specific for the pediatric population. Knowledge of normal ranges is essential. Because cardiac output is dependent on heart rate in infants younger than 6 months, bradycardia (heart rate <100 beats/min for infants) must be treated. In fact, a heart rate less than 60 beats/min in an infant requires performance of CPR. Before administration of drugs, efforts always should be targeted first toward restoring adequate ventilation and oxygenation. For the neonate with a spontaneous heart rate of less than 80 beats/min, epinephrine 0.01 mg/kg IV or IO every 3 to 5 minutes as indicated should be given prior to atropine to elevate the heart rate because stressed neonates quickly deplete their own stores of catecholamines. If these interventions do not produce the desired clinical response, atropine is indicated in the presence of increased vagal tone or AV block. Other pediatric indications for atropine include management of organophosphate toxicity and as pretreatment to prevent bradycardia after succinylcholine administration during rapid-sequence intubation, although this specific indication is currently controversial.

The pediatric dose of atropine is 0.02 mg/kg IV or IO. It is important to be cognizant that in the pediatric population, the minimum single dose is 0.1 mg, and the maximum single dose is 0.5 mg IV. The maximum total pediatric dose is 1 mg in a child and 3 mg in an adolescent (defined as an individual who has reached puberty). Note that when referring to general age groupings of patients, *infants* are considered to be younger than 1 year; a *child* is considered to be age 1 year to adolescence (puberty), and an *adult* is considered to be an adolescent or older. See Chapters 5 and 11 for more information on pediatric medication dosing and monitoring.

Adenosine

Adenosine is the first-line drug of choice to treat **paroxysmal supraventricular tachycardia (PSVT)**, a sudden, uncontrolled, rapid rhythm that exceeds 150 ventricular beats/min in adults and originates above the ventricles. The goal is to convert PSVT to sinus rhythm. Adenosine, a natural substance found in all body cells, slows impulse conduction through the heart's AV node, interrupts dysrhythmia-producing reentry pathways, and restores a normal rhythm in patients with PSVT. Because the half-life is less than 5 seconds, adenosine is best administered rapidly via a peripheral IV site in the port most proximal to the patient as a 6-mg IV bolus over 1 to 3 seconds followed by a 20-mL saline flush. A 12-mg bolus may be given 1 to 2 minutes after the initial dose if PSVT persists. Higher doses are not recommended.

Nursing considerations include continuous cardiac monitoring and frequent assessment of vital signs. Adenosine is inhibited by methylxanthines such as caffeine and theophylline, so higher doses may be needed. Although usually transient, ventricular ectopy, bradycardia, flushing, chest pain, and dyspnea may occur. In addition, a short period of **asystole** may follow injection of adenosine (up to 15 seconds). Spontaneous cardiac activity typically resumes. Adenosine is contraindicated in patients with poison- or drug-related tachycardia, second- and third-degree heart block, and in patients with sick sinus syndrome except those with functioning pacemakers. If the tachycardia originated in the ventricles, the patient could deteriorate and become hypotensive after adenosine administration. See Chapter 37 for more information on antidysrhythmic drugs.

Diltiazem

Diltiazem is a calcium channel blocker, and it is administered as an IV bolus to treat PSVT and to slow the ventricular response rate in atrial fibrillation or flutter. It is considered a second-line agent after adenosine. Diltiazem has less of a negative inotropic effect than other, similar calcium channel blockers, but it has strong negative chronotropic actions. Therefore IV diltiazem is less likely to cause cardiac depression but is very effective in controlling heart rate.

The usual initial bolus dose of IV diltiazem is 0.25 mg/kg given over 2 minutes. If the supraventricular tachycardia does not convert to a normal sinus rhythm in 15 minutes, a second IV bolus of 0.35 mg/kg over 2 minutes may be necessary. For ongoing control of the ventricular rate in patients with atrial fibrillation or flutter, a continuous infusion of diltiazem is indicated at a dose range of 5 to 15 mg/hour, titrated according to the desired heart rate.

The nurse must carefully monitor blood pressure and heart rate and rhythm after administering IV diltiazem. Arrhythmias, bradycardia, heart block, and hypotension may develop. Diltiazem can elevate serum digoxin levels, predisposing the patient to digitalis toxicity. Simultaneous use of calcium channel blockers and beta blockers is contraindicated because their negative inotropic and negative chronotropic effects are synergistic, causing myocardial depression and bradycardia. Other contraindications include preexisting heart failure, Wolff-Parkinson-White syndrome, and heart block or sick sinus syndrome in the patient without a pacemaker.

Amiodarone

The IV form of amiodarone is considered a first-line agent in the ALS algorithms for the treatment of life-threatening ventricular dysrhythmias and cardiac arrest. It has alpha- and beta-adrenergic blocking effects and acts on sodium, potassium, and calcium channels. Indications for use include pulseless ventricular tachycardia and ventricular fibrillation (after defibrillation and epinephrine), hemodynamically stable ventricular tachycardia, PSVT refractory to adenosine, ventricular rate control in atrial fibrillation, and pharmacologic treatment of atrial fibrillation.

Amiodarone is especially good for patients with impaired heart function who have atrial and ventricular dysrhythmias. It has been found to be more effective and to have fewer proarrhythmic properties than other agents with similar actions.

For patients who have a pulse (i.e., those *not* in cardiac arrest), amiodarone 150 mg IV is given over 10 minutes, followed by a continuous infusion of 1 mg/min for 6 hours, then 0.5 mg/min over 18 hours as a maintenance infusion. For patients in cardiac arrest because of pulseless ventricular tachycardia or ventricular fibrillation, a dose of 300 mg diluted in 20 to 30 mL D_5W is given as a rapid infusion followed by a continuous infusion as described earlier. Additional doses of 150 mg may be given by rapid infusion if ventricular fibrillation or ventricular tachycardia recurs. The maximum daily dose is 2.2 g per 24-hour period.

Significant adverse effects include hypotension and bradycardia, therefore the nurse should slow the infusion rate to prevent or treat these effects and should be prepared to administer IV fluids, vasopressors, and agents to increase heart rate. A temporary pacemaker may be needed. Amiodarone has a very long half-life. It should not be given concurrently with pharmacologic drugs that prolong QT interval on electrocardiography (ECG), such as procainamide.

Pediatric Implications

Amiodarone has an off-label use among pediatrics. It is given for pulseless ventricular tachycardia and ventricular fibrillation as a 5-mg/kg rapid IV/IO bolus, which can be repeated up to a maximum dose of 15 mg/kg per 24 hours. For responsive children who have supraventricular (junctional and atrial) tachycardia and ventricular dysrhythmias with pulses present, amiodarone is given as a 5 mg/kg IV/IO loading dose (300 mg maximum) over 20 to 60 minutes and repeated to a maximum daily IV dose of 15 mg/kg per 24 hours.

Lidocaine

As an alternative to amiodarone, lidocaine may be used to treat significant ventricular dysrhythmias, or irregular heartbeats, such as frequent premature ventricular contractions (PVCs), ventricular tachycardia, and ventricular fibrillation. Lidocaine exerts a local anesthetic effect on the heart, thus decreasing myocardial irritability. Typically, a patient with ventricular dysrhythmias is given a 1- to 1.5-mg/kg bolus of lidocaine, followed by 0.5 mg/kg to 0.75 mg/kg every 5 to 10 minutes until the dysrhythmia is controlled or a total dose of 3 mg/kg has been administered via the IV or IO route. A continuous lidocaine infusion is initiated at a rate of 1 to 4 mg/min to maintain a therapeutic serum level. Lidocaine may also be administered via the endotracheal route in doses of 2 to 4 mg/kg.

Important nursing considerations for the patient receiving lidocaine include continuous cardiac monitoring and assessment for signs and symptoms of lidocaine toxicity (e.g., confusion, drowsiness, hearing impairment, cardiac conduction defects, myocardial depression, muscle twitching, and seizures). Because lidocaine is metabolized by the liver, patients with hepatic impairment, heart failure, shock, and advanced age (>70 years) are at higher risk for toxicity. In these patients, the lidocaine dose may need to be reduced by as much as 50% (see Chapter 37). Lidocaine is contraindicated as a *prophylactic* agent to prevent ventricular dysrhythmias following AMI.

Pediatric Implications

Ventricular ectopy is uncommon in children, therefore metabolic causes should be suspected if ventricular dysrhythmias occur. The pediatric dose of lidocaine is 1 mg/kg IV or via the IO route, and the ETT dose is 2 to 3 mg/kg. A maintenance infusion of 20 to 50 mcg/kg/min is recommended following the bolus dose. Prototype Drug Chart 55.1 lists the pharmacologic data for lidocaine.

Procainamide

Procainamide is an antidysrhythmic drug prescribed for ventricular tachycardia, PVCs, and rapid supraventricular dysrhythmias unresponsive to adenosine. The typical IV loading dose of procainamide is 20 to 50 mg/min until the dysrhythmia is successfully treated. Other end points to procainamide administration include a total administration of 17 mg/kg of the drug, development of hypotension, and specific changes on the ECG (e.g., widening of the QRS complex by 50% or more). A continuous maintenance infusion of 1 to 4 mg/min may be ordered following the loading dose.

The nurse must monitor vital signs and the ECG with particular attention to heart rate and rhythm, blood pressure, and the width of the QRS complex. Procainamide administration can cause severe hypotension. Heart block, rhythm disturbances, and cardiac arrest can also occur. Procainamide is contraindicated in patients with torsades de pointes, an unusual polymorphic ventricular tachycardia often associated with a prolonged QT interval. Procainamide is eliminated via the kidneys, therefore patients with renal failure are at higher risk of adverse effects and often require a lower dosage.

PROTOTYPE DRUG CHART 55.1
Lidocaine Hydrochloride

Drug Class	Dosage
Antidysrhythmic, class IB Pregnancy category: C*	A: IV/IO: 1-1.5 mg/kg; may repeat 0.5 mg/kg q5-10min; *max:* 3 mg/kg A: ETT: 2-4 mg/kg A: IV drip: 1-4 mg/min C: IV/IO: Initially: 1 mg/kg; maint: 20-50 mcg/kg/min C: ETT: 2-3 mg/kg Therapeutic range: 2-6 mcg/mL
Contraindications	**Drug-Lab-Food Interactions**
Hypersensitivity, advanced atrioventricular block *Caution:* Liver disease, heart failure, older adults	Drug: Increased effects with phenytoin, quinidine, procainamide, propranolol; increased risk for toxicity with cimetidine, beta-adrenergic blockers
Pharmacokinetics	**Pharmacodynamics**
Absorption: IV Distribution: PB: 60%-80%; concentrates in adipose tissue Metabolism: t½: Initial: 7-30 min; terminal: 9-120 min Excretion: Through the liver	PO: Onset: 45-60 s Peak: 45-60 s Duration: 10-20 min
Therapeutic Effects/Uses	
Antiarrhythmic drug to treat ventricular dysrhythmias such as premature ventricular contractions (PVCs), ventricular tachycardia, and ventricular fibrillation Mode of Action: Decreases automaticity; increases electrical threshold of ventricle	
Side Effects	**Adverse Reactions**
Drowsiness, confusion, dyspnea, lethargy, hypotension, nausea, vomiting	*Life threatening:* Seizures, cardiac arrest

*Pregnancy categories have been revised. See http://www.fda.gov/Drugs/DevelopmentApprovalProcess/DevelopmentResources/Labeling/ucm093307.htm for more information.
A, Adult; *C,* child; *ETT,* endotracheal tube; *IO,* intraosseous; *IV,* intravenous; *maint,* maintenance; *max,* maximum; *min,* minute; *PB,* protein binding; *PO,* by mouth; *q,* every; *s,* seconds; *t½,* half-life.

Pediatric Implications

Procainamide has an off-label use among pediatrics and is given to children for ventricular tachycardia that is recurrent or refractory to other measures and for supraventricular tachycardia. The loading dose is 15 mg/kg IV or IO given over 30 to 60 minutes. The same monitoring guidelines, adverse effects, and contraindications described for adults are relevant in the pediatric population.

Magnesium Sulfate

Magnesium is an essential element in multiple enzymatic reactions in the body, including function of the sodium-potassium adenosine triphosphatase (ATPase) pump. Its physiologic effects can be likened to a calcium channel blocker with neuromuscular blocking properties. Hypomagnesemia is associated with the development of atrial and ventricular dysrhythmias.

The primary indications for emergency administration of magnesium sulfate are refractory ventricular tachycardia, refractory ventricular fibrillation, cardiac arrest associated with hypomagnesemia (low serum magnesium level), and life-threatening ventricular dysrhythmias from digitalis toxicity. It is also the drug of choice for the treatment of torsades de pointes.

Magnesium is administered by diluting 1 to 2 g (2 to 4 mL of a 50% solution) in 10 mL of D5W. For cardiac arrest caused by hypomagnesemia or torsades de pointes, magnesium is given by direct IV push or via the IO route over 5 to 20 minutes. For patients experiencing torsades de pointes who are not in cardiac arrest, a magnesium infusion of 1 to 2 g diluted in 50 to 100 mL of D5W can be given IV/IO over 5 to 60 minutes followed by a continuous infusion of 0.5 to 1 g/h.

Although magnesium toxicity is rare, the nurse should monitor the patient's response to magnesium administration. Hypotension is the most common adverse effect when magnesium is given by rapid IV push. Other effects include mild bradycardia, flush, and sweating. True hypermagnesemia can cause diarrhea, respiratory depression, deep tendon reflex impairment, flaccid paralysis, and circulatory collapse. Because magnesium is eliminated via the kidneys, it should be administered with caution in patients with renal impairment.

Pediatric Implications

Indications for magnesium sulfate in pediatric patients include torsades de pointes, hypomagnesemia, and status asthmaticus that is unresponsive to beta-adrenergic drugs. The magnesium sulfate dose is 25 to 50 mg/kg IV/IO (maximum dose of 2 g) given as a bolus for pulseless ventricular tachycardia, slowly over 10 to 20 minutes for ventricular tachycardia with pulses and over 15 to 30 minutes for status asthmaticus.

Epinephrine

Epinephrine is a catecholamine with alpha- and beta-adrenergic effects. It has multiple uses. Emergency cardiac indications for administration of IV/IO epinephrine include profound bradycardia and hypotension, asystole, pulseless ventricular tachycardia, and ventricular fibrillation. Epinephrine is thought to improve perfusion of the heart and brain in cardiac arrest states by constricting peripheral blood vessels. In addition, epinephrine increases the chances for successful electrical countershock (defibrillation) in ventricular fibrillation. It is important to be aware that epinephrine is available in two primary concentrations: 1:1000 and 1:10,000. The 1:10,000 concentration is used when administering a single IV/IO dose of epinephrine. The 1:1000 form is used when preparing a continuous epinephrine infusion or when giving epinephrine via the intramuscular (IM) route. The subcutaneous (subcut) route should not be used for emergency epinephrine administration because absorption is unpredictable.

For profound bradycardia or hypotension, an epinephrine infusion may be ordered at 0.1 to 0.5 mcg/kg/min. For asystole, pulseless ventricular tachycardia, and ventricular fibrillation, epinephrine is administered in 1-mg doses (1:10,000 solution) IV/IO every 3 to 5 minutes until the desired clinical response—usually return of effective cardiac activity—is achieved. Epinephrine also may be given via the ETT route in doses of 2 to 2.5 mg diluted in 10 mL of normal saline.

Nursing implications for patients receiving epinephrine include constant cardiac and hemodynamic monitoring. Epinephrine can cause myocardial ischemia and cardiac dysrhythmias. It should never be administered in the same site as an alkaline solution, such as with sodium bicarbonate, because alkaline solutions inactivate epinephrine. In addition, the presence of metabolic or respiratory acidosis decreases the effectiveness of epinephrine. All efforts should be made to correct acid-base imbalances in the patient. More drug information about epinephrine and other adrenergic drugs can be found in Chapter 12.

> ### ⚡ PATIENT SAFETY
>
> - Ensure that the correct concentration (1:1000 vs. 1:10,000) is administered. The 1:10,000 preparation is meant to be given intravenously.

Pediatric Implications

The pediatric dose of epinephrine is 0.01 mg/kg (1:10,000 solution) given every 3 to 5 minutes IV/IO for cardiac arrest. The ETT dose of 0.1 mg/kg should be given using the 1:1000 solution every 3 to 5 minutes.

Sodium Bicarbonate

Sodium bicarbonate is prescribed to treat severe metabolic acidosis that may accompany cardiac arrest and the hyperkalemia and acidotic states related to specific drug overdose situations. The current standard in resuscitation is to give sodium bicarbonate only *after* adequate ventilation, chest compressions, IV fluids, and drug therapy fail to correct the acidotic state. Sodium bicarbonate is not considered a first-line drug for the treatment of cardiac arrest; it is preferentially given based on results of arterial blood gas analysis when acidosis is severe. The standard initial IV dose of sodium bicarbonate is 1 mEq/kg. Subsequent dosing depends on arterial blood gas analysis.

Important nursing considerations relevant to sodium bicarbonate include careful monitoring of arterial blood gas analysis results. Sodium bicarbonate administration can lead to metabolic alkalosis, which may be very difficult to reverse and can have deleterious physiologic effects. Catecholamines such as epinephrine, norepinephrine, and dopamine should not be infused in the same site as sodium bicarbonate because they are inactivated by solutions that contain sodium bicarbonate.

Table 55.1 lists emergency cardiac drugs and their dosages, uses, and considerations.

Pediatric Implications

If severe metabolic acidosis persists after attention has been directed at maintaining optimal ventilation and oxygenation, sodium bicarbonate may be given to the pediatric patient in a 1-mEq/kg dose via the IV or IO route. It may also be given as treatment for a tricyclic antidepressant (TCA) overdose. Sodium bicarbonate is hyperosmolar and should be diluted from an 8.4% solution (1 mEq/mL) to a 4.2% solution (0.5 mEq/mL) for infants.

EMERGENCY DRUG FOR INTRACRANIAL HYPERTENSION

Mannitol

Mannitol is an osmotic diuretic used in emergency, trauma, critical care, and neurosurgical settings to treat cerebral edema and to reduce increased intracranial pressure (intracranial hypertension), which may occur following head trauma, neurosurgery, malignancy, and with other types of intracranial pathology (see Chapter 38). Mannitol may be given as an IV bolus or via a continuous drip. The usual initial bolus dose of mannitol is 1 to 2 g/kg IV of a 20% to 25% solution. Subsequent dosing is highly variable and is influenced by serum osmolality. In general, mannitol is held when serum osmolality exceeds 310 to 320 mOsm/kg. Mannitol is highly irritating to veins, and the nurse must use a filter needle when administering the drug because crystals may form in the solution and syringe and can be inadvertently injected. When a filter needle is used to draw up the mannitol, a *new* filter needle *must* be used to administer the mannitol IV. In addition, the nurse should carefully assess the patient's neurologic status; monitor laboratory studies, including electrolytes and serum osmolality; and keep accurate intake and output records to assess fluid volume status because diuresis may be substantial. Prototype Drug Chart 55.2 lists the pharmacologic data for mannitol.

EMERGENCY DRUGS FOR POISONING

Although numerous antidotes exist for specific types of poisoning, the drugs presented in this section are most commonly prescribed in cases of drug overdose and ingestion of toxic substances, and pertinent exceptions are noted. Particular attention must be given to administration guidelines to achieve the best possible clinical outcome for the patient. These drugs are cross-referenced to their specialty chapters.

Naloxone

Naloxone is classified as an opiate antagonist. It reverses the effects of all opiate drugs (e.g., morphine, meperidine, codeine, propoxyphene, heroin) by competitively binding to opiate receptor sites in the body. Naloxone is indicated for individuals who have taken an overdose of opiate drugs, those experiencing respiratory or cardiovascular depression from therapeutic doses

TABLE 55.1	**Emergency Cardiac Drugs**	
Generic	**Route and Dosage****	**Uses and Considerations**
Adenosine	A/C/Adol >50 kg: IV/IO: Initially 6 mg; then 12 mg in 1 to 2 min if needed C/Adol <50 kg: IV/IO: 0.1 mg/kg/dose. May repeat 0.2 mg/kg/dose.	For paroxysmal supraventricular tachycardia Pregnancy category: C*; PB: UK; t½: <10 sec
Amiodarone	A: IV: With pulse: 150 mg over 10 min, then continuous infusion 1 mg/min for 6 h, then 0.5 mg/min over 18 h Cardiac arrest: 300 mg diluted in 20-30 mL D$_5$W rapidly; second dose 150 mg, followed by continuous infusion as above; *max:* 2.2 g/d	Part of ALS algorithm for treatment of both atrial and ventricular dysrhythmias Pregnancy category: C*; PB: UK; t½: 26-107 d
Atropine sulfate	A: IV/IO: 0.5-1 mg; can repeat up to 0.04 mg/kg or 3 mg (max) ETT: 2-3 mg diluted in 10 mL normal saline C/Adol: IV: 0.02 mg/kg/dose, repeat x 1	For symptomatic bradycardia and asystole Pregnancy category: C*; PB: 60%-80%; t½: 2-3 h
Diltiazem	A: IV: 0.25 mg/kg; repeat in 15 min at 0.35 mg/kg IV drip: 5-10 mg/h	For supraventricular tachycardia and atrial fibrillation and flutter Pregnancy category: C*; PB: 80%; t½: 2-5h
Epinephrine	A: IV: 1 mg; may be repeated q3-5min ETT: 2-2.5 mg diluted in 10 mL normal saline C/Adol: IV: 0.01 mg/kg/dose, may repeat q3-5 min C/Adol: ETT: 0.1 mg/kg/dose, may repeat q3-5 min	For cardiac arrest Pregnancy category: C*; PB: UK; t½: UK
Lidocaine	See Prototype Drug Chart 55.1.	
Magnesium sulfate	A: Dilute 1-2 g (2-4 mL of 50% solution) in 10 mL of D$_5$W. Give IV/IO in cardiac arrest over 5-20 min. Torsades de pointes: 1-2 g diluted in 50-100 mL of D$_5$W given IV over 5-60 min followed by continuous infusion of 0.5-1 g/h	For unlabeled use for cardiac arrest due to hypomagnesemia; drug of choice for torsades de pointes after defibrillation in patients with a prolonged QT interval; rapid infusion can cause hypotension. Pregnancy category: D*; PB: 25%-35%; t½: 30 min
Morphine sulfate	A: IV: 1-5 mg q5-30min	For chest pain, unstable angina, pulmonary edema Pregnancy category: C*; PB: 35%; t½: 2-2.5 h
Nitroglycerin	A: SL: 0.3-0.6 mg; translingual aerosol spray: 0.4-0.8 mg metered dose, up to 3 tab/sprays q15min onto or under the tongue A: IV drip: Initially 5 mcg/min; titrate by 5 mcg/min q3-5min; *max rate of* *titration:* 20 mcg/min q3-5 min C: IV drip: Initially 0.25-0.5 mcg/kg/min; titrate 0.5-1 mcg/kg/min q3-5 min	For chest pain, angina, unstable angina, MI; hypotension can occur. *Contraindication:* With drugs for erectile dysfunction (e.g., sildenafil). Pregnancy category: C*; PB: 60%; t½: 1-4 min
Procainamide hydrochloride	A: IV: 20-50 mg/min; *max:* 17 mg/kg; followed by 1-4 mg/min IV drip Recognized end points: Hypotension, QRS widens > 50%, or total of 500 mg administered C: 15 mg/kg over 30-60 min.	For PVCs, ventricular tachycardia, ventricular fibrillation, atrial dysrhythmias Pregnancy category: C*; PB: 20%; t½: 3-4 h
Sodium bicarbonate	A/C >2 y: IV: Initially 1 mEq/kg, then dose based on ABG results	For resp or metabolic acidosis. Not for routine use in cardiac arrest. Pregnancy category: C*; PB: UK; t½: UK

*Pregnancy categories have been revised. See http://www.fda.gov/Drugs/DevelopmentApprovalProcess/DevelopmentResources/Labeling/ucm093
307.htm for more information.
**Other dosing regimens for neonates, infants, and children are available.
A, Adult; *ABG,* arterial blood gas; *ALS,* advanced life support; *Adol,* adolescent; *C,* child; *d,* day; *ETT,* endotracheal tube; *h,* hour; *IO,* intraosseous;
IV, intravenous; *max,* maximum; *MI,* myocardial infarction; *min,* minute; *PB,* protein binding; *PVC,* premature ventricular contraction; *q,* every; *resp,*
respiratory; *SL,* sublingual; *t½,* half-life; *tab,* tablet; *UK,* unknown; *y,* year; *>,* greater than; *<,* less than.

of opiates given in a health care setting, and those brought to the emergency department in a coma of unknown etiology (which may be drug induced). Given the epidemic of opiate overdoses in the general community, there is a widespread effort in many states to make naloxone available to medical first responders and even to members of the lay public who are dealing with drug misuse and abuse.

The typical dose of naloxone for actual or suspected opiate overdose in adults is 0.4 to 2 mg IV administered every 2 minutes until the patient's condition improves to an acceptable level. If there is no improvement within 10 minutes after 10 mg of the drug has been injected, nonopiate drugs or disease must be suspected. Although naloxone should be administered

intravenously in emergency situations, it also may be given via IO, IM, subcut, and intranasal (IN) routes if IV access is not readily obtainable. The adult dose for the IN route is 1 mg per nostril. IN naloxone offers the advantages of a reduced risk of needlestick injuries as well as a readily accessible route of administration for rescuers and laypersons. Naloxone autoinjectors are also now available to facilitate rapid IM administration by rescue personnel and members of the general public.

Because most opiate drugs have a longer duration of action than naloxone, the nurse must monitor the patient closely for signs and symptoms of recurrent opiate effects such as respiratory depression and hypotension. In this situation, naloxone administration may need to be repeated several times, or a

PROTOTYPE DRUG CHART 55.2

Mannitol

Drug Class	Dosage
Osmotic diuretic Pregnancy category: C*	A: IV: Initially 1-2 g/kg, followed by 0.25-1 g/kg q4h Dosing is highly individualized. Hold for serum osmo >320 mOsm/kg.
Contraindications	**Drug-Lab-Food Interactions**
Hypersensitivity, severe dehydration *Caution:* Pregnancy, breastfeeding, current intracranial bleeding	Drug: May decrease effectiveness with lithium
Pharmacokinetics	**Pharmacodynamics**
Absorption: IV Distribution: PB: Confined to extracellular space Metabolism: t½: 100 min Excretion: In urine	Decrease in intracranial pressure: IV: Onset: 30-60 min Peak: 1 h Duration: 6-8 h Diuresis: IV: Onset: 1-3 h Peak: 1 h Duration: 6-8 h
Therapeutic Effects/Uses	
To treat increased intracranial pressure, cerebral edema Mode of Action: Inhibits reabsorption of electrolytes and water by affecting pressure of glomerular filtrate	
Side Effects	**Adverse Reactions**
Temporary volume expansion, hyponatremia/hypernatremia, hypokalemia/hyper-kalemia, dehydration, blurred vision, dry mouth	Pulmonary congestion, fluid/electrolyte imbalances *Life threatening:* Convulsions

*Pregnancy categories have been revised. See http://www.fda.gov/Drugs/DevelopmentApprovalProcess/DevelopmentResources/Labeling/ucm093307.htm for more information.
A, Adult; *h*, hour; *IV*, intravenous; *min*, minute; *osmo*, osmolality; *PB*, protein binding; *q*, every; *t½*, half-life; *>*, greater than

continuous IV infusion may be ordered. Naloxone has no major adverse effects, but it can precipitate withdrawal symptoms in patients addicted to opiate drugs, and rarely, it can cause anaphylaxis. In addition, pulmonary edema has been reported following naloxone administration in patients who have had an overdose of morphine (see Chapter 25). Nurses also must be on guard for combative or violent behavior following naloxone administration, especially in patients who have overdosed on an illicit drug; having security personnel available to stand by is prudent. Prototype Drug Chart 55.3 lists the pharmacologic data for naloxone.

Pediatric Implications

For narcotic reversal in children, give 0.1 mg/kg, repeating the drug as necessary up to 2 mg based upon desired therapeutic effects. Naloxone can be administered as an IV bolus, continuous infusion or via IO, IM, or subcut routes in children.

Flumazenil

Flumazenil is the reversal agent for the respiratory depressant and sedative effects of benzodiazepine drugs (e.g., diazepam, midazolam, chlordiazepoxide). It is administered to counteract the effects of benzodiazepines given as sedative or anesthetic drugs as well as to treat accidental or intentional benzodiazepine overdose. Flumazenil does not reverse the central nervous system (CNS) depressant effects of nonbenzodiazepine agents such as alcohol, opiates, and barbiturates and may not reverse amnesia induced by benzodiazepines.

For suspected benzodiazepine overdose, flumazenil is given IV in an initial dose of 0.2 mg over 15 seconds. A second dose

of 0.3 mg may be given over 30 seconds. A third dose and subsequent doses of 0.5 mg IV may be given every minute until the desired clinical response is achieved or until a total dose of 3 mg is given within an hour. If sedation occurs again, doses of flumazenil may be repeated at 20-minute intervals (not to exceed 1 mg at a time) to a total hourly dose of no more than 3 mg IV.

Nursing considerations include careful assessment of respiratory rate and effort, blood pressure, and mental status. If the benzodiazepine is reversed too rapidly, patients may have emergence reactions in which they become agitated and confused and experience perceptual distortions. Because seizures are precipitated by benzodiazepine withdrawal, seizure precautions must be implemented for patients at risk (those with long-standing benzodiazepine use or abuse) and for those who have a known seizure disorder.

Activated Charcoal

Activated charcoal may be prescribed for poisoning as a means to prevent absorption of toxins into the body if the ingested substance is known to be affected by charcoal in the GI tract. A poison control center should be contacted as soon as possible to help guide medical therapy. In cases of known or suspected poisoning, activated charcoal is prepared as a slurry and is given to the patient orally or via a gastric tube, ideally within 30 minutes to 1 hour of ingestion, sometimes following gastric lavage. The dose is dependent on the amount of poison ingested; the typical adult and pediatric dose is 1 to 2 g/kg/dose. Activated charcoal dosing may need to be repeated for certain types of poisoning, particularly from drugs such as salicylates, slow-release drug preparations, and *Amanita phalloides* (death cap mushrooms), to name a few.

PROTOTYPE DRUG CHART 55.3

Naloxone Hydrochloride

Drug Class	Dosage**
Narcotic antagonist	A: IV/IM/IO/subcut/IN: 0.4-2 mg, repeating every 2-3 min PRN
Pregnancy category: B*	C: IV/IM/subcut/IO: age and weight based: 0.1-2 mg; may repeat q2-3min PRN

Contraindications	Drug-Lab-Food Interactions
Hypersensitivity, respiratory depression	Drug: Naloxone can precipitate withdrawal in patients dependent on narcotic analgesics.
Caution: Opiate-dependent patients, cardiac disease, breastfeeding neonates of opiate-dependent mothers	Lab: Urine vanillylmandelic acid (VMA), 5-hydroxyheptadecatrienoic acid (5-HIAA), urine glucose

Pharmacokinetics	Pharmacodynamics
Absorption: IM/subcut: Well absorbed	IM/IN/subcut: Onset: 2-5 min
Distribution: PB: UK	Peak: UK
Metabolism: t½: Adults: 1-4 h; neonates: 1-3 h	Duration: 1-4 h
Excretion: In urine metabolites	IV/IO: Onset: 1-2 min
	Peak: UK
	Duration: 1-4 h

Therapeutic Effects/Uses

To treat respiratory depression caused by narcotics; to treat narcotic-induced depressant effects and narcotic overdose
Mode of Action: Blocks effects of narcotics by competing for receptor sites

Side Effects	Adverse Reactions
Negligible pharmacologic effect without narcotics in the body	Nausea, vomiting, tremulousness, sweating, tachycardia, elevated blood pressure
	Life threatening: Atrioventricular fibrillation, pulmonary edema (with overdose of morphine)

*Pregnancy categories have been revised. See http://www.fda.gov/Drugs/DevelopmentApprovalProcess/DevelopmentResources/Labeling/ucm093307.htm for more information.
**Other dosing regimens for neonates, infants, and children are available.
A, adult; *C*, child; *h*, Hour; *IM*, intramuscular; *IN*, intranasal; *IO*, intraosseus; *IV*, intravenous; *min*, minute; *PB*, protein-binding; *PRN*, as needed; *q*, every; *subcut*, subcutaneous; *t½*, half-life; *UK*, unknown.

Because vomiting is a common adverse reaction, patients with an impaired gag reflex and/or an impaired mental status are at high risk for aspiration after ingesting activated charcoal. Aspiration pneumonia and death can occur. To promote safety, these patients may need intubation for airway protection followed by administration of the activated charcoal via a gastric tube. Activated charcoal should not be administered with milk products, because they decrease its adsorptive properties. Activated charcoal is ineffective and should not be given to patients who have ingested some forms of pesticides, hydrocarbons, alcohol, acids or alkalis, lithium, solvents, and iron supplements. A cathartic, a purgative that results in bowel movements, may be ordered following administration of activated charcoal to speed elimination of the charcoal-toxin complex from the body. The patient should be told that charcoal produces black stools.

Table 55.2 lists the emergency drugs for poisoning and their dosages, uses, and considerations.

EMERGENCY DRUGS FOR SHOCK

Drugs may be required to elevate blood pressure and to improve cardiac performance in various types of shock states. Therapeutic agents described in this section are primarily indicated in conditions such as cardiogenic, neurogenic, septic, anaphylactic, and insulin shock. A noteworthy exception to the list is hypovolemic shock, that resulting from loss of blood or fluid volume; drugs should never be used as the primary therapy to correct the hypotension associated with this condition. Administration of fluids or blood products or both is the only acceptable initial means to treat hypovolemic shock. However, if hypotension persists after appropriate volume resuscitation, vasoactive drugs may be necessary to elevate and sustain blood pressure. The drugs that follow are cross-referenced to their specialty chapters.

Dopamine

Dopamine is a sympathomimetic agent often used to treat hypotension in shock states (see Chapter 15). Dopamine may also be used to increase heart rate (beta$_1$ effect) in bradycardic rhythms when atropine has not been effective. The typical dose range is 5 to 10 mcg/kg/min. Dopamine enhances cardiac output by increasing myocardial contractility and increasing heart rate (beta$_1$ effect), and it elevates blood pressure through vasoconstriction (alpha-adrenergic effect). Alpha effects predominate at higher doses—vasoconstriction of renal, mesenteric, and peripheral blood vessels occurs. Although sometimes necessary to maintain adequate blood pressure in severe shock, such vasoconstriction can lead to poor organ and tissue perfusion, decreased cardiac performance, and reduction of urine output. The lowest effective dose of dopamine should be used. Patients must be weaned gradually from dopamine; abrupt discontinuation of the infusion can cause severe hypotension.

Dopamine is typically mixed as a concentration of 200 to 800 mg in 250 mL D$_5$W or normal saline solution and is

TABLE 55.2   Emergency Drugs for Poisoning

Generic	Route and Dosage	Uses and Considerations
Flumazenil	A: IV: Initially 0.2 mg over 15 s; additional doses of 0.3-0.5 mg are given over 30 s q1min as indicated. For resedation, may repeat at 20-min intervals to a total dose of no more than 3 mg C/Adol: IV: Initially 0.01 mg/kg over 15 s. May repeat at 1 min interval; *max*. 0.05 mg/kg or 1 mg, whichever is lower.	Reversal agent for benzodiazepine overdose; may precipitate seizures in patients with long-term use or abuse of benzodiazepines and those with seizure disorders; may precipitate emergent reactions. Pregnancy category: C*; PB: 50%; t½: Variable (40-80 min)
Naloxone	See Prototype Drug Chart 55.3.	
Activated charcoal	A/C: PO: 10-100 g/dose. Dose based on age and formulation.	For poisoning. Onset: <1 min. Pregnancy category: C*; PB: NA; t½: NA

*Pregnancy categories have been revised. See http://www.fda.gov/Drugs/DevelopmentApprovalProcess/DevelopmentResources/Labeling/ucm093 307.htm for more information.
A, Adult; *Adol*, adolescent; *C*, child; *IV*, intravenous; *max*, maximum; *min*, minute; *NA*, not applicable; *PB*, protein binding; *PO*, by mouth; *q*, every; *s*, second; *t½*, half-life; <, less than.

PROTOTYPE DRUG CHART 55.4

Dopamine Hydrochloride

Drug Class	Dosage
Adrenergic agonist Pregnancy category: C*	A: IV drip: 5-10 mcg/kg/min; >10 mcg/kg/min may be ordered if lower doses are ineffective. C/Adol: IV: 2-20 mcg/kg/min; titrate in increments of 2.5-5 mcg/kg/min.
Contraindications	**Drug-Lab-Food Interactions**
Hypersensitivity, tachydysrhythmias, ventricular fibrillation, pheochromocytomas *Caution:* Whether this drug is safe in children is unknown.	Drug: May result in hypertensive crisis when used within 2 wk of MAOIs; concurrent IV administration of phenytoin may result in hypotension and bradycardia; sodium bicarbonate solutions inactivate dopamine—do not administer these through the same IV line.
Pharmacokinetics	**Pharmacodynamics**
Absorption: IV Distribution: PB: UK Metabolism: t½: 2 min Excretion: In urine	IV: Onset: 1-2 min Peak: <5 min Duration: <10 min
Therapeutic Effects/Uses	
To treat hypotension in shock states after adequate fluid and/or blood product resuscitation; to increase heart rate in atropine-refractory bradycardia Mode of Action: Stimulates receptors to cause cardiac stimulation; increases systemic vascular resistance	
Side Effects	**Adverse Reactions**
Palpitations, tachycardia, hypertension, ectopic beats, angina, IV line site irritation, piloerection, nausea, vomiting	Cardiac dysrhythmias, azotemia, tissue sloughing (from extravasation) *Life threatening:* MI, gangrene in extremities (from vasoconstriction)

*Pregnancy categories have been revised. See http://www.fda.gov/Drugs/DevelopmentApprovalProcess/DevelopmentResources/Labeling/ucm093307.htm for more information.
A, Adult; *Adol*, adolescent; *C*, child; *IV*, intravenous; *MAOI*, monoamine oxidase inhibitor; *MI*, myocardial infarction; *min*, minute; *PB*, protein binding; *t½*, half-life; *UK*, unknown; *wk*, week; >, greater than; <, less than.

administered intravenously by an electronic infusion device for precision, preferably in a central vein. Sodium bicarbonate will inactivate dopamine, therefore it should not be infused in the same IV line. Continuous heart and blood pressure monitoring is essential. The nurse must carefully document vital signs, cardiac rhythm, and intake and output as prescribed. Significant adverse effects include tachycardia, dysrhythmias, myocardial ischemia, nausea, and vomiting. The IV site must be assessed hourly for signs of drug infiltration; extravasation (escape into tissues) of dopamine can produce tissue necrosis that may necessitate surgical debridement and skin grafting. If extravasation occurs, the site should be injected in multiple areas with phentolamine, 5 to 10 mg diluted in 10 to 15 mL of normal

saline, to reduce or prevent tissue damage. Prototype Drug Chart 55.4 lists the pharmacologic data for dopamine.

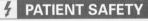

PATIENT SAFETY

Do not confuse...
• **Dopamine** with **dobutamine**

Dobutamine

Dobutamine is a sympathomimetic drug with beta-adrenergic activities (see Chapter 15). The beta₁ effects include enhancing the force of myocardial contraction (positive inotropic effect) and increasing heart rate (positive chronotropic effect). The beta$_2$ effects produce mild vasodilation. Dobutamine is indicated in shock states when improvement in cardiac output and overall cardiac performance is desired. Blood pressure is elevated only through the increase in cardiac output. The usual IV dose range of dobutamine is 2 to 20 mcg/kg/min (titrated) administered via an electronic infusion device for precision. A typical concentration of dobutamine is 250 to 1000 mg mixed in 250 mL of D$_5$W or normal saline. Like dopamine, dobutamine administration should be tapered gradually as the patient's condition warrants; abrupt discontinuation can precipitate clinical deterioration.

Continuous cardiac and blood pressure monitoring is required for patients receiving dobutamine infusions. Adverse effects are dose related and include myocardial ischemia, tachycardia, dysrhythmias, headache, nausea, and tremors. The nurse must carefully monitor intake and output and assess for any signs or symptoms of myocardial ischemia such as chest pain or development of dysrhythmias.

Norepinephrine

Norepinephrine is a catecholamine with extremely potent vasoconstrictor actions (alpha-adrenergic effect) (see Chapter 15). It is used in shock states, often when drugs such as dopamine and dobutamine have failed to produce adequate blood pressure or as an alternative to dopamine. Like high-dose dopamine, the peripheral vasoconstriction that results has the potential to impair cardiac performance and decrease organ and tissue perfusion. In general, 4 mg of norepinephrine are added to 250 mL D$_5$W or normal saline solution for a concentration of 16 mcg/mL and are infused at 0.1 to 0.5 mcg/kg/min (titrated) for adults. Maximum titrated dose is 3.3 mcg/kg/min. Continuous cardiac monitoring and precise blood pressure monitoring are required. The drug must be tapered slowly; abrupt discontinuation can result in severe hypotension.

Nursing actions and considerations are the same as those for dopamine. Norepinephrine should not be used as an initial therapy to treat hypotension in hypovolemic patients; fluid, blood, or both must be administered to restore adequate volume first. Adverse effects of norepinephrine include myocardial ischemia, dysrhythmias, and impaired organ perfusion. Extravasation of norepinephrine causes tissue necrosis, so attention to the IV site is essential. If extravasation occurs, the area should be infiltrated with phentolamine, as was described for dopamine.

Epinephrine

Epinephrine is the drug of choice in the treatment of anaphylactic shock, an allergic response of the most serious type, brought about by an antibody-antigen reaction (see Chapter 15). Anaphylactic shock can be fatal if prompt treatment is not initiated. Severe bronchoconstriction and hypotension resulting from cardiovascular collapse are its hallmarks. Epinephrine is also indicated for an acute, severe asthmatic attack.

Administration of epinephrine causes bronchodilation, enhanced cardiac performance, and vasoconstriction to increase blood pressure. In severe asthma and anaphylactic shock, epinephrine is given in a dose range of 0.3 to 0.5 mg IM for adults (1:1000 solution). The IM route is used because it has a more predictable pattern of absorption than the subcutaneous route. Given the prevalence of severe allergic reactions to foods, drugs, and insect stings, epinephrine autoinjectors in both adult and pediatric formulations are also available to facilitate rapid emergency IM administration of the drug by health care personnel in some settings as well as for self-administration by patients. As an alternative, epinephrine can be given in a dose of 0.1 to 0.25 mg IV over 5 to 10 minutes (1:10,000 solution). Epinephrine administration can be repeated every 5 to 15 minutes if necessary.

The patient who receives epinephrine must be closely monitored for tachycardia, cardiac dysrhythmias, hypertension, and angina. Patients who are given IV epinephrine must be on a cardiac monitor with resuscitation equipment immediately available. Other adverse effects include excitability, fear, anxiety, and restlessness. In addition, the nurse should be alert to the possibility that the anaphylactic response may recur and necessitate repeated treatment. For this reason, antihistamines and steroids are ordered as a standard component of treatment for an allergic reaction along with epinephrine. Diphenhydramine is a commonly prescribed antihistamine and is discussed later. Examples of steroids are hydrocortisone sodium succinate, prednisone, and methylprednisolone. After the initial dose, the steroids are slowly tapered over days to weeks to prevent recurrence.

Patient education should include strict avoidance of the agents responsible for the anaphylactic reaction and follow-up care with a health care provider. For some patients, such as those with severe allergic responses to insect stings or certain foods, the health care provider may prescribe an epinephrine kit, pen, or other type of autoinjector to be carried with the patient for self-medication in the event of contact with the antigen. Proper patient education regarding the use of the kit or pen is essential. See Chapter 8 for more information on patient teaching.

Albuterol

Albuterol is a beta-adrenergic bronchodilator (see Chapter 15) used to reverse bronchoconstriction in anaphylactic shock; asthma, inflammation and narrowing of the airways caused by enhanced responsiveness of the tracheobronchial system to a variety of stimuli; and COPD. In emergency situations, albuterol is typically administered via nebulizer (adults: 2.5 mg in 2.5 mL saline). Albuterol is also supplied as a metered-dose inhaler (MDI), which the patient can carry to self-administer a "rescue" dose of the drug during an acute episode of bronchospasm. The nurse should assess breath sounds before and after administration; effectiveness is evidenced by relief of bronchospasm. In severe bronchospasm, wheezing may not be audible. As the bronchospasm is relieved, wheezing may become more pronounced, indicating that the drug is producing the desired therapeutic effect. Assessment of the patient's subjective feelings of respiratory distress before and after administration is especially important. Adverse effects of albuterol include tachycardia, tremor, nervousness, cardiac dysrhythmias, and hypertension. The patient who is prescribed an albuterol MDI should be taught how to properly use the device and to keep track of the remaining doses. Running out of the drug when a rescue dose is needed can produce life-threatening consequences in a severe asthma attack.

Diphenhydramine Hydrochloride

Diphenhydramine, an antihistamine, is administered with epinephrine to treat anaphylactic shock. This agent is effective for treating the histamine-induced tissue swelling and pruritus common to severe allergic reactions. The standard adult dose is 25 to 50 mg administered via IV or deep IM routes. Oral pill and liquid forms of the drug exist, but the parenteral form is preferred in emergencies. However, the patient may be instructed to keep an oral formulation on hand in the home setting for emergency self-administration during an allergic reaction prior to receiving medical assistance. An important tip for patient teaching is that liquid diphenhydramine is easier to swallow than a pill, especially in the presence of tissue edema in the mouth or throat. Adverse effects include drowsiness, sedation, confusion, vertigo, excitability, hypotension, tachycardia, GI disturbances, and dry mouth (see Chapter 35).

Dextrose 50%

Dextrose 50% is a concentrated, high-carbohydrate solution given to treat severe hypoglycemia, such as insulin-induced hypoglycemia or insulin shock (see Chapter 12). When hypoglycemia is known or suspected, and the patient's state of consciousness is impaired such that oral administration of sugar solutions is contraindicated, 50 mL of dextrose 50% is commonly ordered and is given as an IV bolus. Dextrose 50% is highly irritating to veins and should be administered in a large peripheral or central vein whenever possible; phlebitis can occur, and extravasation of the solution can cause tissue sloughing and necrosis. The nurse must monitor the patient's blood glucose carefully because hyperglycemia is common, especially after rapid injection. Urine output should be accurately recorded, because osmotic diuresis can occur when blood glucose is elevated, and a hyperosmolar state can result. Patient education must be centered on teaching about diabetes, nutrition, physical activity, and properly self-managing insulin or oral hypoglycemic agent administration.

Pediatric Implications

Glycogen stores in infants and children may be quickly depleted in stress states produced by severe illness. Because adequate amounts of glucose are essential to strong myocardial function, hypoglycemia must be corrected to provide the greatest chance for successful resuscitation. After determining that hypoglycemia is present by the fingerstick or heelstick method of rapid blood glucose testing, dextrose 25% or less may be administered per health care provider order. Because glucose is supplied in a 50% concentration, it must be diluted at least 1:1 in sterile water before administration to reduce its osmolarity and prevent sclerosis of peripheral veins. The standard dose is 0.5 to 1 g/kg IV or IO.

Glucagon

Glucagon is a pancreas-produced hormone that elevates blood glucose by stimulating glycogen breakdown (**glycogenolysis**).

Glucagon, like dextrose 50%, is indicated in the treatment of severe hypoglycemia, such as that which results from insulin shock. In an emergency, when dextrose 50% is unavailable or cannot be administered intravenously, glucagon is an effective agent. Glucagon may be given via subcut, IM, or IV routes. The standard dose for adults and children is 1 mg, which can be repeated in 15 minutes for persistent coma. If the coma has not resolved after two doses, dextrose 50% must be administered. Adverse effects from glucagon are uncommon but can include nausea, vomiting, and a hypersensitivity reaction that may produce bronchospasm and respiratory distress. Glucagon can also be used as a drug to reverse the effects of calcium channel blocker and beta-blocker overdose; in this situation, 3.5 to 5 mg IV of glucagon is administered initially, followed by an IV infusion of 1 to 5 mg/h (see Chapter 47).

Table 55.3 lists the emergency drugs for shock and their dosages, uses, and considerations.

EMERGENCY DRUGS FOR HYPERTENSIVE CRISES AND PULMONARY EDEMA

A variety of pharmacologic agents may be prescribed to treat hypertensive crisis, generally defined as a systolic blood pressure that exceeds 180 to 200 mm Hg, a diastolic blood pressure that exceeds 120 mm Hg, and pulmonary edema. Three of the most commonly prescribed drugs are discussed in this section. The drugs are cross-referenced to their specialty chapter.

Labetalol

Labetalol is an alpha- and beta-adrenergic blocker that acts by inhibiting the effects of the sympathetic nervous system (see Chapter 15). Its pharmacologic actions include lowering heart rate, blood pressure, myocardial contractility, and myocardial oxygen consumption and reducing the vasoconstriction that results from sympathetic nervous system stimulation. This drug is indicated for the acute management of clinically significant hypertension in the presence of ischemic and hemorrhagic stroke as well as for hypertensive crisis.

Initially 20 mg of labetalol is administered IV push over 2 minutes. This starting dose can be repeated or doubled every 10 minutes until the desired clinical response is achieved up to a maximum dose of 300 mg. As an alternative approach, a continuous infusion of labetalol mixed with D_5W can be prepared to deliver 1 to 2 mg/min until the target therapeutic response is attained; the maximum dose with this approach is also 300 mg.

Important nursing considerations during the administration of labetalol include the use of an electronic infusion device for accurate continuous-infusion medication delivery, cardiac monitoring, and frequent blood pressure measurement. Documentation of blood pressure may need to be as often as every 5 minutes during IV push dosing or at the initiation of the continuous infusion. Serious adverse effects include hypotension, bradycardia, ventricular dysrhythmias, and bronchospasm. Dizziness is also a frequently reported adverse reaction. Labetalol is contraindicated in patients with bronchial asthma or COPD because of the risk of bronchospasm and in patients with severe bradycardia or apparent heart failure.

TABLE 55.3   Agents for Emergency Treatment of Shock

Generic	Route and Dosage**	Uses and Considerations
Albuterol	A: Nebulizer: 2.5-5 mg q20min x 3 doses; then 2.5-10 mg q1-4h PRN C/Adol: 1.25-5 mg q20min x 3 doses; then 2.5-10 mg q1-4h PRN	For bronchoconstriction secondary to anaphylactic shock, asthma, and COPD. Adverse effects include tachycardia, tremor, nervousness, cardiac dysrhythmias, and hypertension. Pregnancy category: C*; PB: UK; t½: 3.7-5 h
Dextrose 50%	A: IV: 50 mL C: 0.5-1.0 g/kg IV of dextrose 25% sol	For insulin shock, severe hypoglycemia. Pregnancy category: C*; PB: UK; t½: UK
Diphenhydramine	A: IM/IV: 10-50 mg	For anaphylactic shock, acute allergic reaction. Pregnancy category: C*; PB: 98%-99%; t½: 3-8 h
Dobutamine	A: IV drip: 5-10 mcg/kg/min	For low cardiac output. Effects antagonized by beta blockers. Pregnancy category: C*; PB: UK; t½: 2 min
Dopamine hydrochloride	See Prototype Drug Chart 55.4	
Epinephrine	A: IM/Subcut: 0.3-0.5 mg (1:1000 sol); may repeat q5-15 min A: IV/IO: 0.1-0.25 mg (1:10,000 sol); may repeat q5-15 min A: ETT: 2-2.5 mg; may repeat q3-5 min C/Adol: IV: 0.01 mg/kg/dose; may repeat q3-5 min. *Max.* 1 mg/dose C ≥15 kg/Adol: IM/Subcut: weight based: 0.15-0.3 mg/dose; may repeat q5-20min C/Adol: ETT: 0.1 mg/kg/dose; may repeat q3-5 min	For anaphylactic shock, severe acute asthmatic attack. May cause hypertensive crisis with MAOIs, and increased dysrhythmias may occur with cardiac glycosides. Pregnancy category: C*; PB: UK; t½: UK
Glucagon	A: Subcut/IM/IV: 1 mg; may repeat once C/Adol: Subcut/IM/IV: weight based: 0.5-1 mg; may repeat once	Insulin shock, severe hypoglycemia, beta-blocker overdose (reverses effects of beta blockers). Pregnancy category: B*; PB: UK; t½: 3-10 min
Norepinephrine	A: IV: Initially, up to 8-12 mcg/min, titrated in increments of 0.02 mcg/kg/min. *Max.* 3.3 mcg/kg/min	Hypotension not responsive to other therapies. Pregnancy category: D*; PB: UK; t½: UK

*Pregnancy categories have been revised. See http://www.fda.gov/Drugs/DevelopmentApprovalProcess/DevelopmentResources/Labeling/ucm093307.htm for more information.

**Other dosing regimens for neonates, infants, and children are available.

A, Adult; *Adol,* adolescent; *C,* child; *COPD,* chronic obstructive pulmonary disease; *ETT,* endotracheal tube; *h,* hour; *IM,* intramuscular; *IO,* intraosseus; *IV,* intravenous; *MAOIs,* monoamine oxidase inhibitors; *Max,* maximum; *min,* minute; *PB,* protein binding; *PRN,* as needed; *q,* every; *sol,* solution; *subcut,* subcutaneous; *t½,* half-life; *UK,* unknown; ≥, greater than or equal to.

Nitroprusside Sodium

Nitroprusside sodium is an IV agent used to reduce arterial blood pressure in hypertensive emergencies (see Chapter 39). The mechanism of action is immediate, direct arterial and venous vasodilation. Antihypertensive effects end when nitroprusside sodium is discontinued; blood pressure increases as soon as drug administration is stopped. Continuous and accurate blood pressure measurement is required. In general, 50 mg of nitroprusside sodium is mixed in 250 mL D_5W. The typical dose range for adults is 0.25 to 0.3 mcg/kg/min, titrated to the desired clinical response. The maximum dose is 10 mcg/kg/min.

There are several important nursing considerations:

- Nitroprusside sodium is rapidly inactivated by light; the IV bottle or bag must be wrapped with aluminum foil or another opaque material to protect the solution from degradation.
- Although a faint brown tint is typical, blue or brown discoloration of the solution indicates degradation and necessitates that the solution be discarded.
- When nitroprusside sodium therapy is prolonged, or when it is infused at the maximum dose of 10 mcg/kg/min for more than 10 minutes, patients are at risk for toxicity resulting from elevated serum thiocyanate or cyanide levels (by-products of drug metabolism). Signs and symptoms include metabolic acidosis, profound hypotension, dyspnea, dizziness, and

vomiting. Serum thiocyanate levels should be monitored every 24 to 72 hours for patients receiving prolonged infusions of more than 2 mcg/kg/min. Patients with renal insufficiency or failure are at a higher risk because the metabolites are excreted in the urine.

- Patients should be placed on an oral antihypertensive agent as soon as possible so that nitroprusside sodium can be tapered slowly. Drug data for nitroprusside sodium are presented in Prototype Drug Chart 55.5.

Furosemide

Furosemide (Complementary and Alternative Therapies 55.2) is classified as a *loop diuretic* that acts by inhibiting sodium and chloride reabsorption from the ascending loop of Henle and the proximal and distal tubules. It promotes the renal excretion of water, sodium, chloride, magnesium, hydrogen, and calcium, and it depletes potassium (see Chapter 38). Furosemide also has peripheral and renal vasodilating effects that can lower blood pressure. The main indications for use of furosemide as an emergency drug are acute pulmonary edema from left ventricular dysfunction and hypertensive crisis.

Furosemide is given as an initial bolus of 20 to 40 mg IV over 1 to 2 minutes. For patients who take furosemide on a regular basis, the effective dose may be much higher (up to 2 mg/kg).

PROTOTYPE DRUG CHART 55.5

Nitroprusside Sodium

Drug Class	Dosage
Vasodilator Pregnancy category: C*	A/C: IV drip: Initially 0.25-0.3 mcg/kg/min, then titrate to desired response. Usual range is 0.25-10 mcg/kg/min.
Contraindications	**Drug-Lab-Food Interactions**
Hypersensitivity, hypertension (compensatory), decreased cerebral perfusion, coarctation of the aorta *Caution:* Increased intracranial pressure	Drug: Antihypertensives, general anesthetics Note: Do not mix with any other drug in syringe or solution. Lab: Decrease in $PaCO_2$, pH
Pharmacokinetics	**Pharmacodynamics**
Absorption: IV only Distribution: PB: UK Metabolism: t½: <10 min Excretion: In urine	IV: Onset: 1-2 min Peak: Rapid Duration: 1-10 min
Therapeutic Effects/Uses	
To treat hypertensive crisis and to decrease systemic vascular resistance to improve cardiac performance Mode of Action: Stimulates smooth muscle of veins and arteries; produces peripheral vasodilation	
Side Effects	**Adverse Reactions**
Dizziness, headache, nausea, abdominal pain, sweating, palpitations, weakness, vomiting	Thiocyanate toxicity: hypotension, tinnitus, dyspnea, blurred vision, metabolic acidosis *Life threatening:* Severe hypotension, loss of consciousness, profound cardiovascular depression

*Pregnancy categories have been revised. See http://www.fda.gov/Drugs/DevelopmentApprovalProcess/DevelopmentResources/Labeling/ucm093307.htm for more information.
A, Adult; *C,* child; *IV,* intravenous; *min,* minute; *PB,* protein binding; *PaCO2,* partial pressure of carbon dioxide; *t½,* half-life; *UK,* unknown; <, less than.

🌿 COMPLEMENTARY AND ALTERNATIVE THERAPIES 55.2

Furosemide

Ginseng can inhibit the efficacy of furosemide. Licorice can promote potassium loss, which enhances the potential for severe hypokalemia. These products should not be taken concurrently with furosemide.

The vasodilatory effects occur *before* diuresis begins, and they act to lower blood pressure. Central venous pressure is reduced through a decrease in venous return to the heart once vasodilation is achieved. Diuresis should start within 10 minutes of drug administration and may continue for approximately 6 hours.

The most significant adverse effects are severe hypovolemia, dehydration, and electrolyte disturbances (hypokalemia, hypomagnesemia, hyponatremia, and hypochloremia). Patients taking digitalis preparations are at an increased risk of digitalis toxicity from hypokalemia. The patient's fluid and electrolyte status, blood urea nitrogen (BUN), and creatinine must be carefully assessed before and after furosemide administration, including auscultation of breath sounds for rales, strict surveillance of intake and output, and review of laboratory data when available. An indwelling urinary catheter might be necessary. Electrolyte and careful fluid replacement may be required during furosemide therapy to prevent physiologic consequences. The nurse must also exercise caution when giving nephrotoxic agents when furosemide is prescribed and in administering the drug to patients with sulfonamide sensitivity because furosemide is a sulfonamide derivative that can produce an allergic reaction.

Morphine Sulfate

Like furosemide, morphine sulfate is also indicated for acute pulmonary edema because it produces venous vasodilation that decreases cardiac preload, the amount of blood returning to the right ventricle. The net effect is a decrease in pulmonary venous congestion. Morphine was discussed earlier in that subsection under *Emergency Drugs for Cardiac Disorders.*

Table 55.4 lists emergency drugs used for hypertensive crises and pulmonary edema and their dosages, uses, and considerations.

TABLE 55.4	**Emergency Drugs for Hypertensive Crises and Pulmonary Edema**	
Generic	**Route and Dosage***	**Uses and Considerations**
Nitroprusside sodium	See Prototype Drug Chart 55.5.	
Furosemide	A: IM/IV: Initially, 20-40 mg, titrate by 20 mg q2h PRN C: IM/IV: 1-2 mg/kg q6-12h; *max.* 6 mg/kg/dose	For acute pulmonary edema. Adverse effects include hypovolemia, dehydration, and electrolyte disturbances.
Morphine	IV: 1-4 mg q5-30min	For pulmonary edema, chest pain, unstable angina, MI
Labetalol hydrochloride	A: IV: Initially, 20 mg over 2 min; additional doses of 20-80 mg q10 min until desired response A: IV drip: 0.5-2 mg/min; titrate to response; *max:* 300 mg; continuous infusion 2 mg/min	For hypertension in CVA and for hypertensive crisis. Adverse effects include ventricular dysrhythmias, hypotension, and bronchospasm. *Contraindications:* Bronchial asthma, COPD, severe bradycardia, heart failure

*Other dosing regimens for neonates, infants, and children are available.
A, Adult; *C,* child; *COPD,* chronic obstructive pulmonary disease; *CVA,* cerebrovascular accident; *h,* hour; *IM,* intramuscular; *IV,* intravenous; *max,* maximum; *MI,* myocardial infarction; *min,* minute; *PRN,* as needed; *q,* every.

CRITICAL THINKING CASE STUDY

DW, age 19 years, suffered a gunshot wound to the head and a spinal cord injury from a stab wound over the thoracic spine 1 hour ago. He was transported immediately from the injury scene to the trauma center by paramedics. Upon hospital arrival, DW was awake and following simple commands, but his neurologic status has subsequently deteriorated. At this point, he has undergone initial resuscitation and a rapid diagnostic workup. He is now orally intubated, has two functional intravenous (IV) catheters—one peripheral line in the right forearm and one triple-lumen central line in the left subclavian vein—an oral gastric tube, and an indwelling urinary catheter. His current vital signs are blood pressure (BP) 88/56, heart rate (HR) 56, temperature 96.8°F (36°C), and respiratory rate (RR) 16 on a mechanical ventilator. His mother reported that DW is addicted to opioids, including heroin. He also abuses oral diazepam and other street drugs.

DW's diagnoses include a penetrating head injury with intracerebral hemorrhage diagnosed by computed tomography (CT) scan, a penetrating spinal cord injury at the T4 level, and drug abuse. DW opens his eyes spontaneously, does not follow commands, and withdraws to pain with only his upper extremities; his lower extremities do not move.

1. On arrival at the trauma center, should DW have received supplemental oxygen based on his mechanism of injury? What type of oxygen delivery device would be appropriate for DW on his initial presentation, when he was breathing spontaneously?
2. The physician orders 50 g of mannitol to be given now, IV push. On hand are several 50-mL vials of "mannitol, 25%" solution. How many milliliters of mannitol from this vial need to be drawn up into the syringe to administer 50 g?
3. Describe the type of needle that must be used when administering mannitol. Explain your answer. What size syringe

should be used? Which IV line should be used to administer the mannitol?
4. What are the indications for mannitol administration? List at least three nursing considerations when giving mannitol.
5. DW has a history of heroin and diazepam abuse. List the reversal drugs that could be used if the trauma team believes recent illicit drug use may be a contributing factor to his altered mental state.
6. Because of DW's spinal cord injury, he is exhibiting signs of neurogenic shock: bradycardia, warm skin, and hypotension. What is the drug of choice that the nurse should keep at the bedside in case DW requires emergency treatment for symptomatic bradycardia? Name the drug, its mechanism of action, and dosing considerations.
7. The physician orders a dopamine infusion, 800 mg/250 mL D_5W, to be titrated to maintain systolic BP above 110 mm Hg. Which IV site would be the best choice for a continuous dopamine infusion in DW?
8. What is the consequence of dopamine extravasation?
9. Describe the treatment for dopamine extravasation.
10. What vital sign parameters must be monitored while DW receives dopamine? Name at least four adverse effects of dopamine.

Antibiotics are initiated as prophylaxis for infection due to the nature of DW's penetrating injuries. Upon infusion of the antibiotic, a full-body rash, swelling of the lips and tongue, and hypotension develop.

11. After antibiotic administration, what condition has developed in DW?
12. What are the drugs of choice to treat DW's condition now?
13. How can the nurse evaluate the effectiveness of these drugs?

NCLEX STUDY QUESTIONS

1. The nurse is administering atropine 0.3 mg IV to a 75-year-old patient with a heart rate of 45, and his heart rate decreases to 38. What is the most likely explanation?
   a. Atropine exerts its effects by stimulating the vagus nerve.
   b. The ordered dose was too low.
   c. Adenosine was indicated, not atropine.
   d. Atropine typically slows heart rate first and then increases it.

2. An 80-year-old woman with a hip fracture received morphine 3 mg intravenously 20 minutes ago. The patient's son runs to the nurses' station and says that his mother is no longer responding to him. What actions should the nurse take?
   a. Assess the patient; call for additional assistance; support breathing with a bag-valve-mask device as indicated, and prepare to administer flumazenil.
   b. Call the physician and report that the patient most likely suffered a stroke and now has elevated intracranial pressure; prepare to administer mannitol.
   c. Assess the patient; call for additional assistance; support breathing with a bag-valve-mask device as indicated, and prepare to administer naloxone.
   d. Explain to the patient's son that the morphine is taking effect and that unresponsiveness is the desired outcome to best manage her pain.

3. The nurse is caring for a 21-year-old woman with a closed head injury. Her intracranial pressure is 35 (normal <20), and her serum osmolality is 330 mOsm/kg. The nurse should anticipate which action?
   a. Administration of mannitol
   b. Withholding mannitol at this time, but taking other measures to reduce intracranial pressure
   c. Administration of sodium nitroprusside
   d. Taking no action at this time because the patient has a serum osmolality of 330, which will offset the effects of the elevated intracranial pressure

4. A dopamine infusion was started in a patient's antecubital vein during resuscitation after cardiac arrest. The electronic infusion device is now sounding an alert for an occlusion. What is the most important immediate concern for the nurse?
   a. Infiltration with phentolamine will be necessary if there is extravasation.
   b. An interruption in the infusion can produce hypotension in the patient.
   c. The device will need to be reported to the hospital's clinical engineering department for service.
   d. The patient could develop hypertension as a result of the alarm.

5. Adenosine is ordered for a patient in the emergency department. Immediately after intravenous (IV) administration, the nurse observes a short period of asystole on the cardiac monitor that resolves spontaneously. What is the most appropriate initial action for the nurse?
   a. Call for the doctor.
   b. Prepare epinephrine and atropine for intravenous administration.
   c. Initiate cardiopulmonary resuscitation (CPR).
   d. Closely observe the patient and the cardiac monitor.

6. A patient on the medical-surgical unit has suffered an acute anaphylactic reaction during infusion of an IV antibiotic with hives and bronchospasm. The nurse practitioner has written a number of stat drug orders. What is the priority drug to administer first?
   a. Steroid dose pack
   b. Dopamine
   c. Epinephrine
   d. Diphenhydramine

7. The nurse receives a stat order to administer 50% dextrose solution intravenously to a 1-year-old child with hypoglycemia. How should this drug best be prepared for safe administration to the child?
   a. Use a filter needle.
   b. Draw the drug into a tuberculin syringe.
   c. Dilute 1:1 with sterile water to produce dextrose 25%.
   d. Shake the solution vigorously before injection.

8. A 51-year-old woman has been reportedly taking alprazolam for a severe anxiety disorder following her mother's death. She was brought into the emergency department because she became unresponsive while at work in an insurance office. Knowing her history, what should the nurse anticipate administering?
   a. Mannitol
   b. Naloxone
   c. Activated charcoal
   d. Flumazenil

9. A 25-year-old woman was admitted to the emergency department after a successful prehospital resuscitation from cardiac arrest owing to an asthma attack. On arrival, her pulse oximeter reading is 85%. Given her condition, what is the most important initial drug to administer as ordered?
   a. Epinephrine
   b. Sodium bicarbonate
   c. Albuterol
   d. Oxygen

10. The nurse practitioner orders epinephrine 0.3 mg intramuscularly for a severe allergic reaction to a bee sting in an adult patient. Which concentration of epinephrine should the nurse select to administer this particular dose?
   a. 1:10,000
   b. 1:1000
   c. 1:100
   d. 1:10

11. The emergency nurse practitioner orders activated charcoal for a teenage girl who took an intentional overdose of aspirin and several unknown drugs from her parents' drug cabinet. Upon preparing to administer the activated charcoal by mouth, the nurse notes that the patient has become very somnolent and opens her eyes only to a noxious stimulus. Which action by the nurse is most appropriate at this point?
   a. Immediately discuss the change in the patient's mental status with the nurse practitioner so that the plan of care can be reevaluated.
   b. Immediately insert a nasogastric tube and administer the activated charcoal.
   c. Immediately elevate the head of the patient's stretcher, and coax her to drink the activated charcoal while applying noxious stimuli as necessary to keep her awake.
   d. Give only half the dose now, and wait until her mental status improves before giving the remainder of the dose.

12. While getting dressed to go home after minor outpatient surgery on his leg for removal of a mole, a 62-year-old patient notifies the nurse that he has severe chest pain. He is also diaphoretic and complains of shortness of breath. The surgeon is notified and orders administration of aspirin 325 mg by mouth while quickly making arrangements to transfer the patient to the emergency department. Which is the best course of action by the nurse?
   a. Question the aspirin order because the patient just had a surgical procedure and might have bleeding complications.
   b. After checking for drug allergies, first instruct the patient to chew the aspirin tablet and then administer the aspirin.
   c. After checking for drug allergies, instruct the patient to swallow the aspirin tablet whole.
   d. Suggest to the surgeon that the enteric-coated form of aspirin might be better tolerated by the patient to avoid gastrointestinal distress.

Answers: 1, b; 2, c; 3, b; 4, b; 5, d; 6, c; 7, c; 8, d; 9, d; 10, b; 11, a; 12, b.

Activity intolerance: Insufficient physiological or psychological energy to endure or complete required or desired daily activities.

Acute confusion: Abrupt onset of reversible disturbances of consciousness, attention, cognition, and perception that develop over a short period of time.

Acute pain: An unpleasant sensory and emotional experience associated with actual or potential tissue damage, or described in terms of such damage (International Association for the Study of Pain); sudden or slow onset of any intensity from mild to severe with an anticipated or predictable end.

Anxiety: Vague, uneasy feeling of discomfort or dread accompanied by an autonomic response (the source is often nonspecific or unknown to the individual); a feeling of apprehension caused by anticipation of danger. It is an alerting sign that warns of impending danger and enables the individual to take measures to deal with threat.

Autonomic dysreflexia: Life-threatening, uninhibited sympathetic response of the nervous system to a noxious stimulus after a spinal cord injury at T7 or above.

Bathing self-care deficit: Impaired ability to perform or complete bathing activities for self.

Bowel incontinence: Change in normal bowel habits characterized by involuntary passage of stool.

Caregiver role strain: Difficulty in performing family/significant other caregiver role.

Chronic confusion: Irreversible, long-standing, and/or progressive deterioration of intellect and personality characterized by decreased ability to interpret environmental stimuli and decreased capacity for intellectual thought processes, and manifested by disturbances of memory, orientation, and behavior.

Chronic functional constipation: Infrequent or difficult evacuation of feces that has been present for at least three of the prior 12 months.

Chronic low self-esteem: Longstanding, negative self-evaluating/feelings about self or self-capabilities.

Chronic pain: Unpleasant sensory and emotional experience associated with actual or potential tissue damage or described in terms of such damage (International Association for the Study of Pain); sudden or slow onset of any intensity from mild to severe, constant or recurring, without an anticipated or predictable end and a duration of greater than 3 months.

Chronic pain syndrome: Recurrent or persistent pain that has lasted at least 3 months and that significantly affects daily functioning or well-being

Chronic sorrow: Cyclical, recurring, and potentially progressive pattern of pervasive sadness experienced (by a parent, caregiver, or individual with chronic illness or disability) in response to continual loss throughout the trajectory of an illness or disability.

Complicated grieving: A disorder that occurs after the death of a significant other in which the experience of distress accompanying bereavement fails to follow normative expectations and manifests in functional impairment.

Compromised family coping: A usually supportive primary person (family member, significant other, or close friend) provides insufficient, ineffective, or compromised support, comfort, assistance, or encouragement that may be needed by the client to manage or master adaptive tasks related to his or her health challenge.

Constipation: Decrease in normal frequency of defecation accompanied by difficult or incomplete passage of stool and/or passage of excessively hard, dry stool.

Contamination: Exposure to environmental contaminants in doses sufficient to cause adverse health effects.

Death anxiety: Vague, uneasy feeling of discomfort or dread generated by perceptions of a real or imagined threat to one's existence.

Decisional conflict: Uncertainty about course of action to be taken when choice among competing actions involves risk, loss, or challenge to values and beliefs.

Decreased cardiac output: Inadequate blood pumped by the heart to meet the metabolic demands of the body.

Decreased intracranial adaptive capacity: Intracranial fluid dynamic mechanisms that normally compensate for increases in intracranial volumes are compromised, resulting in repeated disproportionate increases in intracranial pressure (ICP) in response to a variety of noxious and nonnoxious stimuli.

Defensive coping: Repeated projection of falsely positive self-evaluation based on a self-protective pattern that defends against underlying perceived threats to positive self-regard.

Deficient community health: Presence of one or more health problems or factors that deter wellness or increase the risk of health problems experienced by an aggregate.

Deficient diversional activity: Decreased stimulation from (or interest or engagement in) recreational or leisure activities.

Deficient fluid volume: Decreased intravascular, interstitial, and/or intracellular fluid. This refers to dehydration or water loss alone without change in sodium level.

Deficient knowledge: Absence or deficiency of cognitive information related to a specific topic.

Delayed surgical recovery: Extension of the number of postoperative days required to initiate and perform activities that maintain life, health, and well-being.

Diarrhea: Passage of loose, unformed stools.

Disabled family coping: Behavior of primary person (family member, significant other, or close friend) that disables his or her capacities and the client's capacities to effectively address tasks essential to either person's adaptation to the health challenge.

Disorganized infant behavior: Disintegrated physiological and neurobehavioral responses of an infant to the environment.

Disturbed body image: Confusion in the mental picture of one's physical self.

Disturbed personal identity: Inability to maintain an integrated and complete perception of self.

Disturbed sleep pattern: Time-limited interruptions of sleep amount and quality due to external factors.

Dressing self-care deficit: Impaired ability to perform or complete dressing activities for self.

Dysfunctional family processes: Psychosocial, spiritual, and physiological functions of the family unit are chronically disorganized, which leads to conflict, denial of problems, resistance to change, ineffective problem solving, and a series of self-perpetuating crises.

Dysfunctional gastrointestinal motility: Increased, decreased, ineffective, or lack of peristaltic activity within the gastrointestinal system.

Dysfunctional ventilatory weaning response: Inability to adjust to lowered levels of mechanical ventilator support that interrupts and prolongs the weaning process.

Excess fluid volume: Increased isotonic fluid retention.

Fatigue: An overwhelming, sustained sense of exhaustion and decreased capacity for physical and mental work at the usual level.

Fear: Response to perceived threat that is consciously recognized as a danger.

Feeding self-care deficit: Impaired ability to perform or complete self-feeding activities.

Frail elderly syndrome: Dynamic state of unstable equilibrium that affects the older individual experiencing deterioration in one or more domains of health (physical, functional, psychological, or social) and leads to increased susceptibility to adverse health effects, particularly disability.

Functional urinary incontinence: Inability of a usually continent person to reach the toilet in time to avoid unintentional loss of urine.

Grieving: A normal complex process that includes emotional, physical, spiritual, social, and intellectual responses and behaviors by which individuals, families, and communities incorporate an actual, anticipated, or perceived loss into their daily lives.

Hopelessness: Subjective state in which an individual sees limited or no alternatives or personal choices available and is unable to mobilize energy on own behalf.

Hyperthermia: Core body temperature above the normal diurnal range due to failure of thermoregulation.

Hypothermia: Core body temperature below normal diurnal range due to failure of thermoregulation.

Imbalanced nutrition: less than body requirements: Intake of nutrients insufficient to meet metabolic needs.

Impaired bed mobility: Limitation of independent movement from one bed position to another.

Impaired comfort: Perceived lack of ease, relief, and transcendence in physical, psychospiritual, environmental, cultural and/or social dimensions.

Impaired dentition: Disruption in tooth development/eruption patterns or structural integrity of individual teeth.

Impaired emancipated decision-making: A process of choosing a health care decision that does not include personal knowledge and/or consideration of social norms, or does not occur in a flexible environment, resulting in decisional dissatisfaction.

Impaired gas exchange: Excess or deficit in oxygenation and/or carbon dioxide elimination at the alveolar-capillary membrane.

Impaired home maintenance: Inability to independently maintain a safe growth-promoting immediate environment.

Impaired memory: Inability to remember or recall bits of information or behavioral skills.

Impaired mood regulation: A mental state characterized by shifts in mood or affect and which is comprised of a constellation of affective, cognitive, somatic, and/or physiological manifestations varying from mild to severe.

Impaired oral mucous membrane: Injury to the lips, soft tissue, buccal cavity, and/or oropharynx.

Impaired parenting: Inability of the primary caretaker to create, maintain, or regain an environment that promotes the optimum growth and development of the child.

Impaired physical mobility: Limitation in independent, purposeful physical movement of the body or of one or more extremities.

Impaired religiosity: Impaired ability to exercise reliance on beliefs and/or participate in rituals of a particular faith tradition.

Impaired resilience: Decreased ability to sustain a pattern of positive responses to an adverse situation or crisis.

Impaired sitting: Limitation of ability to independently and purposefully attain and/or maintain a rest position that is supported by the buttocks and thighs, in which the torso is upright.

Impaired skin integrity: Altered epidermis and/or dermis.

Impaired social interaction: Insufficient or excessive quantity or ineffective quality of social exchange.

Impaired spontaneous ventilation: Decreased energy reserves resulting in an inability to maintain independent breathing that is adequate to support life.

Impaired standing: Limitation of ability to independently and purposefully attain and/or maintain the body in an upright position from feet to head.

Impaired swallowing: Abnormal functioning of the swallowing mechanism associated with deficits in oral, pharyngeal, or esophageal structure or function.

Impaired tissue integrity: Damage to the mucous membrane, cornea, integumentary system, muscular fascia, muscle, tendon, bone, cartilage, joint capsule, and/or ligament.

Impaired transfer ability: Limitation of independent movement between two nearby surfaces.

Impaired urinary elimination: Dysfunction in urine elimination.

Impaired verbal communication: Decreased, delayed, or absent ability to receive, process, transmit, and/or use a system of symbols.

Impaired walking: Limitation of independent movement within the environment on foot.

Impaired wheelchair mobility: Limitation of independent operation of wheelchair within environment.

Ineffective activity planning: Inability to prepare for a set of actions fixed in time and under certain conditions.

Ineffective airway clearance: Inability to clear secretions or obstructions from the respiratory tract to maintain a clear airway.

Ineffective breastfeeding: Difficulty providing milk to an infant or young child directly from the breasts, which may compromise nutritional status of the infant/child.

Ineffective breathing pattern: Inspiration and/or expiration that does not provide adequate ventilation.

Ineffective childbearing process: Pregnancy and childbirth process and care of the newborn that does not match the environmental context, norms, and expectations.

Ineffective community coping: A pattern of community activities for adaptation and problem solving that is unsatisfactory for meeting the demands or needs of the community.

Ineffective coping: Inability to form a valid appraisal of the stressors, inadequate choices of practiced responses, and/or inability to use available resources.

Ineffective denial: Conscious or unconscious attempt to disavow the knowledge or meaning of an event to reduce anxiety and/or fear, leading to the detriment of health.

Ineffective family health management: A pattern of regulating and integrating into family processes a program for the treatment of illness and its sequelae that is unsatisfactory for meeting specific health goals.

Ineffective health maintenance: Inability to identify, manage, and/or seek out help to maintain health.

Ineffective health management: Pattern of regulating and integrating into daily living a therapeutic regimen for the treatment of illness and its sequelae that is unsatisfactory for meeting specific health goals.

Ineffective impulse control: A pattern of performing rapid, unplanned reactions to internal or external stimuli without regard for the negative consequences of these reactions to the impulsive individual or to others.

Ineffective infant feeding pattern: Impaired ability of an infant to suck or coordinate the suck/swallow response resulting in inadequate oral nutrition for metabolic needs.

Ineffective peripheral tissue perfusion: Decrease in blood circulation to the periphery that may compromise health.

Ineffective protection: Decrease in the ability to guard self from internal or external threats such as illness or injury.

Ineffective relationship: A pattern of mutual partnership that is insufficient to provide for each other's needs.

Ineffective role performance: A pattern of behavior and self-expression that does not match the environmental context, norms, and expectations.

Ineffective sexuality pattern: Expressions of concern regarding own sexuality.

Ineffective thermoregulation: Temperature fluctuation between hypothermia and hyperthermia.

Insomnia: A disruption in amount and quality of sleep that impairs functioning.

Insufficient breast milk: Low production of maternal breast milk.

Interrupted breastfeeding: Break in the continuity of providing milk to an infant or young child directly from the breasts, which may compromise breastfeeding success and/or nutritional status of the infant/child.

Interrupted family processes: Change in family relationships and/or functioning.

Labile emotional control: Uncontrollable outbursts of exaggerated and involuntary emotional expression.

Labor pain: Sensory and emotional experience that varies from pleasant to unpleasant, associated with labor and childbirth.

Latex allergy response: A hypersensitive reaction to natural latex rubber products.

Moral distress: Response to the inability to carry out one's chosen ethical/moral decision/action.

Nausea: A subjective phenomenon of an unpleasant feeling in the back of the throat and stomach, which may or may not result in vomiting.

Neonatal jaundice: The yellow-orange tint of the neonate's skin and mucous membranes that occurs after 24 hours of life as a result of unconjugated bilirubin in the circulation.

Noncompliance: Behavior of person and/or caregiver that fails to coincide with a health-promoting or therapeutic plan agreed on by the person (and/or family and/or community) and health care professional. In the presence of an agreed-on, health-promoting, or therapeutic plan, person's or caregiver's behavior is fully or partly non-adherent and may lead to clinically ineffective or partially effective outcomes.

Obesity: A condition in which an individual accumulates abnormal or excessive fat for age and gender that exceeds overweight.

Overflow urinary incontinence: Involuntary loss of urine associated with overdistention of the bladder.

Overweight: A condition in which an individual accumulates abnormal or excessive fat for age and gender.

Parental role conflict: Parental experience of role confusion and conflict in response to crisis.

Perceived constipation: Self-diagnosis of constipation combined with abuse of laxatives, enemas, and/or suppositories to ensure a daily bowel movement.

Post-trauma syndrome: Sustained maladaptive response to a traumatic, overwhelming event.

Powerlessness: The lived experience of lack of control over a situation, including a perception that one's actions do not significantly affect an outcome.

Rape-trauma syndrome: Sustained maladaptive response to a forced, violent, sexual penetration against the victim's will and consent.

Readiness for enhanced breastfeeding: A pattern of providing milk to an infant or young child directly from the breasts, which may be strengthened.

Readiness for enhanced childbearing process: A pattern of preparing for and maintaining a healthy pregnancy, childbirth process, and care of the newborn for ensuring well-being, which can be strengthened.

Readiness for enhanced comfort: A pattern of ease, relief, and transcendence in physical, psychospiritual, environmental, and/or social dimensions, which can be strengthened.

Readiness for enhanced communication: A pattern of exchanging information and ideas with others, which can be strengthened.

Readiness for enhanced community coping: A pattern of community activities for adaptation and problem-solving for meeting the demands or needs of the community, which can be strengthened.

Readiness for enhanced coping: A pattern of cognitive and behavioral efforts to manage demands related to well-being, which can be strengthened.

Readiness for enhanced decision-making: A pattern of choosing a course of action for meeting short- and long-term health-related goals, which can be strengthened.

Readiness for enhanced emancipated decision-making: A process of choosing a healthcare decision that includes personal knowledge and/or consideration of social norms, which can be strengthened.

Readiness for enhanced family coping: A pattern of management of adaptive tasks by primary person (family member, significant other, or close friend) involved with the client's health change, which can be strengthened.

Readiness for enhanced family processes: A pattern of family functioning to support the well-being of family members, which can be strengthened.

Readiness for enhanced fluid balance: A pattern of equilibrium between the fluid volume and chemical composition of body fluids, which can be strengthened.

Readiness for enhanced health management: A pattern of regulating and integrating into daily living a therapeutic regimen for treatment of illness and its sequelae, which can be strengthened.

Readiness for enhanced hope: A pattern of expectations and desires for mobilizing energy on one's own behalf, which can be strengthened.

Readiness for enhanced knowledge: A pattern of cognitive information related to a specific topic, or its acquisition, which can be strengthened.

Readiness for enhanced nutrition: A pattern of nutrient intake, which can be strengthened.

Readiness for enhanced organized infant behavior: A pattern of modulation of the physiological and behavioral systems of functioning (i.e., autonomic, motor, state-organization, self-regulatory, and attentional-interactional systems) in an infant, which can be strengthened.

Readiness for enhanced parenting: A pattern of providing an environment for children or other dependent person(s) to nurture growth and development, which can be strengthened.

Readiness for enhanced power: A pattern of participating knowingly in change for well-being, which can be strengthened.

Readiness for enhanced relationship: A pattern of mutual partnership to provide for each other's needs, which can be strengthened.

Readiness for enhanced religiosity: A pattern of reliance on religious beliefs and/or participation in rituals of a particular faith tradition, which can be strengthened.

Readiness for enhanced resilience: A pattern of positive responses to an adverse situation or crisis, which can be strengthened.

Readiness for enhanced self-care: A pattern of performing activities for oneself to meet health-related goals, which can be strengthened.

Readiness for enhanced self-concept: A pattern of perceptions or ideas about the self, which can be strengthened.

Readiness for enhanced sleep: A pattern of natural, periodic suspension of relative consciousness to provide rest and sustain a desired lifestyle, which can be strengthened.

Readiness for enhanced spiritual well-being: A pattern of experiencing and integrating meaning and purpose in life through connectedness with self, others, art, music, literature, nature, and/or a power greater than oneself, which can be strengthened.

Readiness for enhanced urinary elimination: A pattern of urinary functions for meeting eliminatory needs, which can be strengthened.

Reflex urinary incontinence: Involuntary loss of urine at somewhat predictable intervals when a specific bladder volume is reached.

Relocation stress syndrome: Physiological and/or psychosocial disturbance following transfer from one environment to another.

Risk for activity intolerance: Vulnerable to insufficient physiological or psychological energy to endure or complete required or desired daily activities, which may compromise health.

Risk for acute confusion: Vulnerable to reversible disturbances of consciousness, attention, cognition, and perception that develop over a short period of time, which may compromise health.

Risk for adverse reaction to iodinated contrast media: Vulnerable to noxious or unintended reaction associated with the use of iodinated contrast media that can occur within 7 days after contrast agent injection, which may compromise health.

Risk for allergy response: Vulnerable to exaggerated immune response or reaction to substances, which may compromise health.

Risk for aspiration: Vulnerable to entry of gastrointestinal secretions, oropharyngeal secretions, solids, or fluids to the tracheobronchial passages, which may compromise health.

Risk for autonomic dysreflexia: Vulnerable to life-threatening, uninhibited response of the sympathetic nervous system post-spinal shock, in an individual with spinal cord injury or lesion at T6 or above (has been demonstrated in patients with injuries at T7 and T8), which may compromise health.

Risk for bleeding: Vulnerable to a decrease in blood volume, which may compromise health.

Risk for caregiver role strain: Vulnerable to difficulty in performing the family/significant other caregiver role, which may compromise health.

Risk for chronic functional constipation: Vulnerable to infrequent or difficult evacuation of feces that has been present nearly 3 of the prior 12 months, which may compromise health.

Risk for chronic low self-esteem: Vulnerable to longstanding negative self-evaluating/feelings about self or self-capabilities, which may compromise health.

Risk for complicated grieving: Vulnerable to a disorder that occurs after death of a significant other in which the experience of distress accompanying bereavement fails to follow normative expectations and manifests in functional impairment, which may compromise health.

Risk for compromised human dignity: Vulnerable for perceived loss of respect and honor, which may compromise health.

Risk for constipation: Vulnerable to a decrease in normal frequency of defecation accompanied by difficult or incomplete passage of stool, which may compromise health.

Risk for contamination: Vulnerable to exposure to environmental contaminants which may compromise health.

Risk for corneal injury: Vulnerable to infection or inflammatory lesion in the corneal tissue that can affect superficial or deep layers, which may compromise health.

Risk for decreased cardiac output: Vulnerable to inadequate blood pumped by the heart to meet metabolic demands of the body, which may compromise health.

Risk for decreased cardiac tissue perfusion: Vulnerable to a decrease in cardiac (coronary) circulation, which may compromise health.

Risk for deficient fluid volume: Vulnerable to experiencing decreased intravascular, interstitial, and/or intracellular fluid volumes, which may compromise health.

Risk for delayed development: Vulnerable to delay of 25% or more in one or more of the areas of social or self-regulatory behavior, or in cognitive, language, gross, or fine motor skills, which may compromise health.

Risk for delayed surgical recovery: Vulnerable to an extension of the number of postoperative days required to initiate and perform activities that maintain life, health, and well-being, which may compromise health.

Risk for disorganized infant behavior: Vulnerable to alteration in integration and modulation of the physiological and behavioral systems of functioning (i.e., autonomic, motor, state-organization, self-regulatory, and attentional-interactional systems), which may compromise health.

Risk for disproportionate growth: Vulnerable to growth above the 97th percentile or below the 3rd percentile for age, crossing two percentile channels, which may compromise health.

Risk for disturbed maternal–fetal dyad: Vulnerable to disruption of the symbiotic maternal-fetal dyad as a result of comorbid or pregnancy-related conditions, which may compromise health.

Risk for disturbed personal identity: Vulnerable to the inability to maintain an integrated and complete perception of self, which may compromise health.

Risk for disuse syndrome: Vulnerable to deterioration of body systems as the result of prescribed or unavoidable musculoskeletal inactivity, which may compromise health.

Risk for dry eye: Vulnerable to eye discomfort or damage to the cornea and conjunctiva due to reduced quantity or quality of tears to moisten the eye, which may compromise health.

Risk for dysfunctional gastrointestinal motility: Vulnerable to a decrease in normal frequency of defecation accompanied by difficult or incomplete passage of stool, which may compromise health.

Risk for electrolyte imbalance: Vulnerable to changes in serum electrolyte levels, which may compromise health.

Risk for falls: Vulnerable to increased susceptibility to falling, which may cause physical harm and compromise health.

Risk for frail elderly syndrome: Vulnerable to a dynamic state of unstable equilibrium that affects the older individual experiencing deterioration in one or more domains of health (physical, functional, or social) and leads to increased susceptibility to adverse health effects, in particular disability.

Risk for hypothermia: Vulnerable to a failure of thermoregulation that may result in a core body temperature below the normal diurnal range, which may compromise health.

Risk for imbalanced body temperature: Vulnerable to failure to maintain body temperature within normal parameters, which may compromise health.

Risk for imbalanced fluid volume: Vulnerable to a decrease, increase, or rapid shift from one to the other of intravascular, interstitial, and/or intracellular fluid, which may compromise health. This refers to body fluid loss, gain, or both.

Risk for impaired attachment: Vulnerable to disruption of the interactive process between parent/significant other and child that fosters the development of a protective and nurturing reciprocal relationship.

Risk for impaired cardiovascular function: Vulnerable to internal or external causes that can damage one or more vital organs and the circulatory system itself.

Risk for impaired emancipated decision-making: Vulnerable to a process of choosing a healthcare decision that does not include personal knowledge and/or considerations of social norms, or does not occur in a flexible environment, resulting in decisional satisfaction.

Risk for impaired liver function: Vulnerable to a decrease in liver function, which may compromise health.

Risk for impaired oral mucous membrane: Vulnerable to injury to the lips, soft tissues, buccal cavity, and/or oropharynx, which may compromise health.

Risk for impaired parenting: Vulnerable to inability of the primary caretaker to create, maintain, or regain an environment that promotes the optimum growth and development of the child, which may compromise the well-being of the child.

Risk for impaired religiosity: Vulnerable to an impaired ability to exercise reliance on religious beliefs and/or participate in rituals of a particular faith tradition, which may compromise health.

Risk for impaired resilience: Vulnerable to decreased ability to sustain a pattern of positive response to an adverse situation or crisis, which may compromise health.

Risk for impaired skin integrity: Vulnerable to alteration in epidermis and/or dermis, which may compromise health.

Risk for impaired tissue integrity: Vulnerable to damage to the mucous membrane, cornea, integumentary system, muscular fascia, muscle, tendon, bone, cartilage, joint capsule, and/or ligament, which may compromise health.

Risk for ineffective activity planning: Vulnerable to an inability to prepare for a set of actions fixed in time and under certain conditions, which may compromise health.

Risk for ineffective cerebral tissue perfusion: Vulnerable to a decrease in cerebral tissue circulation, which may compromise health.

Risk for ineffective childbearing process: Vulnerable to not matching environmental context, norms and expectations of pregnancy, childbirth process, and the care of the newborn.

Risk for ineffective gastrointestinal perfusion: Vulnerable to decrease in gastrointestinal circulation, which may compromise health.

Risk for ineffective peripheral tissue perfusion: Vulnerable to a decrease in blood circulation to the periphery, which may compromise health.

Risk for ineffective relationship: Vulnerable to developing a pattern that is insufficient for providing a mutual partnership to provide for each other's needs.

Risk for ineffective renal perfusion: Vulnerable to a decrease in blood circulation to the kidney, which may compromise health.

Risk for infection: Vulnerable to invasion and multiplication of pathogenic organisms which may compromise health.

Risk for injury: Vulnerable to physical damage due to environmental conditions interacting with the individual's adaptive and defensive resources, which may compromise health.

Risk for latex allergy response: Vulnerable to a hypersensitive reaction to natural latex rubber products, which may compromise health.

Risk for loneliness: Vulnerable to experiencing discomfort associated with a desire or need for more contact with others, which may compromise health.

Risk for neonatal jaundice: Vulnerable to the yellow orange tint of the neonate's skin and mucous membranes that occur after 24 hours of life as a result of unconjugated bilirubin in the circulation, which may compromise health.

Risk for other-directed violence: Vulnerable to behaviors in which an individual demonstrates that he or she can be physically, emotionally, and/or sexually harmful to others.

Risk for overweight: Vulnerable to abnormal or excessive fat accumulation for age and gender, which may compromise health.

Risk for perioperative hypothermia: Vulnerable to an inadvertent drop in core body temperature below 36°C (96.8°F) occurring one hour before to 24 hours after surgery, which may compromise health.

Risk for perioperative positioning injury: Vulnerable to inadvertent anatomical and physical changes as a result of posture or equipment used during an invasive/surgical procedure, which may compromise health.

Risk for peripheral neurovascular dysfunction: Vulnerable to disruption in the circulation, sensation, and motion of an extremity, which may compromise health.

Risk for poisoning: Vulnerable to accidental exposure to, or ingestion of, drugs or dangerous products in sufficient doses, which may compromise health.

Risk for post-trauma syndrome: Vulnerable to sustained maladaptive response to a traumatic, overwhelming event, which may compromise health.

Risk for powerlessness: Vulnerable to the lived experience of lack of control over a situation, including a perception that one's actions do not significantly affect the outcome, which may compromise health.

Risk for pressure ulcer: Vulnerable to localized injury to the skin and/or underlying tissue usually over a bony prominence as a result of pressure, or pressure in combination with shear (NPUAP, 2007).

Risk for relocation stress syndrome: Vulnerable to physiological and/or psychosocial disturbance following transfer from one environment to another, which may compromise health

Risk for self-directed violence: Vulnerable to behaviors in which an individual demonstrates that he or she can be physically, emotionally, and/or sexually harmful to self.

Risk for self-mutilation: Vulnerable to deliberate self-injurious behavior causing tissue damage with the intent of causing nonfatal injury to attain relief of tension.

Risk for shock: Vulnerable to an inadequate blood flow to the body's tissues that may lead to life-threatening cellular dysfunction, which may compromise health.

Risk for situational low self-esteem: Vulnerable to developing a negative perception of self-worth in response to a current situation, which may compromise health.

Risk for spiritual distress: Vulnerable to an impaired ability to experience and integrate meaning and purpose in life through connectedness within self, literature, nature, and/or a power greater than oneself, which may compromise health.

Risk for sudden infant death syndrome: Vulnerable to unpredicted death of an infant.

Risk for suffocation: Vulnerable to inadequate air availability for inhalation, which may compromise health.

Risk for suicide: Vulnerable to self-inflicted, life threatening injury.

Risk for thermal injury: Vulnerable to extreme temperature damage to skin and mucous membranes, which may compromise health.

Risk for trauma: Vulnerable to accidental tissue injury (e.g., wound, burn, fracture), which may compromise health.

Risk for unstable blood glucose level: Vulnerable to variation in blood glucose/sugar levels from the normal range, which may compromise health.

Risk for urge urinary incontinence: Vulnerable to involuntary passage of urine occurring soon after a strong sensation or urgency to void, which may compromise health.

Risk for urinary tract injury: Vulnerable to damage of the urinary tract structures from use of catheters, which may compromise health.

Risk for vascular trauma: Vulnerable to damage to vein and its surrounding tissues related to the presence of a catheter and/or infusion solutions, which may compromise health.

Risk-prone health behavior: Impaired ability to modify lifestyle/behaviors in a manner that improves health status.

Sedentary lifestyle: Reports a habit of life that is characterized by a low physical activity level.

Self-mutilation: Deliberate self-injurious behavior causing tissue damage with the intent of causing nonfatal injury to attain relief of tension.

Self-neglect: A constellation of culturally framed behaviors involving one or more self-care activities in which there is a failure to maintain a socially accepted standard of health and well-being (Gibbons, Lauder, & Ludwick, 2006).

Sexual dysfunction: A state in which an individual experiences a change in sexual function during the sexual response phases of desire, excitation, and/or orgasm that is viewed as unsatisfying, unrewarding, or inadequate.

Situational low self-esteem: Development of a negative perception of self-worth in response to a current situation.

Sleep deprivation: Prolonged periods of time without sleep (sustained natural, periodic suspension of relative consciousness).

Social isolation: Aloneness experienced by the individual and perceived as imposed by others and as a negative or threatening state.

Spiritual distress: A state of suffering related to the impaired ability to experience meaning in life through connections with self, others, world, or a superior being.

Stress overload: Excessive amounts and types of demands that require action.

Stress urinary incontinence: Sudden leakage of urine with activities that increase intra-abdominal pressure.

Toileting self-care deficit: Impaired ability to perform or complete self-toileting activities.

Unilateral neglect: Impairment in sensory and motor response, mental representation, and spatial attention of the body, and the corresponding environment, characterized by inattention to one side and overattention to the opposite side. Left-side neglect is more severe and persistent than right-side neglect.

Urge urinary incontinence: Involuntary passage of urine occurring soon after a strong sense of urgency to void.

Urinary retention: Incomplete emptying of the bladder.

Wandering: Meandering, aimless or repetitive locomotion that exposes the individual to harm; frequently incongruent with boundaries, limits, or obstacles.

From Herdman, T. H., & Kamitsuru, S. (Eds.). (2014). *NANDA international nursing diagnoses: Definitions and classification 2015-2017.* Oxford: Wiley Blackwell.

Solution Compatibility Chart

Intravenous Medication	D2½W	D5W	D10W	D5/¼NS	D5/½NS	D5NS	NS	½NS	R	LR	D5R	D5LR	Dextran 6%/D5W/NS	Fruc 10%/W/NS	Invert sug 10%/W/NS	Na Lactate ⅙ M
Acetazolamide	C	C	C	C	C	C	C	C	C	C	C	C	C	C	C	C
Acyclovir		C		C	C	C	C			C						
Aminophylline	C	C	C	C	C	C	C	C	C	C	C	C	C			C
Antithymocyte Globulin	C	C	C	C	C	C	C	C								
Ascorbic Acid	C	C	C	C	C	C	C	C	C	C	C	C	C	C	C	C
Aztreonam		C	C	C	C	C	C		C	C		C				C
Calcium Chloride		C	C	C	C	C	C		C	C	C	C				
Calcium Gluconate		C	C			C	C			C		C		W		C
Cefazolin Na		C	C	C	C	C	C		C	C		C			W	
Cefoperazone Na		C	C	C		C	C			C		C				
Cefotaxime Na		C	C	C	C	C	C			C					W	C
Cefotetan		C					C									
Cefoxitin Na		C	C	C	C	C	C		C	C		C			C	C
Ceftazidime		C	C	C	C	C	C		C	C					W	C
Ceftriaxone Na		C	C			C	C								W	C
Cefuroxime Na		C	C	C	C	C	C		C	C					W	C
Clindamycin		C	C		C	C	C			C	C					
Dexamethasone		C					C									
Dobutamine HCl		C	C		C	C	C	C		C		C				C
Dopamine HCl		C	C		C	C	C			C		C				C
Doxycycline		C					C		C						W	
Epinephrine	C	C	C	C	C	C	C		C	C	C	C	C	C	C	C
Famotidine		C	C				C			C						
Fentanyl		C					C									
Folic Acid		C					C									
Furosemide		C	C			C	C			C		C				C
Gentamicin		C	C				C		C	C						
Heparin Na	C	C*		C	C	C	C*	C	C		C	C	C	C	C	
Hydrocortisone Phosphate		C	C				C	C								
Hydrocortisone Na Succinate	C	C	C	C	C	C	C	C	C	C	C	C	C	C	C	C
Hydromorphone HCl		C	C		C	C	C	C	C	C	C	C			W	C
Imipenem-Cilastatin		C[4]	C[4]	C[4]	C[4]	C[4]	C[10]									
Insulin (Regular)		C[P]	C		C		C[P]			C	C					
Isoproterenol	C	C[P]	C	C	C	C	C[P]		C	C	C	C	C	C	C	C
Kanamycin		C	C			C	C			C						
Labetalol		C		C		C	C		C	C	C	C				
Lidocaine		C[P]			C	C	C	C		C		C				
Magnesium Sulfate		C					C			C						
Meperidine HCl	C	C	C	C	C	C	C	C	C	C	C	C	C	C	C	C
Meropenem		C[1]	C[1]	C[1]		C[1]	C[4]			C[4]	C[4]	C[1]				C[2]

Intravenous Medication	D2½W	D5W	D10W	D5/¼NS	D5/½NS	D5NS	NS	½NS	R	LR	D5R	D5LR	Dextran 6%/D5W/NS	Fruc 10%/W/NS	Invert sug 10%/W/NS	Na Lactate ⅙ M
Metoclopramide HCl		C		C			C		C	C						
Morphine	C	C	C	C	C	C	C	C	C	C	C	C	C	C	C	C
Multivitamin		C	C		C	C				C		C			W	C
Nafcillin Na		C	C	C	C	C	C			C	C	C	C			C
Nitroglycerin		C*			C	C	C*	C		C		C				C
Norepinephrine		C[P]				C[P]	C			C						
Ondansetron HCl		C			C	C	C		C	C						
Oxacillin Na		C	C			C	C			C		C				
Pancuronium		C			C	C	C			C						
Papaverine	C	C	C	C	C	C	C	C	C			C		C	C	C
Penicillin G, K	C	C	C	C	C	C	C	C	C	C	C	C	C	C	C	
Pentobarbital Na	C	C*	C	C	C	C	C	C	C	C	C	C	C	C	C	C
Piperacillin/ Tazobactam		C					C			C*			NS			
Potassium Acetate		C	C				C			C		C				
Potassium Chloride	C	C	C	C	C	C	C	C	C	C	C	C	C	C	C	C
Potassium Phosphate	C	C	C	C	C	C	C	C					C	C	C	C
Prochlorperazine	C	C	C	C	C	C	C	C	C	C	C	C	C	C	C	C
Propranolol		C[P]			C	C	C	C		C						
Pyridoxine HCl		C	C	C	C	C	C		C	C					C	C
Ranitidine		C	C		C					C						
Sodium Acetate		C	C			C	C	C	C			C				
Sodium Bicarbonate	C	C	C	C	C	C	C	C	C		C		C	C	C	C
Sodium Chloride	C	C	C	C	C	C	C	C	C	C	C	C	C	C	C	C
Succinylcholine	C	C	C	C	C	C	C	C	C	C	C	C	C	C	C	C
Thiamine	C	C	C	C	C	C	C	C	C	C	C	C	C	C	C	C
Thiopental	C	C		C	C	C[6]	C	C				C				C
Trace Metals		C	C			C	C			C						
Tranexamic Acid	C	C	C	C	C	C	C		C				C			
Warfarin		C	C		C	C	C*					C				
Zidovudine		C[P]					C									

This chart is not all inclusive. It is based on manufacturer's recommendations and Trissel's.

KEY

C	= Compatible*	D5R	= 5% Dextrose in Ringer's solution
W	= Compatible in water not NS	D5LR	= 5% Dextrose in Lactated Ringer's solution
D2½W	= 2½% Dextrose in water	Dextran 6%/D5W/NS	= Dextran 6% in D5W or normal saline
D5W	= 5% Dextrose in water	Fruc 10%/W/NS	= Fructose 10% in water or normal saline
D10W	= 10% Dextrose in water	Invert sug 10%/W/NS	= Invert sugar 10% in water or normal saline
D5/¼NS	= 5% Dextrose in ¼ normal saline	Na Lactate ⅙ M	= Sodium lactate ⅙ M
D5/½NS	= 5% Dextrose in ½ normal saline	[1]	= Stable for 1 hour
D5NS	= 5% Dextrose in normal saline	[2]	= Stable for 2 hours
NS	= Normal saline	[4]	= Stable for 4 hours
½NS	= ½ Normal saline	[6]	= Stable for 6 hours
R	= Ringer's solution	[10]	= Stable for 10 hours
LR	= Lactated Ringer's solution	[P]	= Preferred diluent

*Compatibility in various concentrations may vary; consult pharmacist.

Immunizations

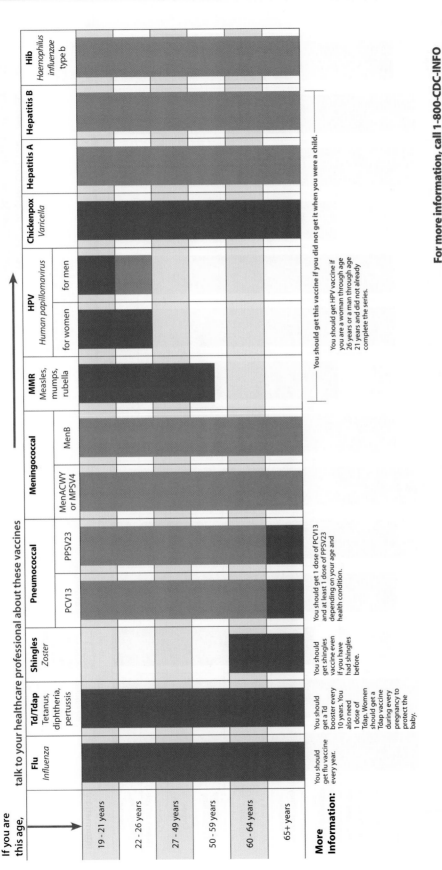

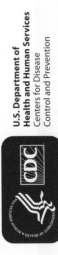

INFORMATION FOR ADULT PATIENTS

2016 Recommended Immunizations for Adults: By Health Condition

If you have this health condition, → talk to your healthcare professional about these vaccines

If you have this health condition	Flu *Influenza*	Td/Tdap Tetanus, diphtheria, pertussis	Shingles *Zoster*	Pneumococcal PCV13	Pneumococcal PPSV23	Meningococcal MenACWY or MPSV4	Meningococcal MenB	MMR Measles, mumps, rubella	HPV for women	HPV for men	Chickenpox *Varicella*	Hepatitis A	Hepatitis B	Hib *Haemophilus influenzae type b*
Pregnancy			SHOULD NOT GET VACCINE					SHOULD NOT GET VACCINE			SHOULD NOT GET VACCINE			
Weakened Immune System														
HIV: **CD4 count less than 200**														
HIV: **CD4 count 200 or greater**														
Kidney disease or poor kidney function														
Asplenia (if you do not have a spleen or if it does not work well)														
Heart disease Chronic lung disease Chronic alcoholism														
Diabetes (Type 1 or Type 2)														
Chronic Liver Disease														

More Information:

Flu: You should get flu vaccine every year.

Td/Tdap: You should get a Td booster every 10 years. You also need 1 dose of Tdap vaccine. Women should get Tdap vaccine during every pregnancy.

Shingles: You should get shingles vaccine if you are age 60 years or older, even if you have had shingles before.

Pneumococcal: You should get 1 dose of PCV13 and at least 1 dose of PPSV23 depending on your age and health condition.

HPV: You should get this vaccine if you did not get it when you were a child. You should get HPV vaccine if you are a woman through age 26 years or a man through age 21 years and did not already complete the series.

Hib: You should get Hib vaccine if you do not have a spleen, have sickle cell disease, or received a bone marrow transplant.

Legend

Recommended For You: This vaccine is recommended for you *unless* your healthcare professional tells you that you cannot safely receive it or that you do not need it.

May Be Recommended For You: This vaccine is recommended for you if you have certain other risk factors due to your age, health, job, or lifestyle that are not listed here. Talk to your healthcare professional to see if you need this vaccine.

YOU SHOULD NOT GET THIS VACCINE

For more information, call 1-800-CDC-INFO (1-800-232-4636) or visit www.cdc.gov/vaccines

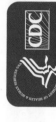

U.S. Department of Health and Human Services
Centers for Disease Control and Prevention

2016 Recommended Immunizations for Children from Birth Through 6 Years Old

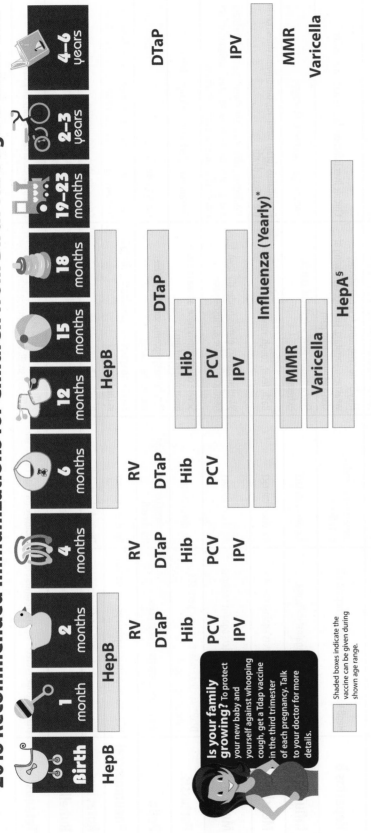

	Birth	1 month	2 months	4 months	6 months	12 months	15 months	18 months	19–23 months	2–3 years	4–6 years
HepB	HepB	HepB			HepB						
RV			RV	RV	RV						
DTaP			DTaP	DTaP	DTaP		DTaP				DTaP
Hib			Hib	Hib	Hib	Hib					
PCV			PCV	PCV	PCV	PCV					
IPV			IPV	IPV	IPV	IPV					IPV
Influenza					Influenza (Yearly)*						
MMR						MMR					MMR
Varicella						Varicella					Varicella
HepA						HepA§					

Shaded boxes indicate the vaccine can be given during shown age range.

Is your family growing? To protect your new baby and yourself against whooping cough, get a Tdap vaccine in the third trimester of each pregnancy. Talk to your doctor for more details.

NOTE: If your child misses a shot, you don't need to start over, just go back to your child's doctor for the next shot. Talk with your child's doctor if you have questions about vaccines.

FOOTNOTES:

*   Two doses given at least four weeks apart are recommended for children aged 6 months through 8 years of age who are getting an influenza (flu) vaccine for the first time and for some other children in this age group.

§   Two doses of HepA vaccine are needed for lasting protection. The first dose of HepA vaccine should be given between 12 months and 23 months of age. The second dose should be given 6 to 18 months later. HepA vaccination may be given to any child 12 months and older to protect against HepA. Children and adolescents who did not receive the HepA vaccine and are at high-risk, should be vaccinated against HepA.

    If your child has any medical conditions that put him at risk for infection or is traveling outside the United States, talk to your child's doctor about additional vaccines that he may need.

SEE BACK PAGE FOR MORE INFORMATION ON VACCINE-PREVENTABLE DISEASES AND THE VACCINES THAT PREVENT THEM.

For more information, call toll free
1-800-CDC-INFO (1-800-232-4636)
or visit
http://www.cdc.gov/vaccines

U.S. Department of Health and Human Services
Centers for Disease Control and Prevention

AMERICAN ACADEMY OF FAMILY PHYSICIANS
STRONG MEDICINE FOR AMERICA

American Academy of Pediatrics
DEDICATED TO THE HEALTH OF ALL CHILDREN™

Vaccine-Preventable Diseases and the Vaccines that Prevent Them

Disease	Vaccine	Disease spread by	Disease symptoms	Disease complications
Chickenpox	Varicella vaccine protects against chickenpox.	Air, direct contact	Rash, tiredness, headache, fever	Infected blisters, bleeding disorders, encephalitis (brain swelling), pneumonia (infection in the lungs)
Diphtheria	DTaP* vaccine protects against diphtheria.	Air, direct contact	Sore throat, mild fever, weakness, swollen glands in neck	Swelling of the heart muscle, heart failure, coma, paralysis, death
Hib	Hib vaccine protects against *Haemophilus influenzae* type b.	Air, direct contact	May be no symptoms unless bacteria enter the blood	Meningitis (infection of the covering around the brain and spinal cord), intellectual disability, epiglottitis (life-threatening infection that can block the windpipe and lead to serious breathing problems), pneumonia (infection in the lungs), death
Hepatitis A	HepA vaccine protects against hepatitis A.	Direct contact, contaminated food or water	May be no symptoms, fever, stomach pain, loss of appetite, fatigue, vomiting, jaundice (yellowing of skin and eyes), dark urine	Liver failure, arthralgia (joint pain), kidney, pancreatic, and blood disorders
Hepatitis B	HepB vaccine protects against hepatitis B.	Contact with blood or body fluids	May be no symptoms, fever, headache, weakness, vomiting, jaundice (yellowing of skin and eyes), joint pain	Chronic liver infection, liver failure, liver cancer
Influenza (Flu)	Flu vaccine protects against influenza.	Air, direct contact	Fever, muscle pain, sore throat, cough, extreme fatigue	Pneumonia (infection in the lungs)
Measles	MMR** vaccine protects against measles.	Air, direct contact	Rash, fever, cough, runny nose, pinkeye	Encephalitis (brain swelling), pneumonia (infection in the lungs), death
Mumps	MMR** vaccine protects against mumps.	Air, direct contact	Swollen salivary glands (under the jaw), fever, headache, tiredness, muscle pain	Meningitis (infection of the covering around the brain and spinal cord), encephalitis (brain swelling), inflammation of testicles or ovaries, deafness
Pertussis	DTaP* vaccine protects against pertussis (whooping cough).	Air, direct contact	Severe cough, runny nose, apnea (a pause in breathing in infants)	Pneumonia (infection in the lungs), death
Polio	IPV vaccine protects against polio.	Air, direct contact, through the mouth	May be no symptoms, sore throat, fever, nausea, headache	Paralysis, death
Pneumococcal	PCV vaccine protects against pneumococcus.	Air, direct contact	May be no symptoms, pneumonia (infection in the lungs)	Bacteremia (blood infection), meningitis (infection of the covering around the brain and spinal cord), death
Rotavirus	RV vaccine protects against rotavirus.	Through the mouth	Diarrhea, fever, vomiting	Severe diarrhea, dehydration
Rubella	MMR** vaccine protects against rubella.	Air, direct contact	Children infected with rubella virus sometimes have a rash, fever, swollen lymph nodes	Very serious in pregnant women—can lead to miscarriage, stillbirth, premature delivery, birth defects
Tetanus	DTaP* vaccine protects against tetanus.	Exposure through cuts in skin	Stiffness in neck and abdominal muscles, difficulty swallowing, muscle spasms, fever	Broken bones, breathing difficulty, death

* DTaP combines protection against diphtheria, tetanus, and pertussis.
** MMR combines protection against measles, mumps, and rubella.

INFORMATION FOR PARENTS | **2016 Recommended Immunizations for Children 7-18 Years Old**

Talk to your child's doctor or nurse about the vaccines recommended for their age.

	Flu *Influenza*	Tdap Tetanus, diphtheria, pertussis	HPV Human papillomavirus	Meningococcal MenACWY	Meningococcal MenB	Pneumococcal	Hepatitis B	Hepatitis A	Inactivated Polio	MMR Measles, mumps, rubella	Chickenpox *Varicella*
7-8 Years											
9-10 Years											
11-12 Years											
13-15 Years											
16-18 Years											

More information:

Preteens and teens should get a flu vaccine every year.

Preteens and teens should get one shot of Tdap at age 11 or 12 years.

Both girls and boys should receive 3 doses of HPV vaccine to protect against HPV-related disease. HPV vaccination can start as early as age 9 years.

All 11-12 year olds should be vaccinated with a single dose of a quadrivalent meningococcal conjugate vaccine (MenACWY). **A booster shot is recommended at age 16.**

Teens, 16-18 years old, **may** be vaccinated with a MenB vaccine.

These shaded boxes indicate when the vaccine is recommended for all children unless your doctor tells you that your child cannot safely receive the vaccine.

These shaded boxes indicate the vaccine is recommended for children with certain health or lifestyle conditions that put them at an increased risk for serious diseases. See vaccine-specific recommendations at www.cdc.gov/vaccines/hcp/acip-recs/index.html

These shaded boxes indicate the vaccine should be given if a child is catching-up on missed vaccines.

This shaded box indicates the vaccine is recommended for children not at increased risk but who wish to get the vaccine after speaking to a provider.

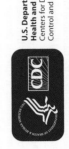
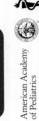

U.S. Department of
Health and Human Services
Centers for Disease
Control and Prevention

American Academy
of Pediatrics
DEDICATED TO THE HEALTH OF ALL CHILDREN™

AMERICAN ACADEMY OF
FAMILY PHYSICIANS
STRONG MEDICINE FOR AMERICA

Vaccine-Preventable Diseases and the Vaccines that Prevent Them

Diphtheria (Can be prevented by Tdap vaccination)

Diphtheria is a very contagious bacterial disease that affects the respiratory system, including the lungs. Diphtheria bacteria can be passed from person to person by direct contact with droplets from an infected person's cough or sneeze. When people are infected, the diphtheria bacteria produce a toxin (poison) in the body that can cause weakness, sore throat, fever, and swollen glands in the neck. Effects from this toxin can also lead to swelling of the heart muscle and, in some cases, heart failure. In serious cases, the illness can cause coma, paralysis, and even death.

Hepatitis A (Can be prevented by HepA vaccination)

Hepatitis A is an infection in the liver caused by hepatitis A virus. The virus is spread primarily person-to-person through the fecal-oral route. In other words, the virus is taken in by mouth from contact with objects, food, or drinks contaminated by the feces (stool) of an infected person. Symptoms can include fever, tiredness, poor appetite, vomiting, stomach pain, and sometimes jaundice (when skin and eyes turn yellow). An infected person may have no symptoms, may have mild illness for a week or two, may have severe illness for several months, or may rarely develop liver failure and die from the infection. In the U.S., about 100 people a year die from hepatitis A.

Hepatitis B (Can be prevented by HepB vaccination)

Hepatitis B causes a flu-like illness with loss of appetite, nausea, vomiting, rashes, joint pain, and jaundice. Symptoms of acute hepatitis B include fever, fatigue, loss of appetite, nausea, vomiting, pain in joints and stomach, dark urine, grey-colored stools, and jaundice (when skin and eyes turn yellow).

Human Papillomavirus (Can be prevented by HPV vaccination)

Human papillomavirus is a common virus. HPV is most common in people in their teens and early 20s. It is the major cause of cervical cancer in women and genital warts in women and men. The strains of HPV that cause cervical cancer and genital warts are spread during sex.

Influenza (Can be prevented by annual flu vaccination)

Influenza is a highly contagious viral infection of the nose, throat, and lungs. The virus spreads easily through droplets when an infected person coughs or sneezes and can cause mild to severe illness. Typical symptoms include a sudden high fever, chills, a dry cough, headache, runny nose, sore throat, and muscle and joint pain. Extreme fatigue can last from several days to weeks. Influenza may lead to hospitalization or even death, even among previously healthy children.

Measles (Can be prevented by MMR vaccination)

Measles is one of the most contagious viral diseases. Measles virus is spread by direct contact with the airborne respiratory droplets of an infected person. Measles is so contagious that just being in the same room after a person who has measles has already

left can result in infection. Symptoms usually include a rash, fever, cough, and red, watery eyes. Fever can persist, rash can last for up to a week, and coughing can last about 10 days. Measles can also cause pneumonia, seizures, brain damage, or death.

Meningococcal Disease (Can be prevented by meningococcal vaccination)

Meningococcal disease is caused by bacteria and is a leading cause of bacterial meningitis (infection around the brain and spinal cord) in children. The bacteria are spread through the exchange of nose and throat droplets, such as when coughing, sneezing or kissing. Symptoms include nausea, vomiting, sensitivity to light, confusion and sleepiness. Meningococcal bacteria also cause blood infections. About one of every ten people who get the disease dies from it. Survivors of meningococcal disease may lose their arms or legs, become deaf, have problems with their nervous systems, become developmentally disabled, or suffer seizures or strokes.

Mumps (Can be prevented by MMR vaccination)

Mumps is an infectious disease caused by the mumps virus, which is spread in the air by a cough or sneeze from an infected person. A child can also get infected with mumps by coming in contact with a contaminated object, like a toy. The mumps virus causes swollen salivary glands under the ears or jaw, fever, muscle aches, tiredness, abdominal pain, and loss of appetite. Severe complications for children who get mumps are uncommon, but can include meningitis (infection of the covering of the brain and spinal cord), encephalitis (inflammation of the brain), permanent hearing loss, or swelling of the testes, which rarely results in decreased fertility.

Pertussis (Whooping Cough) (Can be prevented by Tdap vaccination)

Pertussis is caused by bacteria spread through direct contact with respiratory droplets when an infected person coughs or sneezes. In the beginning, symptoms of pertussis are similar to the common cold, including runny nose, sneezing, and cough. After 1-2 weeks, pertussis can cause spells of violent coughing and choking, making it hard to breathe, drink, or eat. This cough can last for weeks. Pertussis is most serious for babies, who can get pneumonia, have seizures, become brain damaged, or even die. About two-thirds of children under 1 year of age who get pertussis must be hospitalized.

Pneumococcal Disease (Can be prevented by pneumococcal vaccination)

Pneumonia is an infection of the lungs that can be caused by the bacteria called pneumococcus. This bacteria can cause other types of infections too, such as ear infections, sinus infections, meningitis (infection of the covering around the brain and spinal cord), bacteremia and sepsis (blood stream infection). Sinus and ear infections are usually mild and are much more common than the more serious forms of pneumococcal disease. However, in

some cases pneumococcal disease can be fatal or result in long-term problems, like brain damage, hearing loss and limb loss. Pneumococcal disease spreads when people cough or sneeze. Many people have the bacteria in their nose or throat at one time or another without being ill—this is known as being a carrier.

Polio (Can be prevented by IPV vaccination)

Polio is caused by a virus that lives in an infected person's throat and intestines. It spreads through contact with the stool of an infected person and through droplets from a sneeze or cough. Symptoms typically include sore throat, fever, tiredness, nausea, headache, or stomach pain. In about 1% of cases, polio can cause paralysis. Among those who are paralyzed, about 2 to 10 children out of 100 die because the virus affects the muscles that help them breathe.

Rubella (German Measles) (Can be prevented by MMR vaccination)

Rubella is caused by a virus that is spread through coughing and sneezing. In children rubella usually causes a mild illness with fever, swollen glands, and a rash that lasts about 3 days. Rubella rarely causes serious illness or complications in children, but can be very serious to a baby in the womb. If a pregnant woman is infected, the result to the baby can be devastating, including miscarriage, serious heart defects, mental retardation and loss of hearing and eye sight.

Tetanus (Lockjaw) (Can be prevented by Tdap vaccination)

Tetanus is caused by bacteria found in soil, dust, and manure. The bacteria enters the body through a puncture, cut, or sore on the skin. When people are infected, the bacteria produce a toxin (poison) that causes muscles to become tight, which is very painful. Tetanus mainly affects the neck and belly. This can lead to "locking" of the jaw so a person cannot open his or her mouth, swallow, or breathe. Complete recovery from tetanus can take months. One out of five people who get tetanus die from the disease.

Varicella (Chickenpox) (Can be prevented by varicella vaccination)

Chickenpox is caused by the varicella zoster virus. Chickenpox is very contagious and spreads very easily from infected people. The virus can spread from either a cough, sneeze. It can also spread from the blisters on the skin, either by touching them or by breathing in these viral particles. Typical symptoms of chickenpox include an itchy rash with blisters, tiredness, headache and fever. Chickenpox is usually mild, but it can lead to severe skin infections, pneumonia, encephalitis (brain swelling), or even death.

If you have any questions about your child's vaccines, talk to your healthcare provider.

Herb-Drug Interactions

Potential Herb-Drug Interactions for Commonly Used Herbs*

How to Read the Chart

The chart is read from left to right. The information in the Basis of Concern column provides the evidence for the information in the Potential Interaction column. For example, *clinical studies* found that administration of St John's wort resulted in *decreased levels* of cancer chemotherapeutic drugs. (Italicized words represent the information in the Herb-Drug Interaction chart below.)

More details may be provided in the Basis of Concern column. For example, in a clinical study with healthy volunteers administration of St John's wort resulted in increased clearance of the hypoglycemic drug gliclazide, and so may reduce the drug's efficacy, however, glucose and insulin response to glucose loading were unchanged.

A recommended action is suggested on a risk assessment of the information in the Basis of Concern. In these examples:

- It is recommended that St John's wort is contraindicated in patients taking cancer chemotherapeutic drugs.
- In the case of gliclazide, because the trial found little effect on a clinically-relevant outcome, the potential interaction is considered low risk and a caution is recommended: the patient should be monitored, through the normal process of repeat consultations.

For more information on the process used to assess the herb-drug interaction research (and why some research is not included), how the risk of interaction is assessed, with worked examples from the chart: go to www.mediherb.com and view the Herb-Drug Interaction Chart under the 'Literature', then 'Support' tabs, look for the link to 'Assessment of Risk & Recommended Action'.

Health care professionals please note: when a patient presents using any of the drugs listed below and there is a potential interaction with the herb you intend to dispense, it is important that you or your patient discuss the potential interaction with their prescribing physician before you dispense the herb to the patient.

Drug	Potential Interaction	Basis of Concern	Recommended Action
Bilberry *Vaccinium myrtillus*			
Warfarin	Potentiation of bleeding.	**Herb Alone** Antiplatelet activity observed in healthy volunteers (173 mg/day of bilberry anthocyanins).[1] Case report of postoperative bleeding (bilberry extract undefined).[2] **Herb or Constituent and Drug** Uncontrolled trial (600 mg/day of bilberry anthocyanins + 30 mg/day of vitamin C for 2 months then reduced maintenance dose) of 9 patients taking anticoagulant drugs – treatment reduced retinal hemorrhages without impairing coagulation.[3] Case report (patient reported to consume "large amounts of bilberry fruits every day for five years").[4]	**Monitor** at high doses (> 100 mg/day anthocyanins, low level of risk).
Black Cohosh *Actaea racemosa (Cimicifuga racemosa)*			
Statin drugs eg atorvastatin	May potentiate increase in liver enzymes, specifically ALT.	Case report.[5]	**Monitor** (low level of risk).
Bladderwrack *Fucus vesiculosus*			
Hyperthyroid medication eg carbimazole	May decrease effectiveness of drug due to natural iodine content.[6]	Theoretical concern, no cases reported.	**Contraindicated** unless under close supervision.
Thyroid replacement therapies eg thyroxine	May add to effect of drug.	Theoretical concern linked to a case report where "kelp" caused hyperthyroidism in a person not taking thyroxine.[7]	**Monitor** (low level of risk).
Bugleweed *Lycopus virginicus, Lycopus europaeus*			
Radioactive iodine	May interfere with administration of diagnostic procedures using radioactive isotopes.[8]	Case report.	**Contraindicated.**
Thyroid hormones	Should not be administered concurrently with preparations containing thyroid hormone.[9]	Theoretical concern based on deliberations of German Commission E.	**Contraindicated.**
Cat's Claw *Uncaria tomentosa*			
HIV protease inhibitors	May increase drug level.	Case report, in a patient with cirrhosis being evaluated for a liver transplant.[10]	**Monitor** (low level of risk).
Cayenne (Chili Pepper) *Capsicum* spp. (See also Polyphenol-containing herbs)			
ACE inhibitor	May cause drug-induced cough.	Case report (topical capsaicin). Theoretical concern since capsaicin depletes substance P.[11]	**Monitor** (very low level of risk).
Theophylline	May increase absorption and drug level.	Clinical study (healthy volunteers, chili-spiced meal). Absorption and drug level lower than during fasting.[12]	**Monitor** (low level of risk).

Drug	Potential Interaction	Basis of Concern	Recommended Action
Celery Seed *Apium graveolens*			
Thyroxine	May reduce serum levels of thyroxine.	Case reports.[13]	**Monitor** (very low level of risk).
Chinese Skullcap *Scutellaria baicalensis*			
Losartan	May increase drug levels.	Clinical trial with healthy volunteers (water-based extract,[A] dried herb equivalent: 12 g/day).[14]	**Monitor** (low level of risk at typical doses).
Rosuvastatin	May decrease drug levels.	Clinical study with healthy volunteers using 150 mg/day of isolated constituent (baicalin).[15]	**Monitor** (low level of risk).[B]
Coleus *Coleus forskohlii*			
Antiplatelet and anticoagulant drugs	May alter response to drug.	Theoretical concern initially based on *in vitro* antiplatelet activity of active constituent forskolin, and *in vivo* antiplatelet activity in an animal model (oral doses: standardized Coleus extract and forskolin).[16] More recent *in vivo* animal research: standardized Coleus extract reduced the anticoagulant activity of warfarin.[17]	**Monitor** (low level of risk).
Hypotensive medication	May potentiate effects of drug.	Theoretical concern based on ability of high doses of forskolin and standardized Coleus extract to lower blood pressure in normotensive and hypertensive animals.[18,19] Clinical data from weight management trials: no effect on blood pressure in three trials, trend toward lower blood pressure in one small study.[20,21] No experimental or clinical studies conducted with hypotensive medication.	**Monitor** (low level of risk).
Prescribed medication	May potentiate effects of drug.	Theoretical concern based on ability of forskolin to activate increased intracellular cyclic AMP *in vitro*.[22]	**Monitor** (low level of risk).
Cranberry *Vaccinium macrocarpon*			
Midazolam	May increase drug levels.	Clinical trials with healthy volunteers: effect on drug levels conflicting – increased (double-strength juice[c], 240 mL tds; defined as a weak interaction)[23] and no effect (cranberry juice,[E] 200 mL tds).[24]	**Monitor** (low level of risk).
Simvastatin	May increase side effects of drug.	Case report (355–473 mL/day cranberry juice drink (7% juice), rated as 'possible' interaction).[25]	**Monitor** (low level of risk).
Warfarin	May alter INR (most frequently increase).	Case reports (where reported the dosage was often high: up to 2000 mL/day, juice strength undefined; 1.5–2 quarts (1420–1893 mL)/day of cranberry juice cocktail; 113 g/day, cranberry sauce).[26-34] Clinical trials: no significant effect found in atrial fibrillation patients (250 mL/day cranberry juice cocktail),[35] in patients on warfarin for a variety of indications (8 oz (236 mL)/day cranberry juice cocktail),[36] but increase observed in healthy volunteers (juice concentrate equivalent to 57 g of dry fruit/day).[37] No alteration of prothrombin time in patients on stable warfarin therapy (480 mL/day cranberry juice)[38] or of thromboplastin time in healthy volunteers (600 mL/day cranberry juice[F]).[24] See also note C.	**Monitor** (low level of risk at typical doses).
Dong Quai *Angelica sinensis, Angelica polymorpha*			
Warfarin	May potentiate effect of drug.	Case reports: increased INR and PT;[39] increased INR and widespread bruising.[40]	**Monitor** (low level of risk).
Echinacea *Echinacea angustifolia, Echinacea purpurea*			
Antiretroviral drugs **HIV non-nucleoside transcriptase inhibitors** eg etravirine: May alter drug levels.		Clinical trial (*E. purpurea* root; HIV-infected patients): no effect overall, but large interindividual variability occurred (from near 25% decreases to up to 50% increases in drug concentrations). All maintained an undetectable viral load.[41]	**Monitor** (low level of risk).
HIV protease inhibitors eg darunavir: May decrease drug levels.		Clinical trial (*E. purpurea* root; HIV-infected patients): no effect overall, but some patients showed a decrease by as much as 40%. All maintained an undetectable viral load. (Patients were also taking a low dose of ritonavir.)[42]	**Monitor** (low level of risk).
HIV protease inhibitors eg darunavir – *See Antiretroviral drugs above*			
Immunosuppressant medication	May decrease effectiveness of drug.[43,44]	Theoretical concern based on immune-enhancing activity of Echinacea. No cases reported.	**Contraindicated.**
Midazolam	Decreases drug levels when drug administered intravenously.[F]	Clinical study (*E. purpurea* root, 1.6 g/day).[45]	**Monitor** (medium level of risk) when drug administered intravenously.
Eleuthero (Siberian Ginseng) *Eleutherococcus senticosus*			
Digoxin	May increase plasma drug levels.	Case report: apparent increase in plasma level, but herb probably interfered with digoxin assay[G] (patient had unchanged ECG despite apparent digoxin concentration of 5.2 nmol/L).[46] In a later clinical trial no effect observed on plasma concentration.[47]	**Monitor** (very low level of risk).

Drug	Potential Interaction	Basis of Concern	Recommended Action
Evening Primrose Oil *Oenothera biennis*			
Phenothiazines	May decrease effectiveness of drug.	Reports of worsening epilepsy in schizophrenics. No causal association demonstrated and no effect observed in later trials.[48]	**Monitor** (very low level of risk).
Garlic *Allium sativum* (See also Hypoglycemic herbs)			
Antiplatelet and anticoagulant drugs eg aspirin, clopidogrel, warfarin	Aspirin: May increase bleeding time. Warfarin: May potentiate effect of drug. Large doses could increase bleeding tendency.	Concern may be overstated, as antiplatelet drugs are often coadministered eg aspirin and warfarin. **Herb Alone** Case reports of increased bleeding tendency with high garlic intake. In three of the four cases the bleeding occurred after surgery.[49-52] Anecdotal: garlic taken shortly before testing interferes with platelet aggregation in control subjects.[53] *Single-dose studies, and studies demonstrating a beneficial effect on disordered function, including for example, in atherosclerosis, are excluded.* Clinical studies (3 g/day or less of fresh garlic): inhibited platelet aggregation in three trials† (about 2.4–2.7 g/day, patients and healthy volunteers),[54-56] but no effect on platelet aggregation in one trial† (about 1.8 g/day, patients),[57] decreased serum thromboxane in one trial (3 g/day, healthy volunteers)[58]. † *See note H.* Clinical studies (4.2–5 g/day of fresh garlic, patients and healthy volunteers): no effect on platelet aggregation, fibrinogen level, prothrombin time, whole blood coagulation time.[59-61] Clinical studies (8–10 g/day of fresh garlic, healthy volunteers): inhibited platelet aggregation and increased clotting time.[62,63] **Herb and Drug** Aspirin: No published studies. Clopidogrel: Garlic tablet ("odorless", dose undefined) added to improve drug therapy, reduced platelet hyperactivity in two patients.[53] Warfarin: Two cases of increased INR and clotting times, very few details (garlic pearls, garlic tablets: dosage undefined).[54] Clinical trial: no effect in healthy volunteers (enteric-coated tablets equivalent to 4 g/day of fresh garlic).[37]	**Monitor** at doses equivalent to ≥ 3 g/day fresh garlic (low level of risk). **Stop taking** at least one week before surgery.
HIV protease inhibitors eg saquinavir	Decreases drug level.	Two clinical studies (garlic extract, standardized for allicin content) with healthy volunteers[65,66] — large variability (in one study,[66] decrease (15%) was not significant).	**Monitor** (medium level of risk).
Ginger *Zingiber officinale*			
Antacids	May decrease effectiveness of drug.	Theoretical concern since ginger increases gastric secretory activity *in vivo* (animals).[43]	**Monitor** (low level of risk).
Antiplatelet and anticoagulant drugs eg phenprocoumon, warfarin	Phenprocoumon: May increase effectiveness of drug. Warfarin: Increased risk of spontaneous bleeding.	Case report (dosage undefined): increased INR.[67] Concern based on antiplatelet activity and potential to inhibit thromboxane synthetase. **Herb Alone** Clinical studies: inhibition of platelet aggregation (5 g, divided single dose, dried ginger) in healthy volunteers,[68] and coronary artery disease patients (10 g, single dose, dried ginger),[69] but no effect in healthy volunteers (2 g, single dose, dried ginger),[70] or coronary artery disease patients (4 g/day, dried ginger),[69] inhibition of platelet thromboxane production in healthy volunteers (5 g/day, fresh ginger).[71] **Herb and Drug** Case report: bleeding (ginger dosage undefined).[72] No pharmacokinetic or pharmacodynamic effect demonstrated in a clinical trial with healthy volunteers (3.6 g/day, dried ginger).[73] Epidemiological study: ginger (as a complementary medicine) was significantly associated with an increased risk of self-reported bleeding in patients taking warfarin.[74] These results should be viewed cautiously (*see note J*).	**Monitor** at doses equivalent to < 4 g/day dried ginger (low level of risk). **Monitor** at doses equivalent to < 4 g/day dried ginger (very low risk). **Contraindicated** unless under close supervision at doses equivalent to > 4 g/day dried ginger.
Nifedipine	May produce a synergistic antiplatelet effect.	Clinical study (1 g/day, dried ginger) in healthy volunteers and hypertensive patients.[75]	**Contraindicated.**

Ginkgo *Ginkgo biloba*

Drug	Potential Interaction	Basis of Concern	Recommended Action
Anticonvulsant medication eg carbamazepine, sodium valproate	May decrease the effectiveness of drug.	Case reports, two with well-controlled epilepsy,[76] others anecdotal and uncertain.[77-79]	**Monitor** (medium level of risk). Increasing the intake of vitamin B6 may be advisable for patients taking anticonvulsants.[K]
Antiplatelet and anticoagulant drugs eg aspirin, cilostazol, clopidogrel, ticlopidine, warfarin	Prolongation of bleeding and/or increased bleeding tendency.	Concern based on antiplatelet activity. **Herb Alone** Rare case reports of bleeding.[80-82] Meta-analysis of randomized, placebo-controlled trials (healthy volunteers and patients): results indicate standardized Ginkgo extract does not increase the risk of bleeding.[83] **Herb and Drug** Retrospective population-based study in Taiwan: the relative risk of hemorrhage associated with the combined use of ginkgo extract with drugs (clopidogrel, cilostazol, ticlopidine, warfarin) was not significant.[84] Aspirin: Two case reports (bleeding).[80] Clinical studies: no additional effect on platelet function, platelet aggregation or bleeding time.[85-87] Cilostazol: Clinical studies with healthy volunteers (Ginkgo 50:1 extract: single dose 120 mg) — bleeding time prolonged; no change in platelet aggregation or clotting time; and no significant correlation between prolongation of bleeding time and inhibition of platelet aggregation;[88] no effect on pharmacokinetics, platelet aggregation or bleeding time (Ginkgo extract (undefined): 160 mg/day).[89] Clopidogrel: Clinical study with healthy volunteers (Ginkgo 50:1 extract: single dose 120 mg) — no effect on platelet aggregation, bleeding times.[88] Ticlopidine: Case report (bleeding).[81] Clinical study with healthy volunteers (Ginkgo 50:1 extract: single dose 80 mg) – no significant additional effect on bleeding time or platelet aggregation,[90] and at the higher dose (120 mg/day) did not affect drug levels.[91] Warfarin: Case report (bleeding).[80] Clinical studies (healthy volunteers and patients): no additional effect on INR, platelet aggregation, coagulation parameters or plasma drug level.[73,92,93] *See also note L.*	**Monitor** (low level of risk)
Antipsychotic medication eg haloperidol, olanzapine, clozapine	May potentiate the efficiency of drug in patients with schizophrenia.	Randomized, controlled trials (Ginkgo 50:1 extract: 120–360 mg/day).[94-97]	Prescribe cautiously. **Reduce** drug if necessary in conjunction with prescribing physician.
Antiretroviral drugs	**HIV integrase inhibitors** eg raltegravir: May alter drug levels	Clinical study with healthy volunteers (Ginkgo 50:1 extract: 240 mg/day) found an increase in plasma levels, due to large interindividual variability, not considered to be of clinical importance. (The drug's pharmacokinetics are known for considerable intra- and interindividual variability).[98]	**Monitor** (low level of risk).
	HIV non-nucleoside transcriptase inhibitors eg efavirenz: May decrease drug levels.	Case report.[99]	**Monitor** (medium level of risk).
Atorvastatin	May decrease drug levels.	Clinical study with healthy volunteers (Ginkgo 50:1 extract: 360 mg/day). No pharmacodynamic effect was observed.[100]	**Monitor** (low level of risk)
Benzodiazepines eg alprazolam, diazepam, midazolam	May alter drug level.	Alprazolam: Clinical trial in healthy volunteers found no effect (Ginkgo 50:1 extract: 240 mg/day).[101] Diazepam: Clinical trial in healthy volunteers found no effect (Ginkgo 50:1 extract: 240 mg/day).[102] Midazolam: Clinical trials in healthy volunteers found conflicting results on drug levels: increased (defined as a weak interaction)[b], Ginkgo 50:1 extract: 360 mg/day),[103] decreased (Ginkgo 50:1 extract: 240 mg/day)[104] and no effect (Ginkgo 50:1 extract: 240 mg/day).[105]	**Monitor** (low level of risk).
HIV non-nucleoside transcriptase inhibitors eg efavirenz – See Antiretroviral drugs above			
Hypoglycemic drugs eg glipizide, metformin, pioglitazone, tolbutamide	Glipizide: May cause hypoglycemia.	Observation from aborted trial: hypoglycemia occurred in volunteers with normal glucose tolerance within 60 minutes.[106] Ginkgo 50:1 extract was administered as a single dose of 120 mg.[107]	**Monitor** (low level of risk).
	Metformin: May enhance effectiveness of drug.	Clinical trial: elimination half-life was increased at doses of metformin 850 mg, three times a day. Effect not significant at doses to 500 mg, twice a day. Ginkgo 50:1 extract was administered as a single dose of 120 mg.[106]	**Monitor** at doses of metformin > 1 g/day (medium level of risk). **Reduce** drug if necessary in conjunction with prescribing physician.
	Pioglitazone: May increase drug level.	Clinical trial with healthy volunteers (Ginkgo 50:1 extract: 120 mg/day).[108]	**Monitor** (low level of risk).
	Tolbutamide: May decrease effectiveness of drug.	Clinical trials with healthy volunteers: nonsignificant reduction in glucose-lowering effect of drug (Ginkgo 50:1 extract: 360 mg/day);[103] pharmacokinetics not altered (Ginkgo 50:1 extract: 240 and 360 mg/day).[103,105]	**Monitor** (low level of risk).

Drug	Potential Interaction	Basis of Concern	Recommended Action
Nifedipine	May increase drug levels or side effects.	Clinical studies: mixed results found for mean plasma drug level – increase (120 mg/day)[109] and no effect (240 mg/day).[110] However, at the higher dose, maximal plasma drug level and heart rate was increased with adverse drug reactions for participants with highest plasma drug levels (headache, dizziness, hot flashes).[110]	**Monitor** at doses < 240 mg/day (medium level of risk). **Contraindicated** for higher doses.
Omeprazole	May decrease drug levels.	Clinical trials with healthy volunteers found conflicting results on drug levels: decreased (Ginkgo 50:1 extract: 280 mg/day)[111] and no effect (Ginkgo 50:1 extract: 240 mg/day).[105]	**Monitor** (low level of risk).
Talinolol	May increase drug levels.	Clinical trial with healthy volunteers.[112]	**Monitor** (low level of risk).
Golden Seal *Hydrastis canadensis*			
Drugs which displace the protein binding of bilirubin eg phenylbutazone	May potentiate effect of drug on displacing bilirubin.	**Herb Alone** Theoretical concern based on *in vitro* data (displaced bilirubin from albumin) and in animals with high dose of berberine by injection (reduced bilirubin serum protein binding).[113]	**Monitor** (low level of risk).
Midazolam	May increase drug level.	Clinical trial (defined as a weak interaction[)].[114]	**Monitor** (low level of risk).
Green Tea *Camellia sinensis* (See also Polyphenol-containing herbs and Tannin-containing herbs)			
Boronic acid-based protease inhibitors eg bortezomib	May decrease efficacy of drug.	Theoretical concern based on initial *in vitro* data and *in vivo* animal study (green tea constituent: EGCG reduced tumor cell death induced by drug).[115] However, a further *in vivo* animal study found EGCG was not antagonistic to the activity of the drug.[116] *See note M.*	**Contraindicated** at high doses (around 600 mg/day EGCG or 1 g/day green tea catechins).[N] More information required for doses below this level.
Folate	May decrease absorption.	Clinical study with healthy volunteers.[117] Clinical significance unclear, as was a one-day study (ie not ongoing administration), with 50 mg of green tea catechins administered before, during and up to 2 hours after folate (for a total of 250 mg of catechins).	If taken simultaneously, may need to **increase** dose of folate. The effect may be relatively small – more information is required.
Statin drugs eg simvastatin	May increase plasma level and side effect of drug.	One case reported of muscle pain (side effect). Pharmacokinetic evaluation indicated green tea (1 cup) increased the bioavailability of simvastatin in this patient.[118]	**Monitor** (low level of risk).
Sunitinib	May reduce bioavailability of drug.	Case report (effect appeared dose-dependent). Considering the pharmacokinetic data (interaction in mice), the authors recommended avoiding green tea intake or leaving an interval of 4 hours between beverage and drug intake.[119]	**Contraindicated**, unless **taken** at least 4 hours **apart**.
Warfarin	May inhibit effect of drug: decreased INR.	Case report (brewed green tea: 0.5–1 gallon/day).[120]	**Monitor** (very low level of risk).
Hawthorn *Crataegus monogyna, Crataegus laevigata (C. oxyacantha)* (See also Tannin-containing herbs)			
Digoxin	May increase effectiveness of drug.	Clinical studies indicate a (beneficial) synergistic effect.[121,122] Pharmacokinetics not affected in a clinical study (healthy volunteers).[123]	**Monitor** (low level of risk).
Hypotensive drugs	May increase effectiveness of drug.	Controlled trials where drugs known to be taken by all or many heart disease patients: blood pressure decreased significantly (2 trials),[124,125] decreased nonsignificantly (1 trial)[126] and was unchanged (1 trial).[127] Significant decrease in blood pressure observed in diabetics taking hypotensive drugs (1 trial).[128]	**Monitor** (low level of risk).
Hypoglycemic herbs eg *Gymnema sylvestre* (See also Ginkgo, Korean Ginseng, Milk Thistle, St John's Wort)			
Hypoglycemic drugs including insulin	May potentiate hypoglycemic activity of drug.	In uncontrolled trials, high dose, long-term administration of Gymnema extract (equivalent to 10–13 g/day dried leaf) reduced insulin and hypoglycemic drug requirements in diabetics.[129,130] Several trials have found no effect for garlic on blood glucose in type 2 diabetes, although in a double-blind, placebo-controlled trial (using enteric-coated tablets), a reduction in the dosage of oral hypoglycemic drugs was required (these patients had fasting blood glucose above 8.0 mmol/L (144 mg/dL)).[131]	Prescribe cautiously and monitor blood sugar regularly. **Warn** patient about possible hypoglycemic effects. **Reduce** drug if necessary in conjunction with prescribing physician.

Drug	Potential Interaction	Basis of Concern	Recommended Action
Kava *Piper methysticum*			
CNS depressants eg alcohol, barbiturates, benzodiazepines	Potentiation of drug effects.	Theoretical concern based on deliberations of German Commission E[e] and the anxiolytic activity of kava.[43] Two apparent case reports (kava + benzodiazepines (alprazolam, flunitrazepam)).[132,133] Clinical trials with healthy volunteers: no additional side effects observed for kava (extract containing 240 mg/day of kava lactones) + benzodiazepine (bromazepam),[134] and kava (extract containing 210 mg/day of kavalactones) + alcohol.[135] Clinical study with healthy volunteers: no effect on pharmacokinetic parameters of midazolam (extract provided 253 mg/day of kavalactones).[114]	**Monitor** (low level of risk).
L-dopa and other Parkinson's disease treatments	Possible dopamine antagonist effects.	Case reports.[136]	**Contraindicated** unless under close supervision.
Korean Ginseng *Panax ginseng*			
Antihypertensive medications including nifedipine	General: May decrease effectiveness of drug.	Theoretical concern since hypertension is a feature of GAS. Clinical significance unclear.[43] Assessment of 316 hospital patients found Korean ginseng to have a contrary effect only in a very small percentage: blood pressure increase in 5% of hypertensives; increase in 3% and decrease in 2% of normotensives; decrease in 6% of hypotensives.[137] No information on concurrent medications. *Note for clinical trial data below:* Acute, single-dose trials excluded. High doses used in several trials. **Herb Alone** Clinical trials: no significant effects found in healthy volunteers,[138,139] those with metabolic syndrome,[140] type 2 diabetes[141] or glaucoma,[142] although baseline blood pressure may be a factor.[140] **Herb and Drug** Clinical trials: *decreased* blood pressure in essential hypertension,[143] and coronary artery disease[144] but no effect in white coat hypertension[143] and essential hypertension.[145]	**Monitor** (very low level of risk).
	Nifedipine: May increase drug levels.	Clinical trial.[109]	**Monitor** (low level of risk).
Antiplatelet and anticoagulant drugs	General: May potentiate effects of drug.	**Herb Alone** Two epidemiological studies in Korea: long-term intake (3–5 years) prolonged plasma clotting times (APTT),[146,147] and decreased platelet aggregation.[146] (Dosage in Korea is generally high.) Clinical trial (healthy volunteers): inhibited platelet aggregation, but no effect on coagulation (PT, APTT).[148]	**Monitor** (low level of risk).
	Warfarin: May decrease effectiveness of drug.	**Herb and Drug** One case reported (decreased INR)[149] but clinical significance unclear. No effect demonstrated in three clinical trials (healthy volunteers and patients) for INR, prothrombin time and platelet aggregation.[150-152]	**Monitor** (low level of risk).
Cancer chemotherapeutic drugs eg imatinib	May potentiate adverse effect possibly by altered metabolism.	Case report (hepatotoxicity; probable causality).[153]	**Monitor** (low level of risk).
CNS stimulants	May potentiate effects of drug.[43]	Theoretical concern since CNS stimulation is a feature of GAS. Clinical significance unclear.	**Monitor** (low level of risk).
HIV integrase inhibitors eg raltegravir	May potentiate adverse effect possibly by altered metabolism.	Case report (elevated liver enzymes: probable causality; dosage unknown).[154]	**Monitor** (low level of risk).
Hypoglycemic drugs including insulin	May potentiate hypoglycemic activity of drug.[44]	Theoretical concern based on clinically observed hypoglycemic activity of ginseng in newly diagnosed type 2 diabetics.[155] Clinical significance unclear. No effect on insulin sensitivity or beta-cell function after very high doses in newly diagnosed type 2 diabetics or those with impaired glucose tolerance.[156] Korean red ginseng (2.7 g/day) reduced the requirement for insulin in about 40% of diabetics in a small uncontrolled trial.[157] No adverse effects in three trials of type 2 diabetics well controlled with diet and/or oral hypoglycemic drugs.[141,158,189]	**Monitor** (low level of risk).
MAO inhibitors eg phenelzine	May cause side effects such as headache, sleeplessness, tremor.	Case reports.[160-162]	**Contraindicated.**
Midazolam	May decrease drug level.	Clinical study with healthy volunteers (extract providing about 45 mg/day of ginsenosides).[163]	**Monitor** (low level of risk).
Sildenafil	Potentiation of drug possible.	Theoretical concern based on *in vitro* studies which show ginseng increases nitric oxide release from corpus cavernosum tissue.[164,165]	**Monitor** (very low level of risk).

Drug	Potential Interaction	Basis of Concern	Recommended Action
Laxative (anthraquinone-containing) herbs eg cascara (*Frangula purshiana, Rhamnus purshianus*), yellow dock (*Rumex crispus*)			
Antiarrhythmic agents	May affect activity if potassium deficiency resulting from long-term laxative abuse is present.	German Commission E and ESCOP recommendation.[9,166]	**Avoid** excessive doses of laxatives. Maintain patients on a high potassium diet.
Cardiac glycosides	May potentiate activity, if potassium deficiency resulting from long-term laxative abuse is present.	German Commission E and ESCOP recommendation.[9,166]	**Monitor** (low level of risk at normal doses).
Potassium-depleting agents eg thiazide diuretics, corticosteroids, licorice root (*glycyrrhiza glabra*)	May increase potassium depletion.	German Commission E and ESCOP recommendation.[9,166]	**Avoid** excessive doses of laxatives. Maintain patients on a high potassium diet.
Licorice *Glycyrrhiza glabra*			
Antihypertensive medications other than diuretics	General: May decrease effectiveness of drug.	**Herb or Constituent Alone** Hypertension demonstrated in case reports, usually from long-term intake and/or very high dose.[167] Clinical studies (up to 200 g/day of licorice): dose-dependent relationship found between licorice and increase in blood pressure, more pronounced effect in hypertensive patients than in normotensive volunteers, adverse effect greater in women, and effect shown for dose as low as 50 g/day of licorice (75 mg/day of glycyrrhetinic acid = 130 mg/day of glycyrrhizin*) taken for 2 weeks.[168,170] Other studies show variation of effects on blood pressure (see note Q) – renal function may be a factor.[171] The increase in blood pressure after taking glycyrrhetinic acid (874 mg/day of glycyrrhizin) was more pronounced in salt-sensitive than salt-resistant volunteers.[172] Clinical study to establish a no-effect level for glycyrrhizin (healthy female volunteers): significant results (eg blood pressure, serum potassium and aldosterone) compared to controls found for daily dose of 4 mg/kg (220–332 mg/day) but no effect at lower doses of 1–2 mg/kg (55–166 mg/day) of glycyrrhizin.[173] **Herb and Drug** Case report (licorice tea (3 L/day)). Patient still hypertensive despite treatment with drugs.[174]	**Avoid** long-term use at doses > 100 mg/day glycyrrhizin unless under close supervision.[R] Place patients on a high potassium diet.
	ACE-inhibitor: May mask the development of pseudoaldosteronism.	Case report (patient consumed licorice herbal medicine (200–240 mg/day glycyrrhizin)). Drug dosage was reduced, leading to pseudoaldosteronism.[175] *See note S.*	**Avoid** long-term use at doses > 100 mg/day glycyrrhizin unless under close supervision.[R] Place patients on a high potassium diet.
Cilostazol	May cause hypokalemia, which can potentiate the toxicity of the drug.[176]	Case report (patient taking 150 mg/day of glycyrrhizin). Serum potassium levels were stable prior to administration of drug.[176]	**Monitor** (medium level of risk). Place patients on a high potassium diet.

Herb-Drug Interaction Chart: General Prescribing Guidelines

- Exercise great caution when prescribing herbs for patients taking drugs with a narrow therapeutic window. These drugs may become dangerously toxic or ineffective with only relatively small changes in their blood concentrations. Examples include digoxin, warfarin, antirejection (immunosuppressive) drugs, many anti-HIV drugs, theophylline, phenytoin and phenobarbital. These patients need to be monitored on a frequent, regular basis.

- Exercise great caution when prescribing herbs for patients taking drugs:
  - if heart, liver, or kidney function is impaired,
  - in elderly patients,
  - in pregnant women,
  - in those who have received an organ transplant,
  - in those with a genetic disorder that disturbs normal biochemical functions.

  These patients need to be monitored on a frequent, regular basis.

- Care should be exercised with patients who exhibit long-term use of laxative herbs or potassium-losing diuretics.
- Critical drugs should be taken at different times of the day from herbs (and food) to reduce chemical or pharmacokinetic interactions. They should be separated by at least 1 hour, preferably more.
- Stop all herbs approximately 1 week before surgery. Milk thistle may help reduce the toxic after-effects of anesthetic drugs, so it can be taken up to the day before, and then again, after surgery.
- Carefully monitor the effects of drugs such as antihypertensives and antidiabetic drugs when combining with herbal remedies. The herbs may make them more or less effective. In the ideal situation the dose of the drug could be adjusted.
- Interactions may be dose related for the herb and the drug, for example, St John's wort and digoxin.

Reference and further reading: Mills S, Bone K (eds). *The Essential Guide to Herbal Safety.* Churchill Livingstone, USA, 2005.

Drug	Potential Interaction	Basis of Concern	Recommended Action
Corticosteroids eg cortisol (hydrocortisone), prednisolone	Cortisol: May potentiate the action (rather than increase level of drug).	Inhibition of the enzyme 11beta-HSD2 by glycyrrhizin leads to an increased level of cortisol in the kidney. This does not happen in the liver. The plasma half-life of cortisol may be prolonged when herb and drug are coadministered, but drug concentrations remain normal, possibly because of a concomitant fall in cortisol production.[177] Prolonged half-life of cortisol may suggest the potential for licorice to prolong clearance (and hence, activity of the drug). (Studies involving patients with Addison's disease or on hemodialysis are not listed here.) **Herb or Constituent Alone** Clinical studies with healthy volunteers[169,171,178-184] and patients with essential hypertension[169] (ongoing oral administration): increase in urinary excretion of cortisol, but no significant change in plasma cortisol[169,171,178-184] (although plasma cortisone decreased)[178,179,185] and diurnal variation of plasma cortisol was unaffected.[181] Dosage was high: 100-200 g/day of licorice candy (containing glycyrrhizin or glycyrrhetinic acid equivalent to 262-2440 mg/day of glycyrrhizin),[169,180-184] 3.5 g/day of licorice tablets (containing 266 mg/day of glycyrrhizin),[182] 4.8 g/day of licorice extract (containing glycyrrhetinic acid = 587 mg/day of glycyrrhizin),[183] 225 mg/day glycyrrhizin,[178] glycyrrhetinic acid (= 227-874 mg/day glycyrrhizin).[171,179] Clinical study with healthy volunteers and hypertensive patients (single dose, placebo-controlled; oral administration of glycyrrhetinic acid equivalent to 874 mg/day of glycyrrhizin[P]): increased plasma cortisol/cortisone ratio (due mostly to a decrease in plasma cortisone); salivary cortisol increased.[186] Clinical study with healthy volunteers (topical application of a cream containing glycyrrhetinic acid): no effect on plasma cortisol.[187] **Herb or Constituent and Drug** Clinical studies: increased plasma half-life of cortisol (oral administration of licorice candy (200 g/day, containing 580 mg/day glycyrrhizin) + intravenous cortisol to 7 healthy volunteers;[180] oral administration of glycyrrhetinic acid = 227 mg/day of glycyrrhizin[P] + oral cortisol to 2 volunteers).[188,189] See also Note T. Ex vivo study (skin samples from healthy volunteers and patients with psoriasis and eczema; glycyrrhetinic acid and drug topically applied): activity of hydrocortisone potentiated by glycyrrhetinic acid.[190]	**Monitor** (very low level of risk at normal doses).
	Prednisolone: May potentiate the action or increase level of drug.	**Herbal Constituent and Drug** Two clinical studies with healthy volunteers (oral administration of glycyrrhizin or glycyrrhetinic acid;[P] prednisolone administered intravenously): increased drug level[191] and increased prednisolone/prednisone ratio[U] in urine and plasma.[192] Dosage was high: 200 mg/day glycyrrhizin,[191] and 400 mg/day glycyrrhetinic acid (= 700 mg/day glycyrrhizin).[192]	**Monitor** (low level of risk at normal doses) when drug administered intravenously.
Digoxin	May cause hypokalemia which can potentiate the toxicity of the drug.	**Herb Alone** Hypokalemia demonstrated in case reports and clinical studies, usually from long-term intake and/or very high dose, however effect has been demonstrated in sensitive individuals at low doses (licorice containing 100 mg/day of glycyrrhizin). Side effects would be common at 400 mg/day of glycyrrhizin.[167,193,194] **Herb and Drug** Case report (patient taking herbal laxative containing licorice (1.2 g/day) and rhubarb (Rheum spp., 4.8 g/day). In addition to digoxin, patient was also taking a potassium-depleting diuretic.[195]	**Avoid** long-term use at doses > 100 mg/day glycyrrhizin unless under close supervision.[R] Place patients on a high potassium diet.
Diuretics	Spironolactone (potassium-sparing diuretic): Reduce side effects of drug. Thiazide and loop (potassium-depleting) diuretics: The combined effect of licorice and the drug could result in excessive potassium loss.[8]	Clinical study: in women with PCOS addition of licorice extract (containing about 463 mg/day glycyrrhizin) reduced side effects related to the diuretic activity of drug.[196] **Herb or Constituent Alone** Hypokalemia demonstrated in case reports and clinical studies, usually from long-term intake and/or very high dose,[167,193,194] however effect has been demonstrated in patients for ongoing treatment with herbal medicines containing glycyrrhizin at doses of 80-240 mg/day.[197] **Herb and Drug** Case reports, usually from long-term intake and/or very high dose,[174,193,198-204] however effect has been demonstrated for ongoing treatment of glycyrrhizin as low as 80 mg/day.[197] Clinical trial (candy containing 40 mg/day of glycyrrhizin); decreased plasma potassium, with 20% of healthy volunteers hypokalemic in the first week.[205]	**Contraindicated** unless under close supervision at doses > 40 mg/day glycyrrhizin.
Immunosuppressives eg sirolimus	May decrease drug clearance.	Population pharmacokinetic study with 112 Chinese adult renal transplant recipients: clearance of sirolimus decreased in those patients with abnormal ALT values who were taking herbal formulations containing glycyrrhizin (route and dosage unknown).[206]	**Monitor** (medium level of risk) in hepatically-impaired patients.
Midazolam	May decrease drug level.	Clinical study with healthy volunteers (potassium salt of glycyrrhizin, equivalent to 287 mg/day of glycyrrhizin).[207]	**Monitor** (low level of risk at normal doses).

Drug	Potential Interaction	Basis of Concern	Recommended Action
Omeprazole	May decrease drug level.	Clinical study with healthy volunteers (potassium salt of glycyrrhizin, equivalent to 287 mg/day of glycyrrhizin).[208]	**Monitor** (low level of risk at normal doses).
Potassium-depleting drugs other than thiazide and loop diuretics eg corticosteroids, stimulant laxatives	May result in excessive potassium loss.	**Herb Alone** Hypokalemia demonstrated in case reports and clinical studies, usually from candy intake (high dose), however effect has been demonstrated in sensitive individuals at low doses (licorice containing 100 mg/day of glycyrrhizin). Side effects would be common at 400 mg/day of glycyrrhizin.[167,193]	**Avoid** long-term use at doses > 100 mg/day glycyrrhizin unless under close supervision.[R] Place patients on a high potassium diet.
Prednisolone – See Corticosteroids above			
Marshmallow Root Althaea officinalis			
Prescribed medication	May slow or reduce absorption of drugs.	Theoretical concern based on absorbent properties of marshmallow root.	**Take** at least 2 hours **away** from medication.
Meadowsweet Filipendula ulmaria (See also Tannin-containing herbs)			
Warfarin	May potentiate effects of drug.	Theoretical concern based on in vivo animal study demonstrating anticoagulant activity (dosage unavailable).[209]	**Monitor** (very low level of risk).
Milk Thistle Silybum marianum (See also Polyphenol-containing herbs)			
Hypoglycemic drugs including insulin	May improve insulin sensitivity.	Controlled trials: improved glycemic control and reduced insulin requirements in patients with type 2 diabetes and cirrhosis (silymarin: 600 mg/day),[210] although insulin requirements unchanged in another trial (silymarin: 200 mg/day);[211] improved glycemic control in diabetics treated with hypoglycemic drugs (silymarin: 200 and 600 mg/day),[212,213] improved blood glucose, blood insulin and insulin resistance in PCOS patients treated with metformin (silymarin: 750 mg/day),[214] but no effect on glucose metabolism in NAFLD patients including those with insulin resistance (silymarin: 280 and 600 mg/day).[215,216]	Prescribe cautiously and monitor blood sugar regularly. **Warn** patient about possible hypoglycemic effects. **Reduce** drug if necessary in conjunction with prescribing physician.
Immunosuppressives eg sirolimus	May decrease drug clearance.	Population pharmacokinetic study with 112 Chinese adult renal transplant recipients: clearance of sirolimus decreased in those patients with abnormal ALT values who were taking silymarin formulations (route and dosage unknown).[206]	**Monitor** (medium level of risk) in hepatically-impaired patients.
Losartan	May reduce efficacy of drug by inhibiting metabolism.	Clinical study (healthy volunteers): inhibited metabolism of drug; the inhibition was greater in those of a particular CYP2C9 genotype (silymarin: 420 mg/day).[217] See note V.	**Monitor** (low level of risk).
Metronidazole	May decrease absorption of drug, by increasing clearance.	Clinical study with healthy volunteers (silymarin: 140 mg/day).[218]	**Monitor** (medium level of risk).
Nifedipine	May delay the absorption rate of drug.	Clinical study with healthy volunteers (silymarin: 280 mg/day), but bioavailability unchanged.[219]	**Monitor** (low level of risk).
Ornidazole	May increase drug levels.	Clinical study with healthy volunteers (silymarin: 140 mg/day).[220]	**Monitor** (medium level of risk).
Talinolol	May increase drug levels.	Clinical study with healthy volunteers (silymarin: 420 mg/day).[221]	**Monitor** (low level of risk).
Phellodendron Phellodendron amurense			
Drugs that displace the protein binding of bilirubin eg phenylbutazone	May potentiate effect of drug on displacing bilirubin.	**Herb Alone** Theoretical concern based on in vitro data (displaced bilirubin from albumin) and in animals with high dose of berberine by injection (reduced bilirubin serum protein binding).[113]	**Monitor** (low level of risk).

Polyphenol-containing[W] or Flavonoid-containing herbs especially cayenne (*Capsicum annuum*), chamomile (*Matricaria chamomilla* (*Matricaria recutita*)), green tea (*Camellia sinensis*), lime flowers (*Tilia cordata*), milk thistle (*Silybum marianum*), rosemary (*Rosmarinus officinalis*) (See also Tannin-containing herbs)

Drug	Potential Interaction	Basis of Concern	Recommended Action
Immunosuppressives eg cyclosporin	Decreases drug levels, due to impaired absorption or increased metabolism.	Three case reports, in transplant patients (2 L/day of herbal tea; 1–1.5 L/day of chamomile tea; 'large quantities' of fruit tea containing hibiscus extract, and a drink containing black tea). Confirmed by rechallenge in one case, but no signs of rejection.[222]	**Monitor** (medium level of risk). Also advisable not to take simultaneously.
Iron	Inhibition of non-heme iron[X] absorption.	Clinical study (included herb teas (German chamomile, vervain, lime flower, peppermint; all 3 g/300 mL), beverages (e.g. black tea, coffee, cocoa)): effect dependent on polyphenol content (per serving: 20–400 mg).[223] *See also note Y.* Timing of intake may be important. *See also note Z.* Epidemiological study (United States): 1 cup/week of coffee associated with 1% lower serum ferritin in the elderly.[224] Mixed results in other studies (healthy volunteers): rosemary (32.7 mg of polyphenols)[225] and cayenne (high dose: 14.2 g, fresh weight,[AA] containing 25 mg polyphenols)[226] caused inhibition; chamomile[227] and turmeric (2.8 g, fresh weight, containing 50 mg polyphenols)[226] did not. *See also note BB.* Results for green tea have been conflicting: two studies found no effect (healthy volunteers and those with anemia),[228,229] two studies (healthy volunteers) found an effect.[225,230] Drinking green tea (1:100, 1 L/day) lowered serum ferritin in women with low levels of ferritin (< 25 mcg/L) at baseline. No effect in other women or men (vegetarians and omnivores), and no effect on iron status parameters.[231] Two epidemiological studies (French and Japanese populations) found mixed results for serum ferritin and hemoglobin, although risk of iron depletion or anemia was not increased.[232,233] Clinical study (150–300 mg/day EGCG): decreased absorption in healthy women with low iron stores administered together with iron. Results significant only at higher dosage.[234] Concentrated extract of milk thistle reduced iron absorption in hemochromatosis patients.[235]	In anemia and where iron supplementation is required, **do not take simultaneously** with meals or iron supplements.

Schisandra *Schisandra chinensis*

Drug	Potential Interaction	Basis of Concern	Recommended Action
Immunosuppressives eg sirolimus, tacrolimus	May increase drug levels.	Sirolimus: Observations in some liver transplanted recipients. Clinical study: markedly increased drug levels in healthy volunteers[236] given *S. sphenanthera* extract, providing 67.5 mg/day of deoxyschisandrin[CC]. Tacrolimus: Observations in some renal and liver transplanted recipients. Clinical studies: markedly increased drug levels in healthy volunteers[237] and transplant recipients,[238,239] given *S. sphenanthera* extract, providing 67.5 mg/day of deoxyschisandrin[CC].	**Monitor** (low level of risk at normal doses).
Midazolam	May increase drug levels.	Increased drug level (defined as a moderate interaction[D]), increase in sleeping time and increase in mild to moderate adverse effects found in healthy volunteers, given *S. chinensis* extract, providing 22.5 mg/day of deoxyschisandrin[CC].[240]	**Monitor** (medium level of risk at normal doses).
Prescribed medication	May accelerate clearance from the body.	Theoretical concern based on *in vivo* animal studies demonstrating enhanced phase I/II hepatic metabolism.[241,242]	**Monitor** (medium level of risk).
Talinolol	May increase drug levels.	Increased drug level and decreased clearance found in healthy volunteers, given *S. chinensis* extract, providing 33.75 mg/day of deoxyschisandrin[CC].[112]	**Monitor** (low level of risk at normal doses).

Slippery Elm Bark *Ulmus rubra*

Drug	Potential Interaction	Basis of Concern	Recommended Action
Prescribed medication	May slow or reduce absorption of drugs.	Theoretical concern based on absorbent properties of slippery elm.	**Take** at least 2 hours **away** from medication.

Drug	Potential Interaction	Basis of Concern	Recommended Action
St John's Wort[180] *Hypericum perforatum* (See also Tannin-containing herbs)			
Amitriptyline	Decreases drug levels.[243]	Clinical study.	**Monitor** (medium level of risk).
Anticonvulsants eg carbamazepine, mephenytoin, phenobarbitone, phenytoin	May decrease drug levels via CYP induction.[244-246]	Theoretical concern. An open clinical trial demonstrated no effect on carbamazepine pharmacokinetics in healthy volunteers.[247] Case report: increase in seizures in patient taking several antiepileptic drugs, two of which are not metabolized by cytochrome P450.[248] Clinical study (healthy volunteers; clinical significance unclear): increased excretion of a mephenytoin metabolite in extensive metabolizers, but not in poor metabolizers.[249] *See note EE.*	**Monitor** (low level of risk).
Antihistamine eg fexofenadine	Decreases drug levels.	Clinical studies.[250,251]	**Monitor** (medium level of risk).
Antiplatelet and anticoagulant drugs eg clopidogrel, phenprocoumon, warfarin	Clopidogrel: May potentiate effects of drug.	Clinical study: increased responsiveness (decreased platelet aggregation) in hyporesponsive volunteers and patients,[252-254] possibly via the formation of the active metabolite (CYP3A4 activity was increased), thus providing a beneficial effect in these patients. This is a complex situation, with the meaning of clopidogrel resistance/hyporesponsiveness debated.[252,255]	In patients with known clopidogrel resistance: **Monitor** (medium level of risk). In other patients: **Monitor** (risk is unknown).
	Phenprocoumon: Decreases plasma drug levels.	Clinical study.[256]	**Contraindicated.**
	Warfarin: Decreases drug levels and INR.	Case reports (decreased INR (nine cases), increased INR (three cases)), clinical study with healthy volunteers (decreased drug level and INR).[150]	**Contraindicated.**
Benzodiazepines eg alprazolam, midazolam, quazepam	Decreases drug levels, and is probably dependent upon the hyperforin content.[211]	Alprazolam: Mixed results for drug levels in two clinical studies (similarly low amount of hyperforin, ~4 mg/day) – no effect (dried herb equivalent: 1.1 g/day)[261] and decrease.[262]	**Monitor** (medium level of risk).
		Midazolam: Four clinical studies, effect not regarded as clinically relevant for low (< 1 mg/day) hyperforin extracts.[251,260,263,264]	Hyperforin-rich extracts: **Monitor** (medium level of risk). Low-hyperforin extracts: **Monitor** (low level of risk).
		Quazepam: Decreased drug levels, but no effect on pharmacodynamics (sedation).[265]	**Monitor** (low level of risk).
Calcium channel antagonists eg nifedipine, verapamil	Decreases drug levels.	Nifedipine: Clinical studies.[109,266]	**Contraindicated.**
		Verapamil: Clinical study.[267]	**Contraindicated.**
Cancer chemotherapeutic drugs eg irinotecan, imatinib	Decreases drug levels.	Clinical studies.[268-271]	**Contraindicated.**
Clozapine	Decreases drug levels.	Case report.[272]	**Contraindicated.**
Digoxin	Decreases drug levels.	Clinical studies (several studies showed decrease, one study showed no effect)[261,273-275] but effect is dependent upon dose of herb and the hyperforin content.[275]	**Contraindicated** at doses equivalent to > 1 g/day dried herb, especially for high-hyperforin extracts.
Finasteride	May decrease drug levels.	Clinical study with healthy volunteers.[276] Case report: PSA level elevated (due to decreased efficacy of drug?) in patient with benign prostatic hyperplasia.[277]	**Contraindicated.**
HIV non-nucleoside transcriptase inhibitors eg nevirapine	Decreases drug levels.	Case report.[278]	**Contraindicated.**
HIV protease inhibitors eg indinavir	Decreases drug levels.	Clinical study.[279]	**Contraindicated.**
Hypoglycemic drugs eg gliclazide, tolbutamide	Gliclazide: May reduce efficacy of drug by increased clearance.	Clinical study with healthy volunteers, but glucose and insulin response to glucose loading were unchanged.[280]	**Monitor** (low level of risk).
	Repaglinide: May alter metabolism of drug.	Clinical study with healthy volunteers: no effect, and glucose and insulin response to glucose loading were unchanged.[281]	**Monitor** (very low level of risk).
	Tolbutamide: May affect blood glucose.	Two clinical studies (healthy volunteers): no effect on pharmacokinetics,[261,263] but there was an increased incidence of hypoglycemia in the trial using hyperforin-rich extract (33 mg/day).[263]	**Monitor** (low level of risk).
Immunosuppressives eg cyclosporin, tacrolimus	Decreases drug levels.	Cyclosporin: Case reports,[282-290] case series,[291,292] clinical studies.[251,293] Interaction is dependent upon the hyperforin content.[285,293] Tacrolimus: Case report and clinical studies.[294-296]	**Contraindicated** especially for high-hyperforin extracts.
Ivabradine	May decrease drug levels.	Clinical trial with healthy volunteers. No pharmacodynamic effect was observed.[297]	**Monitor** (medium level of risk).

Drug	Potential Interaction	Basis of Concern	Recommended Action
S-ketamine (oral)	May decrease drug levels.	Clinical study with healthy volunteers (high-hyperforin extract). No pharmacodynamic effect was observed (eg analgesic effect not altered).[298]	**Monitor** (medium level of risk).
Methadone	Decreases drug levels, possibly inducing withdrawal symptoms.	Case reports.[299]	**Contraindicated.**
Methylphenidate	May decrease efficacy.	Case report,[300] but clinical significance unclear.	**Monitor** (low level of risk).
Omeprazole	May decrease drug levels.	Clinical trial.[301]	**Monitor** (low level of risk).
Oral contraceptives	May increase metabolism of drug.	Breakthrough bleeding reported which was attributed to increased metabolism of drug.[257,282] Clinical significance unclear. Cases of unwanted pregnancies have been reported.[302,303] Contradictory results for effect on bioavailability, hormone levels and ovulation demonstrated in three clinical studies, although some breakthrough bleeding occurred.[304-306] In one clinical trial an extract low in hyperforin did not affect plasma contraceptive drug levels or cause breakthrough bleeding.[307] Clinical trial: clearance of levonorgestrel at emergency contraceptive doses increased (not statistically significant).[308] Clinical study: antiandrogenic effect of contraceptive not affected.[309]	Hyperforin-rich extracts: **Monitor** (medium level of risk). Low-hyperforin extracts: **Monitor** (very low level of risk).
Oxycodone	Decreases drug levels.	Clinical trial with healthy volunteers.[310]	**Monitor** (medium level of risk).
SSRIs eg paroxetine, trazodone, sertraline **and other serotonergic agents** eg nefazodone, venlafaxine	Potentiation effects possible in regard to serotonin levels.	Case reports: clinical significance unclear.[311-316]	**Monitor** (very low level of risk).
Statin drugs	May decrease effect and/or drug levels.	Atorvastatin: Clinical study, serum LDL-cholesterol increased by 0.32 mmol/L (12.3 mg/dl) which corresponds to a decrease in effect of drug in patients by about 30%. Serum total cholesterol was also increased.[317] Pravastatin: Clinical study, no effect on plasma level in healthy volunteers.[318] Rosuvastatin: Case report.[319] Simvastatin: Two clinical studies, decrease in drug levels in healthy volunteers,[318] and small increases in serum total cholesterol and LDL-cholesterol in patients.[320]	**Monitor** blood cholesterol regularly (medium level of risk).
Talinolol	May decrease drug levels.	Clinical study with healthy volunteers.[321]	**Monitor** (medium level of risk).
Theophylline	May decrease drug levels.	Case report.[322] No effect observed in clinical study.[323]	**Monitor** (low level of risk).
Voriconazole	Decreases drug levels.	Clinical study.[324]	**Monitor** (medium level of risk).
Zolpidem	May decrease drug levels (but with wide interindividual variability).[1F]	Clinical study (healthy volunteers).[325]	**Monitor** (low level of risk).

Tannin-containing or OPC-containing herbs eg grape seed extract (*Vitis vinifera*), green tea (*Camellia sinensis*), hawthorn (*Crataegus* spp.), meadowsweet (*Filipendula ulmaria*), pine bark (*Pinus massoniana*), raspberry leaf (*Rubus idaeus*), sage (*Salvia fruticosa*), St John's wort (*Hypericum perforatum*), uva ursi (*Arctostaphylos uva-ursi*), willow bark (*Salix* spp.) (See also Polyphenol-containing herbs)

Drug	Potential Interaction	Basis of Concern	Recommended Action
Minerals especially iron	Iron: May reduce absorption of non-heme iron[4] from food.	Clinical studies in healthy volunteers, administration during or immediately following the meal.[223,326-333] (black tea, typical strength: 0.8-3.3 g/100 mL;[223,326-332] sorghum[66] (0.15% tannins)[331]), and in women with iron deficiency anemia[334] (black tea: 1-2 x 150 mL of 1:100 infusion containing 78 mg of tannins per 150 mL).[334] Iron absorption reduced to a greater extent in those with iron deficiency anemia (IDA).[334] However, the results from single test meals may exaggerate the effect of iron inhibitors and enhancers.[335] Effects were not significant in a 14-day study.[230] Cases of IDA resistant to treatment: heavy black tea drinkers (2 cases, 1.5-2 L/day).[336,337] Epidemiological studies (12, to 2002) found mixed results, but some evidence of an association between drinking black tea and poor iron status.[335] Clinical study in patients with hemochromatosis (black tea: 250 mL with meal).[338]	**Take** at least 2 hours **away** from food or medication.
	Zinc: May reduce absorption from food.	Clinical studies with healthy volunteers: results conflicting for effect on zinc (undefined tea),[339] black tea[230] consumed at or immediately after food).	**Take** at least 2 hours **away** from food or medication.

Drug	Potential Interaction	Basis of Concern	Recommended Action
Turmeric *Curcuma longa*			
Talinolol	May decrease drug levels.	Clinical study with healthy volunteers (300 mg/day of curcuminoids).[340]	**Monitor** at high doses (≥ 300 mg/day curcumin, low level of risk).
Valerian *Valeriana officinalis*			
CNS depressants or alcohol	May potentiate effects of drug.	Theoretical concern expressed by US Pharmacopeial Convention.[341] However a clinical study found no potentiation with alcohol.[342] Case report of adverse effect with benzodiazepine drug (lorazepam)[343] – herb dosage undefined but likely high (tablet contained valerian and passionflower (*Passiflora incarnata*)). Alprazolam: Clinical study in healthy volunteers found no effect on drug levels (extract provided 11 mg/day total valerenic acids).[344]	**Monitor** (very low level of risk).
Willow Bark *Salix alba, Salix daphnoides, Salix purpurea, Salix fragilis* (See also Tannin-containing herbs)			
Warfarin	May potentiate effects of drug.	**Herb Alone** Clinical study observed very mild but statistically significant antiplatelet activity (extract containing 240 mg/day of salicin).[345]	**Monitor** (low level of risk).

CODE FOR RECOMMENDED ACTION

Contraindicated: Do not prescribe the indicated herb.

Monitor: Can prescribe the indicated herb but maintain close contact and review the patient's status on a regular basis. Note that where the risk is assessed as medium, self-prescription of the herb in conjunction with the drug is not advisable.

ABBREVIATIONS

ACE: angiotensin-converting enzyme; **ALT:** alanine transaminase; **ALT:** alanine transaminase, also known as glutamic pyruvic transaminase (GPT); **AMP:** adenosine monophosphate; **APTT:** activated partial thromboplastin time; **CNS:** central nervous system; **CYP:** cytochrome P450; **ECG:** electrocardiogram/graph; **EGCG:** epigallocatechin gallate; **GAS:** ginseng abuse syndrome; **HIV:** human immunodeficiency virus; **11beta-HSD2:** 11beta-hydroxysteroid dehydrogenase type 2; **IDA:** iron deficiency anemia; **INR:** international normalized ratio; **NAFLD:** nonalcoholic fatty liver disease; **OPC:** oligomeric procyanidin; **PCOS:** polycystic ovary syndrome; **PSA:** prostate specific antigen; **PT:** prothrombin time; **SSRI:** selective serotonin reuptake inhibitors; **tds:** three times per day; **>:** greater than; **≥:** greater than or equal to; **<:** less than.

Health care professionals please note: when a patient presents using any of the drugs listed above and there is a potential interaction with the herb you intend to dispense, it is important that you or your patient discuss the potential interaction with their prescribing physician before you dispense the herb to the patient.

NOTES

* This chart contains information the authors believe to be reliable or which has received considerable attention as potential issues. However, many theoretical concerns expressed by other authors have not been included. Due to the focus on safety, positive interactions between herbs and drugs, and the effect of drugs on the bioavailability of herbs are generally not included.

A. Research paper describes administration of Scutellaria radix. Trial authors confirm this was root of Chinese skullcap (*Scutellaria baicalensis*).[346]

B. Analysis of Chinese skullcap root samples from Japan found the baicalin content varied from 3.5 to 12%. For a dose of 150 mg/day of baicalin, 1.2–4.3 g/day of dried root would be required.[347]

C. Single-strength (freshly squeezed, 100%) cranberry juice is highly acidic and astringent, making it unpalatable. For this reason, cranberry juice is usually diluted and sweetened (often known as cranberry juice drink). Cranberry juice cocktail usually contains 25% cranberry juice, although can be up to 35%. Cranberry juice drinks contain about 10% cranberry juice. Cranberry sauce is about half the strength of cranberry juice cocktail, about the same strength as juice drinks. Cranberry juice can be concentrated to a dry powder (unsweetened and usually up to 25:1) and used in tablets and capsules. Juices can be prepared by diluting juice concentrates yielding a concentrated juice (eg double-strength juice, at twice the strength of single-strength, squeezed juice). It is likely that unless defined, cranberry juice referred to in case reports and clinical studies is juice drink containing around 10% cranberry juice.

D. Refer to Assessment of Risk & Recommended Action (available on www.mediherb.com) for definition of the extent of this interaction.

E. The cranberry 'juice' administered was similar in concentration to a reference cranberry 'juice' containing about 25% cranberry juice,[348] but with a higher concentration of anthocyanins, and lower in catechins and organic acids. *See also note C.*

F. No effect overall when midazolam was administered orally: oral clearance and area under the drug concentration-time curve were unchanged.

G. Eleutherosides (from Eleuthero) and ginsenosides (from Korean ginseng) have some structural similarity with digoxin. Because of this similarity interference with serum digoxin measurements is possible, as confirmed when mice fed these herbs demonstrated digoxin activity in their serum. More specific assays are able to negate the interference.[349]

H. These four trials used tablets containing a concentrated, standardized extract. A dosage of 900 mg/day of dry extract was equivalent to about 2.7 g/day of fresh garlic,[350] and was said to contain 12 mg/day of alliin,[54,62] although there is some doubt as to the amount of allicin released from this brand of tablet from around 1995 to 2000.[351]

J. There may have been variation in patients' interpretations (of bleeding) and the significant association between ginger use and bleeding was based on 7 self-reported events in 25 users.[352]

K. Ginkgotoxin (4'-O-methylpyridoxine) is present in substantial amounts in Ginkgo seed, and convulsions arising from ingestion of Ginkgo seed have been documented in Japan (infants are particularly vulnerable). Ginkgotoxin is known to inhibit vitamin B6 phosphorylation, which may lead to increased neuronal excitability.[353] Poisoning by ginkgotoxin can be counteracted by vitamin B6,[353] in cases of poisoning it is administered by intravenous injection.[354,355] Ginkgotoxin is present in very small amounts in standardized Ginkgo leaf extracts,[356] but is below the detection limits in human plasma after oral doses (240 mg of 50:1 extract, equivalent to 12 g of dried leaf).[357] According to the manufacturer, despite the extensive use of this special extract (more than 150 million daily doses per year for more than two decades) no cases of epileptic seizure have been attributed to this extract.[357] (Ginkgo preparations associated with the above case reports were undefined.) Strictly speaking this is a potential adverse effect (rather than a herb-drug interaction) as there is no pharmacokinetic data indicating an interaction for coadministration of Ginkgo and anticonvulsants in humans. An interaction is suggested though, because Ginkgo has been found to induce CYP2C19 activity (see entry for omeprazole), an enzyme involved in the metabolism of some anticonvulsants.

L. Analysis of over 320 000 patients in a German adverse drug reaction reporting system (1999-2002) found no increase in prevalence of bleeding during Ginkgo intake compared to periods without Ginkgo in those taking anticoagulant or antiplatelet medication.[358] In a trial involving 3069 healthy volunteers treated for an average of 6.1 years, there were no statistically significant differences between placebo and Ginkgo in the rate of major bleeding or the incidence of bleeding in individuals taking aspirin. (Compliance during the trial was however low (at the end of the trial, about 60% were taking Ginkgo/placebo).)[359] In Korea, Ginkgo extract is administered with ticlopidine for the prevention of ischemic stroke or acute coronary syndrome.[360]

M. The *in vitro* reduction by EGCG was overcome when the concentration of the drug was increased (to a level expected clinically ie in plasma from the standard drug dose).[361] A further *in vivo* study found no reduction in the activity of the drug (when EGCG administered by injection to achieve plasma levels of 11–16 microM).[116]

N. The *in vitro* study found a pronounced reduction in the cytotoxic effect of the drug for a concentration of 2.5–5 microM of EGCG, and when applied as green tea polyphenols a very substantial effect occurred at a EGCG concentration of 1 microM (the other polyphenols may contribute to the activity).[115] A pharmacokinetic study with healthy volunteers found a EGCG plasma concentration of 0.7 microM after a dose of 580 mg of EGCG, and a EGCG plasma concentration of 0.5 microM after a dose of 1 g of green tea polyphenols.[362]

P. Glycyrrhetinic acid, is the aglycone of glycyrrhizin. Glycyrrhizin, is the glycoside and contains the aglycone (glycyrrhetinic acid) and a sugar unit.

Q. No effect on blood pressure in healthy volunteers in two studies (130 mg/day of glycyrrhetinic acid = 227 mg/day of glycyrrhizin, for 14 days;[171] licorice tablets (266 mg/day of glycyrrhizin) for 56 days);[182] including where plasma renin levels were high (3.1 ng/mL/h),[182] but in another study, blood pressure increased in healthy volunteers taking 546 mg/day of glycyrrhizin for 4 weeks, only for those with plasma renin activity greater than 1.5 ng/mL/h.[363]

R. This is a guide, based on a recommendation from the German Commission E for long-term consumption of licorice as a flavoring. Glycyrrhizin is also known as glycyrrhizinic acid and glycyrrhizic acid.

S. ACE-inhibitors cause mild natriuresis (an increase in sodium excretion in the urine) and occasionally hyperkalemia. The mechanism of the interaction is not known, although it may involve opposing effects on 11beta-hydroxysteroid dehydrogenase type 2 (glycyrrhizin inhibiting, ACE-inhibitor promoting), thus affecting mineralocorticoid receptor activity. Reduction of drug dosage revealed the existing hypokalemia caused by this dosage of glycyrrhizin.

T. Maximum plasma cortisol (exogenous) was not increased in one volunteer;[189] in the other, plasma (exogenous) cortisone/cortisol ratio decreased,[188] suggesting increased (exogenous) cortisol while (endogenous) cortisol decreased (although statistical and clinical significance is unknown, and may have been within the normal range). In these studies isotope-labelled cortisol was administered, which allowed exogenous and endogenous cortisol to be measured.

U. A higher prednisolone/prednisone ratio indicates decreased conversion of prednisolone (active) to prednisone (inactive).

V. Several variants of CYP2C9 have been identified in humans: the most important mutations are CYP2C9*2 and CYP2C9*3. The CYP2C9*3 variant shows decreased metabolic activity for many drugs metabolized by CYP2C9. CYP2C9 is the main enzyme responsible for transforming losartan to its active metabolite.

W. The word tannin has a long established and extensive usage although it is considered in more recent years to lack precision. Polyphenol is the preferred term when considering the properties at a molecular level. Plant polyphenols are broadly divisible into proanthocyanidins (condensed tannins) and polymers of esters based on gallic and/or hexahydroxydiphenic acid and their derivatives (hydrolyzable tannins).[364] The terms 'tannin' and 'polyphenol' are sometimes used interchangeably. For example, the results of a clinical study are described: "polyphenols present in tea and coffee inhibited iron absorption in a dose-dependent manner". The 'polyphenol' content was measured using a spectrophotometric method for the determination of "tannins and other polyphenolics".[333] Depending on the analytical method used, it is possible that the polyphenol content may actually be the content of tannins or tannins + polyphenols.[365] It is recommended that both sections of this chart be considered: Polyphenol-containing or Flavonoid-containing herbs, and Tannin-containing or OPC-containing herbs.

X. Heme iron is derived from hemoglobin and myoglobin mainly in meat products. Non-heme iron is derived mainly from cereals, vegetables and fruits.

Y. At an identical concentration of total polyphenols, black tea was more inhibitory than all the herb teas excluding peppermint: black tea was of equal inhibition to peppermint tea.[223] The type of polyphenols present, as well as the concentration, may affect iron absorption.

Z. Another clinical study also found a dose-dependent effect, and the reduced absorption was most marked when coffee was taken with the meal or one hour later. No decrease in iron absorption occurred when coffee was consumed one hour before the meal.[332]

AA. Administered in freeze-dried form (4.2 g), which would be expected to have a lower inhibitory effect than with the use of fresh chili, as freeze drying probably decreased the ascorbic acid content (ascorbic acid enhances iron absorption).[226]

BB. The different results for cayenne and turmeric under the same experimental conditions, suggest it is not only the quantity of polyphenol present that determines the inhibition, but also for example, the structure of the polyphenol (and hence mechanism of iron binding).[226]

CC. Fructus Schisandra is defined as the fruit of *Schisandra chinensis* or *Schisandra sphenanthera* in traditional Chinese medicine. The major constituents are dibenzocyclooctene lignans. Several factors including harvest season, origin of herb and extraction solvent affect the levels of the individual lignans. Aqueous or ethanolic extracts of *S. chinensis* are not likely to contain more than 2.5 mg/g of deoxyschisandrin.[366,367] A maximum dose of *S. chinensis* extract equivalent to 4 g/day, would provide 10 mg/day of deoxyschisandrin.

DD. As noted for several drugs, the hyperforin content of the St John's wort preparation, as well as the dosage of herb, affects the extent of the interaction. All types of preparations can contain hyperforin, including dry extracts used in tablets and capsules. Hyperforin is however, unstable – particularly when in solution.[368] Tinctures and liquid extracts made using a standard ethanol content (45%) contain negligible amounts of hyperforin. Liquid extracts using a higher ethanol content (such as 60%) will contain a higher initial amount of hyperforin than standard liquid extracts. Over time the hyperforin content is substantially reduced and after a few months tinctures and liquid extracts contain no hyperforin.[369]

EE. Genetic polymorphisms are important in determining differences in the response to drugs, and may influence interactions. There are many genetic variants of the CYP genes, including the CYP2C19 gene. Phenotypes of CYP2C19 have been classified functionally as extensive metabolizers and poor metabolizers, the latter having a deficiency of CYP2C19 activity.[208,370]

FF. Of the 14 volunteers, in three, a small increase in AUC was observed after administration of St John's wort.

GG. Sorghum also contains phytate. Both phytate and polyphenol inhibit nutrients such as iron.[371,372]

REFERENCES

Braun L. *Herb Drug Interaction Guide for Pharmacists*. FH Faulding, August 2000; Fugh-Berman A. *Lancet* 2000; **355**(9198): 134-138

1 Pulliero G, Montin S, Bettini V et al. *Fitoterapia* 1989; **60**(1): 69-75

2 Duterte M, Waugh S, Thanawala R. *Am J Gastroenterol* 2007; **102**(Suppl 2): S350

3 Neumann L. *Klin Monbl Augenheilkd* 1973; **163**(1): 96-103

4 Aktas C, Senkal V, Sarikaya S et al. *Turk J Geriatr* 2011; **14**(1): 79-81

5 Patel NM, Derkits RM. *J Pharm Pract* 2007; **20**(4): 341-346

6 de Smet PAGM, Keller K, Hansel R et al (eds). *Adverse Effects of Herbal Drugs*, Volume 3. Springer-Verlag, Berlin, 1997.

7 Miller LG. *Arch Intern Med* 1998; **158**(20): 2200-2211

8 de Smet PAGM, Keller K, Hansel R et al (eds). *Adverse Effects of Herbal Drugs*, Volume 2. Springer-Verlag, Berlin, 1993.

9 Blumenthal M et al (eds). *The Complete German Commission E Monographs: Therapeutic Guide to Herbal Medicines*. American Botanical Council, Austin, 1998.

10 Lopez Galera RM, Ribera Pascuet E, Esteban Mur JI et al. *Eur J Clin Pharmacol* 2008; **64**(12): 1235-1236

11 Hakas JF. *Ann Allergy* 1990; **65**(4): 322-323

12 Bouraoui A, Toum A, Bouchoucha S et al. *Therapie* 1986; **41**(6): 467-471

13 Moses G. *Australian Prescriber* 2001; **24**(1): 6

14 Yi SJ, Cho JY, Lim KS et al. *Basic Clin Pharmacol Toxicol* 2009; **105**(4): 249-256

15 Fan L, Zhang W, Guo D et al. *Clin Pharmacol Ther* 2008; **83**(3): 471-476

16 de Souza NJ. *J Ethnopharmacol* 1993; **38**(2-3): 177-180

17 Yokotani K, Chiba T, Sato Y et al. *J Pharm Pharmacol* 2012; **64**(12): 1793-1801

18 de Souza NJ, Dohadwalla AN, Reden J. *Med Res Rev* 1983; **3**(2): 201-219

19 Dubey MP, Srimal RC, Nityanand S et al. *J Ethnopharmacol* 1981; **3**(1): 1-13

20 Sabinsa Corporation. *ForsLean® Product Information*. Available from www.forslean.com. Accessed November 2004.

21 Henderson S, Magu B, Rasmussen C et al. *J Int Soc Sports Nutr* 2005; **2**(2): 54-62

22 Seamon KB, Daly JW. *J Cyclic Nucleotide Res* 1981; **7**(4): 201-224

23 Ngo N, Yan Z, Graf TN et al. *Drug Metab Dispos* 2009; **37**(3): 514-522

24 Lilja JJ, Backman JT, Neuvonen PJ. *Clin Pharmacol Ther* 2007; **81**(6): 833-839

25 Goldenberg G, Khan R, Bharathan T. *Clin Geriatrics* 2012; **20**(8): 38-42

26 Medicines and Healthcare Products Regulatory Agency, Committee on Safety of Medicines. *Current Problems in Pharmacovigilance*, Vol 30, October 2004, p 10.

27 Rindone JP, Murphy TW. *Am J Ther* 2006; **13**(3): 283-284

28 Sylvan L, Justice NP. *Am Fam Physician* 2005; **72**(6): 1000

29 Paeng CH, Sprague M, Jackevicius CA. *Clin Ther* 2007; **29**(8): 1730-1735

30 Welch JM, Forster K. *J Pharm Technol* 2007; **23**(2): 104-107

31 Mergenhagen KA, Sherman O. *Am J Health Syst Pharm* 2008; **65**(22): 2113-2116

32 Griffiths AP, Beddall A, Pegler S. *J R Soc Promot Health* 2008; **128**(6): 324-326

33 Hamann GL, Campbell JD, George CM. *Ann Pharmacother* 2011; **45**(3): e17

34 Haber SL, Cauthon KA, Raney EC. *Consult Pharm* 2012; **27**(1): 58-65

35 Li Z, Seeram NP, Carpenter CL et al. *J Am Diet Assoc* 2006; **106**(12): 2057-2061

36 Ansell J, McDonough M, Zhao Y et al. *J Clin Pharmacol* 2009; **49**(7): 824-830

37 Mohammed Abdul MI, Jiang X, Williams KM et al. *Br J Pharmacol* 2008; **154**(8): 1691-1700

38 Mellen CK, Ford M, Rindone JP. *Br J Clin Pharmacol* 2010; **70**(1): 139-142

39 Page RL, Lawrence JD. *Pharmacotherapy* 1999; **19**(7): 870-876

40 Ellis GR, Stephens MR. *BMJ* 1999; **319**(7210): 650

41 Moltó J, Valle M, Miranda C et al. *Antimicrob Agents Chemother* 2012; **56**(10): 5328-5331

42 Moltó J, Valle M, Miranda C et al. *Antimicrob Agents Chemother* 2011; **55**(1): 326-330

43 Mills S, Bone K. *Principles and Practice of Phytotherapy: Modern Herbal Medicine*. Churchill Livingstone, Edinburgh, 2000.

44 Newall CA, Anderson LA, Phillipson JD. *Herbal Medicines – A Guide for Health-Care Professionals*. Pharmaceutical Press, London, 1996.

45 Gorski JC, Huang SM, Pinto A et al. *Clin Pharmacol Ther* 2004; **75**(1): 89-100

46 McRae S. *Can Med Assoc J* 1996; **155**(3): 293-295

47 Cicero AF, Derosa G, Brillante R et al. *Arch Gerontol Geriatr Suppl* 2004; (9): 69-73

48 Mills S, Bone K *The Essential Guide to Herbal Safety*. Churchill Livingstone, USA, 2005.

49 Rose KD, Croissant PD, Parliament CF et al. *Neurosurgery* 1990; **26**(5): 880-882

50 Burnham BE. *Plast Reconstr Surg* 1995; **95**(1): 213

51 German K, Kumar U, Blackford HN. *Br J Urol* 1995; **76**(4): 518

52 Carden SM, Good WV, Carden PA et al. *Clin Experiment Ophthalmol* 2002; **30**(4): 303-304

53 Manoharan A, Gemmell R, Hartwell T. *Am J Hematol* 2006; **81**(9): 676-683

54 Legnani C, Frascaro M, Guazzaloca G et al. *Arzneim Forsch* 1993; **43**(2): 119-122

55 Kiesewetter H, Jung F, Jung EM et al. *Eur J Clin Pharmacol* 1993; **45**(4): 333-336

56 Kiesewetter H, Jung F, Jung EM et al. *Clin Investig* 1993; **71**(5): 383-386

57 Harenberg J, Giese C, Zimmermann R. *Atherosclerosis* 1988; **74**(3): 247-249

58 Ali M, Thomson M. *Prostaglandins Leukot Essent Fatty Acids* 1995; **53**(3): 211-212

59 Luley C, Lehmann-Leo W, Moller B et al. *Arzneim Forsch* 1986; **36**(4): 766-768

60 Scharbert G, Kalb ML, Duris M et al. *Anesth Analg* 2007; **105**(5): 1214-1218

61 Jain RC. *Am J Clin Nutr* 1977; **30**(9): 1380-1381

62 Lawson LD. *FASEB J* 2007; **21**(6): A1126

63 Gadkari JV, Joshi VD. *J Postgrad Med* 1991; **37**(3): 128-131

64 Sunter W. *Pharm J* 1991; **246**: 722

65 Piscitelli SC, Burstein AH, Welden N et al. *Clin Infect Dis* 2002; **34**(2): 234-238

66 Hajda J, Rentsch KM, Gubler C et al. *Eur J Pharm Sci* 2010; **41**(5): 729-735

67 Kruth P, Brosi E, Fux R et al. *Ann Pharmacother* 2004; **38**(2): 257-260

68 Verma SK, Singh J, Khamesra R et al. *Indian J Med Res* 1993; **98**: 240-242

69 Bordia A, Verma SK, Srivastava KC. *Prostaglandins Leukot Essent Fatty Acids* 1997; **56**(5): 379-384

70 Lumb AB. *Thromb Haemost* 1994; **71**(1): 110-111

71 Srivastava KC. *Prostaglandins Leukot Essent Fatty Acids* 1989; **35**(3): 183-185

72 Lesho EP, Saullo L, Udvari-Nagy S. *Cleve Clin J Med* 2004; **71**(8): 651-656

73 Jiang X, Williams KM, Liauw WS et al. *Br J Clin Pharmacol* 2005; **59**(4): 425-432

74 Shalansky S, Lynd L, Richardson K et al. *Pharmacotherapy* 2007; **27**(9): 1237-1247

75 Young HY, Liao JC, Chang YS et al. *Am J Chin Med* 2006; **34**(4): 545-551

76 Granger AS. *Age Ageing* 2001; **30**(6): 523-525

77 Gregory PJ. *Ann Intern Med* 2001; **134**(4): 344

78 Kupiec T, Raj V. *J Anal Toxicol* 2005; **29**(7): 755-758

79 Bruhn JG. *Phytomedicine* 2003; **10**(4): 358

80 Bent S, Goldberg H, Padula A et al. *J Gen Intern Med* 2005; **20**(7): 657-661

81 Griffiths J, Jordon S, Pilon K. *Canadian Adverse Reaction Newsletter* 2004; **14**(1): 2-3

82 Pedroso JL, Henriques Aquino CC, Escórcio Bezerra ML et al. *Neurologist* 2011; **17**(2): 89-90

83 Kellermann AJ, Kloft C. *Pharmacotherapy* 2011; **31**(5): 490-502

84 Chan AL, Leung HW, Wu JW et al. *J Altern Complement Med* 2011; **17**(6): 513-517

85 DeLoughery TG, Kaye JA, Morris CD et al. *Blood* 2002; **100**(11): Abstract #3809

86 Gardner CD, Zehnder JL, Rigby AJ et al. *Blood Coagul Fibrinolysis* 2007; **18**(8): 787-793

87 Wolf HR. *Drugs R D* 2006, **7**(3): 163-172

88 Aruna D, Naidu MU. *Br J Clin Pharmacol* 2007; **63**(3): 333-338

89 Yeo C, Cho H, Park S et al. *Clin Pharm Ther* 2010; **87**: S43

90 Kim BH, Kim KP, Lim KS et al. *Clin Ther* 2010; **32**(2): 380-390

91 Lu WJ, Huang JD, Lai ML. *J Clin Pharmacol* 2006; **46**(6): 628-634

92 Engelsen J, Nielsen JD, Winther K. *Thromb Haemost* 2002; **87**(6): 1075-1076

93 Lai CF, Chang CC, Fu CH et al. *Pharmacotherapy* 2002; **22**(10): 1326

94 Zhang XY, Zhou DF, Su JM et al. *J Clin Psychopharmacol* 2001; **21**(1): 85-88

95 Zhang XY, Zhou DF, Zhang PY et al. *J Clin Psychiatry* 2001; **62**(11): 878-883

96 Atmaca M, Tezcan E, Kuloglu M et al. *Psychiatry Clin Neurosci* 2005; **59**(6): 652-656

97 Doruk A, Uzun O, Ozsahin A. *Int Clin Psychopharmacol* 2008; **23**(4): 223-237

98 Blonk M, Colbers A, Poirters A et al. *Antimicrob Agents Chemother* 2012; **56**(10): 5070-5075

99 Wiegman DJ, Brinkman K, Franssen EJ. *AIDS* 2009; **23**(9): 1184-1185

100 Guo CX, Pei Q, Yin JY et al. *Xenobiotica* 2012; **42**(8): 784-790

101 Markowitz JS, Donovan JL, Lindsay DeVane C et al. *J Clin Psychopharmacol* 2003; **23**(6): 576-581

102 Zuo XC, Zhang BK, Jia SJ et al. *Eur J Clin Pharmacol* 2010; **66**(5): 503-509

103 Uchida S, Yamada H, Li XD et al. *J Clin Pharmacol* 2006; **46**(11): 1290-1298

104 Robertson SM, Davey RT, Voell J et al. *Curr Med Res Opin* 2008; **24**(2): 591-599

105 Zadoyan G, Rokitta D, Klement S et al. *Eur J Clin Pharmacol* 2012; **68**(5): 553-560

106 Kudolo GB, Wang W, Javors M et al. *Clin Nutr* 2006; **25**(4): 606-616

107 Personal communication from trial author Kudolo GB, 29 February 2008.

108 Wang W, Javors M, Blodgett J et al. *Diabetes* 2007; **56**(Suppl 1): A560

109 Smith M, Lin KM, Zheng MD. *Clin Pharmacol Ther* 2001; **69**(2): P86, Abstract #PIII-89

110 Yoshioka M, Ohnishi N, Koishi T et al. *Biol Pharm Bull* 2004; **27**(12): 2006-2009

111 Yin OQ, Tomlinson B, Waye MM et al. *Pharmacogenetics* 2004; **14**(12): 841-850

112 Fan L, Mao XQ, Tao GY et al. *Xenobiotica* 2009; **39**(3): 249-254

113 Chan E. *Biol Neonate* 1993; **63**(4): 201-208

114 Gurley BJ, Swain A, Hubbard MA et al. *Clin Pharmacol Ther* 2008; **83**(1): 61-69

115 Golden EB, Lam PY, Kardosh A et al. *Blood* 2009; **113**(23): 5927-5937

116 Bannerman B, Xu L, Jones M et al. *Cancer Chemother Pharmacol* 2011; **68**(5): 1145-1154

117 Alemdaroglu NC, Dietz U, Wolffram S et al. *Biopharm Drug Dispos* 2008; **29**(6): 335-348

118 Werba JP, Giroli M, Cavalca V et al. *Ann Intern Med* 2008; **149**(4): 286-287

119 Ge J, Tan BX, Chen Y et al. *J Mol Med* 2011; **89**(6): 595-602

120 Taylor JR, Wilt VM. *Ann Pharmacother* 1999; **33**(4): 426-428

121 Wolkerstorfer H. *MMW* 1966; **108**(8): 438-441

122 Jaursch U, Landers E, Schmidt R et al. *Med Welt* 1969; **27**: 1547-1552

123 Tankanow R, Tamer HR, Streetman DS et al. *J Clin Pharmacol* 2003; **43**(6): 637-642

124 Iwamoto M, Ishizaki T, Sato T. *Planta Med* 1981; **42**(1): 1-16

125 Schmidt U, Kuhn U, Ploch M et al. *Phytomedicine* 1994; **1**(1): 17-24

126 Zick SM, Vautaw BM, Gillespie B et al. *Eur J Heart Fail* 2009; **11**(10): 990-999

127 Dalli E, Colomer E, Tormos MC et al. *Phytomedicine* 2011; **18**(8-9): 769-775

128 Walker AF, Marakis G, Simpson E. *Br J Gen Pract* 2006; **56**(527): 437-443

129 Shanmugasundaram ER, Rajeswari G, Baskaran K et al. *J Ethnopharmacol* 1990; **30**(3): 281-294

130 Baskaran K, Kizar Ahamath B, Radha Shanmugasundaram K et al. *J Ethnopharmacol* 1990; **30**(3): 295-300

131 Sobenin IA, Nedosugova LV, Filatova LV et al. *Acta Diabetol* 2008; **45**(1): 1-6

132 Almeida JC, Grimsley EW. *Ann Intern Med* 1996; **125**(11): 940-941

133 Cartledge A, Rutherford J. Rapid response (electronic letter), *BMJ* 12 Feb 2001. Available from bmj.com/cgi/eletters/322/7279/139#12643, downloaded 21/2/02.

134 Herberg KW, Winter U. 2nd International Congress on Phytomedicine, Munich, September 11-14, 1996, Abstract P-77.

135 Herberg KW. *Blutalkohol* 1993; **30**(2): 96-105

136 Schelosky L, Raffauf C, Jendroska K et al. *J Neurol Neurosurg Psychiatry* 1995; **58**(5): 639-640

137 Yamamoto M, Tamura Y, Kuashima K et al. Cited in: Han KH, Choe SC, Kim HS et al. *Am J Chin Med* 1998; **26**(2): 199-209

138 Caron MF, Hotsko AL, Robertson S et al. *Ann Pharmacother* 2002; **36**(5): 758-763

139 Cherdrungsi P, Rungroeng K. Cited in: Buettner C, Yeh GY, Phillips RS et al. *Ann Pharmacother* 2006; **40**(1): 83-95

140 Park BJ, Lee YJ, Lee HR et al. *Korean J Fam Med* 2012; **33**(4): 190-196

141 Vuksan V, Sung MK, Sievenpiper JL et al. *Nutr Metab Cardiovasc Dis* 2008; **18**(1): 46-56

142 Kim NR, Kim JH, Kim CY. *J Ginseng Res* 2010; **34**(3): 237-245

143 Han KH, Choe SC, Kim HS et al. *Am J Chin Med* 1998; **26**(2): 199-209

144 Chung IM, Lim JW, Pyun WB et al. *J Ginseng Res* 2010; **34**(3): 212-218

145 Rhee MY, Kim YS, Bae JH et al. *J Altern Complement Med* 2011; **17**(1): 45-49

146 Lee JH, Park HJ. *J Ginseng Res* 1998; **22**(3): 173-180

147 Lee JH, Kim SH. *Korean J Nutr* 1995; **28**(9): 862-871

148 Shin KS, Lee JJ, Kim YI et al. *J Ginseng Res* 2007; **31**(2): 109-116

149 Janetzky K, Morreale AP. *Am J Health Syst Pharm* 1997; **54**(6): 692-693

150 Jiang X, Williams KM, Liauw WS et al. *Br J Clin Pharmacol* 2004; **57**(5): 592-599

151 Lee SH, Ahn YM, Ahn SY et al. *J Altern Complement Med* 2008; **14**(6): 715-721

152 Lee YH, Lee BK, Choi YJ et al. *Int J Cardiol* 2010; **145**(2): 275-276

153 Bilgi N, Bell K, Ananthakrishnan AN et al. *Ann Pharmacother* 2010; **44**(5): 926-928

154 Mateo-Carrasco H, Gálvez-Contreras MC, Fernández-Ginés FD et al. *Drug Metabol Drug Interact* 2012; **27**(3): 171-175

155 Sotaniemi EA, Haapakoski E, Rautio A. *Diabetes Care* 1995; **18**(10): 1373-1375

156 Reeds DN, Patterson BW, Okunade A et al. *Diabetes Care* 2011; **34**(5): 1071-1076

157 Okuda H, Yoshida R. *Proceedings of the Third International Ginseng Symposium*. Seoul, Korea. Korea Ginseng Research Institute, September 8-10, 1980, pp 53-57.

158 Ma SW, Benzie IF, Chu TT et al. *Diabetes Obes Metab* 2008; **10**(11): 1125-1127

159 Tetsutani T, Yamamura M, Yamaguchi T et al. *Ginseng Rev* 2000; **28**: 44-47

160 Jones BD, Runikis AM. *J Clin Psychopharmacol* 1987; **7**(3): 201-202

161 Shader RI, Greenblatt DJ. *J Clin Psychopharmacol* 1988; **8**(4): 235

162 Shader RI, Greenblatt DJ. *J Clin Psychopharmacol* 1985; **5**(2): 65

163 Malati CY, Robertson SM, Hunt JD et al. *J Clin Pharmacol* 2012; **52**(6): 932-939

164 Gillis CN. *Biochem Pharmacol* 1997; **54**(1): 1-8

165 Kim HJ, Woo DS, Lee G et al. *Br J Urol* 1998; **82**(5): 744-748

166 *ESCOP Monographs: The Scientific Foundation for Herbal Medicinal Products*, 2nd Edn. ESCOP, European Scientific Cooperative on Phytotherapy, Exeter, 2003.

167 Stormer FC, Reistad R, Alexander J. *Food Chem Toxicol* 1993; **31**(4): 303-312

168 Sigurjonsdottir HA, Franzson L, Manhem K et al. *J Hum Hypertens* 2001; **15**(8): 549-552

169 Sigurjonsdottir HA, Manhem K, Axelson M et al. *J Hum Hypertens* 2003; **17**(2): 125-131

170 Sigurjonsdottir HA, Ragnarsson J, Franzson L et al. *J Hum Hypertens* 1995; **9**(5): 345-348

171 Sobieszczyk P, Borlaug BA, Gornik HL et al. *Clin Sci* 2010; **119**(10): 437-442

172 Ferrari P, Sansonnens A, Dick B et al. *Hypertension* 2001; **38**(6): 1330-1336

173 van Gelderen CE, Bijlsma JA, van Dokkum W et al. *Hum Exp Toxicol* 2000; **19**(8): 434-439

174 Brouwers AJ, van der Meulen J. *Ned Tijdschr Geneeskd* 2001; **145**(15): 744-747

175 Iida R, Otsuka Y, Matsumoto K et al. *Clin Exp Nephrol* 2006; **10**(2): 131-135

176 Maeda Y, Inaba N, Aoyagi M et al. *Intern Med* 2008; **47**(14): 1345-1348

177 Stewart PM, Burra P, Shackleton CH et al. *J Clin Endocrinol Metab* 1993; **76**(3): 748-751

178 Kageyama Y, Suzuki H, Saruta T. *J Endocrinol* 1992; **135**(1): 147-152

179 MacKenzie MA, Hoefnagels WH, Jansen RW et al. *J Clin Endocrinol Metab* 1990; **70**(6): 1637-1643

180 Stewart PM, Wallace AM, Valentino R et al. *Lancet* 1987; **330**(8563): 821-824

181 Epstein MT, Espiner EA, Donald RA et al. *J Clin Endocrinol Metab* 1978; **47**(2): 397-400

182 Mattarello MJ, Benedini S, Fiore C et al. *Steroids* 2006; **71**(5): 403-408

183 Biglieri EG. *Steroids* 1995; **60**(1): 52-58

184 Forslund T, Fyhrquist F, Frøseth B et al. *J Intern Med* 1989; **225**(2): 95-99
185 Stewart PM, Wallace AM, Atherden SM et al. *Clin Sci* 1990; **78**(1): 49-54
186 van Uum SH, Walker BR, Hermus AR et al. *Clin Sci* 2002; **102**(2): 203-211
187 Armanini D, Nacamulli D, Francini-Pesenti F et al. *Steroids* 2005; **70**(8): 538-542
188 Kasuya Y, Yokokawa A, Takashima S et al. *Steroids* 2005; **70**(2): 117-125
189 Kasuya Y, Yokokawa A, Hamura K et al. *Steroids* 2005; **70**(12): 811-816
190 Teelucksingh S, Mackie AD, Burt D et al. *Lancet* 1990; **335**(8697): 1060-1063
191 Chen MF, Shimada F, Kato H et al. *Endocrinol Jpn* 1991; **38**(2): 167-174
192 Conti M, Frey FJ, Escher G et al. *Nephrol Dial Transplant* 1994; **9**(11): 1622-1628
193 Shintani S, Murase H, Tsukagoshi H et al. *Eur Neurol* 1992; **32**(1): 44-51
194 Bernardi M, d-Intimo PE, Trevisani F et al. *Life Sci* 1994; **55**(11): 863-872
195 Harada T, Ohtaki E, Misu K et al. *Cardiology* 2002; **98**(4): 218
196 Armanini D, Castello R, Scaroni C et al. *Eur J Obstet Gynecol Reprod Biol* 2007; **131**(1): 61-67
197 Kurisu S, Inoue I, Kawagoe T et al. *J Am Geriatr Soc* 2008; **56**(8): 1579-1581
198 Heidemann HT, Kreuzfelder E. *Klin Wochenschr* 1983; **61**(6): 303-305
199 Chataway SJ, Mumford CJ, Ironside JW. *Postgrad Med J* 1997; **73**(863): 593-594
200 Folkersen L, Knudsen NA, Teglbjaerg PS. *Ugeskr Laeger* 1996; **158**(51): 7420-7421
201 Famularo G, Corsi FM, Giacanelli M. *Acad Emerg Med* 1999; **6**(9): 960-964
202 Nielsen I, Pedersen RS. *Lancet* 1984; **323**(8389): 1305
203 Conn JW, Rovner DR, Cohen EL. *JAMA* 1968; **205**(7): 492-496
204 Sontia B, Mooney J, Gaudet L et al. *J Clin Hypertens* 2008; **10**(2): 153-157
205 Hukkanen J, Ukkola O, Savolainen MJ. *Blood Press* 2009; **18**(4): 192-195
206 Jiao Z, Shi XJ, Li ZD et al. *Br J Clin Pharmacol* 2009; **68**(1): 47-60
207 Tu JH, He YJ, Chen Y et al. *Eur J Clin Pharmacol* 2010; **66**(8): 805-810
208 Tu JH, Hu DL, Dai LL et al. *Xenobiotica* 2010; **40**(6): 393-399
209 Liapina LA, Koval'chuk GA. *Izv Akad Nauk Ser Biol* 1993; (4): 625-628
210 Velussi M, Cernigoi AM, de Monte A et al. *J Hepatol* 1997; **26**(4): 871-879
211 Jose MA, Abraham A, Narmadha MP. *J Pharmacol Pharmacother* 2011; **2**(4): 287-289
212 Hussain SA. *J Med Food* 2007; **10**(3): 543-547
213 Huseini HF, Larijani B, Heshmat R et al. *Phytother Res* 2006; **20**(12): 1036-1039
214 Taher MA, Atia YA, Amin MK. *Iraqi J Pharm Sci* 2010; **19**(2): 11-18
215 Hashemi SJ, Hajiani E, Sardabi EH. *Hep Mon* 2009; **9**(4): 265-270
216 Deng YQ, Fan XF, Li JP. *Chin J Integr Med* 2005; **11**(2): 117-122
217 Han Y, Guo D, Chen Y et al. *Eur J Clin Pharmacol* 2009; **65**(6): 585-591
218 Rajnarayana K, Reddy MS, Vidyasagar J et al. *Arzneim Forsch* 2004; **54**(2): 109-113
219 Fuhr U, Beckmann-Knopp S, Jetter A et al. *Planta Med* 2007; **73**(14): 1429-1435
220 Repalle SS, Yamsani SK, Gannu R et al. *Acta Pharm Sci* 2009; **51**(1): 15-20
221 Han Y, Guo D, Chen Y et al. *Xenobiotica* 2009; **39**(9): 694-699
222 Nowack R, Nowak B. *Nephrol Dial Transplant* 2005; **20**(11): 2554-2556
223 Hurrell RF, Reddy M, Cook JD. *Br J Nutr* 1999; **81**(4): 289-295
224 Fleming DJ, Jacques PF, Dallal GE et al. *Am J Clin Nutr* 1998; **67**(4): 722-733
225 Samman S, Sandstrom B, Toft MB et al. *Am J Clin Nutr* 2001; **73**(3): 607-612
226 Tuntipopipat S, Judprasong K, Zeder C et al. *J Nutr* 2006; **136**(12): 2970-2974
227 Olivares M, Pizarro F, Hertrampf E et al. *Nutrition* 2007; **23**(4): 296-300
228 Kubota K, Sakurai T, Nakazato K et al. *Nippon Ronen Igakkai Zasshi* 1990; **27**(5): 555-558
229 Mitamura T, Kitazono M, Yoshimura O et al. *Nippon Sanka Fujinka Gakkaai Zasshi* 1989; **41**(6): 688-694
230 Prystai EA, Kies CV, Driskell JA. *Nutr Res* 1999; **19**(2): 167-177
231 Schlesier K, Kuhn B, Kiehntopf M et al. *Food Res Int* 2012; **46**(2): 522-527
232 Mennen L, Hirvonen T, Arnault N et al. *Eur J Clin Nutr* 2007; **61**(10): 1174-1179
233 Imai K, Nakachi K. *BMJ* 1995; **310**(6981): 693-696
234 Ullmann U, Haller J, Bakker GC et al. *Phytomedicine* 2005; **12**(6-7): 410-415
235 Hutchinson C, Bomford A, Geissler CA. *Eur J Clin Nutr* 2010; **64**(10): 1239-1241
236 Li R, Guo W, Fu Z et al. *Can J Physiol Pharmacol* 2012; **90**(7): 941-945
237 Xin HW, Wu XC, Li Q et al. *Br J Clin Pharmacol* 2007; **64**(4): 469-475
238 Jiang W, Wang X, Xu X et al. *Int J Clin Pharmacol Ther* 2010; **48**(3): 224-229
239 Jiang W, Wang X, Kong L. *Immunopharmacol Immunotoxicol* 2010; **32**(1): 177-178
240 Xin HW, Wu XC, Li Q et al. *Br J Clin Pharmacol* 2009; **67**(5): 541-546
241 Ko KM, Ip SP, Poon MK et al. *Planta Med* 1995; **61**(2): 134-137
242 Lu H, Liu GT. *Zhongguo Yao Li Xue Bao* 1990; **11**(4): 331-335
243 Johne A, Schmider J, Brockmoller J et al. *J Clin Psychopharmacol* 2002; **22**(1): 46-54
244 Australian Therapeutic Goods Administration. Media Release, March 2000.
245 Breckenridge A. Message from Committee on Safety of Medicines, 29 February 2000. Medicines Control Agency, London.
246 Henney JE. *JAMA* 2000; **283**(13): 1679
247 Burstein AH, Horton RL, Dunn T et al. *Clin Pharmacol Ther* 2000; **68**(6): 605-612
248 *Drug Safety Update* Volume 1, Issue 4, November 2007, p 7. Available from www.mhra.gov.uk/Publications/Safetyguidance/DrugSafetyUpdate/index.htm. Accessed 18 April 2008.
249 Wang LS, Zhu B, Abd El-Aty AM et al. *J Clin Pharmacol* 2004; **44**(6): 577-581
250 Wang Z, Hamman MA, Huang SM et al. *Clin Pharmacol Ther* 2002; **71**(6): 414-420
251 Dresser GK, Schwarz UI, Wilkinson GR et al. *Clin Pharmacol Ther* 2003; **73**(1): 41-50
252 Lau WC, Gurbel PA, Carville DG et al. *J Am Coll Cardiol* 2007; **49**(9, Suppl 1): 343A-344A
253 Lau WC, Welch TD, Shields TA et al. *J Am Coll Cardiol* 2010; **55**(10, Suppl 1): A171.E1600
254 Lau WC, Welch TD, Shields T et al. *J Cardiovasc Pharmacol* 2011; **57**(1): 86-93
255 Fitzgerald DJ, Maree A. *Hematology Am Soc Hematol Educ Program* 2007; **2007**: 114-120
256 Maurer A, Johne A, Bauer S et al. *Eur J Clin Pharmacol* 1999; **55**(3): A22
257 Yue QY, Bergquist C, Gerden B. *Lancet* 2000; **355**(9203): 576-577
258 Barnes J, Anderson LA, Phillipson JD. *J Pharm Pharmacol* 2001; **53**(5): 583-600
259 Uygur Bayramıçlı O, Kalkay MN, Oskay Bozkaya E et al. *Turk J Gastroenterol* **2011**; 22(1): 115
260 Mueller SC, Majcher-Peszynska J, Uehleke B et al. *Eur J Clin Pharmacol* 2006; **62**(1): 29-36
261 Arold G, Donath F, Maurer A et al. *Planta Med* 2005; **71**(4): 331-337
262 Markowitz JS, Donovan JL, DeVane CL et al. *JAMA* 2003; **290**(11): 1500-1504
263 Wang Z, Gorski JC, Hamman MA et al. *Clin Pharmacol Ther* 2001; **70**(4): 317-326
264 Mueller SC, Majcher-Peszynska J, Mundkowski RG et al. *Eur J Clin Pharmacol* 2009; **65**(1): 81-87
265 Kawaguchi A, Ohmori M, Tsuruoka S et al. *Br J Clin Pharmacol* 2004; **58**(4): 403-410
266 Wang XD, Li JL, Lu Y et al. *J Chromatogr B Analyt Technol Biomed Life Sci* 2007; **852**(1-2): 534-544
267 Tannergren C, Engman H, Knutson L et al. *Clin Pharmacol Ther* 2004; **75**(4): 298-309
268 Mathijssen RH, Verweij J, de Bruijn P et al. *J Natl Cancer Inst* 2002; **94**(16): 1247-1249
269 Mansky PJ, Straus SE. *J Natl Cancer Inst* 2002; **94**(16): 1187-1188
270 Smith PF, Bullock JM, Booker BM et al. *Blood* 2004; **104**(4): 1229-1230
271 Frye RF, Fitzgerald SM, Lagattuta TF et al. *Clin Pharmacol Ther* 2004; **76**(4): 323-329
272 Van Strater AC, Bogers JP. *Int Clin Psychopharmacol* 2012; **27**(2): 121-124
273 Johne A, Brockmoller J, Bauer S et al. *Clin Pharmacol Ther* 1999; **66**(4): 338-345
274 Durr D, Stieger B, Kullak-Ublick GA et al. *Clin Pharmacol Ther* 2000; **68**(6): 598-604
275 Mueller SC, Uehleke B, Woehling H et al. *Clin Pharmacol Ther* 2004; **75**(6): 546-557
276 Lundahl A, Hedeland M, Bondesson U et al. *Eur J Pharm Sci* 2009; **36**(4-5): 433-443
277 Anon. *Reactions Weekly* 2011; **1336**: 22
278 de Maat MMR, Hoetelmans RMW, Mathot RAA et al. *AIDS* 2001; **15**(3): 420-421
279 Piscitelli SC, Burstein AH, Chaitt D et al. *Lancet* 2000; **355**(9203): 547-548
280 Xu H, Williams KM, Liauw WS et al. *Br J Pharmacol* 2008; **153**(7): 1579-1586
281 Fan L, Zhou G, Guo D et al. *Clin Pharmacokinet* 2011; **50**(9): 605-611
282 Bon S, Hartmann K, Kuhn M. *Schweiz Apoth* 1999; **16**: 535-536
283 Ahmed SM, Banner NR, Dubrey SW. *J Heart Lung Transplant* 2001; **20**(7): 795
284 Ruschitzka F, Meier PJ, Turina M et al. *Lancet* 2000; **355**(9203): 548-549
285 Mai I, Kruger H, Budde K et al. *Int J Clin Pharmacol Ther* 2000; **38**(10): 500-502
286 Karliova M, Treichel U, Malago M et al. *J Hepatol* 2000; **33**(5): 853-855
287 Rey JM, Walter G. *Med J Aust* 1998; **169**(11-12): 583-586
288 Barone GW, Gurley BJ, Ketel BL et al. *Transplantation* 2001; **71**(2): 239-241
289 Barone GW, Gurley BJ, Ketel BL et al. *Ann Pharmacother* 2000; **34**(9): 1013-1016
290 Moschella C, Jaber BL. *Am J Kidney Dis* 2001; **38**(5): 1105-1107
291 Beer AM, Ostermann T. *Med Klin* 2001; **96**(8): 480-483
292 Breidenbach T, Kliem V, Burg M et al. *Transplantation* 2000; **69**(10): 2229-2230
293 Mai I, Bauer S, Perloff ES et al. *Clin Pharmacol Ther* 2004; **76**(4): 330-340
294 Bolley R, Zulke C, Kammerl M et al. *Transplantation* 2002; **73**(6): 1009
295 Mai I, Stormer E, Bauer S et al. *Nephrol Dial Transplant* 2003; **18**(4): 819-822
296 Hebert MF, Park JM, Chen YL et al. *J Clin Pharmacol* 2004; **44**(1): 89-94
297 Portoles A, Terleira A, Calvo A et al. *J Clin Pharmacol* 2006; **46**(10): 1188-1194
298 Peltoniemi MA, Saari TI, Hagelberg NM et al. *Fundam Clin Pharmacol* 2012; **26**(6): 743-750
299 Eich-Hochli D, Oppliger R, Golay KP et al. *Pharmacopsychiatry* 2003; **36**(1): 35-37
300 Niederhofer H. *Med Hypotheses* 2007; **68**(5): 1189
301 Wang LS, Zhou G, Zhu B et al. *Clin Pharmacol Ther* 2004; **75**(3): 191-197
302 Information from the MPA (Medical Products Agency, Sweden) and the MCA (Medicines Control Agency, UK), 2000-2002.
303 Schwarz UI, Buschel B, Kirch W. *Br J Clin Pharmacol* 2003; **55**(1): 112-113
304 Murphy PA, Kern SE, Stanczyk FZ et al. *Contraception* 2005; **71**(6): 402-408
305 Hall SD, Wang Z, Huang SM et al. *Clin Pharmacol Ther* 2003; **74**(6): 525-535
306 Pfrunder A, Schiesser M, Gerber S et al. *Br J Clin Pharmacol* 2003; **56**(6): 683-690
307 Will-Shahab L, Bauer S, Kunter U et al. *Eur J Clin Pharmacol* 2009; **65**(3): 287-294
308 Murphy P, Bellows B, Kern S. *Contraception* 2010; **82**(2): 191
309 Fogle RH, Murphy PA, Westhoff CL et al. *Contraception* 2006; **74**(3): 245-248
310 Nieminen TH, Hagelberg NM, Saari TI et al. *Eur J Pain* 2010; **14**(8): 854-859
311 Gordon JB. *Am Fam Phys* 1998; **57**(5): 950, 953
312 Dermott K. *Clinical Psychiatry News* 1998; **26**(3): 28
313 Barbenel DM, Yusuf B, O'Shea D et al. *J Psychopharmacol* 2000; **14**(1): 84-86
314 Lantz MS, Buchalter E, Giambanco V. *J Geriatr Psychiatry Neurol* 1999; **12**(1): 7-10
315 Prost N, Tichadou L, Rodor F et al. *Presse Med* 2000; **29**(23): 1285-1286
316 Waksman JC, Heard K, Jolliff H et al. *Clin Toxicol* 2000; **38**(5): 521
317 Andren L, Andreasson A, Eggertsen R. *Eur J Clin Pharmacol* 2007; **63**(10): 913-916
318 Sugimoto K, Ohmori M, Tsuruoka S et al. *Clin Pharmacol Ther* 2001; **70**(6): 518-524
319 Gordon RY, Becker DJ, Rader DJ. *Am J Med* 2009; **122**(2): e1-e2
320 Eggertsen R, Andreasson A, Andren L. *Scand J Prim Health Care* 2007; **25**(3): 154-159
321 Schwarz UI, Hanso H, Oertel R et al. *Clin Pharmacol Ther* 2007; **81**(5): 669-678
322 Nebel A, Schneider BJ, Baker RK et al. *Ann Pharmacother* 1999; **33**(4): 502
323 Morimoto T, Kotegawa T, Tsutsumi K et al. *J Clin Pharmacol* 2004; **44**(1): 95-101
324 Rengelshausen J, Banfield M, Riedel KD et al. *Clin Pharmacol Ther* 2005; **78**(1): 25-33
325 Hojo Y, Echizenya M, Ohkubo T et al. *J Clin Pharm Ther* 2011; **36**(6): 711-715
326 Rossander L, Hallberg L, Bjorn-Rasmussen E. *Am J Clin Nutr* 1979; **32**(12): 2484-2489
327 Disler PB, Lynch SR, Charlton RW et al. *Gut* 1975; **16**(3): 193-200
328 Brune M, Rossander L, Hallberg L. *Eur J Clin Nutr* 1989; **43**(8): 547-557
329 Derman D, Sayers M, Lynch SR et al. *Br J Nutr* 1977; **38**(2): 261-269
330 Hallberg L, Rossander L. *Hum Nutr Appl Nutr* 1982; **36**(2): 116-123
331 Chung KT, Wong TY, Wei CI et al. *Crit Rev Food Sci Nutr* 1998; **38**(6): 421-464
332 Morck TA, Lynch SR, Cook JD. *Am J Clin Nutr* 1983; **37**(3): 416-420
333 Layrisse M, García-Casal MN, Solano L et al. *J Nutr* 2000; **130**(9): 2195-2159. Erratum in: *J Nutr* 2000; **130**(12): 3106
334 Thankachan P, Walczyk T, Muthayya S et al. *Am J Clin Nutr* 2008; **87**(4): 881-886
335 Nelson M, Poulter J. *J Hum Nutr Diet* 2004; **17**(1): 43-54
336 Gabrielli GB, De Sandre G. *Haematologica* 1995; **80**(6): 518-520
337 Mahlknecht U, Weidmann E, Seipelt G. *Haematologica* 2001; **86**(5): 559
338 Kaltwasser JP, Werner E, Schalk K et al. *Gut* 1998; **43**(5): 699-704
339 Ganji V, Kies CV. *Plant Foods Hum Nutr* 1994; **46**(3): 267-276
340 Juan H, Terhaag B, Cong Z et al. *Eur J Clin Pharmacol* 2007; **63**(7): 663-668
341 USP Drug Information, US Pharmacopeia Patient Leaflet, Valerian (Oral). Rockville: The United States Pharmacopeial Convention, 1998.
342 Herberg KW. *Therapiewoche* 1994; **44**(12): 704-713
343 Carrasco MC, Vallejo JR, Pardo-de-Santayana M et al. *Phytother Res* 2009; **23**(12): 1795-1796
344 Donovan JL, DeVane CL, Chavin KD et al. *Drug Metab Dispos* 2004; **32**(12): 1333-1336
345 Krivoy N, Pavlotzky E, Chrubasik S et al. *Planta Med* 2001; **67**(3): 209-212
346 Personal communication from trial author Yu KS, 2 February 2010.
347 Makino T, Hishida A, Goda Y et al. *Nat Med* 2008; **62**(3): 294-299
348 Product information for Cranberry Classic juice drink. Available from www.oceanspray.com.au. Accessed November 2009.
349 Dasgupta A, Wu S, Actor J et al. *Am J Clin Pathol* 2003; **119**(2): 298-303
350 Warshafsky S, Kamer RS, Sivak SL. *Ann Intern Med* 1993; **119**(7 Pt 1): 599-605
351 Lawson LD, Wang ZJ, Papadimitriou D. *Planta Med* 2001; **67**(1): 13-18
352 De Smet PA, Floor-Schreudering A, Bouvy ML et al. *Curr Drug Metab* 2008; **9**(10): 1055-1062
353 Leistner E, Drewke C. *J Nat Prod* 2010; **73**(1): 86-92
354 Kajiyama Y, Fujii K, Takeuchi H et al. *Pediatrics* 2002; **109**(2): 325-327
355 Hasegawa S, Oda Y, Ichiyama T et al. *Pediatr Neurol* 2006; **35**(4): 275-276
356 Arenz A, Klein M, Fiehe K et al. *Planta Med* 1996; **62**(6): 548-551
357 Kuenick C. *Dtsch Apoth Ztg* 2010; **150**(5): 60-61
358 Gaus W, Westendorf J, Diebow R. et al. *Methods Inf Med* 2005; **44**(5): 697-703
359 DeKosky ST, Williamson JD, Fitzpatrick AL et al. *JAMA* 2008; **300**(19): 2253-2262
360 Kim TE, Kim BH, Kim J et al. *Clin Ther* 2009; **31**(10): 2249-2257
361 Shah JJ, Kuhn DJ, Orlowski RZ. *Blood* 2009; **113**(23): 5695-5696
362 Henning SM, Niu Y, Liu Y et al. *J Nutr Biochem* 2005; **16**(10): 610-616
363 Kageyama Y, Suzuki H, Saruta T. *Endocrinol Jpn* 1991; **38**(1): 103-108
364 Haslam E, Lilley TH. *Crit Rev Food Sci Nutr* 1988; **27**(1): 1-40
365 Price ML, Butler LG. *J Agric Food Chem* 1977; **25**(6): 1268-1273
366 Halstead CW, Lee S, Khoo CS et al. *J Pharm Biomed Anal* 2007; **45**(1): 30-37
367 Zhu M, Chen XS, Wang KX. *Chromatographia* 2007; **66**(1-2): 125-128
368 Ang CYW, Hu L, Heinze TM et al. *J Agric Food Chem* 2004; **52**(20): 6156-6164
369 MediHerb Research Laboratories, 2004.
370 Tomlinson B, Hu M, Lee VW. *Mol Nutr Food Res* 2008; **52**(7): 799-809
371 Lynch SR. *Nutr Rev* 1997; **55**(4): 102-110
372 Gillooly M, Bothwell TH, Charlton RW et al. *Br J Nutr* 1984; **51**(1): 37-46

BIBLIOGRAPHY

About clinical pharmacology. Retrieved from http://www.clinicalpharmac ology.com.

Ageing-related changes affecting medicines use. (2013). Retrieved from http://www.nps.org.au/topics/ages-life-stages/for-individuals/older-people-and-medicines/for-health-professionals/ageing-related-changes.

Agency for Healthcare Research & Quality. (2016). *National guideline clearinghouse.* Retrieved from https://www.guideline.gov/.

Agency for Healthcare Research & Quality. (2014). *Safe meds.* Retrieved from http://archive.ahrq.gov/consumer/safemeds.htm.

AIDS info. (2015). *Clinical guidelines portal.* Retrieved from https://aidsinfo.nih.gov/guidelines.

Alberts, B., Johnson, A., Lewis, J., et al. (2002). *Molecular biology of the cell* (4th ed.). New York: Garland Science. An Overview of the Cell Cycle. Retrieved from http://www.ncbi.nlm.nih.gov/books/NBK26869/.

Alzheimer's Association. www.alz.org.

American Academy of Dermatology. https://www.aad.org/practice-tools/quality-care/clinical-guidelines.

American Botanical Council. (2013). *Terminology.* Retrieved from http://abc.herbalgram.org/site/PageServer?pagename=Terminology.

American Cancer Society. www.cancer.org/cancer/cancerbasics/thehistoryofcancer/the-history-of-cancer-cancer-treatment-targeted-therapy.

American Geriatrics Society 2015 Beers Criteria Update Expert Panel. (2015). American Geriatrics Society 2015 updated Beers criteria for potentially inappropriate medication use in older adults. *Journal of the American Geriatrics Society, 63,* 2227–2246.

American Heart Association. (2015). *Highlights of the 2015 American Heart Association guidelines update for CPR and ECC.* Retrieved from http://eccguidelines.heart.org/wp-content/uploads/2015/10/2015-AHA-Guidelines-Highlights-English.pdf.

American Holistic Nurses Association. (n.d.). Position on the role of nurses in the practice of complementary and alternative therapies. Retrieved from http://www.ahna.org/Resources/Publications/Position-Statements.

American Lung Association. (2016). *E-cigarettes and lung health.* Retrieved from http://www.lung.org/stop-smoking/smoking-facts/e-cigarettes-and-lung-health.html.

American Lung Association. (n.d.). *How to quit smoking.* Retrieved from http://www.lung.org/stop-smoking/i-want-to-quit/how-to-quit-smoking.html.

American Nurses Association. (2010). *Scope and standards of practice* (2nd ed.). Silver Spring, MD. Retrieved from www.nursebook.org.

American Nurses Association. (2015). *Code of ethics for nurses with interpretive statements.* Retrieved from http://nursingworld.org/DocumentVault/Ethics_1/Code-of-Ethics-for-Nurses.html.

American Psychiatric Association. (2013). *Substance-related and addictive disorders.* Retrieved from http://www.dsm5.org/documents/substance%20use%20disorder%20fact%20sheet.pdf.

American Society for Parenteral and Enteral Nutrition (ASPEN). https://www.nutritioncare.org/American.

American Society for Reproductive Medicine. https://www.asrm.org/FACTSHEET_Hyperprolactinemia_Prolactin_Excess/.

American Thyroid Association. http://www.thyroid.org/hyperthyroidism/.

Anastasi, J. K., Chang, M., & Capili, B. (2011). Herbal supplements: Taking with your patients. *Journal for Nurse Practitioners, 7*(1), 29–35. Retrieved from www.medscape.com/viewarticle/735530.

Aspoden, P., Wolcott, J., Bootman, J. L., & Cronewett, L. R. (2007). Preventing medication errors: Quality chasm series. *National Academy of Sciences Executive Summary, 7*(107). Retrieved from http:.www.nap.edu.

Association of Nurses in AIDS Care. (2016). http://www.nursesinaidscare.org/i4a/pages/index.cfm?pageid=4693].

Baker, N. (2013, December/2014, January). The challenges that clinicians and patients face when selecting first-line treatments for multiple sclerosis. *British Journal of Neuroscience Nursing, 9*(6), 267–272. ISSN: 1747–0307.

Balentine, J. R. (2016). *Alcohol intoxication.* Retrieved from http://www.emedicinehealth.com/alcohol_intoxication/article_em.htm.

Bellaz, J. (2015). *This new bill would add $9 billion for medical research. Here are 5 reasons critics are terrified.* Retrieved from http://www.vox.com/2015/7/14/8961923/21st-century-cures-act.

Benowitz, N. L. (2009). Pharmacology of nicotine: Addiction, smoking-induced disease, and therapeutics. *Annual Review of Pharmacology and Toxicology, 49,* 57–71.

Berlin, C. M. (2013). *Pharmacokinetics in children.* Retrieved from https://www.merckmanuals.com/professional/pediatrics/principles-of-drug-treatment-in-children/pharmacokinetics-in-children.

Biological Response Modifier: What Is It? (2015). Retrieved from https://www.verywell.com/what-are-biologics-189483.

Blaise, K., & Hayes, J. (2016). *Professional nursing practice concepts and perspectives* (7th ed.). Upper Saddle River, NJ: Pearson.

Blanco-Reina, E., Ariza-Zafra, G., Ocana-Riola, R., Leon-Ortiz, M., & Bellido-Estevez, I. (2015). Optimizing elderly pharmacotherapy: Polypharmacy vs. undertreatment. Are these two concepts related? *European Journal of Clinical Pharmacology, 71,* 199–207.

Burchum, J., & Rosenthal, L. (2016). *Lehne's pharmacology for nursing care* (9th ed.). St Louis, MO: Elsevier.

Burke, T., Hooper, K., Barlo, S., & Holter, L. (2013, November). Clinical update: Multiple sclerosis. *Amstradan Nursing Federation, 21*(5), 30–33. ISSN: 2202–7114.

Burke, R. M., Leon, J. S., & Suchdev, P. S. (2014). Identification, prevention and treatment of iron deficiency during the First 1000 days. *Nutrients, 6*(10), 4093–4114. doi: 10.3390/nu6104093.

Canada's Food and Drugs Act & Regulations. (2016). Retrieved from http://www.hc-sc.gc.ca/fn-an/legislation/acts-lois/act-loi_reg-eng.php.

Center Watch. http://centerwatch.com/drug-information/fda-approved-drugs/.

Centers for Disease Control and Prevention. (2010). Prevention of perinatal group B streptococcal disease: Revised guidelines from CDC, 2010. *Morbidity and Mortality Weekly Report, 59*(RR10), 1–32.

Centers for Disease Control and Prevention. (2012). *Adults and older adult adverse drug events.* Retrieved from http://www.cdc.gov/MedicationSafety/Adult_AdverseDrugEvents.html.

Centers for Disease Control and Prevention. (2012, August 8). *Basic medication program.* Retrieved from http://www.cdc.gov/MedicationSafety/basics.html.

Centers for Disease Control and Prevention. (2016). *Birth defects.* Retrieved from www.cdc.gov/ncbddd/birthdefects/index.html.

Centers for Disease Control and Prevention. (2016). *National Prevention Information Network.* Retrieved from www.cdcnpin.org.

Chapman, R., & Plaat, F. (2009). Alcohol and anaesthesia. *Continuing Education in Anaesthesia, Critical Care & Pain, 9*(1), 10–13.

Cleveland Clinic. https://my.clevelandclinic.org/health/diseases_conditions/hic_Anemia/hic_erythropoietin-stimulating_agents.

Colhoun, S., Wilkinson, C., Izat, A., White, S., Pull, E., & Roberts, M. (2015, February/March). Multiple sclerosis & disease modifying therapies results of two UK surveys on factors influencing choice. *British Journal of Neuroscience Nursing, 11*(1), 7–13. ISSN: 1747–0307.

Controlled substance schedules. (n.d.). Retrieved from http://www.deadiversion.usdoj.gov/schedules/#define.

Counterfeit drugs: Fake drugs are bad medicine. Retrieved from http://www.ncpc.org/topics/intellectual-property-theft/counterfeit-drugs-1.

de Caen, A. R., Berg, M. D., Chameides, L., et al. (2015). Part 12: Pediatric advanced life support 2015 American Heart Association guidelines update for cardiopulmonary resuscitation and emergency cardiovascular care. *Circulation, 132*(Suppl. 2), S526–S542. Retrieved from http://circ.ahajournals.org/.

Dietary Reference Intakes. https://fnic.nal.usda.gov/dietary-guidance/dietary-reference-intakes/dri-tables-and-application-reports.

Dirckx, J. H. (2014). *Stedman's concise medical dictionary for the health professions* (7th ed.). Baltimore, MD: Lippincott Williams & Wilkins.

Drach-Zahavy, A., Somech, A., Admi, H., Peterfreund, I., Peker, H., & Priente, O. (2014). How do we learn from errors? A prospective study of the link between the wards' learning practices and medication administration errors. *International Journal of Nursing Studies, 51*, 448–457. Retrieved from www.elsevier.com.ijns.

Drugs A-Z. (n.d.). Retrieved from https://www.drugs.com/professionals.html.

Drugs.com. (2016). *Drugs A-Z.* Retrieved from http://www.drugs.com/.

Drugs and medications. (n.d.). Retrieved from http://www.webmd.com/drugs/index-drugs.aspx?show=drugs.

Dunn, S. (2015). Maintaining adequate hydration and nutrition in adult enteral tube feeding. *British Journal of Community Nursing, Supplement,* S16–S23. ISSN: 1462–4753.

Edwards, E. T., Edwards, E. S., Davis, E., et al. (2015). Comparative usability study of a novel auto-injector and an intranasal system for naloxone delivery. *Pain and Therapy, 4,* 89–105. Retrieved from http://link.springer.com/article/10.1007%2Fs40122-015-0035-9.

Fein, J. A., Zempsky, W. T., & Cravero, J. P. (2012). Relief of pain and anxiety in pediatric patients in emergency medical systems. *Pediatrics, 130,* e1391–e1405.

Felicilda-Reynaldo, R. F. (2014). Recognizing signs of prescription drug abuse and addiction, part I. *MedSurg Nursing, 23*(6), 391–396.

Fernandez, E., Perez, R., Hernandez, A., Tejada, P., Arteta, M., & Ramos, J. T. (2011). Factors and mechanisms for pharmacokinetic differences between pediatric population and adults. *Pharmaceutics, 3,* 53–72.

Finely, F. (2014, December). *Patient safety goals: Improving the safety of high-alert medication administration.* Retrieved from http://www.nursingald.com/uploads/publication/pdf/1113/Louisiana_Pelican_12_14.pdf.

Fletcher, J. (2013). Parenteral nutrition: Indications, risks, and nursing care. *Nursing Standard, 27*(46), 50–57. ISSN: 0029–6570.

Fredericks, E. M., & Dore-Stites, D. (2010). Adherence to immunosuppressants: how can it be improved in adolescent organ transplant recipients? *Current Opinions in Organ Transplant, 15*(5), 614–620.

Furdon, S. A., Pfeil, V. C., & Snow, K. (1998). Operationalizing Donna Wong's principle of atraumatic care: Pain management protocol in the NICU. *Pediatric Nursing, 24*(4), 336–342.

Gahart, B., & Nazareno, A. R. (2015). *Intravenous medications* (31st ed.). St. Louis, MO: Elsevier.

Garfin, P. M. (2015). *Posttransplant lymphoproliferative disease.* Retrieved from http://emedicine.medscape.com/article/431364-overview.

Glaser, J., & Rolita, L. (2009). Educating the older adult in over-the-counter medication use. *Geriatrics and Aging, 12*(2), 103–109. Retrieved from www.medscape.com/viewarticle/705665.

Guzman, F. (n.d.). Retrieved from http://pharmacologycorner.com/therapeutic-index/.

Herrell, H. E. (2014). Nausea and vomiting of pregnancy. *American Family Physician, 89*(12), 965–970. Retrieved from http://www.aafp.org/afp/2014/0615/p965.html.

Heuberger, R. (2012). Polypharmacy and food-drug interactions among older persons: A review. *Journal of Nutrition in Gerontology and Geriatrics, 31,* 325–403.

Hewitt, J., Tower, M., & Latimer, S. (2014). An education intervention to improve nursing students' understanding of medication safety. *Nurse Education in Practice, 15*(2015), 17–21.

Horn, J. R., & Hansten, P. D. (2008). *Get to know an enzyme: CYP2D6.* Retrieved from http://www.pharmacytimes.com/publications/issue/2008/2008-07/2008-07-8624.

Horvath, A. T., Misra, K., Epner, A. K., & Cooper, G. M. (n.d.). The diagnostic criteria for substance use disorders (addiction). Retrieved from http://www.amhc.org/1408-addictions/article/48502-the-diagnostic-criteria-for-substance-use-disorders-addiction.

Huang, M., Shen, A., Ding, J., & Geng, M. (2014). Molecularly targeted cancer therapy: Some lessons from the past decade. *Trends in Pharmacological Sciences, 35*(1), 41–50.

Hughes, R. G., & Edgerton, E. A. (2005). First, do no harm: Reducing pediatric medication errors. *American Journal of Nursing, 105*(5), 79–82.

Infectious diseases society of America. (2016). Retrieved from https://www.idsociety.org/Index.aspx.

Institute for Safe Medication Practices. (2001). *Medication safety self-assessment for community/ambulatory pharmacies.* Retrieved from https://www.ismp.org/selfassessments/Book.pdf.

Institute for Safe Medication Practices. (2015). *List of error-prone abbreviations, symbols, and dose designations.* Retrieved from https://www.ismp.org/tools/errorproneabbreviations.pdf

Jawahar, R., Oh, U., Yang, S., & Lapane, K. (2013, October). A systemic revision of pharmacological pain. *Drugs (ADIS), 73,* 1711–1722.

Keane, M. (2014). Recognizing & managing acute hyponatremia. *Emergency Nurse, 21*(9), 32–36.

King, K. (2015). Parenteral nutrition: Reverse nutrient deficiencies. *Today's Dietitian, 17*(9), 12. Retrieved from http://www.todaysdietitian.com/newarchives/ 090115p12.shtml.

Kisch, T., & LoVerde, J. (2015, May–June). Fun with fluids. *MedSurg Nursing, 24*(3), 189–193.

Kramlich, D. (2014). Introduction to complementary, alternative and traditional therapies. *Critical Care Nurse, 34*(6), 50–56. Retrieved from http://ccn.aacnjournals.org/content/34/6/50.full.

Lee, R., & Gabardi, S. (2012). Current trends in immunosuppressive therapies for renal transplant recipients. *American Journal of Health-System Pharmacists, 69*(15), 1961–1975.

Lewis, S., Dirksen, S., Heitkemper, M., & Bucher, L. (2014). *Medical surgical nursing* (9th ed.). St. Louis, MO: Elsevier.

Lexicomp Clinical Drug Information. http://www.wolterskluwercdi.com/lexicomp-online/

Link, M. S., Berkow, L. C., Kudenchuk, P. J., et al. (2015). Part 7: Adult advanced cardiovascular life support 2015 American Heart Association guidelines update for cardiopulmonary resuscitation and emergency cardiovascular care. *Circulation, 132*(Suppl. 2), S444–S464. Retrieved from http://circ.ahajournals.org/.

Lodhi, S. A. (2013). *A clinical guide to successfully managing immunosuppression in solid organ transplantation.* Retrieved from http://www.medscape.org/viewarticle/806307.

Lonsdale, D. O., & Baker, E. H. (2013). Understanding and managing medication in elderly people. *Best Practice & Research Clinical Obstetrics and Gynaecology, 27,* 767–788.

Maher, R. L., Hanlon, J. T., & Hajjar, E. R. (2014). Clinical consequences of polypharmacy in elderly. *Expert Opinion on Drug Safety, 13*(1).

Maja Stojančević, M., Bojić, G., Al Salami, H., & Mikov, M. (2012). The influence of intestinal tract and probiotics on the fate of orally administered drugs. *Current Issues in Molecular Biology, 16,* 55–68. Retrieved from http://www.horizonpress.com/cimb/v/v16/55.pdf.

Manuel, O., Kralidis, G., Mueller, N. J., et al. (2013). Impact of antiviral preventive strategies on the incidence and outcomes of cytomegalovirus disease in solid organ transplant recipients. *American Journal of Transplantation, 13,* 2402–2410.

Mayo Clinic Staff. (n.d.). *Complementary and alternative medicine.* Retrieved from http://www.mayoclinic.org/healthy-lifestyle/consumer-health/in-depth/alternative-medicine/art-20045267.

McCance, K. L., Huether, S. E., Brashers, V. L., & Rote, N. S. (2014). *Pathophysiology: The biologic basis for disease in adults and children* (7th ed.). St. Louis, MO: Elsevier.

Mcilvoy, L. (2014, September). Respiratory failure from a myasthenic crisis. *American Nurse Today, 9*(9), 28–28. ISSN: 1930–5583.

McKenry, L. M., Tessier, E., & Hogan, M. (2006). *Mosby's pharmacology in nursing* (22nd ed.). St. Louis, MO: Elsevier.

Mediherb. https://www.standardprocess.com/Resources/literature#.VvFOa-agvwA.

Medsafe. (2015). *Fruit interactions with common medicines.* Retrieved from http://www.medsafe.govt.nz/profs/PUArticles/March2015FruitInteractions.htm.

Meechan, R., Jones, H., & Valler-Jones, T. (2011). Do medicines OSCE's improve drug administration ability? *British Journal of Nursing, 20*(13), 817–822.

Membrane Diffusion and Animal Cell. (2015). Retrieved from http://vlc.ucdsb.ca/c.php?g=185420&p=1224721.

Mestecky, A. (2013, June/July). Clinical briefing: Myasthenia gravis. *British Journal of Neuroscience Nursing, 9*(3), 110–112. ISSN: 1747-0307.

Meyer, D., Damm, T., & Jensen, K. (2012). Drug dosage adjustments in chronic kidney disease: The pharmacist's role. *Saskatchewan Drug Information Services, College of Pharmacy and Nutrition, U of S.* Retrieved from http://www.rxfiles.ca/rxfiles/uploads/documents/ltc/HCPs/CKD/SDIS.Renal_newsletter.pdf.

Moroney, A. C. (2013). *Drug-receptor interactions.* Retrieved from https://www.merckmanuals.com/professional/clinical-pharmacology/pharmacodynamics/drug%E2%80%93receptor-interactions.

Mosby's dictionary of medicine, nursing & health professions (9th ed.). (2013). St. Louis, MO: Elsevier.

NANDA- Approved Nursing Diagnoses list. (2015-2017). http://www.nanda.org/nanda-international-nursing-diagnoses-definitions-and-classification-2015-17.html.

National Cancer Institute. (n.d.). *Introduction to the endocrine system.* Retrieved from http://training.seer.cancer.gov/anatomy/endocrine/#.

National Cancer Institute. (n.d.). Targeted cancer therapies. Retrieved from http://www.cancer.gov/cancertopics/factsheet/Therapy/targeted.

National Cancer Institute. http://www.cancer.gov/cancertopics/treatment/biologicaltherapy.

National Center for Complementary and Integrative Health. (2016). *Herbs at a glance.* Retrieved from https://nccih.nih.gov/health/herbsataglance.htm.

National Council of State Boards of Nursing. (2014). *What you need to know about substance use disorder in nursing.* Retrieved from https://www.ncsbn.org/SUD_Brochure_2014.pdf.

National Human Genome Research Institute. (2014). *Frequently asked questions about pharmacogenomics.* Retrieved from http://www.genome.gov/27530645.

National Institute for Health & Care Excellence (NICE). http://www.nice.orguk.

National Institute of General Medical Sciences. (2015). *Pharmacogenomics fact sheet.* Retrieved from https://www.nigms.nih.gov/education/Pages/factsheet-pharmacogenomics.aspx.

National Institute on Drug Abuse. (2014). *The science of drug abuse and addiction: The basics.* Retrieved from https://www.drugabuse.gov/publications/media-guide/science-drug-abuse-addiction-basics.

National Institute on Drug Abuse. (2016). *Commonly abused drugs.* Retrieved from https://www.drugabuse.gov/drugs-abuse/commonly-abused-drugs-charts.

National Institutes of Health. National Institute of Child Health and Human Development. www.nichd.nih.gov/womenshealth/.

National Perinatal Association. (n.d.). *Multidisciplinary guidelines for the Care of preterm infants.* http://www.nationalperinatal.org/latepreterm.

Neutropenic precautions. (n.d.). Retrieved from https://www.drugs.com/cg/neutropenic-precautions.html.

Ngan, V. (n.d.). Drug-induced photosensitivity. Retrieved from http://www.dermnetnz.org/reactions/drug-photosensitivity.html.

NICE CG 174. (2014). Guidance notes: intravenous fluid therapy in adults in hospital. *British Journal of Nursing IV Supplement, 23*(8) Mark Allen Publishing LTD.

Office for Human Research Protections (OHRP). (2016). *Informed consent checklist.* Retrieved from http://www.hhs.gov/ohrp/policy/consentckls.html.

Oliver, J., Coggins, C., Compton, P., et al. (2012). American Society for Pain Management Nursing position statement: Pain management in patients with substance use disorders. *Pain Management Nursing, 13*(3), 169–183. Retrieved from http://www.aspmn.org/documents/PainManagementinthePatientwithSubstanceUseDisorders_JPN.pdf.

Online Pharmacy Magazine. (2013). *How do drugs work.* Retrieved from http://pharmacymagazine.blogspot.com/2013/11/how-do-drugs-work.html.

Orbaek, J., Mette, G., Fabricius, P., Lefevre, R., & Moller, T. (2015). Patient safety & technology-driven medication: A qualitative study on how graduate nursing students navigate through complex medication administration. *Nurse Education in Practice, 15,* 203–211.

Parreco, L. K., Ness, E., Galasi, A., & O'Mara, A. M. (2012). Care of clinical trial participants: What nurses need to know. *American Nurse Today, 7*(6). Retrieved from www.americannursetoday.com/care-of-clinical-trial-participants-what-nurses-need-to-know/.

Parry, A., Barriball, K., & While, A. (2015). Factors contributing to registered nurse medication administration error: A narrative review. *International Journal of Nursing Studies, 52,* 403–420.

Parsons, G. (2015). Pain management in patients with a substance use disorder. *Clinical Pharmacist, 7*(9).

Pharmacology 4: Pharmacokinetics – Objectives. (2016). Retrieved from https://quizlet.com/21147360/pharmacology-4-pharmacokinetics-objectives-flash-cards/.

Piccolo, S., & Batlle, E. (2014). Cell cycle, differentiation and disease. *Current Opinion in Cell Biology, 31,* 29–38. Retrieved from http://www.sciencedirect.com/science/article/pii/S0955067414000830.

Pinto, J. C. (n.d.). Pediatric dosage development: Where are we? [PowerPoint slides]. Retrieved from http://www.fda.gov/downloads/NewsEvents/MeetingsConferencesWorkshops/UCM415217.pdf.

Potter, P., & Perry, A. (2009). *Fundamentals of nursing* (7th ed.). St. Louis, MO: Elsevier.

Practice Guidelines for Obstetric Anesthesia. (Feb 2016). An updated report by the American Society of Anesthesiologists Task Force on Obstetric Anesthesia and the Society for Obstetric Anesthesia and Perinatology. The American Society of Anesthesiologists, Inc. Wolters Kluwer Health, Inc. *Anesthesiology 2016, 124* (2).

Pretorius, R., Gataric, G., Swedlund, S. K., & Miller, J. R. (2013). Reducing the risk of adverse drug events in older adults. *American Family Physician, 87*(5). Retrieved from www.aafp.org/afp.

PubMed Health. http://www.ncbi.nlm.nih.gov/pubmedhealth/PMH0072572/.

Quest Diagnostics. (n.d.). *Therapeutic drug monitoring (TDM).* Retrieved from http://www.questdiagnostics.com/home/physicians/testing-services/condition/toxicology/tdm-info.

Reang, P., Gupta, M., & Kohli, K. (2006). Biological response modifiers in cancer. *Medscape.* Retrieved from http://www.medscape.com/viewarticle/545538.

Required daily limits (RDL). https://fnic.nal.usda.gov/sites/fnic.nal.usda.gov/files/uploads/recommended_intakes_individuals.pdf.

Rochon, P. A. (2016). *Drug prescribing for older adults.* Retrieved from http://www.uptodate.com.

Ruscin, J. M., & Linnebur, S. A. (2014). *Pharmacokinetics in the elderly.* Retrieved from https://www.merckmanuals.com/professional/geriatrics/drug-therapy-in-the-elderly/pharmacokinetics-in-the-elderly.

Sample informed consent for a randomized clinical trial of a drug. (n.d.). Retrieved from http://www.aku.edu/research/urc/ethicalreviewcommittee/sampleconsentforms/Pages/sampleconsentforms.aspx.

Sankaranarayanan, J., Collier, D., Furasek, A., et al. (2012). Rurality and other factors associated with adherence to immunosuppressant medications in community-dwelling solid-organ transplant recipients. *Research in Social and Administrative Pharmacy, 8,* 228–239.

Satpathy, H. K. (2015). Labor and delivery, analgesia, regional and local. Retrieved from http://emedicine.medscape.com/article/149337-overview.

Savikko, N., Pitkala1, K., Laurila1, J., et al. (2014). Secular trends in the use of vitamins, minerals & fish-oil. *The Journal of Nutrition, Health & Aging, 18,* 150–154.

Shepherd, A. B. (2013, August). Clinical review: Water everywhere. *Nursing & Residential Care, 15*(8).

Smetzer, J., Vaida, A., Cohen, M., et al. (2003, November). Patient safety findings from the ISMP medication safety self-assessment for hospitals. *Joint Commission Journal on Quality & Safety, 29*(11), 586–597.

Souza de Silva, A. E., Pontes, U. O., Genzini, T., et al. (2014). Integrative review on the role of nurses in post-kidney transplant. *Cogitare Enfermagem, 19*(3), 553–558. Retrieved from http://revistas.ufpr.br/cogitare/article/viewFile/34414/23256.

Stanford Health Care. (n.d.). *Biological response modifiers (BRMs).* https://stanfordhealthcare.org/medical-treatments/i/immunotherapy/types/Biological-response-modifiers.html.

Substance Abuse and Mental Health Services Administration. (2015). *Substance use disorders.* Retrieved from http://www.samhsa.gov/disorders/substance-use.

Substance Abuse and Mental Health Services Administration. (2015). *Treatments for substance use disorders.* Retrieved from http://www.samhsa.gov/treatment/substance-use-disorders.

Symptoms and signs of drug abuse. (n.d.). Retrieved from http://drugabus e.com/library/symptoms-and-signs-of-drug-abuse/.

Taber's cyclopedic medical dictionary (22th ed.). (2010). Philadelphia, PA: F. A. Davis Company.

Teele, M., Scribner-O'Pray, M., & Madhok, M. (2011). Managing pediatric pain in minor injuries. Contemporary Pediatrics. Retrieved from http://contemporarypediatrics.modernmedicine.com/contempor ary-pediatrics/news/modernmedicine/modern-medicine-feature-articles/managing-pediatric-pain?page=full.

The dose response curve and maximal efficacy. Retrieved from http://hom epage.psy.utexas.edu/homepage/class/Psy308/Salinas/Psychopharmac ology/Slide03.gif.

The Joint Commission. www.Joint Commission.org.

Thomas, C. M., & Siela, D. (2011). The impaired nurse. American Nurse Today, 6(8). Retrieved from https://americannursetoday.com/t he-impaired-nurse-would-you-know-what-to-do-if-you-suspected-substance-abuse/.

Turkoski, B. B. (2007). Medicating young or very young patients - part I. Orthopaedic Nursing, 26(2), 134–137.

U.S. Census Bureau. (2015). Older Americans month: May 2015 [Fact sheet]. Retrieved from https://www.census.gov/content/dam/Census/newsroo m/facts-for-features/2015/cb15-ff09_older_american_month.pdf.

U.S. Department of Health and Human Services. (1996). Guidance for industry E6 good clinical practice: Consolidated guidance. Retrieved from http://www.fda.gov/downloads/Drugs/GuidanceComplianceReg ulatoryInformation/Guidances/UCM073122.pdf.

U.S. Department of Veterans Affairs. (2016). HIV/AIDS. Retrieved from http://www.hiv.va.gov/index.asp.

U.S. Food and Drug Administration. (2016). MedWatch: The FDA Safety Information and Adverse Event Reporting Program. Retrieved from http:// www.fda.gov/Safety/MedWatch/default.htm.

U.S. Food and Drug Administration. (2014). The current over-the-counter medicine label: Take a look. Retrieved from http://www.fda.gov/drugs/eme rgencypreparedness/bioterrorismanddrugpreparedness/ucm133411.htm.

U.S. Food and Drug Administration. (2014). Pediatric exclusivity study age group (C-DRG-00909). Retrieved from http://www.fda.gov/Drugs/Dev elopmentApprovalProcess/FormsSubmissionRequirements/Electronic Submissions/DataStandardsManualmonographs/ucm071754.htm.

U.S. Pharmacopeial Convention. (n.d.). USP pictograms. www.usp.org/usp-healthcare-professionals/related-topics-resources/usp-pictograms.

Vallerand, A., Sanoski, C., & Deglin, J. (2016). Davis's drug guide for nurses (14th ed.). Philadelphia, PA: F. A. Davis.

Vogel, W. H. (2010). Infusion reactions: Diagnosis, assessment and management. Clinical Journal of Oncology Nursing, 14(2), E10–E21. Retrieved from http://chemotherapy.vc.ons.org/file_depot/0-10000000/0-10000/3365/folder/87592/Infusion+Reactions+ (Vogel+2010).pdf.

Vorvick, L. J. (2013). Over-the-counter medications. Retrieved from http:// www.nlm.nih.gov/medlineplus/ency/article/002208.htm.

Wang, E. H., Partovi, N., Levy, R. D., et al. (2012). Pneumocystis pneumonia in solid organ transplant recipients: Not yet an infection of the past. Transplant Infectious Disease, 14, 519–525.

Ward-Abel, N., Vernon, K., & Warner, R. (2014, February/March). An exciting era of treatments for relapsing remitting multiple sclerosis. British Journal of Neuroscience Nursing, 10(1), 21–28. ISSN: 1747-0307.

Wilson, B. A., Shannon, M. T., & Shields, K. M. (2016). Pearson nurse's drug guide. Hoboken, NJ: Pearson Education, Inc.

Wong, A., & Townley, S. A. (2011). Herbal medicines and anaesthesia. British Journal of Anesthesia Education, 11(1), 14–17. Retrieved from www.mescape.com/viewarticle/735761.

Woo, T. M. (n.d.). Pediatric pharmacology update. Retrieved from http ://nurse-practitioners-and-physician-assistants.advanceweb.com/article /pediatric-pharmacology-update.aspx.

Wooten, J. M. (2012). Pharmacotherapy considerations in elderly adults. Southern Medical Journal, 105(8), 437–445. Retrieved from http://www .medscape.com/viewarticle/769412_2.

World Health Organization. (2015). Postnatal care for mothers and newborns: Highlights from the World Health Organization 2013 Guide-lines. Retrieved from www.mcsprogram.org.

World Health Organization. (n.d.). Lexicon of alcohol and drug terms published by the World Health Organization. Retrieved from http:// www.who.int/substance_abuse/terminology/who_lexicon/en/.

World Hepatitis Alliance. (n.d.). Prevention, diagnosis, treatment of hepatitis B and C. http://www.worldhepatitisalliance.org/en/viral-hepatitis/prevention-diagnosis-treatment-hepatitis-b-and-c.

Youdim, A. (2013). Nutrient-drug interactions. Retrieved from https://www.merckmanuals.com/professional/nutritional-disorders/ nutrition,-c-,-general-considerations/nutrient-drug-interactions.

GLOSSARY

absorption Movement of a drug into the bloodstream after administration

acetylcholine (ACh) The neurotransmitter located at the ganglions and the parasympathetic terminal nerve endings

acetylcholinesterase (AChE) inhibitor An enzyme responsible for breaking down acetylcholine; also known as *cholinesterase*

acne vulgaris The formation of papules, nodules, and cysts on the face, neck, shoulders, and back that results not from dirt but from keratin plugs at the base of the pilosebaceous (oil) glands near the hair follicles

acquired immunodeficiency syndrome (AIDS) The most advanced stage of human immunodeficiency virus (HIV) infection

acquired resistance Resistance caused by prior exposure to an antibacterial

acromegaly Excessive growth after puberty

activated partial thromboplastin time (aPTT) A medical test that characterizes blood coagulation

active acquired artificial immunity Immunity that occurs when a weakened antigen or immunoglobulin (Ig) is injected into an individual as a vaccination, which then stimulates an immune response

active immunity Immunity that occurs when the body's immune response is stimulated by an antigen or when a pathogen enters the body

active transport A process that requires a carrier, such as an enzyme or protein, to move a drug against a concentration gradient

acute cystitis A lower urinary tract infection (UTI)

acute dystonia Characteristics of this reaction include muscle spasms of the face, tongue, neck, and back; facial grimacing; abnormal or involuntary upward eye movement; and laryngeal spasms that can impair respiration

acute myocardial infarction (AMI) Acute heart attack

acute pharyngitis Inflammation of the throat or "sore throat" caused by a virus, beta-hemolytic streptococci, or other bacteria

acute rhinitis Acute inflammation of the mucous membranes of the nose that usually accompanies the common cold

adequate intake (AI) The consumption and absorption of sufficient food, vitamins, and essential minerals necessary to maintain health

addiction A psychological and physical dependence upon a substance beyond normal voluntary control, usually after prolonged use

Addison disease A decrease in steroid secretion

additive effect When two drugs are administered in combination and the response is increased beyond what either could produce alone

adenohypophysis The anterior pituitary gland

adherence The extent to which a patient continues an agreed-on mode of treatment without close supervision

adjuvant A substance added to a vaccine to increase the body's immune response to the vaccine

adjuvant analgesic A generic term for a medication that is not designed to manage pain

adrenal glands Consist of the adrenal medulla and adrenal cortex

adrenergic agonists A class of G-protein–coupled receptors that are targets of the catecholamines

adrenergic antagonists (adrenergic blockers) Drugs that block either the alpha or the beta receptor

adrenergic neuron antagonists (adrenergic neuron blockers) Drugs that block the release of norepinephrine from the sympathetic terminal neurons

adrenergic receptor Target of the catecholamines

adrenocorticotropic hormone (ACTH) Stimulates the release of glucocorticoids, mineralocorticoids, and androgen from the adrenal cortex and epinephrine and norepinephrine from the adrenal medulla

adsorbents Act by coating the wall of the gastrointestinal tract and adsorbing bacteria or toxins that cause diarrhea

adverse drug event (ADE) Any injury that occurs at the time a drug is used, regardless of whether it is identified as a cause of the injury

adverse drug reaction (ADR) unintentional, unexpected reactions to drug therapy that occur at normal drug dosages

afterload Peripheral vascular resistance

aggregation Clumping together of platelets to form a clot

agonists Drugs that activate receptors and produce a desired response

akathisia A reaction in which the patient has trouble standing still, is restless, paces the floor, and is in constant motion

alcohol toxicity A life-threatening condition that can occur by drinking large amounts of alcohol over a short period of time

alkylating drugs Drugs that damage cellular DNA by cross-linkage of DNA strands, abnormal base pairing, or DNA strand breaks, thus preventing the reproduction of cancer cells

allergic rhinitis Caused by pollen or a foreign substance such as animal dander

alpha antagonists (alpha blockers) Drugs that promote vasodilation, causing a decrease in blood pressure

alternative health therapies The phenomenon of the dominant cultural group borrowing traditional health practices from less dominant groups

alveoli Air sacs

Alzheimer disease A chronic, progressive, neurodegenerative condition with marked cognitive dysfunction

amenorrhea Absence of menstrual periods

American Nurses Association Code of Ethics Developed as a guide for carrying out nursing responsibilities in a manner consistent with quality in nursing care and the ethical obligations of the profession

amphetamines Drugs that stimulate the cerebral cortex of the brain

anabolism Buildup of cellular tissue

analeptic Acts on the brainstem and medulla to stimulate respiration

analgesic A drug prescribed for the relief of pain

anaphylactic shock An allergic response of the most serious type, brought about by an antibody-antigen reaction

anaphylaxis A serious, life-threatening allergic reaction to a specific vaccine or vaccine component

androgen A male sex hormone

anesthetic A drug that causes anesthesia

angina pectoris Acute cardiac pain caused by inadequate blood flow to the myocardium due to either plaque occlusions within or spasms of the coronary arteries

angle-closure glaucoma A condition in which the iris is situated close to the drainage angle, thus blocking the trabecular network

anion A negative charge in ions

anorexiants Drugs thought to suppress appetite by stimulating the satiety center in the hypothalamic and limbic areas of the brain

anovulation Lack of ovulation

anovulatory The absence of ovulation

anoxia Absence of oxygen

antacids Promote ulcer healing by neutralizing hydrochloric acid and reducing pepsin activity

antagonistic effects The negative effect that one chemical or family of chemicals has on other chemicals

antagonists Drugs that prevent receptor activation and block a response

anthelmintics Agents that destroy worms

anthracycline A class of chemotherapeutic agents

antiandrogens Androgen antagonists that block the synthesis or action of androgens

antianginal drugs Medicines that relieve the symptoms of angina pectoris

antibacterials Substances that inhibit bacterial growth or kill bacteria and other microorganisms

antibiotic resistance Biologically occurring short chains of amino acid monomers linked by peptide (amide) bonds

antibodies Defend the body against pathogens

anticoagulants Prevent the formation of clots that inhibit circulation

antidepressants Drugs that treat depression and/or relieve the symptoms

antidiarrheals Agents used for treating diarrhea and decreasing hypermotility

antidiuretic hormone (ADH) A hormone made by the hypothalamus in the brain and stored in the posterior pituitary gland

antidysrhythmics (antiarrhythmics) Drugs that restore the cardiac rhythm to normal

antiemetics Antivomiting agents

antiflatulents Drugs that treat excessive gas in the stomach and intestines

antifungals Drugs used to treat fungal infections

antigen A toxin or other foreign substance that induces an immune response in the body, especially the production of antibodies

antihistamines Compete with histamine for receptor sites and prevent a histamine response

antihyperlipidemics Drugs used to lower lipoproteins

antihypertensives Drugs used to treat hypertension

antimalarials Drugs that provide treatment and prophylaxis for malaria

antimetabolite A chemical that inhibits the use of a metabolite

antimicrobials Substances that inhibit bacterial growth or kill bacteria and other microorganisms

antimuscarinics Agents that block parasympathetic nerve impulses

antimycotic drugs Drugs used to treat fungal infections

antineoplastic drug An agent with antineoplastic properties

antioncogenes Genes that protect other genes

antiplatelets Used to prevent thrombosis in the arteries by suppressing platelet aggregation

antipsychotics Also known as *neuroleptics* or *psychotropics,* but the preferred name for this group is either *antipsychotics* or *neuroleptics*

antiretroviral therapy (ART) The combination of several antiretroviral medicines used to slow the rate at which human immunodeficiency virus (HIV) makes copies of itself in the body

antiseizure drugs Drugs used for epileptic seizures

antispasmodics Agents that block parasympathetic nerve impulses

antitumor antibiotics Instead of treating infection, these agents interfere with DNA replication and RNA transcription of cancer cells

antitussives Agents that act on the cough-control center in the medulla to suppress the cough reflex

antiviral drugs Agents used to prevent or delay the spread of viral infections

anxiolytics Also called *antianxiety drugs* or *sedative-hypnotics*

apolipoprotein A protein that combines with a lipid, such as cholesterol or triglyceride, to form a lipoprotein

apoptosis Cell death

aqueous humor A clear fluid that flows continuously in and out of the chamber of the eye

assessment The phase during which a nurse gathers information from the patient about the patient's health and lifestyle

assimilation Occurs within and among cultural groups, such as when a minority group changes its ways to blend in with the dominant cultural group

asthma An inflammatory disorder of the airway walls associated with a varying amount of airway obstruction

asystole The cardiac rhythm caused by cessation of electrical activity within the heart because the heart is no longer beating

atonic seizure Loss of normal muscle tension; a seizure in which muscles suddenly lose strength

atrial fibrillation Cardiac dysrhythmia with rapid uncoordinated contractions of atrial myocardium

atrial flutter Cardiac dysrhythmia with rapid contractions of 200 to 300 beats/min

attention-deficit/hyperactivity disorder (ADHD) A disorder that might be caused by a dysregulation of the transmitter's serotonin, norepinephrine, and dopamine

attenuated viruses Viruses composed of live, attenuated microorganisms

atypical antidepressants Drugs used for major depression, reactive depression, and anxiety that affect one or two of the three neurotransmitters: serotonin, norepinephrine, and dopamine

atypical antipsychotics The second category of antipsychotics

autonomy The right to self-determination

bactericidal Bacteria killing

bacteriostatic Inhibits bacterial growth; may also be bactericidal (bacteria killing), depending on the drug dose, serum level, and pathogen

balanced anesthesia A combination of drugs frequently used in general anesthesia

barbiturates Long-, intermediate-, short-, and ultrashort-acting sedatives

Beers Criteria for Potentially Inappropriate Medication Use in Older Adults A document developed by a consensus panel of 12 experts in geriatric care to aid health care providers in the safe prescription and administration of drugs to older adults

beneficence The duty to protect research subjects from harm and to assess potential risks and possible benefits to ensure the benefits are greater than the risk

beta antagonists (beta blockers) May inhibit the action of albuterol

bioavailability The percentage of administered drug available for activity

biologic response modifiers (BRMs) A class of pharmacologic drugs used to enhance, direct, or restore the body's immune system

biotransformation The process by which the body chemically changes drugs into a form that can be excreted

bipolar disorder A disorder that involves swings between two moods, the manic and the depressive

Bishop score An objective measurement that assists in predicting whether labor induction may be successful

blackhead A type of noninflammatory acne lesion that is open

blepharitis Infection of the margins of the eyelid

blood-borne pathogens Microorganisms such as viruses or bacteria that are carried in blood and can cause disease in people

blood-brain barrier (BBB) A special endothelial lining in blood vessels in the brain where the cells are pressed tightly together (tight junctions)

blood dyscrasias Blood-cell disorders

bolus The first method used to deliver enteral feedings, by which 250 to 400 mL of solution is rapidly administered through a syringe into the tube four to six times a day

botanicals Additive substances that come from plants

bradycardia A pulse rate below 60 beats/min

bradykinesia Slow movement

brand (trade) name Also known as the *proprietary name,* the name chosen by the drug company; usually a registered trademark

breakthrough bleeding An abnormal flow of blood from the uterus that occurs between menstrual periods

broad-spectrum antibiotics Drugs that can be effective against both gram-positive and gram-negative organisms

bronchial asthma Characterized by bronchospasm, wheezing, mucus secretions, and dyspnea; one of the lung diseases of chronic obstructive pulmonary disease (COPD)

bronchiectasis Abnormal dilation of the bronchi and bronchioles secondary to frequent infection and inflammation

bronchodilators Drugs that relax bronchial muscle and result in expansion of the bronchial air passages

bronchospasm Results when lung tissue is exposed to extrinsic or intrinsic factors that stimulate a bronchoconstrictive response

buccal Administered between the cheek and gum

cadaveric transplantation A healthy organ donated at the time of a person's death that is transplanted into the body of a patient with end-stage organ failure

calcium channel blockers (CCBs) Agents used for the treatment of stable and variant angina pectoris, certain dysrhythmias, and hypertension

cannabinoids The active ingredients in *Cannabis,* approved for clinical use in 1985 to alleviate nausea and vomiting resulting from cancer treatment

capillary leak syndrome A rare disorder characterized by episodes of severe hypotension, hypoalbuminemia, and hemoconcentration

carbonic anhydrase inhibitors (CAIs) Agents that decrease intraocular pressure by decreasing the production of aqueous humor

cardiac dysrhythmia (arrhythmia) Any deviation from the normal rate or pattern of the heartbeat

cardiac glycosides Drugs that inhibit the sodium-potassium pump, which results in an increase in intracellular sodium

catecholamines Chemical structures of a substance, either endogenous or synthetic, that can produce a sympathomimetic response

cathartics Agents used to eliminate fecal matter

cation A positive charge in ions

caudal block An epidural block placed by administering a local anesthetic through the sacral hiatus

cell cycle–nonspecific (CCNS) drugs Drugs that act during any phase of the cell cycle

cell cycle–specific (CCS) drugs Drugs that exert their influence during a specific phase of the cell cycle and are most effective against rapidly growing cancer cells

cellular checkpoints, cellular communication Mechanism by which cell-to-cell communication occurs locally or remotely by signaling molecules to maintain homeostasis, regulate growth and division, develop and organize into tissues, and coordinate cellular functions

central nervous system (CNS) A system that involves the brain and spinal cord and that regulates body functions

cerumen Earwax

ceruminolytics Topical otic agents that soften or break up cerumen so that it can be removed

cervical ripening Softening of the cervix

chalazion Infection of the meibomian glands of the eyelids that may produce cysts, causing blockage of the ducts

chemical name A name that describes the drug's chemical structure

chemoprotectant An agent administered prior to anthracyclines to prevent cardiotoxicity

chemoreceptor trigger zone (CTZ) A major cerebral center that lies near the medulla

chloasma Hyperpigmentation of the skin

cholinergic agonists Drugs that stimulate the parasympathetic nervous system

cholinergic antagonists (blocking agents) Drugs that affect the parasympathetic nervous system

cholinergic crisis Overdosing with acetylcholinesterase (AChE) inhibitors; may complicate myasthenia gravis

cholinergics Medications that produce the same effects as the parasympathetic nervous system

cholinesterase (ChE) May destroy acetylcholine before it reaches the receptor or after it has attached to the site

cholinesterase inhibitors Indirect-acting cholinergics that inactivate the enzyme cholinesterase, which typically breaks down acetylcholine

chronic bronchitis A progressive lung disease caused by smoking or chronic lung infections

chronic obstructive pulmonary disease (COPD) A major category of lower respiratory tract disorders, COPD is caused by airway obstruction with increased airway resistance of airflow to lung tissues

chronotropic An action that decreases heart rate

chylomicrons Large particles that transport fatty acids and cholesterol to the liver

clonic seizure A convulsive seizure

cluster headache Headache characterized by a severe, unilateral, nonthrobbing pain usually located around the eye

colloid A solution that contains protein or other large molecular substances that increase osmolarity without dissolving in the solution

colony-stimulating factors Proteins that stimulate or regulate the growth, maturation, and differentiation of bone marrow stem cells

combination chemotherapy The use of two or more chemotherapy agents to treat cancer

comedones Noninflammatory acne lesions that may be open or closed

common cold The most prevalent type of upper respiratory infection

complementary health therapies Combine traditional and conventional Western health practices

congenital rubella syndrome Transmission of the rubella virus to the fetus via the placenta

congestive heart failure (CHF) Occurs when the heart muscle does not pump blood as well as it should

conjugate vaccines Newer vaccines that require a protein or toxoid from an unrelated organism to link to the outer coating of the disease-causing microorganism

conjunctivitis Inflammation of the membrane covering the eye and inner eyelids

constipation The accumulation of hard fecal material in the large intestine

contact dermatitis A common form of eczema that results when skin is exposed to irritants or allergens

continuous feedings Feedings prescribed for the critically ill and for those who receive feedings into the small intestine

controlled substance A drug or chemical whose manufacture, possession, or use is regulated by government

corticosteroids Any of the steroid hormones made by the outer portion (cortex) of the adrenal gland

cretinism A congenital abnormality caused by severe hypothyroidism and marked by physical stunting and mental retardation

Critical Path Initiative A national strategy "to drive innovation in the scientific processes through which medical products are developed, evaluated, and manufactured"

cross-resistance Tolerance, usually to a toxic substance, that is acquired not as a result of direct exposure but by exposure to a related substance

cross-sensitivity Sensitivity to one substance that predisposes an individual to sensitivity to other substances that are related in chemical structure

cryotherapy A procedure used to destroy tissue of both benign and malignant lesions by the freezing and rethawing process

cryptorchidism Undescended testis

cryptosporidiosis Infection caused by the protozoan parasite *Cryptosporidium*, usually in the bowel mucosa

crystalloid A solution containing fluids and electrolytes that can freely cross capillary walls

crystalluria Crystals in the urine

culturally sensitive Refers to the nurse being alert to the patient's cultural expectations

culture Learned beliefs and behaviors shared by a group of people

Cushing syndrome An increase in steroid secretion

cyclic method A type of continuous feeding infused over 8 to 16 hours daily (day or night)

cyclins A family of proteins that stimulate the cell to move through the cell cycle

cyclooxygenase (COX) The enzyme responsible for converting arachidonic acid into prostaglandins and their products

cyclooxygenase 2 (COX-2) inhibitors Newer nonsteroidal antiinflammatory drugs that block only COX-2 and not COX-1

cycloplegics Drugs that paralyze the muscles of accommodation

cytokine release syndrome A symptom complex associated with the use of anti-T–cell antibody infusions

cytomegalovirus (CMV) Infection caused by a virus that infects the entire body

cytotoxic therapy A treatment that uses drugs to destroy cancer cells

Current Good Manufacturing Practices (CGMPs) U.S. Food and Drug Administration standards requiring that package labels give the quality and strength of all contents and that products be free of contaminants and impurities

decongestants Drugs that stimulate the alpha-adrenergic receptors, producing vascular constriction (vasoconstriction) of the capillaries within the nasal mucosa

delayed puberty Defined clinically by the absence or incomplete development of secondary sexual characteristics bounded by an age at which 95% of children of that sex and culture have begun sexual maturation

dependence A condition in which larger and larger doses of a drug are needed to reproduce the initial response

dependent variable A mathematical variable whose value is determined by that of one or more other variables in a function (outcome, such as clinical effect)

depolarization Myocardial contraction

depression A mood disorder that causes a persistent feeling of sadness and loss of interest

dermatome Where the virus had lain dormant

diabetes insipidus (DI) A rare condition in which the kidneys are not able to conserve water

diabetes mellitus A chronic disease that results from deficient glucose metabolism caused by insufficient insulin secretion from the beta cells

diarrhea Frequent liquid stool

Dietary Supplement Health and Education Act (DSHEA) A U.S. federal act that defined dietary supplements

diffusion Movement across the cell membrane from an area of higher concentration to one of lower concentration

direct-acting cholinergic agonists Drugs that act on receptors to activate a tissue response

disease-modifying antirheumatic drugs (DMARDs) Drugs that help alleviate the symptoms of rheumatic arthritis

distribution Movement from the circulation into body tissues

diuresis Increased urine flow

diuretics Agents used to decrease hypertension and edema

dopamine A neurotransmitter that helps control the brain's reward and pleasure centers

dopamine agonists Drugs that stimulate dopamine receptors

dose-response relationship The body's physiologic response to changes in drug concentration at the site of action

doubling time A factor that plays a major role in how cancer cells respond to anticancer drugs

dromotropic An action that decreases conduction of heart cells

drug diversion The deliberate redirecting of a drug from a patient or facility to the employee for personal use

drug interaction An altered or modified action or effect of a drug as a result of interaction with one or multiple drugs

drug reconciliation The process of identifying the most accurate list of all medications a patient is taking at transitions in care

drug toxicity A condition that occurs when drug levels exceed the therapeutic range

drusen Deposits of extracellular material under the retina

duodenal ulcer Caused by hypersecretion of acid from the stomach passing into the duodenum because of (1) insufficient buffers to neutralize gastric acid in the stomach, (2) a defective or incompetent pyloric sphincter, or (3) hypermotility of the stomach

duration of action The length of time over which a drug exerts its therapeutic effect

dysfunctional uterine bleeding Abnormal uterine bleeding in the absence of organic disease

dyskinesia Impaired voluntary movement

dysmenorrhea Painful periods

dyspareunia Painful sexual intercourse

dysphoria Deep depression

dysrhythmias Irregular heartbeats

dystonia Prolonged muscle contractions with twisting, repetitive movements

dystonic movement Involuntary abnormal movement

e-cigarettes Electronic cigarettes that aerosolize "e-juice," a mixture of flavorings, propylene glycol (a toxic component of antifreeze), glycerin, and nicotine

eclampsia New-onset grand mal seizures in a patient with preeclampsia

ejaculatory dysfunction Impaired ejection of seminal fluid from the male urethra

electroencephalogram (EEG) An electrophysiologic monitoring method to record electrical activity of the brain

electrolytes Substances that separate or dissociate into ions (charged particles) in solution

emetics Drugs used to induce vomiting

emollients Lubricants and stool softeners used to prevent constipation

emphysema A progressive lung disease caused by cigarette smoking, atmospheric contaminants, or lack of the alpha$_1$-antitrypsin protein that inhibits proteolytic enzymes that destroy alveoli

endometriosis The abnormal location of endometrial tissue outside the uterus

endophthalmitis Infection and inflammation of structures of the inner eye

endorphins Neurohormones

enteral nutrition (EN) Delivery of nutrition or fluid via a tube into the gastrointestinal (GI) tract, which requires a functional, accessible GI tract

epidural block Placement of local anesthetic in the epidural space just posterior to the spinal cord or the dura mater

epigenetics The study of environmental influences on genetics

episiotomy An incision made to enlarge the vaginal opening to facilitate childbirth

erectile dysfunction The inability to achieve or maintain an erection satisfactory for sexual performance

ergot alkaloids One of a large group of alkaloids derived from fungi; acts by direct smooth muscle cell–receptor stimulation

ergotism Signs of ergot toxicity

erythema multiforme An erythematous macular, papular, or vesicular eruption that can cover the entire body

erythrocytic phase Invasion of the red blood cells

erythropoietin (EPO) A glycoprotein produced by the kidney; it stimulates red blood cell production in the bone marrow

erythropoietin-stimulating agents (ESAs) Includes epoetin alfa and darbepoetin alfa

esophageal ulcer Results from reflux of acidic gastric secretions into the esophagus as a result of a defective or incompetent cardiac sphincter

essential hypertension The most common type of hypertension, affecting 90% of persons with high blood pressure

estimated average requirement (EAR) The daily intake of a specific nutrient estimated to meet the requirement in 50% of healthy people in an age- and sex-specific group

ethinyl estradiol The most commonly used synthetic estrogen found in CHC products

ethnomedicine Sometimes referred to as *folk medicine* or *traditional medicine,* a focus within medical anthropology that examines the ways in which people from different cultures conceptualize health and illness

ethnopharmacology A subdivision of ethnomedicine that focuses on the use of herbs, powders, teas, and animal products as healing remedies

evaluation The phase of the nursing process during which the nurse determines whether the goals and teaching objectives are being met

excipients Fillers and inert substances such as simple syrup, vegetable gums, aromatic powder, honey, and various elixirs

excretion Elimination of drugs from the body

exfoliative dermatitis Characterized by desquamation, scaling, and itching of the skin

expectorants Agents that loosen bronchial secretions so they can be eliminated by coughing

extrapyramidal syndrome Any of a group of clinical disorders marked by abnormal involuntary movements, alterations in muscle tone, and postural disturbances

extravasation Escape into tissues

facilitated diffusion Relies on a carrier protein to move drug from an area of higher concentration to an area of lower concentration

family-centered care Essential to ensuring safety during and after health care interventions, especially drug administration

fasciculations Involuntary muscle twitching

fat-soluble vitamins Vitamins stored in fatty tissue, liver, and muscle in significant amounts that are metabolized slowly and excreted in the urine at a slow rate; includes vitamins A, D, E, and K

fibrinolysis Fibrin breakdown

first-line drugs Those drugs chosen first for therapy

first-pass effect When drugs are metabolized in the liver to an inactive form and are excreted, thus reducing the amount of active drug available to exert a pharmacologic effect

flatus Intestinal gas

folliculitis Skin inflammation resulting from contact with an irritating substance or allergen

fraction of inspired oxygen (FiO$_2$) The fraction or percentage of oxygen in the space being measured

free drugs Drugs able to exit blood vessels and reach their site of action to cause a pharmacologic response

gastric mucosal barrier (GMB) A thick, viscous, mucous material that provides a barrier between the mucosal lining and acidic gastric secretions

gastric ulcer Frequently occurs because of a breakdown of the gastric mucosal barrier (GMB)

gastroesophageal reflux disease (GERD) Inflammation or erosion of the esophageal mucosa caused by a reflux of gastric acid content from the stomach into the esophagus

gastrostomy tube A gastrointestinal tube used for enteral tube feedings

generic name The official, nonproprietary name for a drug; the name not owned by any drug company and universally accepted as the official drug name

genomes A complete set of chromosomes that make up a cell's DNA

genotoxicity The ability of a compound to damage genetic information in a cell

gestational hypertension Elevated blood pressure without proteinuria after 20 gestational weeks in patients normotensive before pregnancy

gigantism Excessive growth during childhood

gingival hyperplasia Overgrowth of gums or reddened gums that bleed easily

glaucoma A group of eye conditions that damage the optic nerve

glucocorticoids Drugs of the corticosteroid family used to treat respiratory disorders, particularly asthma

Good Clinical Practice (GCP) Consolidated Guideline An international ethical and scientific quality standard for designing, conducting, monitoring, auditing, recording, analyzing, and reporting clinical research

gout An inflammatory condition that attacks joints, tendons, and other tissues

gram The basic unit of measure used in dosage calculations for weight (g, gm, G, Gm)

granulocyte A type of white blood cell with small granules that contain proteins

granulocyte colony–stimulating factor (G-CSF) A glycoprotein that stimulates the bone marrow to produce granulocytes and stem cells and release them into the bloodstream

granulocyte-macrophage colony–stimulating factor (GM-CSF) One of a group of growth factors that support survival, proliferation, and differentiation (maturation) of hematopoietic progenitor cells; induces partially committed progenitor (parent) cells to divide and differentiate in the granulocyte-macrophage pathway

Graves disease The most common type of hyperthyroidism caused by hyperfunction of the thyroid gland

growth fraction A factor that plays a major role in how cancer cells respond to anticancer drugs

gynecomastia Mammary gland enlargement in men

half-life The time it takes for the amount of drug in the body to be reduced by half

hangover Residual drowsiness

healers Individuals who play a role in health practices worldwide; may include priests, shamans, bone setters, herbalists, curanderos, and midwives

health care–acquired infections Infections acquired while patients are hospitalized

heart block A delay in the normal flow of electrical impulses that cause the heart to beat

heart failure A condition that occurs when the heart muscle (myocardium) weakens and enlarges and loses its ability to pump blood through the heart and into the systemic circulation

HELLP syndrome Hemolysis, elevated liver enzymes, and low platelet count

helminthiasis Worm infection

helminths Large parasitic worms that live and lay eggs in warm, moist soil where sanitation and hygiene are poor

hepatotoxicity Liver toxicity

herb Any plant used for culinary or medicinal purposes

herd immunity Occurs when most of the community is immunized against contagious diseases, thus allowing protection of those not immunized

high-density lipoprotein (HDL) One of the five major groups of lipoproteins

high-sensitivity C-reactive protein (hsCRP) A test used to evaluate the risk of developing coronary artery disease

hirsutism Increased hair growth

histamine 2 (H$_2$) receptor antagonists Agents used to treat duodenal ulcers and prevent their return

homocysteine A naturally occurring amino acid found in blood plasma

hordeolum A local infection of eyelash follicles and glands on lid margins, also known as a *stye*

hormone therapy A therapy that significantly improves vasomotor symptoms and vaginal dryness, two frequently encountered symptoms of menopause; also decreases the risk for osteoporosis and osteoporotic fractures

household measurement A measuring system that uses inches and pounds

hybridoma technology A process that makes monoclonal antibodies genetically

hydantoins Inhibit sodium influx, stabilize cell membranes, reduce repetitive neuronal firing, and limit seizures

hydrochloric acid A strongly acidic solution of the gas hydrogen chloride in water

hyperalimentation A form of malnutrition in which the intake of nutrients is oversupplied

hypercalcemia A calcium excess (>10.2 mEq/L)

hypercapnia Increased carbon dioxide in the blood

hyperchloremia An elevated serum chloride level

hyperemesis gravidarum Severe nausea and vomiting that may require hospitalization for hydration and nutrition

hyperglycemia Elevated blood glucose

hyperkalemia A serum potassium level above 5.0 mEq/L

hyperlipidemia A condition that occurs when there is an excess of one or more lipids in the blood

hypermagnesemia A magnesium excess

hypernatremia A serum sodium level above 145 mEq/L

hyperosmolar A fluid that contains more particles than water

hyperoxia Excessive oxygenation

hyperphosphatemia An excess of phosphorus

hypertension Blood pressure greater than 140/90 mm Hg

hypertensive crisis When systolic blood pressure exceeds 180 to 200 mm Hg

hyperthyroidism An increase in circulating T$_3$ and T$_4$ levels, which usually results from an overactive thyroid gland or excessive output of thyroid hormones from one or more thyroid nodules

hypertonic Describes solutions that exert greater osmotic pressure than extracellular fluid (ECF), resulting in a higher solute concentration than the serum

hypertrichosis Darkening of hair

hypnotic effect Not hypnosis but a form of "natural" sleep

hypocalcemia A calcium deficit (<8.6 mEq/L)

hypocarbia Decreased carbon dioxide (CO$_2$)

hypochloremia A decreased serum chloride level

hypoglycemic reaction Occurs when more insulin is administered than is needed for glucose metabolism

hypogonadism The clearest indication for exogenous androgen therapy

hypokalemia Potassium deficit; occurs with serum levels below 3.5 mEq/L

hypomagnesemia Magnesium deficit

hyponatremia A serum sodium level below 135 mEq/L

hypoosmolar Describes fluid that contains fewer particles than water

hypophosphatemia Deficiency of phosphorus

hypophysis The pituitary gland

hypothyroidism A decrease in thyroid hormone secretion

hypotonic Describes solutions that exert less osmotic pressure than extracellular fluid (ECF), which allows water to move into the cell

hypovolemic shock A life-threatening condition that results when you lose more than 20% (one fifth) of your body's blood or fluid supply

hypoxemia Inadequate oxygen in the blood

hypoxia Lack of oxygen to body tissues

idiopathic Of unknown cause

immune globulin The general term used for replacement therapy

immune reconstitution inflammatory syndrome (IRIS) A syndrome related to a disease- or pathogen-specific inflammatory response in patients with antiretroviral therapy being initiated or changed

immune response The reaction of the cells and fluids of the body to the presence of a substance that is not recognized as a constituent of the body itself

immunoglobulins Antibody proteins such as immunoglobulins G and M

immunomodulation The immune system's ability to kill abnormal cells

immunomodulators Agents used to treat moderate to severe rheumatoid arthritis by disrupting the inflammatory process and delaying disease progression

immunosuppression The use of multiple drugs to alter different aspects of the immune system

immunosuppressives Agents used to treat refractory rheumatoid arthritis that does not respond to antiinflammatory drugs

implementation The part of the nursing process in which the nurse provides education, drug administration, patient care, and other interventions necessary to assist the patient in accomplishing the established goals

independent variable A variable that is independent of the other variables in an expression or function and whose value determines one or more of the values of the other variables (e.g., treatment, such as with a drug)

indirect-acting cholinergic agonists Agents that inhibit the action of the enzyme cholinesterase (ChE)

induction therapy Treatment that provides intense immunosuppression with drugs designed to diminish antigen presentation and T-cell response

infection Caused by microorganisms, which results in inflammation

infertility The inability to conceive a child after 12 months of unprotected sexual intercourse

inflammation A response to tissue injury and infection

informed consent Consent to medical treatment or participation in medical experiments after achieving an understanding of what is involved and being apprised of the risks

inhalation Administration of medication via the nasal route

inherent resistance Bacterial resistance can result naturally

inhibited sexual desire Decreased or lacking interest in sexual activity

inotropic Action that increases myocardial contraction stroke volume

insomnia The inability to fall asleep or remain asleep

instillations   Liquid medications usually administered as drops, ointments, or sprays

insulin   A protein secreted from the beta cells of the pancreas that is necessary for carbohydrate metabolism and that plays an important role in protein and fat metabolism

insulin shock   Occurs when more insulin is administered than is needed for glucose metabolism

interferon alfa   An interferon produced by white blood cells that inhibits viral replication, suppresses cell proliferation, and regulates immune response

interferon beta (IFN-β)   A type I interferon produced by fibroblasts, macrophages, and epithelial cells

interferon gamma (IFN-γ)   A type II interferon produced endogenously by activating T lymphocytes and natural killer cells (NKCs), and produced genetically from *Escherichia coli*

interferons (IFNs)   A family of proteins that occur naturally in the body and can be produced in the laboratory

interleukins   A group of signaling-molecule proteins produced by leukocytes, specifically by T lymphocytes

intermittent enteral feedings   Feedings administered every 3 to 6 hours over 30 to 60 minutes by gravity drip or infusion pump

intermittent infusion   Considered an inexpensive method for administering enteral nutrition (EN)

international normalized ratio (INR)   The laboratory test most frequently used to report prothrombin time (PT) results

intradermal   Administered for skin testing

intramuscular (IM)   An administration route used for solutions that are more viscous and irritating for adults, children, and infants

intraocular pressure (IOP)   The pressure within the eyeball that gives it a round, firm shape

intraosseous   Method of drug administration that involves the infusion of medication directly into the bone marrow

intravenous   More rapid injection method than intramuscular or subcutaneous routes

iron   Vital for hemoglobin regeneration

ischemia   Deficient blood flow

isoosmolar   Fluid that has the same weight proportion of particles (e.g., sodium, glucose) and water

isotonic   Describes solutions that have the same approximate osmolality as extracellular fluid (ECF) or plasma

jejunostomy tube   A gastrointestinal route used for enteral tube feedings

Just Culture   An approach that supports encouraging individuals to report drug errors so the system can be repaired and the problem can be fixed

justice   Requires that the selection of research subjects be fair

Kaposi sarcoma   A cancer that causes patches of abnormal tissue to grow under the skin; in the lining of the mouth, nose, and throat; in lymph nodes; and in other organs

keratin   A protein that is part of the skin; may form a plug that results in acne

keratitis   Corneal infection and inflammation

keratolysis   Periodic shedding of the epidermis

ketoacidosis   Diabetic acidosis or diabetic coma

labor augmentation   Stimulation of effective uterine contractions once labor has begun

labor induction   The process of causing or initiating labor

lacrimal duct   Tear ducts

lactation   Production and release of milk by the mammary glands

latency   The establishment and maintenance of latent infection in nerve cell ganglia proximal to the site of infection

latent stage   A period of time after an infection during which symptoms are absent

latent tuberculosis infection   A state of persistent immune response to stimulation by *Mycobacterium tuberculosis* antigens without evidence of clinically manifested active tuberculosis

laxatives   Agents that promote a soft stool; cathartics result in a soft to watery stool with some cramping

lecithin/sphingomyelin (L/S) ratio   Measured in the amniotic fluid, predicts fetal lung maturity and risk for neonatal respiratory distress syndrome (RDS)

ligand-binding domain   The site on the receptor to which drugs bind

lipodystrophy   A disorder of adipose (fatty) tissue characterized by a selective loss of body fat

lipoprotein   Special particles made up of droplets of fats surrounded by a single layer of phospholipid molecules

liposomes   A tiny bubble (vesicle) made out of the same material as a cell membrane

liter   The basic unit of measure for volume used in dosage calculations (L)

living-donor transplantation   An operation in which a kidney or a portion of liver donated by a living person is transplanted into the body of a patient with end-stage kidney or liver disease

loading dose   Administration of a large initial dose

low-density lipoprotein (LDL)   A molecule that is a combination of lipid (fat) and protein; transports cholesterol from the liver to the tissues of the body

lymphokines   Cytokines produced by T cells (lymphocytes) of the immune system

macrophages   Mature monocytes

macules   Flat and nonpalpable, usually less than 10 mm in diameter with varying colors

maximal efficacy   The point at which increasing a drug's dosage no longer increases the desired therapeutic response

menarche   The start of spontaneous menstruation

menopause   The transitional process experienced by women as they move from the reproductive years into the nonreproductive stage of life

menorrhagia   Heavy periods

mestranol   An older form of estrogen found in higher-dose (≥50 mcg) oral combination products

metabolism   The process by which the body chemically changes drugs into a form that can be excreted

metastasis   The spread of the disease to other areas of the body

metastasizing   Spreading to other parts of the body

meter   Basic unit of measure used in dosage calculations for linear measurement (m, M)

metered-dose inhalers (MDIs)   Handheld devices used to deliver a number of commonly prescribed asthma and bronchitis drugs to the lower respiratory tract

metric system   A decimal system based on the power of 10

metrorrhagia   Irregular bleeding between periods, usually heavy

microorganisms   Microscopic organisms that include viruses, fungi, protozoa, and rickettsiae

micturition   Urination

migraine headaches   Characterized by a unilateral throbbing head pain accompanied by nausea, vomiting, and photophobia

mineralocorticoids   A group of hormones, the most important being aldosterone, that regulate the balance of water and electrolytes (ions such as sodium and potassium) in the body

minerals   Substances the body requires in small amounts, such as iron, copper, zinc, chromium, and selenium

miosis   A constriction of the pupil and contraction of the ciliary muscle

mitosis   The process by which the nucleus divides in eukaryotic organisms, producing two new nuclei that are genetically identical to the nucleus of the parent cell

mittelschmerz   Midcycle menstrual pain usually associated with ovulation

Monitoring the Future project   A project that tracks drug use in adolescents and young adults

monoamine oxidase inhibitors (MAOIs)   Agents that inactivate norepinephrine, dopamine, epinephrine, and serotonin

monoclonal antibodies   Antibodies produced by a single clone of cells or a cell line and consisting of identical antibody molecules

mTOR kinase inhibitors   A class of drugs that inhibit the mechanistic target of rapamycin

mucolytics   Agents that act as detergents to liquefy and loosen thick mucous secretions so they can be expectorated

multikinase inhibitors (MKIs)   Chemicals that directly inhibit the activity of multiple kinase enzymes in cancer cells

multiple sclerosis (MS)   A neuromuscular autoimmune disorder that attacks the myelin sheath of nerve fibers, causing lesions known as *plaques*

muscarinic receptors   Receptors that stimulate smooth muscle and slow the heart rate

muscle relaxants   Agents that reduce spasticity of muscles

muscle spasms   Muscle contractions resulting from various causes, including injury or motor neuron disorders associated with conditions such as multiple sclerosis (MS), myasthenia gravis (MG), cerebral palsy, spinal cord injury, cerebrovascular accident, or hemiplegia

myasthenia gravis (MG)   An acquired autoimmune disease that impairs the transmission of messages at the neuromuscular junction, resulting in fluctuating muscle weakness that increases with muscle use

myasthenic crisis   Occurs when muscular weakness in the patient with myasthenia gravis becomes generalized

***Mycobacterium avium* complex (MAC)**   A blood infection caused by bacteria related to *M. tuberculosis,* the pathogen in tuberculosis

mydriasis   An increase in pulse rate

mydriatics   Agents that dilate the pupils

myelosuppression   A condition that occurs when a significant decrease in bone marrow activity results in decreased white blood cells, platelets, and red blood cells

myocardial infarction (MI)   Heart attack

myocardial ischemia   Lack of blood supply to the heart muscle

myxedema   Severe hypothyroidism in the adult

nadir   The low point; in nursing, used to describe the point at which the blood count is at the lowest

narcolepsy   A neurological disorder characterized by falling asleep during normal waking activities, such as while driving a car or talking with someone

narrow-spectrum antibiotics   Tolerance (as of a virus) to a usually toxic substance (as an antibiotic) that is acquired, not as a result of direct exposure, but by exposure to a related substance.

nasoduodenal/nasojejunal   Gastrointestinal routes used for enteral tube feedings

nasointestinal tube   A tube passed through the nose and down through the nasopharynx and esophagus into the intestine

natriuresis   Sodium loss in the urine

natriuretic   An agent with a sodium-losing effect

natural acquired active immunity   Immunity that occurs from exposure to a pathogen or disease

necrosis   Tissue death caused by disease or injury

neoadjuvant chemotherapy   Treatment performed before surgical extraction of a tumor with the objective of reducing the tumor's size

nephrotoxicity   Toxicity to the kidney

nerve block   A pain management technique involving the injection of an anesthetic into the area surrounding an affected nerve

neurohypophysis   The posterior pituitary gland

neuroleptic   Refers to any drug that modifies psychotic behavior and exerts an antipsychotic effect

neuroleptic malignant syndrome (NMS)   A rare but potentially fatal condition associated with antipsychotic drugs

neuropathic pain   An unusual sensory disturbance that often involves neural supersensitivity

neurotransmitters   Substances released as a result of stimulation, such as by amphetamines

neutrophils   The most abundant white blood cells that take part in the inflammatory response system, whose main function it is to detect and destroy harmful bacteria

nicotinic receptors   Receptors that affect the skeletal muscles

nitrates   The first agents used to relieve angina

nociceptors   Sensory receptors for pain

nonopioid analgesics   Drugs that are less potent than opioid analgesics, used to treat mild to moderate pain

non–rapid eye movement (NREM) sleep   A definite stage of sleep

nonselective   A term used to describe drugs capable of affecting multiple receptors

nonspecific   A term used to describe drugs capable of affecting multiple receptor sites

nonsteroidal antiinflammatory drugs (NSAIDs)   Nonopioid analgesics taken for pain and inflammation

normoxemia   Oxygen saturation between 94% and 99%

nursing diagnosis   Diagnosis made based on analysis of the assessment data; determines the type of care the patient will receive

nystagmus   Constant, involuntary, cyclical movement of the eyeball

occlusive   Obstructive

ocular drugs   Drugs designed to be applied to the eyes

off label   Use of a drug for some purpose for which it has not been approved

oligomenorrhea   Very scant periods

oligospermia   Low sperm count

oliguria   A marked decrease in urine output

oncogene   A mutation in a proto-oncogene that affects cellular growth-control proteins and triggers unregulated cell division

onset   The time it takes for a drug to reach the minimum effective concentration (MEC) after administration

open-angle glaucoma   A condition in which the trabecular network is open but becomes clogged

ophthalmia neonatorum   An eye infection among newborns

ophthalmic drugs   Drugs designed to be applied to the eyes

opiates   Analgesic agents that decrease intestinal motility and thereby decrease peristalsis

opioid agonist-antagonists   Medications in which an opioid antagonist is added to an opioid agonist

opioid agonists   Drugs prescribed for moderate and severe pain

opioid antagonist   An agent that blocks the receptor and displaces any opioid that would normally be at the receptor

opportunistic infections   Infections that usually occur in the immunocompromised or debilitated population

oral antidiabetic drugs   Synthetic preparations that stimulate insulin release or otherwise alter the metabolic response to hyperglycemia

oral hypoglycemic drugs   Synthetic preparations that stimulate insulin release or otherwise alter the metabolic response to hyperglycemia

orthostatic hypotension   Low blood pressure that occurs when an individual assumes an upright position from a supine position

osmolality   Describes the concentration of fluids

osmolarity   Describes the concentration of a solution in terms of osmoles of solute per liter of solution

osmole   The number of solutes in a solution, expressed as a unit of measurement

osmotics   Hyperosmolar laxatives

osteopenia   Low bone mineral density

osteoporosis   Loss of bone mass that predisposes patients to fractures

otalgia   Ear pain

otitis externa (OE)   An infection of the external auditory canal that occurs when excess moisture and breaks in the epithelium allow some pathogen, usually bacterial or fungal, to invade the tissues

ototoxicity   Ear poisoning that results from exposure to drugs or chemicals that damage the inner ear or the vestibulocochlear nerve

ounces   A unit of measurement related to mass

over-the-counter (OTC)   Those drugs that have been found to be safe and appropriate for use without the direct supervision of a health care provider and are available for purchase without a prescription

pain threshold   The level of stimulus needed to create a painful sensation

pain tolerance   The amount of pain a person can endure without having it interfere with normal functioning

palliative chemotherapy   Treatment used to relieve symptoms associated with advanced disease

papules   Raised and palpable skin eruptions less than 10 mm in diameter

parasympatholytics   Drugs that affect the parasympathetic nervous system

parasympathomimetics   Drugs that mimic the parasympathetic neurotransmitter acetylcholine

parathyroid hormone (PTH)   A hormone that regulates serum calcium levels

parenteral   Administered via injection

parenteral nutrition (PN)   Administration of nutrients by a route other than the gastrointestinal tract; also called *total parenteral nutrition* (TPN)

paresthesia   A burning or prickling sensation that is usually felt in the hands, arms, legs, or feet but can also occur in other parts of the body

Parkinson disease   A chronic, progressive neurologic disorder that affects the extrapyramidal motor tract, which controls posture, balance, and locomotion

Parkinsonism   A syndrome, or a combination of similar symptoms, whose major features include rigidity, bradykinesia, gait disturbances, and tremors

paroxysmal supraventricular tachycardia (PSVT)   A sudden, uncontrolled, rapid rhythm that exceeds 150 beats/min in adults and originates above the ventricles

partial thromboplastin time (PTT)   A blood test that evaluates how long it takes for blood to clot

passive immunity   Immunity that can be natural, in which case the body produces its own antibodies, or acquired—that is, the body receives antibodies from an outside source

passive transport   Transport that occurs through two processes, diffusion and facilitated diffusion

pathogen   A disease-producing microorganism

patient-controlled analgesia (PCA) An alternative route for opioid administration for self-administered pain relief as needed

peak The point at which a drug reaches its highest concentration in the blood

peak drug level The highest plasma concentration of a drug at a specific time

pelvic inflammatory disease (PID) An infection of the upper genital tract, usually the uterine endometrium, fallopian tubes, or ovaries

pepsin A digestive enzyme activated at a pH of 2

peptic ulcer A broad term for an ulcer that occurs in the esophagus, stomach, or duodenum within the upper gastrointestinal tract

peptides Biologically occurring short chains of amino acid monomers linked by peptide (amide) bonds

percutaneous endoscopic gastrostomy (PEG) tube A tube placed surgically, endoscopically, or radiologically for the purpose of delivering nutrition; requires an intact gastrointestinal system

perinatal transmission Transmission at the time of delivery

peripheral vasodilators Drugs that dilate the distal blood vessels and lower the blood pressure

pharmacodynamics Mechanisms of action and effects of a drug on the body; includes the onset, peak, and duration of effect of a drug

pharmacogenetics The study of genetic factors that influence an individual's response to a specific drug

pharmacogenomics The study of how genetics play a role in a person's response to drugs

pharmacokinetics The process of drug movement throughout the body that is necessary to achieve drug action

phenothiazines Subdivided into three groups— aliphatic, piperazine, and piperidine—which differ mostly in their side effects

photochemotherapy A combination of ultraviolet (UV) radiation and the psoralen derivative methoxsalen; used to decrease proliferation of epidermal cells

photosensitivity A skin reaction caused by exposure to sunlight

phytomedicine A type of medicine that focuses on the therapeutic value of plants

pinocytosis A process by which cells carry a drug across their membrane by engulfing the drug particles in a vesicle

placebo A pill or substance that is given to a patient like a drug but that can be expected to have no lasting physical effect on the patient

placebo effect A drug response not attributed to the chemical properties of the drug

planning The phase during which the nurse uses collected data to set goals or expected outcomes and interventions

plaques Palpable lesions greater than 10 mm in diameter that are depressed or elevated when compared with the skin surface

Pneumocystis jiroveci pneumonia (PJP) A fungal infection that shares biologic characteristics with protozoa that infect the lungs

polycystic ovarian syndrome (PCOS) A form of metabolic syndrome caused by the oversecretion of luteinizing hormone

polydipsia Increased thirst

polydrug use Use of more than one drug

polymorphisms DNA variants that occur within a specific population at a frequency greater than 1%

polyphagia Increased hunger

polypharmacy Use of multiple drugs and/or the administration of drugs above what is clinically warranted

polyuria Increased urine output

postexposure prophylaxis (PEP) The treatment regimen instituted after percutaneous exposure to human immunodeficiency virus (HIV)

potassium-sparing diuretics Diuretics that promote potassium retention

potassium-wasting diuretics Diuretics that promote potassium excretion

potency Refers to the amount of drug needed to elicit a specific physiologic response

preeclampsia Gestational hypertension with proteinuria

preload Amount of blood in the ventricle at the end of diastole

premenstrual syndrome (PMS) A collection of cyclic physical symptoms and perimenopausal mood alterations

preterm labor (PTL) Cervical changes and uterine contractions that occur between 20 and 37 weeks of pregnancy

priapism Painful, continuous erection

primary syphilis Presents with a sore, or chancre, at the site where the infection entered the body, typically the penis in men and outer genitals or inner vagina in women

Principle of Atraumatic Care Provision of therapy using interventions that minimize or eliminate psychological and physical distress experienced by patients, particularly children and their families

progenitor cells Early descendants of stem cells that can differentiate to form one or more kinds of cells but that cannot divide and reproduce indefinitely

progesterone The naturally occurring sex hormone produced in the ovaries of women

progestins Natural or synthetic hormones that have progesterone-like effects

progestogen Any synthetically produced progesterone compound

prolactin (PRL) A protein hormone of the anterior lobe of the pituitary that induces lactation

prophylactic Drugs to prevent tuberculosis (TB) disease in individuals with latent TB infection

prophylaxis Prevention

prostaglandin analogues First-line drugs used primarily in the treatment of open-angle glaucoma and ocular hypertension

prostaglandins Chemical mediators that have been isolated from the exudate at inflammatory sites

proteasome Multienzyme complexes that degrade proteins intracellularly

protein binding Describes how drugs are distributed in the plasma and bind with plasma proteins (albumin, lipoproteins, and alpha-1-acid-glycoprotein [AGP])

prothrombin time (PT) A laboratory test that measures the time it takes blood to clot in the presence of certain clotting factors

proto-oncogenes Normal genes involved in cell differentiation and division; they regulate cell death

pseudoparkinsonism Frequently occurs as an adverse reaction to chlorpromazine, haloperidol, lithium, metoclopramide, methyldopa, and reserpine

psoralen and ultraviolet A (PUVA) Therapy that permits lower doses of methoxsalen and UVA to be given

psoriasis A multisystem disease with predominant skin and joint disorders

psychomotor seizure Occurs in temporal lobe epilepsy; characterized by a temporary impairment of consciousness, loss of judgment, automatic behavior, and abnormal acts

psychosis Loss of contact with reality

puerperium The period from delivery until 6 weeks postpartum

pulse oximetry Provides a digital display of oxygen saturation

purgatives Harsh cathartics that cause a watery stool with abdominal cramping

rapid eye movement (REM) sleep The sleep stage during which people experience most of their recallable dreams, characterized by discernable eye movement

reactive depression Depression that usually has a sudden onset after a precipitating event

rebound nasal congestion Caused by frequent use of decongestants

receptors Found on cell surface membranes or within cells

recombinant DNA The genetic engineering process that combines two human DNA strands artificially

recombinant hepatitis B A three-dose series vaccine for hepatitis B virus (HBV) indicated for HBV prophylaxis in infants

recommended dietary allowance (RDA) The amount of vitamins, minerals, or other essential nutrients that should be ingested every day by a normal person engaged in average activities

repolarization Return of cell membrane potential to resting after depolarization

respect for persons Treating patients as independent persons who are capable of making decisions in their own best interests

respiratory distress syndrome (RDS) A syndrome that can occur because of immature lung development and breathing control and decreased airway muscle tone and surfactant level

restrictive lung disease A decrease in total lung capacity as a result of fluid accumulation or loss of elasticity of the lung

reward circuit A structure that regulates the ability to feel pleasure and other emotions, both positive and negative

Rh sensitization Development of protective antibodies against incompatible Rh-positive blood

Rh$_0$(D) immune globulin A substance routinely administered to women with maternal/fetal blood mixing

rhinorrhea Watery nasal discharge

right assessment Requires the collection of appropriate baseline data before administration of a drug

right documentation Requires the nurse to record immediately the appropriate information about the drug administered

right dose Requires verification by the nurse that the dose administered is the amount ordered and that it is safe for the patient for whom it is prescribed

right drug Requires confirming that a drug is right for the patient prior to its administration

right evaluation Asks whether the medication did for the patient what it was supposed to do

right patient Requires confirmation of a patient's identity with two forms of identification before drug administration

right route Ordered by the health care provider, it indicates the mechanism by which the medication will enter the body

right time The time the prescribed dose is ordered to be administered

right to education Requires that patients receive accurate and thorough information about the drugs they are taking and how each drug relates to their particular condition

right to refuse Refers to the patient's right to decline medication

risk-benefit ratio Identifying physical, psychological, and social risks and weighing them against the benefits

root-cause analysis (RCA) A method of problem solving used to identify potential workplace errors

saddle block Anesthesia given at the lower end of the spinal column to block the perineal area

saluretic Sodium-chloride losing

schizophrenia A chronic psychotic disorder

secondary hypertension Hypertension related to renal and endocrine disorders

secondary syphilis Disease characterized by a skin rash that appears 2 to 8 weeks after the chancre

sedation A state of diminished physical and mental responsiveness

seizure A disorder that results from abnormal electrical discharges from the cerebral neurons, characterized by a loss or disturbance of consciousness and usually involuntary, uncontrolled movements

seizure threshold The point at which a seizure may be induced

selective chloride channel activators A new category of laxatives used to treat idiopathic constipation in adults

selective serotonin reuptake inhibitors (SSRIs) Agents that block the reuptake of serotonin into the nerve terminal of the central nervous system

sentinel event An unanticipated event in a health care setting that results in death or serious harm to a patient unrelated to the natural course of the patient's illness

seroconversion The acquisition of detectable levels of antibodies in the bloodstream

serotonin norepinephrine reuptake inhibitors (SNRIs) Agents that inhibit the reuptake of serotonin and norepinephrine, increasing availability in the synapse

shingles A painful vesicular rash along the region of skin innervated by the nerve root ganglia

side effects Secondary effects of drug therapy

signal transduction A mechanism by which cell-to-cell communication occurs locally or remotely by signal molecules sent to maintain homeostasis, regulate growth and division, develop and organize into tissues, and coordinate cellular functions

signal transduction inhibitors (STIs) Agents that block signals to cancerous cells by blocking signals passed from one molecule to another

sinusitis Inflammation of the mucous membranes of one or more of the maxillary, frontal, ethmoid, or sphenoid sinuses

sloughing Formation of dead tissue that separates from living tissue

small-molecule compounds Chemicals that are small enough to have an intracellular effect, targeting the internal structures of cells

spacer A device used to enhance the delivery of medications from a metered-dose inhaler

spermatogenesis Formation of spermatozoa

spinal anesthesia A local anesthetic injected into the subarachnoid space below the first lumbar space (L1) in adults and the third lumbar space (L3) in children

spinal block Results from the penetration of anesthetic into the subarachnoid space

status epilepticus A rapid succession of epileptic seizures

steady state The plateau drug level

stress ulcer An ulcer that usually follows a critical situation, such as extensive trauma or major surgery

subcutaneous Injections given under the skin only in areas such as the upper outer aspect of the arms; the abdomen, at least 2 inches from the umbilicus; and the anterior thighs

sublingual Given under the tongue

substance use disorder A disorder evidenced by recurrent use of a substance such that it causes considerable impairment, including problems with health and an inability to keep up with family and work responsibilities

superinfection A new infection in a patient with a preexisting infection

suppository A solid medical preparation that is cone or spindle shaped for insertion into the rectum, globular or egg shaped for use in the vagina, or pencil shaped for insertion into the urethra

suppressor gene A gene that suppresses the phenotypic expression of another gene

surfactant A substance that decreases the surface tension of the alveoli to allow the lungs to fill with air and prevent the alveoli from deflating

sympatholytics Drugs that affect the sympathetic nervous system; also called *adrenergic blockers*

sympathomimetics Drugs that affect the sympathetic nervous system; also called *adrenergic agonists*

syndrome of inappropriate antidiuretic hormone (SIADH) A condition in which excessive water retention expands the intracellular volume

synergistic effect Describes what occurs when two or more drugs are given together

tachycardia A condition in which the heart rate is too fast

tachyphylaxis An acute, rapid decrease in response to a drug

tardive dyskinesia A serious adverse reaction that occurs in approximately 20% to 30% of patients who have taken a typical antipsychotic drug for more than 1 year

targeted therapy The cornerstone of precision medicine because it directs the treatment according to the person's genes and proteins

taxanes A drug derived from a yew tree that blocks cell growth by stopping cell division

teratogenic The disturbance of the development of an embryo or fetus

teratogens Substances that cause developmental abnormalities

tertiary syphilis Disease that occurs as early as 1 year after infection or at any time during an untreated person's lifetime

testosterone The principal male sex hormone, an anabolic steroid

therapeutic drug monitoring (TDM) Checking serum drug levels

therapeutic index (TI) The relationship between the therapeutic dose of a drug (ED_{50}) and the toxic dose of a drug (TD_{50})

therapeutic serum level Refers to the dosage range, blood plasma, or serum concentration usually expected to achieve desired therapeutic effects

thromboembolectomy A treatment to dissolve dangerous clots in blood vessels, improve blood flow, and prevent damage to tissues and organs

thromboembolism A clot in a blood vessel

thrombolytics Agents used to promote the fibrinolytic mechanism (converting plasminogen to plasmin, which destroys the fibrin in the blood clot)

thrombosis The formation of a clot in an arterial or venous vessel

thyroid-stimulating hormone (TSH) Stimulates the thyroid gland to release thyroxine (T_4) and triiodothyronine (T_3)

thyrotoxicosis The most common type of hyperthyroidism, caused by hyperfunction of the thyroid gland

thyroxine (T_4) A hormone produced by the thyroid gland that controls metabolism

tinea capitis A fungal infection of the skin, also called *ringworm*

tinea pedis A fungal infection of the feet, also called *athlete's foot*

tissue phase Invasion of body tissue

tocolytic therapy Drug therapy to decrease uterine muscle contractions

tolerable upper intake level (UL) The maximum level of continuing daily nutrient intake that is likely to pose no risk to the health of most of those in the age group for which it has been established

tolerance The need for a larger dose of a drug to obtain the original euphoria

tonic-clonic Convulsive, as with a tonic-clonic seizure

tonic seizure A seizure in which muscles initially stiffen before the sufferer loses consciousness

tonicity Used primarily as a measurement of the concentration of intravenous solutions compared with the osmolality of body fluids

topical Medication applied to the skin, often by painting or spreading it over an area and applying a moist dressing or leaving the area exposed to air

torsades de pointes An unusual polymorphic ventricular tachycardia often associated with a prolonged QT interval

total parenteral nutrition (TPN) The administration of nutrients by a route other than the gastrointestinal tract; also called *parenteral nutrition*

toxoids Inactivated toxins that can no longer produce harmful diseases but do stimulate formation of antitoxins

toxoplasmosis A disease caused by the parasite *Toxoplasma gondii*

transcription factors Substances that enter the nucleus and signal the cell to begin mitosis

transdermal Across the skin; a term used to describe medication stored in a patch and placed on the skin to be absorbed to produce a systemic effect

transplant rejection Occurs when the immune system of the transplant recipient attacks the transplanted organ

trichinosis A disease caused by ingestion of raw or inadequately cooked pork that contains larvae of the *Trichinella spiralis* parasite

tricyclic antidepressants (TCAs) Drugs used to treat major depression

triiodothyronine (T$_3$) A hormone made by the thyroid gland

trough drug level The lowest plasma concentration of a drug, it measures the rate at which the drug is eliminated

type 1 diabetes mellitus A chronic condition in which the pancreas produces little or no insulin

type 2 diabetes mellitus A chronic condition that affects the way the body metabolizes sugar

typical antipsychotics A drug class that is subdivided into *nonphenothiazines*—such as butyrophenones (which block only the neurotransmitter dopamine), dibenzoxazepines, dihydroindolones, and thioxanthenes—and *phenothiazines*, which along with the thioxanthenes block norepinephrine to cause sedative and hypotensive effects early in treatment

tyrosine kinase (TK) An enzyme that activates other substances by adding a phosphate group (PO$_4$) to them, a process known as *phosphorylation*

tyrosine kinase inhibitors (TKIs) Drugs that inhibit tyrosine kinases and primarily exert their effects on an enzyme known as *BCR-ABL tyrosine kinase*

unit dose method Method of dispensing drugs in which drugs are individually wrapped and labeled for single-dose use for each patient

uricosurics Agents that increase the rate of uric acid excretion by inhibiting its reabsorption

urinary analgesics Drugs that relieve pain and burning in the urinary tract

urinary antiseptics/antiinfectives Drugs that prevent microbial infections of any part of the urinary tract

urinary stimulants Agents that increase the tone of urinary muscles

urinary tract infection (UTI) Microbial infection of any part of the urinary tract

urticaria Skin rash caused by an allergic reaction

U.S. Food and Drug Administration (FDA) The U.S. federal agency responsible for approving and regulating drugs

uterine contractility Tightening and shortening of uterine muscles

uterine inertia Uterine inactivity or hypotonic contractions

uveitis Infection of the vascular layer of the eye (ciliary body, choroid, and iris)

vaccination Involves the administration of a small amount of antigen, which although capable of stimulating an immune response does not typically produce the disease

Valsalva maneuver A method to prevent air embolism during dressing and tubing changes in which patients are asked to turn their head in the opposite direction of the insertion site, take a deep breath, hold it, and bear down

vertical transmission The passage of infecting organisms from mother to neonate

very-low-density lipoprotein (VLDL) Contains the highest amount of triglycerides

vesicant A substance that causes tissue blistering

vesicles Clear, fluid-filled blisters smaller than 10 mm in diameter

vinca alkaloids Substances derived from the periwinkle plant

viral load A measurement of the amount of a virus in an organism, typically in the bloodstream, usually stated in virus particles per milliliter

virilization The development of male secondary sex characteristics in women or hypogonadal males

virus An obligate intracellular organism that must reside within a living host cell to survive and reproduce

vitamin K A fat-soluble vitamin given to newborns to prevent vitamin K–deficiency bleeding

vomiting center A major cerebral center that causes vomiting when stimulated

water-soluble vitamins A group of vitamins that includes the B-complex vitamins and vitamin C

whitehead A type of noninflammatory acne lesion that is closed

window period The time delay from infection to a positive test result

withdrawal bleeding Monthly bleeding women experience while using a hormonal birth control method

withdrawal symptoms A wide range of physical or emotional disorders that include nervousness, headaches, and insomnia that occur when an individual who is addicted to a substance (such as drugs or alcohol) stops using the substance

World Health Organization (WHO) An agency of the United Nations with the purpose of monitoring communicable and noncommunicable disease outbreaks globally

xerophthalmia Dry eyes

Z-track technique A technique recommended for administering intramuscular injections to help minimize local skin irritation by sealing the medication in the muscle tissue

INDEX

Page numbers followed by *f*, *t* , and *b* indicate figures, tables, and boxes, respectively.

878

LIST OF FEATURES